COLOR ATLAS AND SYNOPSIS OF CLINICAL DERMATOLOGY

The art of being wise is the art of knowing what to overlook.

William James

take a long time

ECFMG

Thomas B. Fitzpatrick, M.D., Ph.D., D.Sc. (Hon.)

Wigglesworth Professor of Dermatology, Emeritus
Chairman, Emeritus
Department of Dermatology, Harvard Medical School

Chief Emeritus, Dermatology Service
Senior Consultant Dermatologist
Massachusetts General Hospital
Boston, Massachusetts

Richard Allen Johnson, M.D.C.M.

Clinical Instructor in Dermatology
Harvard Medical School

Clinical Associate in Dermatology
Massachusetts General Hospital

Associate Physician (Dermatology)
Brigham and Women's Hospital

Associate in Dermatology
Beth Israel Deaconess Hospital
Boston, Massachusetts

Klaus Wolff, M.D., D.Sc. (Hon.), F.R.C.P.

Professor and Chairman
Department of Dermatology
University of Vienna Medical School

Head, Division of General Dermatology
Vienna General Hospital
Vienna, Austria

Dick Suurmond, M.D.

Professor Emeritus and Chairman
Department of Dermatology, University Hospital
Leiden, The Netherlands

FOURTH EDITION

COLOR ATLAS AND SYNOPSIS OF CLINICAL DERMATOLOGY

COMMON AND SERIOUS DISEASES

Thomas B. Fitzpatrick, M.D.

Richard Allen Johnson, M.D.

Klaus Wolff, M.D.

Dick Suurmond, M.D.

McGraw-Hill
MEDICAL PUBLISHING DIVISION

New York   St. Louis   San Francisco   Auckland   Bogotá
Caracas   Lisbon   London   Madrid   Mexico City   Milan   Montreal
New Delhi   San Juan   Singapore   Sydney   Tokyo   Toronto

Color Atlas and Synopsis of Clinical Dermatology

1234567890   DOC DOC   09876543210

ISBN 0-07-136038-7

This book was set in Times Roman by York Graphic Services, Inc. The editors were Darlene Cooke, Mariapaz Ramos Englis, and John M. Morriss.

The production supervisor was Philip Galea. The text and cover designer was Marsha Cohen of Parallelogram.

The index was prepared by Jerry Ralya.

R. R. Donnelley and Sons, Inc., was printer and binder.

This book is printed on acid-free paper.

Library of Congress Cataloging-in-Publication Data

Fitzpatrick, Thomas B. (Thomas Bernard),
    Color atlas and synopsis of clinical dermatology : common and serious diseases /
    Thomas B. Fitzpatrick, Richard Allen Johnson, Klaus Wolff ; contributing author, Dick
    Suurmond.—4th ed.
        p. ; cm.
    Includes bibliographical references and index.
    ISBN 0-07-136038-7 (alk. paper)
        1. Dermatology—Atlases   I. Johnson, Richard Allen, 1940–   II. Wolff, Klaus, 1935–   III.
    Title.
    [DNLM: 1. Skin Diseases—Atlases. WR 17 F559c 2001]
RL81.C65 2001
616.5—dc21
                                                                                        00-056632

INTERNATIONAL EDITION ISBN 0-07-116295-X
Copyright © 2001. Exclusive rights by The McGraw-Hill Companies, Inc., for manufacture and export. This book cannot be re-exported from the country to which it is consigned by McGraw-Hill. The International Edition is not available in North America.

Available Translations of the *Color Atlas and Synopsis of Clinical Dermatology*

French	(Third Edition)	McGraw-Hill Publishing Company, Maidenhead, U.K.
German	(Third Edition)	McGraw-Hill Publishing Company, Maidenhead, U.K.
Greek	(Third Edition)	Paschalidis Medical Publications, Athens, Greece
Italian	(Third Edition)	McGraw-Hill Libri Italia, s.r.l., Milan, Italy
Korean	(Third Edition)	McGraw-Hill Book Company, Jurong, Singapore
Portuguese	(Third Edition)	McGraw-Hill Interamericana Editores, S.A. de C.V., Mexico City
Russian	(Third Edition)	McGraw-Hill Publishing Co., Maidenhead, U.K.
Spanish	(Third Edition)	McGraw-Hill Interamericana Editores, S.A. de C.V., Mexico City

P A R T   I
DISORDERS PRESENTING IN THE SKIN AND MUCOUS MEMBRANES

P A R T   I I
DERMATOLOGY AND INTERNAL MEDICINE

Section 14 SKIN SIGNS OF VASCULAR INSUFFICIENCY | 452

Section 15 SKIN SIGNS OF SYSTEMIC CANCERS | 478

Section 16 SKIN SIGNS OF HEMATOLOGIC DISEASES | 496

P A R T   I I I
DISEASES DUE TO MICROBIAL AGENTS

P A R T I V
SKIN SIGNS OF HAIR, NAIL, AND MUCOSAL DISORDERS

"Time is change; we measure its passage by how much things alter."

Nadine Godimer

The First Edition of this book appeared 18 years ago (1983) and has been expanded *pari passu* with the major developments that have occurred in dermatology over the past two decades. Dermatology is now one of the most sought after medical specialties because of the large patient population seeking the many new innovative therapies.

For the first time we have effective treatments for the four major diseases: acne, warts, eczema and psoriasis; these four diseases are the most common in the United States.

1) **Acne.** Oral isotretinoin is the first effective therapy for severe acne and is one of the major discoveries in medicine in the past three decades.

2) **Warts.** Genital warts (human papillomavirus) are now manageable with topical imiquimod, which also shows promise for common warts. HPV infections have been one of the major challenges in medicine because of their seriousness (cervical cancer).

3) **Atopic dermatitis.** A hitherto uncontrollable disorder except for topical and oral corticosteroids with their inherent side effects, this is now dramatically turned around with non-steroidal anti-inflammatory topical macrolide immunosuppressants, such as tacrolimus and other ascomycins developed in Japan and Europe, respectively, and soon to be released in the United States.

4) **Psoriasis.** This is a major problem affecting over a million persons in the United States. Modern methods of photochemotherapy (with psoralens) and phototherapy ("broad band" UVB) using computerized irradiators and protocols were first introduced in 1974 and 1982. However, the new UVB source is "narrow-band" UVB (311 nm), which is more effective in the management of psoriasis than broad band UVB, and very recently a monochromatic band at 308 nm obtained from a laser source has been highly effective in localized psoriasis. The patient with psoriasis, therefore, now has options other than oral methotrexate. Finally, a new topical and oral non-steroidal anti-inflammatory drug, an ascomycin derivative recently developed in Vienna, Austria, appears to be as effective as cyclosporine in psoriasis but without serious side effects. This will complete the spectrum of treatment for psoriasis beginning with UVB phototherapy, then PUVA photochemotherapy avoiding the toxic actions of cyclosporine and methotrexate. Oral retinoids are not an option as a long-term monotherapy for psoriasis because of bone toxicity. These new therapeutic options expand the treatments available and will make knowledge of dermatology more important for primary care physicians in order to enable them to take advantage of these new therapies.

The *Color Atlas and Synopsis of Clinical Dermatology* has been used by thousands of primary care physicians and other health care providers principally because it facilitates dermatologic diagnosis by providing large color photographs of the skin lesions and juxtaposed, a succinct summary outline of the major features of common skin disorders as well as the skin signs of serious systemic diseases.

"A picture is worth a thousand words" and this *Atlas* provides both!

In addition, there is a short summary of Management.

The Fourth Edition has been extensively revised with 680 photographs and an updating of the precis.

The *Atlas* has been translated into eight languages.

The Editors

Our secretaries, Renate Kosma and Linda Nolan, worked hard to meet the demands of the writers. Looking back, it was the Dutch Professor M. Polano's initial superb "picture only" Atlas that was the stimulus that led one of us to write the text for the First Edition. More than any person it was the late Patricia Knowles Novak who with her forbearance made possible the publication of the first three editions. J. Dereck Jeffers, Medical Editor, skillfully guided us through the complicated details in the launch of the First Edition.

In the present McGraw-Hill team, we appreciated the counsel of Martin Wonsiewicz, Publisher; Darlene Cooke, Executive Editor; John M. Morriss, Editing Manager; Arlene Stolper Simon and M. Lorraine Andrews; Bob Laffler, Director of Publishing Services; and Phil Galea, Production Manager, who expertly managed the production. We thank Jack Farrell, Publisher and Sales Manager, for his advice about the cover design and the potential markets for this book. But the major force behind this edition and previous editions was Mariapaz Ramos Englis, Senior Managing Editor, whose good nature, good judgment, loyalty to the authors, and most of all, patience, guided the authors to make an even better book.

The following physicians have been consulted for preparation of this Edition: Charles R. Taylor, John Hawk, Joop and Suzanne Grevelink, Arthur R. Rhodes, Richard Langley, Kenneth H. Kraemer, Arthur J. Sober, Hensin Tsao, Arthur Tong, and Martin C. Mihm, Jr.

The authors are very appreciative of the support from 3M Pharmaceuticals, Novartis Pharmaceuticals Corporation, and Roche Pharmaceuticals.

This *Atlas* plus text is proposed as a "field guide" to the recognition of skin disorders. The skin is a treasury of important lesions that can usually be clinically recognized. At present, gross morphology in the form of skin lesions remains the hard core of dermatologic diagnosis. Skin lesions are visible to the unaided eye, just as pulmonary and brain lesions are gross pathology but visible only with imaging. Both types of lesions require a differential diagnosis and both can often lead the clinician to the correct diagnosis—and thus the proper management of the patient.

APPROACH TO DERMATOLOGIC DIAGNOSIS

There are two distinct clinical situations regarding the nature of skin changes:

A. The skin changes are *incidental* findings in *well* people noted during the routine general physical examination

   1. *"Bumps and blemishes"*: See the figures on page 1042 and the inside back cover for the location of many of those lesions that are present in well people, but are not the reason for the visit to the physician; every general physician should be able to recognize each of these diseases and disorders.

   2. *Important skin lesions not* noted by the patient but that cannot be overlooked by the physician:

     Dysplastic nevi
     Melanoma
     Xanthomatoses
     Basal cell carcinoma
     Squamous cell carcinoma
     Café-au-lait macules in von Recklinghausen's disease

B. The skin changes are the *chief complaint* of the patient

   1. Minor problems:
     Localized itchy rash, "rash," warts, common moles, seborrheic keratosis, rash in groin, and so on

2. "4-S" = Serious Skin Signs in Sick Patients:[1]

Generalized Red Rash: with Fever
Measles
Rubella
Rocky Mountain Spotted Fever (Palms and Soles First)
Viral Exanthem

Generalized Red Rash: with Bullae and Prominent Mouth Lesions
Erythema Multiforme (major)
Toxic Epidermal Necrolysis
Pemphigus Vulgaris
Bullous Pemphigoid
Drug Eruptions

Generalized Red Rash: with Pustules
Pustular Psoriasis (von Zumbusch)
Drug Eruptions

Generalized Vesicular Lesions
Disseminated Herpes Simplex
Generalized Herpes Zoster
Varicella
Drug Eruptions

Multiple Bullous Lesions with Mouth Lesions
Pemphigus
Drug Eruptions

Generalized Pustules
Drug Eruptions
Pustular Psoriasis

Generalized Dermatitis over Whole Body
Exfoliative Erythroderma

Facial Inflammatory Edema with Fever
Erysipelas
Lupus Erythematosus

Generalized Purpura
Thrombocytopenia
Purpura Fulminans
Drug Eruptions

Palpable Purpura
Vasculitis
Bacterial Endocarditis

---

[1]Requires complete search for multisystem disease: history, general physical examination, biopsy, basic laboratory studies, possibly immunofluorescence, imaging.

I. EPIDEMIOLOGY

Age, race, sex, etiology, occupation

II. HISTORY

A. Constitutional symptoms
   1. "Acute illness" syndrome: headaches, chills, feverishness, weakness
   2. "Chronic illness" syndrome: fatigue, weakness, anorexia, weight loss, malaise.
B. History of skin lesions. Seven key questions:
   1. When? Onset
   2. Where? Site of onset
   3. Does it itch, or hurt? Symptoms
   4. How has it spread? (Pattern of spread) Evolution
   5. How have individual lesions changed? Evolution
   6. Provacative factors? Heat, cold, sun, exercise, travel history, drug ingestion, pregnancy, season
   7. Previous treatment(s)? Topical and systemic, phototherapy
C. General history of present illness as indicated by clinical situation, with particular attention to constitutional and prodromal symptoms
D. Review of systems as indicated by clinical situation, with particular attention to possible connections between signs and disease of other organ systems (e.g., rheumatic complaints, myalgias, arthralgias, Raynaud's phenomenon, sicca symptoms)
E. Past medical history
   1. Operations
   2. Illnesses (hospitalized?)
   3. Allergies, especially drug allergies
   4. Medications (present and past)
   5. Habits (smoking, alcohol intake, drug abuse)
   6. Atopic history (asthma, hay fever, eczema)
F. Family medical history (particularly of psoriasis, atopy, melanoma, xanthomas, tuberous sclerosis)
G. Social history, with particular reference to occupation, hobbies, exposures, travel
H. Sexual history: history of risk factors of HIV: blood transfusions, IV drugs, sexually active, multiple partners, sexually transmitted disease?

III. PHYSICAL EXAMINATION

A. **Appearance** of patient: uncomfortable, "toxic," well
B. **Vital Signs:** pulse, respiration, temperature

C. **Skin**—four major skin signs: (1) type, (2) shape, (3) arrangement, (4) distribution of lesions
  1. *Type* of lesions (see Appendix A)

Flat Lesion (Usually in the Plane of the Skin)	Elevated Lesion (Above the Plane of the Skin)	Depressed Lesion (Below the Plane of the Skin)
Macule	Papule	Atrophy
Petechiae	Plaque	Sclerosis
Ecchymosis	Nodule	Erosion
Infarct	Wheal	Excoriation
Sclerosis	Vegetation	Fissure
Telangiectasia	Papilloma	Scar
	Vesicle and bulla	Ulcer
	Pustule	Sinus
	Abscess	Gangrene
	Cyst	Sphacelus
	Exudate (crusts)	
	Scales	
	Scar	
	Lichenification	
	Hypertrophies	

Color of lesions or of the skin if diffuse involvement: *"skin color":* white: leukoderma, hypomelanosis; red; erythema; pink; violaceous; brown; hypermelanosis; black; blue; gray; orange; yellow. Red or purple purpuric lesions do not blanch with pressure (diascopy).

Palpation
  Consistency (soft, firm, hard, fluctuant, boardlike)
  Deviation in temperature (hot, cold)
  Mobility
  Presence of tenderness
  Estimate the depth of lesion (i.e., dermal or subcutaneous)
Margination, well-defined (can be traced with the tip of a pencil), ill-defined
  2. **Shape** of individual lesions
  Round, oval, polygonal, polycyclic, annular (ring-shaped), iris, serpiginous (snakelike), umbilicated
  3. **Arrangement** of multiple lesions
  Grouped: herpetiform, zosteriform, arciform, annular, reticulated (net-shaped), linear, serpiginous (snakelike)
  Disseminated: scattered discrete lesions or diffuse involvement (i.e., without identifiable borders)
  4. **Distribution** of lesions
  Extent: isolated (single lesions), localized, regional, generalized, universal
  Pattern: symmetrical, exposed areas, sites of pressure, intertriginous area, follicular localization, random, Blaschko's lines
  Characteristic patterns: secondary syphilis, atopic dermatitis, acne, erythema multiforme, candidiasis, lupus erythematosus, pemphigus, pemphigoid, porphyria cutanea tarda, xanthomas, necrotizing angiitis (vasculitis).

Rocky Mountain spotted fever, Lyme disease, rubella, rubeola, scarlet fever, toxic shock syndrome, typhoid, Kawasaki's disease, herpes zoster, varicella, scalded-skin syndrome, toxic epidermal necrolysis, Kaposi's sarcoma (epidemic), vitiligo

D. **Hair and nails**
E. **Mucous membranes**
F. **General physical examination** as indicated by clinical presentation and differential diagnosis with particular attention to mucous membranes, examine for lymphadenopathy, hepatomegaly, splenomegaly, joints, neurological changes (especially sensation)

IV. LABORATORY EXAMINATIONS

A. **Dermatopathology**
  1. Light microscopy: site, process, cell types
  2. Immunofluorescence
  3. Special techniques: stains, transmission electron microscopy
  4. Microbiologic examination of skin material: scales, crusts, exudate, or tissue
     Direct microscopic examination of skin
        For yeast and fungus: 10% potassium hydroxide preparation
        For bacteria: Gram's stain
        For virus: Tzanck smear
        For spirochetes: dark-field examination
        For parasites: scabies mite from a burrow
     Culture
        Bacterial
        Viral
        Parasitic
        Mycologic
        For granulomas: culture of minced tissue
B. **Laboratory examination of blood**
   Bacteriologic: culture
   Serologic: ANA, STS, serology
   Hematologic: hematocrit or hemoglobin, cells, differential smear
   Chemistry: fasting blood sugar, blood urea nitrogen, creatinine, liver function, and thyroid function tests (if indicated)
C. **Imaging** (x-ray, CT scan, MRI, ultrasound)
D. **Urinalysis**
E. **Stool examination** (for occult blood, e.g., in vasculitis syndromes; for ova and parasites, for porphyrins)
F. **Wood's lamp examination**
   Urine: pink-orange fluorescence in porphyria cutanea tarda (add 1 ml of 5% hydrochloric acid)
   Hair (in vivo): green fluorescence in tinea capitis (hair shaft)
   Skin (in vivo)
      Erythrasma: coral-red fluorescence
      Hypomelanosis: decrease in intensity

Brown hypermelanosis: increase in intensity

Blue hypermelanosis: no change in intensity

G. **Epiluminescence microscopy (dermatoscopy)** for pigmented lesions (see Appendix B)

G. **Patch testing**

H. **Acetowhitening-whitening** of subclinical (i.e., not readily visible) penile warts after application of 5% acetic acid

FINAL DIAGNOSIS

TIME is an important aspect of diagnosis. If the diagnosis is not established at the first visit, the patient should be re-examined in a few days because changes may appear in the eruption with new sites of distribution, new types of lesions (scales, vesicles, bullae, purpura, etc.). The diagnosis may then become possible.

COLOR ATLAS
AND SYNOPSIS
OF
CLINICAL
DERMATOLOGY

DISORDERS OF SEBACEOUS AND APOCRINE GLANDS

ACNE VULGARIS (COMMON ACNE) AND CYSTIC ACNE

Acne is an inflammation of the pilosebaceous units of certain body areas (face and trunk, rarely buttocks) that occurs most frequently in adolescence and manifests itself as comedones *(comedonal acne)*, papulopustules *(papulopustular acne)*, or nodules plus cysts *(nodulocystic acne* and *acne conglobata)*. Pitted, depressed, or hypertrophic scars may follow all types but especially nodulocystic acne and acne conglobata. *Severe acne* includes one or more of the following: persistent or recurrent inflammatory nodules, extensive papulopustular lesions, active scarring, and/or presence of sinus tracts.

EPIDEMIOLOGY

Age of Onset   Puberty—10 to 17 years in females, 14 to 19 in males; may, however, appear first at 25 years or older.

Sex   More severe in males than in females.

Race   Lower incidence in Asians and blacks.

Occupation   Exposure to acnegenic mineral oils, dioxin, others (rarely).

Drugs   Lithium, hydantoin, topical and systemic glucocorticoids, oral contraceptives, androgens may cause exacerbation.

Genetic Aspects   Majority of individuals with cystic acne have parent(s) with a history of severe acne. Multifactorial. Severe acne can be associated with XYY syndrome.

Other Factors   *Endocrine factors* (see Pathogenesis). *Emotional stress* definitely can cause exacerbations. *Occlusion* and *pressure on the skin* by leaning face on hands or on a telephone are *very important* and often unrecognized exacerbating factors (called "acne mechanica") and should be considered in every patient. Acne is not caused by chocolate or fatty foods or, in fact, by any kind of food.

PATHOGENESIS

Acne results from a change in the keratinization pattern in the hair follicle, with the keratinous material becoming more dense and blocking secretion of sebum. The lesions of acne (comedones) are the result of this abnormal keratinization and a complex interaction between hormones (androgens) and bacteria *(Propionibacterium acnes)* in the pilosebaceous units of individuals with appropriate genetic backgrounds. Androgens (which are qualitatively and quantitatively normal) stimulate sebaceous glands to produce larger amounts of sebum. Bacteria contain lipase that converts lipid into fatty acids. Both sebum and fatty acids cause a sterile inflammatory response in the pilosebaceous unit that results in hyperkeratinization of the lining of the follicle with resultant plugging. The enlarged follicular lumen contains inspissated keratin and lipid debris (the whitehead). When the follicle has a portal of entry at the skin, the semisolid mass protrudes, forming a plug (the blackhead). The distended follicle walls may break, and the contents (sebum, lipid, fatty acids, keratin, etc.) may enter the dermis, provoking a foreign-body response (papule, pustule, nodule). Rupture plus intense inflammation leads to scars.

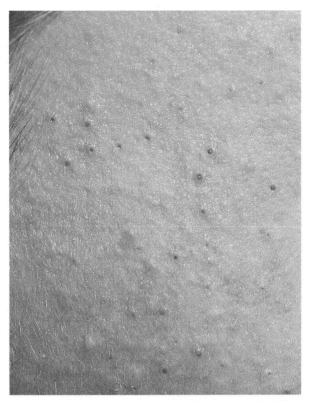

Figure 1-1 Acne vulgaris *Comedones are keratin plugs that form within follicular ostia, frequently associated with surrounding erythema and pustule formation. Comedones associated with small ostia are referred to as closed comedones or "white heads"; those associated with large ostia, open comedones or "black heads." Comedones are best treated with topical retinoids.*

HISTORY

Duration of Lesions   Weeks to months.

Season   Often worse in fall and winter.

Symptoms   Pain in lesions (especially nodulocystic type).

PHYSICAL EXAMINATION

Skin Lesions

Comedones—open (blackheads) or closed (whiteheads) (Fig. 1-1). *Papules and papulopustules*—with (red) (Fig. 1-2) or without inflammation. *Nodules, noduloulcerative lesions, or cysts*—1 to 4 cm in diameter (Fig. 1-3). The soft nodules are not cysts but large secondary comedones from repeated ruptures and reencapsulations with inflammation and ab-scess formation. Round; nodules may coalesce to form linear mounds or sinus tracts. Isolated single lesion (e.g., nodule) or scattered discrete lesions (papules, cysts, nodules) (Fig. 1-4). *Sinuses*—draining epithelial-lined tracts, usually with nodular acne. *Scars*—atrophic depressed (often pitted) or hypertrophic (at times, keloid) scars. *Seborrhea* of the face and scalp is often present and sometimes severe.

Sites of Predilection   Face, neck, upper arms, trunk, buttocks.

Special Forms

Acne in the Adult Woman   Persistent acne in a hirsute female with or without *irregular* menses needs an evaluation for hypersecretion of adrenal and ovarian androgens: total testosterone, free testosterone, and/or dehydro-epianrosterone sulfate (e.g., polycystic ovary syndrome).

Acne Conglobata   Severe cystic acne (Fig. 1-4) with more involvement of the trunk than the face. Coalescing nodules, cysts, and abscesses. Spontaneous remission is long delayed. Rarely, acne conglobata is the type seen in XYY genotype (tall males, slightly mentally retarded, with aggressive behavior) or in the polycystic ovary syndrome.

Acne Fulminans   Young males (ages 13 to 17). *Acute onset* severe cystic acne with concomitant suppuration and always *ulceration;* also, there is malaise, fatigue, fever, generalized arthralgias, leukocytosis, and elevated erythrocyte sedimentation rate (ESR).

Recalcitrant Acne   Can be related to congenital adrenal hyperplasia (11-β- or 21-β hydroxylase deficiencies).

DIFFERENTIAL DIAGNOSIS

Face   *Staphylococcus aureus* folliculitis, pseudofolliculitis barbae, rosacea, perioral dermatitis.

Trunk   *Pityrosporum* folliculitis, "hot-tub" pseudomonas folliculitis, *S. aureus* folliculitis.

Single Painful "Cyst"   Staphylococcal abscess, furuncle, ruptured inclusion cyst, dental sinus cyst.

"Steroid Folliculitis"   From topical or oral glucocorticoids; small papulopustules on the trunk, shoulders, and upper arms *lesions are all in the same stages of development.*

"Mallorca Acne" or Acne Aestivalis   This acne appears after sun exposure, especially in women 20 to 30 years old, on the trunk and shoulders. Resembles steroid acne as the lesions are monomorphous. There are no comedones.

LABORATORY EXAMINATION

Evaluation of Hyperandrogenism and Polycystic Ovary Syndrome

Free testosterone—ovarian source in females, very high in ovarian tumor

FSH and LH—if ratio of LH/FSH is >3:1, highly suggestive (to be done within two weeks before onset of menses and off oral contraceptives)

DHEA-S—adrenal source of androgens

Note: In the overwhelming majority of acne patients, hormone levels are normal.

COURSE

Acne clears often spontaneously by the early twenties but can persist to the fourth decade or older. Flares occur in the winter and with the onset of menses. The only physical sequela is scarring, which should be avoided by proper treatment, *especially with oral isotretinoin early in the course of the disease.*

MANAGEMENT

The psychological impact of acne (perceived cosmetic disfigurement) should be assessed individually in each patient and therapy modified accordingly. The goal of therapy is to remove the plugging of the pilar drainage and to treat the infection with appropriate topical and oral antibiotics.

Mild Acne

Topical antibiotics (clindamycin and erythromycin)

Benzoyl peroxide gels (2%, 5%, or 10%)

Topical retinoids (tretinoin) are effective in comedonal and papulopustular acne but require detailed instructions regarding gradual increases in concentration:

.025% cream **or** .01% gel
$\downarrow$
.05% cream **or** .025% gel
$\downarrow$
.1% cream
$\downarrow$
.05% liquid (rarely given, as this is the most potent of the topical retinoids and is most useful for noninflamed comedones on the nose)
$\downarrow$
lowest effective maintenance

Improvement occurs over a period of months (2 to 5) and may take even longer for noninflamed comedones. Topical retinoids are applied in the evening. Topical antibiotics and benzoyl peroxide gels are applied during the day.

   Combination therapy is best—using benzoyl peroxide–erythromycin gels *plus* topical retinoids (tretinoin) *or* tazarotene gel (1%) used 3 times weekly.

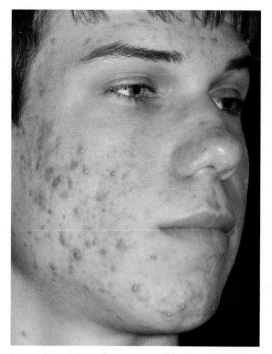

Figure 1-2   Acne vulgaris: papulopustular   *A spectrum of lesions is seen on the face of a 17-year-old male: comedones, papules, pustules, and erythematous macules and scars at site of resolving leisons. The patient was successfully treated with a 4-month course of isotretinoin; there was no recurrence over the next 5 years.*

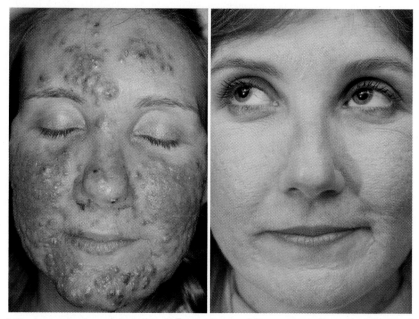

Figure 1-3   Acne vulgaris: nodulocystic   *Inflammatory nodules, cysts, and pustules. Ruptured cysts have coalesced and have led to an intense and painful disfiguring inflammatory reaction. This 23-year-old female was resistant to oral and topical treatment and has developed some scarring (left photograph). The photograph on the right exhibits a remarkable remission of the disfiguring acne following a course of oral isotretinoin, 1 mg/kg, over a period of 4 months.*

Moderate Acne Oral antibiotics are added to the preceding regimen only if topical treatment has failed. The most effective antibiotic is minocycline, 50 to 100 mg bid, and this dose can be tapered to 50 mg/d as acne lessens. Antibiotics are additive and should not be the sole treatment or the beginning treatment. In females, moderate acne can be controlled with high doses of oral estrogens combined with progesterone or antiandrogens. However, recurrences are the rule after cessation of treatment and cerebrovascular disorders are a serious risk.

Severe Acne Scarring, or refractory to treatment. Isotretinoin is a retinoid that inhibits sebaceous gland function and keratinization and has proved to be a very effective treatment for severe acne. It is one of the major discoveries in medical therapeutics and has revolutionized the management of acne.

Indications for Oral Isotretinoin For severe, recalcitrant, nodular acne. The nodules should be ≥5.0 mm; there should be many nodules, not a few; and acne with scarring, as can occur in papulopustular acne. Also, the patient must have been resistant to other acne therapies, including systemic antibiotics.

Contraindications Isotretinoin is a teratogenic drug. Therefore, pregnancy should be prevented. In females who could become pregnant, effective contraception is necessary, i.e., oral. Both tetracycline and isotretinoin may cause pseudotumor cerebri (benign intracranial swelling); therefore, the two medications should never be used together.

Warnings Blood lipids should be determined before therapy is started. About 25% of patients can develop *increased plasma triglycerides.* Also, 15% of patients develop a *decrease in high-density lipoproteins,* and about 7% show an *increase in cholesterol levels.* This may increase the cardiovascular risk. Also, when levels of serum triglycerides rise above 800 mg/μL, the patient may develop acute pancreatitis. Therefore, every attempt should be made to control the triglyceride levels through such measures as weight reduction, dietary fat reduction, restriction of alcohol, and actual reduction of the dose of isotretinoin. Patients should not take vitamin supplements containing vitamin A. *Hepatotoxicity* has been very rarely reported in the form of clinical hepatitis. In one study, 15% of patients developed mild to moderate elevation of hepatic enzyme levels that normalized with reduction of the dose of the drug. Although clinical experience has not confirmed this finding in one large series, hepatic enzyme levels should be determined before beginning therapy. *Eye:* Patients should be advised that *night blindness* has been reported and should be warned about driving at night. Also, patients may have *decreased tolerance to contact lenses* during and after therapy. *Skin:* An eczema-like rash often appears, and this responds dramatically to low potency (class III) topical glucocorticoids. For additional rare possible complications, consult the package insert.

Dosage Isotretinoin, .5 to 2 mg/kg given in divided doses with food for 15 to 20 weeks. Most patients improve with 1 mg/kg. For severe disease, especially on the trunk, a dose of 2 mg/kg may be required. If the nodule count has been reduced by more than 70% in less than 15 to 20 weeks, the drug may be discontinued. After an interval of 2 months, a second course may be given if necessary. As many as three or more courses of isotretinoin have been given in refractory cases.

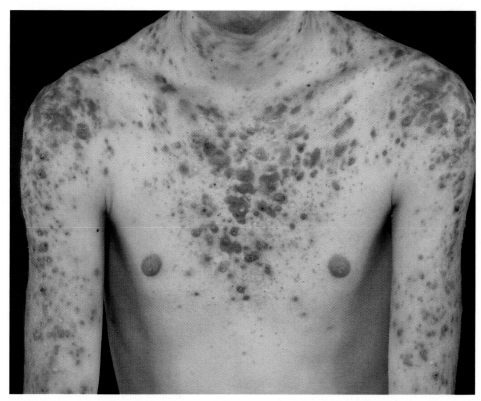

Figure 1-4   Acne vulgaris: acne conglobata   *Inflammatory nodules and cysts have coalesced forming abscesses and even leading to ulceration. There are multiple comedomes and many recent red scars following resolution of inflammatory lesions on the upper chest, neck, arms.*

ROSACEA

Rosacea (Latin: "like roses") is a chronic acneform disorder of the facial pilosebaceous units, coupled with an increased reactivity of capillaries to heat, leading to flushing and ultimately to telangiectasia. Although the disease was previously called *acne rosacea,* it is unrelated to but may coexist with acne, which may have preceded the onset of rosacea. Rosacea is the cause of significant cosmetic disfigurement.

EPIDEMIOLOGY

Age of Onset 30 to 50 years, peak incidence between 40 and 50 years.

Sex Females predominantly; rhinophyma occurs mostly in males.

Race Celtic persons (skin phototypes I and II) but also southern Italians; less frequent or rare in pigmented persons (skin phototypes V and VI, i.e., brown and black)

Other Factors Patients usually have a long history of episodic reddening of the face (flushing) with increases in skin temperature in response to heat stimuli in the mouth (hot liquids), spicy foods; alcohol (cold or hot) may be a precipitating factor, possibly because it causes flushing. Exposure to sun and heat (such as chefs working near a hot stove) may cause exacerbations. Acne may have preceded the onset of rosacea by years; nevertheless, rosacea may and usually does arise de novo without any preceding history of acne or seborrhea.

Stages of Evolution (Plewig and Kligman Classification)

Episodic erythema, "flushing and blushing"— the rosacea diathesis

Stage I: Persistent erythema with telangiectases

Stage II: Persistent erythema, telangiectases, papules, tiny pustules

Stage III: Persistent deep erythema, dense telangiectases, papules, pustules, nodules; may rarely have persistent "solid" edema of the central part of the face, as occurs with acne

HISTORY

Duration of Lesions Days, weeks, months.

Skin Symptoms Patients are concerned about their cosmetic facial appearance; they are often perceived as being alcoholic. Flushing, feeling of "heat" in the face.

PHYSICAL EXAMINATION

Skin Lesions *Early* Pathognomonic: tiny papulopustules (2 to 3 mm), and the pustule is often small (<1 mm) and on the apex of the papule (Fig. 1-5). Nodules. *No comedones.* Red facies, papules, and dusky-red nodules (Figs. 1-5, 1-6, and 1-7). Scattered, discrete lesions.

Late Telangiectases. Chronic rosacea can be associated with marked sebaceous hyperplasia and lymphedema, causing disfigurement of the nose, forehead, eyelids, ears, and chin.

Distribution Characteristic is the symmetrical localization on the face (cheeks, chin, forehead, glabella, nose). Rarely, neck, chest (V-shaped area), back and scalp.

Special Lesions

Rhinophyma (enlarged nose, Fig. 1-8), *metophyma* (enlarged cushion-like swelling of the forehead), *blepharophyma* (swelling of the eyelids) related to marked sebaceous gland hyperplasia, *otophyma* (cauliflower-like swelling of the earlobes), *gnathophyma* (swelling of the chin).

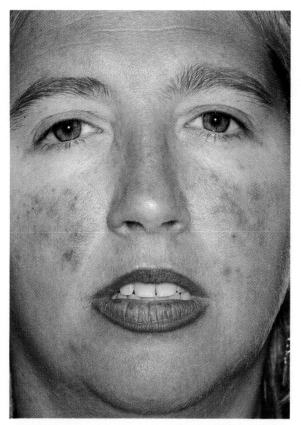

Figure 1-5 **Rosacea** *Moderately severe rosacea in a 29-year-old female in Stage II with persistent erythema, telangiectasia, red papules, and tiny pustules.*

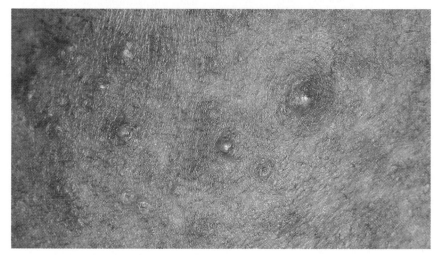

Figure 1-6 **Rosacea** *Tiny 1- to 3-mm pustules, often occurring at the apex of the papules.*

Eye Involvement

"Red" eyes as a result of chronic blepharitis, conjunctivitis, and episcleritis. Rosacea keratitis is a serious problem because corneal ulcers may develop. An ophthalmologist should follow the patient if there is a suspicion of eye involvement.

DIFFERENTIAL DIAGNOSIS

Facial Papules/Pustules

Acne, perioral dermatitis, *Staphylococcus aureus* folliculitis, gram-negative folliculitis, *Demodex folliculorum* infestation.

Facial Flushing/Erythema

Seborrheic dermatitis, prolonged use of topical glucocorticoids, SLE, dermatomyositis.

LABORATORY EXAMINATIONS

Bacterial Culture   Rule out *S. aureus* infection.

Dermatopathology

Stage I: Papules and telangiectases. Nonspecific perifollicular inflammatory infiltrate with occasional foci of "tuberculoid" granulomatous areas: epithelioid cells, lymphocytes, and few giant cells but no caseation. Dilated capillaries surrounded by a nonspecific inflammatory infiltrate

Stage II: Papules and pustules. Foci of neutrophils high and within the follicle

Stage III: Papules, pustules, and nodules. Diffuse hypertrophy of the connective tissue, marked sebaceous gland hyperplasia, epithelioid granuloma without caseation, and many foreign-body giant cells

Rhinophyma   *Glandular Type* Enlarged nose is related to very marked lobular sebaceous hyperplasia. *Fibrous Type* Marked increase in the connective tissue with only a variable amount of sebaceous hyperplasia. *Fibroangiomatous Type* Copper-red nose is related to much enlarged edematous connective tissue with large ectatic veins.

COURSE

Prolonged   Recurrences are common. After a few years, the disease tends to disappear spontaneously. Men and very rarely women may develop rhinophyma, which is treated successfully by surgery or laser surgery.

MANAGEMENT

Prevention   Marked reduction or elimination of alcoholic and hot beverages may be helpful in some patients; it is not the caffeine but the temperature ("hotness") of the tea and coffee that is the culprit. Emotional stress may be a factor in some individuals.

Topical

Metronidazole gel, or cream, .75%, twice daily—very effective.
Metronidazole cream, 1%, once daily.
Sodium sulfacetamide 10 and 5% sulphur lotions
Topical antibiotics (e.g., erythromycin gel) are less effective.

Systemic   If topical treatment fails, or for severe disease, add oral antibiotics:

Tetracycline, 1 to 1.5 g/d in divided doses until clear; then gradually reduce to once-daily doses of 250 to 500 mg.
Minocycline or doxycycline, 50 to 100 mg twice daily, are alternative antibiotics, especially minocycline because doxycycline is a phototoxic drug and its use limits exposure to sunlight in summer.

Maintenance   After control of papulopustules, a dose of 250 to 500 g tetracycline or 50 mg minocycline or doxycycline per day is given.

Oral Isotretinoin   Oral isotretinoin is an alternative in individuals with severe disease (especially stage III) not responding to antibiotics and topical treatments. A low-dose regimen of .1 to .2 mg/kg of body weight per day is effective in most patients but occasionally 1 mg/kg may be required.

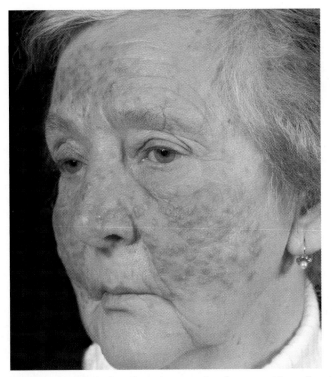

Figure 1-7   Rosacea: Stage III *Typical moderately severe involvement with confluent erythematous papules and pustules on the forehead, cheeks, and nose. Note the absence of comedones that are typically seen with acne vulgaris.*

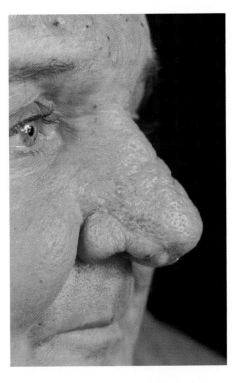

Figure 1-8   Rosacea with rhinophyma *Mild involvement with few erythematous papules and striking erythema, edema, and telangiectasias on the nose (early rhinophyma). Note dilated follicles.*

PERIORAL DERMATITIS

Perioral dermatitis is a pesky facial dermatosis occurring mainly in young women, characterized by discrete erythematous micropapules and micropapulovesicles that often become confluent, forming inflammatory plaques, on the perioral and periorbital skin. *Synonym:* Rosacea-like dermatitis.

EPIDEMIOLOGY

Age of Onset   16 to 45 years; can occur in children.

Sex   Females predominantly.

Etiology   Unknown.

Other Factors   May be markedly aggravated by potent topical (fluorinated) glucocorticoids.

HISTORY

Duration of Lesions   Weeks to months.

Skin Symptoms   Perceived cosmetic disfigurement; occasional itching or burning, feeling of tightness.

PHYSICAL EXAMINATION

Skin Lesions   Papulopustules on an erythematous background (Fig. 1-9) irregularly grouped, symmetric. Initial lesions are erythematous 1- to 2-mm micropapules on a patchy erythematous background. Papules increase in number with central confluence and satellite lesions, including papules, and/or pustules. Confluent plaques may appear eczematous with erythema and scales. There are no comedones.

Distribution   Initial lesions usually perioral. Rim of sparing around the vermilion border of lips. At times, micropapules (1 to 2 mm) and pustules in the periorbital area also occur (Fig. 1-10). Uncommonly, only periorbital involvement is present. Occasionally, glabella and forehead are involved.

DIFFERENTIAL DIAGNOSIS

Small Central Facial Papule

Allergic contact dermatitis, atopic dermatitis, seborrheic dermatitis, rosacea, acne vulgaris, steroid acne.

LABORATORY EXAMINATIONS

Culture   Rule out *Staphylococcus aureus* infection.

DIAGNOSIS

Clinical diagnosis.

COURSE

Appearance of lesions is usually subacute over weeks to months. Perioral dermatitis is, at times, misdiagnosed as an eczematous or a seborrheic dermatitis and treated with a potent topical glucocorticoid preparation, aggravating perioral dermatitis or inducing steroid acne. Untreated, perioral dermatitis fluctuates in activity over months to years but is not nearly as chronic as rosacea.

Topical

Avoid topical glucocorticoids!
Metronidazole, .75% gel two times daily **or** 1% once daily
Erythromycin 2% gel applied twice daily

Systemic

Minocycline, 100 mg bid until clear, then 100 mg daily for 1 month, then 50 mg daily for 1 additional month **or**
Doxycycline 100 mg bid until clear, then 100 mg daily for 1 month, then 50 mg daily for 1 additional month (this is a photosensitizing drug) **or**
Tetracycline, 500 mg bid until clear, then 500 mg daily for 1 month, then 250 mg daily for additional month.

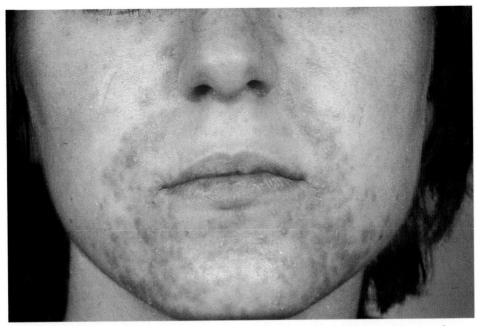

Figure 1-9 Perioral dermatitis *Moderately severe involvement with confluence of tiny papules and a few pustules in a wide perioral distribution. Note typical sparing of the vermilion border (mucocutaneous junction).*

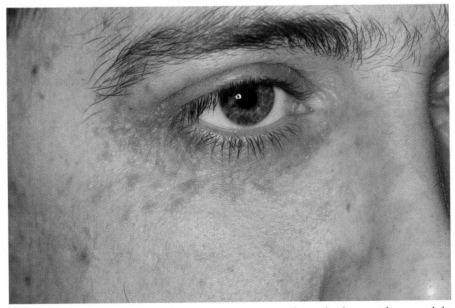

Figure 1-10 Periorbital dermatitis *Note presence of tiny papules and a few pustules around the eye and in the glabella. This is a much less common site than the lesions around the mouth.*

HIDRADENITIS SUPPURATIVA

Hidradenitis suppurativa is a chronic, suppurative, often cicatricial disease of apocrine gland–bearing skin in the axillae, the anogenital region, and rarely, the scalp (called *cicatrizing perifolliculitis*). Sometimes the disease is associated with severe nodulocystic acne and pilonidal sinuses (termed *follicular occlusion syndrome*).

Synonyms: Apocrinitis, hidradenitis axillaris, abscess of the apocrine sweat glands.

EPIDEMIOLOGY

Age of Onset   From puberty to climacteric.

Sex   Affects more females than males; estimated to be 4% of female population. Males more often have anogenital and females axillary involvement.

Race   All races.

Heredity   Although no data are available, mother-daughter transmission has been observed repeatedly. Families may give a history of nodulocystic acne and hidradenitis suppurativa occurring separately or together in blood relatives.

Etiology   Unknown. Predisposing factors: obesity, genetic predisposition to acne, apocrine duct obstruction, secondary bacterial infection.

PATHOGENESIS

The pathogenesis is unknown. The following sequence may be the mechanism of the development of the lesions: keratinous plugging of the apocrine duct → dilatation of the apocrine duct and hair follicle → severe inflammatory changes limited to a single apocrine gland → bacterial growth in dilated duct → ruptured duct/gland resulting in extension of inflammation/infection → extension of suppuration/tissue destruction → ulceration and fibrosis, sinus tract formation.

HISTORY

Symptoms: Intermittent pain and marked point tenderness related to abscess formation in axilla(e) and/or anogenital area.

PHYSICAL EXAMINATION

Skin Lesions   Initial lesion: *very tender,* red inflammatory nodule/abscess (Fig. 1-11) that may resolve or point to surface and drain purulent/seropurulent material; relationship to hair follicle usually not apparent. The same lesion may appear repeatedly in the same location and therefore can be surgically excised. Eventually, sinus tracts may form. Fibrosis, "bridge" scars, hypertrophic and keloidal scars, contractures (Fig. 1-11). Open comedones, and at times unique *double* comedones, form (Fig. 1-11); and these are highly characteristic of the disease. Double comedones, with two adjacent black comedones, may be present even when active nodules are absent, and these are a marker for a patient with hidradenitis suppurativa. Rarely, lymphedema of the associated limb may develop. Lesions moderately to exquisitely tender. Pus drains from opening of abscess and sinus tracts.

Distribution   Axillae, breasts, anogenital area, groin. Often bilateral in axillae and/or anogenital area; may extend over entire back, buttocks (Fig. 1-12), and scalp.

Associated Findings   Cystic acne, pilonidal sinus.

General Examination   Often obesity.

DIFFERENTIAL DIAGNOSIS

Painful papule, molecule, abscess in groin and axilla. *Early:* furuncle, carbuncle, lymphadenitis, ruptured inclusion cyst, cat-scratch disease. *Late:* lymphogranuloma venereum, donovanosis, scrofuloderma, actinomycosis, sinus tracts and fistulas associated with ulcerative colitis and regional enteritis.

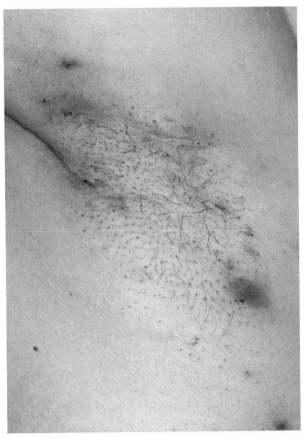

Figure 1-11   Hidradenitis suppurativa   *Many comedones, some of which are paired, are a characteristic finding, associated with several deep exquisitely painful abscesses and old scars in the axilla.*

LABORATORY EXAMINATIONS

Bacteriology Various pathogens may secondarily colonize or "infect" lesions. These include *Staphylococcus aureus,* streptococci, *Escherichia coli, Proteus mirabilis,* and *Pseudomonas aeruginosa.*

Dermatopathology *Early:* keratin occlusion of apocrine duct and hair follicle, ductal/tubular dilatation, inflammatory changes limited to a single apocrine gland. *Late:* destruction of apocrine/eccrine/pilosebaceous apparatus, fibrosis, pseudoepitheliomatous hyperplasia in sinuses.

DIAGNOSIS

Clinical diagnosis:
Stage I: Solitary or multiple isolated tender abscess formation without scarring or sinus tracts
Stage II: Recurrent abscesses, single or multiple, with sinus tract formation and scarring
Stage III: Diffuse or broad involvement across a regional area with sinus tracts and abscesses

COURSE AND PROGNOSIS

The severity of the disease varies considerably. Many patients have only mild involvement with recurrent, self-healing, tender red nodules and do not seek therapy. The disease usually undergoes a spontaneous remission with age (>35 years). In some individuals, the course can be relentlessly progressive, with marked morbidity related to chronic pain, draining sinuses, and scarring, with restricted mobility. Complications (rare): fistulas to urethra, bladder, and/or rectum; anemia, amyloidosis.

MANAGEMENT

Hidradenitis suppurativa is *not* simply an infection, and systemic antibiotics are only part of the treatment program. Combinations of (1) intralesional glucocorticoids, (2) surgery, (3) oral antibiotics, and (4) isotretinoin are used.

Medical Management

Acute Painful Lesions *Nodule* Intralesional triamcinolone (3 to 5 mg/ml).

Abscess Intralesional triamcinolone (3 to 5 mg/ml) into the wall followed by incision and drainage of abscess fluid.

Chronic Low-Grade Disease Oral antibiotics: erythromycin (250 to 500 mg qid), tetracycline (250 to 500 mg qid), or minocycline (100 mg bid) until lesions resolve; may take weeks. Intralesional triamcinolone (3 to 5 mg/ml) into early inflammatory lesions is helpful in hastening resolution of individual lesions.

Prednisone May be given concurrently if pain and inflammation are severe: 70 mg, tapered over 14 days.

Oral Isotretinoin Not useful in severe disease, but it appears to be useful in early disease and when combined with surgical excision of individual lesions.

Surgical Management

- Incise and drain acute abscesses.
- Excise chronic recurrent, fibrotic nodules or sinus tracts. If one or two nodules can be pinpointed with recurrent disease, they can be excised with a good result.
- With extensive, chronic disease, complete excision of axilla or involved anogenital area may be required. Excision should extend down to fascia and requires split skin grafting.

Psychologic Management

These patients need constant reassurance, as they become very depressed because of the nature of the illness and the site of occurrence (anogenital area). Therefore, every effort should be made to deal with the disease, using every modality possible.

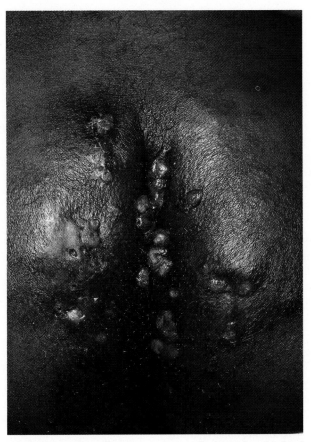

Figure 1-12 Hidradenitis suppurativa *Severe scarring on the buttocks with fistulas and draining sinuses.*

ECZEMA/DERMATITIS

The terms eczema and dermatitis are used interchangeably, denoting a polymorphic inflammatory reaction pattern involving the epidermis and dermis. There are many etiologies and a wide range of clinical findings. Acute eczema/dermatitis is characterized by pruritus, erythema, and vesiculation; chronic eczema/dermatitis, by pruritus, xerosis, hyperkeratosis, ±fissuring. "Dermatitis" is used for exogenous disorders such as irritant or allergic contact dermatitis and "eczema" is more often used to denote endogenous disease such as atopic or constitutional eczema.

CONTACT DERMATITIS

Contact dermatitis is a generic term applied to acute or chronic inflammatory reactions to substances that come in contact with the skin. Irritant contact dermatitis is caused by a chemical irritant; allergic contact dermatitis by an antigen (allergen) that elicits a type IV (cell-mediated or delayed) hypersensitivity reaction.

EPIDEMIOLOGY

Age of Onset No influence on capacity for sensitization; however, allergic contact dermatitis is uncommon in young children.

Occupation This is *the* important cause of disability in industry.

PATHOGENESIS

Contact (nonallergic) dermatitis (Fig. 2-1) may occur in normal skin or cause an exacerbation of preexisting dermatitis as a result of exposure to, for example, croton oil, kerosene, or detergents. *Contact (allergic) dermatitis,* more commonly called *contact eczematous dermatitis,* is a classic, delayed, cell-mediated hypersensitivity reaction. Exposure to a strong sensitizer such as poison ivy resin results in sensitization in a week or so, while exposure to a weak allergen may take months to years for sensitization. The antigen is taken up by a specialized dendritic cell in the epidermis, the Langerhans cell, which processes the antigen and migrates from the epidermis to the draining lymph nodes, where it presents the processed antigen in association with MHC class II molecules to T cells that then proliferate. Sensitized T cells leave the lymph node and enter the blood circulation. Thus, all the skin becomes hypersensitive to the contact allergen. The specially sensitized T-effector lymphocytes home to the skin and produce or mediate the release by other cells of a variety of cytokines after being presented with the same specific antigen.

HISTORY

Duration of Lesion(s) Acute contact—days, weeks; chronic contact—months, years.

Skin Symptoms Pruritus, burning, smarting.

Constitutional Symptoms "Acute illness" syndrome, including fever, in severe allergic contact dermatitis (e.g., poison ivy).

PHYSICAL EXAMINATION

Skin Lesions

Type *Acute* Well-demarcated plaques of erythema and edema (Fig. 2-1) on which are superimposed closely spaced, nonumbilicated vesicles (Fig. 2-3), punctate erosions exuding serum, and crusts (Fig. 2-4).

Subacute Plaques of mild erythema showing small, dry scales or superficial desquamation, sometimes associated with small, red, pointed or rounded, firm papules (Fig. 2-2).

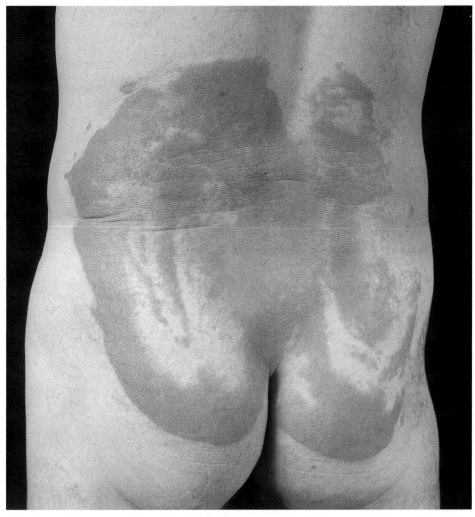

Figure 2-1   Irritant contact dermatitis of back, acute: croton oil   *Erythema and edema with spared areas on the back at sites in contact with irritant in 30-year-old male.*

Chronic   Plaques of lichenification (thickening of the epidermis with deepening of the skin lines in parallel or rhomboidal pattern), scaling (Fig. 2-2) with satellite, small, firm, rounded or flattopped papules, excoriations, and pigmentation or mild erythema.

Arrangement   Often linear, with artificial patterns, an "outside job." Plant contact often re-sults in linear lesions, as in plant (e.g., Rhus) dermatitis (Fig. 2-5).

Distribution   *Extent*   Isolated, localized to one region (e.g., shoe dermatitis), or generalized (e.g., plant dermatitis).

Pattern   Random or on exposed areas (as in airborne allergic contact dermatitis).

LABORATORY EXAMINATIONS

Dermatopathology

Inflammation with intraepidermal intercellular edema (spongiosis) and monocyte and histiocyte infiltration in the dermis suggests allergic contact dermatitis, while more superficial vesicles containing polymorphonuclear leukocytes suggest a primary irritant dermatitis. In chronic contact dermatitis there is lichenification (hyperkeratosis, acanthosis, elongation of rete ridges, and elongation and broadening of papillae).

Patch Tests

In allergic contact dermatitis sensitization is present on every part of the skin; therefore, application of the allergen to any area of normal skin provokes inflammation. A positive patch test shows erythema and papules, as well as possibly vesicles confined to the test site. Patch tests should be delayed until the dermatitis has subsided at the selected site of application for at least 2 weeks. (See Appendix B.)

COURSE

Evolution of Contact Dermatitis Reaction

Toxic Irritant Contact Dermatitis

Acute Erythema with a dull, nonglistening surface (Fig. 2-1)→vesiculation (or blister formation)→erosion→crusting–shedding of crusts and scaling.

Chronic Inflammatory thickening of skin→scaling→fissures→crusting (Fig. 2-2). Toxic irritant dermatitis heals spontaneously if exposures are not repeated, chronic toxic irritant contact dermatitis evolves when the noxious agent continues to come into contact with the skin. Chronic inflammation with thickening, fissuring, scaling, and crusting results (Fig. 2-2). A previously sharp margination gives way to an ill-defined border, lichenification.

Allergic Contact Dermatitis

Acute Erythema→papules→vesicles→erosions→crusts→scaling (Figs. 2-3, 2-4).
Note: In the acute forms of contact dermatitis papules occur only in the allergic form.

Chronic Papules→scaling→lichenification→excoriations.

Note: Contact dermatitis is always confined to the site of exposure to the allergen. Margination is originally sharp in allergic contact dermatitis; however, it spreads in the periphery beyond the actual site of exposure. If strong sensitization has occurred, spreading to other parts of the body and generalization occur. The main differences between toxic irritant and allergic contact dermatitis are summarized in Table 2-1.

General Notes on Contact Dermatitis The acute form of toxic contact dermatitis, which in severe cases may even lead to necrosis, occurs after a single exposure to the offending agent that is toxic to the skin (e.g., croton oil, phenols, kerosene, organic solvents, sodium and potassium hydroxide, lime acids) (Fig. 2-1). It is thus dependent on concentration of the offending agent and occurs in everyone, depending, of course, on the permeability and thickness of the stratum corneum. There is a threshold concentration for these substances above which they cause acute dermatitis and below which they do not. This sets it apart from acute allergic contact dermatitis, which is dependent on sensitization and thus occurs only in sensitized individuals (Table 2-2). Depending on the degree of sensitization, minute amounts of the offending agents may elicit a reaction. Since toxic irritant contact dermatitis is a toxic phenomenon, it is confined to the area of exposure, and it is therefore always sharply marginated and never spreads. Allergic contact dermatitis is an immunologic reaction that tends to involve the surrounding skin (spreading phenomenon) and may even spread beyond affected sites. Generalization occurs.

Chronic Toxic Contact Dermatitis of the Hands This contact dermatitis results from repeated exposures to toxic or subtoxic concentrations of offending agents and is usually associated with a chronic disturbance of the barrier function that allows even subtoxic concentrations of offending agents to penetrate into the skin and elicit a chronic inflammatory response. It is thus often the result of repeated exposure to alkaline detergents and organic solvents, which, if applied only once in normal skin, do not elicit a reaction. Injury, (e.g., repeated rubbing of the skin), prolonged soaking in water, or chronic contact with corrosive agents fosters the evolution of chronic toxic contact dermatitis. A typical example is the hand eczema of bricklayers, mechanics, and painters. In these persons, hand eczema is usually a combination of chronic toxic contact der-

---

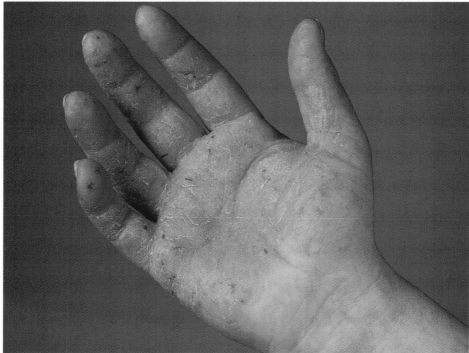

Figure 2-2 Irritant contact dermatitis of hand: subacute/chronic *Erythema, edema, scaling, fissuring, crusting of the palmar aspect of the hand and wrist; the other hand had similar involvement. The patient is atopic, a housewife, and has some element of lichen simplex chronicus.*

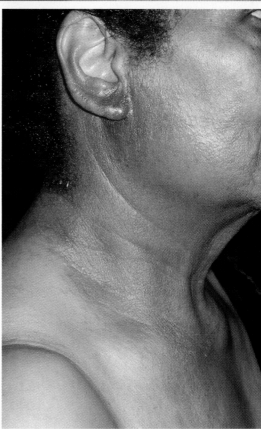

Figure 2-3 Allergic contact dermatitis of ear and neck: neomycin *Erythema, edema microvesiculation. Most severe on the ear and adjacent neck associated with severe pruritus in a 64-year-old female. The patient was allergic to neomycin applying neomycin-containing otic drops for two weeks.*

matitis (alkaline medium of cement, sand, rubbing) and allergic contact dermatitis due to chromates in cement (see Irritant Contact Dermatitis below).

MANAGEMENT

Acute

Identify and remove the etiologic agent.
Larger vesicles may be drained, but tops should *not* be removed.
Wet dressings with gauze soaked in Burow's solution, changed every 2 to 3 h.

Topical class I glucocorticoid preparations.
In severe cases, systemic glucocorticoids may be indicated.
Prednisone: 2-week course, 70 mg initially, tapering by 5 mg daily.

Subacute and Chronic If the lesions are not bullous, it is possible to use a short course of one of the potent topical glucocorticoid preparations, betamethasone dipropionate or clobetasol propionate. No doubt the newer topical anti-inflammatory preparations (e.g., tacrolimus or ascomycins) will replace the glucocorticoids for all stages of contact allergic dermatitis.

Table 2-1 DIFFERENCES BETWEEN TOXIC (IRRITANT) AND ALLERGIC CONTACT DERMATITIS

		Toxic/Irritant CD	Allergic CD
Lesions	Acute	Erythema→vesicle→ erosion→crust→ scaling	Erythema→papules→ vesicles→erosions →crusts→scaling
	Chronic	Papules, plaques, fissures, scaling, crusts	Papules, plaques, scaling, crusts
Margination and Site	Acute	Sharp, strictly confined to site of exposure	Sharp, confined to site of exposure but spreading in the periphery, usually tiny papules, may become generalized
	Chronic	Ill-defined	Ill-defined, spreads
Evolution	Acute	Rapid (few hours after exposure)	Not so rapid (12 to 74 h after exposure)
	Chronic	Months to years of repeated exposure	Months or longer; exacerbation after every reexposure
Causative Agent		Dependent on concentration of agent; occurs only above threshold level	Relatively independent of amount applied; usually very low concentrations sufficient but depends on degree of sensitization
Incidence		May occur in practically everyone	Occurs only in the sensitized

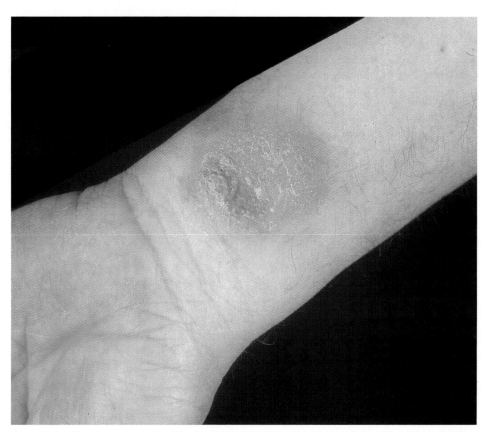

Figure 2-4 Allergic contact dermatitis of wrist: nickel *An acute eczematous patch on the wrist at the site of contact with a watch band clasp containing nickel.*

Table 2-2 COMMON CONTACT ALLERGENS

Neomycin (Fig. 2-3)	Usually contained in creams, ointments
Procaine, benzocaine	Local anesthetics
Sulfonamides	
Terpentine	Solvents, shoe polish, printer's ink
Balsam of Peru	Topical medications
Thiuram	Rubber
Formalin	Disinfectant, curing agents, plastics
Mercury	Disinfectant, impregnation
Chromates	Cement, antioxidants, industrial oils, matches
Nickel sulfate (Fig. 2-4)	Metals, metals in clothing, jewelry, catalyzing agents
Cobalt sulfate	Cement, galvanization, industrial oils, cooling agents, eye shades
p-Phenylene diamine	Black or dark dyes of textiles, printer's ink
Parahydroxybenzoic acid ester	Conserving agent in foodstuffs

IRRITANT CONTACT DERMATITIS

Irritant contact dermatitis (ICD) is caused by exposure of the skin to chemical or other physical agents which are capable of irritating the skin, acutely or chronically. Severe irritants can cause toxic reactions even after a short exposure. Most cases, however, are caused by chronic cumulative exposure to one or more irritants. The hands are the most commonly affected area (Fig. 2-2). In addition to dermatitis, irritant contact responses of the skin include: subjective irritancy, transient irritant reactions, persistent irritant reactions, toxic (caustic) burn. Irritant contact responses of skin appendages and pigmentary system include: follicular and acneform eruptions, miliaria, pigmentary changes (hypo- and hyperpigmentation), granulomatous reactions, and alopecia.

EPIDEMIOLOGY

Etiologic Agents in Irritant Contact Dermatitis:

- Abrasives.
- Cleaning agents, solvents, alkalis (e.g., cement), acids, detergents, soaps, solvents (organic), cutting oils.
- Oxidizing agents (e.g., sodium hypochlorite); reducing agents (e.g., phenols, hydrazine, aldehydes, thiophosphates).
- Plants (e.g., spurge, *Boracinaceae, Ranunculaceae*).
- Animal enzymes, secretions.
- Dessicant powders, dust, soils.
- Water.

Predisposing Factors Atopics with a history of atopic dermatitis are at highest risk for ICD. White skin. Temperature (low), climate (low humidity), occlusion, mechanical irritation. Cement ICD tends to flare in summer in hot humid climates.

Occupational Exposure Individuals engaged in the following occupations/activities are at risk for ICD: housekeeping (Fig. 2-2); hairdressing; medical, dental, and veterinary services; cleaning; floral arranging; agriculture; horticulture; forestry; food preparation and catering; printing; painting; metal work; mechanical engineering; construction; fishing.

PATHOGENESIS

Both chemical and physical agents can be irritants, causing cell damage if applied for sufficient time and in adequate concentration. ICD occurs when defense or repair capacity of the skin is unable to maintain normal skin integrity

and function or when penetration of chemical(s) induces an inflammatory response. Lesser irritants cause reaction only after prolonged exposure. The initial reaction is usually limited to the site of contact with irritant, the concentration of irritant diffusing outside the area of contact almost always falls below the critical threshold necessary to provoke a reaction. Individuals with an atopic diathesis are predisposed to irritant dermatitis; chronic rubbing and scratching compounds both irritant and atopic dermatitis. The majority of workers with significant occupational ICD are atopic; other contributory factors include car maintenance, gardening, adverse climatic or environmental conditions.

HISTORY

Symptoms In some individuals, subjective symptoms (itching, burning, stinging, smarting) may be the only manifestations. Paintful sensations can occur within seconds after exposure (immediate-type stinging) to acids, chloroform, and methanol. Delayed-type stinging occurs within 1 to 2 minutes, peaking at 5 to 10 minutes, fading by 30 minutes, and is caused by agents such as aluminum chloride, phenol, and propylene glycol. Both immediate- and delayed-type stinging occurs most commonly on the face, especially the eyelids, and is more common in atopics.

PHYSICAL EXAMINATION

Skin Findings The spectrum of changes ranges from mild xerosis (dryness), to erythema/chapping to frank eczematous dermatitis (Figs. 2-1 and 2-2) to acute caustic burn and vesiculation.

Additional Findings Chemical burns, erosions, ulcerations, folliculitis, acneform eruption, miliaria, granulomatous dermatitis, edema, pigmentary change, contact urticaria, allergic contact dermatitis.

Secondary Changes Secondary infection with *Staphylococcus aureus* or group A streptococcus (impetigo, ecthyma, folliculitis, soft tissue infection); excoriations, lichenification, hyper- and/or hypopigmentation, scarring.

DIFFERENTIAL DIAGNOSIS

Plaques on exposed skin sites Atopic eczema (acute, subacute, chronic), allergic contact dermatitis, photodermatitis, contact urticaria, pellagra, thermal injury, ionizing radiation damage.

LABORATORY EXAMINATIONS

Patch Tests Rule out allergic contact dermatitis.

Microbiology Rule out secondary *S. aureus* or GAS infection.

COURSE

Healing usually occurs within 2 weeks of removal of noxious stimuli; in more chronic cases, 6 weeks or longer may be required. In the setting of occupational ICD, only one-third of individuals have complete remission; atopic individuals have a worse prognosis. In cases of chronic subcritical levels or irritant, some workers develop tolerance or "hardening."

MANAGEMENT

Prevention
- Avoid irritant or caustic chemical(s) by wearing protective clothing (i.e., goggles, shields, gloves).
- If contact does occur, wash with water or weak neutralizing solution.
- Barrier creams.
- In occupational ICD which persists in spite of adherence to the above measures, change of job may be necessary.

Topical Treatment

For acute exudative ICD, wet dressings using gauze soaked in Burow's solution changed every 2 to 3 hours.

Corticosteroids

Topical Corticosteroid Preparations Class I preparations may be effective in nonexudative, nonbullous ICD.

Systemic Corticosteroids Indicated if severe (i.e., if patient cannot perform usual daily functions, cannot sleep) for exudative lesions. Prednisone beginning at 70 mg (adults) tapering by 5 to 10 mg/d over a 2- to 1-week period.

ALLERGIC CONTACT DERMATITIS DUE TO PLANTS

Allergic contact dermatitis associated with plants, termed *allergic phytodermatitis* (APD), occurs in sensitized individuals after exposure to a wide variety of plant allergens and is characterized by an acute, very pruritic, eczematous dermatitis, often with blisters arising in a linear arrangement at the site of plant contact. In the United States, poison ivy/oak are by far the most common plants implicated in APD. In contrast, phytophotodermatitis is a photosensitive reaction occurring in any individual with a photosensitizing plant-derived chemical on the skin after sun exposure (see Section 8).

Synonyms: Poison oak dermatitis, poison ivy dermatitis, toxicodendron dermatitis.

EPIDEMIOLOGY

Age of Onset Occurs in individuals of all ages. Very young and very old are less likely to be exposed to plants. No influence on capacity for sensitization. Allergic contact dermatitis, however, is uncommon in young children. Sensitization is life-long.

Etiology Pentadecylcatechols, which are present in the Anacardiaceae plant family, are the most common sensitizers and the most common cause of allergic contact dermatitis in the United States. Pentadecylcatechols cross-react with other phenolic compounds such as resorcinol, hexylresorcinol, and hydroxyquinones.

Plants
Anacardiaceae Family Poison ivy (*Toxicodendron radicans*) and poison oak (*T. querifolium, T. diversilobum*) are the most common causes of APD in the United States. Also caused by exposure to poison sumac (*T. vernix*). Plants related to poison ivy group: Brazilian pepper, cashew nut tree, ginkgo tree, Indian marker nut tree, lacquer tree, mango tree, rengas tree.

Geography Poison ivy occurs throughout the United States (except extreme southwest) and southern Canada. Poison oak occurs on the West Coast (west of Cascade and Sierra Nevada Mountains, from Puget Sound area to Mexico). Poison sumac and poison dogwood grow only in woody, swampy areas.

Race Dark-skinned individuals may be less susceptible to APD.

Susceptibility >70% of individuals can be sensitized.

Exposure Telephone and electrical workers who work in the out-of-doors with transmission lines are commonly exposed to poison oak/ivy. Leaves, stems, seeds, flowers, berries, root of plants contain milky sap that turns to a black resin on exposure to air.

Cashew oil: unroasted cashew nut (heat destroys hapten); cashew oil in wood (Haitian voodoo dolls, swizzle sticks), resins, printer's ink. Mango rind. Marking nut tree of India: laundry marker (dhobi itch). Furniture lacquer from Japanese lacquer tree.

Season In the eastern United States, APD usually occurs in the spring, summer, and fall; can occur year round if exposed to stems or roots. In southwest, occurs year round.

PATHOGENESIS

All *Toxicodendron* plants contain identical allergens, causing identical APD. Hapten is present in milky sap in leaves, stems, seeds, flowers, berries, and roots. The oleoresins of Anacardiaceae plants are referred to as urushiol. The haptens in oleoresins are the pentadecylcatechols(1,2-hydroxybenzenes with a 15-carbon side chain in position three). Washing with soap and water removes oleoresins.

Genetically, >70% of individuals can be sensitized to *Toxicodendron* haptens. After first exposure to the oleoresin, sensitization and dermatitis occur 7 to 12 days later. In a previously sensitized person (may be many decades before), dermatitis can occur (especially on face or genitalia) in <12 h after reexposure. Difference in clinical course among individuals varies with individual reactivity, inoculum of hapten on skin, regional variation of cutaneous reactivity.

Misconceptions about Poison Ivy/Oak Dermatitis Contrary to Widely Held Belief:

- Blister fluid does not contain hapten and cannot spread the dermatitis.
- Exposure to smoke from the burning plant is harmless; dermatitis can occur if particulate matter from the plant in the smoke can produce dermatitis.
- Mucous membranes uncommonly experience allergic dermatitis after antigen exposure; ingestion of urushiol can produce allergic contact dermatitis of the anus and perineum as it is passed in feces.

HISTORY

Exposure

Posion Ivy/Oak Dermatitis Direct plant exposure: Plant brushes against exposed skin giving rise to linear lesions; resin usually is not able to penetrate the thick stratum corneum of palms/soles. Blotting of oleoresin from hands to other sites: APD commonly arises on areas with thin stratum corneum. Clothing: wearing clothing previously contaminated with resin can reexpose the skin. Pets: oleoresin on fur can be transferred to skin.

Food Containing Urushiol Eating unpeeled mango with rind can expose lips to oleoresin. Eating unroasted cashew nuts can expose lips.

Skin Symptoms Pruritus is often sensed before any detectable skin changes. Pruritus, mild to severe. Pain in some cases. Secondary infection can be associated with local tenderness or pain.

Constitutional Symptoms Sleep deprivation due to pruritus.

PHYSICAL EXAMINATION

Skin Lesions

Sites of Exposure Exposure can be by direct contact of the plant with exposed skin or indirectly from the hands, clothing, fur of a pet, etc. Initially, well-demarcated patches of erythema. Sites of direct contact can have characteristic linear lesions (Fig. 2-5). Erythematous areas rapidly evolve into edematous papules, nodules, plaques mimicking urticaria or angioedema; may be severe especially on face and/or genitals, resembling cellulitis (Fig. 2-6). Blisters:

initially microvesiculation in erythematous plaques; may evolve to vesicles and/or bullae. Erosions, crusts: after rupture of blisters. With resolution, erythematous plaques ±scale, ±erosion, ±crusting. Post-inflammatory hyperpigmentation is common in darker skinned individuals.

Distribution Most commonly on exposed extremities, where direct contact with the plant occurs; blotting can transfer to any exposed site; palms/soles are usually spared, however, lateral fingers can be involved.

Clothing-protected Sites Oleoresin can penetrate damp clothing onto covered skin.

Nonexposed Sites "Id"-like reaction or some systemic absorption can be associated with disseminated urticarial, erythema multiforme-like, or scarlitiniform lesions away from sites of exposure in some individuals with well-established APD.

DIFFERENTIAL DIAGNOSIS

Red, Warm, Edematous Plaque—Single Soft-tissue infection (cellulitis, erysipelas), insect bite, atopic dermatitis, inflammatory epidermal dermatophytosis, early herpes zoster, fixed drug eruption.

Red, Warm, Edematous Plaque—Multiple Urticaria/angioedema, inflammatory pityriasis rosea, inflammatory epidermal dermatophytosis.

LABORATORY EXAMINATIONS

Culture/Gram Stain Rule out secondary *S. aureus* or group A streptococcal infection if lesions purulent or tender.

Dermatopathology See Contact Dermatitis.

Patch Tests with Pentadecylcatechols Contraindicated. Can sensitize the individual to hapten.

DIAGNOSIS

By history and clinical findings.

COURSE

The duration of APD varies among individuals, resolving in some in 1 to 2 weeks.

MANAGEMENT

Termination of Exposure to Allergen Identify and remove the etiologic agent.

Topical Therapy Class I topical glucocorticoid ointments/gels are effective for early nonbullous lesions. Larger vesicles may be drained, but tops should not be removed. Wet dressings with cloths soaked in Burow's solution changed every 2 to 3 h.

Systemic Therapy In patients with blisters, topical glucocorticoids are ineffective. Prednisone, 1 mg/kg (40 to 70 mg/d) reduced over 1 to 2 weeks, is very effective with minimal side effects. A convenient dosing schedule (given as a single A.M. dose) is 70 mg as the initial dose, tapering by 10 or 5 mg each day over 1 to 2 weeks. There is no risk of side effects with this short dosing schedule.

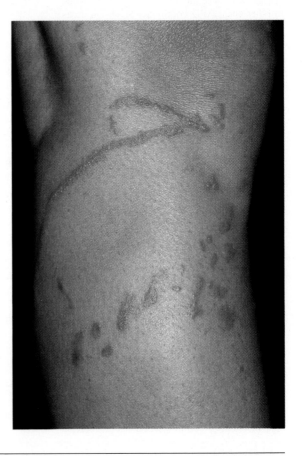

Figure 2-5 Allergic phytodermatitis of leg: poison ivy *Linear vesicular lesions with erythema and edema on the calf at sites of direct contact of the skin 5 days after exposure with the poison ivy leaf.*

ECZEMA/DERMATITIS

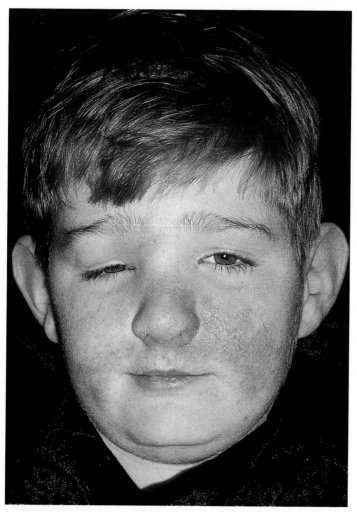

Figure 2-6   Allergic phytodermatitis of face: poison ivy   *Very pruritic erythema, edema, microvesiculation of the cheeks and periorbital area in a previously sensitized seven-year-old boy, occurring 3 days after exposure.*

ATOPIC DERMATITIS

Atopic dermatitis (AD) is a acute, subacute or chronic relapsing skin disorder that usually begins in infancy and is characterized principally by marked pruritus, which with rubbing and scratching leads to lichenification (hyperplasia of the skin.) The diagnosis is based on clinical findings, although the serum IgE level is usually (85%) elevated. AD is often associated with a personal or family history of AD, allergic rhinitis and asthma; 35% of infants with AD develop asthma later in life. Treatment of AD is fraught with problems: dependence on glucocorticoids, a necessity in some patients, results in atrophy, tachyphylaxis, hypertrichosis.

Synonyms: IgE dermatitis, "eczema," atopic eczema.

EPIDEMIOLOGY

Age of Onset   First two months of life and by the first years in 60% of patients.

Gender   Slightly more common in males than females.

Prevalence   7 to 15% reported in population studies in Scandinavia and Germany.

Genetic Aspects   The inheritance pattern has not been ascertained. However, in one series, 60% of adults with AD had children with AD. The prevalence in children was higher (81%) when both parents had AD.

Eliciting Factors   Subset of infants and children have flares of AD with *foods:* eggs, milk, peanuts, soybeans, fish, and wheat. *Inhalants* (specific aeroallergens, especially dust mites) have been shown to cause exacerbations of AD. *Microbial agents:* Exotoxins of *Staphylococcus aureus* may act as superantigens and stimulate activation of T cells and macrophages. *S. aureus* infection can usually be assumed to be present in severe cases, and systemic antibiotic treatment is indicated for 4 to 5 days. Recurrent herpes simplex is not uncommon and may take the form of disseminated vesicles rather than herpetiform arrangements.

Other Exacerbating Factors   *Skin dehydration* by frequent bathing and hand washing; bathing must be considered an important exacerbating factor. *Hormonal:* pregnancy, menstruation, thyroid. *Infections:* S. aureus is almost always present in severe cases; group A streptococcus; herpes simplex virus; rarely fungus (dermatophytosis, candidiasis). *Season:* in temperate climates, usually improves in summer, flares in winter. *Clothing:* pruritus flares *after* taking off clothing; wool clothing or blankets directly in contact with skin. *Emotional stress* that results from the disease or is itself an exacerbating factor in flares of the disease.

PATHOGENESIS

Type I (IgE-mediated) hypersensitivity reaction occurring as a result of the release of vasoactive substances from both mast cells and basophils that have been sensitized by the interaction of the antigen with IgE (reaginic or skin-sensitizing antibody). The role of IgE in AD is still not fully clarified, but it has been shown that epidermal Langerhans cells possess high-affinity IgE receptors through which an eczema-like reaction could be mediated.

HISTORY

Onset   Most patients are affected between infancy and age 12, with 60% by first year; 30% are seen for the first time by age 5, and only 10% develop AD between 6 and 20 years of age. Rarely atopic dermatitis has an adult onset.

Duration of Lesions   Untreated involved sites persist for months or years.

Skin Symptoms   Patients have dry skin. Pruritus is the sine qua non of atopic dermatitis—"Eczema is the itch that rashes." The constant scratching leads to a vicious cycle of itch→scratch→rash→itch (the rash being lichenification of the skin).

Other Symptoms of Atopy   Allergic rhinitis, characterized by sneezing, rhinorrhea, obstruc-

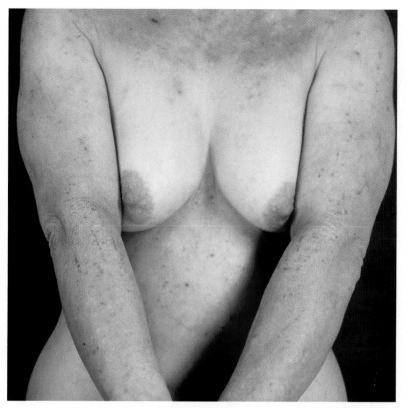

Figure 2-7 Atopic dermatitis: chronic *Chronic eczematous dermatitis with sparing under the bra. Note lichenification and numerous long excoriations. One does not have to take a history to realize that this condition itches severely.*

tion of nasal passages, conjunctival and pharyngeal itching, and lacrimation; may be seasonal when associated with lacrimation allergens such as pollen.

PHYSICAL EXAMINATION

Skin Lesions

Acute Poorly defined erythematous patches, papules, and plaques with or without scale. Edema with widespread involvement; skin appears "puffy" and edematous (Fig. 2-9). Erosions: moist, crusted. Excoriations: result from scratching. Secondarily infected sites: *S. aureus.* Pustules (usually follicular). Crusts.

Chronic Lichenification (Fig. 2-7) (thickening of the skin with accentuation of skin markings) that results from repeated rubbing or scratching; follicular lichenification (especially in brown and black persons) (Fig. 2-8). Fissures: painful, especially on palms, fingers, and

soles. Alopecia: lateral one-third of the eyebrows as a result of rubbing the eyelids. Periorbital pigmentation: also as a result of compulsively rubbing the eyelids. Characteristic infraorbital fold in the eyelids (Dennie-Morgan sign).

Distribution Predilection for the flexures, front and sides of the neck, eyelids, forehead, face, wrists, and dorsa of the feet and hands. Generalized in severe disease.

Special Features Related to Ethnicity In blacks, so-called follicular eczema is common and is characterized by discrete follicular papules involving all hair follicles of the involved site (Fig. 2-8).

Special Features Related to Age

Infantile AD The lesions present as red skin, tiny vesicles on "puffy" surface (especially the face, sparing the mouth). Scaling, exudation with wet crusts and cracks (fissures) (Fig. 2-9).

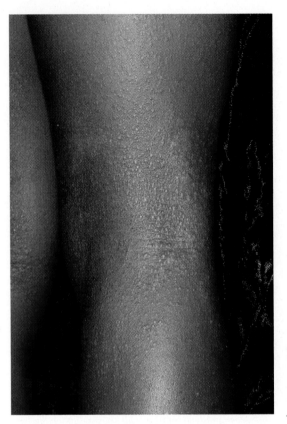

Figure 2-8 Atopic dermatitis in black child: follicular *Pruritic follicular papules on the posterior leg. Follicular eczema is a reaction pattern which occurs more commonly in African and Asian children. Some patients have an associated nickel allergy to the metal fastener in jeans.*

Skin lesions seem to be a reaction to itching and rubbing. In *childhood-type AD*, the lesions are papular, lichenified plaques, erosions, crusts, especially on the antecubitol and popliteal fossae (Fig. 2-10), the neck and face. In *adult-type AD*, there is a similar distribution with lichenification and exoriations being the most conspicuous symptoms (Fig. 2-7).

Associated Findings

"White" dermatographism on stroking is a special and unique feature of involved skin; delayed blanch to cholinergic agents. Ichthyosis vulgaris and keratosis pilaris occur in 10% of patients. Cataracts in a small percentage.

DIFFERENTIAL DIAGNOSIS

Pruritic Plaques Seborrheic dermatitis, contact dermatitis (allergic and irritant), psoriasis, nummular eczema, dermatophytosis, early stages of mycosis fungoides. Rarely, acrodermatitis enteropathica, gluten-sensitive en-

teropathy, glucagonoma syndrome, histidinemia, phenylketonuria; also, some immunologic disorders including Wiskott-Aldrich syndrome, X-linked agammaglobulinemia, hyper-IgE syndrome, Letterer-Siwe disease, and selective IgA deficiency.

LABORATORY EXAMINATIONS

Bacterial Culture Colonization with *S. aureus* is very common in the nares and in the involved skin; almost 90% of patients with severe AD are secondarily colonized/infected.

Viral Culture Rule out HSV infection in crusted lesions (eczema herpeticum).

Blood Studies Increased IgE in serum.

Dermatopathology Various degrees of acanthosis with rare intraepidermal intercellular edema (spongiosis). The dermal infiltrate is composed of lymphocytes, monocytes, and mast cells with few or no eosinophils.

ECZEMA/DERMATITIS

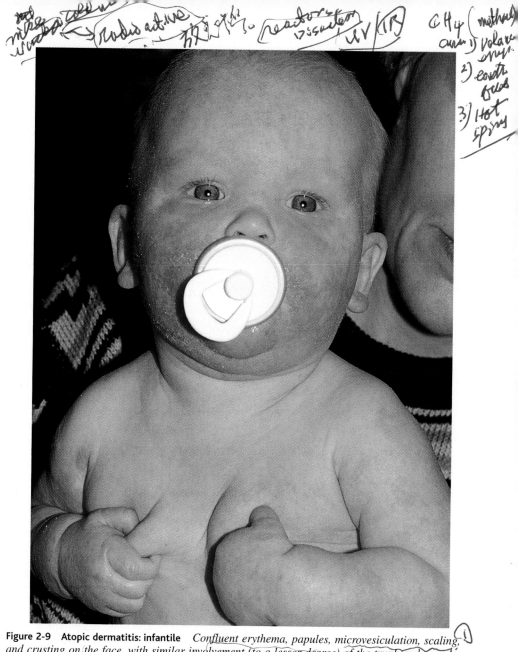

Figure 2-9 Atopic dermatitis: infantile *Confluent erythema, papules, microvesiculation, scaling, and crusting on the face, with similar involvement (to a lesser degree) of the trunk and arms. The facial involvement is more severe due to easier access to scratching. The baby is squeezing the breast skin to relieve the intense pruritus.*

DIAGNOSIS

History in infancy, clinical findings (typical distribution sites, morphology of lesions, white dermatographism).

COURSE AND PROGNOSIS

Spontaneous, more or less complete remission during childhood occurs in >40% with occasional, more severe recurrences during adolescence. In many patients, the disease persists for 15 to 20 years, but is less severe. From 30 to 50% of patients develop asthma and/or hay fever. Adult-onset AD often runs a severe course. *S. aureus* infection leads to extensive erosions and crusting, and herpes simplex infection to eczema herpeticum, which may be life-threatening (see Section 23).

MANAGEMENT

Education of the patient to avoid rubbing and scratching is most important. Topical antipruritic (menthol/camphor) lotions are helpful in controlling the pruritus but are useless if the patient continues to scratch and rub the plaques.

An allergic workup is rarely helpful in uncovering an allergen; however, in patients who are hypersensitive to house dust, mites, various pollens, and animal hair proteins, exposure to the appropriate allergen may cause flares. Atopic dermatitis is considered by many to be related, at least in part, to emotional stress.

Warn patients of their special problems with herpes simplex and the frequency of superimposed staphylococcal infection, for which oral antibiotics are indicated. Antiviral drugs for herpes simplex are indicated if HSV infection is suspected.

Acute

1. Wet dressings and topical glucocorticoids; topical antibiotics (mupirocin ointment) when indicated.
2. Hydroxyzine, 10 to 100 mg qid for pruritus.
3. Oral antibiotics (dicloxacillin, erythromycin) to eliminate *S. aureus*. (See Bacterial Infection.)

Subacute and Chronic

1. Oral H_1 antihistamines are useful in reducing itching.

2. Topical ointments containing H_1 and H_2 blockers (doxepin) are useful for pruritus, if it is not controlled by hydroxyzine.
3. Hydration (oilated baths or baths with oatmeal powder) followed by application of unscented emollients (e.g., hydrated petrolatum) is a basic daily treatment needed to prevent xerosis. Soap showers are permissible to wash the body folds, but soap seldom should be used on the other parts of the skin surface. 12% ammonium lactate or 10% α-hydroxy acid lotion is very effective for the xerosis often seen in AD.
4. Topical anti-inflammatory agents such as glucocorticoids, hydroxyquinoline preparations, and tar are the mainstays of treatment. Of these, glucocorticoids are the most readily accepted by the patient.
5. Systemic glucocorticoids should be avoided, except in rare instances for only short courses. They are widely overused. Osteopenia and cataracts are complications. For severe intractable disease, prednisone, 60 to 80 mg daily for two days, then halving the dose each two days for the next six days. Glucocorticoids should be given with meals and in divided doses. Patients with AD tend to become dependent on oral glucocorticoids. Often, small doses (5 to 10 mg) make the difference in control and can be reduced gradually to even 2.5 mg/d, as is often used for the control of asthma. Intramuscular glucocorticoids are risky and should be avoided.
6. Patients should learn and use stress management techniques.
7. UVA-UVB phototherapy (combination of UVA plus UVB and increasing the radiation dose each treatment, with a frequency of two to three times weekly). Narrow band UV (311 nm), PUVA photochemotherapy also effective, if available.
8. In severe cases of adult-onset AD and in normotensive healthy persons without renal disease, cyclosporin A (cyclosporine) treatment (starting dose 5 mg/kg/d) is indicated when all other treatments fail, but should be monitored closely. Treatment is limited to 3 to 6 months because of potential side effects, including hypertension and reduced renal function. Blood pressure should be checked weekly and chemistry panels biweekly. Nifedipine should be used for moderate increases in blood pressure.
9. Since the advent of topical glucocorticoids, the problem has lost much of its serious

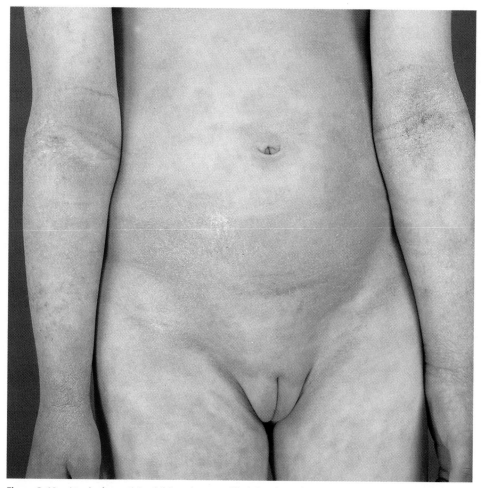

Figure 2-10 Atopic dermatitis: childhood-type *Ill-defined erythema, papules, excoriations, lichenification (thickening of the skin with accentuation of the skin lines) in the antecubital fossae, with less severe changes on the trunk and thighs.*

ness. Yet use of class I (potent) glucocorticoids is to be avoided on the face. Newer topical nonsteroidal preparations such as tacrolimus ointment (not available yet in the United States but available in Japan) or topical ascomycins show great promise for control without the disturbing side-effects of glucocorticoids. Prompt response to potent glucocorticoids; after improvement, use low-potency glucocorticoids or emol-

lients. For recurrence, return for a short period to the stronger glucocorticoids. Beware of skin atrophy. With sensible use, no danger of suppression of pituitary-adrenal axis. For extra security, monitor growth curve. Tar baths, ointments, pastes, and gels are also effective. Newer nonsteroidal anti-eczema preparations may soon be available and will replace topical glucocorticoids. Reassure parents.

LICHEN SIMPLEX CHRONICUS

Lichen simplex chronicus (LSC) is a special localized form of lichenification usually occurring in circumscribed plaques. Lichenification is a characteristic feature of atopic dermatitis, whether generalized or localized. Lichen simplex can last for decades unless the rubbing and scratching is stopped by treatment of the lichenified skin.

EPIDEMIOLOGY

Age of Onset   Older than 20 years.

Sex   More frequent in women.

Race   A possibly higher incidence in Asians.

Factors   Emotional stress in some cases. It becomes a habit and may persist for months to years, with resulting marked lichenification.

PATHOGENESIS

A special predilection of the skin to respond to physical trauma by epidermal hyperplasia; skin becomes highly sensitive to touch, a fact probably related to proliferation of nerves in the epidermis. The very abnormal itching hyperexcitability of lichenified skin arises in response to minimal external stimuli that would not elicit an itch response in normal skin.

HISTORY

Duration of Lesion(s)   Weeks to months to years.

Skin Symptoms   Pruritus, often in paroxysms. The lichenified skin is like an erogenous zone—it becomes a pleasure (orgiastic) to scratch. Often the areas on the feet are rubbed at night with the heel and the toes. The rubbing becomes automatic and reflexive and an unconscious habit.

Most patients with LSC give a history of itch attacks starting from minor stimuli: putting on clothes; removing ointments; clothes rubbing the skin; and when they go to bed, the skin becomes warmer and the warmth precipitates itching.

PHYSICAL EXAMINATION

Skin Lesions   A solid plaque of lichenification, arising from the confluence of small papules (Fig. 2-11); scaling is minimal except in nuchal lichen simplex. Lichenified skin is palpably thickened; skin markings (barely visible in normal skin) are accentuated and can be seen readily (see also Fig. 2-7). Excoriations are often present. Lightly stroking the involved skin with a cotton swab generates a strong desire to scratch the skin; the same reflex is not present in uninvolved skin. Usually dull red, later brown or black hyperpigmentation, especially in skin phototypes IV, V, and VI. Round, oval, linear (following path of scratching). Usually sharply defined.

Distribution   Isolated single lesion or several randomly scattered plaques. Nuchal area (female) (Fig. 2-11), scalp, ankles, lower legs, upper thighs, exterior forearms, vulva, pubis, anal area, scrotum, and groin.

Special Features Related to Ethnicity   In black skin, lichenification may assume a special type of pattern—there is not a solid plaque, but the lichenification consists instead of a multitude of small (2- to 3-mm) lichenified papules—i.e., a "follicular" pattern (as in Fig. 2-8).

DIFFERENTIAL DIAGNOSIS

Chronic Pruritic Plaque   Psoriasis vulgaris, early stages of mycosis fungoides, contact dermatitis (irritant or allergic), epidermal dermatophytosis, Schamberg's disease.

LABORATORY EXAMINATIONS

KOH Preparation   Rule out dermatophytosis.

Dermatopathology   Hyperplasia of all components of epidermis: hyperkeratosis, acanthosis, and elongated and broad rete ridges. Spongiosis is infrequent. In the dermis there is a chronic inflammatory infiltrate.

DIAGNOSIS

Made on basis of the history and physical findings.

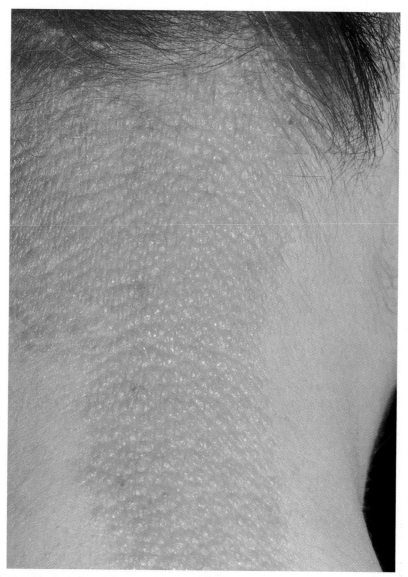

Figure 2-11 Lichen simplex chronicus *Confluent, papular, follicular eczema, creating a plaque of lichen simplex chronicus of the posterior neck and occipital scalp. Condition had been present for many years as a result of chronic rubbing of the area.*

MANAGEMENT

Difficult! Repeatedly explain to the patient that the rubbing and scratching must be stopped. It is important to apply occlusive bandages at night to prevent rubbing and to facilitate penetration of topical glucocorticoids.

Topical Therapy

Topical Glucocorticoid Preparations Covered by continuous dry occlusive gauze dressings.

Intralesional Triamcinolone Often highly effective (3 mg/mL; higher concentrations may cause atrophy).

Tar Preparations Combinations of 5% crude coal tar in zinc oxide paste plus class II glucocorticoids covered by occlusive cloth dry dressings are effective for body areas where this approach is feasible (e.g., legs, arms).

Occlusive Dressings Glucocorticoid preparations are usually applied first, followed by an occlusive dressing. The dressing alone, however, prevents the patient from scratching and is an effective treatment. Glucocorticoids incorporated in adhesive plastic tape are very effective and can be left on for 24 h.

Unna Boot A gauze roll dressing impregnated with zinc oxide paste is wrapped around a large lichenified area such as the calf. The dressing can be left on for up to 1 week.

Antihistamines

Topical Preparations Doxepin 5% ointment may be effective in some patients.

Oral Hydroxyzine, 25 to 50 g at night, may be helpful.

Prurigo Nodularis

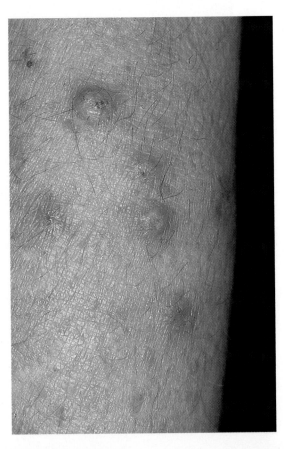

Figure 2-12 Prurigo nodularis *Multiple, firm, excoriated nodules arising at sites of chronically picked or excoriated skin. Often occurring in patients with atopy but also without it. Usually in younger or middle-aged females, who often exhibit signs of neurotic stigmatization. Starts with piercing pruritus that leads to picking and scratching. Note that in this particular patient—a 36-year-old female—prurigo nodules occur in the context of lichenified atopic dermatitis. Lesions persist for months after the trauma has been discontinued.*

DYSHIDROTIC ECZEMATOUS DERMATITIS

Dyshidrotic eczema is a special vesicular type of hand and foot dermatitis. It is an acute, chronic, or recurrent dermatosis of the fingers, palms, and soles, characterized by a sudden onset of many deep-seated pruritic, clear "tapioca-like" vesicles; later, scaling fissures, and lichenification occur. Although implied by the name "dyshidrosis," there are no abnormalities of sweat gland function.

Synonyms: Pompholyx, vesicular palmar eczema.

EPIDEMIOLOGY

Age of Onset Majority under 40 years (range 12 to 40 years).

Gender Equal in males and females.

PATHOGENESIS

Despite the name *dyshidrotic eczema,* there is no evidence that sweating plays a role in the pathogenesis. About half the patients have an atopic background. Emotional stress is possibly a precipitating factor. Many patients claim the eruption recurs only in hot, humid weather.

HISTORY

Duration of Lesions Outbreaks usually last for several weeks. And then the skin is completely clear of lesions.

Skin Symptoms Pruritus at sites of new vesicles. Pain in fissures and secondarily infected lesions.

PHYSICAL EXAMINATION

Skin Lesions *Early* Vesicles, usually small (1 mm), deep-seated, appearing like "tapioca" in clusters, especially along the sides of the fingers. Bullae, occasionally (Fig. 2-13). *Later* Papules, scaling, lichenification, *painful fissures,* and erosions, which result from coalescing ruptured vesicles and may be quite extensive. Crusts. Secondarily infected lesions are characterized by pustules, crusts, cellulitis, lymphangitis, and painful lymphadenopathy.

Vesicles often deep-seated, grouped in clusters, like "tapioca."

Distribution Hands (80%) and feet. Sites of predilection: initially, lateral aspects of fingers, palms, soles; later, dorsa of fingers.

DIFFERENTIAL DIAGNOSIS

Contact (allergic or irritant) dermatitis, atopic dermatitis of hands/feet, palmar/plantar pustulosis, bullous tinea pedis, "id" reaction (vesicular reaction to active dermatophytosis on the feet or stasis dermatitis), scabies.

LABORATORY EXAMINATIONS

Bacterial Culture Rule out *Staphylococcus aureus* infection.

KOH Preparation Rule out epidermal dermatophytosis.

Dermatopathology Eczematous inflammation (spongiosis and intraepidermal edema) with intraepidermal vesicles.

COURSE AND PROGNOSIS

Recurrent attacks are the rule. Spontaneous remissions in 2 to 3 weeks. Interval between attacks is weeks to months. Secondary infection may complicate the course.

Uncommonly, the disease may be disabling because of severe, frequently recurring outbreaks.

MANAGEMENT

Wet Dressing For early vesicular stage: Burow's wet dressings. Large bullae should be drained with a puncture but not unroofed.

Fissures Disabling and painful. Can be readily "healed" with topical application of flexible collodion.

Glucocorticoids

Topical High-potency glucocorticoids with plastic occlusive dressings for 1 to 2 weeks to involved areas only.

Intralesional Injection Very effective for small areas of involvement; triamcinolone, 3 mg/mL.

Systemic In severe cases, a short, tapered course can be given: prednisone, 70 mg, tapering by 10 or 5 mg/d over 7 or 14 days.

Systemic Antibiotic For suspected (localized pain) or documented secondarily infected lesions (usually *S. aureus;* less commonly group A streptococcus) (See Impetigo.) Oral antibiotics are indicated even without the typical crusts being present.

PUVA Oral or topical as "soaks." Successful in many patients if given over prolonged periods of time and worth trying, especially in severe cases.

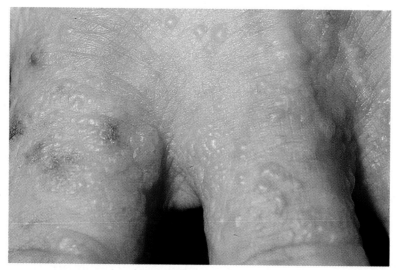

Figure 2-13 Dyshidrotic eczema *Confluent tapioca-like vesicles and crusted (excoriated) erosions on the dorsum of fingers.*

NUMMULAR ECZEMA

Nummular eczema is a chronic, pruritic, inflammatory dermatitis occurring in the form of coin-shaped plaques composed of grouped small papules and vesicles on an erythematous base, especially common on the lower legs of older males during winter months; often seen in atopic individuals.

Synonym: Discoid eczema.

EPIDEMIOLOGY

Age of Onset Two peaks in incidence: young adulthood and old age.

Season Fall and winter.

PATHOGENESIS

Unknown. Unrelated to atopic diathesis; IgE levels are normal. Incidence peaks in winter, when xerosis is maximal.

HISTORY

Duration of Lesions Weeks to months.

Skin Symptoms Pruritus, often intense.

PHYSICAL EXAMINATION

Skin Lesions Closely grouped, small vesicles and papules that coalesce into plaques (Fig. 2-14), often more than 4 to 5 cm in diameter, with an erythematous base with distinct borders. Plaques may become exudative and crust. Excoriations secondary to scratching. Dry scaly plaques that may be lichenified. Round or *coin-shaped,* hence the adjective *nummular* (Latin: *nummularis,* "like a coin"). Margins often more pronounced than center.

Distribution Regional clusters of lesions (e.g., on legs or trunk) or generalized, scattered. Lower legs (older men), trunk, hands and fingers (younger females).

DIFFERENTIAL DIAGNOSIS

Scaling Plaques Epidermal dermatophytosis, contact dermatitis (allergic or irritant), psoriasis vulgaris, early stages of mycosis fungoides, impetigo, familial pemphigus.

LABORATORY EXAMINATIONS

Bacterial Culture Rule out *Staphylococcus aureus* infection.

Dermatopathology Subacute inflammation with acanthosis and spongiosis.

COURSE AND PROGNOSIS

Chronic. Often difficult to control even with potent topical glucocorticoid preparations.

MANAGEMENT

Skin Hydration "Moisturize" involved skin after bath or shower with hydrated petrolatum or other moisturizing cream. (See Ichthyosis Vulgaris.)

Glucocorticoids *Topical Preparations* Potent ointment (classes I and II) applied bid until lesions have resolved. Steroid impregnated tape.

Intralesional Triamcinolone, 3 mg/mL, is very effective.

Crude Coal Tar 2 to 5% crude coal tar ointment daily. May be combined with glucocorticoid preparation. Tar baths are useful in patients with refractory lesions.

Systemic Therapy Systemic antibiotics if *S. aureus* is present, which is usually the case.

PUVA or UVB 311-nm Therapy Very effective.

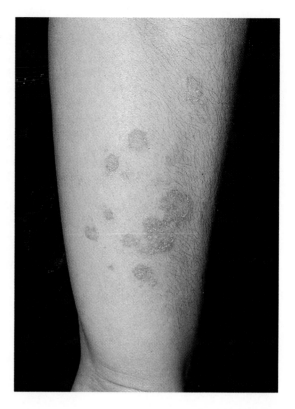

Figure 2-14 Nummular eczema *Pruritic, round, nummular (coin-shaped) plaques with erythema, scales, and crusts on the forearm.*

AUTOSENSITIZATION DERMATITIS

This term refers to an often unrecognized pruritic dermatitis on the trunk; however, the rash is directly related to a primary dermatitis on the legs. For example, a patient with venous stasis dermatitis on the lower legs may develop pruritic, symmetrical, scattered, erythematous, maculopapular, or papulovesicular lesions on the forearms, thighs, legs, and especially the trunk. The eruption persists and spreads until the basic underlying primary dermatitis on the legs is controlled. The itching on the trunk may be severe and intractable, and disappears only when the leg dermatitis is treated. Similarly, autosensitization may occur as an "id" reaction in inflammatory tinea pedis and manifests as a dyshidrosiform, vesicular eruption on the feet and hands (Fig. 2-15) and papulovesicular eczematoid lesions on the trunk.

The phenomenon results from the release of cytokines that develop in the primary dermatitis, as a result of sensitization. These cytokines circulating in the blood could heighten the sensitivity of the distant skin areas. The diagnosis of autosensitization dermatitis is often *post hoc,* that is, the distant eruption disappears when the primary dermatitis is controlled. with topical corticosteroids which are known to ablate cytokines. Oral corticosteroids hasten the disappearance of the lesions.

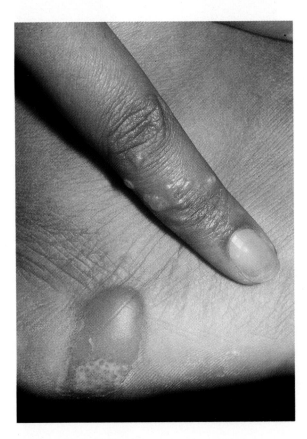

Figure 2-15 Autosensitization dermatitis ("id" reaction): dermatophytid *Vesicles and bullae on the finger and the lateral foot of a 21-year-old female. Bullous (inflammatory) tinea pedis was present and was associated with dermatophytid reaction. Prednisone was given for two weeks; pruritus and vesiculation resolved.*

ECZEMA/DERMATITIS

SEBORRHEIC DERMATITIS

Seborrheic dermatitis (SD) is a very common chronic dermatosis characterized by redness and scaling occurring in regions where the sebaceous glands are most active, such as the face and scalp, the presternal area, and in the body folds. Mild scalp SD causes flaking, i.e., dandruff. Chronic recurrent seborrheic dermatitis is a challenge for the clinician because of the lack of safe and effective treatments. Generalized seborrheic dermatitis, failure to thrive, and diarrhea in an infant should bring to mind Leiner's disease with a variety of immunodeficiency disorders.

Synonyms: "Cradle cap" (infants), pityriasis sicca (dandruff).

EPIDEMIOLOGY

Age of Onset   Infancy (within the first months), puberty, most between 20 and 50 years or older.

Sex   More common in males.

Incidence   2 to 5% of the population.

Predisposing and Exacerbating Factors   In immunocompetent patients there is often a hereditary diathesis, the so-called "seborrheic state," with marked seborrhea and marginal blepharitis. May be associated with psoriasis as a pre-psoriasis state in which the patient later develops psoriasis, or in some patients a mix of lesions (superficial scales on the scalp and eyebrows and polycyclic scaling patches on the trunk) suggests the use of the term seborrhiasis. There is reputedly an increased incidence in Parkinson's disease, and facial paralysis. Also, some neuroleptic drugs are possibly a factor, but the disease is so common that it has not been proved. Emotional stress is a putative factor in flares.

HIV-infected individuals have an increased incidence, and severe intractable seborrheic dermatitis should be a clue to the existence of HIV disease.

PATHOGENESIS

Pityrosporon ovale is said to play a role in the pathogenesis, and the response to topical ketoconazole and selenium sulfide is some indication that this yeast may be pathogenic as well as the frequency of SD in immunosuppressed patients (HIV, cardiac transplants). SD-like lesions are seen in nutritional deficiencies such as zinc deficiency (as a result of IV alimentation) and experimental niacin deficiency and in Parkinson's disease (including drug-induced). SD develops in experimental pyridoxine deficiency in humans.

HISTORY

Duration of Lesions   Gradual onset.

Seasonal Variations   Some patients are worse in a winter dry, indoor environment. Sunlight exposure causes SD to flare in a few patients and promotes improvement of the condition in others.

Skin Symptoms   Pruritus is variable, often increased by perspiration.

PHYSICAL EXAMINATION

Skin Lesions

Yellowish-red or gray-white skin, often with "greasy" or white dry scaling macules and papules of varying size (5 to 20 mm) (Fig. 2-16), rather sharply marginated (Fig. 2-17). Sticky crusts and fissures are common in the folds behind the external ear. On the scalp there is mostly marked scaling ("dandruff"). Nummular, polycyclic, and even annular on the trunk. Scattered, discrete on the face and trunk; diffuse involvement of scalp.

Distribution and Major Types of Lesions (Based on Localization and Age)

Hairy Areas of Head   Scalp, eyebrows, eyelashes (blepharitis), beard (follicular orifices); "cradle cap" (Fig. 2-16).

Face   The flush ("butterfly") areas, on forehead ("corona seborrheica"), nasolabial folds, eyebrows, glabella (Fig. 2-17). Ears: retroauricular, meatus. Simulating lesions of tinea facialis.

Trunk Simulating lesions of pityriasis rosea or pityriasis versicolor; yellowish-brown patches over the sternum is common.

Body Folds Axillae, groins, anogenital area, submammary areas, umbilicus—presents as a diffuse, exudative, sharply marginated, brightly erythematous eruption; fissures are common.

Genitalia Often with yellow crusts and psoriasiform lesions.

DIFFERENTIAL DIAGNOSIS

Red Scaly Plaques

Common Mild psoriasis vulgaris (the two diseases can sometimes be indistinguishable, impetigo, dermatophytosis (tinea capitis, tinea facialis, tinea corporis), pityriasis versicolor, candidiasis (intertriginous), subacute lupus erythematosus.

Rare Langerhans cell histiocytosis (occurs in infants, usually associated with perifollicular purpura), acrodermatitis enteropathica, zinc deficiency, pemphigus foliaceus, glucagonoma syndrome.

LABORATORY STUDIES

Dermatopathology Focal parakeratosis, with few pyknotic neutrophils, moderate acanthosis, spongiosis (intercellular edema), nonspecific inflammation of the dermis. The most characteristic feature is neutrophils at the tips of the dilated follicular openings, which appear as crusts/scales.

DIAGNOSIS

Made on clinical findings.

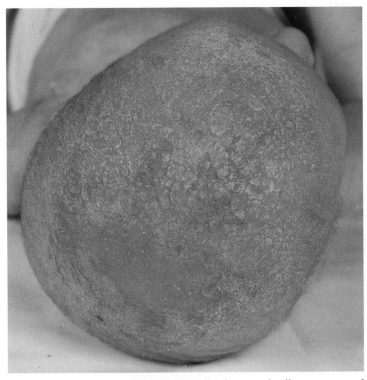

Figure 2-16   Seborrheic dermatitis of scalp: infantile   *Erythema and yellow-orange scales and crust on the scalp of an infant ("cradle cap"). Eczematous lesions are also present on the arms and trunk.*

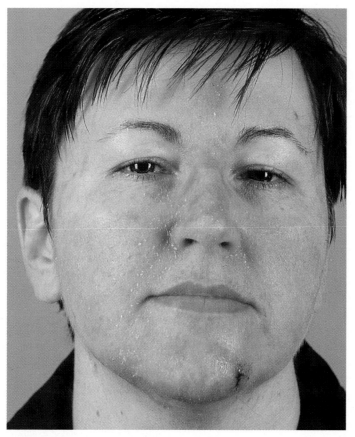

Figure 2-17   Seborrheic dermatitis of face: adult   *Erythema and yellow-orange scaling of the forehead, cheeks, nasolabial folds, and chin. Scalp and retroauricular areas were also involved.*

COURSE AND PROGNOSIS

SD is very common, affecting the majority of individuals at some time during life. UV radiation is beneficial for many individuals; the condition improves in the summer and flares in the fall. Recurrences and remissions, especially on the scalp, may be associated with alopecia in severe cases. Infantile and adolescent SD disappears with age. Seborrheic erythroderma may occur. *Seborrheic erythroderma with diarrhea and failure to thrive (Leiner's disease) is associated with a variety of immunodeficiency disorders including defective yeast opsonization, C3 deficiency, severe combined immunodeficiency, hypogammaglobulinemia, and hyperimmunoglobulinemia.*

MANAGEMENT

SD is a chronic disorder that requires initial therapy followed by chronic maintenance therapy and is a therapeutic challenge. Topical glucocorticoid preparations are effective but can cause atrophy and erythema and telangiectasia, especially on the face, or initiation/exacerbation of perioral dermatitis or rosacea. UV radiation is beneficial for many individuals with SD as the condition improves in the summer and flares in the fall.

Initial Topical Therapy

Scalp

Adults

Shampoo Effective OTC shampoos containing selenium sulfide, zinc pyrithione, are helpful. By prescription (U.S.), 2% ketoconazole shampoo, used initially to treat and subsequently to control the symptoms; lather can be used on face and chest during shower. Tar shampoos (OTC) are equally effective in many patients.

Glucocorticoids Low-potency glucocorticoid solution, lotion, or gels following a medicated shampoo (ketoconazole or tar) for more severe cases.

Infants ("Cradle Cap")

Removal of crusts with warm olive oil compresses, followed by baby shampoo, 2% ketoconazole shampoo, and application of 1 to 2.5% hydrocortisone creams, 2% ketoconazole cream.

Face and Trunk *Ketoconazole shampoo 2%* Lather face during shower.

Ketoconazole Cream: Glucocorticoid cream and lotions: initially 1 or 2.5% hydrocortisone.

More Potent Glucocorticoid Lotions (e.g., clobetasol propionate) may be used for *initial* control and are used along with the medicated shampoos.

Eyelids

Seborrheic blepharitis is managed by gentle removal of the crusts in the morning with a baby shampoo (a cotton ball is dipped in a diluted shampoo); the scales are gently removed from the eyelids. Then the lids are covered with 10% sodium sulfacetamide in a suspension containing .2% prednisolone and .12% phenylephrine; this commercially available formulation should be used cautiously because it contains glucocorticoids, which may precipitate glaucoma. Sodium sulfacetamide ointment alone is also effective and should be used initially to avoid the glucocorticoid problems in the eye. Also, 2% ketoconazole cream is effective.

Intertriginous Areas *Ketoconazole, 2%* If uncontrolled with these treatments, Castellani's paint for dermatitis of the body folds is often very effective, but staining is a problem.

Systemic Therapy

In severe cases, 13-cis retinoic acid orally, 1 mg/kg, is highly effective. Contraception should be used in females of child-bearing age.

Maintenance Therapy

Ketoconazole 2% shampoo. Tar shampoos may be equally effective. Ketoconazole cream; or if this does not work, then the old "standard," 3% sulfur precipitate and 2% salicylic acid in an oil-in-water base is very effective; this must be properly compounded. Also, 1 to 2.5% hydrocortisone cream qd; will work but patients should be monitored for signs of atrophy. We clearly need a new approach to the pesky persistent problem of chronic SD. Possibly, some of the newer topical anti-inflammatory agents will be effective.

ASTEATOTIC DERMATITIS

Synonym: Eczema craquelé (*craquelé* is French, meaning "marred with cracks," such as in old china and ceramic tile).

Asteatotic dermatitis is a common pruritic dermatitis that occurs especially in older persons, in the winter in temperate climates—related to the low humidity of heated houses. It is often unrecognized. The sites of predilection are the legs (Fig. 2-18), arms, and hands, but also the trunk. The eruption is characterized by dry, "cracked," fissured skin with slight scaling. There may be histologic changes similar to eczema (spongiosis) and, in fact, the incessant pruritus can lead to lichenification, which can persist when the environmental conditions have been corrected; the lichenification persists for weeks to months, if scratching is continued. The disorder results from too frequent bathing in hot soapy baths or showers and/or in older persons living in rooms with a high environmental temperature and low relative humidity (as in a heated room in temperate climates). The disorder is managed by avoiding overbathing with soap, especially tub baths, and increasing the ambient humidity, preferably above 50%; room humidifiers (in the bedroom) are helpful; also, using tepid water baths *without* soap and containing bath oils for hydration, followed by immediate liberal application of emollient ointments, such as hydrated petolatum. The treatment of xerosis involves, first, wetting the skin and then immediately applying emollients. Also helpful is the use of medium-potency corticosteroid ointments, applied twice daily until the eczematous component has resolved.

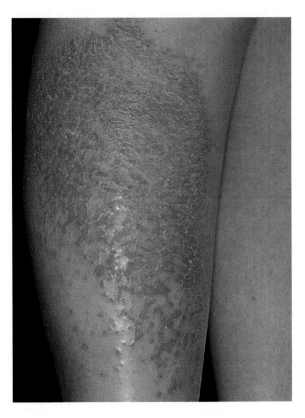

Figure 2-18   Asteatotic dermatitis (eczema craquelé)   *Erythema with a tessellated (tilelike) pattern arising in fissures on an area of xerosis of the lower leg of a 46-year-old female. Occurred in midwinter.*

PSORIASIS AND ICHTHYOSIFORM DERMATOSES

PSORIASIS VULGARIS

(New Latin from Greek words: *psor-* (itching) -*iasis* (condition)

Psoriasis vulgaris is a challenge for the physician, because chronic generalized psoriasis is one of the "miseries that beset mankind," causing shame and embarrassment and a compromised lifestyle. The "heartbreak of psoriasis" is no joke. As the writer John Updike (who himself has psoriasis) so poignantly said about being a person with psoriasis, "I am silvery, scaly. Puddles of flakes form wherever I rest my flesh. Lusty, though we are loathsome to love. Keen-sighted, though we hate to look upon ourselves. The name of the disease, spiritually speaking, is Humiliation."

Psoriasis, which affects 1.5 to 2% of the population in western countries, is a hereditary disorder of skin with several clinical expressions. The most frequent type is *psoriasis vulgaris,* which occurs as chronic, recurring, scaling papules and plaques in characteristic sites on the body. Clinical presentation varies in individuals from presenting with only a few localized plaques or with generalized skin involvement. Disease activity is reflected as scaling in stationary plaques and as inflammation in the eruptive, guttate lesions.

CLASSIFICATION

Nonpustular Psoriasis
  Psoriasis vulgaris
  Psoriatic erythroderma

Pustular Psoriasis
  Pustular psoriasis of von Zumbusch
  Pustulosis palmaris et plantaris
  Pustular psoriasis, annular type
  Acrodermatitis continua
  Impetigo herpetiformis

EPIDEMIOLOGY

Age of Onset *Early* Peak incidence occurs at 22.5 years of age (in children, the mean age of onset is 8 years). *Late* Presents about age 55.

These two age-related peaks seem to separate into two types of psoriasis: *early onset* predicts a more severe disease and a positive family history of psoriasis.

Incidence In the United States, there are 3 to 5 million persons with psoriasis. Most have localized psoriasis, but approximately 300,000 persons have generalized psoriasis requiring specialized approaches with ultraviolet radiation, PUVA photochemotherapy, methotrexate, or cyclosporin.

Sex Equal incidence in males and females.

Race Low incidence in West Africans, Japanese, and Eskimos; very low incidence or absence in North and South American Indians.

Heredity Polygenic trait. When one parent has psoriasis, 8% of offspring develop psoriasis; and when both parents have psoriasis, 41% develop psoriasis. HLA types most frequently associated with psoriasis are HLA-B13, -B17, Bw57 and, most importantly, HLA-Cw6.

Trigger Factors *Physical trauma* (Koebner's phenomenon) is a major factor in eliciting lesions; rubbing and scratching stimulate the psoriatic proliferative process. *Infections:* acute streptococcal infection precipitating guttate psoriasis. *Stress:* a factor in flares of psoriasis as high as 40% in adults and higher in children. *Drugs:* systemic glucocorticoids, class I topical glucocorticoids, oral lithium, antimalarial drugs, systemic interferon, and β-adrenergic blockers can flare existing psoriasis and cause a psoriasiform drug eruption; alcohol ingestion is a putative trigger factor.

> **Type**   Two types: eruptive, inflammatory type with multiple small (guttate or nummular) lesions and a greater tendency toward spontaneous resolution (Fig. 3-2); and a chronic, stable plaque-type (Figs. 3-1 and 3-4).

PATHOGENESIS

The principal abnormality in psoriasis is an alteration of the cell kinetics of keratinocytes. The major change is a shortening of the cell cycle from 311 to 36 h, which results in 28 times the normal production of epidermal cells. The epidermis and dermis appear to respond as an integrated system: the changes in the germinative zone of the epidermis and the inflammatory changes in the dermis, which may "trigger" the epidermal changes. Immunologic phenomena recently have been proved to be a major factor in the pathogenesis of psoriasis inasmuch as immunosuppressive drugs such as cyclosporine are dramatically effective in causing a total remission of the disease. There are many T cells present in psoriatic lesions surrounding the upper dermal blood vessels, and the cytokine spectrum is that of a T_H1 response. Therapies for psoriasis are based in part on suppression of T cells. Maintenance of psoriatic lesions is considered as an ongoing autoreactive immune response.

HISTORY

Duration of Lesions   Usually, indolent lesions are present for months but may be of sudden onset, as in acute guttate psoriasis and generalized pustular psoriasis (von Zumbusch syndrome).

Skin Symptoms   Pruritus is reasonably common, especially in scalp and anogenital psoriasis.

Constitutional Symptoms   Joint pain in special type of arthritis, i.e., *psoriatic arthritis.* In von Zumbusch syndrome (acute onset of generalized pustular psoriasis), there is an "acute illness" syndrome with weakness, chills, and fever.

PHYSICAL EXAMINATION

Skin Lesions

Salmon-pink papules and plaques, sharply marginated with marked silvery-white scale (Fig. 3-1). Scales are lamellar, loose, and easily removed by scratching. Removal of scale results in the appearance of minute blood droplets. Lesions are round, oval (Fig. 3-1), polycyclic, annular, linear, and arranged in arciform, serpiginous patterns or are scattered (Fig. 3-2).

Distribution   *Extent*   Single lesion or lesions localized to one area (e.g., penis, nails), regional involvement (scalp), generalized or universal (entire skin) There may be only a "pinking" erythema in the gluteal cleft as a clue to a patient with, for example, nail involvement alone.

Pattern   (1) Bilateral, often symmetrical; often spares exposed areas; favors elbows (Fig. 3-1), knees, scalp, and intertriginous areas (see Figure 3-I); facial region is *uncommonly* involved, and when the face is involved, it is usually associated with a refractory type of psoriasis. (2) Disseminated small lesions without predilection of site (guttate psoriasis) (Fig. 3-2).

Erythroderma

This is a condition in which psoriasis involves practically the entire skin. A serious condition that is discussed in Section 6.

Arthritis

Psoriatic arthritis is included among the seronegative spondyloarthropathies, which include ankylosing spondylitis, enteropathic arthritis and Reiter's syndrome. Asymmetric peripheral joint involvement of upper extremities and especially smaller joints. Associated with MHC class I antigens, while rheumatoid arthritis is associated with MHC class II antigens. Incidence is 5 to 8%. Rare before age 20. *May be present (in 10%*

of individuals) without any visible psoriasis; then search for a family history.

Three types: (1) "Distal"—seronegative, without subcutaneous nodules, and involving, asymmetrically, a few distal interphalangeal joints of the hands and feet: an asymmetric oligoarthritis (Fig. 3-7). (2) Multilating psoriatic arthritis with bone erosion and osteolysis and, ultimately, ankylosis. (3) "Axial"—especially involving the sacroiliac, hip, and cervical areas with ankylosing spondylitis; seen especially in erythrodermic and pustular psoriasis.

DIFFERENTIAL DIAGNOSIS

Scaling Plaques *Seborrheic dermatitis*—may be indistinguishable in sites involved and morphology; sometimes termed *seborriasis*. *Lichen simplex chronicus*—may complicate psoriasis as a result of pruritus. *Candidiasis*—especially in intertriginous psoriasis. *Psoriasiform drug eruptions*—especially beta blockers, gold, and methyldopa. *Glucagonoma syndrome* —an im-

portant differential because this is a serious disease (malignant tumor of the pancreatic islet cells). The lesions have to be distinguished from intertriginous psoriasis and assay for glucagon should be performed in "atypical" psoriasis. *Tinea corporis*—rarely a problem except in single lesions; KOH exam is mandatory in these lesions. *Mycosis fungoides*—scaling plaques can be an initial stage of mycosis fungoides.

LABORATORY EXAMINATIONS

Dermatopathology There is (1) marked thickening (acanthosis); thinning of the epidermis acanthosis over elongated dermal papillae; (2) increased mitosis of keratinocytes, fibroblasts, and endothelial cells; (3) parakeratotic hyper-keratosis (nuclei retained in the stratum corneum); and (4) inflammatory cells in the dermis (usually lymphocytes and monocytes) and in the epidermis (polymorphonuclear cells), forming microabscesses of Munro in the stratum corneum.

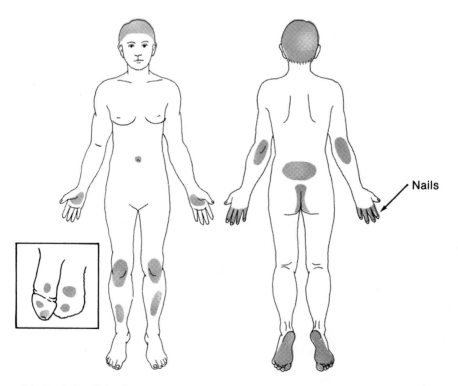

Nails

Figure 3-1 Psoriasis *Vulgaris.*

PSORIASIS AND ICHTHYOSIFORM DERMATOSES

Serology Sudden onset of psoriasis may be associated with HIV infection. Determination of HIV serostatus is indicated in at-risk individuals: homosexual and bisexual males and females, persons who have received blood transfusions. Serum uric acid is increased in 50% of patients, usually correlated with the extent of the disease; there is an increased risk of gouty arthritis. The levels of uric acid decrease as therapy is effective.

MANAGEMENT

Factors Influencing Selection

1. Age: childhood, adolescence, young adulthood, middle age, >60 years.
2. Type of psoriasis: guttate, plaque, palmar and pustular, generalized pustular psoriasis, erythrodermic psoriasis.
3. Site and extent of involvement: *localized* to palms and soles, scalp, anogenital area, scattered plaques but <5% involvement; *generalized* and >30% involvement.

4. Previous treatment: ionizing radiation, systemic glucocorticoids, PUVA, cyclosporine, arsenics, methotrexate.
5. Associated medical disorders (e.g., HIV disease).

Ideally all patients with suspected psoriasis should be seen at least once by a dermatologist to establish the diagnosis and select the best available treatment regimen. Localized psoriasis (covering <5% of the body surface) can be managed by the primary care physician if a proper regimen is selected. Psoriasis of all other types, especially generalized psoriasis, should be managed by a dermatologist who has access to all therapies, as "rotational" therapy shifting from ultraviolet to PUVA to methotrexate is necessary in most patients. Finally, it is important to emphasize that in all types of psoriasis new lesions may be induced on "normal" skin by physical trauma, including rubbing and scratching psoriatic spots.
In the following pages managment of psoriasis is discussed in the context of types of psoriasis, sites, and extent of involvement.

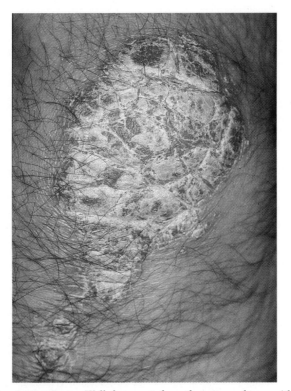

Figure 3-1 Psoriasis vulgaris: elbow *Well-demarcated, erythematous plaque with a thick whitish scale, which has arisen from the coalescence of smaller papular lesions.*

Localized Psoriasis

This consists of a limited number of chronic stable psoriasis plaques (Fig. 3-1) on the predelectious sites (Fig. 3-I) or elsewhere.

TOPICAL TREATMENT

1. Topical fluorinated glucocorticoids (betamethasone valerate, fluocinolone acetonide, betamethasone propionate, clobetasol propionate) in *ointment* base applied after the scales are removed by soaking in water. The ointment is applied to the wet skin, covered with plastic wrap, and left on overnight. Glucocorticoid-impregnated tape (Cordran tape) is useful for small plaques.
2. Hydrocolloid dressing, left on for 24 to 48 h, is helpful, effective, and prevents scratching. During the day, classes I and II fluorinated glucocorticoid creams can be used without occlusion. Patients develop tolerance (tachyphylaxis) after long periods. *Caveat:* Prolonged application of the fluorinated glucocorticoids leads to atrophy of the skin, permanent striae, and unsightly telangiectasia. Clobetasol-17-propionate is stronger and active even without occlusion. To avoid systemic effects of this class I glucocorticoid: maximum of 50 g ointment per week.
3. For small plaques (≤4 cm), triamcinolone acetonide aqueous suspension 3 mg/ml diluted with normal saline is injected into the lesion. The injection should be intradermal rather than subcutaneous; *if the injection does not require some pressure to inject, it is not going into the dermis. Warning:* Hypopigmentation at the injection site can result; this is more apparent in brown and black skin, but it is reversible.
4. Topical anthralin preparations are excellent when used properly. Follow directions on the package insert with attention to details.
5. Vitamin D analogues (calcipotriene, 0.005%, ointment and cream) are good nonsteroidal antipsoriatic topical agents and are not associated with cutaneous atrophy. They are not as potent as class I glucocorticoids (e.g., clobetasol propionate) but can be combined with them, using the class I glucocorticoids only on weekends and calcipotriene ointment or cream during the week. Calcipotriene should not be applied to more than 40% of the body surface and not more than 100 g per week to avoid hypercalcemia.
6. Tazarotene (a new topical retinoid) is another alternative to topical glucocorticoids or can be best combined with class II (medium strength) topical glucocorticoids, as tazarotene can cause irritation. Also there is some indication, but no proof, that topical retinoids such as tazarotene may prevent cutaneous atrophy.
7. When there is more than 10% (palm of the hand = 1%) involvement with psoriatic plaques, it is preferable to combine these topical treatments with UVB 311-nm phototherapy or PUVA photochemotherapy.

Table 3-1   TREATMENT OF LOCALIZED PSORIASIS (EXCLUDING SCALP AND ANOGENITAL AREAS)

Treatment
1. Calcipotriene ointment; if this fails, move to:
2. Calcipotriene plus highest-potency glucocorticoids
3. Highest potency corticosteroids under occlusion.

Maintenance
Calcipotriene plus medium- or low-potency glucocorticoids ± occlusion with plastic dressings

Other Helpful Agents
Triamcinolone suspension (3 mg/mL in saline) injections to small (<3cm) plaques
Glucocorticoid-impregnated tape for small lesions
Anthralin tazarotene tar

Eruptive (Guttate) Psoriasis

Guttate psoriasis, which is relatively rare (<2.0% of all psoriasis), is similar to an exanthem: a shower of lesions appears rather rapidly and in young adults, often but not always following streptococcal pharyngitis. Guttate psoriasis may, however, be persistent, recurring, and unrelated to streptococcal infection. It may evolve into chronic, stable plaque psoriasis.

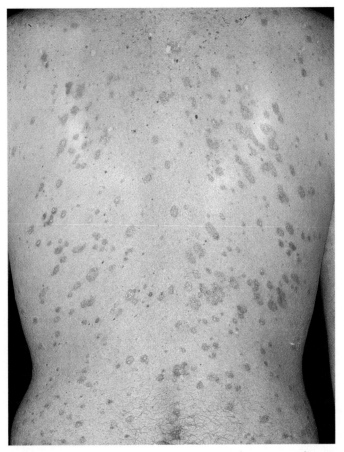

Figure 3-2 Psoriasis vulgaris: trunk (guttate type) *Discrete, erythematous scaling, small papules and plaques on the trunk, appearing after a group A streptococcal pharyngitis. There was a family history of psoriasis.*

PHYSICAL EXAMINATION

Skin Lesions (Fig. 3-2) Salmon pink papules 2.0 mm to 1.0 cm. Guttate (Latin: "gutta-=drop"). Scattered discrete lesions. Generalized, usually sparing the palms and soles and concentrating on the trunk, less on the face, scalp, and nails.

DIFFERENTIAL DIAGNOSIS

Multiple Small Scaling Plaques Psoriasiform drug eruption, secondary syphilis, pityriasis rosea, tinea corporis, secondary syphilis.

LABORATORY EXAMINATIONS

Serologic An increased antistreptolysin titer in those patients with antecedent streptococcal infection.

Culture Throat culture for group A β hemolytic streptococcus infection.

COURSE AND PROGNOSIS

Appears rapidly, a generalized "rash". Sometimes this type of psoriasis disappears spontaneously in a few weeks without any treatment. More often, guttate psoriasis requires phototherapy or PUVA photochemotherapy.

MANAGEMENT

The resolution of lesions can be accelerated by phototherapy. For persistent lesions, treatment is the same as for generalized plaque psoriasis. Penicillin VK or erythromycin if group A β-hemolytic streptococcus on throat culture.

Psoriasis Vulgaris: Scalp

Psoriasis of the scalp presents a special therapeutic problem similar to that of anogenital psoriasis. Both areas are inaccessible for treatment with phototherapy and are often pruritic, which results in lichenification and koebnerization.[1] Patients need to understand that new lesions may be induced in "normal" skin by physical trauma, including rubbing and scratching the normal skin or the psoriasis lesions. This must be emphasized to patients being treated for all types of psoriasis, or the treatment will be ineffective, as the constant trauma will reverse the therapy given for the lesions. Psoriasis of the scalp may be part of generalized plaque psoriasis, may coexist with isolated plaques, or may be the only site involved.

HISTORY

Duration   Months to years.

Relationship to Season   Does not go into remission with phototherapy or with sunlight exposure, as does the exposed psoriatic skin.

Skin Symptoms   Mild to severe pruritus, which often causes compulsive and subconscious scratching and which is a major cause of failure of the scalp therapy.

PHYSICAL EXAMINATION

Skin Lesions   Plaques, often with thick, adherent scales (Fig. 3-3). Lichenification (often superimposed on the basic psoriatic lesions and resulting from rubbing and scratching). Exudation and fissures, especially behind the ears. Scattered discrete plaques or diffuse involvement of the entire scalp. (*Note:* Paradoxically, psoriasis of the scalp does not lead to hair loss, even after years of thick, plaque-type involvement. Thus, the condition is not exposed to public view, and this may be one reason why patients learn to live with it and do not seek treatment.)

DIFFERENTIAL DIAGNOSIS

Red Scaling Plaques on Scalp   Seborrheic dermatitis of the scalp may be almost indistinguishable from psoriasis. Some have called this *seborriasis*. Also consider *tinea capitis, atopic dermatitis, lichen simplex chronicus.*

MANAGEMENT

Mild   Superficial scaling and lacking thick plaques:

- Tar or ketoconazole shampoos *followed by*
- Betamethasone valerate, 1% lotion; if refractory, clobetasol propionate, .05% scalp application.

Severe   Thick, adherent plaques:

- Removal of plaques before active treatment. Topical applications are virtually useless unless the thick scale is removed by applications of 10% salicylic acid in mineral oil, covered with a plastic cap, and left on overnight.
- After scales have been removed (in one to three treatments followed by shampooing), fluocinolone cream or lotion is applied, and the scalp is covered with plastic sheets or a shower cap, which is left on overnight or for 6 h.
- When the thickness of the plaques is reduced, clobetasol propionate, .05% lotion, or calcipotriene lotion can be used for maintenance.

COURSE AND PROGNOSIS

The prognosis for control is good; after treatment as outlined above, the scalp lesions may undergo a remission for several months to years. The habit of scratching and rubbing the scalp must be avoided to maintain the remission.

---

[1]The phenomenon of induction of new lesions on "normal" skin by physical trauma, including rubbing and scratching.

PSORIASIS AND ICHTHYOSIFORM DERMATOSES

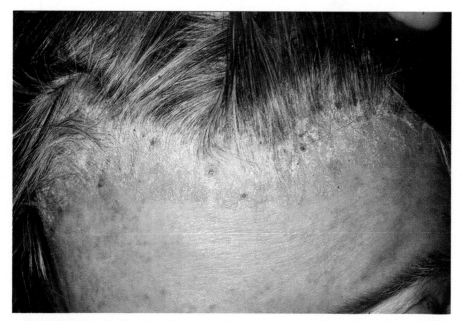

Figure 3-3 Psoriasis vulgaris: scalp *Erythema of the forehead with adjacent hyperkeratotic plaque with crusted excoriations on the scalp.*

Psoriasis Vulgaris: Widespread Plaque-Type

This is a chronic, stable plaque-type psoriasis with sharply demarcated salmon-red or brownish-red plaques with silvery white lamellar scaling that can easily be removed or, when the lesion is extremely chronic, tightly adheres to the underlying inflammatory and infiltrated skin. Lesions are round, polycyclic and confluent, forming geographic patterns (Fig. 3-4).

MANAGEMENT

The management of generalized plaque-type psoriasis (Figs. 3-4 and 3-5 *A*, *B*) is the province of the dermatologist or of a psoriasis center where the major options are available: (1) phototherapy with emollients, (2) PUVA photochemotherapy, (3) methotrexate (given weekly), (4) combination therapy with etretinate (or other retinoids such as acitretin or isotretinoin) or methotrexate with PUVA (such combinations are perhaps the ideal treatment available at the present time), or (5) cyclosporine, only as a *last* option.

Up to 50% of patients with thin-plaque psoriasis respond well to phototherapy when given according to a published protocol. The same percentage of patients also respond to topical calcipotriene as long as no more than 40% of the body surface is involved and not more than 100 g per week is used. Response is slow. Those with thick plaques or who do not respond to UVB or 311 nm phototherapy are treated with oral PUVA photochemotherapy or, ideally, with a combination of retinoids plus PUVA. For males, combination treatment with etretinate and oral PUVA photochemotherapy (so-called Re-PUVA) is the most effective therapy. For females, isotretinoin can be used, but contraception is mandatory during and 2 months after treatment is completed. Methotrexate is used only in older patients (>50 years) or when combination phototherapy or photochemotherapy (retinoids plus PUVA or retinoids plus UVB, 311 nm plus emollients) has failed to bring about a remission or cannot be performed.

Oral PUVA Photochemotherapy Treatment consists of oral ingestion of 8-methoxypsoralen (8-MOP) (.6 mg 8-MOP kilogram of body weight) and exposure to doses of UVA that are adjusted to the sensitivity of the patient. Approximately 1 to 2 h after ingestion of the psoralen, UVA is given, starting at a dose of 1 J/cm², adjusted upward for skin phototype. Alternatively, phototoxicity testing can be done, which permits a better adjustment of the UVA dose to the individual's sensitivity to PUVA. The UVA dose is increased at successive treatment sessions. Treatments are performed 2 or 3 times a week or, with a more intensive protocol, 4 times a week. Most patients clear after 19 to 25 treatments, and the amount of UVA needed ranges from 100 to 245 J/cm². Long-term side effects: PUVA keratoses and squamous cell carcinomas in some patients who receive an excessive number of treatments. Re-PUVA reduces the total number of treatments.

In patients with recalcitrant plaque-type psoriasis, etretinate (in males) or isotretinoin (in females) may be combined with other antipsoriatic therapy, e.g., PUVA, UVB, 311 nm, topical glucocorticoids, or anthralin. These combination modalities reduce the length of treatments as well as the total amount of antipsoriatic drug necessary for clearing. Topical glucocorticoids, calcipotriene ointments, anthralin, oral methotrexate, and oral etretinate, combined with either PUVA or UVB, 311 nm are all effective in reducing the dose of one another.

Table 3-2 TREATMENT OF GENERALIZED PSORIASIS (EXCLUDING SCALP AND ANOGENITAL AREAS)

Thin Plaques
UVB, 311 nm + emollients

Thick Plaques
1. UVB, 311 nm + emollients;
   if this fails, move to:
2. PUVA photochemotherapy;
   if this fails, move to:
3. Retinoids + PUVA photochemotherapy;
   if this fails, move to:
4. Methotrexate, 2.5 to 5 mg by mouth every 12 h for a total of three doses, once weekly

---

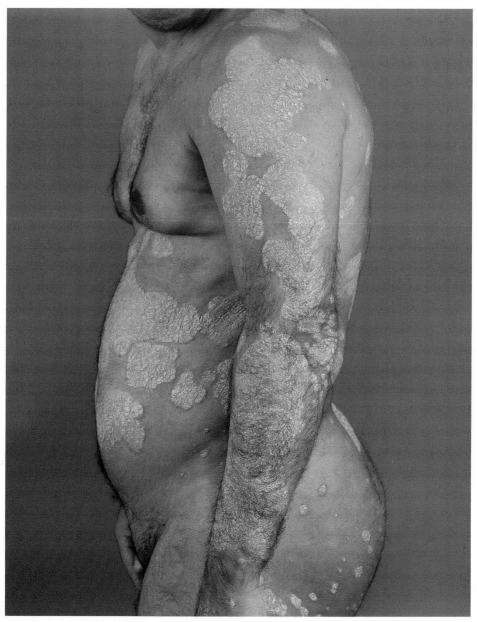

Figure 3-4 Psoriasis vulgaris: chronic stable type *Multiple large hyperkeratotic plaques on the trunk, arm, buttocks, and abdomen. Lesions are polycyclic and confluent forming geographic patterns. This patient was cleared by acitretin/PUVA combination treatment.*

Silver like?"

Psoriasis Day-Care Centers These facilities have available phototherapy or UVB, 311 nm plus tar (Goeckerman regimen) and PUVA. The patient remains in the phototherapy unit during the day and goes home at night. In these centers there is a camaraderie among the patients with psoriasis and the staff, which no doubt has a positive effect on the course of the disease and ensures compliance with the therapy. There are more day-care centers in Europe than in the United States.

Methotrexate Therapy Oral methotrexate (MTX) is one of the most effective treatments and certainly the most convenient treatment for generalized plaque-type psoriasis (Fig. 3-5). Nevertheless, MTX is a potentially dangerous drug, principally because of liver toxicity that can occur after prolonged use. Hepatic toxicity occurs after cumulative doses in normal persons (1.5 g), but other risk factors include a history of alcohol intake, abnormal liver chemistries, IV drug use, and obesity. Inasmuch as hepatic toxicity is related to total life dose, this therapy should, in general, not be given to young patients who may face many years of therapy. There is some evidence that the disease in older patients can be controlled with lower doses of MTX because of slower excretion of the drug by the kidney.

Schedule of Methotrexate Therapy with the Triple-Dose Regimen (preferred by most over the single-dose MTX once weekly). Begin with a test dose of 5 mg (2.5-mg tablet followed 24 h later with a second 2.5-mg tablet); this dose will ascertain whether there is a special sensitivity to MTX. A complete blood count (CBC) is obtained after 1 week and every 1 to 4 weeks thereafter as the dose of MTX is increased. If the CBC is normal at 1 week, 2.5 mg (1 tablet) is given every 12 h for a total of three doses of 7.5 mg once a week (1/1/1 tablet schedule). Some patients respond to this dose;

but if not, the dose is increased after 2 weeks to 2/2/2 or 15 mg total dose. This regimen achieves an 80% improvement but not total clearing, and higher doses increase the risk of toxicity. The dose of MTX can be reduced by one or two tablets periodically. In the summer the dose of MTX may be decreased or the treatment discontinued.

Monitoring CBC (at beginning of therapy and every 1 to 4 weeks; after on a stable dose, once monthly). Platelet count must also be closely watched as it may decrease before the white blood cell count (WBC).

Renal and Liver Function Obtain liver function tests just prior to first MTX dose, at start and every 3 months; creatinine at start and every 2 to 4 months.

A pretreatment liver biopsy is required only in patients with a history of liver disease or in patients with abnormal liver chemistries. In patients with normal liver chemistries and no risk factors present, a liver biopsy should be done after a cumulative dose of approximately 1500 mg MTX; if the post-MTX liver biopsy is normal, repeat liver biopsy should be done after further therapy with an additional 1000 to 1500 mg MTX.[2] Be aware of the various drug interactions with MTX.

Cyclosporin A (CyA) Therapy CyA treatment is highly effective at a dose of 3 to 5 mg/kg per day. As the patient responds, the dose is tapered to the lowest effective maintenance dose. Monitoring blood pressure and serum creatinine is mandatory because of the known nephrotoxicity of the drug. *CyA should be employed only in patients without risk factors.* (For details and drug interactions see MJ Mihatsch, K Wolff: Consensus Conference on Cyclosporin A for Psoriasis. Br J Dermatol 126:621, 1992.

The efficacy and toxicity of treatments for generalized psoriasis are compared in Table 3-3.

---

[2]For details regarding MTX therapy of psoriasis, see HH Roenigk Jr et al: Methotrexate in psoriasis: Revised guidelines. J Am Acad Dermatol 19:145, 1988.

PSORIASIS AND ICHTHYOSIFORM DERMATOSES

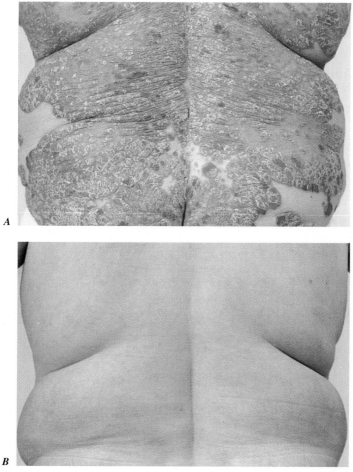

A

B

Figure 3-5   Psoriasis vulgaris: trunk   A. *Near-complete involvement of the trunk with erythematous hyperkeratotic plaques.* B. *Several months after initiation of oral methotrexate, all lesions had resolved with only slight residual erythema.*

Table 3-3 EFFICACY AND TOXICITY OF TREATMENTS FOR GENERALIZED PSORIASIS VULGARIS

Therapy	Efficacy	Toxicity[a]
Phototherapy (UVB, 311 nm + emollients)	Good	A
PUVA photochemotherapy	Good to excellent	A, B
Methotrexate	Excellent	C
Retinoids	Poor to fair	D
Methotrexate + PUVA	Excellent	A, B, E
Retinoids + PUVA (re-PUVA)	Excellent	A, B, E
Cyclosporin A (CSA)	Good to excellent	F, G, H

[a]Toxicity:

A. Phototoxicity leading to induction of new lesions.
B. Development of lentigines in 30% of patients. Dermatoheliosis, related to total dose. Nonmelanoma skin cancer in high-risk populations (patients with skin phototypes I and II and those previously treated with ionizing radiation, including grenz rays) and in patients who undergo prolonged treatment.
C. Hepatic cirrhosis related to total cumulative dose; risk increase with obesity or alcohol consumption.
D. Hyperostosis related to total cumulative dose. Teratogenicity, hypertriglyceridemia.
E. Combination treatment reduces toxicity compared to retinoid, methotrexate, or PUVA monotherapy.
F. Renal tubular toxicity.
G. Elevated blood pressure.
H. Lymphoma.

Psoriasis Vulgaris: Palms and Soles

This disease is a major therapeutic challenge. The palms and soles may be the only areas involved. There is massive silvery white or yellowish hyperkeratosis and scaling, which in contrast to lesions on the trunk, is not easily removed (Fig. 3-6). Desquamation of hyperkeratosis will, however, reveal an inflammatory plaque at the base unlike chronic hand dermatitis that is always sharply demarcated (Fig. 3-6). There may be cracking and painful fissures and bleeding. Topical glucocorticoids with plastic occlusion are only moderately effective. UVB phototherapy is not often effective.

MANAGEMENT

Effective treatments available are as follows:

1. PUVA photochemotherapy, administered in specially designed hand and foot lighting cabinets that deliver UVA. PUVA "soaks" of hands and feet are being used more frequently. In this treatment the hands and feet are immersed in a solution of 8-methoxypsoralen (10 mg/L of warm water) for 15 min and then exposed to hand and foot UVA phototherapy units.

2. Retinoids (etretinate) given alone orally are effective in removing the thick hyperkeratosis of the palms and soles; however, combination with PUVA (Re-PUVA) is much more efficacious. Combinations of oral retinoids and PUVA improve the efficacy of each and permit a reduction of the dose and duration of each (page 58).

3. In disease that is very refractory to treatment, MTX should be considered.

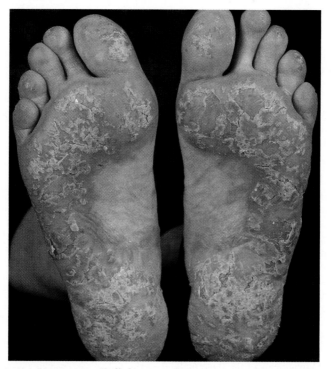

Figure 3-6 Psoriasis vulgaris: soles *Well-demarcated, erythematous plaques with thick, yellowish scale and desquamation on sites of pressure arising on the plantar feet; similar lesions were present on the palms.*

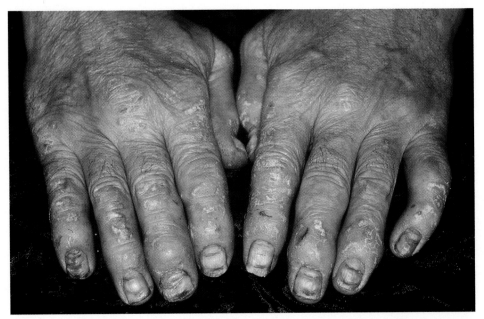

Figure 3-7 Psoriasis vulgaris: hands with nail involvement; and psoriatic arthritis *Striking joint swelling of the distal interphalangeal and several metacarpophalangeal joints with associated severe nail dystrophy. The transverse nail ridges are associated with psoriatic involvement of the nail matrix.*

Psoriasis Vulgaris: Nail Apparatus

Psoriasis of the nails is quite common (25% of patients with psoriasis), varies in severity of involvement, and often disappears spontaneously or pari passu with treatment of psoriasis of the skin, especially with the three major treatments: UVB, 3ll nm phototherapy, PUVA photochemotherapy, and methotrexate. (See also Nails, Section 28.)

PHYSICAL EXAMINATION

Nail Findings Fingernails and toenails frequently (25%) involved, especially with concomitant arthritis (Fig. 3-7). Nail changes include pitting, subungual hyperkeratosis, onycholysis (also nonspecific), and yellowish-brown spots under the nail plate—the *oil spot* (pathognomonic).

MANAGEMENT

Specially directed treatments of the fingernails (inasmuch as the nails are disfiguring and a nuisance) are unsatisfactory. Injection of the nail fold with intradermal triamcinolone acetonide (3 mg/mL) may be quite effective but is impractical when all nails are involved. PUVA photochemotherapy is somewhat effective; the UVA is administered in special hand and foot lighting units providing high-intensity UVA. Long-term systemic retinoids (acitretin, .5 mg/kg) are also effective as are systemic methotrexate and cyclosporin A (cyclosporine) therapy. Since a diseased nail (plate) cannot be cured, therapy of nails aims at securing *regrowth* of a normal nail plate. It therefore depends on the speed of nail growth that is slow and thus requires a long time. This should be taken into account when a treatment is considered that may cause side effects when administered over a prolonged period of time.

PSORIASIS AND ICHTHYOSIFORM DERMATOSES

Chronic Psoriasis of the Perianal and Genital Regions and of the Body Folds

The anogenital area is a site that can be the locus of rubbing and scratching. The patient needs to understand that new lesions may be induced in "normal" skin by physical trauma, including rubbing and scratching the normal skin or the psoriasis lesions. Due to the warm and moist environment in these regions psoriatic plaques in the body folds are usually not scaly, but are bright red, and fissured. The sharp demarcation permits distinction from intertrigo, candidiasis, contact dermatitis, tinea cruris, and the symmetry from extramammary Paget's disease.

MANAGEMENT

Psoriasis of the body folds (inguinal area, umbilicus, axillae, inframammary, intergluteal fold) (Fig. 3-8), and of the male and female genitalia is especially vulnerable to the development of steroid-induced skin atrophy; low-potency steroids are recommended but are not very effective. The fact that anthralin and tar preparations are irritating in these areas poses a difficult problem in control. Castellani's paint is sometimes useful in genital and perianal psoriasis. The topical vitamin D_3 preparation, calcipotriene ointment, and tazarotene are moderately effective in these areas and there is no risk of skin atrophy or tachyphylaxis. Irritation may occur but is worth the nuisance as the treatment is safe and effective. Tar baths may be very effective.

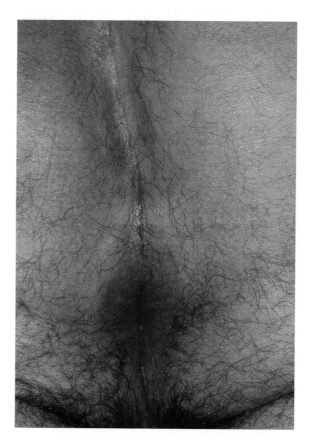

Figure 3-8 Psoriasis vulgaris: inverse pattern *Well-demarcated, erythematous plaque (so-called "pinking") of the intergluteal fold (may be only skin manifestation), perianal area, and medial raphe of a 30-year-old male with psoriasis of elbows, knees, and fingernails. So-called inverse pattern psoriasis occurs in moist intertriginous sites (skin touching skin): in the axillae, inframammary region, umbilicus, and intergluteal/inguinal folds and is commonly mistaken for candidiasis or tinea corporis, seborrheic and intertriginous dermatitis.*

PALMOPLANTAR PUSTULOSIS

Palmoplantar pustulosis is a chronic, relapsing eruption limited to the palms and soles and characterized by numerous very typical sterile, yellow, deep-seated pustules that evolve into dusky-red crusts. It is considered by some as a localized form of pustular psoriasis (Barber type) and by others as a separate entity.

EPIDEMIOLOGY

Age of Onset 50 to 60 years.

Incidence Low.

Sex More common in females (4:1).

HISTORY

Duration of Lesions Months.

PHYSICAL EXAMINATION

Skin Lesions Pustules in stages of evolution, 2 to 5 mm, deep-seated, develop into dusky-red macules and crusts; present in areas of erythema and scaling or normal skin (Fig. 3-9). Eruptions come and go, in waves.

Distribution Limited to palms and soles, may be only a localized patch on the sole or hand, but may involve both hands and feet with a predilection of thenar and hypothenar, flexor aspects of fingers, heels, and insteps; acral portions of the fingers and toes usually spared.

DIFFERENTIAL DIAGNOSIS

Palmar/Plantar Dermatosis Epidermal dermatophytosis (tinea manus, tinea pedis), dyshidrotic eczematous dermatitis, HSV infection.

LABORATORY EXAMINATIONS

KOH Preparations To exclude dermatophytosis.

Bacterial and Viral Culture To exclude *Staphylococcus aureus* infection and HSV infection if lesions are localized to one site.

Dermatopathology Edema and exocytosis of mononuclear cells that appear first form a vesicle, and later myriads of neutrophils, which form a unilocular spongiform pustule and acanthosis.

PROGNOSIS

Persistent for years and characterized by unexplained remissions and exacerbations; rarely psoriasis vulgaris may develop elsewhere.

MANAGEMENT

The condition is recalcitrant to treatment, but persistence in treatment can be rewarding.

PUVA "Soaks" of Hands and Feet Ideal for this condition. The hands and feet are immersed in a solution of 8-methoxypsoralen (10 mg/L warm water) for 15 min and then exposed to special hand and foot UVA phototherapy units. Re-PUVA is highly efficacious.

Topical Glucocorticoids, Dithranol, and Coal Tar Ineffective. Strong glucocorticoids under plastic occlusion (e.g., for the night) may be effective, but do not prevent recurrences. Methotrexate (see page 58) for recalcitrant cases.

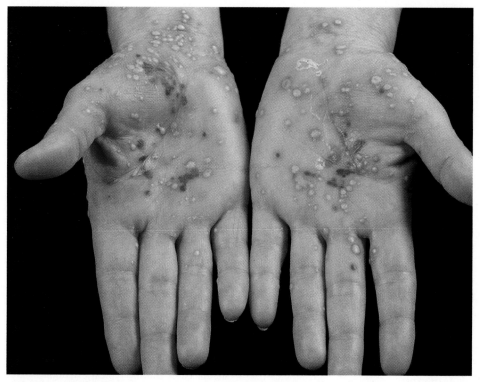

Figure 3-9 Palmar pustulosis *Deep-seated, dusky-red macules and creamy-yellow pustules progress to hyperkeratotic/crusted papules. Lesions are confined to the palms and/or soles and/or a single digit. Because of the pustules, the disorder is commonly mistaken for a bacterial or herpetic infection.*

GENERALIZED ACUTE PUSTULAR PSORIASIS (VON ZUMBUSCH)

This disorder can be a life-threatening medical problem with an abrupt onset. The skin involvement is distinctive and starts with a burning erythema that spreads in hours to result in large areas of fiery-red skin. Pinpoint pustules appear in clusters, peppering the red areas of skin; these pustules become confluent and form "lakes" filled with purulent fluid. Fever, generalized weakness, severe malaise, and a leukocytosis are prominent features in almost every patient.

EPIDEMIOLOGY

Age of Onset   Adults, rarely children.

Precipitating Factors   There are no known precipitating factors, and the patient may or may not have had a stable plaque-type psoriasis in the past.

PATHOGENESIS

The fever and leukocytosis result from the release of cytokines and chemokines from the epidermis.

HISTORY

Onset of Lesions   The constellation of fiery-red erythema followed by formation of pustules and "lakes" occurs over a period of less than 1 day. Waves of pustules may follow each other; as one set dries, another appears.

Skin Symptoms   Marked burning, tenderness.

Constitutional Symptoms

Acute   Headache, chills, feverishness, marked fatigue, severe malaise.

PHYSICAL EXAMINATION

Appearance of Patient   Frightened, "toxic."

Vital Signs   Fast pulse, rapid breathing, fever that may be high.

Skin Lesions   There is a sequence of burning erythema followed by the appearance of clusters of tiny, nonfollicular, and very superficial pustules that usually become confluent, forming circinate lesions and "lakes" of pus (Fig. 3-10). Removal of the top yields superficial, oozing erosions, and there will be crusting. Once crusts are shed, new crops of pustules may appear in the same site. The eruption is generalized.

Hair and Nails   Nails become thickened, and there is onycholysis; subungual "lakes" of pus lead to shedding of nails; hair loss of the telogen defluvium type may develop in 2 or 3 months.

DIFFERENTIAL DIAGNOSIS

Widespread Erythema with Pustules   The abrupt onset and the typical evolution of erythema followed by pustulation are highly characteristic. Nevertheless, blood cultures always should be obtained because of possible superinfection, especially with staphylococcal bacteremia. Generalized herpes simplex has umbilicated pustules, and the Tzanck tests and viral cultures establish the diagnosis. Generalized pustular drug eruptions (e.g., after furosemide, amoxicillin/clavulanic acid, and other drugs) may be clinically indistinguishable, but patients are less toxic.

LABORATORY EXAMINATIONS

Dermatopathology   Large spongiform pustules resulting from the migration of neutrophils to the upper stratum malpighii, where they aggregate within the interstices between the degenerated and thinned keratinocytes.

Bacterial Culture of Tissue   Rule out *S. aureus* infection.

Hematologic   Polymorphonuclear leukocytosis—WBC as high as 20,000.

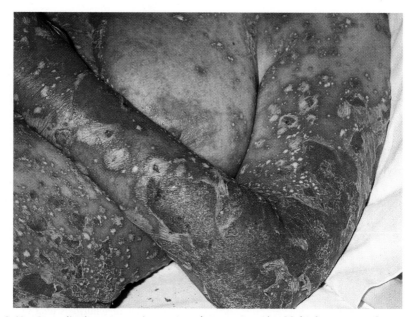

Figure 3-10 Generalized acute pustular psoriasis (von Zumbusch) *Multiple, creamy-white pustules on an erythematous base coalesced to form lakes of pus. These primary lesions ruptured, resulting in large areas of secondary erosion. Fever and neutrophilic leukocytosis were also present.*

SIGNIFICANCE

These patients are often brought to the emergency rooms of hospitals, and there is a serious question of overwhelming bacteremia until a dermatologist is consulted and the blood cultures are shown to be negative.

COURSE AND PROGNOSIS

Relapses and remissions may occur over a period of years. May follow, evolve into or be followed by psoriasis vulgaris.

Acrodermatitis continua of Hallopeau This is a chronic recurrent pustulation of nail folds, nail bed and distal fingers leading to loss of nails. It can occur alone or in association with pustular psoriasis of Zumbusch.

MANAGEMENT

Acutely ill patients with generalized rash should be hospitalized and treated in the same manner as patients with extensive burns, toxic epidermal necrolysis or exfoliative erythroderma—in a specialized unit: isolation, fluid replacement, and repeated blood cultures.

Systemic Therapy Some patients undergo a rapid, spontaneous remission without any therapy; and if they have had a previous spontaneous remission and are having a recurrence, specific systemic treatment is often omitted. For new patients, most are started on IV antibiotics pending the results of the blood culture. Systemic glucocorticoids should be avoided and may be indicated only in the initial toxic phases of an eruption. First-line therapy of generalized pustular psoriasis is oral etretinate or acitretin, .5 to 1 mg/kg of body weight per day. It results in rapid cessation of pustular eruptions but has to be continued for a considerable time to prevent recurrence.

PUVA Photochemotherapy Highly effective, but often difficult to perform in a toxic patient with fever. It is therefore added to etretinate once systemic symptoms have improved and pustulation has come to a halt.

Parenteral Methotrexate 15 to 25 mg once a week. A second-line choice.

ICHTHYOSES

The ichthyoses are a group of hereditary disorders characterized by an excess accumulation of cutaneous scale, whose severity varies from very mild and asymptomatic to life-threatening. A relatively large number of types of ichthyoses exist; most are extremely rare and often part of multiorgan syndromes. Only the four most common and important types are discussed below.

CLASSIFICATION

Dominant ichthyosis vulgaris (DIV)
X-linked ichthyosis (XLI)
Lamellar ichthyosis (LI)
Epidermolytic hyperkeratosis (EH)

PATHOGENESIS

In the various forms of ichthyosis, individual keratin genes may not be expressed or may result in the formation of abnormal keratins. LI shows increased germinative cell hyperplasia and increased transit rate through the epidermis, and there is a transglutaminase deficiency. In DIV and XLI, formation of thickened stratum corneum is caused by increased adhesiveness of the stratum corneum cells and/or failure of normal cell separation. Abnormal stratum corneum formation results in variable increases in transepidermal water loss. The etiology of the most common ichthyosis, DIV, is unknown; in XLI, there is a steroid sulfatase deficiency. In EH, there are mutations in the genes encoding keratin 1 or 10; here the disturbance of epidermal differentiation and the expression of abnormal keratin genes result in vacuolization of the upper epidermal layers, blistering, and hyperkeratosis.

HISTORY

All four types of ichthyosis tend to be worse during the dry, cold winter months and improve during the hot, humid summer. Patients living in tropical climates may remain symptom-free but may experience appearance or worsening of symptoms on moving to a temperate climate.

DIAGNOSIS

Usually made on clinical findings.

Ichthyosis Vulgaris

Ichthyosis vulgaris is characterized by usually mild generalized hyperkeratosis with xerosis most pronounced on the lower legs and by perifollicular hyperkeratosis (keratosis pilaris) and is frequently associated with atopy.

EPIDEMIOLOGY

Age of Onset 3 to 12 months.

Sex Equal incidence in males and females.

Mode of Inheritance Autosomal dominant.

PATHOGENESIS

Etiology unknown. There is reduced or absent filaggrin. Epidermis proliferates normally, but keratin is retained with a resultant thickened stratum corneum.

HISTORY

Very commonly associated with atopy, i.e., atopic dermatitis, allergic rhinitis, intrinsic asthma. Xerosis and pruritus worse in winter months. Keratosis pilaris and, less commonly, xerosis are of cosmetic concern to many patients. Occasionally, however, hyperkeratosis may be severe.

PSORIASIS AND ICHTHYOSIFORM DERMATOSES

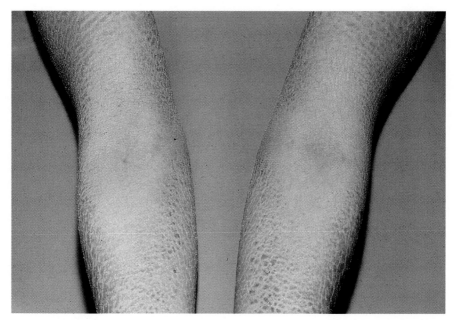

Figure 3-11 Ichthyosis vulgaris: arms *Fish scale-like hyperkeratosis of the arms with sparing of the antecubital fossae.*

PHYSICAL EXAMINATION

Skin Lesions Xerosis (dry skin) with fine, powdery scaling but also larger, firmly adherent scales in a fish-scale pattern that is most apparent on the shins. These are tacked-down scales with superficial fissuring at the margins (Fig. 3-11). There is usually diffuse involvement, accentuated on the shins, arms, and back but also on the buttocks and lateral thighs; The axillae and the fossae (anticubital and popliteal) are spared (Fig. 3-11); the face is usually also spared; but the cheeks and forehead may be involved (see Figure 3-II). *Keratosis pilaris* is perifollicular hyperkeratosis with little, spiny hyperkeratotic follicular papules of normal skin color that are either grouped or disseminated and appear mostly on the extensor surfaces of the extremities (Fig. 3-12). In childhood, when keratosis pilaris is most common, it may also be prominent on the cheeks. Hands and feet are usually spared, but palmoplantar markings are more accentuated (hyperlinear); occasional keratoderma.

Associated Diseases More than 50% of individuals with DIV also have atopic dermatitis, and rarely keratopathy can occur.

DIFFERENTIAL DIAGNOSIS

Xerosis/Hyperkeratosis Xerosis; acquired ichthyosis (may be a paraneoplastic syndrome; must be distinguished from DIV); drug-induced ichthyosis (triparanol); X-linked ichthyosis; lamellar ichthyosis; widespread, epidermal dermatophytosis.

LABORATORY EXAMINATIONS

Dermatopathology Compact hyperkeratosis; reduced or absent granular layer; germinative layer flattened. Electron microscopy: small, poorly formed keratohyalin granules.

DIAGNOSIS

Usually by clinical findings; electron microscopic finding of abnormal keratohyalin granules.

COURSE AND PROGNOSIS

May show improvement in the summer, in humid climates, and in adulthood. Keratosis pilaris occurring on the cheeks during childhood usually improves during adulthood.

MANAGEMENT

Hydration of Stratum Corneum Pliability of stratum corneum is a function of its water content. Hydration is best accomplished by immersion in a bath followed by the application of petrolatum. Urea-containing creams may help bind water in the stratum corneum.

Keratolytic Agents Propylene glycol–glycerin–lactic acid mixtures are effective without occlusion. Another effective preparation is 6% salicylic acid in propylene glycol and alcohol, which is used under plastic occlusion. Alpha-hydroxy acids such as lactic acid or glycolic acid bind or control scaling. Urea-containing preparations (2 to 10%) are effective; some preparations contain both urea and lactic acid.

Systemic Retinoids Isotretinoin, acitretin, and etretinate are effective, but careful monitoring for toxicity is required. Only severe cases may require intermittent therapy over long periods of time.

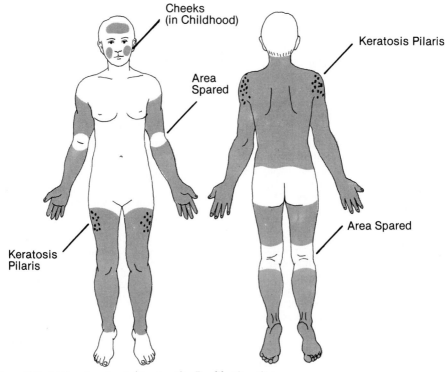

Figure 3-11   Ichthyosis vulgaris (dominant)   *Predilection sites.*

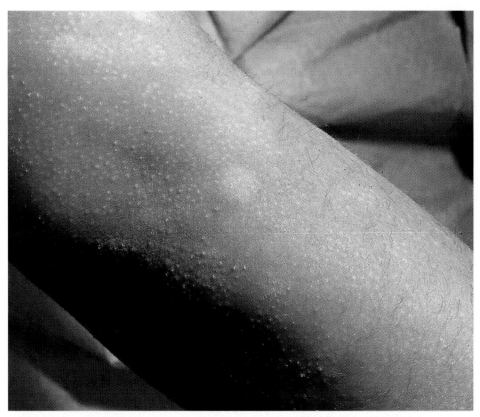

Figure 3-12 Keratosis pillaris: arm *Small, follicular, horny spines occur as a manifestation of mild ichthyosis vulgaris; arising mostly on the shoulders, upper arms, and thighs.*

X-linked Ichthyosis

X-linked ichthyosis (XLI) occurs only in males and is characterized by prominent, dirty brown scales occurring on the neck, extremities, trunk, and buttocks, with onset soon after birth.

EPIDEMIOLOGY

Age of Onset   Birth or infancy.

Sex   Males.

Mode of Inheritance   X-linked recessive; gene locus Xp22.32.

Genetic Defect   Steroid sulfatase deficiency.

Incidence   1:2000 to 1:6000.

PATHOGENESIS

Steroid sulfatase deficiency is associated with failure to shed senescent keratinocytes normally, resulting clinically in retention hyperkeratosis associated with normal epidermal proliferation.

HISTORY

Onset of skin abnormality 2 to 6 weeks of age; corneal opacities develop during the second to third week. Usually asymptomatic; may also be present in female carriers of XLI. Discomfort due to xerosis. Cosmetic disfigurement due to the dirty brown scales.

PHYSICAL EXAMINATION

Skin Lesions   Large adherent scales (not powdery as in ichthyosis vulgaris) that appear brown or dirty (Fig. 3-13) and are most pronounced on posterior neck, extensor arms, antecubital and popliteal fossae, and trunk with relative sparing of flexural areas. Note absence of palm/sole and face involvement.

Eye Lesions   Comma-shaped stromal corneal opacities in 50% of adult males. Present in some female carriers.

Genitourinary Abnormality   Cryptorchidism in 20% of individuals.

DIFFERENTIAL DIAGNOSIS

Lamellar ichthyosis, ichthyosis vulgaris, epidermolytic hyperkeratosis, contiguous gene syndromes.

LABORATORY EXAMINATIONS

Chemistry   Determine cholesterol sulfate level, which is elevated. Increased mobility of β-lipoproteins in electrophoresis.

Dermatopathology   Hyperkeratosis; granular layer present, sometimes hypergranulosis.

DIAGNOSIS

By family history and clinical findings.

Prenatal Diagnosis   Via amniocentesis and chorionic villus sampling; steroid sulfatase assay detects enzyme deficiency.

COURSE AND PROGNOSIS

No improvement with age. Usually worse in temperate climates and in winter season. With placental sulfatase deficiency, failure of labor to begin or progress may occur in mother carrying affected fetus.

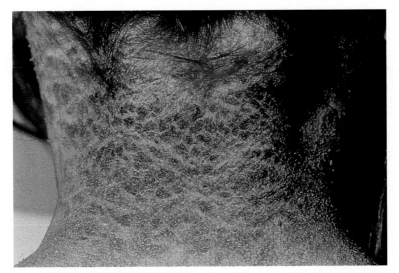

Figure 3-13 X-linked ichthyosis: neck *Dark-brown hyperkeratosis of the neck gives a dirty appearance to the area.*

MANAGEMENT

TOPICAL THERAPY

Emollients Hydrated petrolatum.

Keratolytics *Propylene glycol* 44 to 60% in water applied half strength (h.s.) after bath and occluded with a plastic suit worn as pajamas. When excess scaling has been removed, repeat once weekly as necessary.

Other agents: Salicylic acid, urea, and α-hydroxy acids (glycolic acid, lactic acid) in various vehicles.

Systemic Treatment

Acitretin, .5 to 1 mg/kg orally (PO) until marked improvement, then taper dose to maintenance level. Continuous laboratory monitoring and, in long-term regimens, x-rays for calcifications and DISH syndrome are mandatory.

Lamellar Ichthyosis

Lamellar ichthyosis often presents at birth with the infant encased in a collodion-like membrane (collodion baby) (page 80) that is soon shed, with subsequent formation of large, coarse scales involving the entire body including all flexural areas as well as the palms and soles. During childhood and adulthood, the skin is encased in this platelike scale, which causes significant cosmetic disfigurement.

EPIDEMIOLOGY

Age of Onset At birth, usually as collodion baby.

Sex Equal.

Mode of Inheritance Autosomal recessive; gene locus is 14q11 in some families.

Incidence ≤1:300,000.

PATHOGENESIS

Mutation in the gene encoding transglutaminase 1, an enzyme that catalyzes the cross-linking of proteins during the formation of cornified envelopes of corneocytes.

HISTORY

Heat intolerance, usually during exercise and hot weather because of inability to sweat. Water loss (excess)/dehydration due to fissuring of stratum corneum. Increased nutritional requirements for young children due to rapid growth and shedding of stratum corneum. Painful palmar/plantar fissures.

PHYSICAL EXAMINATION

Skin Lesions

Newborn Collodion baby, encased in a translucent collodion-like membrane (Fig. 3-16); shed in few weeks. Ectropion; eclabion. Generalized erythroderma.

Child/Adult Large parchment-like scales develop over the entire body (Figure 3-14), fracturing of the hyperkeratotic plate results in a tessellated (tilelike) pattern. Scales are large and very thick and brown, over most of the body, accentuated on lower extremities, and involving the flexural areas. Hyperkeratosis around joints may be verrucous. Hands/feet: keratoderma; accentuation of palmar/plantar creases.
Erythroderma may develop.

Hair Bound down by scales; frequent infections may result in scarring alopecia.

Nails Dystrophy secondary to nail fold inflammation.

Mucous Membranes Usually spared. Ectropion may result in secondary infection.

Eye Lesions Ectropion.

DIFFERENTIAL DIAGNOSIS

X-linked ichthyosis, epidermolytic hyperkeratosis, congenital ichthyosiform erythroderma, Netherton's syndrome, trichothiodystrophy.

LABORATORY EXAMINATIONS

Culture Rule out secondary infection and sepsis, especially in newborns.

Dermatopathology Hyperkeratosis; granular layer present; acanthosis. Epidermal transglutaminase ↓.

COURSE AND PROGNOSIS

Collodion membrane present at birth is shed within first few days to weeks (Fig. 3-16). Newborns are at risk for hypernatremic dehydration, secondary infection, and sepsis. Disorder persists throughout life. No improvement with age. Hyperkeratosis results in obstruction of eccrine sweat glands with resultant impairment of sweating.

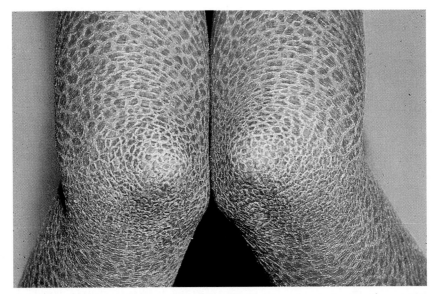

Figure 3-14 Lamellar ichthyosis: arms *Tessellated (tilelike) hyperkeratosis gives the appearance of reptilian scales on the arms around the elbows. The entire body was involved and there was ectropium.*

MANAGEMENT

Newborn Care in neonatal intensive care unit. High-humidity chamber. Emolliation. Monitor electrolytes, fluids. Follow for signs of local or systemic infection.

Child/Adult *Emollients* Hydrated petrolatum.

Keratolytics Propylene Glycol 40 to 60% in water applied h.s. after bath and occluded with a plastic suit worn as pajamas. When excess scaling has been removed, repeat once weekly as necessary.

Other agents: Salicylic acid, urea, and α-hydroxy acids (glycolic acid, lactic acid) in various vehicles.

Overheating Parents and affected individuals should be instructed about overheating and heat prostration that can follow exercise, high environmental temperatures, and fever. Repeated application of water to skin can replace function of sweating, cooling the body.

Retinoids Etretinate, acitretin, and, to a lesser degree, isotretinoin (.5 to 1 mg/kg) are effective as in XLI. Monitor continously for serum triglycerides, transaminases and bony toxicities if given over prolonged period of time. Teratogenicity requires effective contraception.

Support Groups Such as Foundation for Ichthyosis and Related Skin Types (FIRST) exist.

Epidermolytic Hyperkeratosis

Epidermolytic hyperkeratosis presents at or shortly after birth with blistering. With time, the skin becomes keratotic and even verrucous, particularly in the flexural areas, knees, and elbows.

EPIDEMIOLOGY

Age of Onset   Birth or shortly thereafter.

Sex   Equal incidence in males and females.

Mode of Inheritance   Autosomal dominant.

Incidence   Very rare.

PATHOGENESIS

Mutations of genes that encode the epidermal differentiation keratins, keratin 1 and 10.

HISTORY

Blistering may recur periodically, leading to denuded areas, secondary infection, and sepsis. Hyperkeratotic lesions become verrucous, particularly in the flexural areas, and are associated with an unpleasant odor.

PHYSICAL EXAMINATION

Skin Lesions   Blistering at birth or shortly thereafter. Generalized or localized. Denuded areas develop that heal with normal-appearing skin. With time, the skin becomes keratotic and verrucous (Fig. 3-15), particularly in the flexural areas, knees, and elbows. Hyperkeratotic scales adhere to underlying skin, often in a mountain range–like appearance; they may be quite dark in color and are associated with an unpleasant odor (like rancid butter). Recurrent blisters in hyperkeratotic areas (Fig. 3-15) and also shedding of hyperkeratotic masses result in circumscribed areas of skin that are relatively normal in appearance. This normal-appearing skin in hyperkeratotic areas is a valuable diagnostic sign. Secondary pyogenic infections, especially impetigo.

Generalized distribution with prominent involvement of flexural areas. Palmar and plantar involvement (hyperkeratosis). (*Note:* A variant of epidermolytic hyperkeratosis is localized to palms and soles and is genetically distinct from the generalized form.)

Hair and Nails   Hair is normal, but involvement of the nails may produce abnormal nail plates.

Mucous Membranes   Spared.

LABORATORY EXAMINATIONS

Dermatopathology   Giant, coarse keratohyalin granules and vacuolization of the granular layer, resulting in cell lysis and subcorneal multiloculated blisters. Papillomatosis, acanthosis, and hyperkeratosis.

COURSE AND PROGNOSIS

Blister formation and massive hyperkeratosis are prone to bacterial superinfection, which is probably also responsible for the unpleasant odor. Palmar involvement can adversely affect manual dexterity.

MANAGEMENT

Topical application of α-hydroxy acids, systemic retinoids. Antimicrobial therapy. Systemic retinoids (etretinate, acitretin) may transiently lead to a worsening of the condition because of increased blister formation but later improve the skin dramatically owing to a relative normalization of epidermal differentiation. Determine dose carefully, and monitor for side effects.

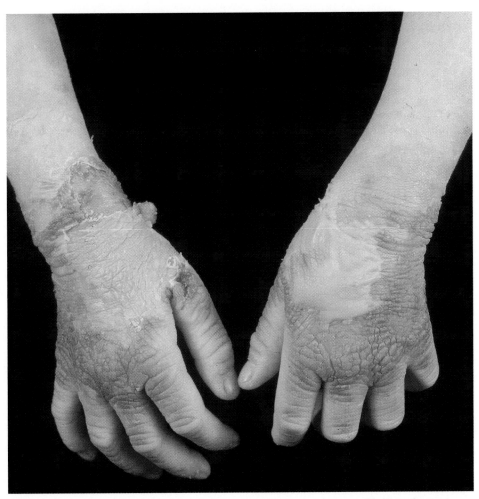

Figure 3-15 Epidermolytic hyperkeratosis: arms and hands *Mountain range-like hyperkeratosis of the dorsum of hands with blistering that results in erosions and shedding of large sheets of keratin.*

Ichthyosis in the Newborn (Collodion Baby)

Ichthyosis in the newborn presents most commonly as the collodion baby. Encasement in a transparent parchment-like membrane (Fig. 3-16A) may impair respiration and sucking. Breaking and shedding of the hyperkeratotic collodion membrane may lead initially to difficulties in thermoregulation and increased risk of infection. Skin is bright red and moist. After healing, the skin appears normal for some time until signs of ichthyosis develop. Collodion baby may be the initial presentation of lamellar ichthyosis or some less common forms of ichthyosis not discussed here. Collodion baby also may be a form of ichthyosis which, after the collodion membrane is shed and the resultant erythema has cleared, will progress to normal skin for the rest of the child's life (Figure 3-16B).

MANAGEMENT

Children should be kept in an incubator in which the air is saturated with water. Careful monitoring of the child's temperature and parenteral fluids and nutrient replacement may be necessary for some time. Infection of the skin and lungs is an important problem, and aggressive antibiotic therapy may be indicated.

Harlequin Fetus

Harlequin fetus is a condition in which the child is born with very thick plates of stratum corneum separated by deep cracks and fissures. Eclabium, ectropion, absence of ears, or rudimentary ears give the newborn a grotesque appearance. These children usually die shortly after birth, but there are reports of survival for weeks to several months. This condition is different from collodion baby and the other forms of ichthyosis with an unusual fibrous protein within the epidermis.

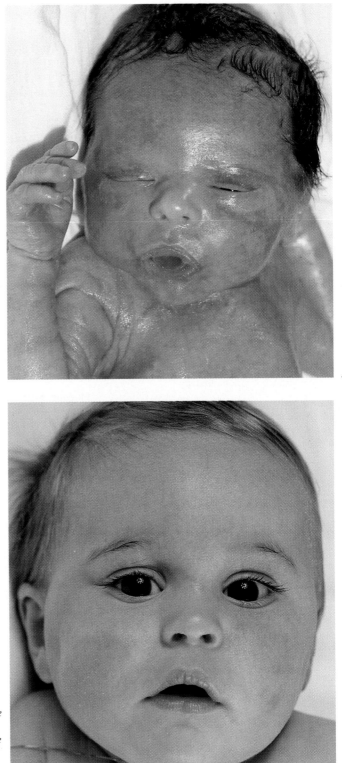

Figure 3-16 Ichthyosis in the newborn A. *"Collodion baby" shortly after birth with a parchment-like membrane covering the entire skin. The eyes and lips pucker outward, i.e., ectropion and eclabion. B. At six months of age, the same infant is a beautiful baby with minimal residual scale and erythema on the cheeks.*

A

B

ACANTHOSIS NIGRICANS

Acanthosis nigricans (AN) is a diffuse, velvety thickening and hyperpigmentation of the skin, chiefly in axillae and other body folds, the etiology of which may be related to factors of heredity, associated endocrine disorders, obesity, drug administration, and in one form, malignancy (see Section 15, Skin Signs of Systemic Cancers).

CLASSIFICATION

Type 1: Hereditary Benign AN   No associated endocrine disorder.

Type 2: Benign AN   Various endocrine disorders associated with insulin resistance: insulin-resistant diabetes mellitus, hyperandrogenic states, acromegaly/gigantism, Cushing's disease, hypogonadal syndromes with insulin resistance, Addison's disease, hypothyroidism.

Type 3: Pseudo-AN   Complication of obesity; more common in patients with darker pigmentation. Obesity produces insulin resistance.

Type 4: Drug-induced AN   Nicotinic acid in high dosage, stilbestrol in young males, glucocorticoid therapy, diethylstilbestrol/oral contraceptive, growth hormone therapy.

Type 5: Malignant AN   Paraneoplastic, usually adenocarcinoma of GI or GU tract; less commonly, lymphoma (see Section 15, Skin Signs of Systemic Cancers).

EPIDEMIOLOGY

Age of Onset   Type 1: during childhood or puberty.

Etiology   Dependent on associated disorder.

PATHOGENESIS

Epidermal changes may be caused by hypersecretion of pituitary peptide or nonspecific growth-promoting effect of hyperinsulinemia.

HISTORY

Usually insidious onset; first visible change is darkening of pigmentation.

PHYSICAL EXAMINATION

Skin Lesions   *All types of AN:* Darkening of pigmentation, skin appears dirty (Fig. 3-17). As skin thickens, appears velvety; skin line further accentuated; surface becomes rugose, mammillated. *Type 3:* velvety patch on inner, upper thigh at site of chafing; often has many skin tags in body folds, especially axillae, groins, neck. *Type 5:* hyperkeratosis and hyperpigmentation more pronounced. Hyperkeratosis of palms/soles, involvement of oral mucosa and vermilion border of lips. Accentuation of normal pigmentation. Velvety feel.

Distribution   Most commonly, axillae, neck (back, sides) (Fig. 3-17); also, groins, anogenitalia, antecubital fossae, knuckles, submammary umbilicus.

Mucous Membranes   Oral mucosa: velvety texture with delicate furrows. *Type 5:* Mucous membranes and mucocutaneous junctions commonly involved; warty papillomatous thickenings periorbitally, periorally.

General Examination   Examine for underlying endocrine disorder in benign AN, and search for malignancy in malignant AN.

DIFFERENTIAL DIAGNOSIS

Dark Thickened Flexural Skin   Confluent and reticulated papillomatosis (Gougerot-Carteaud syndrome), pityriasis versicolor, X-linked ichthyosis, retention hyperkeratosis, nicotinic acid ingestion.

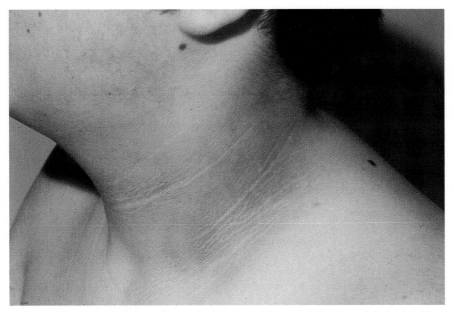

Figure 3-17   Acanthosis nigricans *Velvety, dark-brown epidermal thickening of the neck with prominent skin fold and feathered edges in a 25-year-old obese woman with a family history of acanthosis nigricans. Changes had been stable for more than five years. There were similar changes in the axillae, antecubital fossae, and dorsum of the knuckles.*

LABORATORY EXAMINATIONS

Chemistry   Rule out diabetes mellitus.

Dermatopathology   Papillomatosis, hyperkeratosis; epidermis thrown into irregular folds, showing various degrees of acanthosis.

Imaging   Rule out associated carcinoma.

Endoscopy   Rule out associated carcinoma.

DIAGNOSIS

Clinical findings.

COURSE AND PROGNOSIS

Type 1: Accentuated at puberty and, at times, regresses when older. *Type 2:* Depending on underlying disturbance. *Type 3:* May regress after significant weight loss. *Type 4:* Resolves when causative drug is discontinued. *Type 5:* AN may precede other symptoms of malignancy by 5 years; removal of malignancy may be followed by regression of AN.

MANAGEMENT

Symptomatic   Treat   associated   disorder. Pseudoacanthosis nigricans may regress with weight loss.

BULLOUS DISEASES

HEREDITARY EPIDERMOLYSIS BULLOSA

Hereditary epidermolysis bullosa (EB) is the term applied to a spectrum of rare genodermatoses in which a disturbed coherence of the epidermis of skin and mucous membranes leads to blister formation following trauma. Hence, the designation mechano-bullous dermatoses; there are more than 20 different types. Disease manifestations range from very mild to severely mutilating and even lethal forms that differ in mode of inheritance, clinical manifestations, and associated findings. The best classification is based on the site of blister formation and distinguishes among three main groups: epidermolytic or EB simplex (EBS), junctional EB (JEB), and dermolytic or dystrophic EB (DEB) (Table 4-1). In each of these groups there are several distinct types of EB based on clinical, genetic, histologic, and biochemical evaluation (Table 4-2).

EPIDEMIOLOGY

The overall incidence of hereditary EB is placed at 19.6 live births per one million births in the United States. Stratified by subtype, the incidences are 11 for EBS, 2 for JEB, and 5 for DEB. The estimated prevalence in the United States is 8.2 per million, but this figure probably represents only the most severe cases and does not include the majority of very mild disease going unreported.

CLINICAL PHENOTYPES

EB Simplex

EBS is defined as trauma-induced, intraepidermal blistering, based in most cases on keratin gene mutations. Different subgroups have considerable phenotypic variations (Table 4-3), and there are 11 distinct forms, seven of which are dominantly inherited. The two most common are dominantly inherited and described below.

Generalized EBS Generalized EBS is the so-called Koebner variant, with onset at birth to early infancy. There is generalized blistering following trauma with a predilection for traumatized body sites such as feet, hands, elbows, knees. Blisters are tense or flaccid at first and lead to erosions (Fig. 4-1). There is rapid healing and only minimal scarring at sites of repeated blistering. Palmoplantar hyperkeratoses may be present. Nails, teeth, and oral mucosa are usually spared.

Localized EBS Also called the Weber-Cockayne subtype. Has an onset in childhood or later in life and is the most common form of EBS. Often the disease may not present itself until adulthood, when thick-walled blisters on the feet and hands occur after excessive exercise, manual work or military training. Hyperhydrosis of palms and soles, is associated and secondary infection of blistered lesions often occurs.

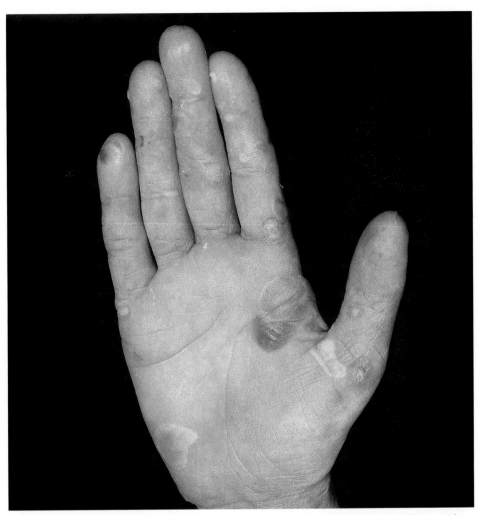

Figure 4-1 Generalized EBS *This 22-year-old male has had blistering since early infancy with a predilection for traumatized body sites such as the palms and soles, but also the elbows and knees. Blistering also occurs on the trunk. His initial aspiration to become a mechanic had to be dropped because severe blistering on the palms occurred every time he handled tools. The present eruption occurred after the patient helped his mother in the garden using a shovel. Note, that despite multiple blistering episodes, there is hardly any evidence of scarring on this palm.*

Junctional EB

All forms of JEB share the pathologic feature of blister formation within the lamina lucida of the basement membrane. This trait is autosomal recessive and comprises clinical phenotypes depending on the type of genetic lesion and environmental factors. There are at least six clinical subtypes, and the three principal forms are described below.

JEB Gravis (Herlitz EB)   Patients with JEB gravis often do not survive infancy; the mortality rate is 40% during the first year of life. There is generalized blistering at birth (Fig. 4-2) with clinically distinctive and severe periorificial granulation tissue, loss of nails, and involvement of most mucosal surfaces. The skin of these children may be completely denuded, representing oozing painful erosion; and associated findings include all symptoms resulting from epithelial blistering with respiratory, gastrointestinal, and genitourinary organ systems involved.

JEB Mitis   These children may have moderate or severe JEB at birth but survive infancy and clinically improve with age. Periorificial non-healing erosions during childhood.

Generalized Atrophic Benign Epidermolysis Bullosa (GABEB)   GABEB is a separate JEB that presents at birth with generalized cutaneous blistering and erosions not only on the extremities but also on the trunk, face, and scalp. Survival to adulthood is the rule, but blistering on traumatized areas continues (Fig. 4-3). It is particularly pronounced with increased ambient temperature, and there is atrophic healing of the lesions. Nail dystrophy, non-scarring or scarring alopecia, mild oral mucous membrane involvement, and enamel defects occur. Mutations are in the gene for bullous pemphigoid antigen 2 and laminin 5.

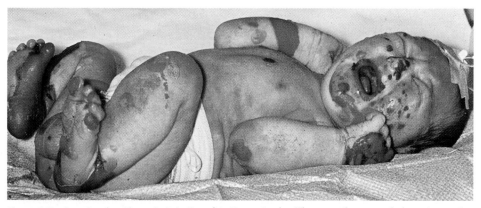

Figure 4-2 Junctional epidermolysis bullosa (Herlitz variant) *There are large eroded, oozing and bleeding areas that occurred intrapartum. When this newborn is lifted up, dislodgment of epidermis as well as erosions occur due to manual handling.*

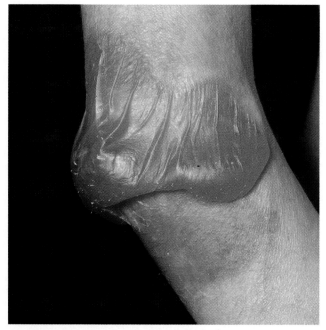

Figure 4-3 Generalized atrophic benign epidermolysis bullosa (GABEB) *This 17-year-old boy has had generalized cutaneous blistering since birth, with blisters and erosions arising on the elbows and knees but also on the trunk and face. Note, large flaccid bulla in an area of atrophy over the elbow; milia can also be seen on the trunk.*

Dystrophic Epidermolysis Bullosa

DEB is a spectrum of dermolytic diseases where blistering occurs below the basal lamina, and therefore healing after blister formation is usually accompanied by scarring and milia formation—hence, the name dystrophic. There are four principal subtypes, and all are due to mutations in anchoring fibril type 7 collagen. Anchoring fibrils are therefore only rudimentary or absent. The four main types of dermolytic EB are shown in Table 4-2, but only two of these are described below.

Dominant DEB Dominant DEB is also called Cockayne-Touraine's disease. Onset in infancy or early childhood with acral blistering and nail dystrophy; milia and scar formation, which may be hypertrophic or hyperplastic. Oral lesions are uncommon, and teeth are usually normal.

Recessive DEB Recessive DEB (RDEB) comprises a larger spectrum of clinical phenotypes. There is a localized, less severe form (RDEB mitis) that occurs at birth, shows acral blistering, atrophic scarring, and little or no mucosal involvement. Generalized, severe RDEB is mutilating and is called the Hallopeau-Siemens variant. There is generalized blistering at birth,

and progression and repeated blistering at the same sites (Fig. 4-4) result in remarkable scarring, syndactyly with mitten-like deformities of hands and feet (Fig. 4-5), flexion contractures, and massive scarring over pressure sites on the trunk and the extremities. There are enamel defects with caries and parodontitis, strictures and scarring in the oral mucous membrane and esophagus, urethral and anal stenosis, and ocular surface scarring. Malnutrition, growth retardation, and anemia result; and the most serious complication is squamous cell carcinoma in chronic recurrent erosions. The pathology is a sublamina densa plane of blister cleavage, and the molecular pathology rests on mutations of the gene coding for type 7 collagen.

PATHOGENESIS

A mutation of the genes for keratin 5 and 14 results in a disturbance of the stability of the keratin filament network within keratinocytes; this event causes cytolysis of basal keratinocytes after trauma and thus leads to blister formation. Histologically, therefore, the cleft occurs within the basal cell layer.

Table 4-3 CLINICAL PHENOTYPE—MOLECULAR DEFECT CORRELATIONS IN EPIDERMOLYSIS BULLOSA

Disease[a]	Genes[b]	Proteins
EBS-DM	KRT5, 14	Keratins 5, 14
EBS-WC	KRT5, 14	Keratins 5, 14
EBS-K	KRT5, 14	Keratins 5, 14
Recessive EBS-MD	PLEC1	Plectin
JEB-lethal	LAMA3, B3, C2	Laminin $5\alpha_3$, β_3, γ_2
JEB-PA	ITGA6, B4	Integrin α_6, β_4
GABEB	COL17A1, LAMB3	BP180, laminin
DDEB	COL7A1	Type VII collagen
RDEB	COL7A1	Type VII collagen

[a] Disease categories reflect clinical phenotypes of individual EB patients studied.

[b] Genes indicated represent candidate genes identified by DNA mutation analysis as correlating with disease phenotype. Examples of genetic defects include: KRT5 or 14 heterozygous missense or in-frame deletions in dominant forms of EBS; KRT5 or 14 homozygous missense or premature termination codons (PTC) in recessive EBS; PLEC1 homozygous in-frame deletion or PT in EBS-MD; LAMA3, B3, C2 homozygous PTC in Herlitz JEB; ITGA6 or B4 heterozygous PTC/in-frame deletion or homozygous PTC in JEB-PA; COL17A1 heterozygous PTC/missense or homozygous PT in GABEB; COL7A1 heterozygous gly substitution in DDEB; COL7A1 homozygous PT or gly substitution in RDEB-HS; COL7A1 homozygous missense or gly substitution or heterozygous PTC/gly substitution in RDEB mitis.

NOTE: EBS-DM, EB simplex, Dowling-Meara type; EBS-WC, EB simplex, Weber-Cockayne type; EBS-K, EB simplex, Koebner type; recessive EBS-MD, EB simplex associated with muscular dystrophy; JEB-lethal, junctional EB, Herlitz type; JEB-PA, JEB associated with pyloric atresia; GABEB, generalized atrophic benign EB; DDEB, dominant dystrophic EB; RDEB, recessive dystrophic EB.

SOURCE: From MP Marinkovich et al, Hereditary epidermolysis bullosa, in IM Freedberg, AZ Eisen, K Wolff, KF Austen, LA Goldsmith, SI Katz, TB Fitzpatrick (eds): *Fitzpatrick's Dermatology in General Medicine*, 5th ed. New York, McGraw-Hill, 1999.

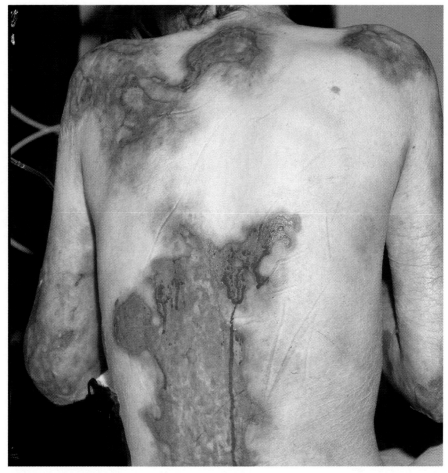

Figure 4-4   Generalized recessive dystrophic epidermolysis bullosa   *This is a severe disease with generalized blistering, often in the same sites, as in this 14-year-old girl. Erosions have become ulcers that have a low tendency to heal; and when healing occurs, it results in scarring. This girl also has enamel defects with caries, strictures in the esophagus, growth retardation and severe anemia. Any time the skin is even slightly traumatized, new blisters will appear. It is obvious that these large wounds are portal entries for systemic infection.*

DIAGNOSIS

Based on clinical appearance and history. Histopathology determines the level of cleavage, which is further defined by electron microscopy and/or immunohistochemical mapping. A molecular technique including Western blot, Northern blot, restriction fragment length polymorphism (RFLP) analysis and DNA sequences may then identify the mutated gene.

MANAGEMENT

There is no therapy for EB. Management, therefore, has to be tailored to the severity and extent of skin involvement and consists of supportive skin care, supportive care for other organ systems, and systemic therapies for complications. Wound management, nutritional support, and infection control are key to the management of all EB patients.

In EBS, maintenance of a cool environment and use of soft, well-ventilated shoes, are important. Blistered skin is treated by saline compresses and topical antibiotics or, in the case of inflammation, with topical steroids. More severely affected JEB and DEB patients are treated like patients in a burn unit. Gentle bathing and cleansing are followed by protective emollients and nonadherent dressings.

Management of cutaneous infection is important, and surgical treatment is often required in the management of patients with DEB for the release of fused digits and correction of limb contractures.

Although rare, EB and, in particular, JEB and DEB pose a major health and socioeconomic problem. Organizations such as the Dystrophic Epidermolysis Bullosa Research Association (DEBRA) offer assistance that includes patient education and support.

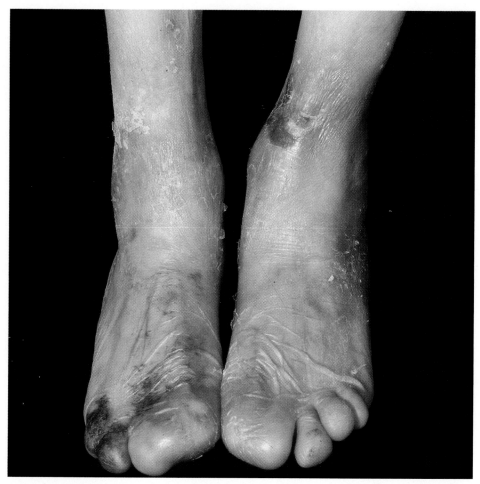

Figure 4-5 Generalized recessive dystrophic epidermolysis bullosa *Loss of toenails and mitten-like deformities of the feet due to repeated blistering, reepithelialization and scarring. This is the same patient as shown in Figure 4-4.*

FAMILIAL BENIGN PEMPHIGUS

Familial benign pemphigus or Hailey-Hailey's disease is a rare genodermatosis with dominant inheritance that is classically described as a blistering disorder but actually presents as an erythematous, erosive, oozing condition with cracks and fissures localized to the nape of the neck, axillae (Fig. 4-6), submammary regions, unguinal folds, and scrotum. The underlying pathologic process is acantholysis whereby the fragility of the epidermis is probably due to a defect in the adhesion complex between desmosomal proteins and tonofilaments. Onset is usually between the third and fourth decade, and the disease is often mistaken for intertrigo, candidiasis, frictional or contact dermatitis. Individual lesions consists of microscopically small flaccid vesicles on an erythematous background that soon turn into eroded plaques with the described, highly characteristic, fissured appearance (Fig. 4-6). Crusting, scaling, and hypertrophic vegetative growths may occur. Histology explains the clinical appearance as epidermal cells lose their coherence with acantholysis throughout the epithelium, giving the appearance of a dilapidated brick wall.

Colonization of the lesions, particularly by Staphylococcus aureus is a trigger for further acantholysis and maintenance of the pathologic process. Secondary colonization by Candida has a similar effect.

Treatment rests on anti-infective agents, administered both topically and systemically; systemically tetracyclines seem to work better than most. Topical glucocorticoids depress the anti-inflammatory response and accelerate healing. In severe cases, dermabrasion or carbon dioxide laser vaporization leads to healing with scars, which are resistant to recurrences. The condition becomes less troublesome with age.

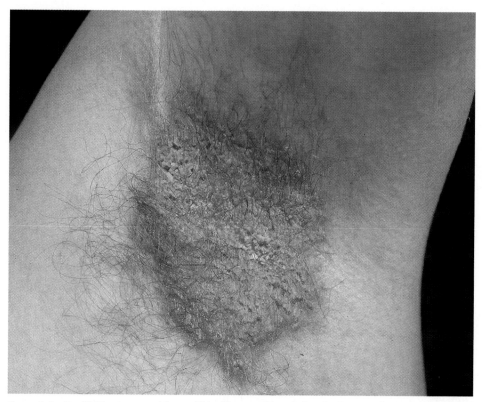

Figure 4-6   Familial benign pemphigus   *This 46-year-old male has had oozing lesions in both axillae, occasionally in the groins and sometimes also on the nape of the neck, for several years. Eruptions worsen during the summer months. The father and sister have similar lesions that wax and wane. Lesions are painful and show typical cracks and fissures within an erosive erythematous plaque. Although classified among the blistering diseases, familial benign pemphigus hardly ever shows intact vesicles and is often mistaken for intertrigo.*

FAMILIAL BENIGN PEMPHIGUS

PEMPHIGUS VULGARIS

Pemphigus vulgaris (PV) is a serious, acute or chronic, bullous, autoimmune disease of skin and mucous membranes that is often fatal unless treated with immunosuppressive agents. It is the prototype of the pemphigus family, a group of autoimmune acantholytic blistering diseases (Table 4-4).

EPIDEMIOLOGY

Age of Onset   40 to 60 years.

Sex   Equal incidence in males and females.

Etiology   Autoimmune disorder.

PATHOGENESIS

A loss of the normal cell-to-cell adhesion in the epidermis occurs as a result of circulating antibodies of the IgG class; these antibodies bind to cell surface glycoproteins (pemphigus antigens; desmoglein 3, a member of the cadherin superfamily) of the epidermis and induce acantholysis, probably by the activation of serine proteases.

HISTORY

PV usually starts in the oral mucosa, and months may elapse before skin lesions occur; lesions may be localized for 6 to 12 months, after which generalized bullae occur. Less frequently there may be a generalized, acute eruption of bullae from the beginning. No pruritus, but burning and pain. Painful and tender mouth lesions may prevent adequate food intake. Epistaxis, hoarseness, dysphagia. Weakness, malaise, weight loss (with prolonged mouth involvement).

Table 4-4   CLASSIFICATION OF PEMPHIGUS

Pemphigus vulgaris
  Pemphigus vegetans: localized
  Drug-induced
Pemphigus foliaceus
  Pemphigus erythematosus: localized
  Fogo selvagem: endemic
  Drug-induced
Paraneoplastic pemphigus

PHYSICAL EXAMINATION

Skin Lesions   Round or oval vesicles and bullae with serous content (Fig. 4-7), flaccid (flabby), easily ruptured, and weeping, arising on normal skin, randomly scattered, discrete. Localized (e.g., to mouth) or generalized with a random pattern. Extensive erosions that bleed easily (Fig. 4-8), crusts particularly on scalp. *Note:* Since blisters rupture so easily, only erosions are seen in many patients. These are very painful.

Nikolsky's Sign   Dislodging of epidermis by lateral finger pressure in the vicinity of lesions, which leads to an erosion. Pressure on bulla leads to lateral extension of blister.

Sites of Predilection   Scalp, face, chest, axillae, groin, umbilicus. In bed-ridden patients, there is extensive involvement of back (Fig. 4-8).

Mucous Membranes   Bullae rarely seen, erosions of mouth (see Section 29) and nose, pharynx and larynx, vagina).

LABORATORY EXAMINATIONS

Dermatopathology   Light microscopy (select early small bulla or, if not present, margin of larger bulla or erosion): (1) loss of intercellular cohesion in lower part of epidermis, leading to (2) acantholysis (separation of keratinocytes) and to (3) bulla that is split just *above* the basal cell layer and contains separated, rounded-up (acantholytic) keratinocytes.

Immunofluorescence (IF)   Direct IF staining reveals IgG and often C3 deposited in lesional and paralesional skin in *the intercellular substance of the epidermis.*

Serum   Autoantibodies (IgG) detected by indirect immunofluorescence. Titer usually correlates with activity of disease process. Autoantibodies are directed against a 130-kDa glycoprotein designated desmoglein 3.

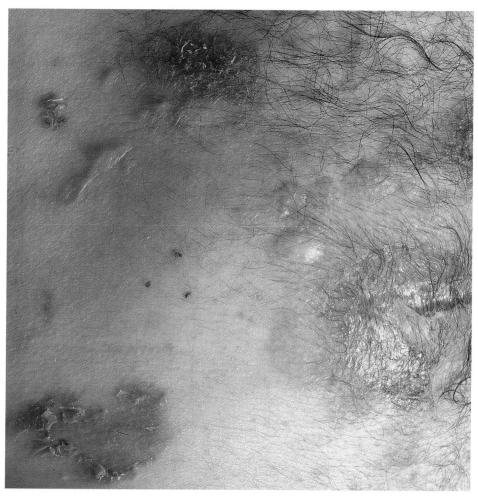

Figure 4-7 Pemphigus vulgaris *This 56-year-old male patient noticed areas of increased skin fragility on his trunk; and only when examined more closely, were flaccid bullae seen that easily ruptured and turned into erosions. The patient previously had erosive and very painful stomatitis for over six months and was treated unsuccessfully with topical remedies by his dentist. When skin lesions as shown in this picture appeared, he consulted a dermatologist who made the correct diagnosis.*

DIAGNOSIS

Can be a difficult problem if only mouth lesions are present. Biopsy of the skin and mucous membrane, direct immunofluorescence, and demonstration of circulating autoantibodies confirm a high index of suspicion.

COURSE

The disease inexorably progresses to death unless treated aggressively with immunosuppressive agents. The mortality rate has been markedly reduced since treatment has become available.

Variants (Table 4-4)

Pemphigus Vegetans (PVeg) Usually confined to intertriginous regions, perioral area, neck, and scalp. Granulomatous vegetating purulent plaques that extend centrifugally. Suprabasal acantholysis with intraepidermal abscesses containing mostly eosinophils, pseudoepitheliomatous hyperplasia of the epidermis, exuberant granulation tissue with abscess formation. IgG autoantibodies as in PV. PV may evolve into PVeg and vice versa.

Pemphigus Foliaceus (PF)

Most commonly on face, scalp, upper chest, and abdomen but may involve entire skin, presenting as exfoliative erythroderma. Superficial form of pemphigus with acantholysis in the granular layer of the epidermis. Bullae hardly ever present; lesions consist of erythematous patches and erosions covered with crusts. PF is also mediated by circulating autoantibodies to a 160-kDa intercellular (cell surface) antigen, desmoglein I, in the desmosomes of keratinocytes. PV (130 kDa) and PF (160 kDa) antigens differ. This explains the different sites of acantholysis and thus the different clinical appearances of the two conditions.

Brazilian Pemphigus (Fogo Selvagem) A distinctive form of pemphigus foliaceus endemic to south central Brazil. Clinically, histologically, and immunopathologically identical to PF. Patients improve when moved to urban areas but relapse after returning to endemic regions. It is speculated that the disease is somehow related to an arthropod-borne infectious agent. More than 1000 new cases per year are estimated to occur in the endemic regions.

Pemphigus Erythematosus (PE) *Synonym:* Senear-Usher syndrome. A localized variety of PF largely confined to seborrheic sites. Erythematous, crusted, and erosive lesions in the "butterfly" area of the face, forehead, presternal, and interscapular regions. Despite clinical, histopathologic, and immunopathologic similarity to PF, PE may be unique, since patients have immunoglobulin and complement deposits at the dermal-epidermal junction, in addition to intercellular pemphigus antibody in the epidermis, and antinuclear antibodies, as is the case in lupus erythematosus. In addition, PE may be associated with thymoma and myasthenia gravis.

Drug-Induced Pemphigus A PV- and PF/ PE-like syndrome can be induced by D-penicillamine and less frequently by captopril and other drugs. In most, but not all, instances the eruption resolves after termination of therapy with the offending drug.

Paraneoplastic Pemphigus (PNP)

Mucous membranes primarily and most severely involved. Lesions combine features of pemphigus vulgaris and erythema multiforme, clinically and histologically (Section 15).

MANAGEMENT

Glucocorticoids 2 to 3 mg/kg of body weight of prednisone until cessation of new blister formation and disappearance of Nikolsky's sign. Then rapid reduction to about half the initial dose until patient is almost clear, followed by very slow tapering of dose to minimal effective maintenance dose.

Concomitant Immunosuppressive Therapy Immunosuppressive agents are given concomitantly for their glucocorticoid-sparing effect:

Azathioprine, 2 to 3 mg/kg of body weight until complete clearing; tapering of dose to 1 mg/kg. Azathioprine alone is continued even after cessation of glucocorticoid treatment and may have to be continued for many months. Clinical freedom from disease and a negative pemphigus antibody titer for at least 3 months permit cessation of therapy.

Methotrexate, either orally (PO) or intramuscularly (IM) at doses of 25 to 35mg/week. Dose adjustments are made as with azathioprine.

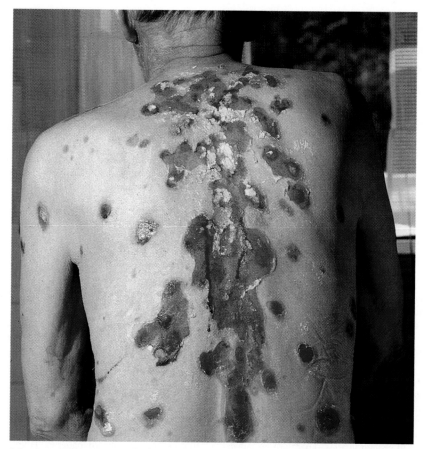

Figure 4-8 Pemphigus vulgaris *Widespread, confluent erosions on the back of a patient who has a generalized eruption including the scalp and the mucous membranes. Due to the fragility of the blisters—some of which can still be recognized on the left lower back—pemphigus vulgaris presents as erosions which are extremely painful and tend to bleed with minimal trauma.*

Cyclophosphamide, 100 to 200 mg daily, with reduction to maintenance doses of 50 to 100 mg/d. Alternatively, cyclophosphamide "bolus" therapy with 1000 mg intravenously (IV) once a week or every 2 weeks in the initial phases, followed by 50 to 100 mg/d PO as maintenance.

Plasmapheresis, in conjunction with glucocorticoids and immunosuppressive agents in poorly controlled patients, in the initial phases of treatment to reduce antibody titers.

Gold therapy, for milder cases. After an initial test dose of 10 mg IM, 25 to 50 mg of gold sodium thiomalate is given IM at weekly intervals to a maximum cumulative dose of 1 g.

Mycophenolate mofetil has been reported to be beneficial, and clinical studies are ongoing.

High dose intravenous immunoglobulin (HIVIG) has been reported to have a glucocorticoid-sparing effect.

Other measures: cleansing baths, wet dressings, topical and intralesional glucocorticoids, antibiotics to combat bacterial infections. Correction of fluid and electrolyte imbalance.

Monitoring Clinical, for improvement of skin lesions and development of drug-related side effects. Laboratory monitoring of pemphigus antibody titers and for hematologic and metabolic indicators of glucocorticoid- and/or immunosuppressive-induced adverse effects.

BULLOUS PEMPHIGOID

Bullous pemphigoid is an autoimmune disorder presenting as a chronic bullous eruption mostly in patients over 60 years of age.

EPIDEMOLOGY

Age of Onset 60 to 80 years.

Sex Equal incidence in males and females.

PATHOGENESIS

Interaction of autoantibody with bullous pemphigoid antigen on the surface of basal keratinocytes (extending into the lamina lucida of basement membrane) is followed by complement activation and attraction of neutrophils and eosinophils. Bullous lesion results from interaction of multiple bioactive molecules released by mast cells and eosinophils.

HISTORY

Often starts with a prodromal eruption (urticarial, papular lesions) and evolves in weeks to months to bullae that may appear suddenly as a generalized eruption. Initially no symptoms except moderate or severe pruritus; later, tenderness of eroded lesions. There are no constitutional symptoms, except in widespread, severe disease.

PHYSICAL EXAMINATION

Skin Lesions Erythematous, papular or urticarial-type lesions, not unlike the lesions in erythema multiforme (Fig. 4-9), may precede bullae formation by months. Bullae, large, tense, firm-topped, oval or round (Fig. 4-10); may arise in normal or erythematous skin and contain serous or hemorrhagic fluid. The eruption may be localized or generalized, usually scattered but also grouped in arciform and serpiginous patterns. Bullae rupture less easily as in pemphigus; but sometimes large, bright red, oozing, and bleeding erosions become a major problem. Usually, however, the originally tense bullae collapse and transform into crusts (Fig. 4-10).

Sites of Predilection Axillae; medial aspects of thighs, groins, abdomen; flexor aspects of forearms; lower legs (often first manifestation).

Mucous Membranes Mouth, anus, vagina rare; less severe and painful than in pemphigus, the bullae less easily ruptured.

LABORATORY EXAMINATIONS

Dermatopathology

Light Microscopy Neutrophils in "Indian-file" alignment at dermal-epidermal junction; neutrophils, eosinophils, and lymphocytes in papillary dermis; *subepidermal* bullae.

Electron Microscopy Junctional cleavage, i.e., split occurs in lamina lucida of basement membrane.

Immunopathology IgG deposits along the basement membrane zone. Also, C3, which may occur in the absence of IgG.

Serum Circulating anti-basement membrane IgG antibodies detected by indirect immunofluorescence in 70% of patients. Titers do not correlate with course of disease. Autoantibodies in bullous pemphigoid recognize two types of antigens. BP-Ag1 is a 230-kDa glycoprotein (gene on short arm of chromosome 6) that has high homology with desmoplakin I/II and is part of hemidesmosomes. BP-Ag2 is a transmembranous 180-kDa polypeptide (type XVII collagen) encoded by a gene on the long arm of chromosome 10.

Hematology Eosinophilia (not always).

DIFFERENTIAL DIAGNOSIS

Histopathology and immunology permit a differentiation from pemphigus, erythema multiforme, or dermatitis herpetiformis.

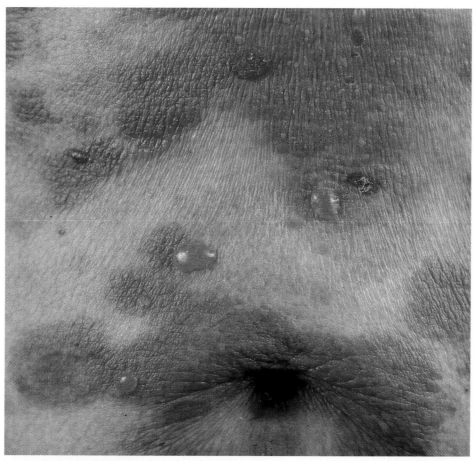

Figure 4-9 Bullous pemphigoid *This 17-year-old female had a severely pruritic generalized eruption that consisted of urticarial, inflammatory plaques, papules and crusted lesions. Originally diagnosed as generalized eczema by the family doctor, the patient was eventually referred to us; and upon close inspection, small vesicles and occasional bullae were seen arising not only in normal but also, and most prominently, in the inflammatory plaques. The diagnosis of bullous pemphigoid, was verified by biopsy and immunofluorescence studies. Note that in contrast to pemphigus vulgaris (Figure 4-7), where blisters arise exclusively in normal appearing skin, bullous pemphigoid shows blistering in inflammed areas as well; and these blisters are tense.*

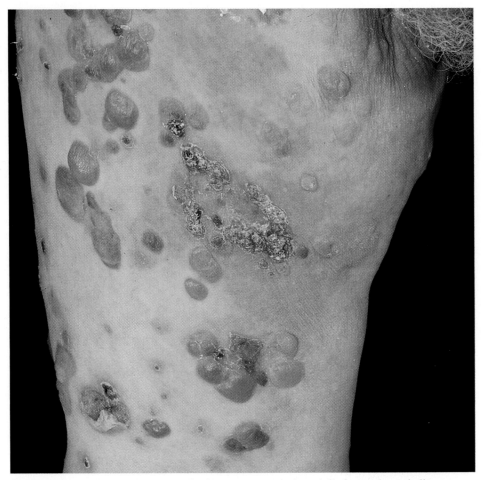

Figure 4-10   Bullous pemphigoid   *Multiple tense serous and partially hemorrhagic bullae are seen on the thigh of this elderly female. There is crusting where lesions have ruptured. Postinflammatory tan discoloration is present at sites of prior erythematous urticarial-type lesions.*

DIAGNOSIS

Clinical, confirmed by histopathology and immunopathology.

MANAGEMENT

Systemic prednisone with starting doses of 50 to 100 mg/d continued until clear, either alone or combined with azathioprine, 150 mg daily, for remission induction and 50 to 100 mg for maintenance; in milder cases, sulfones (dapsone), 100 to 150 mg/d. In very mild cases and for local recurrences, topical glucocorticoid therapy may be beneficial. Tetracycline ± nicotinamide has been reported to be effective in some cases.

Patients often go into a permanent remission and do not require therapy; local recurrences can sometimes be controlled with topical glucocorticoids.

CICATRICIAL PEMPHIGOID

Cicatricial pemphigoid is a rare disease, largely of the elderly, that leads to blisters that rupture easily and also to primary erosions resulting from epithelial fragility in the mouth, oropharynx, and, more rarely, the nasopharyngeal, esophageal, genital, and rectal mucosae. Ocular involvement may initially manifest as unilateral or bilateral conjunctivitis with burning, dryness, and foreign body sensation as the first symptoms. Chronic involvement results in scarring, symblepharon (Fig. 4-11), and, in severe disease, fusing of the bulbar and palpebral conjunctiva. Entropion and trichiasis result in corneal irritation, superficial punctate keratinopathy, corneal neovascularization, ulceration, and blindness. Scarring also occurs in the larynx and supraglottis; esophageal involvement results in stricture formation leading to dysphagia or dynophagia. The skin is involved in roughly 30% of patients. *Brunsting-Perry pemphigoid* describes a subset of patients whose skin lesions recur at the same sites, mainly on the head and neck, and also lead to scarring. Autoantigens in patients with cicatricial pemphigoid include bullous pemphigoid antigen (BPAg) 2, type 7 collagen, integrin subunit b4, LAD antigen, and laminin a3.

Management: Most patients respond to dapsone in combination with low-dose prednisone. Some patients may require more aggressive immunosuppressive treatment with cyclophosphamide or azathioprine, in combination with glucocorticosteroids. In addition, surgical intervention for scarring and supportive measures.

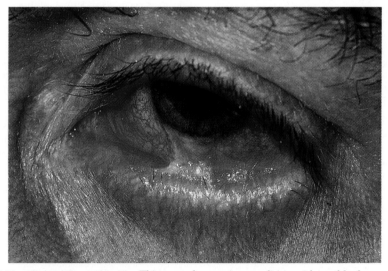

Figure 4-11   Cicatricial pemphigoid   *This severely scarring condition with symblepharon and fusion of the bulbar and palpebral conjunctiva in a 75-year-old female started as bilateral conjunctivitis with foreign body sensation as the first symptom. The conjunctiva then became erosive with scarring and fibrous tracts between the eyelids and the eye. The patient also had esophageal involvement with strictures and dysphagia.*

DERMATITIS HERPETIFORMIS

Dermatitis herpetiformis (DH) is a chronic, recurrent, intensely pruritic eruption occurring symmetrically on the extensor surfaces of the extremities and the trunk and comprising three types of lesions: tiny vesicles, papules, and urticarial plaques that are arranged in groups and are severely pruritic. It is associated with gluten sensitive enteropathy.

EPIDEMIOLOGY

Age of Onset   20 to 60 years, but most common at 30 to 40 years; may occur in children.

Sex   Male:female ratio 2:1.

PATHOGENESIS

The relationship of the gluten-sensitive enteropathy to the skin lesions is not completely worked out. Circulating immune complexes are found in patients with dermatitis herpetiformis. It is not known whether IgA binds to antigens in the bowel and complexes then circulate to bind in the skin or whether IgA has specificity for skin proteins. In skin, IgA is associated with microfibrils. IgA and complement mediate a cascade of events (possibly through the alternative complement pathway) leading to tissue injury by chemotaxis of neutrophils and release of enzymes.

HISTORY

Pruritus, intense, episodic; burning or stinging of the skin; rarely, pruritus may be absent. Symptoms often precede the appearance of skin lesions by 8 to 12 h. Ingestion of iodides and overload of gluten are exacerbating factors.

Systems Review   Laboratory evidence of small-bowel malabsorption is detected in 10 to 20%. Gluten-sensitive enteropathy occurs in nearly all patients and is demonstrated by small-bowel biopsy. There are usually no systemic symptoms.

PHYSICAL EXAMINATION

Skin Lesions   Lesions consist of erythematous papules or wheal-like plaques; tiny firm-topped vesicles, sometimes hemorrhagic; occasionally bullae (Fig. 4-12). Lesions are arranged in groups (hence the name herpetiformis), and the distribution is strikingly symmetric. Scratching results in excoriations, crusts (Fig. 4-12). Postinflammatory hyper- and hypopigmentation at sites of healed lesions.

Sites of Predilection   Extensor areas—elbows, knees. Buttocks, scapular and sacral areas. Scalp, face, and hairline.

LABORATORY EXAMINATIONS

Immunogenetics   Association with HLA-B8, HLA-DR3, and HLA-DQw2.

Dermatopathology   Biopsy is best from early erythematous papule. Microabscesses (polymorphonuclear cells and eosinophils) at the tips of the dermal papillae. Fibrin accumulation and necrosis occur also. Dermal infiltration (severe) of neutrophils and eosinophils. *Subepidermal vesicle.*

Immunofluorescence   (of perilesional skin, best on the buttocks) Granular IgA deposits in tips of papillae that correlate well with small-bowel disease. Granular IgA is found in most patients and is diagnostic.

Circulating Autoantibodies   Circulating antibasement membrane zone antibodies are generally not detectable in the sera of dermatitis herpetiformis patients but have been found in a few. Antireticulin antibodies of the IgA and IgG types can be present, and antimicrosomal antibodies and antinuclear antibodies have all been detected. Immune complexes are present in 20 to 40% of patients. IgA antibodies binding to the intermyofibril substance of smooth muscles (*antiendomysial antibodies*) are present in most patients and seem to correlate with the severity of the intestinal disease.

Malabsorption Studies   Steatorrhea (20 to 30%) and abnormal D-xylose absorption (10 to 73%).

Hematology   Anemia secondary to iron or folate deficiency.

Imaging Small bowel: in the proximal areas of the small intestine there is blunting and flattening of the villi (80 to 90%), as in celiac disease. Lesions are focal and best seen by endoscopy. Verification by small-bowel biopsy.

DIAGNOSIS

Biopsy of early lesions is usually diagnostic, but immunofluorescence detecting IgA deposits in normal-appearing or perilesional skin is the best confirming evidence.

DIFFERENTIAL DIAGNOSIS

Allergic contact dermatitis, atopic dermatitis, scabies, neurotic excoriations, papular urticaria, bullous pemphigoid, herpes gestationis.

COURSE

Prolonged, for years, with a third of the patients eventually having a spontaneous remission.
Note: A subset of patients clinically identical with classical dermatitis herpetiformis, but usually showing more vesiculation and even blisters and who have *linear* IgA deposits at the dermal-epidermal junction, have a different disease, termed linear IgA dermatosis (page 104).

MANAGEMENT

Systemic Therapy *Dapsone* 100 to 150 mg daily with gradual reduction to 50 to 25 mg and often as low as 50 mg twice a week. There is a dramatic response, often within hours. Obtain G-6-PD level before starting sulfones; obtain methemoglobin levels in the initial two weeks, and follow blood counts carefully for the first few months.

Sulfapyridine 1 to 1.5 g/d, with plenty of fluids, if dapsone contraindicated or not tolerated. Monitor for casts in urine and kidney function.

Diet A gluten-free diet *may* completely suppress the disease or allow reduction of the dosage of dapsone or sulfapyridine, but response is very slow.

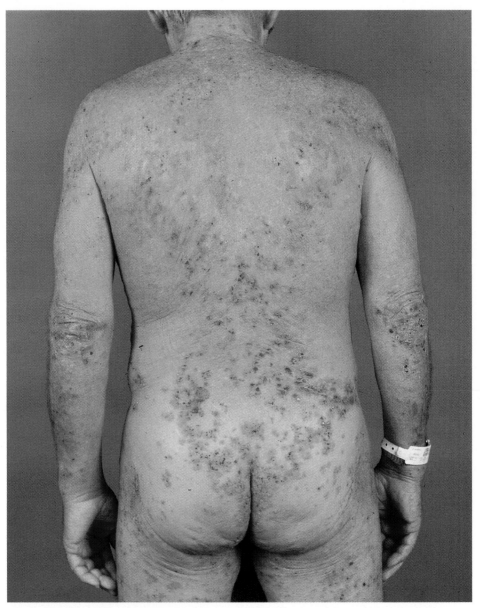

Figure 4-12 Dermatitis herpetiformis *In this 56-year-old male patient with a generalized highly pruritic eruption, the diagnosis can be made upon first sight by the distribution of the lesions. Most heavily involved are the elbows, the scapular, sacral and gluteal areas and (not seen in this picture) the knees. Upon close inspection there are grouped papules, small vesicles, crusts and erosions on an erythematous base and there is postinflammatory hypo- and hyperpigmentation. The patient had previously been diagnosed with atopic dermatitis, scabies and allergic contact dermatitis and had responded only poorly to topical corticosteroids. This particular eruption occurred after he had spent a vacation on the Dalmation coast, having been told that sunbathing would be good for his condition, where his meals consisted of seafood (iodides) and white bread (gluten).*

LINEAR IgA DERMATOSIS

Linear IgA dermatosis is a rare, immune-mediated, subepidermal blistering skin disease defined by the presence of homogeneous linear deposits of IgA at the cutaneous basement membrane. It is clearly separate from dermatitis herpetiformis (DH) on the basis immunopathology, immunogenetics, and lack of association with gluten-sensitive enteropathy. It is probably identical with chronic bullous disease of childhood (CBDC), which is a rare blistering disease that occurs predominantly in children younger than 5 years and has an identical pattern of homogeneous linear IgA deposits at the epidermal basement membrane. Linear IgA dermatosis most often occurs after puberty. Clinical manifestations are very similar to those of DH, but there is more blistering. Patients present with combinations of annular or grouped papules, vesicles, and bullae (Fig. 4-13) that are distributed symmetrically on extensor surfaces including elbows, knees, and buttocks. The lesions are very pruritic but less severe than those of DH. Mucosal involvement is important and ranges from large asymptomatic oral erosions and ulceration to severe oral disease alone, or severe generalized cutaneous involvement and oral disease similar to that in cicatricial pemphigoid. Circulating autoantibodies against the epidermal basement membrane have been found.

Management: Patients respond to dapsone or sulfapyridine but in addition, most may require low-dose prednisone. Patients do not respond to a gluten-free diet.

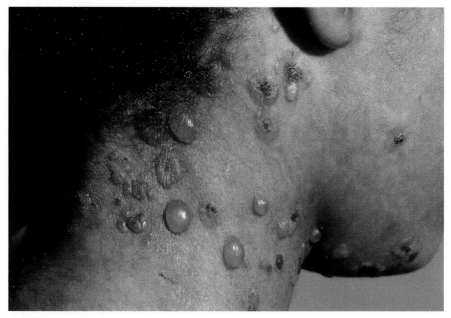

Figure 4-13   Linear IgA dermatosis *Annular and grouped vesicles, bullae. Initially, they are tense, but become flaccid after they have ruptured.*

SECTION 5

MISCELLANEOUS INFLAMMATORY DISORDERS

PITYRIASIS ROSEA

Pityriasis rosea is an acute exanthematous eruption with a distinctive morphology and often with a characteristic self-limited course. First, a single (primary or "herald" plaque) lesion develops, usually on the trunk, and 1 or 2 weeks later a generalized secondary eruption develops in a typical distribution pattern; the entire process remits spontaneously in 6 weeks without any therapy. Atypical forms also occur.

EPIDEMIOLOGY

Age of Onset   10 to 43 years, but can occur rarely in infants and old persons.

Season   Spring and fall.

Etiology   Herpes 7 is suspected.

HISTORY

Duration of Lesions   A single herald patch precedes the exanthematous phase. The exanthematous phase develops over a period of 1 to 2 weeks. Pruritus—absent (25%), mild (50%), or severe (25%).

PHYSICAL EXAMINATION

Skin Lesions   *Herald Patch*   (80% of patients) oval, slightly raised plaque 2 to 5 cm, bright red, fine collarette scale at periphery may be multiple (Fig. 5-1).

Exanthem   Fine scaling papules and plaques with characteristic 1 marginal collarette (Fig. 5-1). Dull pink or tawny (exanthem). Oval lesions are characteristic. Scattered discrete lesions.

Distribution   Characteristic pattern of lesions—the long axes of the lesions follow the lines of cleavage in a "Christmas tree" distribution (Figure 5-I). Lesions usually confined to trunk and proximal aspects of the arms and legs. Rarely on face.

Atypical Pityriasis Rosea   Lesions may be present only on the face and neck. The primary plaque may be absent, may be the sole manifestation of the disease, or may be multiple. Most confusing are the examples of pityriasis rosea with vesicles, or simulating erythema multiforme but occurring in the typical distribution of pityriasis rosea. This usually results from irritation and sweating, often as a consequence of inadequate treatment (pityriasis rosea irritata).

DIFFERENTIAL DIAGNOSIS

Multiple Small Scaling Plaques   *Drug eruptions* (e.g., captopril, barbiturates); *secondary syphilis* (obtain serology, and it is always positive); *guttate psoriasis* (no marginal collarette); *erythema migrans* with secondary lesions, season, and history; *erythema multiforme;* and *tinea corporis.*

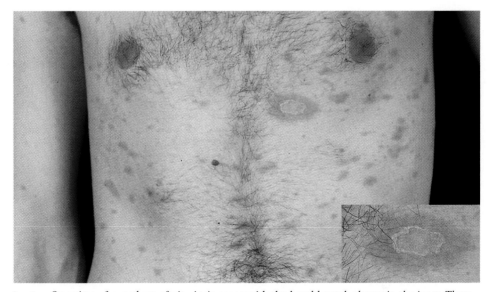

Inset: *Overview of exanthem of pityriasis rosea with the herald patch shown in the inset. There are papules and small plaques with oval configuration that follow the lines of cleavage. The fine scaling of the salmon-red papules cannot be seen at this magnification, while the collarette of the herald patch is quite obvious.* **Inset: herald patch** *An erythematous (salmon-red) plaque with scale apparent in the central portion of the lesion. The scale forms a collarette on the trailing edge of the advancing border. Collarette means that scale is attached at periphery and loose toward the center of the lesion.*

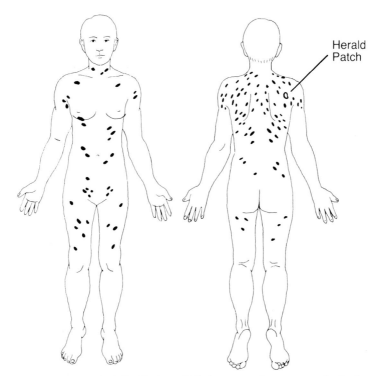

Herald Patch

Figure 5-1 Pityriasis rosea: typical distribution *"Christmas tree" pattern on the back.*

LABORATORY EXAMINATIONS

Dermatopathology Patchy or diffuse parakeratosis, absence of granular layer, slight acanthosis, focal spongiosis, microscopic vesicles. Occasional dyskeratotic cells with an eosinophilic homogenous appearance. Edema of dermis, homogenization of the collagen.

Perivascular infiltrate mononuclear cells.

COURSE

Spontaneous remission in 6 to 12 weeks or less. If the eruption persists for >6 weeks, a skin biopsy should be done. Recurrences are uncommon.

MANAGEMENT

Symptomatic Oral antihistamines and/or topical antipruritic lotions for relief of the pruritus. Topical corticosteroids.

Pruritus may be improved by UVB phototherapy or natural sunlight exposure if treatment is begun in the first week of eruption. The protocol is five consecutive exposures, starting with 80% of the minimum erythema dose and increasing by 20% on each exposure. Phototherapy is not always efficacious for shortening the course of the eruption. Short course of corticosteroids.

PARAPSORIASIS EN PLAQUES

Two types are now generally recognized. (1) "Small-plaque" parapsoriasis (also known as digitate dermatosis or chronic superficial dermatitis). Small-plaque parapsoriasis is not regarded as a lesion in which mycosis fungoides (cutaneous T cell lymphoma, CTCL) can occur. (2) "Large-plaque" parapsoriasis is an important disorder to follow carefully with repeated biopsies to rule out early mycosis fungoides.

SMALL-PLAQUE PARAPSORIASIS (DIGITATE DERMATOSIS)

HISTORY

Gradual development over months. Multiple lesions. Rare pruritus. Middle age.

PHYSICAL EXAMINATION

Skin Lesions Round, oval, erythematous, yellowish, only slightly elevated plaques, <5 cm in diameter (Fig. 5-2). Slight scale and wrinkled surface with cigarette-paper appearance. Finger-like (digitate shapes), on trunk, proximal extremities, and buttocks, following lines of cleavage, giving appearance of a hug that left fingerprints (Fig. 5-2).

DIFFERENTIAL DIAGNOSIS

Pityriasis rosea, large-plaque parapsoriasis.

LABORATORY EXAMINATIONS

Dermatopathology Spongiform dermatitis with focal areas of hyperkeratosis, parakeratosis, and exocytosis. In the dermis there is a mild superficial vascular lymphohistiocytic infiltrate and dermal edema.

MANAGEMENT

No treatment necessary, reassurance of patient. Disease may be treated with lubricant or topical steroids. UVB 311 nm, or broad band phototherapy. PUVA is highly effective.

LARGE-PLAQUE PARAPSORIASIS (PARAPSORIASIS EN PLAQUES)

HISTORY

Gradual development over months and years, starting with 1 or 2 plaques. Pruritus is rare, and the lesions may disappear after exposure to sun. Middle age.

PHYSICAL EXAMINATION

Skin Lesions Barely elevated, erythematous, dusky-red, sometimes yellowish plaque (Fig. 5-3) with or without slight atrophy and smooth or slight scaling surface. Lesions are circular, >10 cm in diameter, and randomly scattered on trunk, buttocks, breasts (females), or extremities (Fig. 5-3).

DIFFERENTIAL DIAGNOSIS

Scaling Plaques "Premycotic" stage of CTCL (mycosis fungoides) parapsoriasis-like lesions. The development of "infiltration" in the lesions, atrophy, and *poikilodermatous changes* are clues to early mycosis fungoides. Repeated biopsies may be necessary to establish the diagnosis of prelymphomatous disease.

LABORATORY EXAMINATIONS

Dermatopathology Nonspecific or, later, a bandlike mononuclear cell infiltrate with atrophy of the epidermis, vacuolization of the basal cell layer, capillary dilatation. There are no atypical lymphocytes. Mild exocytosis. Lymphocytes infiltrating epidermis are CD4$^+$.

Peripheral Blood Monoclonal T helper cells with skin–homing specificity can be detected.

COURSE AND PROGNOSIS

The lesions persist for life and can progress to CTCL.

Topical   Temporary remission with topical glucocorticoids.

Phototherapy   Good responses to PUVA photochemotherapy.

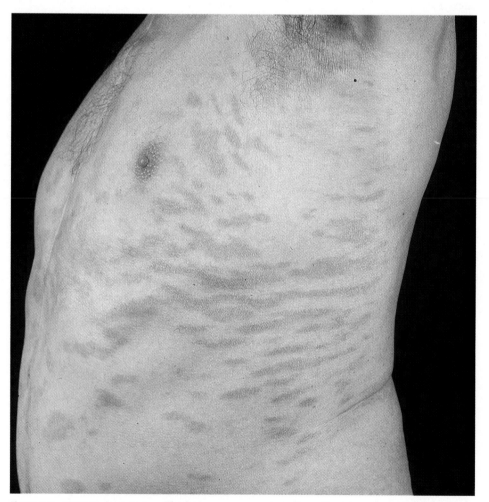

Figure 5-2   Digitate dermatosis   *The lesions are asymptomatic, yellowish or fawn-colored, very thin, slightly scaly plaques. The lesions follow the lines of cleavage of the skin, giving the appearance of a "hug" that left fingerprints on the trunk. The long axis of these lesions often reaches more than 5 cm.*

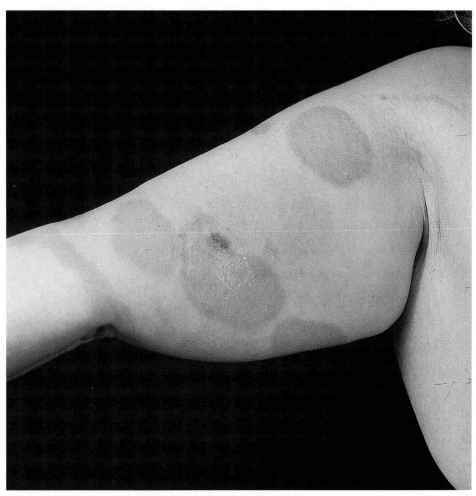

Figure 5-3 Large plaque parapsoriasis (parapsoriasis en plaques) *The lesions are asymptomatic, slightly scaly, thin plaques. The lesions are most often larger than 10 cm and are light red-brown or salmon-pink. There may be atrophy in some areas. The lesions here are located on the extremities but they are more commonly noted on the trunk. These lesions must be carefully followed and repeated biopsies are necessary to detect mycosis fungoides. Some regard this entity as premycotic mycosis fungoides.*

GROVER'S DISEASE

Grover's disease (GD), or transient acantholytic dermatosis, is a pruritic dermatosis primarily affecting middle-aged men, located principally on the trunk, and occurring as crops of discrete papular and papulovesicular lesions, sparse or numerous. Pruritus can be a major problem. As the name implies, the principal histopathologic feature of the lesions is the presence of acantholysis. GD is self-limited but not always transient, since the course may last for weeks to several months or more.

EPIDEMIOLOGY

Age of Onset   Middle age and older, mean age 50 years.

Sex   Males>females.

Precipitating Factors   Heavy, sweat-inducing exercise, excessive solar exposure, persistent fever, exposure to heat and persistent fever; also may occur in bedridden patients, with heat and sweating as factors.

HISTORY

Onset   Usually abrupt onset of pruritus and simultaneouly the appearance of crops of lesions (papules and papulovesicles) possibly correlated with heavy exercise, excessive sun exposure, or high fever.

Skin Symptoms   Pruritus that is out of proportion to the exent of the eruption.

PHYSICAL EXAMINATION

Skin Lesions   Skin-colored or reddish papules (small, 3 to 5 mm, some with slight scale or smooth) (Figure 5-4), papulovesicles, and erosions. Upon palpation, smooth or warty (Fig. 5-4). Scattered, discrete on central trunk and proximal extremities (Fig. 5-4).

DIFFERENTIAL DIAGNOSIS

Small Discrete Pruritic Papules on Chest Darier-White disease, heat rash (miliaria rubra), papular urticaria, scabies, dermatitis herpetiformis (there is grouping and the lesions are symmetric), *Pityrosporum* or eosinophilic folliculitis, insect bites, and drug eruptions.

LABORATORY EXAMINATIONS

Dermatopathology   Acantholysis and spongiosis, focal acantholytic dyskeratosis with different patterns occurring at the same time and simulating Darier's disease, pemphigus foliaceus, and Hailey-Hailey disease; in the dermis there is a superficial infiltrate of eosinophils, lymphocytes, and histiocytes.

DIAGNOSIS

The diagnosis of GD may be difficult, and a biopsy is required; the histologic findings are diagnostic.

COURSE AND PROGNOSIS

The disease is by no means always transient, and there appear to be two types: acute ("transient") and chronic relapsing. The mean duration in one series was 47 weeks.

MANAGEMENT

Topical   Class II topical glucocorticoids under plastic (e.g., dry-cleaning plastic suit bags with holes cut for arms)) are used for 4 h.

Systemic   Oral glucocorticoids and dapsone have been used with success, but relapses occur after withdrawal.

Phototherapy   UVB or PUVA photochemotherapy is useful for patients who do not respond to topical glucocorticoids under occlusion.

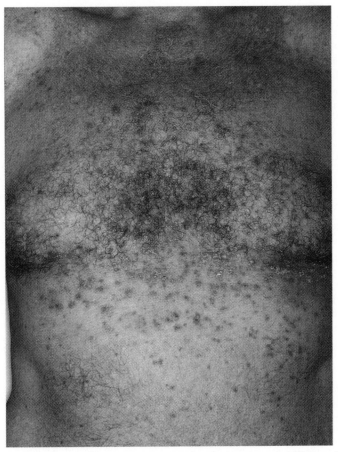

Figure 5-4 Grover's disease *A rash consisting of reddish hyperkeratotic scaling and/or crusted papules with a sandpaper feel upon palpation. Papules are discrete, scattered on the central trunk and are extremely pruritic.*

LICHEN PLANUS

Lichen planus (LP) is an acute or chronic inflammatory dermatosis involving skin and/or mucous membranes, characterized by flat-topped (Latin: *planus*, "flat"), pink to violaceous, shiny, pruritic polygonal papules on the skin and milky white reticulated papules in the mouth. The features of the lesions have been designated as the four Ps—purple, polygonal, pruritic, papule.

EPIDEMIOLOGY

Age of Onset 30 to 60 years.

Sex Females>males.

Race Hypertrophic LP more common in blacks.

Etiology Idiopathic in most cases. Drugs, metals (gold, mercury), or infection (HCV) resulting in alteration in cell-mediated immunity. There could be HLA-associated genetic susceptibility that would explain a predisposition in certain persons.

HISTORY

Onset Acute (days) or insidious (over weeks). Lesions last months to years, asymptomatic or pruritic, sometimes severe pruritus lesions. Mucous membrane lesions are painful, especially when ulcers are present.

PHYSICAL EXAMINATION

Skin Lesions Papules, flat-topped, 1 to 10 mm, sharply defined, shiny (Figs. 5-5, 5-6, and 5-7). Violaceous, with white lines (Wickham's striae), (Fig. 5-5), seen best with hand lens after application of mineral oil. In dark-skinned individuals, postinflammatory hyperpigmentation is common. Polygonal or oval. Grouped, (Figs. 5-5 and 5-6) linear (isomorphic phenomenon), annular, or disseminated scattered discrete lesions when generalized (Fig. 5-7).

Sites of predilection Wrists (flexor), lumbar region, eyelids, shins (thicker, hyperkeratotic lesions), scalp, and glans penis, mouth, penis.

Variants

Hypertrophic Large thick plaques arise on the foot (Fig. 5-6) and shins; more common in black males. Although typical lichen planus papule is smooth, hypertrophic lesions may become hyperkeratotic.

Follicular Individual keratotic-follicular papules and plaques that lead to cicatricial alopecia. Spinous follicular lesions, typical skin and mucous membrane lichen planus, and cicatricial alopecia of the scalp are called *Graham Little syndrome.*

Vesicular Vesicular or bullous lesions may develop within lichen planus patches or independent of them within normal-appearing skin. In the latter there are direct immunofluorescence findings consistent with bullous pemphigoid, and the sera of these patients contain bullous pemphigoid IgG autoantibodies. (See Section 4.)

Actinicus Papular LP lesions arise in sun-exposed sites, especially the dorsum of hands and arms.

Ulcerative Lichen planus may lead to therapy-resistant ulcers, particularly on the soles, requiring skin grafting.

Mucous Membranes 40 to 60% of individuals with LP have oropharyngeal involvement.

Recticular LP: reticulate (netlike) pattern of lacy white hyperkeratosis on buccal mucosa (see Fig. 29-7), lips (Fig. 5-8), tongue, gingiva; the most common pattern of oral LP. *Plaque-type* LP: leukoplakia with Wickham's striae; arises on buccal mucosa. *Atrophic LP:* shiny red plaque, often with Wickham's striae in surrounding mucosa. *Erosive or ulcerative LP:* superficial erosion with overlying fibrin clot; occurs on tongue and buccal mucosa; shiny red painful erosion of gingiva (desquamative gingivitis) (see Fig. 29-8). *Bullous LP:* intact blisters up to several centimeters in diameter; rupture results in erosive LP. Milky-white papules, with white lacework on the buccal mucosa. May become erosive and painful. Carcinoma may very rarely develop in mouth lesions.

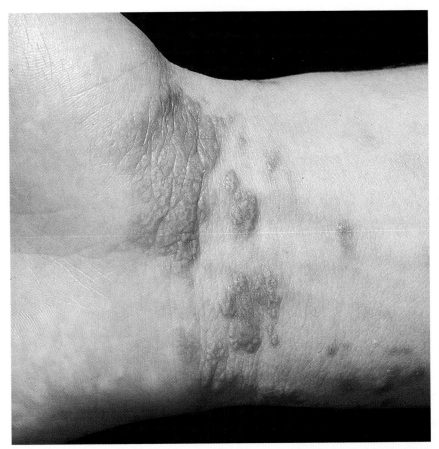

Figure 5-5 Lichen planus *Flat-topped, polygonal, sharply defined papules of violaceous color, grouped and confluent. Surface is shiny and upon close inspection or a hand lens, reveals fine white lines (Wickham's striae), which can be further enhanced by applying a drop of mineral oil to the lesions.*

Genitalia Papular, annular, or erosive lesions arise on penis (especially glans), scrotum, labia majora, labia minora, vagina.

Hair and Nails

Scalp Atrophic scalp skin with scarring alopecia.

Nails Destruction of nail fold and nail bed with longitudinal splintering.

LICHEN PLANUS-LIKE ERUPTIONS

Lichen planus-like eruptions closely mimic typical lichen planus, both clinically and histologically. They occur as a clinical manifestation of chronic graft-versus-host disease, in dermatomyositis, and as cutaneous manifestations of malignant lymphoma but also may develop as the result of therapy with certain drugs and after industrial use of certain compounds (Table 5-1).

DIFFERENTIAL DIAGNOSIS

Papular LP Chronic cutaneous lupus erythematosus, psoriasis, pityriasis rosea, eczematous dermatitis, lichenoid graft-versus-host disease, superficial basal cell carcinoma, Bowen's disease (in situ squamous cell carcinoma).

Hypertrophic LP Psoriasis vulgaris, lichen simplex chronicus, prurigo nodularis, stasis dermatitis, Kaposi's sarcoma.

Drug-Induced LP See Table 5-1.

Mucous Membrane Leukoplakia, pseudomembranous candidiasis (thrush), HIV-associated hairy leukoplakia, lupus erythematosus, bite trauma, mucous patches of secondary syphilis, pemphigus vulgaris, bullous pemphigoid.

Table 5-1 AGENTS REPORTED TO INDUCE CUTANEOUS DISORDERS THAT VERY CLOSELY RESEMBLE TYPICAL LICHEN PLANUS

Types of Agents	Specific Agents
Angiotensin-converting enzyme inhibitors	Captopril
	Enalapril
Antiarthritic	Gold
Antibiotic	Streptomycin
	Tetracycline
Antimalarial	Quinacrine
	Chloroquine
	Quinine isomer, quinidine
Antitubercular	*p*-Amino salicylic acid
Ataractic	Phenothiazine derivatives
	Metopromazine
	Levomepromazine
Chelator	Penicillamine
Color film developer	*p*-Phenylenediamine salts
	2-Amino-5-diethylaminotoluene monochloride (CD2)
	4-Amino-*N*-diethyl-aniline sulfate (TTS)
	Antimony trioxide
Diuretic	Chlorothiazide
	Hydrochlorothiazide
Hypoglycemic agents	Chlorpropamide
	Tolazamide

SOURCE: From KA Arndt, Lichen planus, in TB Fitzpatrick, et al (eds): *Dermatology in General Medicine,* 4th ed. New York, McGraw-Hill, 1993, pp. 1134–1144.

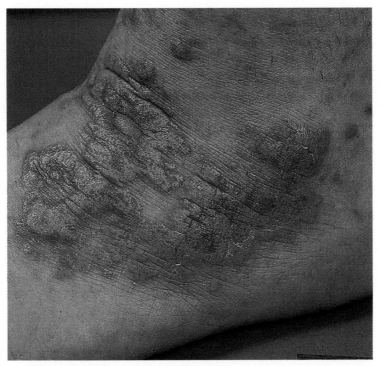

Figure 5-6 Lichen planus *Violaceous color of flat-topped, confluent papules that form plaque is particularly evident in this figure. This color is highly characteristic. Note also that lesions are thicker than in Figure 5-5, which is due to their location on a dependent site (foot). These lesions will later evolve into hypertrophic lichen planus.*

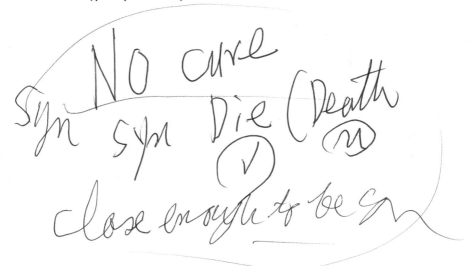

LABORATORY EXAMINATIONS

Dermatopathology Inflammation with hyperkeratosis, increased granular layer, irregular acanthosis, liquefaction degeneration of the basal cell layer, and bandlike mononuclear infiltrate that hugs the epidermis. Lymphocytes are predominantly CD4+ helper inducer cells. Degenerate keratinocytes (colloid, Civatte bodies) are found at the dermal-epidermal junction. Direct immunofluorescence reveals heavy deposits of fibrin at the junction and IgM and less frequently IgA, IgG, and C3 in the colloid bodies.

DIAGNOSIS

Clinical findings confirmed by histologic findings.

COURSE

Cutaneous LP usually persists for months, but in some cases, for years; hypertrophic LP on the shins and oral LP often persists for decades. The incidence of oral cancer (squamous cell carcinoma) in individuals with oral LP is increased by 5%; patients should be followed at regular intervals.

MANAGEMENT

Topical Therapy

Glucocorticoids Topical glucocorticoids with occlusion for cutaneous lesions. Intralesional triamcinolone (3 mg/mL) is helpful for symptomatic cutaneous or oral mucosal lesions and lips.

Cyclosporine The solution can be used as a retention "mouthwash" for severely symptomatic oral LP.

Systemic Therapy

Cyclosporine In very resistant and generalized cases, 5 mg/kg/d will induce rapid remission, quite often not followed by recurrence.

Glucocorticoids Oral prednisone is effective for individuals with symptomatic pruritus, painful erosions, dysphagia, or cosmetic disfigurement. A short, tapered course is preferred: 70 mg initially, tapered by 5 mg.

Systemic Retinoids (Acitretin or Etretinate) 1 mg/kg/d is helpful as adjunctive measure in severe (oral, hypertrophic) cases, but usually additional topical treatment is required.

PUVA Photochemotherapy Indicated in symptomatic individuals with generalized LP or cases resistant to topical therapy.

Reports of Other Successful Treatment Mycophenolate mofetil, heparin analogues (enoxaparin) in low doses have antiproliferative and immunomodulatory properties, azathioprine.

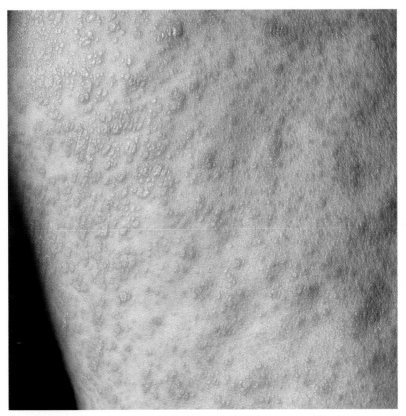

Figure 5-7 Generalized lichen planus *Small, flat-topped, violaceous papules, some groups and some disseminated, becoming confluent on the trunk.*

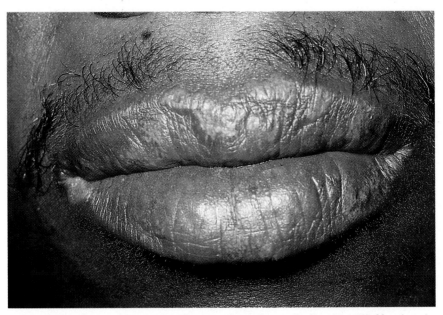

Figure 5-8 Lichen planus *Silvery white flat-topped papules on the lips. Note Wickham's striae. In Africans these lesions can lead to considerable disfigurement.*

GRANULOMA ANNULARE

Granuloma annulare (GA) is a self-limited, asymptomatic, chronic dermatosis of the dermis that exhibits papules in an annular arrangement, commonly arising on the dorsa of the hands and feet, elbows, and knees, and which sometimes becomes generalized in distribution.

EPIDEMIOLOGY

Age of Onset   Children and young adults.

Sex   Female:male ratio 2:1.

Etiology   Unknown. An immunologically mediated inflammation that surrounds blood vessels, and the collagen and elastic tissue are altered. The lesions are sometimes indistinguishable from necrobiosis lipoidica. Generalized GA may be associated with diabetes mellitus.

PATHOGENESIS

A necrotizing inflammatory reaction occurs around blood vessels, altering collagen and elastic tissues. This vaculitis is not leukocytoclastic vasculitis. The nature of the antigen is unclear.

HISTORY

Duration of Lesions   Months to years.

Skin Symptoms   Usually asymptomatic. Cosmetic disfigurement.

PHYSICAL EXAMINATION

Skin Lesions   Firm, smooth, shiny dermal papules and plaques, 1 to 5 cm (Figs. 5-9 and 5-10). Keratotic papules and nodules in *perforating* granuloma annulare. Nodules, subcutaneous: large, painless, skin-colored, deep dermal or subcutaneous, solitary or multiple. Skin-colored, erythematous, violaceous. Dome-shaped, annular arciform.

Distribution   Isolated lesion, particularly on dorsum of hand (Fig. 5-9), multiple lesions in certain regions (Fig. 5-10), or generalized (older patients). Subcutaneous lesions are located near joints, palms and soles, buttocks.

Variants

- *Perforating* lesions are rare and mostly on the hands; central umbilication followed by crusting and ulceration; this type was associated with diabetes in one series.
- GA associated with necrobiosis lipoidica can be confusing, as some patients can have both diseases at the same time.
- May rarely involve fascia and tendons causing sclerosis.
- Generalized GA and in this form a search for diabetes mellitus should be made.

DIFFERENTIAL DIAGNOSIS

Papular Lesions   Necrobiosis lipoidica, papular sarcoid, lichen planus, lymphocytic infiltrate of Jessner.

Subcutaneous Nodules   Rheumatoid nodules: confusion can occur because of the same pathology of GA and rheumatic nodule or rheumatoid nodules.

Annular Lesions   Dermatophytosis, erythema migrans, sarcoid, lichen planus.

LABORATORY EXAMINATIONS

KOH Preparation   Rule out epidermal dermatophytosis.

Dermatopathology   Foci of chronic inflammatory and histiocytic infiltrations in superficial and middermis with necrobiosis of connective tissue surrounded by a wall of palisading histiocytes and multinucleated giant cells.

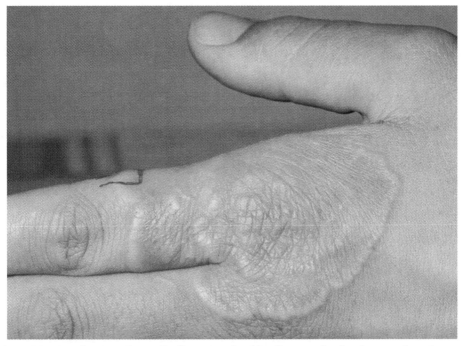

Figure 5-9 Granuloma annulare *Confluent, pearly white, firm papules forming two rings, 1 cm and 5 cm in diameter on the dorsum of hand which is a site of predilection. Lesions are firm and asymptomatic. Note there is no scaling.*

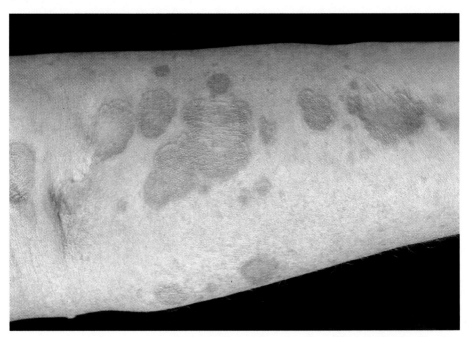

Figure 5-10 Granuloma anulare *Multiple annular and semicircular plaques with central regression on the arm. When located in sites other than the dorsa of the hands, granuloma annulare may acquire a reddish or brownish color and then is very difficult to distinguish from sarcoidosis.*

COURSE

The disease disappears in 75% of patients in 2 years. Recurrences are common (40%), but they also disappear.

MANAGEMENT

Patients should be reassured that GA is a local skin disorder and not a marker for internal disease and that spontaneous remission is the rule. *No treatment is an option if the lesions are not disfiguring.*

Topical Therapy *Topical Glucocorticoids* Applied under plastic occlusion or hydrocolloid.

Intralesional Triamcinolone 3 mg/mL into lesions is effective.

Cryospray Superficial lesions respond to liquid nitrogen, but atrophy may occur.

PUVA Photochemotherapy Effective in generalized GA.

MORPHEA

Morphea is a localized cutaneous sclerosis characterized by early violaceous, later ivory-colored plaques, which may be solitary, linear, generalized, and rarely, accompanied by atrophy of underlying structures.

Synonyms: Localized scleroderma, circumscribed scleroderma.

EPIDEMIOLOGY

Age of Onset 75% have their onset between the ages of 20 and 50; in linear morphea the onset is earlier. Pansclerotic morphea, a disabling disorder in children, usually starts before age 14.

Sex Females are affected about 3 times as often as males, including children. Linear scleroderma is the same in males and females

Etiology Unknown. However, there is evidence that at least some patients (predominantly in Europe) with classic morphea have sclerosis due to *Borrelia burgdorferi* infection and, if not too sclerotic, the lesions can disappear with prolonged courses of oral antibiotics. Pigmentation, however, persists. Morphea has been noted after x-irradiation for breast cancer.

Incidence Rare.

CLASSIFICATION OF VARIOUS TYPES OF LOCALIZED SCLERODERMA

Circumscribed or localized: plaques or bands.
Linear scleroderma: upper or lower extremity.
Frontoparietal (*en coup de sabre*): linear scleroderma occurring on the head with or without hemiatrophy of face.
Generalized morphea.
Pansclerotic: involvement (trunk, extremities, face, and scalp, with sparing of fingertips and toes) of dermis, fat, fascia, muscle, bone.

HISTORY

Symptoms Usually none. No history of Raynaud's phenomenon. Pansclerotic morphea involving the lower extremities can result in major facial or limb asymmetry, flexion contractures, and disability.

PHYSICAL EXAMINATION

Skin Findings *Plaques*—initially indurated, but poorly defined areas; 2 to 15 cm in diameter, round or oval, and often better felt than seen. In time, surface becomes smooth and shiny (Fig. 5-11); hair follicles and sweat duct orifices disappear. *Purpura, telangiectasia,* and very rarely, *bullae* may be seen later in course. Deep involvement of tissue may be associated with atrophy of muscle and bone, with resultant growth disturbance in children and flexion contracture; pseudoinhuman-like lesion may occur circumferentially on limb with subsequent distal edema. Scalp involvement results in scarring alopecia. Usually multiple, bilateral, asymmetric (Fig. 5-12). May be linear on extremity (Fig. 5-13) or scalp.

Color Initially, purplish or mauve; after months to years, may be hyperpigmented. Ivory with lilac-colored edge (Fig. 5-11). In lesions of rapid onset, may be erythematous. May have hyperpigmentation in involved sclerotic areas, and, in addition, large areas of brown macules but *without* sclerosis may coexist on the trunk away from the sclerotic plaques.

Palpation Indurated, hard, or not palpable (brown macules). May be hypesthetic. Rarely, lesions become atrophic without going through a sclerotic stage (atrophoderma of Pasini and Pierini).

Distribution

Circumscribed Trunk (Fig. 5-11), limbs, face, genitalia; less commonly, axillae, perineum, areolae.

Linear Usually on extremity (Fig. 5-13).

Frontoparietal Scalp and face.

Generalized Initially on trunk (upper, breasts, abdomen) (Fig. 5-12), thighs.

Mouth With linear morphea of head, may have associated hemiatrophy of tongue.

Hair and Nails Scarring alopecia with scalp plaque, generalized, or frontoparietal morphea. Nail dystrophy in linear lesions of extremity or in pansclerotic morphea.

General Examination

Involvement around joints may lead to flexion contractures, especially of hands and feet. Deeper involvement of tissue is associated with atrophy and fibrosis of muscle. Extensive involvement may result in restricted respiration. With linear morphea of the head, may have associated atrophy of ocular structures and atrophy of bone.

DIFFERENTIAL DIAGNOSIS

Sclerotic Plaque Sclerotic plaque associated with *B. burgdorferi* infection, acrodermatitis chronica atrophicans, progressive systemic sclerosis, lichen sclerosus et atrophicus, eosinophilic fasciitis, eosinophilia-myalgia syndrome associated with L-tryptophan ingestion, scleredema, Parry-Romberg syndrome (hemiatrophy).

LABORATORY EXAMINATIONS

Serology Appropriate serologic testing to rule out *B. burgdorferi* infection.

Dermatopathology Epidermis appears normal to atrophic with loss of rete ridges. Initially dermis edematous with swelling and degeneration of collagen fibers; later these become homogeneous and eosinophilic. Slight infiltrate, perivascular or diffuse; lymphocytes, plasma cells, macrophages. Later, dermis thickened with few fibroblasts and dense collagen; inflammatory infiltrate at dermal-subcutis junction; dermal appendages disappear progressively. Pansclerotic lesions show fibrosis and disappearance of subcutaneous tissue, fibrosis broadening, as well as sclerosis of fascia. Silver stains should be performed to rule out *B. burgdorferi* infection.

DIAGNOSIS

Clinical diagnosis, usually confirmed by skin biopsy.

COURSE

May be slowly progressive, but spontaneous remissions can occur.

MANAGEMENT

There is no effective treatment for morphea, but some reports of treatment are as follows:

Morphea-Like Lesions Associated with Lyme Borreliosis In patients with early involvement, there may be a reversal of sclerosis with high-dose parenteral penicillin or ceftriaxone treatment given in several courses over a time span of several months. Best response if combined with oral corticosteroids.

Phototherapy with UVA-1 (340 to 400 nm) The mechanism of action of UVA-1 is thought to be by the induction of interstitial collagenase [matrix metalloproteinase 1 (MMP-1)]. Collagenase initiates degradation of types I and III collagen and plays a key role in the remodeling of dermal collagen. UVA-1 phototherapy, however, can induce a variety of cytokines and soluble factors, resulting in immunomodulation. In our experience, the treatment is not easy or very successful because of the prolonged irradiation times and the disfiguring hyperpigmentation of the irradiated areas.

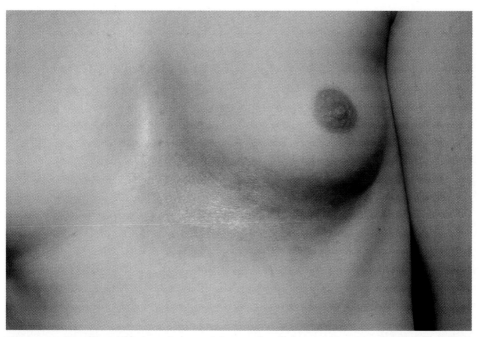

Figure 5-11 Morphea *This is an indurated, ivory-colored plaque with a lilac-colored, ill-defined border. Typically localized on the trunk, below the breast, this lesion is better felt than seen and since it is hard and close to the breast, it is of considerable concern to the patient.*

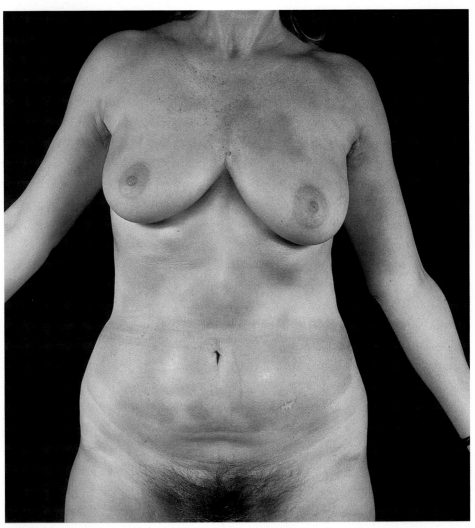

Figure 5-12 Morphea *Generalized lesions on trunk. Ill-defined, indurated; some being hypo- or hyperpigmented. If the hyperpigmented lesions are just atrophic and cannot be felt, they are called atrophoderma of Pasini and Pierini.*

MISCELLANEOUS INFLAMMATORY DISORDERS

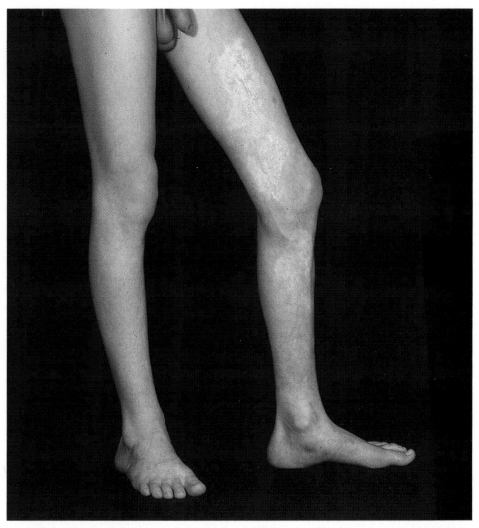

Figure 5-13   Linear morphea   *Indurated, ivory-white lesion extending from upper thigh to dorsum of foot. If induration is pronounced and extends to fascia (pansclerotic morphea), it will severely limit movements of joints.*

LICHEN SCLEROSUS

Lichen sclerosus (LS) is a chronic atrophic disorder of the anogenital skin of females and males and the general skin. It is characterized by white, angular, well-defined, indurated papules and plaques and characteristic follicular keratotic plugs, known as *dells*. The disorder affects the vulva, penis, and also the general skin, especially the trunk.
Synonyms: Lichen sclerosus et atrophicus (LSA).

EPIDEMIOLOGY

Age of Onset   A disease of adults, but occurs in children 1 to 13 years of age. Mean age: 50 years in females, 43 in males.

Sex   Female:male ratio 10:1.

Etiology   Unknown.

Borrelia in Morphea and Lichen Sclerosus Reports from Europe have documented an association between *Borrelia* spp., morphea, and LS. Studies from the United States have not confirmed these findings. In the most recent European study, skin biopsy specimens (19 morphea and 34 LS) were obtained from patients in the United States, Japan, and Germany. Genotype-specific sequences in the flagellin gene for *B. burgdorferi* were determined, sensu strictu *B. garinii,* and *B. afzelii.* Five cases of morphea and two cases of LS in Germany and Japan yielded positive results for *B. garinii* or *B. afzelii;* however, DNA for these spirochetes was not detected in any of the American samples.

HISTORY

Duration of Lesions   May be present for years before detection. May first be noted by gynecologist or internist doing pelvic examination.

Symptoms

Nongenital Usually asymptomatic. *Genital* Often asymptomatic, even with striking clinical changes. In females, vulvar lesions may be sensitive, especially while walking; pruritus; painful, especially if erosions are present; dysuria; dyspareunia. In males, acquired phimosis, recurrent balanitis; in boys, may be discovered on pathologic examination of prepuce removed during circumcision.

PHYSICAL EXAMINATION

Skin Lesions   *Macules and papules:* Whitish, ivory or porcelain-white, sharply demarcated, individual lesions may become confluent, forming *plaques* (Fig. 5-14). Surface of lesions may be elevated or in the same plane as normal skin; older lesions may be depressed. Dilated pilosebaceous or sweat duct orifices filled with keratin plugs (dells); if plugging is marked, surface appears verrucous. *Bullae and erosions:* may heal with fusion of labia minora. *Purpura* is often a characteristic and identifying feature; *telangiectasia.* On vulva, hyperkeratotic plaques may become macerated; vulva may become atrophic, shrunken, especially clitoris and labia minora, with vaginal introitus reduced in size. Fusion of labia minora and majora. In uncircumcised males, prepuce becomes sclerotic and cannot be retracted (*phimosis*). Ivory or porcelain-white; semitransparent, resembling mother-of-pearl.

Distribution

Genital   Females: vulva and perianal regions as well as the perineum; inverted keyhole or figure-of-eight in anogenital area; inguinal line. Males: undersurface of prepuce and glans.

Nongenital Trunk, especially upper back, periumbilical, neck, axillae; flexor surface of wrists; rarely palms and soles.

Oral Mucosa   Bluish-white plaques on buccal or palatal mucosa; tongue. Superficial erosions. Hyperkeratotic, macerated lesions may have reticulate pattern resembling lichen planus.

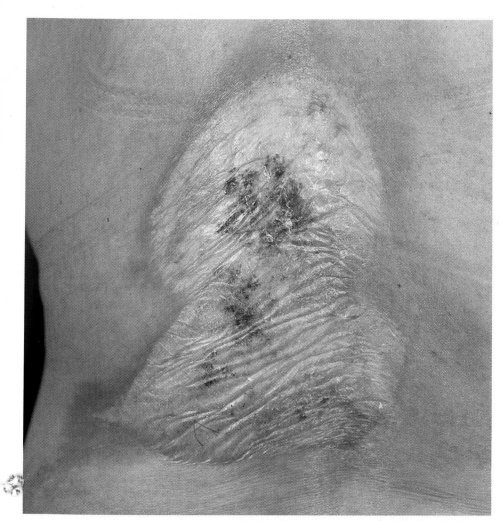

Figure 5-14   Lichen sclerosus et atrophicus   *An ivory-white, indurated but superficially atrophic plaque on the lower back that has arisen from the confluence of multiple whitish papules (best seen on left border). In the center there is superficial petechial hemorrhage, and the border is surrounded by a hyperpigmented ring of normal-appearing skin.*

DIFFERENTIAL DIAGNOSIS

Sclerotic/Atrophic Plaque Morphea (may coexist with LSA), lichen simplex chronicus, chronic cutaneous lupus erythematosus, leukoplakia, lichen planus, intraepithelial neoplasia (bowenoid papulosis), extramammary Paget's disease, intertrigo, candidiasis. In children may appear first as "vitiligo" of the vulva, which then gradually develops the typical lesions of LSA.

LABORATORY EXAMINATIONS

Dermatopathology Early in course, *epidermis:* variably thickened, hyperkeratotic, follicular plugging; later, atrophic. *Dermis:* band of homogenization of dermal collagen below epidermis; structureless, edematous; lymphocytic infiltrate, bandlike subepidermal in early lesions, later below the edematous, structureless, subepidermal zone. Dilated capillaries, hemorrhage.

DIAGNOSIS

Clinical diagnosis at times confirmed by biopsy.

COURSE AND PROGNOSIS

Waxes and wanes. In girls, may undergo spontaneous resolution. At times, coexisting lesions of morphea and vitiligo may be present. Patients should be followed every 12 months to check for occurrence of squamous cell carcinoma of the vulva. Also, males can develop squamous cell carcinoma (5%); they need to be monitored and the phimosis corrected with circumcision. Extragenital lesions in adults are more likely to undergo remission.

MANAGEMENT

Management is very important, as this disease can cause a devastating atrophy of the labia minora and clitoral hood. In males phimosis should be corrected by circumcision.

Topical Glucocorticoids Potent topical glucocorticoid preparations (clobetasol propionate) have proved effective for genital LS and should be used for 6 to 8 weeks only. Patients should be monitored for signs of glucocorticoid-induced atrophy

Topical Androgens Less used now because of the efficacy of clobetasol. Androgens can sometimes cause a clitoral hypertrophy.

Systemic Therapy Hydrochloroquine, 125 to 150 mg/d for weeks to a few months (monitor for ocular side effects).

Circumcision In males, circumcision relieves symptoms of phimosis and in some cases can result in remission.

PIGMENTED PURPURIC DERMATOSES

Pigmented purpuric dermatoses are distinguished by their clinical characteristics, having identical dermatopathologic findings, and include:

- Schamberg's disease, also known as progressive pigmented purpuric dermatosis and progressive pigmentary purpura
- Majocchi's disease, also known as purpura annularis telangiectodes
- Gougerot-Blum disease, also known as pigmented purpuric lichenoid dermatitis and purpura pigmentosa chronica
- Lichen aureus, also known as lichen purpuricus

Clinically, each entity shows recent pinpoint cayenne pepper–colored hemorrhages associated with older hemorrhages and hemosiderin deposition. Capillaritis histologically. Pigmented purpuric dermatoses are significant only if they are a cosmetic concern to the patient; they are often mistaken as manifestations of vasculitis or thrombocytopenia. *Synonym:* Capillaritis of unknown cause.

EPIDEMIOLOGY

Age of Onset 30 to 60 years; uncommon in children.

Sex More common in males.

Etiology Unknown. Primary process believed to be cell-mediated immune injury with subsequent vascular damage and erythrocyte extravasation. Other etiologic factors: pressure, trauma, eczematous dermatitis, drugs (acetaminophen, ampicillin—carbromal, diuretics, meprobamate, nonsteroidal anti-inflammatory drugs, zomepirac sodium).

HISTORY

Onset and Duration Insidious, slow to evolve—except drug-induced variant, which may develop rapidly and be more generalized in distribution. Persists for months to years. Most drug-induced purpuras resolve more quickly after discontinuation of the drug.

Symptoms Usually asymptomatic, but may be mildly pruritic.

PHYSICAL EXAMINATION

Schamberg's Disease Discrete clusters of pinhead-sized macules (fresh hemorrhages) become confluent, coalescing into patches (Fig. 5-15). Reddish-brown, "cayenne pepper." New lesions are red, representing pinpoint hemorrhages. Older lesions are tan to brown, representing degradation of extravasated erythrocytes with the formation of hemosiderin. Discrete clusters of macules and patches that can become confluent.

Distribution of Lesions Lower extremities (especially pretibial and on ankles) but may extend proximally to lower trunk and to upper extremities. Usually bilateral but may be unilateral. Uncommonly, generalized.

Majocchi's Disease Essentially an annular form of Schamberg's disease with telangiectasias (Fig. 5-16). An arciform variant also has been described.

Gougerot-Blum Disease Lichenoid papules, plaques, macules in association with lesions of Schamberg's disease.

Lichen Aureus Solitary or few patches or plaques, rust-colored, purple, or golden, arising on the extremities or trunk.

DIFFERENTIAL DIAGNOSIS

Nonpalpable Purpura Chronic venous insufficiency with clotting abnormalities, glucocorticoid usage, cutaneous T cell lymphoma, dysproteinemias, nummular eczema, old fixed drug eruption, parapsoriasis, poikiloderma vasculare atrophicans, primary amyloidosis, scurvy, senile purpura, stasis dermatitis, thrombocytopenia, trauma.

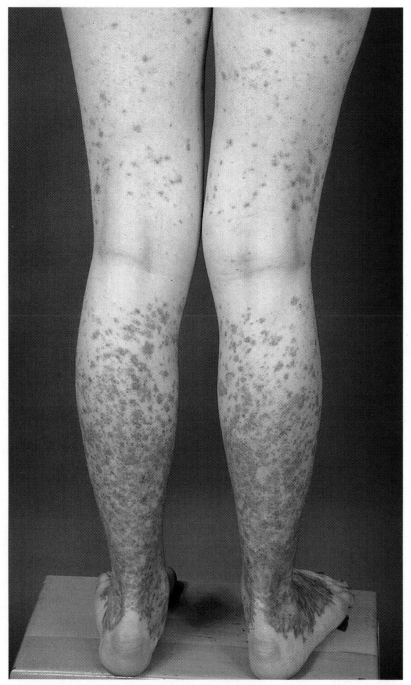

Figure 5-15 Pigmented purpuric dermatosis: Schamberg's disease *Multiple, discrete, and confluent nonpalpable, nonblanching purpuric lesions of many months' duration on the legs. Acute microhemorrhages resolve with deposition of hemosiderin, creating a disfiguring dark-brown stain.*

MISCELLANEOUS INFLAMMATORY DISORDERS

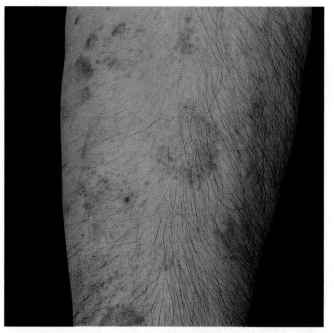

Figure 5-16   Pigmented purpuric dermatosis: Majocchi's disease   *Multiple non-palpable, non-blanching purpuric lesions arranged in annular configurations and associated with tiny telangiectasias. Note brownish discoloration of older lesions.*

Palpable Purpura   Atheroembolism, collagen vascular disease, cryoglobulinemias, infections, leukocytoclastic vasculitis.

LABORATORY EXAMINATIONS

Dermatopathology   Epidermal involvement varies, but dermal pathology (capillaritis) is common to all. Epidermis is normal in lichen aureus and drug-induced eruptions; in some cases there is vacuolar degradation of basal layer, spongiosis, and/or lymphocytic exocytosis. Dermal features present in all variants: extravasation of erythrocytes, hemosiderin pigment-laden macrophages (more extensive in lichen aureus), mild perivascular and interstitial lymphohistiocytic infiltrate in reticular dermis (more dense and bandlike lichenoid infiltrate in lichen aureus and Gougerot-Blum disease).

Immunohistochemistry   Immunofluorescence is variable and nonspecific. Most common pattern: deposits in superficial dermal vessels of fibrinogen, IgM, and/or C3; keratinocytes express HLA-DR; CD4 cells are the predominant lymphocytes in the dermis and bear HECA-452-recognized antigen; B cells are ab-

sent or rare, suggesting that the role of humoral immunity is minimal.

DIAGNOSIS

Usually made on clinical findings.

COURSE

Chronic (months to years), slow to evolve and resolve; spontaneous resolution has occurred. In lesions of long standing, hemosiderin deposits resolve very slowly (months to years). Almost all cases due to drugs clear within months after discontinuation of the offending agent.

MANAGEMENT

Symptomatic   Long-standing lesions may be cosmetically disfiguring, and patients may choose to treat these lesions. Topical low- and middle-potency glucocorticoid preparations inhibit new purpuric lesions. Systemic tetracycline or minocycline (50 mg bid) are effective. PUVA is effective in severe forms.

PITYRIASIS LICHENOIDES (ACUTE AND CHRONIC)

Pityriasis lichenoides (PL) is an eruption of unknown etiology, characterized clinically by successive crops of a wide range of morphologic lesions, i.e., macules, papules, vesicles, pustules, and crusts in the acute form, and by reddish-brown papules with adherent central scale in the chronic form.

Synonym: Guttate parapsoriasis.

EPIDEMIOLOGY

Age of Onset   Adolescents and young adults.

Sex   More common in males than females.

Etiology   Unknown.

CLASSIFICATION

PL has been classified into an acute form, pityriasis lichenoides et varioliformis acuta (PLEVA) (Mucha-Habermann disease), and a chronic form, pityriasis lichenoides chronica (PLC) (guttate parapsoriasis of Juliusberg); however, most patients have lesions of PLEVA and PLC simultaneously.

HISTORY

Duration of Lesions   Lesions tend to appear in crops over a period of weeks or months.

Symptoms   Uncommonly, patients with an acute onset of the disorder may have symptoms of an acute infection with fever, malaise, and headache. Cutaneous lesions are usually asymptomatic, but may be pruritic or sensitive to touch. Lesions may heal with significant scarring and postinflammatory pigmentation.

PHYSICAL EXAMINATION

Skin Lesions   Initially, randomly distributed, red edematous papules (i.e., lichenoides). Less commonly, vesicles-to-bullae, which undergo necrosis with central vesiculation and hemorrhagic crusting (i.e., varioliformis) (Fig. 5-17). In the chronic form, scaling papules of reddish-brown color and mica-like scale are seen (Fig. 5-18). Postinflammatory hypo- or hyperpigmentation often present after lesions resolve. May heal with depressed or elevated scars. Acutely, pink-to-erythematous. Chronic lesion, reddish-brown. Scars may be hypopigmented or depigmented.

Arrangement   Randomly arranged.

Distribution   Most commonly, trunk, proximal extremities. Lesions may occur in a generalized distribution, including palms and soles.

Oral and Genital Mucosa   Inflammatory papules and necrotic lesions may occur.

DIAGNOSIS

Clinical diagnosis, which is confirmed by skin biopsy.

DIFFERENTIAL DIAGNOSIS

Disseminated papules ± crust   Varicella, lichen planus, guttate psoriasis, prurigo nodularis, lymphomatoid papulosis.

LABORATORY EXAMINATIONS

Dermatopathology   *Epidermis:* spongiosis, keratinocyte necrosis, vesiculation, ulceration; exocytosis or erythrocytes within epidermis. *Dermis:* Edema, chronic inflammatory cell infiltrate in wedge shape extending to deep reticular dermis; hemorrhage; vessels congested with blood; endothelial cells swollen.

COURSE AND PROGNOSIS

New lesions appear in successive crops. PL tends to resolve spontaneously after 6 to 12 months. In some cases, relapses after many months or years.

MANAGEMENT

Most patients do not require any therapeutic intervention. Both topical glucocorticoid preparations and oral erythromycin and tetracycline are reported to be effective in some cases. Ultraviolet radiation, whether natural sunlight or broad band UVB, UVB 311 nm, and PUVA are the treatment of choice if the oral antibiotics fail after a 2-week trial.

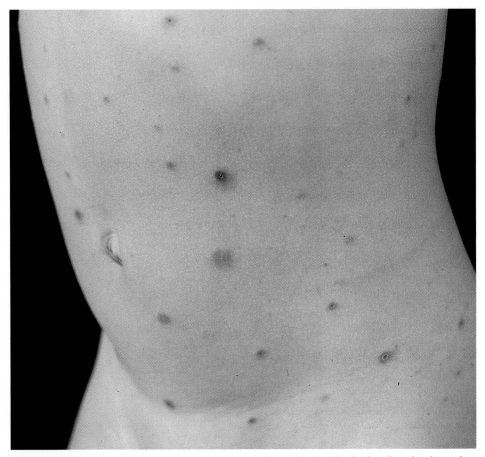

Figure 5-17 Pityriasis lichenoides et varioliformis acuta (PLEVA) *Randomly distributed red papules of different size, some of which show central hemorrhagic crusting. In this 5-year-old child the eruption appeared in crops over a period of ten days. Since individual lesions showed minimal signs of vesiculation and lesions were of different age, the eruption was mistaken for varicella.*

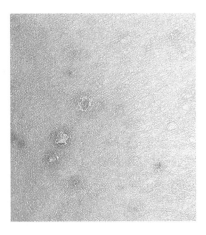

Figure 5-18 Pityriasis lichenoides chronica (PLC) *Discrete papules with fine, mica-like scales on the trunk of a 19-year-old adolescent. Note, in contrast to PLEVA (Figure 5-17), there is no hemorrhagic crusting.*

ERYTHEMA MULTIFORME SYNDROME

This reaction pattern of blood vessels in the dermis with secondary epidermal changes is exhibited clinically as characteristic erythematous iris-shaped papules and vesicolobullous lesions typically involving the extremities (especially the palms and soles) and the mucous membranes.

EPIDEMIOLOGY AND ETIOLOGY

Age of Onset   50% under 20 years.
Sex   More frequent in males than in females.

ETIOLOGIES

Drugs   Sulfonamides, phenytoin, barbiturates, phenylbutazone, penicillin, allopurinol.

Infection Especially following herpes simplex, *Mycoplasma*.

Idiopathic >50%.

HISTORY

Evolution of Lesions   Several days. May have history of prior episode of erythema multiforme (EM).

Skin Symptoms   May be pruritic or painful.

Mucous Membrane Symptoms   Mouth lesions are painful, tender.

Constitutional Symptoms   Fever, weakness, malaise.

PHYSICAL EXAMINATION

Skin Lesions   Lesions may develop over 10 days or more. Macule (48 hours)→papule, 1 to 2 cm; (Fig. 5-19). Vesicles and bullae (in the center of the papule) (Fig. 5-20). Dull red. Iris or targetlike lesions are typical (Figs. 5-19 and 5-20).

Arrangement   Localized to hands, face (Fig. 5-20), or generalized (Fig. 5-21).

Distribution   Bilateral and often symmetric.

Sites of Predilection   Dorsa of hands, palms (Fig. 5-19), and soles; forearms; feet; face (Fig. 5-20); elbows and knees; penis (50%) and vulva (see Figure 5-II).

Mucous Membranes   Erosions with fibrin membranes: lips, oropharynx, nasal, conjunctival, vulvar, anal.

Other Organs   Pulmonary, eyes with corneal ulcers, anterior uveitis.

DIFFERENTIAL DIAGNOSIS

Acute Erythematous Plaques   Drug eruption, psoriasis, secondary syphilis, urticaria.

Acute Oral Erosions   Primary herpes, pemphigus, acute lupus erythematosus.

COURSE

Mild Forms (EM Minor)   Little or no mucous membrane involvement, vesicles but no bullae or systemic symptoms. Eruption usually confined to extensor aspects of extremities, classic target lesions (Figure 5-20). Recurrent EM minor is usually associated with an outbreak of herpes simplex preceding it by several days. Chronic suppressive acyclovir therapy prevents recurrence of herpes as well as EM.

Severe Forms   (EM Major) Most often occurs as a drug reaction, always with mucous membrane involvement, severe, extensive, tendency to become confluent and bullous, positive Nikolsky sign in erythematous lesions, systemic symptoms, fever, prostration (see Fig. 5-24). Cheilitis and stomatitis interfere with eating; vulvitis and balanitis, with micturition. Conjunctivitis can lead to keratitis and ulceration; lesions also in pharynx, larynx, and trachea.

Maximal Variant   Life-threatening. In addition to the preceding, necrotizing tracheobronchitis, meningitis, renal tubular necrosis (Stevens-Johnson syndrome, see below).

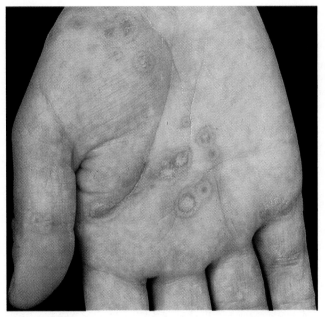

Figure 5-19   Erythema multiforme   *Iris and targetlike patterns with concentric macules and papules on the palm.*

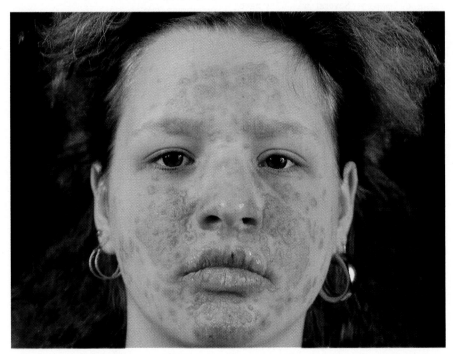

Figure 5-20   Erythema multiforme   *Multiple, confluent targetlike papules and vesicles on the central facies. Bullae are seen on the lips and were also present on the buccal mucosa.*

ERYTHEMA MULTIFORME SYNDROME

DERMATOPATHOLOGY

Site Epidermis and dermis.

Process Inflammation characterized by perivascular mononuclear infiltrate, edema of the upper dermis; if bulla formation, there is eosinophilic necrosis of keratinocytes with subepidermal bulla formation. In severe cases, complete necrosis of epidermis as in toxic epidermal necrolysis.

DIFFERENTIAL DIAGNOSIS

The targetlike lesion and the symmetry are quite typical, and the diagnosis is not difficult. In the absence of skin lesions, the mucous membrane lesions may present a difficult differential diagnosis: bullous diseases, fixed drug eruption, and primary herpetic gingivostomatitis. Urticaria.

MANAGEMENT

Prevention Control of herpes simplex using oral acyclovir may prevent development of recurrent erythema multiforme.

Corticosteroids In severely ill patients, systemic corticosteroids are usually given (prednisone 50 to 80 mg/d in divided doses, quickly tapered), but their effectiveness has not been established by controlled studies.

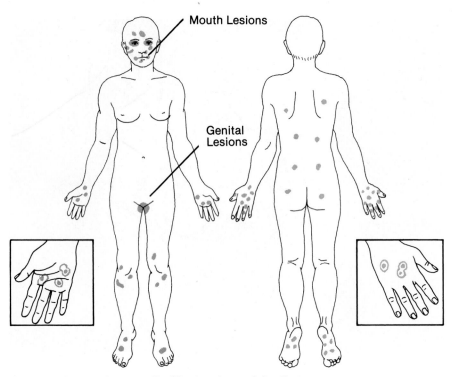

Mouth Lesions

Genital Lesions

Figure 5-II Erythema multiforme *Predilection sites and distribution.*

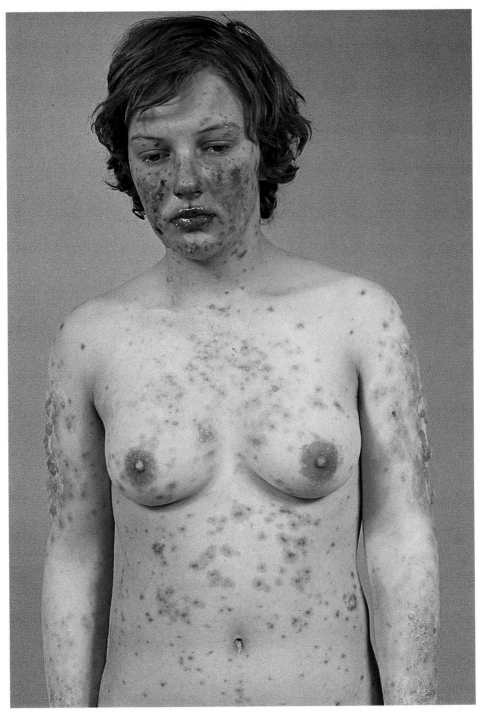

Figure 5-21 Erythema multiforme: major *Erythematous iris and target-like papules, plaques, bullae, and erosions on the trunk, arms, neck, and face. Mucosal involvement is manifested by erosive lip lesions and conjunctivitis.*

STEVENS-JOHNSON SYNDROME AND TOXIC EPIDERMAL NECROLYSIS

Stevens-Johnson syndrome (SJS) and toxic epidermal necrolysis (TEN) are mucocutaneous drug-induced or idiopathic reaction patterns characterized by skin tenderness and erythema of skin and mucosa, followed by extensive cutaneous and mucosal exfoliation, and are potentially life-threatening due to multisystem involvement.
Synonym: TEN: Lyell's syndrome.

EPIDEMIOLOGY

Age of Onset Any age, but most common in adults >40 years.

Sex Equal incidence.

Incidence *TEN:* .4 to 1.2 per million person-years. *SJS:* 1.2 to 6 per million person-years.

Risk Factors Systemic lupus erythematosus, HLA-B12, HIV disease.

Etiology *TEN:* 80% of cases have strong association with specific medication; <5% of patients report no drug use. Also: chemicals, *Mycoplasma* pneumonia, viral infections, immunization. *SJS:* 50% are associated with drug exposure; etiology often not clear-cut.

Drugs most frequently implicated Sulfa drugs (sulfadoxine, sulfadiazine, sulfasalazine, cotrimazole), allopurinol, hydantoins, carbamazepine, phenylbutazone, piroxicam, chlormezanone, amithiozone, aminopenicillins.

Drugs also implicated Cephalosporins, fluoroquinolones, vancomycin, rifampin, ethambutol, fenbufen, tonoxicam, tiaprofenic acid, diclofenac, sulindac, ibuprofen, ketoprofen, naproxen, thiabendazole.

Definition of SJS and TEN Not clearly defined. SJS is considered by most a maximal variant of erythema multiforme (major) and TEN a maximal variant of SJS. Both can start with target-like lesions; however, about 50% of TEN do not, and in these the condition evolves from diffuse erythema and immediate necrosis and detachment.

SJS <10% epidermal detachment.

SJS/TEN overlap 10% to 30% epidermal detachment.

TEN >30% epidermal detachment.

PATHOGENESIS

Unknown but consistent with immunologic mechanisms, i.e., cell-mediated cytotoxic reaction against epidermal cells. Epidermis infiltrated by activated lymphocytes, mainly CD8 cells, and macrophages. Cytokines produced by activated mononuclear cells and keratinocytes probably contribute to local cell death, fever, and malaise.

HISTORY

Time from First Drug Exposure to Onset of Symptoms 1 to 3 weeks. Occurs more rapidly with rechallenge.

Prodrome Fever, influenza-like symptoms 1 to 3 days prior to mucocutaneous lesions. Mild to moderate skin tenderness, conjunctival burning or itching.

Skin Symptoms Skin pain, burning sensation, tenderness, paresthesia.

Mucous Membrane Symptoms Mouth lesions are painful, tender.

General Symptoms Impaired alimentation, photophobia, painful micturition, anxiety.

Drug Ingestion Occurs after days of ingestion of the drug; newly added drug is most suspect.

PHYSICAL EXAMINATION

Skin Lesions

Types *Prodromal Rash* Morbilliform, erythema multiforme-like; diffuse erythema.

Early Necrotic epidermis first appears as macular areas (Fig. 5-22) with crinkled surface that enlarge and coalesce.

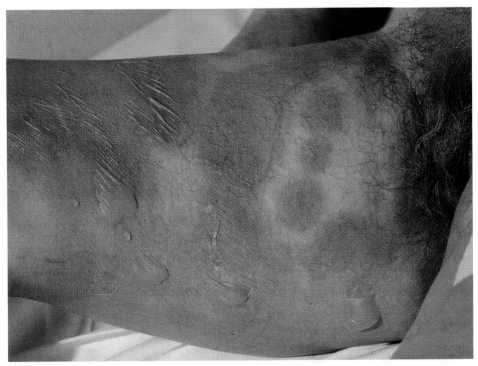

Figure 5-22 Stevens-Johnson syndrome *Generalized eruption of lesions that initially had a target-like appearance but then became confluent, brightly erythematous, and bullous. The patient had extensive mucous membrane involvement and tracheobronchitis.*

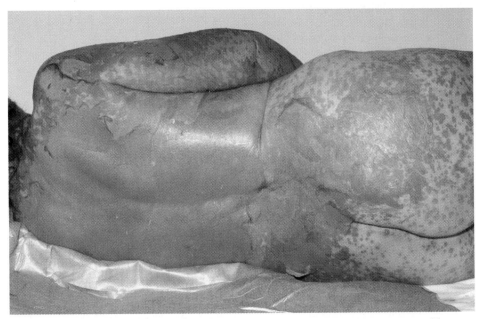

Figure 5-23 Toxic epidermal necrolysis *Generalized, macular eruption with some target-like lesions which rapidly developed epidermal necrosis, positive Nikolsky's sign, bulla formation, and denuded erosive areas. This eruption was due to sulfonamide.*

Later Sheet-like loss of epidermis. Raised flaccid blisters (Fig. 5-22 and 5-23) that spread with lateral pressure (Nikolsky's sign) on erythematous areas. With trauma, full-thickness epidermal detachment yields exposed, red, oozing dermis (Fig. 5-23).

Recovery Regrowth of epidermis begins within days; completed in 3 weeks. Pressure points and periorificial sites exhibit delayed healing. Skin that is not denuded acutely is shed in sheets, especially palms/soles. Nails and cilia may shed.

Color Very early lesions pink-red. Later, dusky cyanotic (Fig. 5-22). Red and glistening following epidermal sloughing (Figure 5-23).

Palpation Even early lesions are tender.

Distribution Initial erythema on face, extremities, becoming confluent over a few hours or days. Epidermal sloughing may be generalized, resulting in large denuded areas, resembling a second-degree thermal burn. Denudation most pronounced over pressure points. Scalp, palms, soles may be less severely involved or spared. *SJS:* widely distributed with prominent involvement of trunk and face. *TEN:* generalized, universal (Fig. 5-23).

Mucous Membranes 90% of patients have mucosal lesions, i.e., erythema, painful erosions: lips, buccal mucosa, conjunctiva, genital and anal skin.

Eyes 85% have conjunctival lesions: hyperemia, pseudomembrane formation; synechiae between eyelids and conjunctiva; keratitis, corneal erosions.

Sequelae in Skin Scarring, irregular pigmentation, eruptive nevomelanocytic nevi, abnormal regrowth of nails.

Eyes Common, including Sjögren-like sicca syndrome with deficiency of mucin in tears; entropion, trichiasis squamous metaplasia, neovascularization of conjunctiva and cornea; symblepharon, punctate keratitis, corneal scarring; persistent photophobia, burning eyes, visual impairment, blindness.

Anogenitalia Phimosis, vaginal synechiae.

General Findings Fever usually higher in TEN (>38°C) than in SJS. Usually mentally alert. In distress due to severe pain. Tubular necrosis. Acute renal failure; erosions in lower respiratory tract, gut. Epithelial erosions of trachea, bronchi, GI tract.

DIFFERENTIAL DIAGNOSIS

Early Exanthematous or pustular drug eruptions, erythema multiforme (EM) major, scarlet fever, phototoxic eruptions, toxic shock syndrome, graft-versus-host disease (GVHD).

Fully Evolved EM major (see typical target-like lesions, predominantly on extremities), GVHD (may mimic TEN; less mucosal involvement), thermal burns, phototoxic reactions, staphylococcal scalded-skin syndrome (in young children, rare in adults), generalized bullous fixed drug eruption, exfoliative dermatitis.

LABORATORY EXAMINATIONS

Hematology Anemia, lymphopenia; eosinophilia uncommon. Neutropenia correlates with poor prognosis.

Dermatopathology

Early Vacuolization/necrosis of basal keratinocytes and individual cell necrosis throughout the epidermis.

Late Full-thickness epidermal necrosis and detachment with formation of subepidermal split above basement membrane. Little or no inflammatory infiltrate in dermis. Immunofluorescence studies unremarkable, ruling out other blistering disorders.

DIAGNOSIS

Clinical findings confirmed by biopsy.

COURSE AND PROGNOSIS

Average duration of progression is <4 days. Course similar to that of extensive thermal burns. Prognosis related to extent of skin necrosis. Transcutaneous fluid loss large and varies with area of denudation; associated electrolyte abnormalities. Prerenal azotemia common. Bacterial colonization common, and associated with sepsis. Other complications include hypermetabolic state and diffuse interstitial pneumonitis. Mortality rate for TEN 30%, mainly in elderly; for SJS, 5%. Mortality related to sepsis, GI hemorrhage, fluid/electrolyte imbalance. If the patient survives the first episode of SJS or TEN, reexposure to the causative drug may be followed by recurrence within hours to days, more severe than the initial episode.

MANAGEMENT

Acute SJS/TEN

- Early diagnosis and withdrawal of suspected drug(s) are very important.
- Patients are best cared for in a burn or intensive care unit.
- Manage replacement of IV fluids and electrolytes as for patient with a third-degree thermal burn.
- Systemic corticosteroids are probably *not* helpful in reducing morbidity or mortality but this has not been proven. Some claim beneficial effects particularly if corticosteroids are given in high doses and early.
- High dose IV immunoglobulins have recently been shown to halt progression of TEN if administered early.
- Pentoxiphyllin IV by continuous drip early on in the eruption has been anecdotally reported to be beneficial.
- Conjunctival erythromycin ointment.
- Suction frequently with oropharyngeal involvement to prevent aspiration pneumonitis.
- Debride only frankly necrotic skin.
- Diagnose and treat complicating infections, including sepsis (fever, hypotension, change in mental status).

Prevention   The patient must be aware of the likely offending drug and that other drugs of the same class can crossreact. These drugs must never be readministered. Patient should wear a medical alert bracelet.

ERYTHEMA NODOSUM SYNDROME

Erythema nodosum is an important acute inflammatory/immunologic reaction pattern of the panniculus characterized by the appearance of painful nodules on the lower legs and caused by multiple and diverse etiologies.

EPIDEMIOLOGY

Etiology The age of onset is from 15 to 30 years, but age distribution is related to etiology. Erythema nodosum is three times more common in females than in males. Etiologic associations include infections, drugs, and other inflammatory/granulomatous diseases, notably sarcoidosis (Table 5-2).

HISTORY

Painful, tender lesions, usually of a few days duration, are accompanied by fever, malaise and arthralgia (50%), most frequently of ankle joints. Other symptoms depending on etiology.

PHYSICAL EXAMINATION

Skin Lesions Indurated but very tender nodules (3 to 20 cm), not sharply marginated (Fig. 5-24), deep seated, mostly on the anterior lower legs, bilateral but not symmetric. Nodules are bright to deep red, are located in the subcutaneous fat, and are appreciated as such only upon palpation. The term "erythema nodosum" best describes the skin lesions: they look like erythema but feel like nodules (Fig. 5-24). Lesions are oval, round, arciform; as they age, they become violaceous, brownish, yellowish, green, like resolving hematomas. Lesions are scattered, discrete, and may also occur on knees and arms but only rarely on the face and on the neck.

LABORATORY EXAMINATIONS

Hematology Elevated ESR, C-reactive protein, elevated, leukocytosis.

Bacterial Culture Culture throat for group A β-hemolytic streptococcus (GABHS), stool for *Yersinia*.

Imaging Radiologic examination of the chest is important to rule out sarcoidosis.

Dermatopathology Acute (polymorphonuclear) and chronic (granulomatous) inflammation in the panniculus and around blood vessels in the septum and adjacent fat. It is a septal panniculitis.

COURSE

Spontaneous resolution occurs in 6 weeks, with new lesions erupting during that time. Course depends on the etiology. Lesions never break down or ulcerate and heal without scarring.

DIAGNOSIS AND DIFFERENTIAL DIAGNOSIS

Diagnosis rests on clinical criteria, may be supported by histopathology. Differential diagnosis includes all other forms of panniculitis, panarteritis nodosa, nodular vasculitis, pretibial myxedema, nonulcerated gumma, and lymphoma.

MANAGEMENT

Symptomatic Bed rest or compressive bandages (lower legs), wet dressings.

Anti-inflammatory Treatment Salicylates, NSAIDs.

Systemic Glucocorticoids Response is rapid, but their use is indicated only when the etiology is known (and infectious agents are excluded).

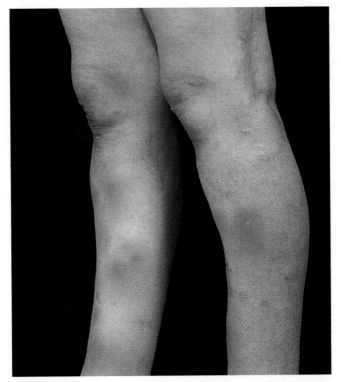

Figure 5-25   Erythema nodosum   *Indurated, very tender inflammatory nodules mostly in the pretibial region. Lesions are seen as red, ill-defined erythemas but palpated as deep-seated nodules, hence the designation. In this 45-year-old patient there was also fever and arthritis of ankle joints following an upper respiratory tract infection. Throat cultures yielded β-hemolytic streptococci.*

Table 5-2   ETIOLOGY OF ERYTHEMA NODOSUM

Sarcoidosis
Streptococcal infections
Tuberculosis
Other bacterial infections
   Yersinia enterocolitica
   Salmonella enteritidis
   Mycoplasma pneumoniae
   Leprosy
   Leptospirosis
   Tularemia
Fungal infections
   Coccidioidomycosis
   Blastomycosis
   Histoplasmosis
   Dermatophytes
Viruses and *Chlamydia* agents
   Paravaccinia
   Infectious mononucleosis
   Lymphogranuloma venereum
   Cat-scratch disease
   Psittacosis
   Hepatitis B

Drug-induced
   Sulfonamides
   Bromides
   Oral contraceptives
Enteropathies
   Ulcerative colitis
   Crohn's disease
Malignant disease
   Lymphogranuloma and leukemia
   Carcinoma
   Postradiation therapy
Behçet's syndrome
Sweet's syndrome

SOURCE: From EF Bondi et al, Panniculitis; in IM Freedburg, AZ Eisen, K Wolff, KF Austen, LA Goldsmith, SI Katz, TB Fitzpatrick (eds): Dermatology in General Medicine, 5th ed. New York, McGraw-Hill, 1999.

OTHER PANNICULITIDES

Panniculitis is the term used to describe diseases where the major focus of inflammation is in the subcutaneous tissue. In general, panniculitis presents as erythematous or violaceous nodule in the subcutaneous fat that may be tender or not, that may ulcerate or heal without scarring, and that may be soft or hard on palpation. Thus, the term panniculitis describes a wide spectrum of disease manifestations, although diagnostic clues can be derived from the history, distribution, or characteristics of the lesions. An accurate diagnosis requires an ample deep skin biopsy that should reach down to or even beyond the fascia.

The panniculitides are classified histologically as lobular or septal depending on where the disease process begins. Panniculitis may also be associated with vasculitis or in most cases without vasculitis. A simplified classification of panniculitis is given in Table 5-3.

Only idiopathic lobular panniculitis (Pfeiffer-Weber-Christian disease), pancreatic panniculitis, and α_1 antitrypsin–deficiency panniculitis are briefly discussed here. Other diseases in which panniculitis occurs are referred to in the table, and the reader is also referred to *Fitzpatrick's Dermatology in General Medicine*, 5th ed.[1]

Idiopathic lobular panniculitis, which occurs predominantly in females 30 to 60 years of age, manifests as subcutaneous inflammatory nodules, primarily on the lower extremities but also on the trunk and elsewhere, that erupt in crops and are usually tender. New waves of lesions appear at intervals. Occasionally, lesions can break down, discharging an oily yellow-brown liquid; and these inflammatory nodules are generally accompanied by malaise, fatigue, fever, arthralgia, and myalgia. Due to systemic involvement there may be focal necrosis in the intravisceral and perivisceral fat of internal organs, including the mesenteric and omental fat, pericardium, and pleura. Organ involvement may present as hepatomegaly, abdominal pain, nausea, and vomiting.

Leukocytosis and an elevated erythrocyte sedimentation rate are further characteristics of this disease, of which the etiology is unknown. The course and prognosis are variable; the prognosis is good in patients who have only cutaneous involvement, but lobular panniculitis associated with prominent visceral involvement may lead to death. There is no uniform effective therapy recognized; fibrinolytic agents, chloroquine, azathioprine, thalidomide, cyclophosphamide, and cyclosporine have been tried.

α_1 *antitrypsin–deficiency panniculitis* is also characterized by recurrent tender, erythematous, subcutaneous, ulcerating nodules ranging from 1 to 5 cm and located predominantly on the trunk and the proximal extremities, very much like those shown in Figure 5-25. Nodules break down and discharge a clear serous or oily fluid. Diagnosis is substantiated by a decrease in the level of serum α_1 antitrypsin, and treatment consists of oral dapsone in doses up to 200 mg/d. The intravenous infusion of human α_1-proteinase inhibitor concentrate has been shown to be very effective.

Pancreatic panniculitis is characterized clinically by painful erythematous nodules that may occur at any site. It is frequently accompanied by arthritis and polyserositis and is associated with either pancreatitis or pancreatic carcinoma. This form of panniculitis affects middle-aged to elderly individuals, males more often than females. The history usually reveals alcoholism, abdominal pain, weight loss, or recent-onset diabetes mellitus. Skin lesions are tender, warm, erythematous nodules and plaques that may fluctuate and occur at any site (Fig. 5-25) with a predilection for legs, buttocks, and abdomen. Skin biopsy reveals lobular panniculitis, and after biopsy of a lesion, liquefied fat drains from the biopsy site. General examination may reveal pleural effusion, ascites and arthritis, particularly of the ankles.

Laboratory examinations show eosinophilia, hyperlipasemia, hyperamylasemia, and increased excretion of amylase and/or lipase in the urine. The pathophysiology is probably a break down of subcutaneous fat caused by enzymes (amylase, trypsin, lipase) released into the circulation from a diseased pancreas. The course and prognosis depend on the type of pancreatic disease. Treatment is directed at the underlying pancreatic disorder.

[1]IM Freedberg, AZ Eisen, K Wolff, KF Austen, LA Goldsmith, SI Katz, TB Fitzpatrick (eds): *Fitzpatrick's Dermatology in General Medicine*, 5th ed. New York, McGraw-Hill, 1999.

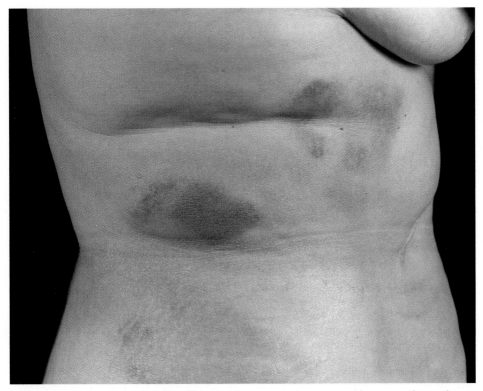

Figure 5-25 Pancreatic panniculitis *Three erythematous, subcutaneous plaques on the trunk. Hemorrhage within the lesions produces various color changes associated with extravasated blood: red, violet, and yellow-green. This 53-year-old female had a history of recent onset diabetes and alcoholism. Lesions were warm, tender and later started to fluctuate; and when one of these was biopsied, liquefied fat drained from the biopsy site. The patient had pancreatitis with hyperlipasemia, hyperamylasemia and an increased excretion of pancreatic enzymes in the urine.*

Table 5-3 SIMPLIFIED CLASSIFICATION OF PANNICULITIS

	Lobular Panniculitis	Septal Panniculitis
Neonatal:	Sclerema neonatorum, neonatal subcutaneous fat necrosis	Erythema nodosum
Physical:	Cold, trauma	Eosinophilic fasciitis
Drugs:	Post-steroid panniculitis	
Idiopathic:	Idiopathic lobular panniculitis (Pfeiffer-Weber-Christian) syndrome	Eosinophilia myalgia syndrome
Pancreatic:	With pancreatitis or carcinoma of the pancreas	Scleroderma
α_1 Antitrypsin–deficiency panniculitis systemic disease:	LE, sarcoidosis, lymphoma, histiocytic cytophagic panniculitis	
With vasculitis:	Nodular vasculitis	Thrombophlebitis, panarteritis nodosa

PYODERMA GANGRENOSUM

Pyoderma gangrenosum (PG) is a rapidly evolving, idiopathic, chronic, and severely debilitating skin disease. It occurs most commonly in association with a systemic disease, especially chronic ulcerative colitis, and is characterized by the presence of irregular, boggy, blue-red ulcers with undermined borders surrounding purulent necrotic bases.

ETIOLOGY

Unknown.

HISTORY

Acute onset with painful hemorrhagic pustule or painful nodule either de novo or after minimal trauma.

PHYSICAL EXAMINATION

Skin Lesions Starts as deep-seated nodule or superficial hemorrhagic pustule surrounded by erythematous halo; very painful. Breakdown of this lesions occurs with ulcer formation whereby ulcer borders are dusky-red or purple, irregular and raised, undermined, boggy with perforations that drain pus (Fig. 5-26). The base of the ulcer is purulent with hemorrhagic exudate, partially covered by necrotic eschar (Fig. 5-27), with or without granulation tissue. Pustules may be seen at the advancing border and in the ulcer base, and a halo of erythema spreads centrifugally at the advancing edge of the ulcer (Fig. 5-26). Lesions are usually solitary but may be multiple and form in clusters that coalesce. Most common sites: lower extremities (Fig. 5-26) >buttocks>abdomen>face (Fig. 5-27). Healing of ulcers results in thin atrophic cribriform scars.

Mucous Membranes Rarely, aphthous stomatitis-like lesions; massive ulceration of oral mucosa and conjunctivae.

General Examination Patient may appear ill.

Associated Systemic Diseases Up to 50% occur without associated disease. Remainder of cases associated with large- and small-bowel disease (Crohn's disease, ulcerative colitis), diverticulosis (diverticulitis), arthritis, paraproteinemia and myeloma, leukemia, active chronic hepatitis, Behçet's syndrome.

DIFFERENTIAL DIAGNOSIS

Progressive synergistic gangrene, ecthyma gangrenosum, atypical mycobacterial infection, clostridial infection, deep mycoses, amebiasis, bromoderma, pemphigus vegetans, stasis ulcers, Wegener's granulomatosis.

LABORATORY EXAMINATIONS

ESR Variably elevated.

Dermatopathology Not diagnostic. Neutrophilic inflammation with abscess formation and necrosis.

DIAGNOSIS

Clinical findings plus course of illness.

COURSE AND PROGNOSIS

Untreated, course may last months to years but spontaneous healing can occur. Ulceration may extend rapidly within a few days or slowly. Healing may occur centrally with peripheral extension. New ulcers may appear as older lesions resolve. Pathergy, i.e. slight trauma initiating new PG lesion noted at sites of minor trauma, biopsy, or needle sticks.

MANAGEMENT

With Associated Underlying Disease Treat underlying disease.

For PG High doses of oral glucocorticoids or IV glucocorticoid pulse therapy (1 to 2 g prednisolone per day) may be required. ±Intralesional triamcinolone. Sulfasalazine (particularly in cases associated with Crohn's disease), sulfones, and cyclosporine have been shown to be effective in uncontrolled studies.

Figure 5-26 Pyoderma gangrenosum *This extremely painful, boggy ulcer developed from a hemorrhagic pustule in the course of only three days. The patient had ulcerative colitis and had experienced similar lesions previously. Note dusky-red peripheral rim; bullous detachment of epidermis at the lower margin; and irregular, undermined border with pustules on top. Pus is also seen at the base of the ulcer.*

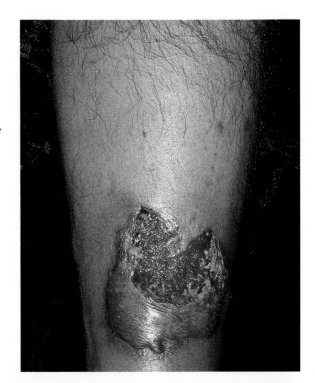

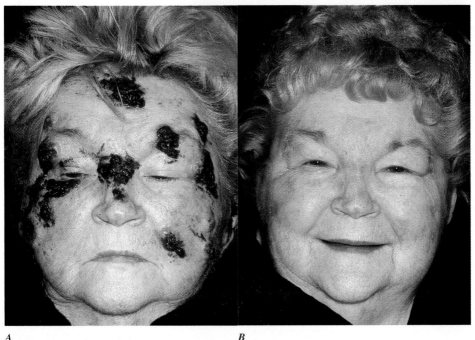

A   B

Figure 5-27 Bullous pyroderma gangrenosum *A 68-year-old female with multiple myeloma for several years presented with disseminated lesions of several weeks' duration. A. Multiple large hemorrhagic bullae on the face. B. After a 14-day tapered course of prednisone beginning at 70 mg/d, all lesions resolved without scarring.*

SWEET'S SYNDROME

Sweet's syndrome (SS) is an uncommon, recurrent skin disease characterized by painful plaque-forming inflammatory papules and associated with fever, arthralgia, and peripheral leukocytosis. *Synonym:* Acute febrile neutrophilic dermatosis.

EPIDEMIOLOGY

Age of Onset   Most 30 to 60 years.

Sex   Women>men.

Etiology   Unknown, possibly hypersensitivity reaction. In some cases associated with *Yersinia* infection.

Associated Disorders   Febrile upper respiratory tract infection. Hematologic malignancy.

HISTORY

Prodromes are febrile upper respiratory tract infections. GI symptoms (diarrhea), tonsillitis, influenza-like illness, 1 to 3 weeks before skin lesions. Lesions tender/painful. Fever (not always present), headache, arthralgia, general malaise.

PHYSICAL EXAMINATION

Skin Lesions   Bright red, smooth, tender papules (2 to 4 mm in diameter) that coalesce to form irregular, sharply bordered, inflammatory plaques (Fig. 5-28). Pseudovesiculation: intense edema gives the appearance of vesiculation. Lesions arise rapidly, and as they evolve, central clearing may lead to annular or arcuate patterns (Fig. 5-28). Tiny, superficial pustules may occur. If associated with leukemia, bullous lesions may occur (Fig. 5-29), and lesions may mimic pyoderma gangrenosum. May present as a single lesion or multiple lesions, asymmetrically distributed (Fig. 5-28). Most commonly on face and neck, upper extremities (Fig. 5-28) but also lower extremities where lesions may be deep in the panniculus and thus mimic panniculitis or erythema nodosum. Truncal lesions are uncommon but widespread, and generalized forms occur.

Mucous Membranes   ±Conjunctivitis, episcleritis.

General Examination   Patient may appear ill.

DIFFERENTIAL DIAGNOSIS

Very Edematous Acute Plaques   Erythema multiforme, erythema nodosum, prevesicular herpes simplex infection, preulcerative pyoderma gangrenosum.

LABORATORY EXAMINATIONS

CBC   Leukocytosis with neutrophilia.

ESR   Elevated.

Dermatopathology   Epidermis usually normal but may show subcorneal pustulation. Massive edema of papillary body, dense leukocytic infiltrate with starburst pattern in mid-dermis, consisting of neutrophils with occasional eosinophils/lymphoid cells. Leukocytoclasia, nuclear dust, but other signs of vasculitis absent. ±Neutrophilic infiltrates in subcutaneous tissue.

DIAGNOSIS

Clinical impression plus skin biopsy confirmation.

COURSE AND PROGNOSIS

Untreated, lesions enlarge over a period of days or weeks and eventually resolve without scarring. With oral prednisone, lesions resolve within a few days. Recurrences occur in 50% of patients, often in previously involved sites. Some cases follow *Yersinia* infection or are associated with acute myelocytic leukemia, transient myeloid proliferation, various malignant tumors, ulcerative colitis, benign monoclonal gammopathy.

MANAGEMENT

Rule out sepsis.

Prednisone   30 to 50 mg/d, tapering in 2 to 3 weeks; some but not all patients respond to dapsone, 100 mg/d, or to potassium iodide.

Antibiotic Therapy   Clears eruption in *Yersinia*-associated cases; in all other cases antibiotics are ineffective.

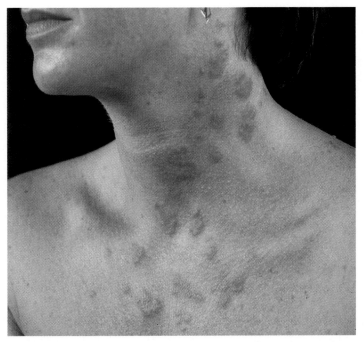

Figure 5-28   Sweet's syndrome   *Edematous, erythematous papules coalesce to form irregular, inflammatory, mammillated (covered with nipple-like protuberances) plaques on the neck and upper chest. Note arciform configuration. The eruption occurred in a 33-year-old female following an upper respiratory infection. The patient also had fever and leucocytosis.*

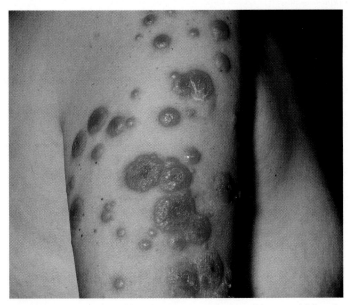

Figure 5-29   Sweet's syndrome   *A sudden, painful eruption in a 50-year-old female who was febrile and had general malaise. There are multiple very edematous and erythematous papules and plaques, most of which upon first sight, appear as if they were vesicles or bullae but are firm upon palpation (pseudovesiculation). However, the confluent lesions in the lower part of the picture are indeed bullous and here there is also exudation and crusting. Systems review in this patient revealed myelocytic leukemia.*

ERYTHRODERMA AND RASHES IN THE ACUTELY ILL PATIENT

EXFOLIATIVE ERYTHRODERMA SYNDROME

The exfoliative erythroderma syndrome (EES) is a serious, at times life-threatening reaction pattern of the skin characterized by generalized and uniform redness and scaling involving practically the entire skin and associated with systemic "toxicity," generalized lymphadenopathy, and fever. Two stages, acute and chronic, merge one into the other. In the acute and subacute phases, there is rapid onset of generalized vivid red erythema and fine branny scales; the patient feels hot and cold, shivers, and has fever. In the chronic EES, the skin thickens, and scaling continues and becomes lamellar. There is a loss of scalp and body hair, the nails become thickened and separated from the nail bed (onycholysis), and there may be hyperpigmentation or patchy loss of pigment in patients whose normal skin color is brown or black. About 50% of the patients with EES have a history of a preexisting dermatosis, which is recognizable only in the acute or subacute stages. The most frequent preexisting skin disorders are (in order of frequency) psoriasis, eczematous dermatitis (atopic, allergic contact), adverse cutaneous drug reaction, lymphoma, and pityriasis rubra pilaris (Table 6-1) Drugs most commonly implicated in erythroderma are found in Table 6-2. In 10 to 20% of patients it is not possible to identify the cause by history or histology. (See Sézary's Syndrome, for a special consideration of this form of EES.)

EPIDEMIOLOGY

Age of Onset >50 years; in children, EES usually results from pityriasis rubra pilaris or atopic dermatitis.

Sex Males >females.

PATHOGENESIS

The metabolic response to exfoliative dermatitis may be profound. Large amounts of warm blood are present in the skin due to the dilatation of capillaries, and there is considerable heat dissipation through insensible fluid loss and by convection. Also, there may be high output cardiac failure; the loss of scales through exfoliation can be considerable, up to 9 g/m^2 of body surface per day, and this may contribute to the reduction in serum albumin and the edema of the lower extremities so often noted in these patients.

HISTORY

Depending on the etiology, the acute phase may develop rapidly, as in a drug reaction, lymphoma, eczema, or psoriasis. At this early acute stage it is possible to identify the preexisting dermatosis. There is pruritus, fatigue, weakness, anorexia, weight loss, malaise, feeling cold.

Table 6-1 ETIOLOGY OF EXFOLIATIVE DERMATITIS IN ADULTS

Cause	Average Percent[a]
Undetermined or unclassified	23
Psoriasis	23
Atopic dermatitis, eczema	16
Drug allergy	15
Lymphoma, leukemia	11
Allergic contact dermatitis	5
Seborrheic dermatitis	5
Stasis dermatitis with "id" reaction	3
Pityriasis rubra pilaris	2
Pemphigus foliaceus	1

[a]As collated from the literature.

SOURCE: Abbreviated from IM Freedberg, in IM Freedberg, AZ Eisen, K Wolff, KF Austen, LA Goldsmith, SI Katz, TB Fitzpatrick (eds): *Fitzpatrick's Dermatology in General Medicine*, 5th ed. New York, McGraw-Hill, 1999. p 535.

Table 6-2 DRUGS REPORTED IN ASSOCIATION WITH EXFOLIATIVE DERMATITIS— SPECIFIC AND GROUPS

Allxopurinol	Isoniazid
Aminoglycosides	Isotretinoin
Amiodarone	Lithium
Antimalarials	Mephenytoin
Arsenic	Mercurials
Aspirin	Mercury
Aztreonam	Mexiletine
BAL	Minocycline
Babiturates	Neomycin
Calcium channel blockers	Penicillin
Captopril	Phenindione
Carbamazepine	Phenothiazines
Cephalosporins	Phenytoin
Chlorpromazine	Quinacrine
Chlorpropamide	Quinidine
Cimetidine	Ranitidine
Cisplatin	Rifampin
Codeine	Streptomycin
Dapsone	Sulfonamides
Diltiazem	Sulfonylureas
Diphenylhydantoin	Terbutaline
Ethylenediamine	Thalidomide
Fluorouracil	Thiazides
Gold	Trimethadione
Indinavir	Trimethoprim
Iodine	Vancomycin

SOURCE: IM Freedberg, in IM Freedberg, AZ Eisen, K Wolff, KF Austen, LA Goldsmith, SI Katz, TB Fitzpatrick (eds): *Fitzpatrick's Dermatology in General Medicine,* 5th ed. New York, McGraw-Hill, 1999. p 535.

PHYSICAL EXAMINATION

Appearance of Patient Frightened, red, "toxic."

Skin Lesions Skin is red, thickened, scaly. Dermatitis is uniform involving the entire body surface (Figs. 6-1, 6-2, and 6-3), except for pityriasis rubra pilaris, where EES spares sharply defined areas of normal skin. Thickening leads to exaggerated skin folds (Figures 6-2 and 6-3); scaling may be fine and branny, and may be barely perceptible or large, up to .5 cm, and lamellar (Figure 6-1).

Palms and Soles Usually involved, with massive hyperkeratosis and deep fissures in pityriasis rubra pilaris, Sézary's syndrome, and psoriasis.

Hair Thinning of hair, even alopecia, except for EES arising in eczema or psoriasis.

Nails Onycholysis, shedding of nails.

General Examination Lymph nodes generalized, rubbery, and usually small; enlarged in Sézary's syndrome. Edema of lower legs and ankles.

LABORATORY EXAMINATIONS

Chemistry Low serum albumin and increase in gammaglobulins; electrolyte imbalance; acute-phase proteins increased.

Hematology Leukocytosis.

Bacterial Culture *Skin:* rule out secondary *Staphylococcus aureus* infection. *Blood:* rule out sepsis.

Dermatopathology Depends on type of underlying disease. Parakeratosis, inter- and intracellular edema, acanthosis with elongation of the rete ridges, and exocytosis of cells. There is edema of the dermis and a chronic inflammatory infiltrate.

Imaging CT scans or MRI should be used to find evidence of lymphoma.

Lymph Node Biopsy When there is suspicion of lymphoma.

DIAGNOSIS

Diagnosis is not easy, and the history of the pre-existing dermatosis may be the only clue. Also, pathognomonic signs and symptoms of the pre-existing dermatosis may help, e.g., dusky-red color in psoriasis and yellowish-red in pityriasis rubra pilaris; typical nail changes of psoriasis; lichenification, erosions, and excoriations in atopic dermatitis and eczema; diffuse, relatively nonscaling palmar hyperkeratoses with fissures in CTCL and pityriasis rubra pilaris; sharply demarcated patches of noninvolved skin within the erythroderma in pityriasis rubra pilaris; massive hyperkeratotic scale of scalp, usually without hair loss in psoriasis and with hair loss in CTCL and pityriasis rubra pilaris; in the latter and in CTCL, ectropion may occur.

COURSE AND PROGNOSIS

Guarded, depends on underlying etiology. Despite the best attention to all details, patients may succumb to infections or, if they have cardiac problems, to cardiac failure ("high output" failure) or to the effects of the prolonged glucocorticoid therapy that may be required.

MANAGEMENT

This is an important medical problem that should be dealt with in a modern inpatient dermatology facility with experienced personnel. The patient should be hospitalized in a single room, at least for the beginning workup and during the development of a therapeutic program. The hospital room conditions (heat and cold) should be adjusted to the patient's needs; most often these patients need a warm room with many blankets.

Topical Water baths with added bath oils, followed by application of bland emollients.

Systemic Oral glucocorticoids for remission induction and for maintenance (except in psoriatic EES); systemic and topical therapy as required by underlying condition.

Supportive Supportive cardiac, fluid, electrolyte, protein replacement therapy as required.

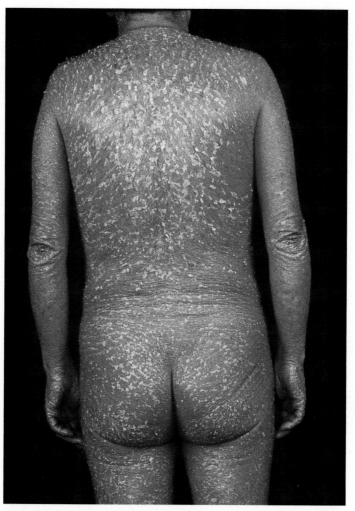

Figure 6-1 Erythroderma *There is universal erythema, thickening of the skin, and heavy scaling. This patient had psoriasis as suggested by the large silvery white scales and the scalp and nail involvement not seen in this illustration. The patient had fatigue, weakness, malaise and was shivering. It is quite obvious that such massive scaling can lead to protein loss, and the maximal dilatation of skin capillaries to considerable heat dissipation and high output cardiac failure.*

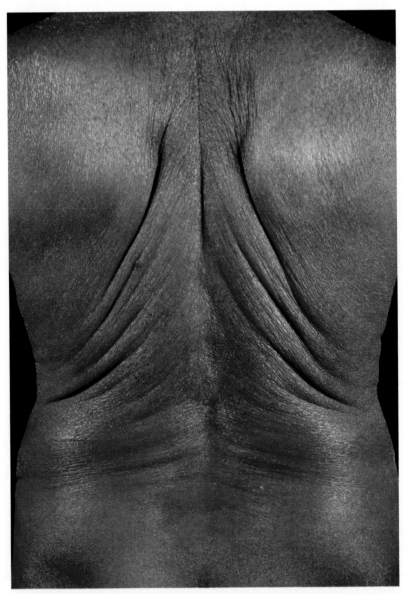

Figure 6-2 Erythroderma: drug-induced *This is generalized erythroderma with thickening of skin resulting in increased skin folds, universal redness, a fine brawny scaling. This patient had developed erythroderma following the injection of gold salts for rheumatoid arthritis.*

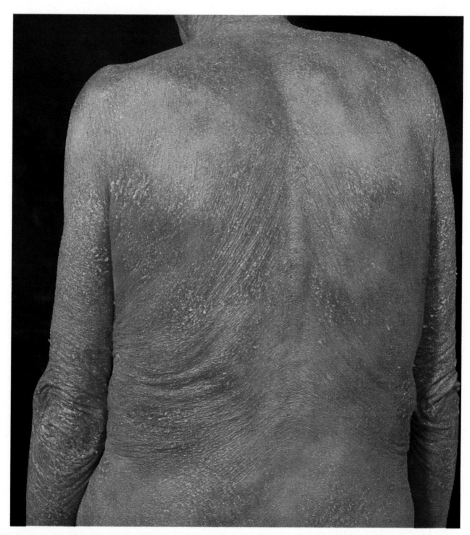

Figure 6-3 Erythroderma: cutaneous T cell lymphoma *There is universal erythema, thickening, and scaling. Note, that in contrast to erythroderma shown in Figures 6-1 and 6-2 the degree of erythema and thickness is not uniform and the redness has a brownish hue. In addition, this elderly patient had hair loss, massive involvement of palms and soles with diffuse hyperkeratoses, cracks, and fissures. Generalized lymphadenopathy was also present.*

RASHES IN THE ACUTELY ILL FEBRILE PATIENT

The sudden appearance of a rash and fever is frightening for the patient. Medical advice is sought immediately and often in the emergency units of hospitals; about 10% of all patients seeking emergency medical care have a dermatologic problem.

The diagnosis of an acute rash with a fever is a clinical challenge. Rarely do physicians have to "lean" on their eyes as much as when confronted by an acutely ill patient with fever and a skin eruption. If a diagnosis is not established promptly in certain patients (e.g., those having septicemia), lifesaving treatment may be delayed.

The cutaneous findings alone may be diagnostic before confirmatory laboratory data are available. As in problems of the acute abdomen, the results of some laboratory tests, such as microbiologic cultures, may not be available immediately. On the basis of a differential diagnosis, appropriate therapy—whether antibiotics or corticosteroids—may be started. Furthermore, prompt diagnosis and isolation of the patient with a contagious disease, which may have serious consequences, prevent spread to other persons. For example, varicella in adults rarely can be fatal. Contagious diseases presenting with rash and fever as the major findings include *viral infections* (rubella, enterovirus, and parvovirus infections) and *bacterial infections* (streptococcal, staphylococcal, meningococcal, typhoid, and syphilis).

The physical diagnosis of skin eruptions is a discipline mainly based on precise identification of the type of skin lesion. The physician must not only identify and classify the *type* of skin lesion but also look for additional morphologic clues such as the *configuration* (annular? iris?) of the individual lesion, the *arrangement* (zosteriform? linear?) of the lesions, the distribution pattern (exposed areas? centripetal or centrifugal? mucous membranes?). In the *differential diagnosis* of exanthems it is important to determine, by history, the *site of first appearance* (the rash of Rocky Mountain spotted fever characteristically appears first on the wrists and ankles), and very important is the *temporal evolution* of the rash (measles spreads from head to toes in a period of 3 days, while the rash of rubella spreads rapidly in 24 to 48 hours from head to toes and then sequentially clears—first face, then trunk, and then limbs).

Although there may be some overlap, the differential diagnostic possibilities may be grouped into four main categories according to the type of lesion (Table 6-3).

LABORATORY TESTS AVAILABLE FOR QUICK DIAGNOSIS

The physician should make use of the following laboratory tests immediately or within 8 hours:

1. *Direct smear from the base of a vesicle.* This procedure, known as the *Tzanck test,* is performed by unroofing an intact vesicle, gently scraping the base with a curved scalpel blade, and smearing the contents on a slide. After air drying, the smear is stained with Wright's or Giemsa's stain and examined for acantholytic cells, giant acanthocytes, and/or multinucleated giant cells.

2. *Viral culture,* negative stain for infections with herpes viruses.

3. *Gram's stain of aspirates or scraping.* This is essential for proper diagnosis of pustules. Organisms can be seen in the lesions of acute meningococcemia, rarely in the skin lesions of gonococcemia and ecthyma gangrenosum.

4. *Touch preparation.* This is especially helpful in deep fungal infections and leishmaniasis. The dermal part of a skin biopsy specimen is touched repeatedly to a glass slice; the touch preparation is *immediately* fixed in 95% ethyl alcohol. Special stains are then performed and the slide examined for organisms in the cytology laboratory.

5. *Biopsy of the skin lesion.* All purpuric lesions should be biopsied. Inflammatory dermal nodules and most ulcers should be biopsied and a portion of tissue minced and cultured for bacteria and fungi. A 3- to 4-mm trephine and local anesthesia are used. In many laboratories the biopsy specimen can be processed within 8 hours if necessary.

6. *Blood and urine examinations.* Blood culture, rapid serologic tests for syphilis, and serology for lupus erythematosus require 24 hours. Examination of urine sediment may reveal red cell casts in allergic vasculitis.

7. *Dark-field examination.* In the skin lesions of secondary syphilis, repeated examination of papules may show *Treponema pallidum*. The dark-field examination is not reliable in the mouth because nonpathogenic organisms are almost impossible to differentiate from *T pallidum*, but a lymph node aspirate can be subjected to dark-field examination.

Table 6-3 RASH AND FEVER IN THE ACUTELY ILL PATIENT: DIAGNOSIS ACCORDING TO TYPE OF LESION

Diseases Manifested by Macules, Papules, Nodules, or Plaques	Diseases Manifested by Vesicles, Bullae, or Pustules	Diseases Manifested by Purpuric Macules, Purpuric Papules, or Purpuric Vesicles	Diseases Manifested by Widespread Erythema ± Edema Followed by Desquamation	Diseases Manifested by Macules, Papules, Nodules, or Plaques
Drug hypersensitivities	Drug hypersensitivities	Drug hypersensitivities	Drug hypersensitivities	German measles
Sweet's syndrome	Allergic contact	Bacteremia[b]	Staphylococcal scalded-	(rubella)[c]
Eosinophilia-myalgia	dermatitis from plants	Meningococcemia	skin syndrome	Enterovirus infections
syndrome	Rickettsialpox	(acute or chronic)	Toxic shock syndrome	(echovirus and
				Coxsackie)
Streptococcal cellulitis	Gonococcemia	Gonococcemia	Kawasaki's syndrome	Adenovirus infections
Erythema migrans of	Varicella	Staphylococcemia	Toxic epidermal	Typhoid fever
Lyme disease	(chickenpox)[a]	*Pseudomonas*	necrolysis	Secondary syphilis
Meningococcemia	Herpes zoster	bacteremia	Graft-versus-host	Typhus, murine
HIV, primary infection	Herpes simplex[a]	Subacute bacterial	reaction	(endemic)
Erythema infectiosum	Eczema herpeticum[a]	endocarditis	von Zumbusch	Rocky Mountain spotted
(parvovirus B19)	Enterovirus infections	Enterovirus infections	pustular psoriasis	fever (early lesions)[c]
Cytomegalovirus,	(echovirus and	(echovirus and	Erythroderma	Other spotted fevers
primary infection	Coxsackie), including	Coxsackie)	(exfoliative dermatitis)	Disseminated deep fungal
Epstein-Barr virus,	hand-foot-and-mouth	Rickettsial diseases:	Cellulitis (streptococcal	infection in
primary infection	disease	Rocky Mountain	and staphylococcal)	immunocompromised
Exanthem subitum	Toxic epidermal	spotted fever		patients
(human herpesvirus	necrolysis	Typhus, louse-		Pityriasis rosea (fever,
type 6)	Staphylococcal scalded-	borne (epidemic)		rare)
Measles (rubeola)	skin syndrome	"Allergic" vasculitis[b]		Erythema multiforme
Measles (rubeola),	Erythema multiforme	Disseminated		Erythema marginatum
atypical	bullosum	intravascular		Systemic lupus
German measles	Kawasaki's disease	coagulation		erythematosus
(rubella)[c]		(purpura fulminans[d])		Dermatomyositis
Scarlet fever		Vibrio infections		"Serum sickness"
Still's disease				(manifested only as
Ehrlichiosis				wheals and
				angioedema)
				Urticaria, acute (viral
				hepatitis)
				Gianotti-Crosti
				syndrome

[a]One characteristic lesion of these exanthems is an umbilicated papule or vesicle.
[b]Often present as infarcts.
[c]May have arthralgia or musculoskeletal pain.
[d]Leading to large areas of black necrosis.

BENIGN NEOPLASMS AND HYPERPLASIAS

DISORDERS OF MELANOCYTES

Acquired Melanocytic Nevocellular Nevi

Melanocytic nevocellular nevi (NCN) are small (<1 cm), circumscribed, acquired pigmented macules, papules, or nodules composed of groups of melanocytic nevus cells located in the epidermis, dermis, and rarely, subcutaneous tissue.

EPIDEMIOLOGY

One of the most common acquired new growths in Caucasians (most adults have about 20 nevi), less common in blacks or pigmented persons, and sometimes absent in persons with red hair and marked freckling.

Race Blacks and Asians have more nevi on the palms, soles, nail beds.

Heredity Common acquired nevi occur in family clusters. Dysplastic nevi (Clark's nevi), which are putative precursor lesions of malignant melanoma, occur in virtually every patient with familial cutaneous melanoma and in 30 to 50% of patients with sporadic nonfamilial primary melanoma.

Sun Exposure A factor in the induction of nevi on the exposed areas.

Significance Risk of melanoma is related to the numbers of common nevi and to dysplastic nevi, even if only a few lesions are present.

HISTORY

Duration of Lesions These lesions, which are commonly called *moles,* appear in early childhood and reach a maximum in young adulthood. There is a gradual involution of lesions, and most disappear by age 60 (the dermal melanocytic NCN does not disappear). Dysplastic nevi continue to appear throughout life and are believed not to involute (see Section 10).

Skin Symptoms Nevocellular nevi are asymptomatic. If a lesion persistently itches or is tender, it should be followed carefully or excised, since *pruritus* may be an early indication of malignant change.

CLASSIFICATION

Nevocellular nevi can be classified according to the site of the clusters of nevus cells.

Junctional Melanocytic NCN Cells at the dermal-epidermal junction above the basement membrane (Fig. 7-1)
Compound Melanocytic NCN A combination of the histologic features of the junctional and dermal (Fig. 7-2)
Dermal Melanocytic NCN Cells exclusively in the dermis (Fig. 7-3)

EVOLUTION

Melanocytic NCN develop during childhood and usually have reached their final number by adolescence, even though some NCN may arise during adulthood. NCN undergo a predetermined evolution, which usually results in involution and fibrosis in time.

1. *Junctional melanocytic NCN:* These arise at the dermal-epidermal junction, on the epidermal site of the basement membrane; in other words, they are intraepidermal.
2. *Compound melanocytic NCN:* Nevus cells invade the papillary dermis, and nevus cell nests are now found both intraepidermally and dermally.
3. *Dermal melanocytic NCN:* These represent the last stage of the evolution of NCN.

"Dropping off" (*Abtropfung*) into the dermis is now completed, and the nevus grows or remains intradermal. With progressive age, there will be gradual fibrosis.

Since common melanocytic NCN lose their capacity for melanization the further the nevus cells penetrate into the dermis, the lesser is the intensity of pigmentation with the increase in the dermal proportion of the nevus. Purely dermal NCN are therefore almost always without pigment.

Junctional Melanocytic Nevocellular Nevi

Skin Lesions Macule, or only very slightly raised (Fig. 7-1) If >1 cm, the mole is a congenital nevomelanocytic nevus or a dysplastic nevus. Uniform tan, brown, or dark brown. Round or oval with smooth, regular borders. Scattered discrete lesions.

Distribution Random, but predilection for the sun-exposed areas. Trunk, upper extremities, face, lower extremities, occasionally palmar and plantar.

DIFFERENTIAL DIAGNOSIS

Tan/Brown/Black Macule Solar lentigo, lentigo maligna, dyplastic nevus.

Compound Melanocytic Nevocellular Nevi

Compound melanocytic NCN represent a combination of junctional and dermal NCN and are usually darkly pigmented, elevated, and may be nodular due to the dermal component.

Skin Lesions Papules or nodules (Fig. 7-2). Dark brown, sometimes even black; color may become mottled as progressive conversion into dermal NCN occurs. Round, dome-shaped, smooth, occasionally papillomatous or hyperkeratotic. May have hairs.

Distribution Face, trunk, extremities, scalp.

DIFFERENTIAL DIAGNOSIS

Tan/Brown/Black Papule Seborrheic keratosis, dermatofibroma, dysplastic nevus, Spitz nevus, blue nevus, and nodular melanoma.

Figure 7-1 Junctional nevomelanocytic nevus *Two uniformly brown small macules, round in shape with smooth regular borders.*

Dermal Melanocytic Nevocellular Nevi

Skin Lesions Papule or nodule. Skin-colored, tan, brown, or flecks of brown, often with telangiectasia. Round, dome-shaped (Fig. 7-3).

Distribution More common on the face and neck but can occur on the trunk or extremities.

Other Features Usually present in the second or third decade. Older lesions, mostly on the trunk, may become papillomatous or pedunculated and do not disappear spontaneously. May be hairy.

DIFFERENTIAL DIAGNOSIS

Skin-Colored Papule Basal cell carcinoma, neurofibroma, trichoepithelioma, sebaceous hyperplasia, dermatofibroma.

MANAGEMENT

Indications for removal of acquired melanocytic NCN are the following:

Site Lesions on the scalp (difficult to follow), mucous membranes, anogenital area.

Color If color is or becomes variegated.

Border If irregular borders are present or develop.

Symptoms If lesion begins to persistently itch, hurt, or bleed.

If criteria for melanoma or very atypical dysplastic nevus are detected by epiluminescence microscopy.

Melanocytic NCN rarely become malignant because of manipulation or trauma. If there is an indication for the removal of an NCN, the nevus always should be excised for histologic diagnosis and for definite treatment (particularly applicable to and decisive in ruling out congenital, dysplastic, or blue nevi).

Removal of papillomatous, compound, or dermal NCN for cosmetic reasons by electrocautery requires that a nevus be unequivocally diagnosed as benign NCN and histology be performed. If an early melanoma cannot be excluded with certainty, an excision for histologic examination is obligatory but can be performed with narrow margins.

The criteria listed above are based on anatomic sites at risk for change of acquired nevi to malignant melanoma or changes in individual lesions (color, border) that indicate the development of a focus of cells with dysplasia, the precursor of malignant melanoma. Clark's dysplastic melanocytic nevi may become usually > 6 mm, with distinctive variegation of color (tan, brown) and irregular borders. These lesions occur over the trunk and upper extremities but also on the buttocks, groin, scalp, and female breasts and may arise de novo during adulthood.

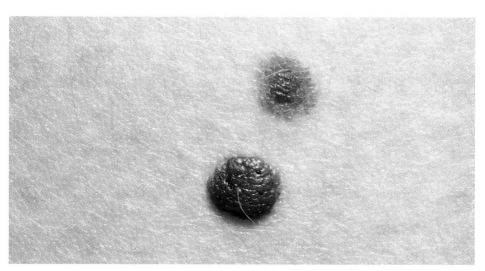

Figure 7-2   Compound nevomelanocytic nevus   *Uniformly pigmented papule and domed nodule, tan (with a more elevated, darker center) and chocolate brown, dark brown to sometimes black papules. The larger lesion is older; the smaller is younger and has a predominantly junctional component at the periphery.*

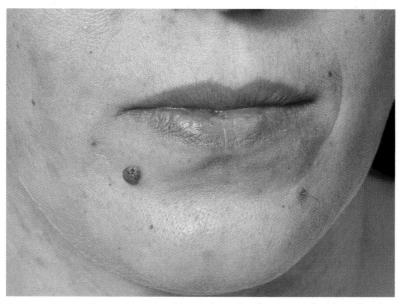

Figure 7-3   Dermal nevomelanocytic nevus   *Dome-shaped, soft, tan papule. A smaller dermal nevus is seen on the opposite side.*

Halo Nevomelanocytic Nevus

This lesion is a nevomelanocytic nevus that is encircled by a halo of leukoderma or depigmentation. The leukoderma is based on a decrease of melanin in melanocytes or disappearance of melanocytes at the dermal-epidermal junction. Halo nevi often undergo spontaneous involution, often with regression of the centrally located pigmented nevus.

Synonym: Sutton's leukoderma acquisitum centrifugum.

EPIDEMIOLOGY

Age of Onset First three decades.

Incidence Occurs in patients with vitiligo (18 to 26%). May herald vitiligo.

Race and Sex All races, both sexes.

Family History Halo nevi occur in siblings and with history of vitiligo in family.

Associated Disorders Vitiligo, metastatic melanoma (around metastatic lesions and around NCN). The leukoderma that occurs in patients with melanoma may surround a nevus.

PATHOGENESIS

Immunologic phenomena are responsible for the dynamic changes through the action of circulating cytotoxic antibodies and/or cytotoxic lymphocytes. This phenomenon awaits a reevaluation with newer techniques.

HISTORY

Three Stages

1. Development (in months) of halo around preexisting NCN. Halo may be preceded by faint erythema
2. Disappearance (months to years) of NCN
3. Repigmentation (months to years) of halo

PHYSICAL EXAMINATION

Skin Lesions Papular brown NCN (5 mm) with halo of sharply marginated hypomelanosis (Fig. 7-4). The nevus is *centrally* located. Oval or round hypomelanosis. Scattered discrete lesions (1 to 90).

Distribution Trunk (same as distribution of NCN)

DIFFERENTIAL DIAGNOSIS

"Halo" Depigmentation around Other Lesions Can occur around blue nevus, congenital garment NCN, Spitz's juvenile nevus, verruca plana, primary melanoma, dermatofibroma, and neurofibroma.

LABORATORY EXAMINATIONS

Dermatopathology Junctional dermal or compound nevus surrounded by lymphocytic infiltrate (lymphocytes and histiocytes) around and between nevus cells. Nevus cells develop evidence of cell damage and disappear. "Halo" shows decrease or total absence of melanin and melanocytes (as shown by electron microscopy).

DIAGNOSIS

If clinical findings atypical: the nevus has variegation of color and/or irregular borders, confirm histologically.

COURSE

The lesions undergo spontaneous resolution, in stages: first the nevus becomes depigmented and then disappears, then the halo becomes repigmented to a normal skin color. Nevus cell nevi within the halo always must be evaluated for clinical criteria of malignancy (variegation of pigment and irregular borders) because a halo can and does occasionally develop around primary malignant melanoma.

MANAGEMENT

Reassurance.

Excision If the features of the nevus are atypical: variegation of color, irregular borders.

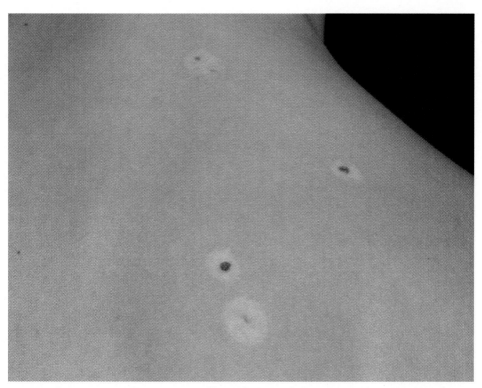

Figure 7-4   Halo nevomelanocytic nevus   *White depigmented halos surround several compound nevomelanocytic nevi on the upper back; in time, the nevus may disappear leaving only the white macular portion.*

Blue Nevus

A blue nevus is an acquired, benign, firm, dark-blue to gray-to-black, sharply defined papule or nodule representing a localized proliferation of melanin-producing dermal melanocytes.
Synonyms: Blue neuronevus, dermal melanocytoma.

EPIDEMIOLOGY

Age of Onset Childhood and late adolescence.

Sex Equal distribution.

Variants Three types: common blue nevus, cellular blue nevus, combined blue nevus–nevomelanocytic nevus.

PATHOGENESIS

Probably represents accumulations of melanin-producing melanocytes in the dermis during their migration from neural crest to sites in the skin.

HISTORY

Nearly always asymptomatic, occasionally of cosmetic concern.

PHYSICAL EXAMINATION

Skin Lesions Papules to nodules usually 10 mm in diameter (Fig. 7-5). Cellular nevi are larger (1 to 3 cm). Blue, blue-gray, blue-black. Occasionally has target-like pattern of pigmentation. Usually round to oval.

Sites of Predilection Most commonly small lesions are located on the dorsa of hands or feet (50%); cellular blue nevi occur on the buttocks, lower back, scalp and face.

DIFFERENTIAL DIAGNOSIS

Blue/Gray Papule Dermatofibroma, glomus tumor, primary (nodular) or metastatic mela-

noma, pigmented spindle cell (Spitz) nevus, traumatic tattoo, angiokeratoma, pigmented basal cell carcinoma.

LABORATORY EXAMINATIONS

Dermatopathology Melanin-containing wavy dermal melanocytes with long thin dendrites grouped in irregular bundles admixed with melanin-containing macrophages in the upper or middle dermis: excessive fibrous tissue production in upper reticular dermis. Epidermis normal.

DIAGNOSIS

Usually made on clinical findings, at times confirmed by excision and dermatopathologic examination to rule out nodular melanoma.

COURSE AND PROGNOSIS

Most remain unchanged. Malignant melanoma rarely develops in blue nevi.

MANAGEMENT

Blue nevi smaller than 10 mm in diameter and stable for many years usually do not need excision. Sudden appearance or change of an apparent blue nevus warrants surgical excision and dermatopathologic examination. Cellular blue nevi (1 to 3 cm) are usually excised to rule out melanoma.

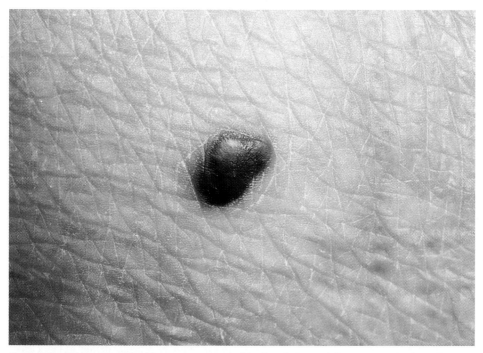

Figure 7-5 Blue nevus *The blue nevus presented in the photograph has some quite irregular borders and is solidly blue-black in color. Therefore, the differential diagnosis must include nodular melanoma. If the lesion has been present for years, then biopsy is not necessary; if the lesion was noted only a few months ago, excision biopsy is required to rule out nodular melanoma. Epiluminescence microscopy greatly facilitates clinical differential diagnosis.*

Spitz Nevus

Spitz nevus is a benign, dome-shaped, hairless, small (<1 cm in diameter) nodule, most often pink or tan. The clinical presentation is distinctive, and there is often a history of recent rapid growth. However, the pathology of Spitz nevus is misleading, consisting of spindle and epithelioid nevus cells, some of which may be atypical. Differentiation from nodular malignant melanoma may require the help of a dermatopathologist who is familiar with pigment-cell neoplasms.

Synonyms: Pigmented and epithelioid spindle-cell nevus.

EPIDEMIOLOGY

Age of Onset Occurs at all ages. A third of the patients are children younger than 10 years, a third are 10 to 20 years old, and a third are older than 20; rarely seen in persons 40 years of age or older.

Incidence 1.4:100,000 (Australia).

HISTORY

Onset of Lesions Recent (within months). The large majority of the lesions (> 90%) are acquired.

Skin Symptoms None.

PHYSICAL EXAMINATION

Skin Lesions Papule or dome-shaped or relatively flat nodule, smooth-topped, hairless. Uniform pink (Fig. 7-6), tan, brown, dark brown (Fig. 7-7). Firm nodule. Round, dome-shaped, well-circumscribed.

Distribution Head and neck.

DIFFERENTIAL DIAGNOSIS

Pink or Tan Papule The tumor is deeply pigmented, and often surrounded by a lighter brown regular rim. Other lesions in the differential diagnosis are pyogenic granuloma, hemangioma, molluscum contagiosum, juvenile xanthogranuloma, mastocytoma, dermatofibroma, atypical melanocytic nevi, nodular melanoma, and dermal melanocytic nevus.

LABORATORY EXAMINATIONS

Dermatopathology

Hyperplasia of epidermis, and of melanocytes, dilatation of capillaries. Admixed large epithelioid cells, large spindle cells with abundant cytoplasm, occasional mitotic figures; there are sometimes bizarre cytologic patterns; nests of large cells extend from the epidermis ("raining down") into the reticular dermis as fascicles of cells form an "inverted triangle," with the base lying at the dermal epidermal junction and the apex in the reticular dermis.

DIAGNOSIS

Although the clinical appearance and recent growth are characteristic of a Spitz nevus, histologic examination must be done to confirm the clinical diagnosis.

COURSE AND PROGNOSIS

Excision in its entirety is important because the condition recurs in 10 to 15% of all cases in lesions that have not been excised completely. This tumor poses some special problems in cytologic diagnosis. Atypical lesions are worrisome. Although most Spitz nevi are benign,

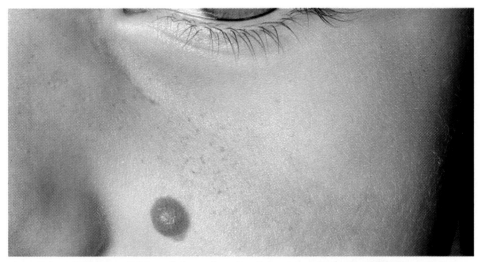

Figure 7-6 Spitz nevus *Bright red dome-shaped nodule on the cheek of a child, developing abruptly within the previous few months; the lesion is easily mistaken for a hemangioma.*

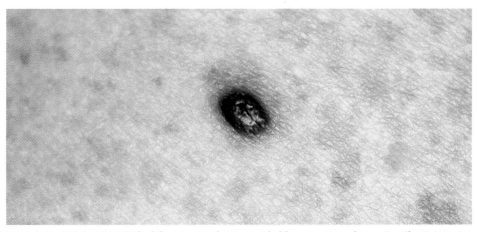

Figure 7-7 Spitz nevus *A dark brown papule surrounded by a tan macular region (lentiginous) developed within a few months on the back of a young female; the lesion was excised and the diagnosis confirmed histologically. The differential diagnosis includes superficial spreading and nodular melanoma.*

there can be a histologic similarity between Spitz nevi and melanoma. Also, atypical Spitz nevi can occur and even have occasional "metastases" from such lesions. Melanoma has been reported to arise rarely in Spitz nevi.

Spitz tumors probably do not involute, as do common acquired nevomelanocytic nevi. However, some lesions have been observed to transform into common compound NCN, some undergo fibrosis and in late stages may resemble dermatofibromas.

MANAGEMENT

Excision with a border of 5 mm. Follow-up in 6 to 12 months is advised, especially for atypical lesions.

Nevus Spilus

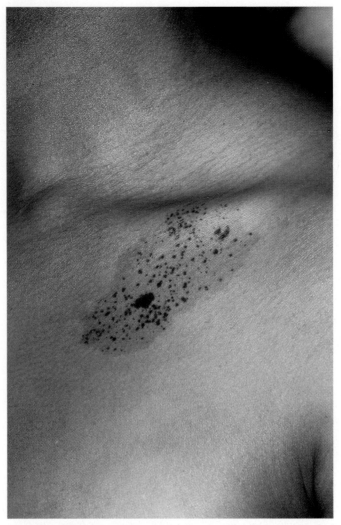

Figure 7-8 **Nevus spilus** *This is a rather common disorder of melanocyte morphology that consists of a varying-sized, light brown pigmented macule from a few centimeters to a very large area (>15 cm); the distinctive feature of this lesion is the many dark brown small macules (2 to 3 mm) or papules scattered throughout the pigmented background. The term* spilus *(Latin: "spot") refers to these spots. These can be either flat (macules) or slightly raised (papules). The pathology of the background of the macular pigmented lesion is the same as lentigo simplex, i.e., increased numbers of melanocytes, while the flat or raised lesions scattered throughout are either junctional or compound nevi. Rarely, these are dysplastic melanocytic junctional or compound nevi. The lesions are not as common as junctional or compound nevi but are not at all rare. In one series in a large dermatology practice, the nevus spilus was present in 3% of white patients. Malignant melanoma very rarely arises in these lesions.*

Mongolian Spot

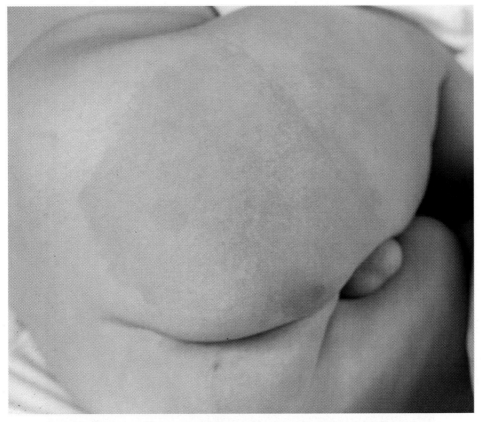

Figure 7-9 Mongolian spot *These* congenital *gray-blue macular lesions, which are characteristically located on the lumbosacral area, also can occur on the scalp or anywhere on the skin. There is usually a single lesion, but rarely, several truncal lesions can be present at birth. Melanocytes are not normally present in the dermis, and it is believed that these ectopic melanocytes represent pigment cells that have been interrupted in their migration from the neural crest to the epidermis. Mongolian spots disappear in early childhood, in contrast to Nevus of Ota (Figure 7–10). As the term* Mongolian *implies, these lesions are found almost always (99 to 100%) in infants of Asiatic and Amerindian origin; however, they have been reported in black and, rarely, in white infants. No melanomas have been reported to occur in these lesions.*

Nevus of Ota

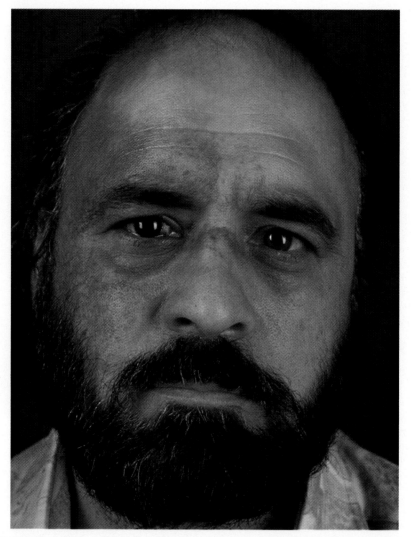

Figure 7-10   Nevus of Ota   *This pigmentary disorder is very common in Asiatic populations and is said to occur in 1% of outpatient visits in Japan. It has been reported in East Indians, blacks, and, rarely, whites. The pigmentation, which can be quite subtle or markedly disfiguring, consists of a mottled, dusky admixture of blue and brown hyperpigmentation of the skin. The pigmentation mostly involves the skin and mucous membranes innervated by the first and second branches of the trigeminal nerve. The blue hue results from the presence of ectopic melanocytes in the dermis. It can occur in the hard palate, and in the conjunctivae, sclerae, and tympanic membranes. It may be congenital but is not hereditary; more often it appears in early childhood or during puberty and remains for life, in contrast to the Mongolian spot, which disappears in early childhood. Treatment with lasers is an effective new modality for this disfiguring disorder. Malignant melanoma can occur but is rare.*

BENIGN NEOPLASMS AND HYPERPLASIAS

DISORDERS OF BLOOD VESSELS

CLASSIFICATION OF VASCULAR "BIRTHMARKS"[1]

Hemangiomas of Infancy (Strawberry Nevus, Angiomatous Nevus)

Benign vascular proliferations of endothelial lining that undergo spontaneous involution.

Vascular Malformations

Capillary Malformations (Nevus Flammeus or Port-Wine Stain) Capillary malformations that do not undergo spontaneous involution.

Venous Malformations (Cavernous Hemangioma) Venous malformations *without* endothelial proliferation, and may be combinations of capillaries, veins, arteries, lymphatics; these disorders do not undergo spontaneous involution.

Capillary Hemangioma of Infancy

A capillary hemangioma of infancy (CHI) is a soft, bright-red to deep-purple, vascular nodule-to-plaque that develops at birth or soon after birth and disappears spontaneously by the fifth year. *Synonyms:* Nevus or mark, angiomatous nevus.

EPIDEMIOLOGY

Incidence 1 to 2%.

PATHOGENESIS

CHI is a localized proliferation of angioblastic mesenchyme.

HISTORY

Duration of Lesions Lesion appears as a pale patch within the first month of life in most patients and always by the ninth month. They enlarge rapidly during the first year.

PHYSICAL EXAMINATION

Skin Lesions Nodule, plaque, 1 to 8 cm (Fig. 7-11). With the onset of spontaneous regression, a white-to-gray area appears on the surface of the central part of the lesion. Ulceration may occur with rapid regression. Ulcerated lesions may become secondarily infected. Multiple CHI may be associated with hemangiomas of CNS, GI tract, and/or liver. Often resolve with minimal scarring. The superficial CHI is bright red (Fig. 7-11); the deeper CHI is purple and lobulated. Soft or moderately firm, depending on the proportionate amounts of vascular and fibrous elements. On diascopy, does not blanch completely.

Distribution Localized or extending over an entire region. Head and neck 50%, trunk 25%. Face, trunk, legs, oral mucous membrane.

DIFFERENTIAL DIAGNOSIS

Red/Purple Nodule/Tumor/Plaque The distinction between a CHI and a *cavernous angioma* is based on color and depth. Mixed angiomas (both superficial and deep) may occur.

LABORATORY EXAMINATIONS

Dermatopathology Proliferation of endothelial cells in various amounts in the dermis and/or subcutaneous tissue; there is more endothelial proliferation in the superficial type and little or no endothelial proliferation in the deep angiomas.

[1]This classification was proposed by Mulliken and Glowacki as a more rational basis for these disorders (JB Mulliken, J Glowacki; Hemangioma and vascular malformation in infants and children: A clarification based on endothelial characteristics. Plast Reconstr Surg 69:412, 1982).

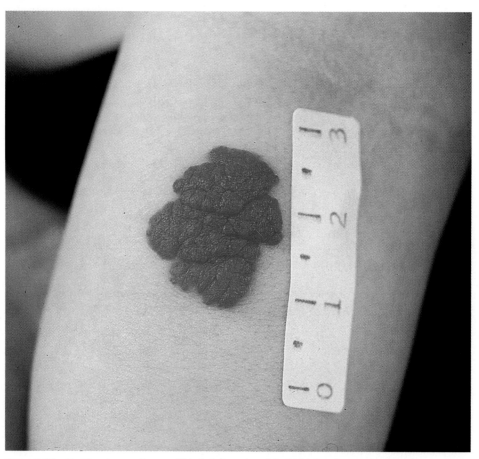

Figure 7-11 Capillary hemangioma *This bright red nodule is frightening to the parents, but caution is needed to prevent scarring from the treatment itself. The lesions disappear spontaneously, with only 20% there can be residual atrophy, depigmentation.*

DIAGNOSIS

Made on clinical findings and MRI.

COURSE AND PROGNOSIS

CHI spontaneously involutes by the fifth year, with some few percent disappearing only by age 10 (Figs. 7-12 A and 7-12 B). There is virtually no residual skin change at the site in most lesions (80%); in the rest there is residual atrophy, depigmentation, and infiltration. Deeper lesions, especially those involving mucous membranes, may not involute completely. Synovial involvement may be associated with hemophilia-like arthropathy. Large CHI, usually associated with cavernous hemangiomas, may have platelet entrapment, thrombocytopenia (Kasabach-Merritt syndrome) and even disseminated intravascular coagulation. Rarely, morbidity associated with CHI occurs secondary to hemorrhage or high-output heart failure.

MANAGEMENT

Each lesion must be judged individually regarding the decision to treat or not to treat and the selection of a treatment mode. Surgical and medical interventions include continuous wave or pulsed dye laser, cryosurgery, and systemic glucocorticoids. When possible, treatment should be avoided because spontaneous resolution gives the best cosmetic results (Fig. 7-12).

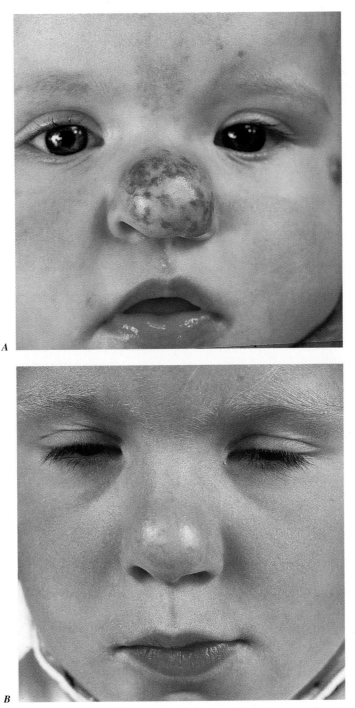

Figure 7-12 Capillary hemangioma *Most lesions disappear without therapy of any type, by the fifth year as in this child.*

Port-Wine Stain

A port-wine stain (PWS) is an irregularly shaped, red or violaceous, macular, vascular malformation of dermal blood vessels that is present at birth and never disappears spontaneously except for the salmon patch (see below); the malformation is usually confined to the skin but may be associated with vascular malformations in the eye and leptomeninges (Sturge-Weber syndrome). *Synonym:* Nevus flammeus.

EPIDEMIOLOGY

Age of Onset Congenital.

Incidence .3%.

Clinical Variants

Nevus flammeus nuchae ("stork bite," erythema nuchae, salmon patch) occurs in approximately one-third of infants on the nape of the neck and tends to regress spontaneously. Similar lesions occur on eyelids and glabella.
Sturge-Weber syndrome (SWS) is the association of PWS with vascular malformations in the eye (glaucoma) and leptomeninges and superficial calcifications of the brain.
Klippel-Trénaunay-Weber syndrome may have an associated PWS overlying the deeper vascular malformation of soft tissue and bone.
PWS on the midline back may be associated with an underlying arteriovenous malformation of the spinal cord.

HISTORY

Skin Symptoms None.

Systemic Symptoms SWS may be associated with contralateral hemiparesis, muscular hemiatrophy, epilepsy, mental retardation; glaucoma and ocular palsy may occur.

PHYSICAL EXAMINATION

Skin Lesions In infancy and childhood, PWS are macular (Fig. 7-13). With increasing age of the patient, papules or nodules (Fig. 7-14) often develop, leading to significant disfigurement. Varying hues of pink to purple (Figs. 7-13 and 7-14). Large lesions follow a dermatomal distribution and rarely cross the midline.

Distribution Unilateral (85%) (Fig. 7-13) but not always (Fig. 7-14). Most commonly involve the face but may occur at any cutaneous site. In SWS, PWS occurs in the distribution of the trigeminal nerve, usually the superior and middle branches; mucosal involvement of conjunctiva and mouth may occur. PWS in trigeminal distribution is common and does not necessarily indicate the presence of SWS.

DIAGNOSIS

Made on clinical findings. All patients should be screened for glaucoma and for CNS involvement.

LABORATORY EXAMINATIONS

Dermatopathology Developmental defect leading to ectasia of capillaries. No proliferation of endothelial cells.

Imaging In SWS, skull x-rays show characteristic calcifications of angiomas or localized linear calcification along cerebral convolutions. CT scan should be done.

COURSE AND PROGNOSIS

PWSs do not regress spontaneously. The area of involvement tends to increase in proportion to the size of the child. In adulthood, PWSs usually become raised with papular and nodular areas and are the cause of significant progressive cosmetic disfigurement (Fig. 7-14).

MANAGEMENT

During the macular phase, PWS can be covered with makeup such as Covermark. Treatment with tunable dye or copper vapor lasers is very effective.

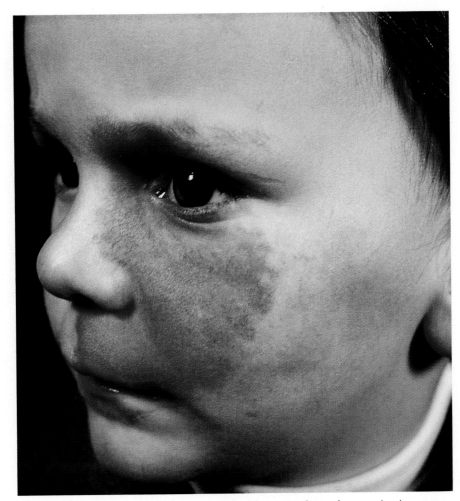

Figure 7-13 Port-wine stain *Sharply marginated, port-wine red macule occurring in a distribution of the second branch (maxillary) of the trigeminal nerve in a young child.*

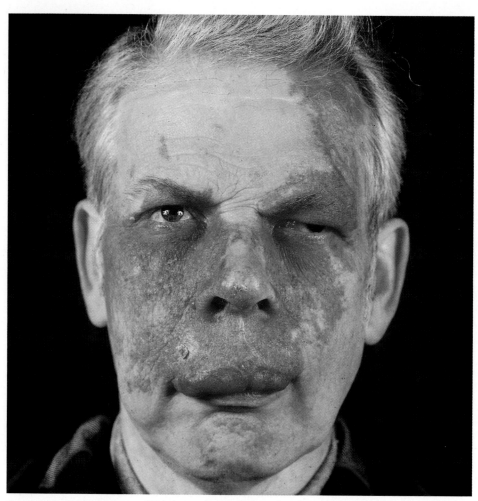

Figure 7-14   Port-wine stain   *With increasing age, the color deepens and papular and nodular hemangiomas develop within the previously macular lesion causing progressively increasing disfigurement.*

Capillary/Venous/Lymphatic (CVL) Malformations

CVL malformations are deep vascular malformations, characterized by soft compressible deep-tissue swelling, which, at times, is associated with varicosities, arteriovenous shunts, and nevus flammeus-like changes.

Synonym: Cavernous hemangioma.

EPIDEMIOLOGY

Age of Onset Lesions are not apparent at birth but become so during childhood.

HISTORY

Lesions usually asymptomatic. Limb hypertrophy may interfere with function.

PHYSICAL EXAMINATION

Skin Lesions Soft tissue swelling, dome-shaped or multinodular (Fig. 7-15). When vascular malformation extends to the epidermis, surface may be verrucous. Borders poorly defined. Considerable variation in size. Often, normal skin color. Nodular portion blue to purple. Easily compressed, fills promptly when pressure released. Some types may be tender.

Variants

Vascular Hamartomas CVL with deep soft-tissue involvement and resultant swelling or diffuse enlargement of extremity. May involve skeletal muscle with muscle atrophy. Cutaneous changes include dilated tortuous veins and arteriovenous fistulas.

Klippel-Trénaunay-Weber Syndrome Local overgrowth of soft tissue and bone with resultant enlargement of an extremity. Associated cutaneous changes include phlebectasia, arteriovenous aneurysms, and nevus flammeus-like cutaneous telangiectasia. Associated developmental abnormalities: nevus unius lateris, syndactylism, polydactylism.

Blue Rubber Bleb Nevus Spontaneously painful and/or tender, compressible, soft, blue swelling in dermis and subcutaneous tissue. Size ranges from a few millimeters to several centimeters. May exhibit localized hyperhidrosis over CVL. Occur, often multiply, on trunk and upper arms. Similar vascular lesions can occur in GI tract and may be a source of hemorrhage.

Marfucci's Syndrome CVL associated with dyschondroplasia, manifested as hard nodules on fingers or toes, bony deformities. Some CVL may be blue rubber bleb variant.

DIAGNOSIS

Clinical diagnosis, at times confirmed by arteriography.

LABORATORY EXAMINATIONS

Dermatopathology Dilated, blood-filled vascular spaces lined with flattened endothelial cells. Vessels may be of cavernous, capillary, venous, and lymphatic types.

COURSE AND PROGNOSIS

CVL may be complicated by ulceration and bleeding, scarring, secondary infection, and high-output heart failure in large lesions. Platelet sequestration and destruction may result in thrombocytopenia (Kasabach-Merritt syndrome) in mucous membranes of mouth, pharynx, and larynx. May interfere with food intake or breathing. If located on eyelids or vicinity of eyes, it will obstruct vision in an instant and may lead to blindness.

MANAGEMENT

There is no satisfactory treatment except compression. In larger lesions—if organ function is compromised—surgical procedures, intravascular coagulation. High-dose systemic glucocorticoids, interferon-α, may be effective.

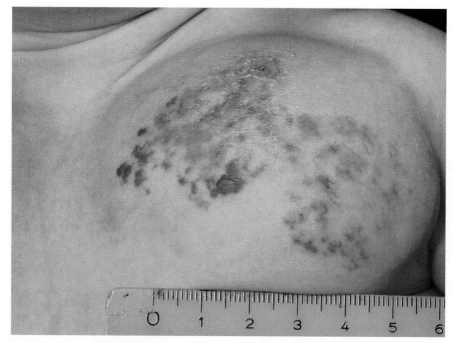

Figure 7-15 Cavernous hemangioma *Large, soft, hemispheric blue-tinged swelling of the dermis and subcutaneous tissue; superficial telangiectases are present in the upper dermis.*

Venous Lake

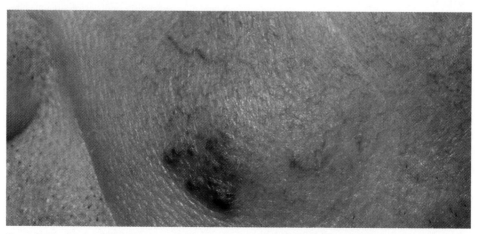

Figure 7-16 Venous lake *A venous lake is a dark blue to violaceous, asymptomatic, soft papule resulting from a dilated venule, occurring on the face, lips, and ears of patients over 50 years of age. The etiology is unknown, although it has been thought to be related to solar exposure. These lesions are few in number and remain for years. The lesion results from a dilated cavity lined with a single layer of flattened endothelial cells and a thin wall of fibrous tissue filled with red blood cells. The lesion may be confused with nodular melanoma or pyogenic granuloma. The use of epiluminescence microscopy permits an easy diagnosis as a vascular lesion and not a pigment cell neoplasm such as a melanoma. The management is for cosmetic reason and can be accomplished with electrosurgery or laser or, rarely, with surgical excision.*

Cherry Angioma

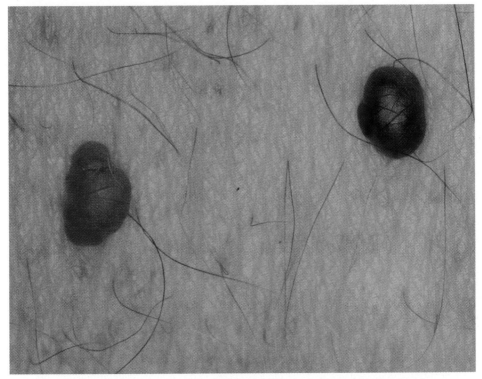

Figure 7-17 Cherry angioma Synonyms: *Campbell de Morgan spots, senile (hem)angioma. Cherry angiomas are exceedingly common, asymptomatic, bright-red to violaceous, domed vascular lesions, or they can occur as myriads of tiny red spots simulating petechiae. They are found principally on the trunk. The differential diagnosis includes angiokeratoma (especially on genital skin), venous lake, pyogenic granuloma, nodular melanoma, and metastatic carcinoma (especially hypernephroma) to skin. The lesions appear first at about 30 and increase in number over the years. The histology consists of numerous moderately dilated capillaries lined by flattened endothelial cells; stroma is edematous with homogenization of collagen. They are of no consequence other than their cosmetic appearance. Management is electro- or laser coagulation if indicated cosmetically for small lesions, excision for larger lesions. Cryosurgery is not effective.*

Spider Angioma

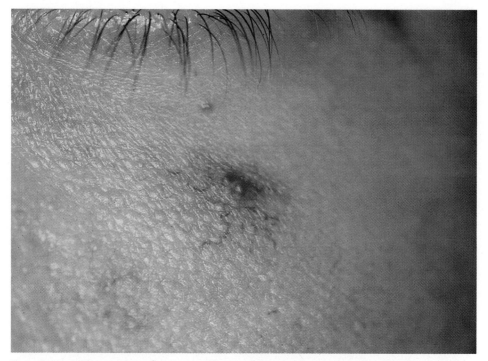

Figure 7-18 Spider angioma Synonyms: *Nevus araneus, spider nevus, arterial spider, spider telangiectasia, vascular spider. A spider angioma is red and is a focal telangiectatic network of dilated capillaries radiating from a central arteriole (punctum). The central papular punctum is the site of the feeding arteriole with macular radiating telangiectatic vessels. Up to 1.5 cm in diameter. Usually solitary. On diascopy, the radiating telangiectasia blanches and the central arteriole may pulsate. Most commonly occurs on the face, forearms, and hands. It not infrequently occurs in normal persons and is more common in females. It may be associated with hyperestrogenic states, such as pregnancy (one or more in two-thirds of pregnant women) or in patients receiving estrogen therapy, e.g., oral contraceptive use, or in hepatocellular disease such as subacute and chronic viral hepatitis and alcoholic cirrhosis. The lesion can occur in young children without any significance. Spider angioma arising in childhood and pregnancy may regress spontaneously. The lesion may be confused with hereditary hemorrhagic telangiectasia, ataxia-telangiectasia, or telangiectasia in systemic scleroderma. Lesions may be treated easily with electro- or laser surgery.*

Angiokeratoma

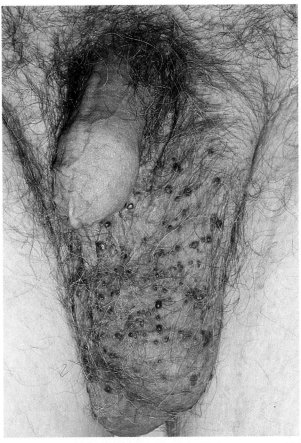

Figure 7-19 Angiokeratoma *The term* angio *("blood vessel")* keratoma *would imply a vascular tumor with keratotic elements. In fact, this term has been used to describe several quite distinctive conditions, each with its own characteristic features. The most common is* angiokeratoma of Fordyce; *this disease involves the scrotum and vulva; the lesions are dilated venules 4 mm in size and dark red in color, present in quite large numbers (Fig. 7-19);* Angiokeratoma of Mibelli *comprises pink to dark red papules that occur on the elbows, knees, and dorsa of the hands. This autosomal dominant disease is rare and occurs in young females.* Angiokeratoma corporis diffusum *(Fabry's disease), an X-linked recessive disease (virtually only occurring in males), is an inborn error of metabolism in which there is a deficiency of alpha-galactosidase A leading to an accumulation of neutral glycosphingolipid ceramide trihexoside in endothelial cells, fibrocytes, and pericytes in the dermis, heart, kidneys, and autonomic nervous system. The lesions of Fabry's disease are numerous dark red, punctate, and tiny (<1 mm), located on the lower half of the body: lower abdomen, genitalia, and buttocks, although lesions also may occur on the lips. The homozygous males have not only the skin lesions but also symptoms related to involvement of other organ systems: acroparesthesias, excruciating pain, transient ischemic attacks, and myocardial infarction. Heterozygous females may have corneal opacities.*

Pyogenic Granuloma

Pyogenic granuloma is a rapidly developing hemangioma, at times arising at sites of minor trauma, characterized as a solitary eroded vascular nodule that bleeds spontaneously or after minor trauma. *Synonym:* Granuloma telangiectaticum.

EPIDEMIOLOGY

Age of Onset <30 years old.

HISTORY

Duration of Lesions Days or months.

Skin Symptoms Recurrent bleeding from the lesion occurs frequently.

PHYSICAL EXAMINATION

Skin Lesions Nodule with smooth surface, with or without crusts, with or without erosion (Fig. 7-20). Bright red, dusky red, violaceous, brown-black. Less than 1.5 cm in diameter. Dome-shaped, sessile, or pedunculated. On palmar and soles: epidermal collarette at base; but also anywhere on the body.

Distribution Isolated single lesion: fingers, lips, mouth, trunk, toes.

DIFFERENTIAL DIAGNOSIS

Red Nodule Nodular malignant melanoma (especially amelanotic), squamous cell carcinoma, glomus tumor, nodular basal cell carcinoma, metastatic carcinoma, bacillary angiomatosis.

LABORATORY EXAMINATIONS

Dermatopathology Proliferation of capillaries with prominent endothelial cells embedded in edematous, gelatinous stroma; epidermis commonly eroded. Dense infiltrate of neutrophilia common.

DIAGNOSIS

Clinical findings confirmed by histologic findings. The need for histologic confirmation cannot be emphasized enough, especially to rule out amelanotic melanoma.

COURSE AND PROGNOSIS

Lesions persist for many months, bleeding frequently. A significant percentage of lesions treated with removal and ablation of the base recur, requiring additional therapy. Recurrence after surgical excision is uncommon.

MANAGEMENT

In that pyogenic granuloma cannot be distinguished from primary or secondary (metastatic) carcinoma or amelanotic melanoma, the lesion should be sent for histologic examination.

Surgical Excision The lesion can be excised surgically after removal of the major portion of the lesion by curettage, parallel-plane with a scalpel, or scissors excision (for histopathologic examination), the base of the lesion can be destroyed by electrodesiccation or (pulse-dye) laser surgery. Cosmetic results are excellent. In children, an eutectic mixture of local anesthetics (EMLA) should always be used.

Pyogenic Granuloma

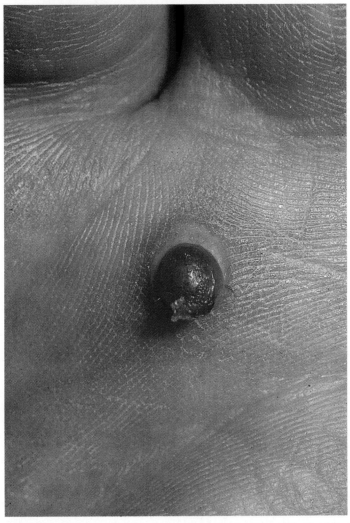

Figure 7-20   Pyogenic granuloma   *This is a solitary eroded vascular nodule that bleeds spontaneously or after minor trauma. The lesions have a smooth surface, with or without crusts, with or without erosion. They appear as bright red, dusky red, violaceous, brown-black, and occur on the fingers, lips, mouth, trunk, and toes.*

Glomus Tumor

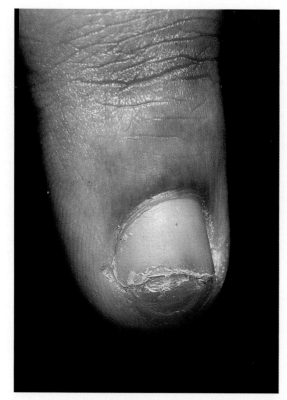

Figure 7-21 Glomus tumor Synonym: *glomangioma. This is a tumor of the* glomus body. *The* glomus body *is an anatomic and functional unit composed of specialized smooth muscle, the* glomus cells, *that surround thin-walled endothelial spaces; this anatomic unit functions as an A-V shunt linking arterioles and venules. The glomus cells surround the narrow lumen of the Sucquet-Hoyer canal that branches from the arteriole and leads to the collecting venule segment that acts as a reservoir. Glomus bodies are present on the pads and nail beds of the fingers and toes and also on the volar aspect of hands and feet, in the skin of the ears, and in the center of the face. The glomus tumor presents as an exquisitely tender subungual papule or nodule. Glomus tumors are characterized by paroxysmal painful attacks, especially elicited by exposure to cold. They are most often present as solitary* solid *subungual tumors but may rarely occur as multiple papules or nodules. These do not only occur under the nail but are noted, especially in children, as discrete papules or sometimes plaques anywhere on the skin surface. They are mostly vascular and not solid as are the solitary glomus tumors.*

Lymphatic Malformation (Lymphangioma)

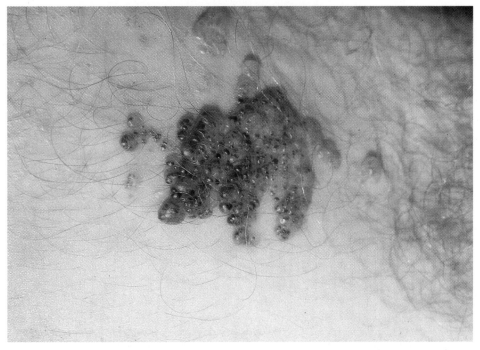

Figure 7-22 Lymphatic malformation (lymphangioma) *The term lymphatic malformation is the new terminology for what was formerly called "lymphangioma." These typical lesions are comprised of multiple small macroscopic vesicles filled with clear or serosanguinous fluid ("frog-spawn"). This is a microcystic lesion (lympangioma) as opposed to a macrocystic lesion (cystic hygroma) The lesion is present at birth or appears in infancy or even in childhood. It does not spontaneously disappear. Bacterial infection may occur. The lesion can be excised if feasible or treated with sclerotherapy.*

MISCELLANEOUS CYSTS AND PSEUDOCYSTS

Epidermoid Cyst

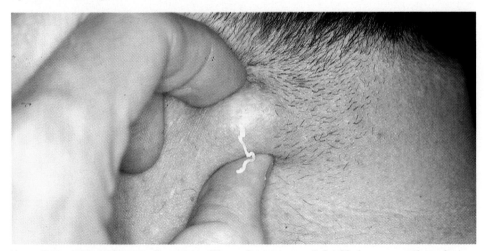

Figure 7-23   Epidermoid cyst   Synonyms: *Wen, sebaceous cyst, infundibular cyst, epidermal cyst. An epidermal cyst is the most common cutaneous cyst, derived from epidermis or the epithelium of the hair follicle, and is formed by cystic enclosure of epithelium within the dermis that becomes filled with keratin and lipid-rich debris; because of their thin walls, rupture is common and accompanied by a painful inflammatory mass. It occurs in young to middle-aged adults. The lesions occur on the face, neck, upper trunk, and scrotum. The lesion, which is usually solitary but may be multiple, is a dermal-to-subcutaneous nodule, .5 to 5 cm, which often connects with the surface by keratin-filled pores. The cyst has an epidermal-like wall (stratified squamous epithelium with well-formed granular layer); the content of the cyst is keratinaceous material— cream-colored with a pasty consistency and the odor of rancid cheese. Scrotal lesions may calcify. The cyst wall is relatively thin. Following rupture of the wall, the irritating cyst contents initiate an inflammatory reaction, enlarging the lesion manyfold; the lesion is now associated with a great deal of pain.*

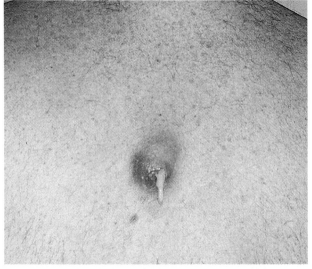

Figure 7-24   Epidermoid cyst
Ruptured cysts are often misdiagnosed as being infected rather than ruptured.

Trichilemmal Cyst

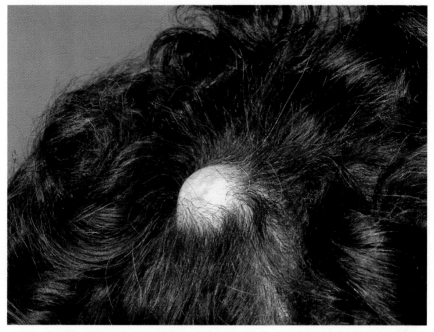

Figure 7-25 Trichilemmal cyst Synonyms: *Pilar cyst, isthmus catagen cyst.* Archaic terms: *Wen, sebaceous cyst. A trichilemmal cyst is the second most common type of cutaneous cyst (the most common being the epidermoid cyst) and is seen most often on the scalp and, in middle age, more frequently in females. It is often familial. Occurs frequently as multiple lesions. These are smooth, firm, dome-shaped, .5- to 5-cm nodules to tumors* (lacks the central punctum *seen in epidermoid cysts). Over 90% occur on the scalp, and the overlying scalp hair is usually normal but may be thinned if cyst is large. Not connected to epidermis. The cyst wall is usually thick; it can be removed intact. The wall is a stratified squamous epithelium with a palisaded outer layer resembling that of outer root sheath of hair follicle. The inner layer is corrugated without a granular layer. The cyst contains keratin, very dense, pink, homogeneous. Often calcified, cholesterol clefts. If cyst ruptures, may be inflamed and very painful.*

Epidermal Inclusion Cyst

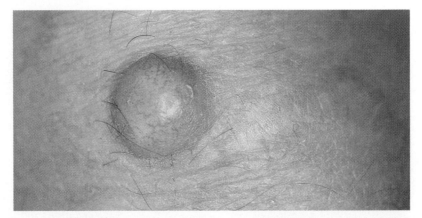

Figure 7-26 Epidermal inclusion cyst Synonym: *Traumatic epidermoid cyst. An epidermal inclusion cyst occurs secondary to traumatic implantation of epidermis within the dermis. Traumatically grafted epidermis grows in the dermis, with accumulation of keratin within the cyst cavity, enclosed in a stratified squamous epithelium with a well-formed granular layer. The lesion appears as a dermal nodule and most commonly occurs on the palms and soles. It should be excised.*

Milium

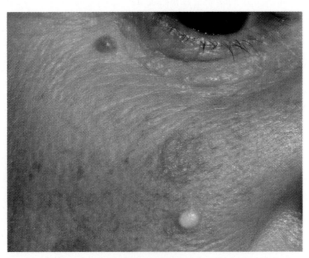

Figure 7-27 Milium *A milium is a 1- to 2-mm, superficial, white to yellow, keratin-containing epidermal cyst, occurring multiply, located on the eyelids, cheeks, and forehead in pilosebaceous follicles and at sites of trauma. The lesions can occur at any age, even in infants. Milia arise from pluripotential cells in epidermal or adnexal epithelium either de novo, especially around the eye, or in association with various dermatoses with subepidermal bullae or vesicles (pemphigoid, porphyria cutanea tarda, bullous lichen planus, epidermolysis bullosa) and skin trauma (abrasion, burns, dermabrasion, radiation therapy). Incision and expression of contents are the method of treatment.*

Digital Myxoid Cyst

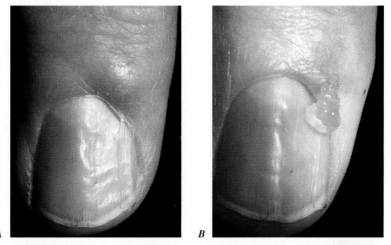

Figure 7-28   Digital myxoid cyst   Synonyms: *Mucous cyst, synovial cyst, myxoid pseudocyst. A digital myxoid cyst is a pseudocyst occurring over the distal interphalangeal joint and the base of the nail of the finger* (A) *or toe, often associated with Heberden's (osteophytic) node. The lesion occurs in older patients, usually >60 years of age. It is usually a solitary cyst, rubbery, translucent. A clear gelatinous viscous fluid may be extruded from the opening* (B). *When the myxoid cyst is over the nail matrix, a nail plate dystrophy occurs in the form of a 1- to 2-mm groove that extends to the length of the nail* (A). *The lesion is easy to recognize, but many physicians are not acquainted with the entity. Various methods of management have been advocated, including surgical excision, incision and drainage, injection of sclerosing material, and injection of a triamcinolone suspension. A simple and most effective method is to use firm compression (daily) of the lesion over a period of weeks.*

MISCELLANEOUS BENIGN NEOPLASMS AND HYPERPLASIAS

Seborrheic Keratosis

The seborrheic keratosis is perhaps the most common of the benign epithelial tumors. These lesions, which are hereditary, do not appear until age 30 and continue to occur over a lifetime, varying in extent from a few scattered lesions to literally thousands in some very elderly patients.

EPIDEMIOLOGY

Age of Onset   Rarely before 30 years.

Sex   Slightly more common and more extensive involvement in males.

Other Features   Probably autosomal dominant inheritance.

HISTORY

Duration of Lesions   Usually months to years.

Skin Symptoms   Rarely pruritic; tender if secondarily infected.

PHYSICAL EXAMINATION

Skin Lesions *Early*   Small, 1- to 3-mm, barely elevated papule or plaque (Figs. 7-29 and 7-30) with or without pigment. The surface often shows, with 7 to 10× magnification, fine stippling like the surface of a thimble. *Late*   Plaque with warty surface and "stuck on" appearance (Fig. 7-31), "greasy"; with a hand lens (7 to 10×), horn cysts often can be seen. Size from 1 to 6 cm. Nodule. Brown, gray, black, skin-colored. Round, oval. Scattered, discrete lesions.

Distribution   Isolated lesion or generalized. Face, trunk (Fig. 7-32), upper extremities.

DIFFERENTIAL DIAGNOSIS

"Tan Macules"   The early "flat" lesions of seborrheic keratosis may be confused with solar lentigo or spreading pigmented actinic keratosis (the surface of seborrheic keratosis is more verrucous; also, horn cysts are present).

Skin-Colored/Tan/Black Verrucous Papules/ Plaques   Larger pigmented lesions are easily mistaken for pigmented basal cell carcinoma or malignant melanoma (only biopsy will settle this or ELM will be of assistance in making a differential diagnosis, q.v.); verruca vulgaris may be similar in clinical appearance but thrombosed capillaries are present in verrucae.

LABORATORY EXAMINATIONS

Dermatopathology   Proliferation of keratinocytes (with marked papillomatosis) and melanocytes, formation of horn cysts. Some lesions can exhibit atypia of keratinocytes, mimicking Bowen's disease or squamous cell carcinoma, and these should be excised.

COURSE AND PROGNOSIS

The lesion starts as a *macule,* a skin-colored or light tan lesion (Fig. 7-29), and in the course of time becomes more pigmented; at this time the lesion has a "stuck on" appearance in the form of a *plaque* (Figs. 7-30 and 7-31); further on in their course, the surface appears "warty," and there are multiple plugged follicles or "horn cysts" that are very characteristic of seborrheic keratosis and are virtually pathognomonic of this lesion (Fig. 7-32).

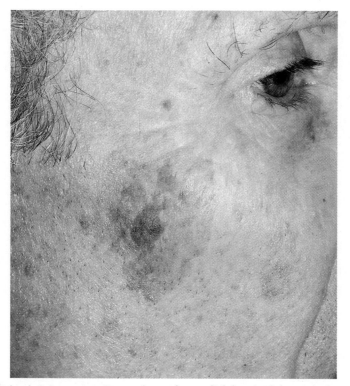

Figure 7-29   Seborrheic keratosis, solitary   *A very large, slightly raised, keratotic, brown, flat plaque on the zygomatic region in an older female. The differential diagnosis includes lentigo maligna and lentigo maligna melanoma.*

MANAGEMENT

Light electrocautery permits the whole lesion to appear to be easily rubbed off. Then the base can be lightly cauterized to prevent recurrence. This, however, precludes histopathologic verification of diagnosis and should be done only by an experienced diagnostician. Cryosurgery with liquid nitrogen spray is excellent, but recurrences are possibly more frequent. Best approach is curettage after slight freezing with cryosurgery; this also permits histopathologic examination. In solid black lesion without horn cysts a shave biopsy is mandatory to rule out malignant melanoma.

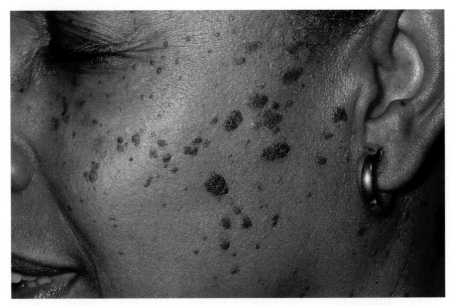

Figure 7-30   Seborrheic keratosis (dermatosis papulosa nigra)   *This consists of myriads of tiny black lesions, some enlarging to more than a centimeter. This is seen in Black Africans and African Americans. Treatment is a problem because white spots may be produced in lieu of the black papules.*

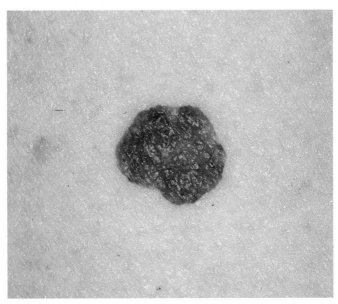

Figure 7-31   Seborrheic keratosis   *This has a "stuck on" appearance but is very dark and quite irregular and may pose a problem in the differential diagnosis of nodular melanoma. The examination with epiluminescence microscopy reveals "horn cysts" that are virtually (not 100%) pathognomonic of seborrheic keratosis. If in doubt, a shave biopsy should be obtained for diagnosis.*

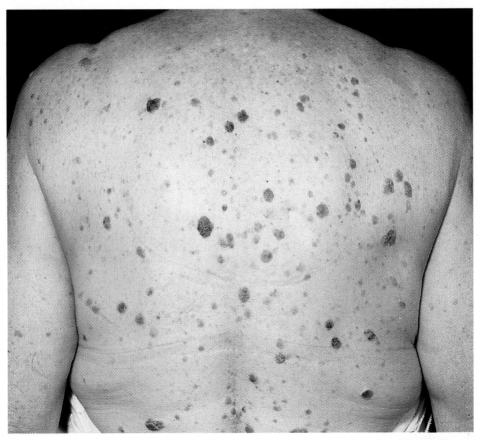

Figure 7-32 Seborrheic keratoses, multiple *Multiple brown, warty papules and nodules on the back, having a "stuck on" appearance.*

Keratoacanthoma

Keratoacanthoma (KA) is a special lesion, a pseudocancer, occurring as an isolated nodule, usually on the face. It presents as a dome-shaped nodule with a central keratinous plug that mimics squamous cell carcinoma. Unique features are its rapid growth rate, much faster than that of a squamous cell carcinoma, and also its spontaneous remission over a period of several months. Still, in every solitary KA, tissue must be obtained to rule out squamous cell carcinoma.

EPIDEMIOLOGY

Age of Onset   Over 50 years; rare below 20 years.

Sex   Male:female ratio 2:1.

PATHOGENESIS

HPV-9, -16, -19, -25, and -37 have been identified in keratoacanthomas. Other possible etiologic factors include ultraviolet radiation and chemical carcinogens (industrial: pitch and tar).

HISTORY

Onset   Rapid growth, achieving a size of 2.5 cm within a few weeks.

Duration of Lesions   Untreated, months to years.

Skin Symptoms   Usually none. Cosmetic disfigurement. Occasional tenderness.

PHYSICAL EXAMINATION

Skin Lesions   Nodule, dome-shaped, often with a central keratotic plug (Figs. 7-33 and 7-34). Skin-colored or slightly red, tan/brown. Firm but not hard. 2.5 cm (range 1 to 10 cm), round. Removal of keratotic plug results in a crater.

Distribution   Isolated single lesion. Uncommonly, may be multiple, eruptive. On exposed skin: cheeks, nose, ears, hands (dorsa).

DIFFERENTIAL DIAGNOSIS

Solitary KA   Squamous cell carcinoma (SCC), hypertrophic actinic keratosis, verruca vulgaris.

LABORATORY EXAMINATIONS

Dermatopathology   A representative biopsy that extends through the entire lesion to present the architecture of the nodule is required. Central, large, irregularly shaped crater filled with keratin. The surrounding epidermis extends in a liplike manner over the sides of the crater. The keratinocytes are atypical and many are dyskeratotic. Differentiation of KA from SCC may not be possible, in which case the lesion is best regarded and treated as SCC.

DIAGNOSIS

Clinical findings confirmed by dermatopathologic findings.

COURSE AND PROGNOSIS

Spontaneous regression in 2 to 6 months or sometimes more than 1 year.

MANAGEMENT

Surgery   Surgical excision is recommended in that KA cannot always be distinguished from SCC on clinical findings.

Multiple KAs   Systemic retinoids and methotrexate have been used.

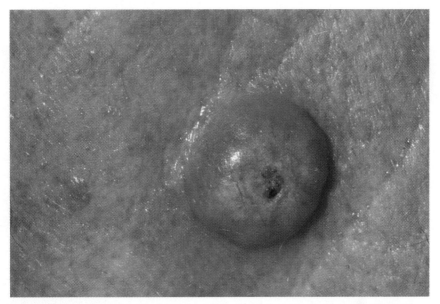

Figure 7-33 Keratoacanthoma *Erythematous, dome-shaped, tumor, 1 cm in diameter with a keratinaceous plug in the center, developing on facial skin exhibiting moderate dermatoheliosis.*

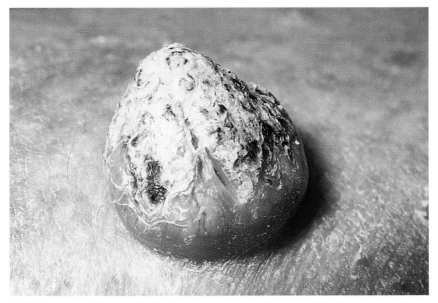

Figure 7-34 Keratoacanthoma *Erythematous, dome-shaped, tumor with a large, central, keratotic plug arising on the upper trunk and of 6-weeks duration. The lesion cannot be distinguished clinically from squamous cell carcinoma.*

Becker's Nevus

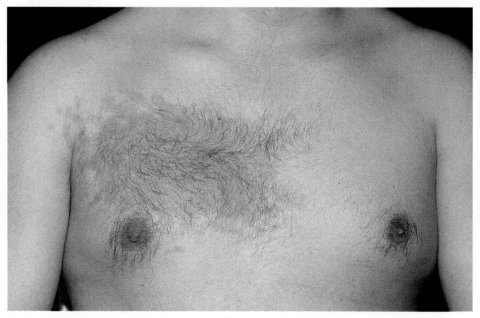

Figure 7-35 Becker's nevus *Becker's nevus (BN) is a distinctive asymptomatic clinical lesion that needs to be recognized by dermatologists and pediatricians. It is a pigmented hamartoma—that is, a developmental anomaly comprised of changes in pigmentation, hair growth, and most important, a slightly elevated smooth verrucous surface as part of the presentation. It occurs mostly in males, in all races. It appears not at birth but usually before 15 years of age and sometimes after age 15. The lesion is predominantly a macule but with a papular verrucous surface not unlike the lesion of acanthosis nigricans. It is light brown in color and has a geographic pattern (like the coast of Maine) with sharply demarcated borders. Commonest locations are the shoulders and the back. The increased hair growth follows the onset of the pigmentation and is localized to the areas that are pigmented. The pigmentation is related to increased melanin in basal cells and not to an increased number of melanocytes. It is differentiated from a hairy congenital melanocytic nevus because BN is not usually present at birth, and from Albright's pigmentation, which is also present at birth and there is no increased hair growth. The lesion extends for a year or two and then remains stable, only rarely fading. Coarse hairs may develop. There is rarely hypoplasia of underlying structures, e.g., shortening of the arm or reduced breast development in areas under the lesion.*

BENIGN NEOPLASMS AND HYPERPLASIAS

Trichoepithelioma

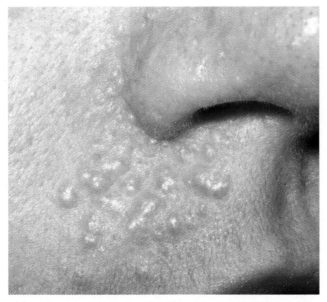

Figure 7-36   Trichoepithelioma   *Trichoepitheliomas are benign appendage tumors with hair differentiation. The lesions, which appear at puberty, occur on the face and less often on the scalp, neck, and upper trunk. The lesions, which may be only a few small pink or skin-colored papules at first, gradually increase in number and may become quite large and be confused with basal cell carcinoma. Trichoepitheliomas can also appear as solitary tumors, which may be nodular, or appear as ill-defined plaques like sclerodermiform BCC!*

Syringoma

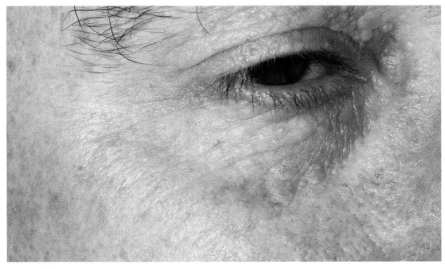

Figure 7-37   Syringoma   *Syringoma is a benign adenoma of the eccrine ducts. They are 1- to 2-mm, skin-colored or yellow, firm papules that occur mostly in women beginning at puberty and may be familial. The lesions, most often multiple rather than solitary, occur most frequently around the eyelids and on the face, axillae, umbilicus, upper chest, and vulva. The lesions have a specific histologic pattern: many small ducts in the dermis with comma-like tails with the appearance of "tadpoles." The lesions are considered to be disfiguring, and most patients want them removed; this can be done easily with electrosurgery.*

Sebaceous Hyperplasia

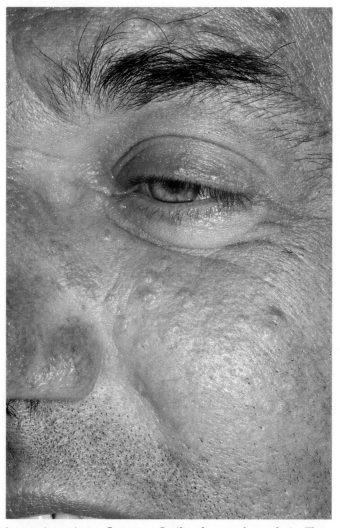

Figure 7-38   Sebaceous hyperplasia   Synonym: *Senile sebaceous hyperplasia. These are very common lesions in older persons and are confused with basal cell carcinomas (BCC). The lesions are 1 to 3 mm in diameter and have both telangiectasia and central umbilication. Two distinguishing features from BCC: sebaceous hyperplasia is soft to palpation, not firm as in BCC, and second, with firm lateral compression it is often possible to elicit a very small globule of sebum in the valley of the umbilicated portion of the lesion. Sebaceous hyperplasias can be destroyed with light electrocautery.*

Nevus Sebaceous

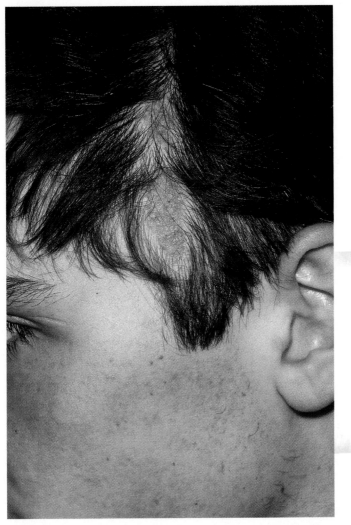

Figure 7-39 Nevus sebaceous Synonym: *Organoid nevus. This congenital malformation of sebaceous differentiation occurs on the scalp or, rarely, on the face. The lesion appears on the scalp and has a distinctive morphology: a hairless, thin, elevated, 1- to 2-cm plaque with a characteristic orange color. About 10% of patients can be expected to develop basal cell carcinoma in the lesion. Excision is recommended at around puberty for cosmetic reasons and also to prevent the occurrence of basal cell carcinoma.*

Epidermal Nevus

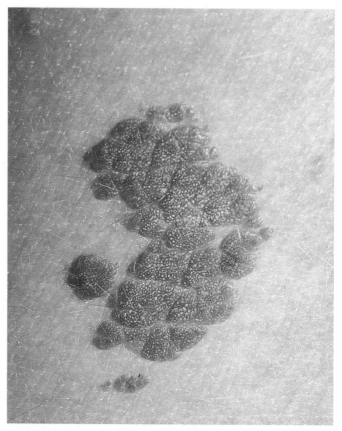

Figure 7-40   Epidermal nevus   *As the name* nevus *implies this is a developmental (hamartomatous) disorder characterized by hyperplasia of epidermal structures (epidermis and adnexa). There are no nevocellular nevus cells (melanocytes). This is usually present at birth or occurs in infancy, and rarely develops in puberty. All epidermal nevi on the head are present at birth.*

There are several variants of epidermal nevi. The verrucous epidermal nevus *may be localized or multiple. The lesions are skin-colored, brown or grayish brown. The lesions are composed of closely set verrucous papules, well circumscribed and are often in a linear arrangement—especially on the leg—or they may appear in Blaschko's lines on the trunk. Excision is the best treatment, if feasible. Biopsy of the lesions should be considered to rule out basal cell carcinoma.*

When the lesions are extensive they are termed systematized epidermal nevus *and when they are located on half the body they are termed* nevus unius lateris. *The lesions can exhibit erythema, scaling and crusting and then are called* inflammatory linear verrucous epidermal nevus *(ILVEN). The lesions gradually enlarge and in adolescence become stable.*

Extensive epidermal nevi are called epidermal nevus syndrome *and are multisystem disorders and may be associated with developmental abnormalities (bone cysts, hyperplastia of bone, scoliosis, spina bifida, kyphosis) and Vitamin D-resistant rickets, and neurologic associations (mental retardation, seizures, cortical atrophy, hydrocephalus). These patients require a complete examination, including the eyes (cataracts, optic nerve hypoplasia) and cardiac studies to rule out aneurysms, patent ductus arteriosus).*

BENIGN DERMAL AND SUBCUTANEOUS NEOPLASMS AND HYPERPLASIAS

Lipoma

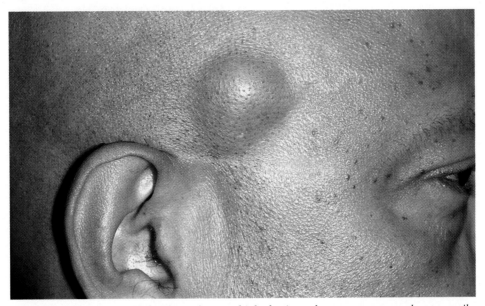

Figure 7-41 Lipoma *Lipomas are single or multiple, benign subcutaneous tumors that are easily recognized because they are soft, rounded, or lobulated and movable against the overlying skin. Many lipomas are small but also may enlarge to >6 cm. They occur especially on the neck, trunk, and on the extremities. Lipomas are composed of fat cells that have the same morphology as normal fat cells. There may, however, in some lesions, be a connective tissue framework in many lipomas. Single and/or few lipomas should be excised when they are small as they can reach a very large size, as large as 12 cm, and then are much more difficult to excise.* Familial lipoma syndrome, *an autosomal dominant trait appearing in early adulthood consists of hundreds of slowly growing nontender lesions. Multiple tender lipomas may arise in adult life and this is then called* adipositas dolorosa *or* Dercum's disease *and occurs in women in middle age; there are multiple tender circumscribed but more commonly diffuse fatty deposits. Benign symmetric* lipomatosis, *which affects middle-aged men consists of several large nontender, coalescent poorly circumscribed lipomas mostly on the trunk and upper extremities; they coalesce on the neck and may lead to a "horse-collar" appearance.*

Dermatofibroma

A dermatofibroma is a very common, button-like dermal nodule, usually occurring on the extremities, important only because of its cosmetic appearance or its being mistaken for other lesions, such as malignant melanoma when it is pigmented. The lesion may be tender.
Synonyms: Solitary histiocytoma, sclerosing hemangioma.

EPIDEMIOLOGY

Age of Onset   Adults.

Sex   Females > males.

Etiology   Unknown.

HISTORY

Symptoms   Usually asymptomatic.

PHYSICAL EXAMINATION

Skin Lesions   Papule or nodule (Fig. 7-42), 3 to 10 mm in diameter. Surface variably domed but may be depressed below plane of surrounding skin. Texture of surface may be dull, shiny, or scaling. Top may be crusted or scarred secondary to excoriation or shaving. Borders ill-defined, fading to normal skin. *Color variable*: skin-colored, pink, brown, tan, dark chocolate brown (Fig. 7-44). Usually darker at center, fading to normal skin color at margin. Often center shows postinflammatory hypo- or hyperpigmentation secondary to repeated trauma. Firm dermal button- or pealike papule or nodule. *Dimple sign:* lateral compression with thumb and index finger (Fig. 7-43) produces a depression or "dimple."

Distribution   Legs>arms>trunk. Hardly ever occurs on head, palms, soles. Usually solitary, may be multiple, and are randomly scattered.

DIFFERENTIAL DIAGNOSIS

Firm Dermal Papule/Nodule   The "dimple sign" is quite specific, but there are other lesions that can result in depression with lateral pressure, e.g., papulonodular lesions containing mucin, primary malignant melanoma, scar, blue nevus, pilar cyst, metastatic carcinoma, Kaposi's sarcoma, dermatofibrosarcoma protuberans.

LABORATORY EXAMINATIONS

Dermatopathology   Whorling fascicles of spindle cells with small amounts of pale blue cytoplasm and elongate nuclei. Some tumors extend to the panniculus. Pigmented dermatofibromas (Fig. 7-44) contain lipids or hemosiderin pigment in the histiocytes. Variable increase in vascular spaces. Overlying epidermis frequently hyperplastic.

DIAGNOSIS

Clinical findings, "dimple" sign (Fig. 7-43).

COURSE AND PROGNOSIS

Lesions appear gradually over several months, may persist without increase in size for years to decades, and may regress spontaneously.

MANAGEMENT

Surgical removal is not usually indicated, as the resulting scar is often less cosmetically acceptable than the dermatofibroma. Indications for excision include repeated trauma, unacceptable cosmetic appearance, or uncertainly of clinical diagnosis.

Cryosurgery   Cryosurgery with a cotton-tip applicator is often effective and produces a cosmetically acceptable scar in most patients.

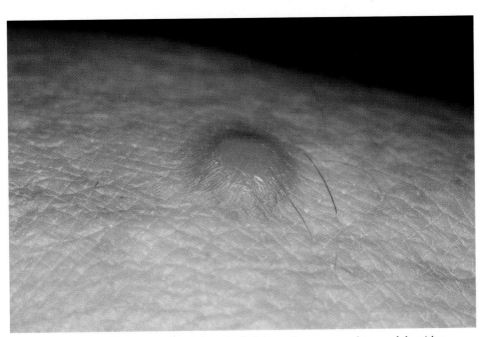

Figure 7-42 **Dermatofibroma** *A dome-shaped, slightly erythematous and tan nodule with a button-like, firm consistency.*

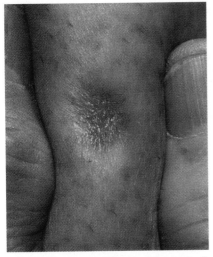

Figure 7-43 **Dermatofibroma: "dimple sign"** *Dimpling of the lesion is seen when pinched between two fingers.*

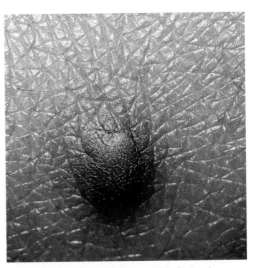

Figure 7-44 **Dermatofibroma** *This lesion is pigmented! Confused with blue nevus or even nodular melanoma. The pigment is melanin and hemosiderin.*

Hypertrophic Scars and Keloids

Hypertrophic scars and keloids are exuberant fibrous repair tissues after a cutaneous injury. A *hypertrophic scar* remains confined to the site of original injury; a *keloid,* however, extends beyond this site, often with clawlike extensions. May be cosmetically very unsightly and pose a serious problem for the patient if the lesion is large and on the ear or face.

EPIDEMIOLOGY

Age of Onset   Third decade, but all ages.

Sex   Equal incidence in males and females.

Race   Much more common in blacks and in persons with blood group A.

Etiology   Unknown. Usually follow injury to skin, i.e., surgical scar, laceration, abrasion, cryosurgery, electrocoagulation, as well as vaccination, acne, etc. May also arise spontaneously, without history of injury, usually in presternal site.

HISTORY

Skin Symptoms   Usually asymptomatic. May be pruritic or painful if touched.

PHYSICAL EXAMINATION

Skin Lesions   Papules to nodules (Fig. 7-46) to large tuberous lesions. Most often the color of the normal skin but also bright red, bluish. May be linear after traumatic or surgical injury (Fig. 7-45). Hypertrophic scars tend to be elevated and are confined to approximately the site of the original injury. Keloids, however, may extend in a clawlike fashion far beyond any slight original injury or may be nodular; tumor-like. Firm to hard; may be tender, surface smooth (Fig. 7-46).

Distribution   Earlobes, shoulders, upper back, chest.

DIFFERENTIAL DIAGNOSIS

Scar, dermatofibroma, dermatofibrosarcoma protuberans, desmoid tumor, scar with sarcoidosis, foreign-body granuloma.

LABORATORY EXAMINATIONS

Dermatopathology   *Hypertrophic Scar* Whorls of young fibrous tissue and fibroblasts in haphazard arrangement. **Keloid**   Features of hypertrophic scar with added feature of thick, eosinophilic, acellular bands of collagen.

DIAGNOSIS

Clinical diagnosis; biopsy not warranted unless there is clinical doubt, because another biopsy may induce new hypertrophic scarring.

COURSE AND PROGNOSIS

Hypertrophic scars tend to regress, in time becoming flatter and softer. Keloids, however, may continue to expand in size for decades.

MANAGEMENT

This is a real challenge, as no treatment is highly effective. Possibly, methods that induce collagenase will be forthcoming; UVA-1 (340 to 400 nm) is said to be effective by this mechanism.

Prevention   Individuals prone to hypertrophic scars or keloids should be advised to avoid cosmetic procedures such as ear piercing.

Intralesional Glucocorticoids   Intralesional injection of triamcinolone acetonide (10 to 40 mg/mL) every month may reduce pruritus or sensitivity of lesion, as well as reduce its volume and flatten it. This works quite well in small hypertrophic scars, such as occur with acne, but less well in keloids.

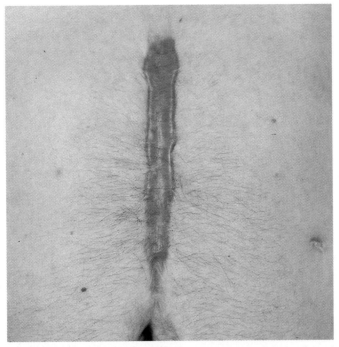

Figure 7-45 Hypertrophic scar *A broad, raised scar developing at the site of surgical incision with large telangiectatic blood vessels and a shiny atrophic epidermis.*

Combined Cryotherapy and Intralesional Triamcinolone The lesion is initially frozen with liquid nitrogen spray, allowed to thaw for 15 min, and then injected with triamcinolone acetonide (10 to 40 mg/mL). After freezing, the lesion becomes edematous and is much easier to inject.

Surgical Excision Lesions that are excised surgically often recur larger than the original lesion. Excision with immediate postsurgical radiotherapy is beneficial.

Silicone Cream and Silicone Gel Sheet Reported to be beneficial in keloids and is painless and noninvasive.

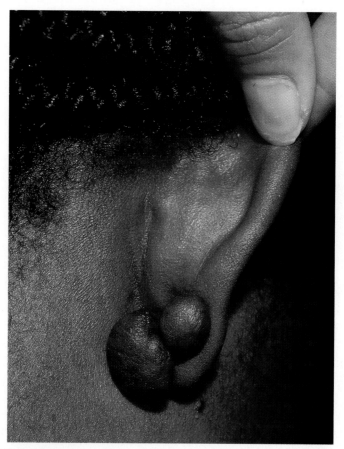

Figure 7-46 Keloid, following ear piercing *Persons with susceptibility to developing keloids should not have their ears pierced! There is no consensus on the management of keloids at this time: intralesional glucocorticoids before and after surgery, excision, and postoperative radiation.*

Skin Tag

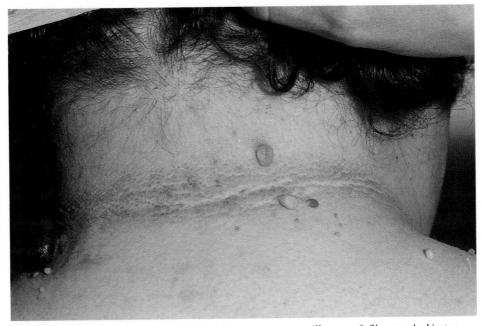

Figure 7-47 Skin tag Synonyms: *Acrochordon, cutaneous papilloma, soft fibroma. A skin tag is a very common, soft, skin-colored or tan or brown, round or oval, pedunculated papilloma (polyp); it is usually constricted at the base and may vary in size from >1 mm to as large as 10 mm. Histologic findings include an epidermis that is thinned and which contains a loose fibrous tissue stroma. It occurs more often in the middle aged and in the elderly. The lesion is asymptomatic but occasionally may become tender following trauma or torsion and may become crusted or hemorrhagic. The lesion is more common in females and in obese patients. It is most often noted in intertriginous areas (axillae, inframammary, groin) but is common on the neck and the eyelids. It may be confused with a pedunculated seborrheic keratosis, dermal or compound melanocytic nevus, solitary neurofibroma, or molluscum contagiosum. Lesions tend to become larger and more numerous over time, especially during pregnancy. Following spontaneous torsion, autoamputation can occur. Management is accomplished with simple snipping with a scissors or with electrodesiccation.*

PHOTOSENSITIVITY AND PHOTO-INDUCED DISORDERS

SKIN REACTIONS TO SUNLIGHT

CLASSIFICATION OF PHOTO-INDUCED

Acute

Phototoxicity
  Sunburn
  Drug-induced
  Plant-induced (phytophotodermatitis)
Photoallergy
  Drug-induced
  Solar urticaria
Idiopathic
  Polymorphic light eruption
  Actinic prurigo
  Hydroa vacciniforme
  Solar urticaria

Chronic

Dermatoheliosis ("photoaging")
Chronic actinic dermatitis
DNA repair-deficient photodermatoses
Solar lentigo
Solar keratosis
Skin cancer
  Basal cell carcinoma
  Squamous cell carcinoma
  Malignant melanoma
Metabolic and nutritional
  Porphyria cutanea tarda
  Variegate porphyria
  Erythropoietic protoporphyria
  Xeroderma pigmentosum
  Pellagra

When a confusing eruption is approached, the discovery of a clue to the etiology is always exciting—this finding narrows the differential diagnostic list. This could be a positive KOH or an eruption localized in the light-exposed areas. Once the etiologic role of light is established, there is, moreover, a possibililty of control of the disorder by discontinuing drugs or by topical or systemic treatment. The term *photosensitivity* describes an abnormal response to light, usually sunlight, occurring within minutes, hours, or days of exposure and lasting up to weeks and months.

Two broad types of *acute* photosensitivity are:

1. A *sunburn*-type response with the development of morphologic skin changes simulating a normal sunburn: erythema, edema, vesicles, bullae. Examples are phototoxic reactions to drugs and phytophotodermatitis, e.g., lime contact and sunlight.
2. A *rash* response to light exposure with development of varied morphologic expressions: macules, papules, plaques, eczematous dermatitis, urticaria. Examples are polymorphous light eruption, photoallergic drug reaction to sulfonamides.

Chronic repeated sun exposures over time result in polymorphic skin changes that have been termed *dermatoheliosis* or photoaging.

ACUTE SUN DAMAGE (SUNBURN)

Sunburn is an acute, delayed, and transient inflammatory response of the skin after exposure to ultraviolet radiation (UVR) from sunlight or artificial sources. Sunburn is characterized by erythema and, if severe, by vesicles and bullae, edema, tenderness, and pain; in normal sunburn there are never "rashes," i.e., scarlatiniform macules, papules, or plaques that occur in abnormal reactions to UVR. UVR in photomedicine is divided into two principal types: UVB (290 to 320 nm), the "sunburn spectrum," and UVA (320 to 400 nm). UVA has been subdivided into UVA-1 (340 to 400 nm) and UVA-2 (320 to 340 nm). The unit of measurement of sunburn is the *minimum erythema dose* (MED), which is the minimum ultraviolet exposure that produces a clearly marginated erythema in the irradiated site after a single exposure. The MED is expressed in the amount of energy per unit area: mJ/cm^2 (UVB) or J/cm^2 (UVA). The MED for UVB in Caucasians is 20 to 40 mJ/cm^2 (for a skin phototype I or II, about 20 min in northern latitudes at noon in June) and for UVA is 15 to 20 J/cm^2 (about 120 min in northern latitudes at noon in June). UVB erythema develops in 6 to 24 h and fades within 72 to 120 h. UVA erythema peaks between 4 to 16 h and fades within 48 to 120 h.

Variations in Sun Reactivity in Normal Persons : Phototypes

Skin Phototypes (Table 8-1)   Sunburn is seen most frequently in individuals who have pale white or white skin and a limited capacity to develop *facultative* or inducible melanin pigmentation (tanning) after exposure to UVR. Basic skin color (*constitutive* melanin pigmentation) is divided into white, brown, and black. Not all persons with white skin have the same capacity to develop tanning, and this fact is the principal basis for the classification of "white" persons into four *skin phototypes* (SPT). The SPT is based on the basic skin color (Table 8-1) *and* on a *person's own estimate* of sunburning and tanning. One question permits the identification of the SPT: "Do you tan easily?" Persons with SPT I or II will say immediately, "No," and those with SPT III or IV will say, "Yes." Persons with SPT I or II are regarded as "melanocompromised" and those with SPT III or IV as "melanocompetent."

SPT I persons usually have pale white skin color, blond or red hair, and blue eyes; but, in fact, they may have dark brown hair and brown eyes, while their skin color is pale white. SPT I persons sunburn easily with short exposures, and SPT IV persons tan with ease and do not sunburn with short exposures. SPT IV persons may have blond hair and blue eyes but more often have brown hair and brown eyes and light tan (beige) constitutive skin color.

SPT II persons are a subgroup of SPT I and

sunburn easily but *tan with difficulty,* whereas SPT III persons have some sunburn with short exposures but can develop, over time, marked tanning. It is estimated that about 25% of white-skinned persons in the United States are SPT I and II. Persons with constitutive brown skin are termed SPT V and with black skin SPT VI.

Race   *Skin phototypes are not solely based on ethnicity*. The SPT of various races has not yet been determined. However, it is known that some Asiatic and Hispanic individuals have SPT I and II; and these persons have white not brown skin, although the hair and eye color may be black and brown, respectively.

Age   Very young children and elderly persons are said to have a reduced capacity to sunburn, although this has not been thoroughly documented.

Geography   Sunburn can occur at any latitude; it may be observed less frequently in the indigenous populations near the equator who respect the sun. Sunburn is seen more often in people who frequent beaches or who travel to sunny vacation areas.

PATHOGENESIS

The chromophores (molecules that absorb UVR) for UVB sunburn erythema are not known, but damage to DNA possibly may be the initiating event. The damage to DNA, in

Table 8-1   CLASSIFICATION OF SKIN PHOTOTYPES (SPT)

SPT	Basic Skin Color	Response to Sun Exposure
I	Pale white	Do not tan, burn easily
II	White	Tan with difficulty, burn easily
III	White	Tan after initial sunburn
IV	Light brown	Tan easily
V	Brown	Tan easily
VI	Black	Become darker

Questionnaire for estimating the skin phototype in *white* persons
Question: "Do you tan easily?"

Three possible answers:	Skin phototype
"No, I burn easily."	I and II
"I burn first and then tan."	III
"Yes, I tan easily."	IV

fact, results in excision of pyrimidine dimers which *sui generis* initiates a protective tanning response. The mediators that cause the erythema include histamine for both UVA and UVB. In UVB erythema, other mediators include serotonin, prostaglandins, lysosomal enzymes, and kinins. However, the cytokine interleukin 6 (IL-6) that peaks at 12 h is probably the main mediator of the sunburn reaction in humans.

HISTORY

Relationship of Sunburn to Medications   An "exaggerated" sunburn response can occur in persons who are taking *phototoxic* drugs: sulfonamides (chlorothiazides, furosemide), tetracyclines, doxycycline, phenothiazines, nalidixic acid, amiodarone, naproxen, psoralens.

Skin Symptoms   Pruritus may be severe even in mild sunburn; pain and tenderness occur with severe sunburn.

Constitutional Symptoms   Headache, chills, feverishness, and weakness are not infrequent in severe sunburn; some SPT I and II persons develop headache and malaise even after short exposures.

Family History   Skin phototypes are genetically determined.

PHYSICAL EXAMINATION

General Appearance   In severe sunburn, the patient is "toxic"—with fever, weakness, and lassitude.

Vital Signs   In severe sunburn, pulse rate is rapid.

Skin Lesions   Confluent bright erythema (Fig. 8-1), edema, vesicles, and bullae confined to areas of exposure; no "rash" is present as occurs in most photoallergic reactions. Edematous areas are raised and tender.

Distribution   Strictly confined to areas of exposure; sunburn can occur in areas covered with clothing, depending on the degree of UV transmission through clothing, the level of exposure, and the SPT of the person.

Mucous Membranes   Sunburn of the tongue can occur rarely in mountain climbers who hold their mouth open "panting"; is frequent on the vermilion border of the lips.

DIFFERENTIAL DIAGNOSIS

Sunburn   Obtain history of *medications* that can induce phototoxic erythema; *systemic lupus erythematosus* (SLE) can cause a sunburn-type erythema. *Erythropoietic protoporphyria* causes erythema, vesicles, edema, purpura and, only rarely, urticarial wheals.

LABORATORY EXAMINATIONS

Dermatopathology

Light Microscopy   "Sunburn" cells (apoptotic keratinocytes); also, exocytosis of lymphocytes, vacuolization of melanocytes and Langerhans cells. *Dermis:* endothelial cell swelling of superficial blood vessels and in the subcutaneous fat. Dermal changes are more prominent with UVA erythema with a denser mononuclear infiltrate and more severe vascular changes.

Serology ANA

To rule out SLE.

Hematology

Leukopenia may be present in SLE.

DIAGNOSIS

History of UVR exposure and sites of reaction on exposed areas.

COURSE AND PROGNOSIS

History of "blistering" sunburns in youth is definitely a risk factor for development of malignant melanoma and also basal cell carinoma of the skin years later. Repeated sunburns result in dermatoheliosis, or "photoaging," over time.

Sunburn, unlike thermal burns, cannot be classified on the basis of depth, i.e., first-second-, and third-degree. Third-degree burns after UVR do not occur and none of the features of third-degree thermal burns are seen: scarring, loss of sensation, loss of sweating, hair loss. The only permanent reaction from severe ultraviolet burns is depigmentation, probably related to the destruction of melanocytes.

MANAGEMENT

Prevention There are now many highly effective topical chemical filters (sunscreens) in lotion, gel, and cream formulations. Persons with SPT I or II should avoid sunbathing, especially between 1100 and 1400 h. Clothing: UV-screening cloth garments. It is still not clear whether regular use of topical sunscreens can prevent melanoma of the skin, but there is a general belief that topical sunscreens reduce the induction of solar keratoses and, probably, squamous cell carcinoma.

Moderate Sunburn

Topical Cool wet dressings, topical glucocorticoids.

Systemic Acetylsalicylic acid, indomethacin.

Severe Sunburn Bed rest. If very severe, a "toxic" patient is best managed in a specialized "burn unit" for fluid replacement, prophylaxis of infection, etc.

Topical Cool wet dressings, topical glucocorticoids.

Systemic Oral glucocorticoids are often given, but their efficacy has not been established by controlled studies.

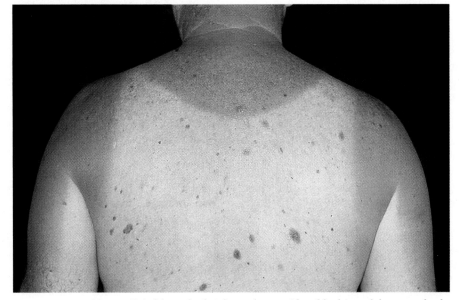

Figure 8-1 Acute sunburn *Painful, tender bright erythema with mild edema of the upper back with sharp demarcation between the sun-exposed and sun-protected white areas. Note large atypical melanocytic nevi. The patient is at risk for developing malignant melanoma.*

DERMATOHELIOSIS ("PHOTOAGING")

Repeated solar injuries over many years ultimately can result in the development of a skin syndrome, *dermatoheliosis*. Dermatoheliosis (DHe) results from excessive and/or prolonged exposure of the skin to ultraviolet radiation (UVR) in persons with SPT I to III and in persons with SPT IV who have heavy exposure to sunlight, such as lifeguards and outdoor workers. The syndrome results from the cumulative effects of sun exposure after the first exposures in early life. DHe describes a polymorphic response of various components of the skin (especially cells in the epidermis, the vascular system, and the dermal connective tissue) to prolonged and/or excessive sun exposure. As stated previously, the severity of DHe depends principally on the duration and intensity of sun exposure and on the indigenous (constitutive) skin color and the capacity to tan (facultative melanin pigmentation).

EPIDEMIOLOGY

Age of Onset   DHe is observed most often in persons older than 40 years; young white children (age 10) living in southern Borneo (cool climate with high UVR) have been observed to have DHe, including solar keratoses.

Sex   Higher incidence in males.

Skin Phototype   Persons with SPT I and II are most susceptible, but persons with SPT III and IV and even V (brown skin color) can develop DHe.

Incidence   In persons of SPT I to IV who have had *prolonged* exposure to sunlight or UVR from artificial sources. The population most susceptible to development of DHe consists of persons with SPT I and II, who comprise about 25% of the white population in the United States.

Occupation   Farmers ("farmer's skin"), telephone linemen, sea workers ("sailor's skin"), construction workers, lifeguards, swimming instructors, sportspersons, and "beach bums"; persons who spend considerable time in mountain or sea resorts.

Geography   DHe is more severe in white populations living in areas with high solar UVR (at high altitudes or in low latitudes).

PATHOGENESIS

While UVB is the most obvious damaging UVR, UVA in high doses can produce connective tissue changes in mice. In addition, visible (400 to 700 nm) and infrared (1000 to 1,000,000 nm) radiations have been implicated. The action spectrum for DHe is not known for certain; there is some experimental evidence in mice that infrared radiation is implicated, in addition to UVB and UVA.

HISTORY

Personal History   There is a history of intensive exposure to sun in youth (younger than 20 years), even though sun exposure may have been quite limited in later adult life. Sun exposure in youth is a risk factor for melanoma, basal cell carcinoma.

Family History   Because skin phototypes are genetically determined, there is often a family history of DHe.

PHYSICAL EXAMINATION

General Appearance   Wrinkled, wizened, leathery, "prematurely aged," or "looks old but is young." Persons with brown and black skin color are deceptively young looking because of the virtual absence of DHe. Persons with black skin who are albinos can develop DHe and sun-induced skin cancers, but, curiously, only rarely develop malignant melanoma.

Skin Findings

Epidermis

Keratinocytes   Epidermal atrophy: with increased translucence. Solar keratosis (Fig. 8-2). Xerosis (dryness).

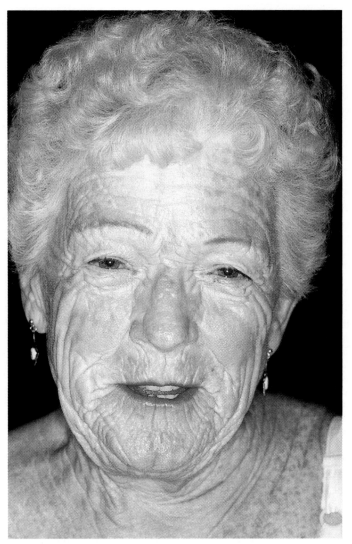

Figure 8-2 Dermatoheliosis *Severe fine (periorbital skin above the upper lip) and deep wrinkling (cheeks and neck). The skin appears waxy, papular with a yellowish hue (actinic elastosis). It shows some tan spots that are dry and scaling (actinic keratoses). This 68-year-old Irish-American female with skin phototype I lived in New England near the sea and in her youth spent hours in the sun—during an era in which it was believed that "sun was good for you!"*

Melanocytes Solar lentigo (Figs. 8-3 and 8-4). Ephelides (freckles) of "old age" (less seasonal dependency than juvenile ephelides). Guttate hypomelanosis, especially on the shins.

Dermis

Vascular System Permanent dilatation of vessels (telangiectasia). Purpura, easy bruising.

Connective Tissue Wrinkling (fine surface, deep furrows), roughness, and elastosis (fine nodularity and inelasticity), yellow dermal papules and plaques (Fig. 8-2).

Pilosebaceous Unit Comedones (especially periorbital) (Favre-Racouchet disease).

Distribution of Lesions Exposed areas. Scalp (bald males). Nuchal area: cutis rhomboidalis ("red neck") with rhomboidal furrows; periorbital and perioral areas: wrinkling.

LABORATORY EXAMINATIONS

Dermatopathology Acanthosis of epidermis, increased horny layer. Flattening of the dermal-epidermal junction. Atypia of the keratinocytes. Marked alteration in microcirculation with loss of small vessels in the papillary dermis. Elastosis: degraded elastic tissue with formation of coarse amorphous masses and increase in glycosaminoglycans. Increase in fibroblasts, but a decrease in collagen and an increase in elastin.

DIFFERENTIAL DIAGNOSIS

Wrinkled/Freckled Dry Skin *Xeroderma pigmentosum* exhibits severe DHe in addition to skin cancers (squamous cell and basal cell carcinomas, melanoma, fibrosarcoma, angiosarcoma); however, the disorder is present at a very young age. In *progeria* there is little or no wrinkling, but atrophy of skin and subcutis with marked increase in translucency of the epidermis. There are no pigmentary changes and no xerosis of the skin or solar keratoses.

COURSE AND PROGNOSIS

There is evidence based on case control studies that severe sunburns in youth can lead to the development of malignant melanoma two or three decades later in life. This may result from sun-induced mutations in the gene regulating melanocytes present in common acquired nevomelanocytic and in dysplastic melanocytic nevi. The appearance of DHe marks a relatively young person as "old," a state that everyone tries to delay. There is a current wave to prevent skin cancers and to prevent the development of DHe with the use of protective sunblocks, a change of behavior in the sun, and the use of topical chemotherapy (tretinoin) that reverses some of the changes of DHe (solar keratoses, solar lentigo, vascular and connective tissue changes).

DHe is inexorably progressive and irreversible, but some repair of connective tissue effects can occur if the skin is protected. Some processes leading to DHe continue to progress, however, even when sun exposures are severely restricted in later life; solar keratoses and lentigo develop in the sun-damaged skin that is now being protected by avoidance and sunblocks. Yet, there are documented examples of spontaneous reversal of solar keratoses.

MANAGEMENT

Topical Treatment *Tretinoin* in lotions, gels, and creams in varying concentrations has been demonstrated in controlled studies to effect a reversal (clinical and histologic) of some aspects of DHe, especially the connective tissue and vascular changes. There is a current notion that topical tretinoin can alter the progression of incipient epithelial skin cancers. *5-Fluorouracil* in lotions and creams is highly effective in causing a disappearance of solar keratoses.

Prevention Persons of SPT I and II should be identified early in life and advised that they are susceptible to the development of DHe and skin cancers, including melanoma. These persons should never sunbathe and should, from an early age, adopt a daily program of self-protection using sunfiltering clothing and substantive and effective topical sun-protective solutions, gels, or lotions that can filter DNA-damaging UVB; UVA filters are less effective. SPT I and II persons should avoid the peak hours of UVB intensity, which are the 2 h before and after solar noon (1200 GMT).

CAUTION: There is experimental evidence that while sunscreens protect from sunburn, they do not protect from UV-induced local immunosuppression. Prevention of sunburn may lure individuals into exposing themselves to the sun for prolonged periods, which may abrogate immunosurveillance mechanisms in the skin. This has been linked to the rising incidence of melanoma.

Solar Lentigo

Solar lentigo is a circumscribed 1- to 3-cm brown macule resulting from a localized proliferation of melanocytes due to chronic exposure to sunlight.

EPIDEMIOLOGY

Usually older than 40 years but may occur at 30 years in sunny climates and in susceptible persons. Most common in Caucasians but seen also in Asians. Generally correlated with skin phototypes I to III and duration and intensity of solar exposure.

PHYSICAL EXAMINATION

Skin Lesions

Strictly macular (Fig. 8-3), 1 to 3 cm, as large as 5 cm (Fig. 8-4). Light yellow, light brown, or dark brown; variegated mix of brown and not uniform color (Fig. 8-4), as in café-au-lait macules. Round, oval, with slightly irregular border. Often scattered, discrete lesions (Fig. 8-3).

Distribution Exclusively exposed areas: forehead, cheeks, nose, dorsa of hands and forearms, upper back, chest, shins.

LABORATORY EXAMINATIONS

Dermatopathology Club-shaped elongated rete ridges that show hypermelanosis and an increased number of melanocytes in the basal layer.

DIFFERENTIAL DIAGNOSIS

Brown Macules "Flat," acquired, brown lesions of the exposed skin of the face, which may on cursory examination appear to be similar, have distinctive features: solar lentigo, seborrheic keratosis, pigmented solar keratosis (SPAK) lentigo maligna.

MANAGEMENT

Cryosurgery or laser surgery are effective. No more than 10 seconds of liquid nitrogen should be administered; otherwise depigmentation of normal skin will occur.

Solar Keratosis

These single or multiple, discrete, dry, rough, adherent scaly lesions occur on the habitually sun-exposed skin of adults.
Synonym: Actinic keratosis.

EPIDEMIOLOGY

Age of Onset Middle age, although in Australia and southwestern United States solar keratoses may occur in persons younger than 30 years.

Sex More common in males.

Race Skin phototypes (SPT) I, II, and III; rare in SPT IV; almost never in blacks or East Indians.

Occupation Outdoor workers (especially farmers, ranchers, sailors) and outdoor sportspersons (tennis, golf, mountain climbing, deep-sea fishing).

PATHOGENESIS

Prolonged and repeated solar exposure in susceptible persons (SPT I, II, and III) leads to cumulative damage to keratinocytes by the action of ultraviolet radiant energy, principally, if not exclusively, UVB (290 to 320 nm).

HISTORY

Duration of Lesions Months to years.

Skin Symptoms Some lesions may be tender.

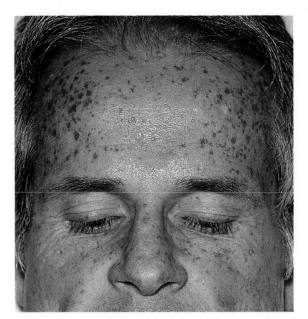

Figure 8-3 Dermatoheliosis: solar lentigines *Multiple dark-brown macules on the forehead occurred after a sunburn.*

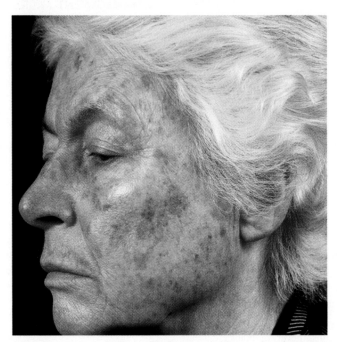

Figure 8-4 Dermatoheliosis: solar lentigines *Moderate wrinkling, solar elastosis (creamy yellowing), and dyschromia (solar lentigines) with multiple, variegated, tan-to-dark-brown macules on the malar and frontal area in the face. Solar lentigines are not the same as ephelides (freckles)—they do not fade in the winter as freckles do. They remain for life; freckles largely disappear or become inapparent in older people. (The winner of the freckle contest in Charlestown, MA, at age 11, has very few freckles on his face 25 years later.) Also, in solar lentigo there is melanocytic proliferation; in freckles there is no increase in the number of melanocytes, but there is increased pigment in the freckle melanocytes.*

PHYSICAL EXAMINATION

Skin Lesions Adherent hyperkeratotic scale, which is removed with difficulty and pain. May be papular or nodular. Skin-colored, yellow-brown, or brown; often there is a reddish tinge. Rough, like coarse sandpaper, "better felt than seen" on palpation with a finger. Most commonly <1 cm, oval or round (Fig. 8-5A and B).

Distribution Isolated single lesion or scattered discrete lesions. Face (forehead, nose, cheeks (Fig. 8-5), temples, vermilion border of lower lip), ears (in males), neck (sides), forearms, and hands (dorsa), shins, and the scalp in bald males.

DIFFERENTIAL DIAGNOSIS

Small Keratotic Pink Macules in Sun-Exposed Sites Chronic cutaneous LE, irritated seborrhea keratosis, flat warts, SCC in situ, superficial BCC.

LABORATORY EXAMINATIONS

Dermatopathology Large bright-staining keratinocytes, with mild to moderate pleomorphism in the basal layer, parakeratosis, and atypical (dyskeratotic) keratinocytes.

DIAGNOSIS

Usually made on clinical findings. Hyperkeratotic lesions may require biopsy to rule out squamous cell carcinoma (in situ or invasive).

COURSE AND PROGNOSIS

Solar keratoses may disappear spontaneously, but in general they remain for years. The actual incidence of squamous cell carcinoma in pre-existing solar keratoses is unknown but has been estimated at one squamous cell carcinoma developing annually in each 1000 solar keratoses.

MANAGEMENT

Prevention Afforded by use of highly effective UVB/UVA sunscreens, which should be applied daily to the face, neck, and ears during the summer in northern latitudes for SPT I and SPT II persons and for those SPT III persons who sustain prolonged sunlight exposures.

Topical Therapy

Cryosurgery Light spray or with cotton-tipped applicator is effective in most cases. Longer freeze periods may affect the dermal vasculature and cause a permanent white macule (scar).

5-Fluorouracil (5-FU) Cream 5% Effective, but difficult for many individuals. Treatment of facial lesions causes significant erythema and erosions, resulting in temporary cosmetic disfigurement. Apply bid for 2 to 4 weeks on face; may require longer period of therapy on dorsum of hands or lower legs. Efficacy can be increased and duration of treatment can be shortened if applied under occlusion and/or combined with topical tretinoin. This, however, leads to confluent erosions and may require hospitalization. Re-epithelialization occurs after treatment is discontinued. Pretreatment with light cryosurgery to hyperkeratotic lesions may improve efficacy of 5-FU cream.

Retinoids Used chronically, may be effective for treatment of dermatoheliosis and solar keratoses.

Facial Peels Trichloroacetic acid (5 to 10%) effective for widespread lesions.

Laser Surgery Erbium or carbon dioxide lasers. High cost. Usually effective for individual lesions. For extensive facial lesions, facial resurfacing is effective.

System Therapy

Retinoids Acitretin or isotretinoin are effective in reducing the number of solar keratoses and SCC in situ in patients with advanced dermatoheliosis, many solar keratoses, SCCs in situ, and invasive SCCs, especially if immunocompromised. Lesions recur once therapy is discontinued.

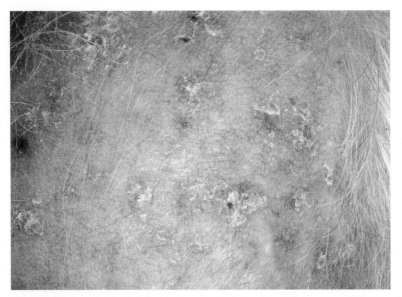

Figure 8-5A   Solar keratosis   *Erythematous macules and papules with coarse, adherent scale becomes confluent on the forehead, arising in a background of dermatoheliosis. Gently abrading lesions with a fingernail usually induces pain, even in early subtle lesions, a helpful diagnostic finding.*

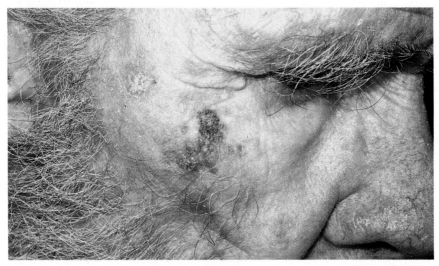

Figure 8-5B   Spreading pigmented actinic keratosis (SPAK)   *This is a rather uncommon variant of actinic keratosis. The distinctive features of SPAK include size (1.5 cm or larger), pigmentation (brown to black and variegated), and history of lateral spreading, especially the verrucous surface. The lesion is important because it can mimic lentigo maligna (LM). It is, however, easily distinguished from LM because LM is completely flat without evidence of verrucous change. The epidermal change in SPAK may appear as a slightly verrucous surface perceptible only with a hand lens and oblique lighting. Biopsy is necessary to confirm the clinical diagnosis. The lesion responds to a combination of cryosurgery (a very light freeze) followed by application of 5% 5-fluorouracil ointment for 10 to 12 days; the application of the ointment is begun 3 days following the cryosurgery, after the scale falls off.*

PHYTOPHOTODERMATITIS (PLANT + LIGHT = DERMATITIS)

Phytophotodermatitis (PPD) is an inflammation of the skin caused by contact with certain plants during recreational or occupational exposure to sunlight. The inflammatory response is a phototoxic reaction to photosensitizing chemicals in several plant families; a common type of PPD is due to exposure to limes.
Synonyms: Berloque dermatitis, lime dermatitis.

EPIDEMIOLOGY

Age of Onset   PPD can occur at any age; in children, exposure to plants in the grassy meadows near beaches may occur.

Race   All skin colors; brown- and black-skinned persons may develop only marked spotty dark pigmentation without erythema or bullous lesions.

Occupation   Celery pickers, carrot processors, gardeners [exposed to carrot greens or to "gas plant" (*Dictamnus albus*)], and bartenders (lime juice) who are exposed to sun in outside bars.

Etiology   The phototoxic reaction is caused by the presence of photoactive chemicals, psoralens contained in the plants.

HISTORY

The patient gives a history of exposure to certain plants (lime, lemon, wild parsley, celery, giant hogweed, parsnips, carrot greens, figs). Lime juice is a frequent cause: making lime drinks, hair rinses with lime juice. Women who use perfumes containing oil of bergamot (which contains bergapten, 5-methoxypsoralen) may develop only streaks of pigmentation in areas where the perfume was applied, especially the sides of the neck, upper anterior chest, and wrists. This is called *berloque dermatitis* (*berloque,* French: "pendant"). Persons walking on beaches containing meadow grass develop phytophotodermatitis on the legs; meadow grass contains agrimony.

Relationship of Skin Lesions to Season   Occur most often during the summer months in northern latitudes or all year in tropical climates.

Skin Symptoms   Marked pruritus.

PHYSICAL EXAMINATION

Skin Lesions   Acute: erythema, vesicles, and bullae (Fig. 8-6), but not an eczematous dermatitis as in rhus dermatitis. Residual dark hyperpigmentation in bizarre streaks (Fig. 8-7). Bizarre streaks, artificial patterns that indicate an "outside job."

Distribution and Arrangement   Scattered areas on the sites of contact, especially the arms, legs, and face.

SPECIAL EXAMINATIONS

Wood's Lamp Examination   The sites of involvement can be detected by the enhancement of the erythema and pigmentation.

DIAGNOSIS

Easily made if the pattern is recognized and a careful history is taken.

COURSE

May be an important occupational problem, as in celery pickers.
  The acute eruption fades spontaneously, but the pigmentation may last for many weeks. In contrast to rhus dermatitis, the process has a short life and has only a vesiculobullous response; eczematous reactions are never observed as they are in plant dermatitis from *Rhus*.

MANAGEMENT

Wet dressings may be indicated in the acute vesicular stage. Topical glucocorticoids.

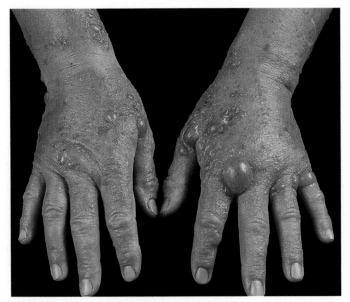

Figure 8-6 Phytophotodermatitis (plant + light): acute with blisters *These bullae were the result of exposure to both lime juice and the sun. This 50-year-old bartender was making drinks in an outside bar on a beach in the Bahamas. Lime contains bergapten (5-methoxypsoralen), which is a potent topical phototoxic chemical.*

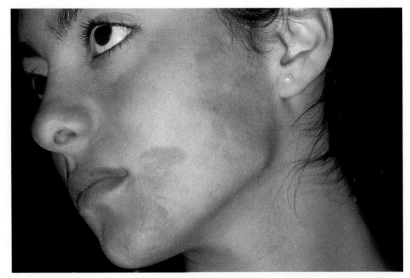

Figure 8-7 Phytophotodermatitis: hyperpigmentation *The patient had the oil from the rind of a lime on her fingers, which she then touched to her face while sunbathing ("lime" disease).*

DRUG-INDUCED PHOTOSENSITIVITY (TABLE 8-2)

Drug-induced photosensitivity describes an adverse reaction of the skin that results from simultaneous exposure to certain drugs (via ingestion, injection, or topical application) and to ultraviolet radiation (UVR) or visible light. The chemicals may be therapeutic, cosmetic, industrial, or agricultural. There are two types of reaction: (1) *phototoxic*, which can occur in all individuals and is essentially an exaggerated sunburn response (erythema, edema, vesicles, etc.), and (2) *photoallergic*, which involves an immunologic response and in which the eruption is papular, vesicular, eczema-like, and occurs only in the previously sensitized.

Phototoxic Drug-Induced Photosensitivity

EPIDEMIOLOGY

Age of Onset   Any age.

Race   All types of skin color: black, white, and brown.

Incidence   Phototoxic drug reactions are more frequent than photoallergic drug sensitivity.

Etiology   Amiodarone, thiazides, coal tar and derivatives, doxycycline, furosemide, nalidixic acid, demethylchlortetracycline, oxytetracycline, phenothiazines, piroxicam, psoralens (furocoumarins), sulfonamides. (See Table 8-2.) Some drugs causing phototoxic reaction can also elicit photoallergic reactions (see below).

PATHOGENESIS

Formation of toxic photoproducts such as free radicals or reactive oxygen species such as singlet oxygen. The principal sites of damage are nuclear DNA or cell membranes (plasma, lysosomal, mitochondrial). The action spectrum is UVA.

HISTORY

There are three patterns of phototoxic reaction: (1) immediate erythema and urticaria, (2) delayed sunburn-type pattern developing within 16 to 24 h or later (48 to 72 h in psoralen-related phototoxic reactions), or (3) delayed (72 to 96 h) melanin hyperpigmentation.

Skin Symptoms   Pruritus, burning, or stinging.

PHYSICAL EXAMINATION

Skin Lesions   The skin lesions are those of an "exaggerated sunburn." In phototoxic drug reactions there is erythema, edema (Fig. 8-8), and vesicle and bulla formation (e.g., pseudoporphyria). An eczematous reaction pattern is not seen in phototoxic reactions. Marked brown epidermal melanin pigmentation may occur in the course of the eruption; and especially with certain drugs (chlorpromazine and amiodarone), a gray dermal melanin pigmentation develops. After repeated exposure, some scaling and lichenification can develop.

Distribution   Confined exclusively to areas exposed to light (distribution pattern of light eruptions, Figure 8-I).

Nails   Photoonycholysis can occur with certain drugs (psoralens, demethylchlortetracycline, and benoxaprofen).

DIFFERENTIAL DIAGNOSIS

Acute Photosensitivity   Phototoxic reactions due to excess of endogenous porphyrins; photosensitivity due to other diseases, e.g., systemic lupus erythematosus.

LABORATORY EXAMINATIONS

Dermatopathology   Inflammation, "sunburn cells" in the epidermis, epidermal necrobiosis, intraepidermal and subepidermal vesiculation. Absence of eczematous changes.

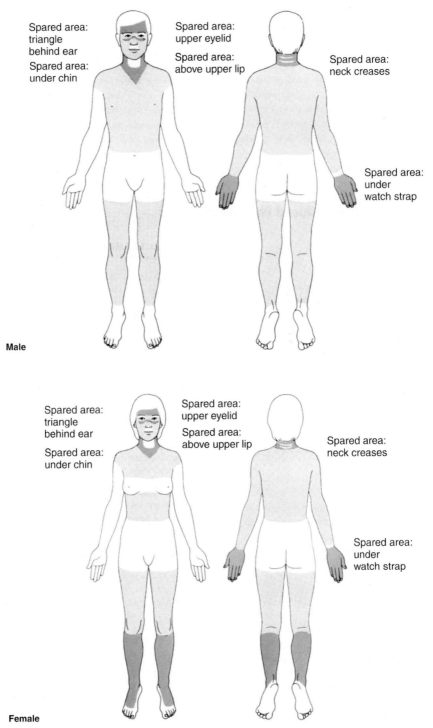

Figure 8-I *Variations in solar exposure on different body areas:* ☐, *Rarely or never exposed (including doubly covered areas);* ▨, *often exposed;* ▮, *habitually exposed.*

PHOTOSENSITIVITY AND PHOTO-INDUCED DISORDERS

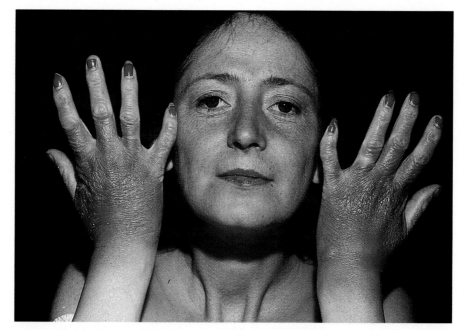

Figure 8-8 Phototoxic drug-induced photosensitivity *An acute sunburn is seen on the dorsum of the hands of an individual who was treated with demethylchlortetracycline, which is used for acne. She had attended a sporting event and wore a hat that protected her head and neck; but she was holding onto a rail, thus increasing the exposure of her hands.*

Phototesting For verification of incriminated agent, template test sites are exposed to increasing doses of UVA (phototoxic reactions are almost always due to UVA) while patient is on the incriminated drug. The UVA minimum erythema dose (MED) will be much lower than that for normal individuals of the same skin phototype. After drug is excreted and then eliminated from the skin, a repeat UVA phototest will reveal an *increase* in the UVA MED. This test may be important if patient was on multiple potentially phototoxic drugs.

DIAGNOSIS

History of exposure to drugs is most important as well as the types of morphologic changes in the skin characteristic of phototoxic drug eruptions: confluent erythema, edema, vesicles, bullae.

COURSE AND PROGNOSIS

Phototoxic drug sensitivity is a major problem, since the abnormal reactions seriously limit or exclude the use of important drugs: diuretics, antihypertensive agents, drugs used in psychiatry. It is not known why some individuals show phototoxic reactions to a particular drug and others do not. Phototoxic drug reactions disappear after cessation of drug.

Table 8-2 DRUGS THAT CAUSE PHOTOSENSITIVITY

Antibiotics
Amoxicillin
Ciprofloxacin
Clofazimine
Dapsone
Demeclocycline
Doxycycline
Enoxacin
Flucytosine
Griseofulvin
Lomefloxacin
Minocycline
Nalidixic acid
Norfloxacin
Ofloxacin
Oxyfloxacin
Oxytetracycline
Pyrazinamide
Sulfonamide
Tetracycline
Trimethoprim

Anticancer drugs
Dacarbazine (DTIC)
Fluorouracil
Flutamide
Methotrexate
Vinblastine

Antidepressants
Amitriptyline
Amoxapine
Clomipramine
Desipramine
Doxepin
Fluoxetine
Imipramine
Maprotiline
Nortriptyline
Phenelzine
Protriptyline
Trazodone
Trimipramine

Antihistamines
Astemizole
Cimetidine
Cyproheptadine
Diphenhydramine
Ranitidine
Terfenadine

Antihypertensives
β blockers
Captopril
Diltiazem
Methyldopa
Minoxidil
Nifedipine

Antiparasitics
Chloroquine
Quinine
Thiabendazole

Antipsychotic drugs
Chlorpromazine
Fluphenazine
Haloperidol
Perphenazine
Prochlorperazine
Thioridazine
Thiothixene
Trifluoperazine
Triflupromazine

Diuretics
Acetazolamide
Amiloride
Bendroflumethiazide
Benzthiazide
Chlorothiazide
Furosemide
Hydrochlorothiazide
Hydroflumethiazide
Methyclothiazide
Metolazone
Polythiazide
Triamterene
Trichlormethiazide

Hypoglycemics
Acetohexamide
Chlorpropamide
Glipizide
Glyburide
Tolazamide
Tolbutamide

**Nonsteroidal anti-
inflammatory drugs**
Benoxaprofen
Diclofenac

Diflunisal
Fenbufen
Ibuprofen
Indomethacin
Ketoprofen
Nabumetone
Naproxen
Phenylbutazone
Piroxicam
Sulindac

Sunscreens
Aminobenzoic acid
Avobenzone
Benzophenones
Cinnamates
Homosalate
Methyl anthranilate
PABA

**Miscellaneous
photosensitizing agents**
Alprazolam
Amantadine
Amiodarone
Benzocaine
Bergamot oil, oils of citron,
   lavender, lime, sandalwood,
   cedar
Carbamazepine
Chlordiazepoxide
Clofibrate
Contraceptives, oral
Desoximetasone
Disopyramide
Etretinate
Fluorescein
Gold salts
Griseofulvin
Hexachlorophene
Isotretinoin
6-Methylcoumarin
Musk ambrette
Promethazine
Quinine sulfate and gluconate
Tretinoin
Trimeprazine

SOURCE: Adapted from: Drugs that cause photsensitivity. Med Lett Drugs Ther 37:35, 1995.

Photoallergic Drug-Induced Photosensitivity

In photoallergic drug photosensitivity, the chemical agent (drug) present in the skin absorbs photons and forms a photoproduct; this photoproduct then binds to a soluble or membrane-bound protein to form an antigen. Since photoallergy depends on individual immunologic reactivity, it develops in only a small percentage of persons exposed to drugs and light.

EPIDEMIOLOGY

Age of Onset Probably more common in adults.

Race All skin phototypes: black, white, and brown.

Incidence Photoallergic drug reactions occur much less frequently than do phototoxic drug reactions.

Etiology Halogenated salicylanilides, phenothiazines, sulfonamides; PABA esters, benzocaine, neomycin, benzophenones, and 6-methylcoumarin in sunscreens; musk ambrette in aftershave lotions; and stilbenes in whiteners.

PATHOGENESIS

Formation of photoproduct that conjugates with protein producing an antigen. The action spectrum involved is almost always UVA.

HISTORY

The history may be unclear in that initial exposure induces sensitization to delayed-type hypersensitivity reactions, and the eruption occurs on subsequent exposure. Topically applied photosensitizers are the most frequent cause of photoallergic eruptions, e.g., halogenated salicylanilides, benzocaine (in soaps and other household products used to inhibit bacterial overgrowth), or musk ambrette used in aftershave lotions; photoallergy also results from the systemic administration of a drug.

Skin Symptoms Pruritus.

PHYSICAL EXAMINATION

Skin Lesions The morphology of the skin reaction is much different from that in phototoxic drug sensitivity. Acute photoallergic reaction patterns resemble (1) allergic contact eczematous dermatitis (Fig. 8-9) similar to allergic contact dermatitis (see also Eczema/Dermatitis, Section 2) or (2) lichen planus-like eruptions. In chronic drug photoallergy, there is scaling, lichenification, and marked pruritus mimicking atopic dermatitis or chronic contact eczematous dermatitis (Fig. 8-10). (See also Eczema/Dermatitis, Section 2.)

Distribution Confined primarily to areas exposed to light (distribution pattern of photosensitivity), but there may be spreading onto adjacent nonexposed skin; therefore, not so well circumscribed as in phototoxic reactions.

LABORATORY EXAMINATIONS

Dermatopathology Acute and chronic delayed-type hypersensitivity reaction: epidermal spongiosis with lymphocytic infiltration.

DIAGNOSIS

History of exposure to drug is most important, as well as the types of morphologic changes in the skin that are characteristic of photoallergic drug reactions; this is essentially a contact eczematous pattern, while phototoxic drug eruptions mimic an exaggerated sunburn. In essence, the differential diagnosis between phototoxic and photoallergic drug-induced photosensitivity is identical to that described for toxic/irritant and allergic contact dermatitis (see also Eczema/Dermatitis, Section 2).

COURSE AND PROGNOSIS

Photoallergic drug reactions are difficult to diagnose and require the use of patch and photopatch tests. Photopatch tests are done in duplicate because photoallergens also can cause contact hypersensitivity. As in patch tests for contact hypersensitivity, photoallergens are applied to the skin and covered. After 24 h, one set of the duplicate test sites is exposed to UVA while the other set remains covered, and test

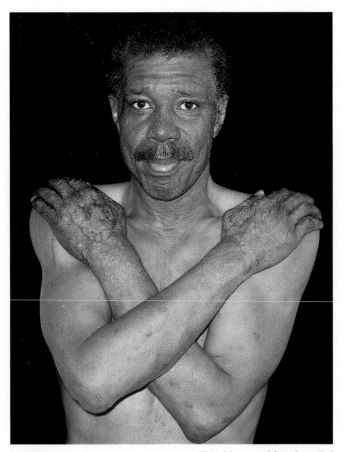

Figure 8-9   Photoallergic drug-induced photosensitivity   *This 51-year-old male with brown normal skin with advanced HIV disease shows an eczematous dermatitis with hyperpigmentation in the sun-exposed sites (face, neck, dorsum of hands and wrist). He was taking trimethoprim-sulfamethoxazole as primary prophylaxis of* Pneumocystis carinii *pneumonia (PCP).*

sites are read for reactions after 48 to 96 h. An eczematous reaction in the irradiated site but not in the nonirradiated site confirms photoallergy to the particular agent tested.

Photoallergic dermatitis can persist for months to years. This is known as *persistent light reaction (chronic actinic dermatitis)* (Fig. 8-10) and was first observed in soldiers in World War II in whom topical sulfonamides were used and in patients with chronic chlorpromazine photoallergy. The classic generalized persistent light reactions were caused by exposure to topical salicylanilides. In the persistent light reaction, the action spectrum usually broadens to involve UVB, and the condition persists despite discontinuation of the causative photoallergen

with each new UV exposure aggravating the condition. Chronic eczema-like lichenified and itching confluent plaques result (Fig. 8-10), which lead to gross disfigurement and a distressing situation for the patient. As the condition is now independent of the original photoallergen and is aggravated by each new solar exposure, avoidance of photoallergen does not cure the disease.

MANAGEMENT

In severe cases, immunosuppression (azathioprine plus glucocorticoids or oral cyclosporine) is required.

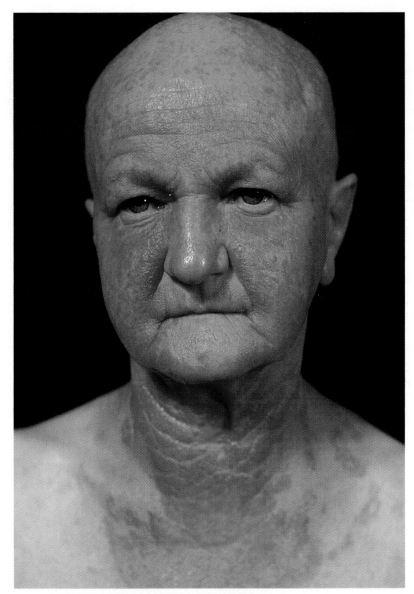

Figure 8-10   Drug-induced photosensitivity: persistent light eruption   *Thick erythematous plaques confined to the scalp, face, and exposed chest, sparing areas shaded by the nose. There is excruciating pruritus.*

POLYMORPHOUS LIGHT ERUPTION

Polymorphous light eruption (PMLE) is a term that describes a group of heterogeneous, idiopathic, acquired, acute recurrent photodermatoses characterized by delayed abnormal reactions to ultraviolet radiation (UVR) and manifested by varied lesions. The various morphologic types include erythematous macules, papules, plaques, and vesicles. However, in each patient the eruption is consistently monomorphous. By far the most frequent morphologic types are the papular and papulovesicular eruptions.

EPIDEMIOLOGY

Age of Onset   Average age is 23 years.

Sex   Much more common in females.

Race   All races, including brown and black peoples. In American Indians (North and South America) there is a hereditary type of PMLE that is also called *actinic prurigo.*

Incidence   Most common of the photodermatoses.

Skin Phototype (SPT)   More often seen in SPT I, II, III, and IV.

Geography   PMLE is less frequently observed in areas that have high solar intensity throughout the year and in persons who have adapted to persistent sun exposures. In fact, PMLE often occurs for the first time in persons traveling for short vacations to tropical areas in winter from northern latitudes. Even in these persons, the face, which has been persistently exposed, is rarely involved and the eruption appears on the trunk, arms, and legs, which have been less habitually exposed.

PATHOGENESIS

A delayed-type hypersensitivity reaction to an antigen induced by UVR is possible because of the morphology of the lesions and the histologic pattern, which shows an infiltration of T cells. Immunologic studies thus far have not been rewarding except to suggest that a delayed-type hypersensitivity is the probable immunologic basis for PLE. More commonly, UVA is the action spectrum, but PLE lesions have been evoked with UVB and with both UVA and UVB.

HISTORY

Onset and Duration of Lesions   PMLE appears in spring or early summer, and not infrequently the eruption does not recur by the end of summer, suggesting a "hardening." PMLE most often appears within 18 to 24 h of exposure and, once established, persists for 7 to 10 days, thereby limiting the vacationer's subsequent time in the sun.

Special Features   The eruption is elicited most frequently by exposure to UVA, but also can be caused by UVB or by both. Since UVA is transmitted through window glass, PMLE can be precipitated while riding in a car. In patients who travel to sunny vacation areas such as the Caribbean, the eruption will occur, yet is not noted even during the summer months in the northern latitudes; presumably the "threshold" for elicitation occurs with higher solar intensities. Also, areas of the skin habitually exposed (face and neck) are often spared, despite severe involvement of the arms, trunk, and legs.

Skin Symptoms   Pruritus (may precede the onset of the rash) and paresthesia (tingling).

Systems Review   Negative.

Family History   PMLE in American Indians is hereditary (actinic prurigo) and is characterized by papules, plaques, and nodules (mostly on the face) that can cause disfigurement.

PHYSICAL EXAMINATION

Lesions   The papular and papulo-vesicular types (Figs. 8-11 and 8-12) are the most frequent. Less common are plaques or urticarial plaques. The lesions are pink to red. In the individual patient, lesions are quite monomorphous, i.e., papulovesicular or urticarial plaques. Recurrences follow the original pattern.

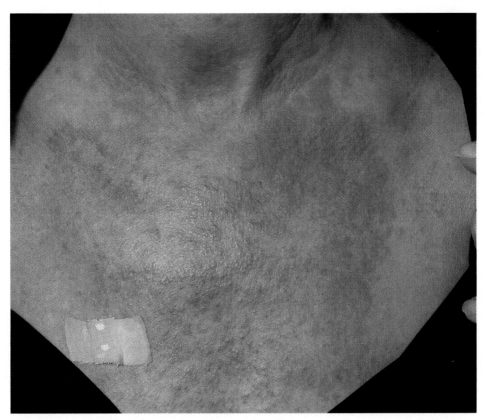

Figure 8-11 Polymorphic light eruption *Clusters of confluent, extremely pruritic papules and vesicles on the exposed chest, occurred the day following the first sun exposure of the season. The eruption also involved the dorsum of the arms, but spared the face and dorsal hands.*

Distribution The eruption often spares the face and appears most frequently on the forearms, V area of the neck (Fig. 8-11), and arms (Fig. 8-12). The lesions may also occur on the trunk if there has not been previous exposure, i.e., the relatively unexposed areas that are covered in winter, such as the upper chest and arms.

DIFFERENTIAL DIAGNOSIS

Rashes in Light-Exposed Areas *Lupus erythematosus* is the most important disease to exclude. Serologic study of antinuclear antibodies (ANA) and anti-Ro and anti-La antibodies are necessary in plaque-type PMLE. Photosensitivity eruptions caused by systemic or topical drugs and cosmetics can be ruled out by history.

LABORATORY EXAMINATIONS

Dermatopathology In papular and eczematous lesions there is edema of the epidermis, spongiosis, vesicle formation, and mild liquefaction degeneration of the basal layer but no atrophy or thickening of the basement membrane. A dense lymphocytic infiltrate is present in the dermis, with occasional neutrophils. There is edema of the papillary dermis and endothelial swelling.

Immunofluorescence (Direct) Negative.

Serology ANA is negative.

Hematology There is no leukopenia.

DIAGNOSIS

The diagnosis is not difficult: delayed onset of eruption, characteristic morphology, histopathologic changes that rule out lupus erythematosus, and the history of disappearance of the eruption in days. In plaque-type PMLE, a biopsy and immunofluorescence studies are mandatory to rule out lupus erythematosus. *Phototesting* is done with both UVB and UVA. Test sites are exposed daily, starting with 2 MEDs of UVB and UVA, respectively, for 1 week to 10 days, using increments of the UV dose. In 50% of patients, a PMLE-like eruption will occur in the test sites, confirming the diagnosis. This also helps to determine whether the action spectrum is UVB, UVA, or both.

COURSE AND PROGNOSIS

This is a pesky problem that severely limits recreational or occupational exposure to the sun. As it may occur first on vacations, it virtually limits the time outdoors for the balance of the vacation.

The course is chronic and recurrent and may, in fact, become worse each season. Although some patients may develop "tolerance" by the end of the summer, the eruption usually recurs again the following spring and/or when the person travels to tropical areas in the winter. However, spontaneous improvement or even cessation of eruptions occurs after years.

MANAGEMENT

Prevention Sunblocks, even the potent UVA-UVB sunscreens, are not always effective but should be tried first in every patient.

Systemic β-Carotene, 60 mg tid for 2 weeks before going in the sun and while in the sun; this has not been very effective but can be tried before antimalarials. Antimalarials (hydroxychloroquine, 200 mg bid 1 day before and daily while on vacation or on weekends) are quite effective drugs for the treatment of PMLE in some patients and should be used in selected patients not helped by topical sunblocks or oral β-carotene.

PUVA Photochemotherapy This treatment given in early spring induces "tolerance" for the following summer. It is highly effective, but has to be performed *before* the sunny season or before taking a trip to a sunny region. PUVA treatments are given three times weekly for 4 weeks. It is not known whether their effectiveness is based on the production of an increase in the "filtering" capacity of the epidermis (increase in the stratum corneum and in melanin content of the epidermis) or to an effect of PUVA on T cells. PUVA treatments have to be repeated each spring but are usually not necessary for more than 3 or 4 years.

Narrow band UVB-311 nm has been used with success but there are not enough patients to make a comparison with PUVA. We have had both failures and successes with hydroxychloroquine and with prophylactic use of PUVA.

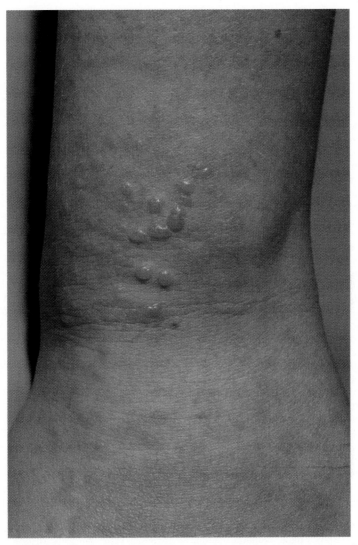

Figure 8-12 Polymorphic light eruption *Clusters of pruritic papules and vesicles on the dorsal wrist and arm, and an erythematous plaque on the dorsum of the hand following first sun exposure of the season. The face is typically spared.*

DIAGNOSIS OF PHOTOSENSITIVITY SYNDROMES*

HISTORY

The patient's history is often essential in making a diagnosis, especially because the eruption may have cleared by the time the patient is seen in consultation (Table 8-3). The persons most easily recognized as photosensitive are those whose intermittent skin eruptions have an obvious temporal relationship to sun exposure. Others, who complain of an apparent allergic reaction to sunscreens, may instead be suffering from photosensitivity for which their sunscreens are not providing adequate protection—for example, a reaction to UVA exposure, against which most current sunscreens are not fully effective. A patient taking a thiazide diuretic might present with a chronic persistent rash on exposed sites, not recognizing it as light-induced. Much less commonly, generalized erythroderma might indicate UV exposure in the context of light-sensitive psoriasis or chronic actinic dermatitis.

The age of onset of the eruption is important because certain types of photosensitivity—for example, actinic prurigo—typically begin in childhood, whereas others, such as polymorphic light eruption, can occur at any age. It is also essential to ascertain the time course of the eruption, since reactions may occur minutes (e.g., erythropoietic protoporphyria) or days (e.g., polymorphic light eruption) after exposure; they may last only a few hours (e.g., solar urticaria) or several weeks (e.g., polymorphic light eruption). Symptoms such as itching (as in polymorphic light eruption, actinic prurigo, solar urticaria, photoallergic dermatitis) or pain/burning (as in erythropoietic protoporphyria) should be noted. A rash that also occurs near an oven or open fire suggests that heat rather than UV radiation may be the exacerbating agent. A history of an eruption confined to the sunshine months is helpful when present, but some photodermatoses may occur at other times of the year. An eruption confined to the summer months suggests that UVB (290 to 320 nm) has a role; a perennial eruption suggests that UVA (320 to 400 nm) and/or visible radi-

* We acknowledge the contributions of Drs. Charles R. Taylor and John Hawk.

ation (400 to 800 nm) may be important. Another clue is to ask if the eruption can be induced by sunlight transmitted through window glass; if so, this suggests a UVA component; if not, UVB.

Other factors of importance in the history are exposure to chemicals and drugs (Table 8-2)—systemic, such as certain antipsychotic medications or antibiotics, or topical, such as sunscreens or cosmetics. A careful drug history should include both current medications and drugs to which the patient was exposed at the time the photosensitivity started, since some degree of photosensitivty occasionally can persist for months after discontinuation of an offending agent. Also important is whether occupational or recreational exposure to UV radiation or plants has occurred. For example, a patient with lupus erythematosus who works as a welder or who sits in an office under fluorescent lighting may be chronically exposed to UV radiation if protection is not used. Questions should be asked about avocations such as gardening. Finally, a review of systems should include consideration of connective tissue disease symptoms and the neurologic signs occasionally associated with some of the porphyrias.

PHYSICAL EXAMINATION

Distribution Pattern The most important clinical feature common to all the photosensitivity disorders is the distribution of skin lesions. The eruption predominantly affects sun-exposed skin, generally sparing shaded sites. Classic photodermatoses involve the forehead, malar region, nose, rim of the ears, sides and back of the neck, the V area of the chest, and the extensor surfaces of the extremities. Areas of sparing are also very important diagnostically. These usually include the recessed areas of the eyelids, the nasolabial lines, the web spaces of the fingers, and the areas behind the ears, under the nose, and under the chin (Fig. 8-1). There may be a sharp cutoff at clothing margins or at sites of jewelry. However, although the distribution is often limited to sun-exposed areas, it may not involve all exposed areas, because of protection induced by chronic UV exposure and perhaps by consequent tanning

Table 8-3 CLINICAL EVALUATION FOR PHOTOSENSITIVITY SYNDROMES

	Actinic prurigo	Chronic actinic dermatitis	Hydroa vacciniforme	Polymorphic light eruption	Solar urticaria	Hereditary coproporphyria	Porphyria cutanea tarda	Variegate porphyria	Congenital porphyria	Erythropoietic protoporphyria	Bloom's syndrome	Cockayne's syndrome	Rothmund-Thompson syndrome	Xeroderma pigmentosum	Chemical/drug-induced
	Idiopathic					Metabolic									
SIGNS AND SYMPTOMS															
Pain alone				R						◆					O
Erythema				O	M					◆	◆	◆	◆	A	O
Swelling				S						◆				A	O
Papules	◆		E	◆											O
Wheals					◆										O
Petechiae										O					O
Vesicles			◆	O		◆	◆	◆	◆	S			A		O
Scarring	◆		◆			◆	◆	◆	◆	◆				◆	O
Scaly patches	◆	◆													O
Erythroderma		◆													O
Hyperpigmentation	◆					◆	◆	◆	◆					◆	O
Other morphology	◆								◆			◆	◆	◆	
TIMING															
Exposure interval															
Minutes				R	◆			A		◆					O
Hours				◆							◆	◆	◆	A	◆
Uncertain	◆	◆	◆	O		◆	◆	◆	◆						O
Persistence															
1–2 h					◆										
Hours to days			◆	◆				A		◆					◆
Indefinite	◆	◆				◆	◆	◆	◆		◆	◆	◆	◆	
Season															
Spring/summer			◆	◆	O	◆	◆	A	◆	◆					
Year-round	◆	◆			O					◆	O				
Age of onset															
Child	◆		◆						◆	◆	◆	◆	◆	◆	
Young adult				◆		◆		◆							
Older adult		◆						◆							
Sex															
Male		◆													
Female	◆			◆											
HISTORY															
Family history															
Usual						◆		◆	◆				O		
Sometimes				◆			◆			O					
Chemical/drug															
Exposure	O					◆	◆	◆							◆

◆ = many cases   A = acute cases   M = mild cases   S = severe cases
O = occasional cases   E = early cases   R = rare cases

SOURCE: TB Fitzpatrick, J Clin Dermatol. 3:14, 1996.

CHART INFORMATION COMPILED BY JOHN L. M. HAWK, MD

or local immunologic tolerance. By contrast, nonexposed areas sometimes may be affected, because clothing is not always completely protective or because the photosensitivty may be so severe that the disease extends beyond the exposed skin, in very rare cases to erythroderma. Usually patients with such extensive disease initially develop their eruption only on exposed areas.

Types of Lesions The morphologic changes encountered with photosensitivity include combinations of erythema, papules, plaques, vesicles, urticaria, bullae, eczema, and altered pigmentation. Infrequently, petechiae, purpura, erythroderma, and scarring may be seen. Confluent erythema is typical of sunburn and occasionally may be the only sign of drug phototoxicity. Erythema and edema, especially if patchy on exposed sites, may suggest polymorphic light eruption—or, if they are confluent, solar urticaria or erythropoietic protoporphyria. Pruritic papules and less often plaques in a sunexposed distribution, but often with sparing of some sun-exposed sites, are typical of polymorphic light eruption. Eczematous dermatitis may be seen in chronic actinic dermatitis, light-aggravated atopic or seborrheic dermatitis, photocontact dermatitis, or occasionally, photosensitivity induced by drugs (e.g., thiazides). Blistering may be seen with porphyria cutanea tarda, polymorphic light eruption, photocontact dermatitis, solar urticaria, and drug phototoxicity.

Laboratory Studies (Table 8-4) First-line laboratory investigations for all photosensitive patients generally should include a routine assessment of complete blood count with platelets, liver function tests, renal function, and particularly serum ANA/Ro/La and possibly histology. Skin biopsy is adjunctive and often nondiagnostic, used mainly to confirm a suspected diagnosis or to classify a clinically atypical eruption. Usually these biopsies are from lesional skin, whether sun-exposed or not. If systemic lupus erythematosus is suspected, lesional biopsies from both sun-exposed and sunprotected skin may be needed, along with a nonlesional biopsy from a sun-protected area for histology and direct immunofluorescence.

Second-line investigations may be available only in specialized centers. In patients with a suggestive history or with signs of a porphyria—or in doubtful cases—screening of blood, urine, and stool porphyrins, or preferably of the plasma by spectrofluorometry, is necessary. If an abnormality is found, the porphyrin should then be quantified. Cutaneous phototesting is very important if photosensitivity is suspected; monochromatic or broad-spectrum testing may be used—the former to define an abnormal action spectrum, most reliably in solar urticaria and chronic actinic dermatitis, and the latter to attempt to reproduce the eruption for diagnosis on clinical and histologic grounds, which is sometimes difficult. Patch and photopatch testing are indicated in an eczematous photosensitivity, particularly in chronic actinic dermatitis, where contact factors are often suspected of promoting the eruption.

MANAGEMENT

General treatment principles for all photosensitive patients require removal of any offending agent(s) such as the causative drug or allergen and instruction concerning restriction of sun exposure between the hours of 11 A.M. and 3 P.M., high sun protection factor sunscreens, and appropriate protective clothing, including a hat. Patients with UVA sensitivity need to be aware that many sunblocks have until recently provided only minimal protection in the UVA range and that there is thus a greater need to restrict sun exposure and use protective clothing. Therapy for the eruptions themselves is generally similar to that for other inflammatory dermatoses and involves topical glucocorticoids in mild cases and prophylactic courses of low-dose phototherapy, whether UVB or PUVA, systemic glucocorticoids, or immunosuppressive therapy, in severe chronic actinic dermatitis. The majority of patients can be helped significantly.

Table 8-4 LABORATORY TESTS FOR PHOTOSENSITIVITY

The diagnosis of a photosensitivity syndrome is frequently made on the basis of a careful history and physical examination. Laboratory investigations serve to support the clinical suspicion. Generally, serology (ANA, Ro, La) is indicated for all patients with photosensitivity. Because of the possibility of overlapping syndromes (for example, solar urticaria and erythropoietic protoporphyria) many specialized centers will obtain the following laboratory studies and utilize the panel of positive and negative results to define the photosensitivity.

Blood, Urine, and Stool Porphyrin Testing
Useful in suspected light sensitivity

Blood cell and plasma
- Congenital porphyria (raised uroporphyrin and coproporphyrin)
- Erythropoietic protoporphyria (raised protoporphyrin)

Urine
- Congenital porphyria (raised uroporphyrin and coproporphyrin)
- Hereditary coproporphyria (raised coproporphyrin; raised aminolevulinic acid and porphobilinogen during attacks only)
- Porphyria cutanea tarda (raised uroporphyrin)
- Variegate porphyria (raised aminolevulinic acid and porphobilinogen during attacks only)

Stool
- Congenital porphyria (raised uroporphyrin and coproporphyrin)
- Erythropoietic protoporphyria (raised protoporphyrin)
- Hereditary coproporphyria (raised coproporphyrin)
- Porphyria cutanea tarda (occasionally positive with coproporphyrin)
- Variegate prophyria (raised protoporphyrin and coproporphyrin)

Antinuclear Factor, Anti-SSA, and Anti-SSB Titer Estimations
Essential in lupus suspected light sensitivity

Phototesting
Essential in suspected light sensitivity, especially eczematous variety

Used to make diagnosis of chronic actinic dermatitis or eczematous chemical/drug-induced photosensitivity. Determines action spectrum; broadbased testing may establish reduced minimal erythema dose photosensitivities; repeated photoprovocation testing may induce actual eruption, especially in polymorphic light eruption.

Helpful in suspected:
- Solar urticaria—to induce wheals and to determine action spectrum (preferably monochromatic testing); wheals induced by UVB, UVA, visible light, or combination
- Xeroderma pigmentosum, Cockayne's syndrome—to make diagnosis (delayed and persistent appearance of minimal erythema dose photosensitivity for 48–72 h)

Often helpful in suspected:
- Actinic prurigo
- Hydroa vacciniforme
- Light-exacerbated dermatoses (preferably using a solar simulator)
- Polymorphic light eruption

Occasionally helpful in suspected:
- Cutaneous porphyrias, for which monochromator may induce erythema and, less often, wheal, pigmentation, or petechiae at 400–500 nm.

Patch and Photopatch Testing
Essential in eczematous suspected light sensitivity.

Undertaken on clear skin of back to standard patch and photopatch test series; sometimes shows precipitating or exacerbating allergen or photoallergen.
- Chemical/drug-induced photosensitivity
- Chronic actinic dermatitis

Lesional Skin Biopsy
May provide supporting evidence for photosensitivity diagnosis
- Cutaneous porphyrias
- Hydroa vacciniforme
- Lupus erythematosus
- Polymorphic light eruption
- Porphyria cutanea tarda
- Severe chronic actinic dermatitis

Assessment of DNA Repair
Useful for early diagnosis of xeroderma pigmentosum

Direct immunofluorescence
May provide strong or supporting evidence for:
- Lupus erythematosus

Porphyria Cutanea Tarda

Porphyria cutanea tarda (PCT), as the name implies, occurs mostly in adults rather than children. Patients do not present with characteristic photosensitivity but with complaints of "fragile skin," vesicles, and bullae, particularly on the dorsa of the hands, especially after minor trauma; the diagnosis is confirmed by the presence of a pinkish-red fluorescence in the urine when examined with a Wood's lamp. PCT is distinct from variegate porphyria (VP) and acute intermittent porphyria (AIP) in that patients with PCT do not have acute life-threatening attacks (abdominal pain, peripheral autonomic neuropathy, and respiratory failure). Furthermore, the drugs that induce PCT (ethanol, estrogens, and chloroquine) are fewer than the drugs that induce VP and AIP. For classification of the porphyrias, see Table 8-5.

Table 8-5 CLASSIFICATION OF THE PORPHYRIAS

	Erythropoietic Porphyrias		Hepatic Porphyria		
	Congenital Erythropoietic Porphyria	Erythropoietic Protoporphyria	Porphyria Cutanea Tarda	Variegate Porphyria	Intermittent Acute Porphyria
Inheritance	Autosomal recessive	Autosomal dominant	Autosomal dominant (familial form)	Autosomal dominant	Autosomal dominant
Signs and symptoms					
Photosensitivity	Yes	Yes	Yes	Yes	No
Cutaneous lesions	Yes	Yes	Yes	Yes	No
Attacks of abdominal pain	No	No	No	Yes	Yes
Neuropsychiatric syndrome	No	No	No	Yes	Yes
Laboratory abnormalities	+	+	+	+	+
Red blood cells					
Fluorescence	+	+	−	−	−
Uroporphyrin	+++	N	N	N	N
Coproporphyrin	++	+	N	N	N
Protoporphyrin	(+)	+++	N	N	N
Plasma					
Fluorescence	+	+	−	−	−
Urine		−			
Fluorescence	−	−	+	±	−
Porphobilinogen	N	N	N	(+++)	(+++)
Uroporphyrin	+++	N	+++	+++	+++
Feces					
Protoporphyrin	+	++	N	+++	N

NOTE: N, normal; +, above normal; ++, moderately increased; +++, markedly increased; +++, frequently increased—depends on whether patient has an attack or is in remission; (+), increased in some patients.

EPIDEMIOLOGY

Age of Onset 30 to 50 years, rarely in children; females on oral contraceptives (18 to 30 years); males on estrogen therapy for prostate cancer (older than 60 years).

Sex Equal in males and in females.

Heredity Most PCT patients have *type I (acquired)* induced by drugs, especially alcohol, or chemicals (e.g., hexachlorobenzene fungicide). *Type II (hereditary)*—possibly these patients actually have VP, but this is not yet resolved. There is also a "dual" type with VP and PCT in the same family.

Enzyme abnormality UROGEN decarboxylase in both types I and II.

Chemicals and Drugs That Induce PCT Ethanol, estrogen, hexachlorobenzene (fungicide), chlorinated phenols, iron, tetrachlorodibenzo-*p*-dioxin. High doses of chloroquine may lead to clinical manifestations in "latent" cases (low doses, 125 mg twice weekly, are used as treatment).

Other Predisposing Factors Diabetes mellitus (25%), hepatitis C virus.

PATHOGENESIS

In some patients there is a reduction in the liver enzyme uroporphyrin decarboxylase, which catalyzes decarboxylation of the four acetate groups to methyl groups. This reduction of enzyme may occur in familial or nonfamilial PCT.

HISTORY

Duration of Lesions No acute skin changes but gradual onset, and patients may present with bullae on the hands and feet based on a photosensitivity reaction to sun and yet will have a suntan.

Symptoms Pain from erosions in easily traumatized skin ("fragile skin").

Systems Review In VP there is autonomic neuropathy with acute abdominal pain and peripheral neuropathy. In erythropoietic protoporphyria and PCT there can be hepatic disease. Associated diseases may lead to multisystem alterations (see Differential Diagnosis, below).

PHYSICAL EXAMINATION

Skin Lesions Tense bullae on normal-appearing skin (Fig. 8-13).

Erosions: in the sites of the vesicles and bullae; erosions slowly heal to form pink atrophic scars at sites of erosions. Milia, 1 to 5 mm. Hypertrichosis of the face (may be a presenting complaint). Scleroderma-like induration.
Purple-red suffusion ("heliotrope") of central facial skin (Fig. 8-14), especially periorbital areas. Brown hypermelanosis, diffuse, on exposed areas (Fig. 8-14).

Distribution Dorsa of hands and feet (toes), nose (vesicles, bullae, and erosions).
Scleroderma-like changes, diffuse or circumscribed, waxy yellowish white areas on exposed areas of face, neck, and trunk, sparing the doubly clothed area of the breast in females.
Hypertrichosis: dark brown or black hair on the temples and cheeks and, in severe disease, on the trunk and extremities.

DIAGNOSIS

By clinical features, pink-red fluorescence of urine and elevated urinary porphyrins.

DIFFERENTIAL DIAGNOSIS

Bullae on Dorsa of Hands and Feet

Pseudo-PCT A distinctive syndrome with blisters and erosions clinically indistinguishable from PCT. Drugs (naproxen, ibuprofen, tetracyclines, nalidixic acid, dapsone, amiodarone, bumetanide, cyclosporine, etretinate, furosemide, chlorthalidone, diazide, pyridoxine). Chronic renal failure with hemodialysis. Tanning salon radiation (visible and UVA). Other associated conditions: hepatoma, SLE, sarcoidosis, Sjögren's syndrome, hepatitis C. May occasionally resemble dyshidrotic eczema but bullae are on the dorsa. *Epidermolysis bullosa acquisita* has the same clinical picture (increased skin fragility, easy bruising, and light-provoked bullae) and some of the histology (subepidermal bullae with little or no dermal inflammation). (See Variegate porphyria, page 242.)

LABORATORY EXAMINATIONS

Dermatopathology Bullae, subepidermal with "festooned" (undulating) base. PAS reveals thickened vascular walls. Paucity of an inflammatory infiltrate.

Immunofluorescence IgG and other immunoglobulins at the dermal-epidermal junction and in and around blood vessels, in the sun-exposed areas of the skin. Thickening of vessel walls is due to multiple reduplications of vas-

cular basement membrane and deposits of immunoglobulins and fibrin.

Chemistry

Plasma iron may be increased

Blood glucose   Increased in those patients
with diabetes mellitus (25% of patients).

Porphyrin Studies in Stool and Urine
(Tables 8-5 and 8-6)
Increased uroporphyrin (I isomer, 60%) in urine
and plasma.
Increased isocoproporphyrin (type III) and 7-
carboxylporphyrin in the feces.
No increase in δ-aminolevulinic acid or porphobilinogen in the urine.
Wood's lamp examination of the urine. To enhance the orange-red fluorescence, add a few
drops of 10% hydrochloric acid.
It is important to obtain levels of porphyrins in
the stool to rule out VP, which has markedly elevated fecal protoporphyrin as the diagnostic
hallmark.

Liver Biopsy   Reveals porphyrin fluorescence
and often fatty liver.

MANAGEMENT

1. Avoid ethanol. Stop drugs that could be in-
    ducing PCT, such as estrogen, and elimi-
    nate exposure to chemicals (chlorinated
    phenols, tetrachlorodibenzo-*p*-dioxin). In
    some patients, complete avoidance of
    ethanol ingestion will result in a clinical
    and biochemical remission and in depletion
    of the high level of iron stores in the liver.
2. Phlebotomy is done by removing 500 ml of
    blood at weekly or biweekly intervals until
    the hemoglobin is decreased to 10 g. Clin-
    ical and biochemical remission occurs
    within 5 to 12 months after regular phle-
    botomy. Relapse within a year is uncom-
    mon (5 to 10%).
3. Chloroquine is used to induce remission of
    PCT in patients in whom phlebotomy is
    contraindicated because of anemia. Since
    chloroquine can exacerbate the disease and,
    in higher doses, may even induce hepatic
    failure in these patients, this treatment re-
    quires considerable experience. However,

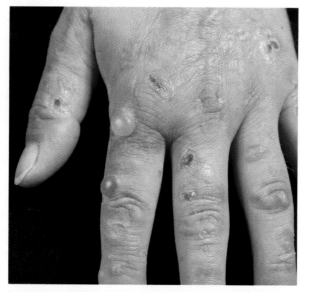

Figure 8-13   Porphyria cutanea tarda   *Bullae and atrophic depigmented scars on the knuckles and
milia of the left hand. This is not an acute reaction to initial sun exposure but develops over time
with repeated sun exposure. The patient presents with a history of "fragile" skin, and bullae. The
hand changes developed in mid-summer while this patient was on a fishing trip during which he
noticed that the skin on the backs of his hands were easily damaged, with the skin slipping in
spots. This condition is called the "fisherman's disease," in which there are three etiologic
factors present: alcohol (beer drinking while fishing), sun exposure (while in a boat), and trauma
to the backs of the hands (reeling in the fish).*

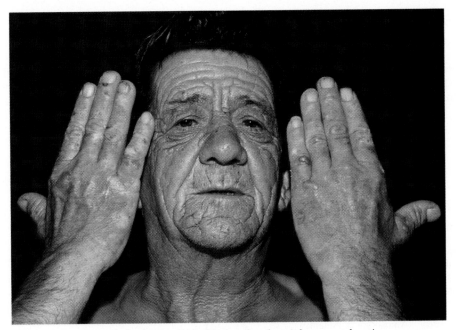

Figure 8-14 Porphyria cutanea tarda *Periorbital and malar violaceous coloration, hyperpigmentation, and hypertrichosis on the face; bullae, crust, and scars on the dorsa of the hands.*

long-lasting remissions and, in a portion of patients, clinical and biochemical "cure" can be achieved.

The best approach currently used by one of us (K. W.) is to start with a course of three consecutive phlebotomies every other day followed by 150 mg of chloroquine PO/d. Close clinical and laboratory (transaminases, porphyrin excretion in urine) is required to adjust the chloroquine dose which is eventually tapered to 150 mg twice a week and continued for several months.

Table 8-6 LABORATORY DIFFERENTIAL DIAGNOSIS OF HEPATIC PORPHYRIAS

	Porphyria Cutanea Tarda	Variegate Porphyria
Urine tests		
During acute attacks		
PBG	N	++
URO	++	++
COPRO	+	++
Between acute attacks		
PBG	N	N
URO	++	N
COPRO	+	N
Ratio URO/COPRO	>1	<1
Stool tests		
COPRO	++	++
PROTO	+	++
URO	+	N

ABBREVIATIONS: N, normal; +, mild elevation; ++, marked elevation; URO, uroporphyrin; COPRO, coproporphyrin; PBG, porphobilinogen

Variegate Porphyria

Variegate porphyria (VP) is a serious autosomal dominant disorder of heme biosynthesis characterized by skin lesions that are identical to those of PCT (vesicles and bullae, skin fragility, milia, and scarring of the dorsa of the hands and fingers), acute attacks of abdominal pain, neuropsychiatric manifestations, and increased excretion of porphyrins; especially characteristic are high levels of protoporphyrin in the feces.

Synonym: Porphyria variegata.

EPIDEMIOLOGY

Age of Onset   Second to fourth decades.

Race   All races; especially common in white South Africans (3:1000) (a large proportion of the present white population was descended from an early Dutch settler who emigrated to South Africa from Holland in 1680 to where VP can be traced). It is increasingly recognized in Europe (Finland) and the United States.

Heredity   Autosomal dominant.

Precipitating Factors   See Table 8-7.

PATHOGENESIS

The basic metabolic defect is accentuated by ingestion of certain drugs (sulfonamides, barbiturates, phenytoin, estrogens, alcohol, and others) (Table 8-7), with the resultant precipitation of acute attacks of abdominal pain and neuropsychiatric disorders (delirium, seizures, personality changes). There is an enzyme defect resulting in a reduction of protoporphyrin oxidase, with accumulation of protoporphyrinogen in the liver, which is excreted in the bile and is nonenzymatically converted to protoporphyrin; this accounts for the high fecal protoporphyrin.

HISTORY

Change with Seasons   Skin lesions occur during the summer season but may persist throughout the winter; lesions result from exposure to sunlight.

Skin Symptoms   Painful erosions, skin fragility.

Constitutional Symptoms   None.

Systems Review   Acute attacks of abdominal pain, constipation, nausea and vomiting, muscle weakness, seizures, confusional state, psychiatric symptoms (depression, coma); rarely, cranial nerve involvement, bulbar paralysis, sensory loss, and paresthesias.

Drug Exposure   See Table 8-7.

PHYSICAL EXAMINATION

Skin Lesions   Vesicles or, more commonly, bullae (Fig. 8-15); erosions, milia; sclerosis (scleroderma-like changes); scars (pink, atrophic). Periorbital heliotrope hue, diffuse melanoderma on exposed areas.

Distribution   Localization to dorsa of hands, fingers, and feet (exposed areas).

Hair   Hypertrichosis (especially in sunny climates).

Miscellaneous Findings   Neurologic, especially peripheral neuropathy.

DIFFERENTIAL DIAGNOSIS

Pseudoporphyria, scleroderma, epidermolysis bullosa (acquired-type), hereditary coproporphyria, hepatoerythropoietic porphyria.

LABORATORY EXAMINATIONS

Dermatopathology

Site   Dermal-epidermal interface and dermis.

Process   Subepidermal bullae formation (festooning); PAS-positive, diastase-resistant depositions in and around blood vessels of the upper dermis.

General   Laboratory   Examination *Porphyrins*   See Table 8-6.

Plasma   Distinctive plasma fluorescence with emission maximum at 626 nm.

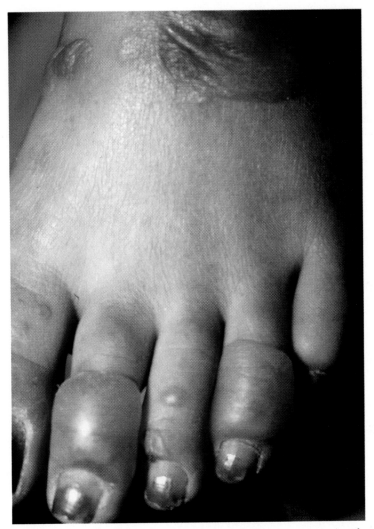

Figure 8-15 Variegate porphyria *Bulllae on the dorsum of the foot, a common site of sun exposure in patients wearing open footwear. This 42-year-old female was diagnosed with porphyria cutanea tarda. The lesions in porphyria cutanea tarda are identical to the lesions in variegate porphyria. This patient, however, gave a history of recurrent attacks of abdominal pain, which was a clue to the diagnosis of variegate porphyria; this diagnosis was established by the detection of elevated stool protoporphyrins. Variegate porphyria (or South African porphyria) is akin to acute porphyria, in which a fatal outcome may occur with ingestion of certain drugs (see Table 8-7). In South Africa every patient who is scheduled for major surgery must have laboratory tests for porphyrins since variegate porphyria is common in that country.*

Urine   Increased porphobilinogen during acute attacks.

Stools   High protoporphyrin.

COURSE AND PROGNOSIS

Lifetime disease with onset after puberty and peak incidence in the second to fourth decades. Skin manifestations not provoked by drugs that precipitate abdominal and neuropsychiatric symptoms, except for estrogens, which provoke cholestatic hepatitis, diverting porphyrin from the bile to the blood, with resulting increased porphyrin deposition in the skin.

Good, if exacerbating factors are avoided (certain drugs, alcohol, infection). Rarely, death can occur after ingestion or injection of drugs (e.g., barbiturates, general anesthesia) that induce increased amounts of cytochrome P450 and create a demand for increased synthesis of heme.

MANAGEMENT

None; oral β-carotene may or may not control the skin manifestations but has no effect on porphyrin metabolism or the important systemic manifestations.

Table 8-7   DRUGS HAZARDOUS TO PATIENTS WITH VARIEGATE PORPHYRIA

Anesthetics: barbiturates and halothane	Imipramine
Anticonvulsants: hydantoins, carbamazepine, ethosuximide, methsuximide, phensuximide, primidone	Methyldopa
	Minor tranquilizers: chlordiazepoxide, diazepam, oxazepam, flurazepam, meprobamate
Antimicrobial agents: chloramphenicol, griseofulvin, novobiocin, pyrazinamide, sulfonamides	Pentazocine
	Phenylbutazone
Ergot preparations	Sulfonylureas: chlorpropamide, tolbutamide
Ethyl alcohol	Theophyline
Hormones: estrogens, progestins, oral contraceptive preparations	

Erythropoietic Protoporphyria

This hereditary metabolic disorder of porphyrin metabolism is unique among the porphyrias in that porphyrins or porphyrin precursors are not excreted in the urine. Also, erythropoietic protoporphyria (EPP) is characterized by an acute sunburn-like photosensitivity, in contrast to the other common porphyrias (porphyria cutanea tarda or variegate porphyria), in which obvious acute photosensitivity is *not* a presenting complaint.

Synonym: Erythrohepatic protoporphyria.

EPIDEMIOLOGY

Age of Onset Acute photosensitivity begins early in childhood; rarely, late onset in early adulthood.

Sex Equal in males and females.

Race All ethnic groups, including blacks.

Heredity Autosomal dominant with variable penetrance.

Incidence Not uncommon; series reported from Europe (in The Netherlands, 1:100,000; Austria, United Kingdom), and the United States.

PATHOGENESIS

The specific enzyme defect occurs at the step in porphyrin metabolism in which protoporphyrin is converted to heme by the enzyme ferrochelatase. This leads to an accumulation of protoporphyrin that is highly photosensitizing.

HISTORY

Duration of Onset of Lesions Stinging, burning, and itching may occur *within a few minutes* of sunlight exposure; later, erythema and edema appear after 1 to 8 h. Not always easy to elicit a history of photosensitivity: subtle history with burning on the hands while on the steering wheel that have been exposed through the front glass plate, while driving into the sun.

Seasonal Changes Photosensitivity is less common in the winter months in temperate areas.

Symptoms Burning or "stinging" sensation within minutes may be the only abnormality. Children may choose not to go out in the direct sunlight after a few painful episodes, which may cause serious sociopsychologic problems. Symptoms occur when exposed to sunlight through window glass.

Systems Review Biliary colic, even in children.

PHYSICAL EXAMINATION

Skin Changes in Acute Reactions to Sunlight Exposure Bright red erythema, later edema (swelling of hands especially), urticaria (less common), purpura [especially on the nose (Fig. 8-16) and tips of ears]. Vesicles or bullae rarely occur. These changes appear within 1 to 8 h and subside after several hours or days without obvious scarring.

Skin Changes After Chronic Recurrent Exposures Shallow, often linear scars, especially on the nose and dorsa of the hands ("aged knuckles"). Diffuse wrinkling of the skin of the face (nose, around the lips, cheeks) with obvious thickening of the skin and a waxy color (Fig. 8-17). Crusted, erosive lesions may occur on the nose and lips. In contrast to PCT absence of sclerodermoid changes, hypertrichosis, or hyperpigmentation.

General Medical Findings Hemolytic anemia with hypersplenism (rare). Cholelithiasis (12%), even in children; stones contain large amounts of protoporphyrin. Liver disease may result from massive deposition of protoporphyrin in the hepatocytes; fatal hepatic cirrhosis is rare, but occurs.

LABORATORY EXAMINATIONS

Porphyrin Studies Increased protoporphyrin in red blood cells (RBCs), plasma, and stools but no excretion in the urine except in the rare cases with fatal hepatic cirrhosis. Decreased activity of the enzyme, ferrochelatase, in the bone marrow, liver, and skin fibroblasts (Table 8-5).

Liver Function Tests for liver function are indicated. Liver biopsy has demonstrated portal and periportal fibrosis and deposits of brown pigment and birefringent granules in hepatocytes and Kupffer cells. With electron microscopy, needle-like crystals are observed. About 20 patients have been reported with cirrhosis and portal hypertension.

Special Examination for Fluorescent Erythrocytes RBCs in a blood smear exhibit a characteristic *transient* fluorescence when examined with a fluorescent microscope with a mercury or tungsten-iodide lamp that emits 400-nm radiation.

Dermatopathology

Marked eosinophilic homogenization and thickening of the blood vessels in the papillary dermis; there is an accumulation of an amorphous, hyaline-like eosinophilic substance in and around blood vessels.

Radiography Gallstones may be present.

DIAGNOSIS

In EPP there is photosensitivity but no "rash," only an exaggerated sunburn response that appears much earlier than ordinary sunburn erythema. Also, the skin changes occur behind window glass. Finally, there are virtually no photosensitivity disorders in which the symptoms appear so rapidly (minutes after exposure to sunlight). Porphyrin examination establishes the diagnosis with elevated free protoporphyrin levels in the RBCs and in the stool. The fecal protoporphyrin is most consistently elevated. The urinary porphyrins are not elevated. In chronic cases, the waxy thickening and wrinkling of facial skin is diagnostic.

COURSE AND PROGNOSIS

EPP persists throughout life, but the photosensitivity may become less apparent in late adulthood. Liver cirrhosis may become manifest in adults. Rarely, fatal outcome due to hepatic failure.

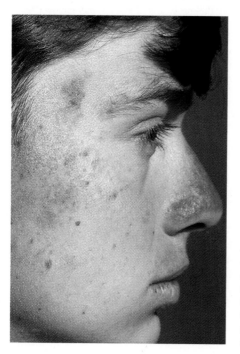

Figure 8-16 Erythropoietic protoporphyria
Diffuse erythematous infiltration of the nose with edema, petechial hemorrhage, and scattered atrophic scars on the side of the face with telangiectasia. There are no porphyrins in the urine. A clue to the diagnosis is the history of tingling and burning within 4 to 5 minutes of sun exposure, so that children will not play outdoors.

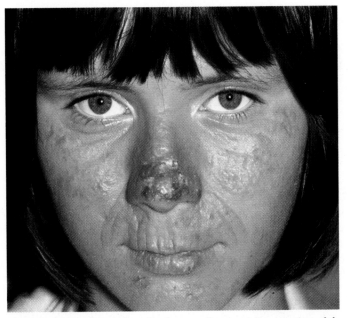

Figure 8-17 Erythropoietic protoporphyria *Erythema, edema, erosion, crusting of the nose with less severe changes on the chin of a 15-year-old female. Deep wrinkling and a peculiar waxy thickening on the upper lip and cheeks similar to dermatoheliosis in photoaged skin.*

MANAGEMENT

There is no treatment for the basic metabolic abnormality, but symptomatic relief of the photosensitivity can be achieved in many patients with oral β-carotene in divided doses of 180 mg/d. Therapeutic levels of carotenoids are achieved in 1 to 2 months. This treatment brings about an amelioration of the photosensitivity but does not completely eliminate the problem of photosensitivity. Patients on β-carotene can remain outdoors longer by a factor of 8 to 10 but still burn if exposures are too long. Nevertheless, many patients can participate in outdoor sports for the first time. There is no toxicity with prolonged treatment with β-carotene. Protection by β-carotene can be considerably enhanced by PUVA-induced tanning.

PRECANCEROUS LESIONS AND CUTANEOUS CARCINOMAS

EPIDERMAL PRECANCERS AND CANCERS

Cutaneous epithelial cancers [nonmelanoma skin cancer (NMSCa)] are the most easy of all cancers to diagnose and treat. They originate most commonly in the epidermal germinative keratinocytes or adnexal structures (e.g., sweat apparatus, hair follicle, or nail apparatus). Squamous cell carcinoma (SCC) often has its origin in an identifiable dysplastic in situ lesion that can be treated before frank invasion occurs. In contrast, in situ basal cell carcinoma (BCC) does not occur, however, minimally invasive "superficial" BCCs are common. Solar keratoses are the most common precursor lesions of squamous cell carcinoma in situ (SCCIS) and invasive SCC, occurring at sites of chronic sun exposure in individuals of northern European heritage (see Section 8). Identification and treatment of precursor lesions prevents progressive cancers. NMSCa can also arise within the epithelium of adnexal structures such as sweat duct glands (e.g. porocarcinoma) and from specialized cells within the epidermis, i.e., Merkel cell carcinoma.

The two principal NMSCas are BCC and SCC. The most common etiology of NMSCa in fair skinned individuals is sunlight, ultraviolet radiation (UVR) and human papillomavirus (HPV). HPV and UVR cause the spectrum of changes ranging from epithelial dysplasia to SCCIS to invasive SCC of cutaneous epithelium. Much less commonly, NMSCa can be caused by ionizing radiation (arising in sites of chronic radiation damage), chronic inflammation, hydrocarbons (tar), and chronic ingestion of inorganic arsenic; these tumors can be much more aggresive than those associated with UVR or HPV. In the increasing population of immunosuppressed individuals (those with HIV disease, organ transplant recipients, etc.), UVR- and HPV-induced SCCs are much more common, and can be more aggressive.

Epithelial Precancerous Lesions and SCCIS

Dysplasia of epidermal keratinocytes in epidermis and squamous mucosa can involve the lower portion of the epidermis (e.g., solar keratosis, squamous intraepithelial lesion) or the full thickness (e.g., squamous cell carcinoma). Basal cells are affected by agents such as ultraviolet radiation (UVR) or human papillomavirus (HPV) infection, and mature into dysplastic keratinocytes with retention of nuclear DNA in the corneocytes resulting in a hyperkeratotic papule, nodule, or plaque, clinically identified as "keratoses". A continuum of dysplasia exists from dysplasia to squamous cell carcinoma in situ (SCCIS) to invasive SCC. These lesions have various associated eponyms such as Bowen's disease, erythroplasia of Queyrat, etc., which as descriptive morphological terms are helpful but are mainly of historical interest. Terms such as UVR- or HPV-associated SCCIS, however, are more meaningful, but can be used only for those lesions with known etiology.

Precancerous keratinocyte lesions (intraepithelial dysplasias and squamous cell carcinoma in situ)

UVR-induced
Solar (actinic) keratosis
Hypertrophic actinic keratosis
Spreading pigmented actinic keratosis (SPAK)
Proliferative actinic keratosis
Lichenoid actinic keratosis
Bowenoid actinic keratosis
SCCIS (Bowen's disease)
HPV-induced
Low-grade squamous intraepithelial lesion (LSIL)
High-grade squamous intraepithelial lesion (HSIL)
SCCIS (bowenoid papulosis)
Arsenical keratoses
Palmoplantar keratoses
Bowenoid arsenical keratoses
Hydrocarbon (tar) keratoses
Bowenoid tar keratoses

Thermal keratoses
Bowenoid thermal keratoses
Keratoses in chronic radiation dermatitis
Bowenoid radiation keratoses
Chronic cicatrix (scar) keratoses
Bowenoid tar keratoses
Squamous cell carcinoma in situ (Bowen's disease)
URV-associated
HPV-associated (bowenoid papulosis)
Solitary genital lesions (erythroplasia of Queyrat); may or may not be HPV-associated
The terms *leukoplakia* or *erythroplakia* are archaic, having no precise clinical or histologic meaning. A precancerous lesion is implied, but many white or red lesions such as lichen planus are benign inflammatory lesions. Lesions should be biopsied and diagnosis made as to whether the process is benign, precancerous, or cancerous. (See Section 29.)

Solar Actinic Keratosis

These single or multiple, discrete, dry, rough, adherent scaly lesions occur on the habitually sun-exposed skin of adults.

Synonym: Actinic keratosis.

For a full discussion of this condition, see Section 8.

Cutaneous Horn

A cutaneous horn (CH) is a clinical entity having the appearance of an animal horn such as that of a rhinoceros, with a macular, papular, or nodular base with a keratotic cap of various shapes and lengths. Multiple disorders can result in the formation of a CH. They most commonly represent hypertrophic solar keratoses. In situ or invasive squamous cell carcinoma (SCC) can arise within solar keratoses and present as CHs. CHs which represent solar keratoses, SCCIS, or invasive SCC and usually arise within areas of photoaging (dermatoheliosis) on the face, ear, dorsum of hands, or forearms. CH formation can also occur in seborrheic keratoses, warts, and keratoacanthomas.

Clinically, CHs vary in size from a few millimeters to several centimeters (Fig. 9-1). The horn may be white, black, or yellowish in color, and straight, curved, or spiral in shape. Histologically, CH shows solid hyperkeratosis and parakeratosis. The granular layer may be present under the hyperkeratotic areas ± variable acanthosis (thickening or hyperplasia of the viable epidermis) and usually solar keratosis, SCCIS, or invasive SCC at the base. Because of the possibility of invasive SCC, a CH should be excised.

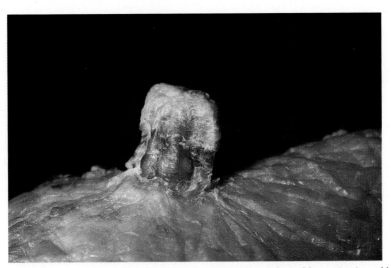

Figure 9-1 Cutaneous horn, hand: hypertrophic actinic keratosis *A horn-like projection of keratin on a slightly raised base in the setting of advanced dermatoheliosis in an 83-year-old female. Excision showed actinic keratosis at the base.*

RADIATION DERMATITIS[1]

Radiation dermatitis is defined as skin changes resulting from exposure to ionizing radiation. There are *reversible effects,* i.e., erythema, epilation, suppression of sebaceous glands, and pigmentation that lasts for weeks to months to years, and *irreversible effects,* i.e., acute and chronic radiation dermatitis and radiation-induced cancers.

Type of Exposure

Result of therapy (for cancer, formerly also used for acne and psoriasis), accidental, or occupational (e.g., formerly, in dentists who held the film in the mouth with their fingers). The radiation causing radiodermatitis includes superficial and deep x-ray radiation, electron-beam therapy, and grenz-ray therapy. It is a prevailing myth among some dermatologists that grenz rays are "soft" and not carcinogenic; it has been estimated that SCC can appear from more than 5000 cGy of grenz rays.

Types of Reactions

Acute Temporary erythema that lasts 3 days and then main erythema, which reaches a peak in 2 weeks (Fig. 9-2); pigmentation appears about day 20; a late erythema also can occur beginning on day 35 to 40, and this lasts 2 to 3 weeks. Massive reactions lead to blistering and ulceration. Permanent scarring may result.

Chronic After *fractional* but relatively intensive therapy with total doses of 3000 to 6000 rad, there develops an epidermolytic reaction in 3 weeks. This is repaired in 3 to 6 weeks, and scars and hypopigmentation develop; there is loss of all skin appendages and atrophy of the epidermis and dermis. During the next 2 to 5 years, the atrophy increases; there is hyper- and hypopigmentation (poikiloderma), telangiectasia, and superficial venules become ectatic (Fig. 9-3). There are hyperkeratoses (x-ray keratoses), but necrosis and ulceration (Fig. 9-3) are rare except by accidental exposure or error in dose: either one or a few accidentally high doses or multiple small doses at frequent intervals (monthly or weekly). When necrosis occurs, it is leathery, yellow, and adherent, and the base and surrounding skin are extremely painful. Ulcerations have a very poor tendency to heal and usually require surgical intervention

(Fig. 9-3). Accidental exposure occurs mostly in occupational exposure and affects the hands, feet, and face. There is a destruction of the fingerprint pattern, xerosis, scanty hair, atrophy of sebaceous and sweat glands, and development of keratoses. Persistent painful ulcers may appear.

Generalized Exanthems These occur beyond the irradiated area and usually follow deep x-ray therapy for internal cancers given through multiple ports. There may be fever and a dermatosis mimicking erythema multiforme or urticaria.

PHYSICAL EXAMINATION

Skin Lesions See preceding descriptions of acute and chronic radiation dermatitis. Sharp borders, rectangular, square (when result of therapy).
  Diffuse involvement (when the result of prolonged, repeated exposures, as on the hands).

Distribution Hands and fingers (in professional personnel, in dentists, or in physicians using fluoroscopy). Any site of previous therapy with ionizing radiation.

Nails Longitudinal striations (Fig. 9-5) (in chronic radiodermatitis—after repeated exposures). Thickening, dystrophy.

LABORATORY EXAMINATIONS

Dermatopathology (Chronic Radiation Dermatitis)

Atrophy of epidermis, with loss of hair follicles, sebaceous glands, and alteration of sweat glands. Hyalinization, loss of nuclei, fusion of collagen and elastic tissue. Vessel changes, including telangiectatic dilatation and fibrous thickening of the arterial wall.

[1]We acknowledge the contribution of Prof. F. Urbach and Prof. A. Wiskemann.

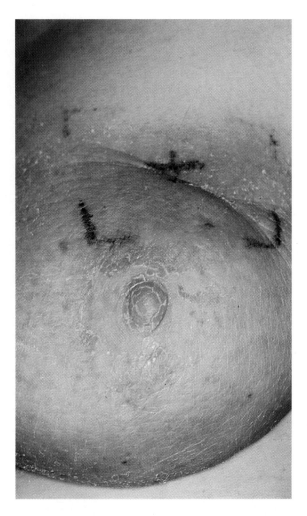

Figure 9-2　Radiodermatitis: acute
*Localized area of erythema and
edema in the radiation portal
occurring at the end of a course of
radiotherapy for breast cancer.*

COURSE, PROGNOSIS, AND MANAGEMENT

Chronic radiation dermatitis is permanent, progressive, and irreversible. Squamous cell carcinoma (SCC) may develop in 4 to 39 years (Figs. 9-3 and 9-4), with a median of 7 to 12 years, almost exclusively from the chronic repeated types of exposures. SCC always develops within the area of radiodermatitis, never in normal skin. The tumors are often multiple and metastasize late in about 25%; despite extensive surgery (excision, grafts, etc.), the prognosis is poor, and recurrences are common. In recent years there has been about an equal incidence of SCC and basal cell carcinoma (BCC). BCC appears mostly in patients formerly treated with x-rays for acne vulgaris and acne cystica or epilation (tinea capitis). The tumors may appear 40 to 50 years after exposure. Excision and grafting is often possible before the cancer develops.

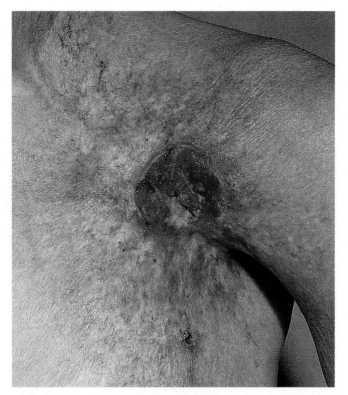

Figure 9-3 Radiation dermatitis: chronic with invasive squamous cell carcinoma of chest wall
Atrophy, fibrosis, poikiloderma, and telangiectasis on the chest wall, 20 years after radical mastectomy and axillary lymph node dissection. The ulceration is due to radionecrosis and is characterized by leathery adherent necrosis. The border of the ulcer is elevated and firm and represents SCC arising in this radiation dermatitis.

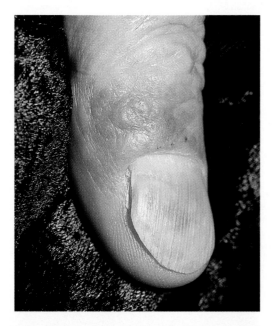

Figure 9-4 Nail changes in site of radiation exposure *Note the linear striations resulting from damage to the nail matrix. At the nailfold and extending proximally on the thumb, there is an irregular erythematous plaque which represents mostly SCCIS, but focally, also invasive SCC.*

SQUAMOUS CELL CARCINOMA IN SITU

Squamous cell carinoma in situ (SCCIS) is most often caused by ultraviolet radiation (UVR) or human papillomavirus (HPV) infection, presenting as solitary or multiple macules, papules, or plaques, which may be scaling or hyperkeratotic. SCCIS commonly arises in epithelial dysplastic lesions such as solar keratoses or HPV-induced squamous intraepithelial lesions (SIL). (See Sexually Transmitted Diseases, Section 25; Diseases of Oropharynx, Section 29).

Synonyms: These lesions have various associated eponyms such as Bowen's disease or erythroplasia of Queyrat. While terms such as UVR- or HPV-associated SCCIS are more meaningful to all specialties of medicine, Bowen's disease or erythroplasia are well defined morphological entities and thus helpful to the dermatologist.

EPIDEMIOLOGY

ETIOLOGY

UVR, HPV, arsenic, tar, chronic heat exposure, chronic radiation dermatitis, scar.

HISTORY

Lesions are most often asymptomatic, but may bleed. Nodule formation within SCCIS suggests progression to invasive SCC.

PHYSICAL EXAMINATION

Skin Findings Appears as a sharply demarcated, scaling, or hyperkeratotic macule, papule, or plaque (Fig. 9-5). Solitary or multiple lesions are often pink or red in color and have a slightly scaling surface, small erosions, and can be crusted. Such lesions are always well-defined and are called Bowen's disease (Fig. 9-5). Red, sharply demarcated, glistening macular or plaque-like SCCIS on the glans penis or labia minora are called erythroplasia (see Disorders of the Genitalia, Perineum, and Anus, Section 30). Anogenital HPV-induced SCCIS may be tan, brown, or black in color and are referred to as bowenoid papulosis. Eroded lesions may have areas of crusting (see Disorders of the Genitalia, Perineum, and Anus, Section 30). SCCIS may be mistaken for a patch of eczema or psoriasis and go undiagnosed for years, resulting in large lesions with annular or polycyclic borders (Fig. 9-7).

Distribution UVR-induced SCCIS commonly arise within a solar keratosis in the setting of photoaging (dermatoheliosis). HPV-induced SCCIS arises within an area of low-grade or high-grade SIL; multiple areas of SIL are usually present in the area. HPV-induced lesions arise periungually (Fig. 9-7), most commonly on the thumb, or in the nail bed.

Associated Findings Depending on the etiology, dermatoheliosis, actinic keratoses, condyloma acuminatum, SIL, poikiloderma congenita, epidermal nevus, porokeratosis, epidermodysplasia verruciformis.

DIFFERENTIAL DIAGNOSIS

Well-dermarcated Pink-red Plaques(s) Nummular eczema, other eczemas, psoriasis, lichen planus, seborrheic keratosis, solar keratosis, verruca vulgaris, verruca plana, condyloma acuminatum, superficial basal cell carcinoma, melanoma, Merkel cell carcinoma, Paget's disease.

LABORATORY EXAMINATIONS

Dermatopathology Keratinocytes show loss of polarity, atypia, and increased mitotic rate with involvement of the entire thickness of the epidermis from basal layer to stratum corneum. The basement membrane remains intact. The epidermis may be thickened (acanthosis) with elongation and thickening of the rete ridges. Individual cell keratinization may occur appearing as large and rounded with eosinophilic cytoplasm and a pyknotic nucleus (in some cases, multinucleated); horn pearls may occur. Depending on the etiology, associated findings include an associated solar keratosis, dermatoheliosis, evidence of HPV infection, etc.

DIAGNOSIS

Dermatopathologic findings.

COURSE AND PROGNOSIS

Untreated, invasive SCC may arise within SCCIS. Lymph node metastasis can occur without demonstrable invasion. SCCIS associated with arsenic ingestion may be associated with internal malignancies.

MANAGEMENT

Topical Chemotherapy 5-fluorouracil cream applied qd or bid with or without tape occlu-

sion is effective in some cases arising in the trunk or extremities.

Cryosurgery Effective in some cases. Lesions are usually treated more aggressively than solar keratoses and less aggressively than basal cell carcinoma.

Surgical Excision Has the highest cure rate but the greatest chance of causing cosmetically disfiguring scars.

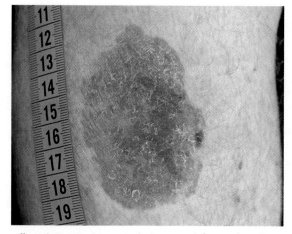

Figure 9-5 Squamous cell carcinoma in situ: Bowen's disease *A large, sharply demarcated, scaly, erythematous plaque simulating a psoriatic lesion on the calf.*

INVASIVE SQUAMOUS CELL CARCINOMA

Invasive squamous cell carcinoma (SCC) is a malignant tumor of keratinocytes, arising in the epidermis, skin appendages, and stratified squamous mucosa. In contrast to basal cell carcinoma (BCC), invasive SCC usually arises in epidermal precancerous lesions (see above). Invasive SCC varies in its aggressiveness. The majority of ultraviolet radiation (UVR)-induced lesions have a low rate of distant metastasis in otherwise healthy individuals. More aggressive SCC occur in immunosuppressed individuals with a greater incidence of metastasis.

Squamous Cell Carcinoma of the Epidermis

Squamous cell carinoma (SCC) is a malignant tumor of squamous cells, arising in the epidermis and stratified squamous mucosa. The most common etiologies of epidermal SCC are ultraviolet radiation (UV) and human papillomavirus (HPV) infection. In many cases, a precursor to invasive SCC exists associated with both these etiologic agents. Treatment of precursor lesions prevents invasive SCC.

EPIDEMIOLOGY

ETIOLOGY

Ultraviolet Radiation

Age of Onset   Older than 55 years of age in the United States; in Australia and New Zealand, in the twenties and thirties.

Sex   Males>females, but SCC can occur more frequently on the legs of females.

Exposure   Sunlight. Phototherapy with oral PUVA (oral psoralen + UVA). Photochemotherapy can lead to promotion of SCC in patients with skin phototypes I and II and in those patients who have had an excessive number of PUVA treatment sessions, or a history of previous exposure to ionizing radiation (electron beam, grenz rays) or a history of methotrexate treatment for psoriasis.

Incidence   Continental United States: 12 per 100,000 white males; 7 per 100,000 white females. Hawaii: 62 per 100,000 whites.

Race   Persons with white skin and poor tanning capacity (skin phototypes I and II) (see Section 8). Brown- or black-skinned persons can develop SCC from numerous etiologic agents other than the UVR.

Geography   Most common in areas that have many days of sunshine annually, i.e., in Australia and southwestern United States.

Occupation   Persons working outdoors—farmers, sailors, lifeguards, telephone line installers, construction workers, dock workers.

Human Papillomavirus

Oncogenic HPV type-16, -18, -31, -33, -35, -45, etc, are associated with epithelial dysplasia, SCC in situ (SCCIS), and invasive SCC.

Other Etiologic Factors

Immunosuppression   Solid organ transplant recipients, individuals with chronic immunosuppression of inflammatory disorders, and those with HIV disease are associated with an increased incidence of UVR- and HPV-induced SCCIS and invasive SCCs. SCCs in these individuals are most common, and may be much more aggressive than in nonimmunosuppressed individuals. UVR-induced SCC occur in fair-skinned individuals with a history of much UVR prior to immunosuppression.

Chronic Inflammation   Chronic cutaneous lupus erythematosus, chronic ulcers, burn scars, chronic radiation dermatitis.

Industrial Carcinogens   Pitch, tar, crude paraffin oil, fuel oil, creosote, lubricating oil, nitrosoureas.

Inorganic Arsenic   Trivalent arsenic had been used in the past in medications such as Asiatic pills, Donovan's pills, Fowler's solution (used as a treatment for psoriasis). Arsenic is still present in drinking water in some geographic regions.

HISTORY

Slowly evolving—any isolated keratotic or eroded papule or plaque in a suspect patient that persists for over a month is considered a carcinoma until proved otherwise. Also, a nodule evolving in a plaque that meets the clinical criteria of SCCIS (Bowen's disease), a chronically eroded lesion on the lower lip, or nodular lesions evolving in or at the margin of a chronic venous ulcer, or a nodule within chronic radiation dermatitis should be biopsied. Note that SCC is always asymptomatic. Potential carcinogens often can be detected only after detailed interrogation of the patient.

PHYSICAL EXAMINATION

For didactic reasons, two types can be distinguished:

1. Highly differentiated SCCs, which practically always show signs of keratinization either within or on the surface of the tumor. These are firm or hard upon palpation.
2. Poorly differentiated SCCs, which do not show signs of keratinization and clinically appear fleshy, granulomatous, amd consequently are soft upon palpation.

Differentiated SCC

Lesions Indurated papule, plaque, or nodule (Fig. 9-6); adherent thick keratotic scale or hyperkeratosis; when eroded or ulcerated, the lesion may have a crust in the center and a firm, hyperkeratotic, elevated margin. Horny material may be expressed from the margin or the center of the lesion (Fig. 9-7). Erythematous, yellowish, skin color. Hard. Polygonal, oval, round, or umbilicated and ulcerated.

Distribution Usually isolated but may be multiple. Exposed areas. Sun-induced keratotic and/or ulcerated lesions especially on the face [cheeks, nose, lips (Fig. 9-6)], tips of ears (Fig. 9-7), preauricular area, scalp (in bald men), dorsa of the hands, and forearms, trunk, and shins (females)

Miscellaneous other skin changes Evidence of chronic skin exposure, termed *dermatoheliosis*: telangiectasia, freckling, dry scaly atrophic skin, small hypopigmented macules.

Other physical findings Regional lymphadenopathy due to metastases.

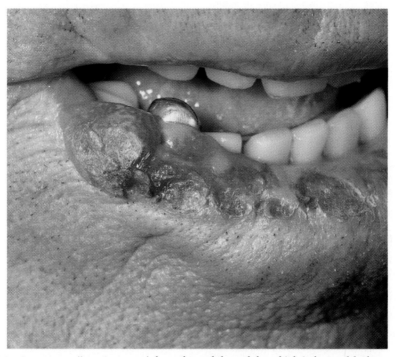

Figure 9-6 Squamous cell carcinoma *A large but subtle nodule, which is better felt than seen, on the vermillion border of the lower lip with areas of hyperkeratosis and erosion, arising in the setting of dermatoheliosis of the lip (cheilitis actinica).*

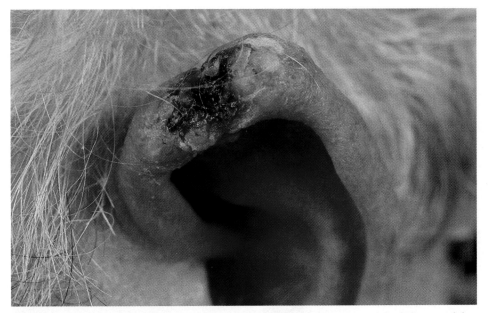

Figure 9-7 **Squamous cell carcinoma** *A large notch on the superior aspect of the helix, a nodule of SCC with hyperkeratosis and ulceration.*

Special features SCCs of the lips develop from leukoplasia or actinic cheilitis; in 90% of cases they are found on the lower lip (Fig. 9-6). In chronic radiodermatitis they arise from radiation-induced keratoses; in individuals with a history of chronic intake of arsenic from arsenical keratoses. SCCs in scars from burns or in chronic stasis ulcers of long duration are often difficult to identify. Suspicion is indicated when nodular lesions are hard and show signs of keratinization.

Histopathology SCCs with various grades of anaplasia and keratinization within the parenchyma or on its surface.

Undifferentiated SCC

Lesions Fleshy, granulating, easily vulnerable, erosive papules and nodules and papillomatous vegetations (Fig. 9-8). Ulceration with a necrotic base and soft, fleshy margin. Hemmorhage, crusting. Red. Soft. Polygonal, irregular, often cauliflower-like.

Distribution Isolated but also multiple, particularly on the genitalia, where they arise from erythroplasia (Fig. 9-9) and on the trunk, lower extremities (Fig. 9-8), or face (rare), where they arise from Bowen's disease.

Miscellaneous other skin changes Lymphadenopathy as evidence of regional matas-

tases is far more common than with differentiated, hyperkeratotic SCCs.

Histopathology Anaplastic SCC with multiple mitoses and little evidence of differentiation and keratinization.

DIFFERENTIAL DIAGNOSIS

As stated previously, any persistent nodule, plaque, or ulcer, but especially when these occur in sun-damaged skin, on the lower lips, in areas of radiodermatitis, in old burn scars, or on the genitalia, must be examined for SCC. *In situ* SCC: nummular eczema, psoriasis, Paget's disease, superficial multicentric BCC.

MANAGEMENT

Surgery Depending on localization and extent of lesion, excision with primary closure, skin flaps, or grafting.

Microscopically controlled surgery in difficult sites.

Radiotherapy should be performed only if surgery is not feasible.

Carcinoma *in situ* Cryotherapy, 5-fluororacil topically.

COURSE AND PROGNOSIS

SCC has an overall remission rate after therapy of 90%. Those tumors which are induced by ionizing radiation, or following inorganic trivalent arsenic, or in an old burn scar, or on the lip or genitalia, are more likely to metastasize. SCC in patients with arsenical ingestion can also have primary SCC of the lung and the bladder. SCC in the skin has an overall metastatic rate of 3 to 4%, with those lesions arising in solar keratoses having the lowest potentiol for metastasis. Cancers arising in chronic osteomeyelitis sinus tracts and in burn scars and sites of radiation dermatitis have a much higher metastatic rate (31, 20, and 18%, respectively).

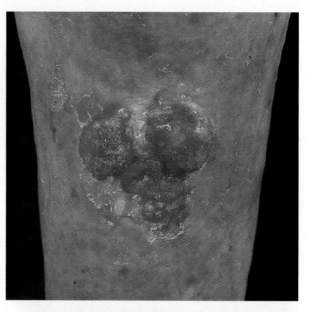

Figure 9-8   Squamous cell carcinoma: undifferentiated *Large, eroded friable, red nodules arising within an old leg scar resemble granulation tissue, lacking the hyperkeratotic surface of a more well-differentiated SCC.*

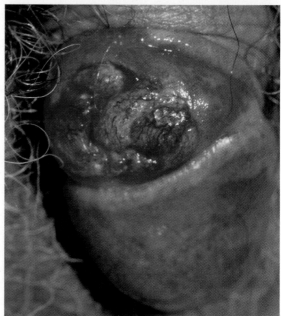

Figure 9-9   Squamous cell carcinoma arising from erythroplasia of Queyrat undifferentiated: *A large, ulcerated, fungating soft nodule arising within an area of SCC in situ (erythroplasia of Queyrat) of the preputial sac. Note the absence of keratinization.*

BASAL CELL CARCINOMA

Basal cell carcinoma (BCC) is the most common type of skin cancer. This malignant tumor is locally invasive, aggressive, and destructive, but there is a limited capacity to metastasize. The reason for this characteristic is the tumor's growth dependency on its stroma, which on invasion of tumor cells into the vessels is not disseminated with the tumor cells. When tumor cells lodge at distant sites, they do not multiply and grow because of the absence of growth factors derived from the stroma of the tumor. Exceptions occur when a BCC shows signs of dedifferentiation, for instance, after inadequate radiotherapy. BCC usually arises only from epidermis that has a capacity to develop (hair) follicles. Therefore, BCCs rarely occur on the vermilion border of the lips or on the genital mucous membranes.

Most lesions are readily controlled by various surgical techniques or cryotherapy. Serious problems, however, may occur with BCC arising in certain locations on the face: around the eyes, in the nasolabial folds, around the ear canal, or in the posterior auricular sulcus. In these sites the tumor may invade deeply, cause extensive destruction of muscle and bone, and even invade to the dura mater. In such cases, death may result from hemorrhage of eroded large vessels or infection (meningitis).

EPIDEMIOLOGY

Age of Onset   Older than 40 years.

Sex   Males more than females.

Incidence   United States: 500 to 1000 per 100,000, higher in the sunbelt; >400,000 new patients annually.

Race   Rare in brown- and black-skinned persons.

Predisposing Factors   White-skinned persons with poor tanning capacity (skin phototypes I and II) and albinos are highly susceptible to develop BCC with prolonged sun exposure. Previous therapy with x-rays for facial acne greatly increases the risk of BCC, even in those persons with a good ability to tan (skin phototypes III and IV). Superficial multicentric BCC occurs 30 to 40 years after ingestion of arsenic but also without apparent cause. Recent evidence of a history of heavy sun exposure in youth predisposing the skin to the development of BCC later in life puts BCC in the same category as malignant melanoma, in which sun exposure before age 14 sets a pattern for development of melanoma 30 to 40 years later.

PHYSICAL EXAMINATION

Skin Lesions

Four clinical types   Nodular, ulcerating, sclerosing (cicatricial), superficial, pigmented.

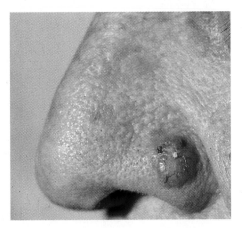

Figure 9-10   Basal cell carcinoma: nodular type
A solitary, shiny, red nodule with large telangiectatic vessels on the ala nasi, arising on skin with dermatoheliosis (solar elastosis).

Nodular Papule or nodule, translucent or "pearly" (Figs. 9-10 and 9-11).

Ulcerating Ulcer (often covered with a crust) with a rolled border (rodent ulcer) (Fig. 9-12). **Cicatricial BCCs** appear as scars (Fig. 9-13). **Superficial multicentric BCC** appear as thin plaques (Figs. 9-14 and 9-15). Pink or red; characteristic fine threadlike telangiectasia can be seen with the aid of a hand lens. **Pigmented BCC** may be brown to blue or black (Fig. 9-16). Smooth, glistening surface; hard, firm; cystic lesions may occur, however. Round, oval shape, depressed center ("umbilicated").

Distribution Isolated single lesion; multiple lesions are not infrequent. Search carefully for "danger sites": medial and lateral canthi (Fig. 9-11), nasolabial fold, behind the ears (Fig. 9-16).

Sclerosing (Sclerodermiform or Morphea-like) BCC (Fig. 9-13) In this infiltrating type of BCC there is an excessive amount of fibrous stroma. The lesion therefore appears as a whitish, sclerotic patch with ill-defined borders and only occasional pearly papules at the periphery. Histologically, finger-like strands of tumor extend far into the surrounding tissue, and excision therefore requires wide margins by the use of Mohs surgery, which should always be done.

Superficial BCC (Figs. 9-14 and 9-15) These superficial lesions are usually multiple, occur on the trunk, and often have no relation to sun exposure. They appear as erythematous, slightly scaly thin plaques, often but not always with a fine, rolled, pearly border. These lesions can mimic psoriasis, seborrheic keratosis, Bowen's disease, and tinea corporis.

Pigmented BCC (Fig. 9-16) These may occur in skin phototypes IV and V and are easily confused with primary malignant melanoma, especially nodular melanoma. Pigmented BCC is usually hard, whereas nodular melanoma is firm. Epiluminescence microscopy (ELM) easily permits a clinical diagnosis of BCC versus malignant melanoma, and this is reassuring to the patient until the pathology is confirmed. Thus, ELM saves anguish while awaiting the pathology report.

LABORATORY EXAMINATIONS

Dermatopathology

Solid tumor consisting of proliferating atypical basal cells, large, oval, deep-blue staining on

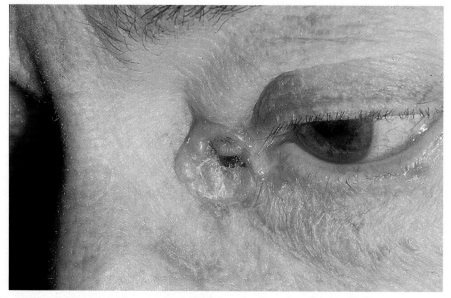

Figure 9-11   Nodular basal cell carcinoma in "danger" zone   *Smooth, glistening, pearly tumor with telangiectasia. Basal cell carcinomas arising in the central area of the face, in the nasolabial folds, around the eye, and in the sulcus behind the ear ("danger zones") must be removed with Moh's surgery to prevent unmanageable recurrences, as these tumors move deeply along the fascial planes.*

PRECANCEROUS LESIONS AND CUTANEOUS CARCINOMAS

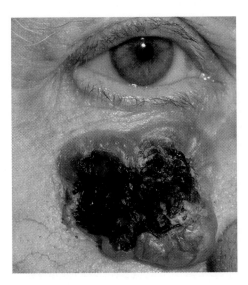

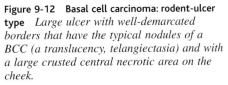
Figure 9-12 Basal cell carcinoma: rodent-ulcer type *Large ulcer with well-demarcated borders that have the typical nodules of a BCC (a translucency, telangiectasia) and with a large crusted central necrotic area on the cheek.*

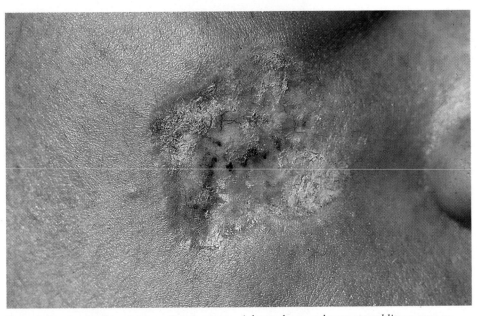

Figure 9-13 Basal cell carcinoma: sclerosing type *A large depressed area resembling a scar or morphea; many small areas of pigmentation typical of BCC and telangiectasia are seen with the lesion, the lateral margin is slightly raised.*

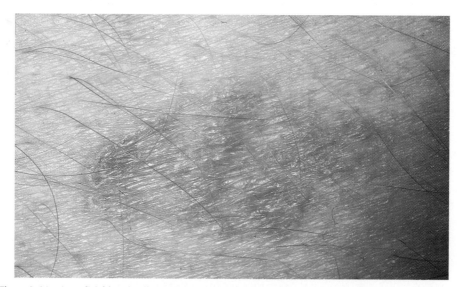

Figure 9-14 Superficial basal cell carcinoma: solitary lesion *This bright red lesion has a slightly elevated rolled border that can be detected with "side lighting"; although this lesion is typical enough to be diagnosed clinically, a biopsy is necessary to establish the diagnosis.*

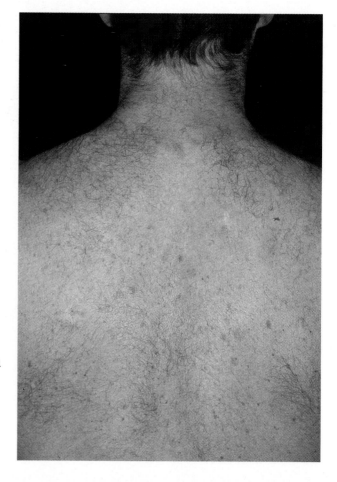

Figure 9-15 Multiple superficial basal cell carcinomas
Many superficial basal cell carcinomas on the trunk. They appear as brightly erythematous, often scaling, flat lesions often without a rolled border.

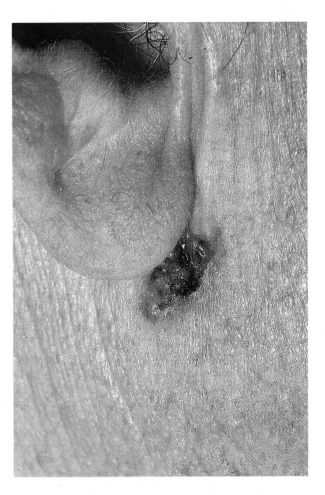

Figure 9-16   Basal cell carcinoma, pigmented *A nodule with irregular borders and variegation of melanin hues, easily confused with a malignant melanoma. Features indicating BCC are the areas of translucency and surface telangiectasia.*

H&E; but with little anaplasia and infrequent mitoses; palisading arrangement at periphery, variable amounts of mucinous stroma.

DIAGNOSIS

Serious BCCs occurring in the danger sites [central part of the face (Fig. 9-11), behind the ears] are readily detectable by careful examination with good lighting, a hand lens, and careful palpation.

MANAGEMENT

Excision with primary closure, skin flaps, or grafts. Cryosurgery and electrosurgery are options, but not in the danger sites or on the scalp.

For lesions in the danger sites (nasolabial area, around the eyes, in the ear canal, in the posterior auricular sulcus, in sclerosing BCC, and on the scalp) microscopically controlled surgery (Mohs surgery) is the best approach. Radiation therapy is an alternative only when disfigurement may be a problem with surgical excision (e.g., eyelids or large lesions in the nasolabial area).

There are a variety of topical treatments that can be used for superficial basal cell carcinomas but only for those tumors below the neck; this is because these therapies are not always definitive in removing all the neoplastic cells, and recurrences on the head and neck may be difficult to manage because of the invasion along the fascial planes. Nevertheless, these modalities do save the need for surgery with its resultant scarring and are worthwhile but only when used on the arms, legs, and trunk. Some patients prefer *cryosurgery*, but this treatment leaves a white spot that remains for life. Electrocautery and curettage is another popular treatment, but it leaves scars. Topical 5-fluorouracil ointment and imiquimod cream are effective and do not cause scars. Some new modalities are promising, such as PDT (photodynamic dye + visible light), and this does not leave a scar.

BASAL CELL NEVUS SYNDROME (BCNS)

This autosomal dominant disorder affects skin [multiple BCCs and palmoplantar pits] and has a variable expression of abnormalities in a number of systems, including skeletal malformations (mandibular "keratocysts"), soft tissue, eyes, CNS, and endocrine organs. Synonym: Gorlin's syndrome, nevoid basal cell carcinoma syndrome.

EPIDEMIOLOGY

Age of Onset BCCs may begin in late childhood, although several abnormalities are congenital.

Race Mostly white, but also occurs in African Americans and Asians.

Sex Equal incidence.

Incidence Frequency not known, but the condition is not rare.

Heredity Autosomal dominant with variable penetrance.

Precipitating Factors There appear to be more BCCs on the sun-exposed areas of the skin, but they can occur in covered areas also.

ETIOLOGY AND PATHOGENESIS

BCNS is caused by mutations in the PATCHED (PTCH) gene. It resides on chromosome 9q (9q22).

HISTORY

Duration of Lesions BCCs begin to appear singly in childhood or early adolescence and continue to appear throughout life.

Systems Review Congenital anomalies include undescended testes; hydrocephalus; blindness from coloboma, cataracts, and glaucoma.

PHYSICAL EXAMINATION

General Appearance There may be hundreds of lesions. Characteristic facies, with frontal bossing, broad nasal root, and hypertelorism.

Skin Lesions

Principal Lesions Basal cell carcinomas (translucent, 1- to 10-cm papules and nodules with and without ulcers) that are skin-colored or pigmented. Invasive tumors are uncommon, but do occur. Tumors on the eyelids, axillae, and neck tend to be pedunculated, occur bilaterally, often symmetric on the face (Fig. 9-17), neck, upper trunk, axillae, usually sparing scalp and extremities.

Palmoplantar Lesions (Fig. 9-18) Present in 50%, and these pits are pinpoint to several millimeters in size and 1 mm deep. There may be hundreds, especially on the lateral surfaces of the palms, soles, and fingers. The pits are the result of premature shedding of the horny layer. There may rarely be a BCC, and there are almost always telangiectases at the bottom of the pit.

Extracutaneous Lesions *Bone* Mandibular jaw odontogenic keratocysts, which are multiple and may be unilateral or bilateral. Other bone lesions include defective dentition, bifid or splayed ribs, pectus excavatum, short fourth metacarpals, scoliosis, and kyphosis.

Eye Strabismus, hypertelorism, dystopia canthorum, and congenital blindness.

Central Nervous System Agenesis of the corpus callosum, medulloblastoma; mental retardation is rare. Calcification of the lamellar falx.

Internal Neoplasms Fibrosarcoma of the jaw, ovarian fibromas, teratomas, and cystadenomas.

LABORATORY EXAMINATIONS

Dermatopathology All types of basal cell carcinomas: solid, adenoid, cystic, ulcerating, superficial, and sclerodermiform.

Imaging Lamellar calcification of the falx is a useful diagnostic sign.

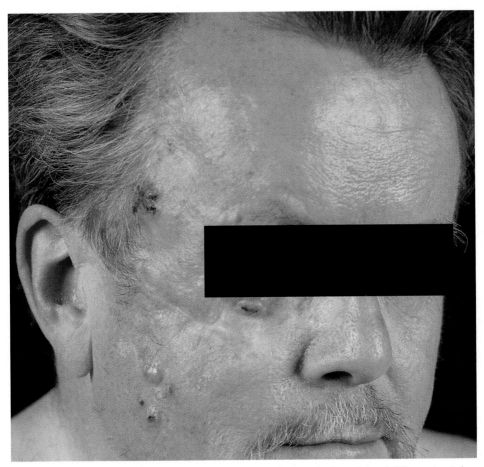

Figure 9-17 Basal cell nevus syndrome: basal cell carcinomas *Multiple nodular BCCs on the right side of the face, frontal bossing, and a large scar on the right cheek at the site of excision of an odontogenic cyst.*

DIAGNOSIS

The disease is often discovered by oral surgeons or dentists because of the mandibular bone cysts; and the patient is referred to a dermatologist, who detects the palmar pits, observes the characteristic facies, and confirms the tumors to be BCC.

SIGNIFICANCE

The large number of skin cancers create a lifetime problem of vigilance on the part of the patient and the physician. The multiple excisions can cause considerable scarring.

COURSE AND PROGNOSIS

The tumors continue throughout life, and the patient must be followed carefully to detect early lesions in order to prevent disfiguring scars.

MANAGEMENT

Surgical excision and Mohs surgery for cancers in certain locations such as the central areas of the face and behind, in, and around ears. Small lesions *on the trunk or extremities* but not on the face or scalp can be treated with electrocautery, or with combined topical tretinoin and 5% fluorouracil for 25 to 30 days.

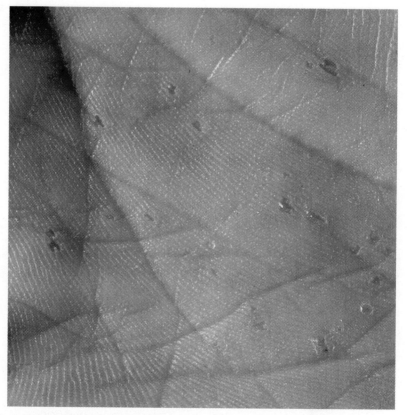

Figure 9-18 Basal cell nevus syndrome: palmar pits *Palmar surface of hand showing 1- to 2-mm, sharply marginated, depressed red lesions, i.e., palmar pits.*

Malignant Appendage Tumors

Carcinomas of the eccrine sweat gland are rare, and include eccrine porocarcinoma, syringoid eccrine carcinoma, mucinous carcinoma, and clear cell eccrine carcinoma. Carcinomas of the apocrine glands is rare, arising in axillae, nipples, vulva, and eyelids. Carcinomas of the sebaceous glands are equally rare, most commonly arising on the eyelids. These lesions are clinically indistinguishable from other carcinomas. They are usually more aggressive than other invasive cutaneous SCCs.

MERKEL CELL CARCINOMA

Merkel cell carcinoma (MCC) (cutaneous neuroendocrine tumor) is a rare malignant solid tumor thought to be derived from a specialized epithelial cell, the Merkel cell. It is a non-dendritic, nonkeratizing, "clear" cell present in the basal cell layer of the epidermis, free in the dermis, and around hair follicles as the hair disk of Pinkus. The etiology is unknown, but may be related to chronic ultraviolet radiation (UVR) damage. The tumor may be solitary or multiple and occurs on the head and on the extremities. There is a high rate of recurrence following excision, but, more important, it spreads to the regional lymph nodes in more than 50% of the patients and can be disseminated to the viscera and CNS.

HISTORY

Clinically, MCC usually grows rapidly within one year. Only 8% occur before the age of 50.

PHYSICAL EXAMINATION

Skin Lesions

Present as a cutaneous to subcutaneous papule, nodule, or tumor (.5 to 5 cm) (Fig. 9-19). Overlying skin usually intact; larger lesions may be ulcerated. Pink, red-to-violet, or reddish-brown. Solitary. Firm. Dome-shaped.

Distribution   Head and neck (50%), extremities (35%, mostly the lower), trunk (10%).

LABORATORY EXAMINATIONS

Dermatopathology   Variable but with two main patterns; nodular and/or diffuse pattern mimicking lymphoma (small cell type), or sheets of cells forming nests, cords, trabeculae (trabecular type), or may be mixed type. Electron microscopy reveals characteristic organelles, immunocytochemistry: cytokeratin and neurofilament markers, chromogranin A and neuron-specific enolase.

Course   Recurrence rates are high, with a 5-month average for local recurrence. Patients are followed monthly for the first 6 months, every 3 months for the next 2 years, and then biannually. Survival rates: 1-year, 88%; 2-year; 72%, 3-year, 55%; 5-year, 64 to 30%.

MANAGEMENT

Excision by Mohs' surgery and prophylactic regional node dissection are advocated because of the high rate of regional metastases. In one series, *even without a local recurrence*, a large number of patients (60%) developed regional node metastases, and in those patients with local recurrence, 86% developed regional node metastases. Therefore, the excision should be followed by prophylactic radiotherapy to the nodal areas.

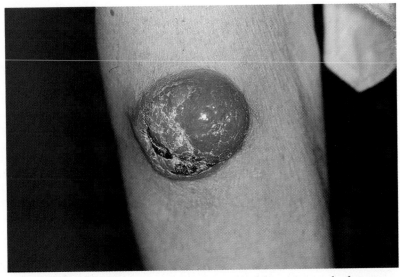

Figure 9-19   Merkel cell carcinoma   *Large, eroded tumor nodule arising on the forearm.*

MELANOMA PRECURSORS AND PRIMARY CUTANEOUS MELANOMA

PRECURSORS OF MELANOMA

Melanoma of the Skin Is Approaching Epidemic Proportions

Melanoma arising in the skin in white persons is not a rare tumor in the United States—47,000 new primary melanomas in 1999, and 7300 deaths—1 in 90 individuals will develop melanoma. In males age 30 to 49, melanoma of the skin is the second most prevalent cancer (the first being cancer of the testis), and in slightly older males (age 50 to 59), melanoma is the fourth most prevalent cancer, exceeded only by bladder, lung, and rectal cancer (in that order). Primary melanoma of the skin is therefore a disease affecting the young and middle-aged.

Mortality rates of primary melanoma for single years from 1976 to 1987 rose at the rate of 3% per year for men and 1% per year for women. Early accessibility to physicians is especially important in primary melanoma because curability is directly related to the size and depth of invasion of the tumor. Even with a rising mortality rate, there has been an encouraging increase in the detection of early melanoma, with very high 5-year survival rates (approaching 98%) for thin (<.75 mm) primary melanoma and an 83% rate for all stages. The trend over the past three decades illustrates the dramatic increased overall survival of melanoma patients: In 1960 to 1963 the 5-year survival rate for melanoma was 60%, and by 1989 to 1994 this rate had increased to 88%.

Early Recognition and Excision of Primary Melanoma = Virtual Cure

Cancer education programs in the 1970s stressed the "danger signs of cancer"; the markers of a dangerous pigmented lesion were "bleeding or ulcer" in a mole. These are now regarded as features of advanced disease, the melanoma being incurable only <50% of the time by excision surgery. Cutaneous melanoma education in the 2000s stresses the detection of early melanoma, with high cure rates after surgical excision.

Of all the cancers, melanoma of the skin is the most rewarding for detection of early curable primary tumors, thereby preventing metastatic disease and death from melanoma. At the present time, the most critical tool for conquering this disease is, therefore, the identification of early "thin" melanomas by clinical examination. Total skin examination for melanoma and its precursors should be done routinely. Special attention should be given to the back above the waist; the legs, between the knees and ankles in women; the scalp; the toes and soles of black- and brown-skinned persons; and the skin around body orifices (mouth, anus, vulva).

About 30% of melanomas arise in a preexisting melanocytic lesion; 70% arise in normal skin. Almost all melanomas show an initial radial growth phase followed by a subsequent vertical growth phase. Radial growth phase refers to a mostly intraepidermal, preinvasive, or minimally invasive growth pattern; vertical growth refers to growth into the dermis and thus into the vicinity of vessels that serve as avenues for metastasis. Since melanomas represent proliferating malignant melanocytes that in most melanomas produce melanin pigment, even preinvasive melanomas in their radial growth phase are clinically detectable by their color patterns. The prognostic difference among the clinical types relates mainly to the duration of the radial growth phase, which may last from years to decades in lentigo maligna melanoma, from months to 2 years in superficial spreading melanoma, and 6 months or less in nodular melanoma. Since metastasis occurs only infrequently (or some believe not ever) during the radial growth phase, detection of early melanomas (i.e., "thin" melanomas) during this phase is essential.

All Physicians and Nurses Have the Responsibility of Detecting Early Melanoma

Early detection of primary melanoma assures increased survival; advanced primary melanoma has a poor prognosis and survival. The survival rate plummets when there is regional metastasis to lymph nodes. The seriousness of this disease thus places the responsibility on the health care provider in the pivotal role: not to overlook pigmented lesions. This is especially true for the primary care physician, the nurse, the physical therapist, or a health care provider who sees the total skin of the body. It must be remembered that most melanomas are not visible in fully dressed persons because the most common sites are the back of both males and females. It is, therefore, recommended that in clinical practice, no matter what is the presenting complaint (e.g., a wart on the finger, hand eczema, etc.), total examination of the body should be requested of all nonpigmented (i.e., white) patients at the time of the first encounter. As some persons are reluctant to get into a gown when the chief problem is a lesion on the face or the hands, we use the following approach: All patients fill out a questionnaire listing the risk factors (Table 10-1). If they discover that they themselves have one or more of the six risk factors for melanoma, they then are usually willing to have a total body examination in search of melanoma or the important melanoma precursor lesions, i.e., dysplastic melanocytic nevi.

Table 10-1   MMRISK[a]

A mnemonic device for promoting melanoma risk awareness among physicians and patients. Each letter represents one of the major risk factors for melanoma of the skin.

M   Moles: atypical (dysplastic or Clark nevus) (>5)
M   Moles: common moles (numerous, >50)
R   Red hair and freckling (often these persons have few or no moles)
I   Inability to tan: skin phototypes I and II
S   Sunburn: severe sunburn especially before age 14 relevant (only in nevus-associated melanoma)
K   Kindred: family history of melanoma (Family history must be documented with photographs or clear history from the parent that the lesion was present before the age of 4 years. Many confuse "skin cancer" with melanoma when it was actually non-melanoma skin cancer that was remembered. Also, family history is irrelevant in lentigo maligna melanoma, acrolentiginous melanoma, and melanoma arrising in congenital melanocytic nevi.)

[a]The original presentation was in 1997 in Dublin at the inaugural meeting of The Brendan Society and was simulcast on Skindex (www.skindex.com).

CLASSIFICATION OF CUTANEOUS MELANOMA AND PRECURSORS

Melanoma

A. *Most Common*
   1. Melanoma arising in dysplastic melanocytic nevus
   2. Melanoma in situ
   3. Superficial spreading melanoma
   4. Nodular melanoma
   5. Lentigo maligna melanoma
B. *Less Common*
   6. Acral lentiginous melanoma
   7. Melanoma of the mucous membranes
   8. Melanoma arising in congenital melanocytic nevus
C. *Rare*
   9. Desmoplastic melanoma

Precursors of Cutaneous Melanoma

1. Congenital nevomelanocytic nevus (giant *or* small)
2. Clark's (dysplastic) melanocytic nevus

The Clark Melanocytic Nevus (Dysplastic Melanocytic Nevus, Atypical Nevus)

Clark melanocytic nevi (CMN) are a special type of acquired, circumscribed, pigmented lesions that represent disordered proliferations of variably atypical melanocytes. CMN arise de novo or as part of a compound melanocytic nevus. CMN are clinically distinctive from common acquired nevi: larger and more variegated in color, asymmetric in outline, irregular borders; they also have characteristic histologic features. CMN are regarded as potential precursors of superficial spreading melanoma and also as markers of persons at risk for developing primary malignant melanoma of the skin, within the dysplastic nevus or on "normal" skin.

EPIDEMIOLOGY

Age of Onset Children and adults.

Sex Equal in males and females.

Prevalence CMN occur in almost every patient with familial cutaneous melanoma and in 30 to 50% of patients with sporadic nonfamilial primary melanomas of the skin. CMN are, moreover, present in 5% of the general white population.

Race White persons. Data on persons with brown or black skin are not available; CMN are rarely seen in the Japanese population.

Transmission Autosomal dominant.

PATHOGENESIS

Multiple loci, including 1p36 and 9p21, have been implicated in familial melanoma/dysplastic nevus syndrome. The abnormal clone of melanocytes can be activated by exposure to sunlight. Immunosuppressed patients (renal transplantation) with dysplastic nevi have a higher incidence of melanoma. Dysplastic nevi favor the exposed areas of the skin, and this is related to the degree of sun exposure. Dysplastic nevi may, however, occur on the covered areas (e.g., hairy scalp or groin).

HISTORY

Duration of Lesions CMN usually arise later in childhood than common acquired nevomelanocytic nevi, appearing first in late childhood, just before puberty. New lesions continue to develop over many years in affected persons; in contrast, common acquired nevomelanocytic nevi do not appear after middle age and disappear entirely in older persons. CMN are thought not to undergo spontaneous regression at all or at least much less than common acquired nevomelanocytic nevi.

Precipitating Factors Exposure to sunlight is regarded by some as an inducing agent for CMN; nevertheless, CMN are not infrequently observed in completely covered areas such as the scalp and anogenital areas.

Skin Symptoms Asymptomatic.

Family History In the familial setting, family members can develop melanoma without the presence of CMN.

PHYSICAL EXAMINATION

See Comparative Clinical Features of Three Pigmented Neoplasms, Table 10-2 (Figs. 10-1 and 10-2). Melanoma arising in a CMN appears initially as a small papule (often of a different color) within the precursor lesion (Figs. 10-3 and 10-4).

Wood's Lamp This will markedly accentuate the epidermal hyperpigmentation of the individual lesions.

Epiluminescence Microscopy This noninvasive technique allows for clinical improvement of diagnostic accuracy in CMN by 25 to 30% (Epiluminescence Microscopy, page 1015).

DIFFERENTIAL DIAGNOSIS

Congenital nevomelanocytic nevi, common acquired nevomelanocytic nevi, superficial spreading malignant melanoma, melanoma in situ, lentigo maligna, Spitz nevus, pigmented basal cell carcinoma.

LABORATORY EXAMINATIONS

Dermatopathology Hyperplasia and proliferation of melanocytes in a single-file, "lentiginous" pattern in the basal cell layer either as spindle cells or as epithelioid cells and as irregular and dyshesive nests.

1. Melanocytes are "atypical," larger than normal size, exhibiting both pleomorphism of nuclei and cell bodies and hyperchromasia of nuclei.
2. Increased number of melanocytes with a tendency for dyshesive and irregular nesting; "bridging" between rete ridges by melanocytic nests; spindle-shaped melanocytes oriented parallel to skin surface.
3. Lamellar fibroplasia and concentric eosinophilic fibrosis (not a constant feature).
4. Proliferation of blood vessels (not a constant feature).
5. Sparse or dense lymphocytic infiltrate (not a constant feature).

Association Most CMN arise in contiguity with a compound melanocytic nevus (rarely, a junctional nevus) that is centrally located; i.e., CMN often have extension of intraepidermal melanocytic hyperplasia beyond the shoulder of the dermal nevus component; some CMN may not have a dermal nevus component.

DIAGNOSIS

The diagnosis of CMN is made by clinical recognition of typical distinctive lesions, and diagnostic accuracy is considerably improved by epiluminescence microscopy; one of these lesions should be excised for histologic confirmation of the diagnosis of CMN. The clinicopathologic correlations are now well documented. Siblings, children, and parents also should be examined for CMN once the diagnosis is established in a family member.

Anatomic association (in contiguity) of dysplastic nevi has been observed in 36% of sporadic primary melanomas, in about 70% of familial primary melanomas, and in 94% of melanomas with familial melanoma and dysplastic nevi. The lifetime risks of developing primary malignant melanoma are estimated to be as follows:

General population	.8%
Familial dysplastic nevus syndrome with *two* blood relatives with melanoma	100%
All other patients with dysplastic nevi	18%

The presence of *one* dysplastic nevus doubles the risk for development of melanoma; with ten or more dysplastic nevi the risk increases 12-fold.

Table 10-2   COMPARATIVE CLINICAL FEATURES OF THREE PIGMENTED NEOPLASMS (IN WHITES)

Lesion	Common Acquired Nevomelanocytic Nevus	Dysplastic (Clark) Melanocytic Nevus	Cutaneous Melanoma (Early)
Number	One or many, average in white adults is 12 to 15; 10–30% have no nevi	One or many, especially in familial melanoma	Single lesion (1–2% have multiple primaries)
Distribution	Predominant on trunk and extremities	Mostly on the trunk, arms, legs; rarely on the face. Exposed and covered areas, including scalp. Dorsa of feet and buttocks often involved	Anywhere, but predominant on upper back, legs (females), trunk, arms (Fig. 10-29)
Types	Small lesions (junctional nevi) are macules; compound and dermal nevi are uniformly elevated papules or plaques	Macules (Figs. 10-1 and 10-2) with obviously raised or only slightly elevated portions, especially in the center	Plaque [superficial spreading melanoma (SSM); melanoma in situ or lentigo maligna melanoma (LMM)] Nodule (SSM, LMM, and nodular) Most ≥5 mm, 30% <6 mm
Diameter	Most lesions, despite elevation, are rarely >10 mm in diameter, usually <5 mm. 10% of whites have one or two nevi ≥5 mm	Usually ≥5 mm, but may be smaller. May be up to 15 mm or larger. Pigmented nevi or lesions >15 mm are dysplastic melanocytic or congenital nevomelanocytic nevi or melanoma	Any size, usually ≥5 mm, but, of course, starts smaller
Shape	Round, oval, papillomatous	Round, oval, ellipsoid	Round, oval, ellipsoid, asymmetric
Border	Regular Sharply demarcated	Irregular May have distinct margin when target-like. Usually indistinct margin, "fuzzy" margins	Irregular Distinct border in nodular melanomas, SSM and most other varieties. May be indistinct in LM and ALM
Color	Brown (medium or dark), tan	Brown (dark, light, or medium), tan, pink, or red	Brown (dark, light), black, red, gray, blue, white
Pattern	Uniform or orderly pattern	Irregular display (variegation) of color	Marked variegation

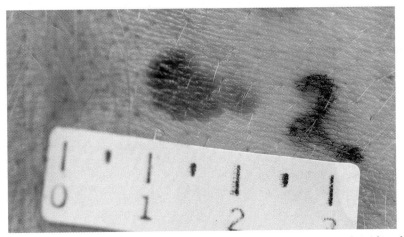

Figure 10-1 Clark melanocytic nevus *A large (1.2 cm), variegated, brown macule with a slightly raised area (10 o'clock), fuzzy margins, and oval shape.*

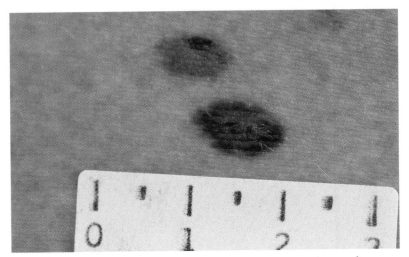

Figure 10-2 Clark melanocytic nevi *Two large, variegated, brown oval flat papules.*

MANAGEMENT

Surgical excision of lesions with minimal margins. Laser or other types of physical destruction should never be used because they do not permit histopathologic verification of diagnosis. The following guidelines for selection of lesions to be excised are suggested:

- Lesions that are changing (increase in size, change in pigmentation pattern, changes in shape and/or border).
- Lesions that cannot be closely followed by the patient by self-examination (on the scalp, genitalia, upper back).

Patients with dysplastic nevi in the familial melanoma setting need to be followed carefully: in familial dysplastic nevi, every 3 months; in sporadic dysplastic nevi, every 6 months to one year. Search for changes in existing dysplastic nevi and development of new nevi. Photographic follow-up is important with Polaroid prints of the trunk and extremities; also Polaroid prints (1:1) of larger lesions (>6 mm) and all lesions that have some variegation. Patients should be given color-illustrated pamphlets that depict the clinical appearance of CMN, malignant melanoma, and common acquired nevomelanocytic nevi. Patients with dysplastic nevi (familial and nonfamilial) should not sunbathe and should use sunscreens when outdoors. They should not use tanning parlors. Family members of the patient should also be examined regularly.

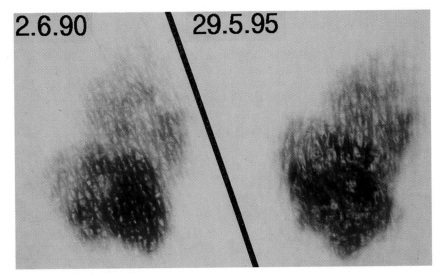

Figure 10-3 Melanoma in situ: evolving in Clark melanocytic nevus *(Left) Image (2 June 1990) variegation of pigmentation and irregular borders. Five years later (29 May 1995), the lesion (right) shows darkening of melanin pigmentation, more irregularity in shape, and elevation in the most darkly pigmented region. Histologically, the lesion showed dysplastic nevus evolving into melanoma in situ. Evolution of dysplastic nevi into in situ and/or invasive melanoma can occur within a period of months or many years.*

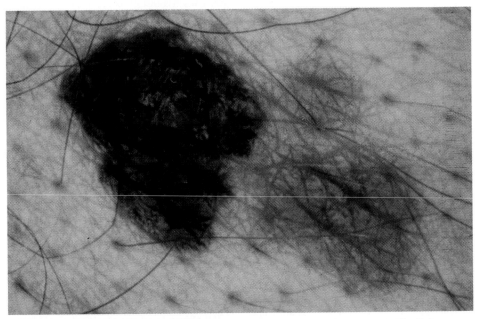

Figure 10-4 Superficial spreading melanoma: arising with a Clark melanocytic nevus *The lighter macular portion of this lesion is a dysplastic lesion on the upper back; the blue-black plaque is a superficial spreading melanoma (1.2 mm thickness) arising within the dysplastic nevus. The patient was a 34-year-old internist who died 36 months following detection and excision of this lesion.*

Congenital Nevomelanocytic Nevus

Congenital nevomelanocytic nevi (CNN) are pigmented lesions of the skin usually present at birth; rare varieties of CNN can develop and become clinically apparent during infancy. CNN may be any size from very small to very large. CNN are benign neoplasms composed of cells called *nevomelanocytes,* which are derived from melanoblasts. All CNN, regardless of size, may be precursors of malignant melanoma.

EPIDEMIOLOGY

Age of Onset Present at birth (congenital). Some CNN become visible only after birth (*tardive*), "fading in" as a relatively large lesion over a period of weeks. Large nevomelanocytic nevi (i.e., >1.5 cm) that are historically "acquired" should be regarded as tardive CNN or dysplastic melanocytic nevi.

Sex Equal prevalence in males and females.

Race All races.

Prevalence Present in 1% of white newborns—majority <3 cm in diameter. Larger varieties of CNN are present in 1:2000 to 1:20,000 newborns. Lesions ≥9.9 cm in diameter have a prevalence of 1:20,000, and giant CNN (occupying a major portion of a major anatomic site) occur in 1:500,000 newborns.

PATHOGENESIS

Congenital and acquired nevomelanocytic nevi are presumed to occur as the result of a developmental defect in neural crest–derived melanoblasts. This defect probably occurs after 10 weeks in utero but before the sixth uterine month; the occurrence of the "split" nevus of the eyelid is an indication that nevomelanocytes migrating from the neural crest were in place in this site before the eyelids split (24 weeks).

PHYSICAL EXAMINATION

Small and Large CNN CNN have a rather wide range of clinical features, but the following are typical (Figs. 10-5 to 10-7): CNN usually distort the skin surface to some degree and are therefore a plaque with or without coarse terminal dark brown or black hairs. Sharply demarcated or merging imperceptibly with surrounding skin (Fig. 10-6); regular or irregular contours. Large lesions may be "wormy" or soft (Fig. 10-7), but are not normally firm except in desmoplastic types of CNN (rare). May or may not have altered skin surface ["pebbly," mamillated, rugose, cerebriform, bulbous, tuberous, or lobular (Fig. 10-7)]. These surface changes are observed more frequently in lesions that extend into the reticular dermis (so-called *deep CNN*).

Color Light or dark brown. When examined with a 10× magnification lens (under oil), a fine speckling of a darker hue with a lighter surrounding brown hue is seen; often the pigmentation is follicular. A "halo" similar to the type that is observed in leukoderma acquisitum centrifugum (so-called *halo nevus*) may occur rarely.

Size Small (Fig. 10-5) large (Fig. 10-6) or giant (Fig. 10-7). Nevomelanocytic nevi >1.5 cm in diameter should be regarded as probably CNN when a history is not available; dysplastic melanocytic nevi must, however, be excluded.

Shape Oval or round.

Distribution of Lesions Isolated, discrete lesion in any site (Figs. 10-5 and 10-6). Fewer than 5% of CNN are multiple. Multiple lesions are more common in association with large CNN. Numerous small CNN occur in patients with giant CNN, in whom there may be numerous small CNN on the trunk and extremities away from the site of the giant CNN (Fig. 10-7).

Very Large ("Giant") CNN (Fig. 10-7) Giant CNN of the head and neck may be associated with involvement of the leptomeninges with the same pathologic process; this presentation may be asymptomatic or manifested by seizures, focal neurologic defects, or obstructive hydrocephalus.

Number of Lesions While small CNN usually occur as single lesions (95%) (Fig. 10-5), giant CNN often present as a single very large lesion and multiple smaller lesions (Fig. 10-7).

Type of Lesion Usually a plaque with at least some surface distortion, often with focal nod-

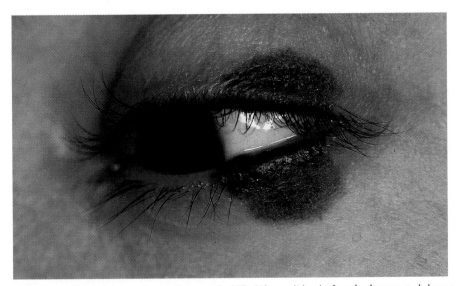

Figure 10-5 Congenital nevomelanocytic nevus; "split" of the eyelid *A sharply demarcated, brown plaque, involving the upper and lower eyelids in a 45-year-old Asian female. Nevomelanocytes migrate from the neural crest to the skin after the 10th week in utero but before 24 weeks when splitting of eyelids occurs.*

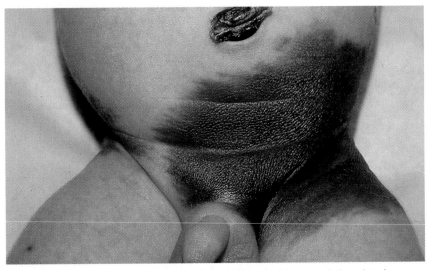

Figure 10-6 Congenital nevomelanocytic nevus, large *Sharply demarcated chocolate-brown hairless plaque with smudged borders in a newborn. With increasing age, lesions usually become elevated and hairy.*

ules and papules on a background of a raised plaque, often with coarse, usually dark hair. Entire segments of the trunk, extremities, head, or neck. Oval or round, bizarre shapes. Borders may be regular or irregular.

Distribution of Lesions Present on any region of the body and localized or widespread.

Melanoma in CNN A papule or nodule arises within CNN (Fig. 10-8). Often melanoma arises in dermal or subcutaneous nevomelanocytes and can be far advanced when detected.

DIFFERENTIAL DIAGNOSIS

Common acquired nevomelanocytic nevi, dysplastic melanocytic nevi, congenital blue nevus, nevus spilus, Becker's nevus, pigmented epidermal nevi, and café-au-lait macules should be considered in the differential diagnosis of CNN. Small CNN are virtually indistinguishable clinically from common acquired nevomelanocytic nevi except for size, and lesions >1.5 cm may be presumed to be either CNN or dysplastic melanocytic nevi. Without a good history or photographs, it may not be possible to ascertain the age of onset of a nevomelanocytic nevus <1.5 cm in diameter.

LABORATORY EXAMINATIONS

Histopathology

Nevomelanocytes occur as well-ordered clusters (*theques*) in the epidermis and in the dermis as sheets, nests, or cords. *A diffuse infiltration of strands of nevomelanocytes in the lower one-third of the reticular dermis and subcutis is, when present, quite specific for CNN.*

Small and large CNN: Unlike the common acquired nevomelanocytic nevus, the nevomelanocytes in CNN tend to occur in the skin appendages (eccrine ducts, hair follicles, sebaceous glands) and in nerve fascicles and/or arrectores pilorum muscles, blood vessels (especially veins), and lymphatic vessels and extend into the lower two-thirds of the reticular dermis and deeper.

Very large or giant CNN: A similar histopathology to small and large CNN, but the nevomelanocytes may extend into the muscle, bone, dura mater, and cranium.

COURSE AND PROGNOSIS

By definition, CNN appear at birth, but varieties of CNN may arise during infancy (so-called *tardive CNN*). The life history of CNN is not documented, but CNN have been observed in elderly persons, an age when the common acquired nevomelanocytic nevi have disappeared.

Very large or giant CNN: The lifetime risk for development of melanoma in large CNN has been estimated to be at least 6.3% In 50% of patients who develop melanoma in large CNN, the diagnosis is made between the ages of 3 and 5 years. Melanoma that develops in a large CNN has a poor prognosis.

Small CNN: The lifetime risk of developing malignant melanoma is 1 to 5%.

Based on the detection of congenital nevi in association with melanoma by means of histology and a careful history, a significantly increased risk is apparent for developing melanoma in persons with small congenital nevus cell nevi (SCNN). This risk is as high as 21-fold based on history and 3- to 10-fold based on histology. Of 134 patients with primary cutaneous melanoma, 15% stated that the melanoma arose in a congenital nevus. Of 234 primary melanomas, 8.1% had nevus cell nevi with congenital features. The expected association of SCNN and melanoma is less than 1:171,000 based on chance alone. Nonetheless, all SCNN should be considered for prophylactic excision at puberty if there are no atypical features (variegated color and irregular borders); SCNN with atypical features should be excised immediately.

MANAGEMENT

Small Nevi Nevi <1.5 cm that are not known to be present at birth should be assumed to be acquired and be managed according to the appearance and growth pattern. Atypical-appearing CNN should be removed. Small CNN should be removed before age 12 years.

Large Nevi Nevi >1.5 cm that are not obviously dysplastic melanocytic nevi should be managed as CNN when the history is not available.

Alternatives Prophylactic excision, periodic follow-up for life, or patient's parents or patient advised to see physician only if a change (color, pattern, size) in the lesion.

Surgical Excision Surgical excision is the only acceptable method.

Small and large CNN: Excision, with full-thickness skin graft, if required; swing flaps, tissue expanders for large lesions.

Giant CNN: Risk of development of melanoma is significant even in the first 3 to 5 years of age, and thus giant CNN should be removed as soon as possible. Individual considerations are necessary (size, location, degree of loss of function, or amount of mutilation). New surgical techniques utilizing the patient's own normal skin grown in tissue culture can now be used to facilitate removal of very large CNN. Also, tissue expanders can be used.

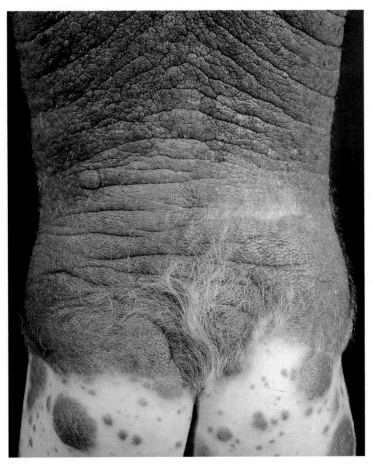

Figure 10-7 Congenital nevomelanocytic nevus, giant *The lesion involves the majority of the skin, with complete replacement of normal skin on the back and multiple smaller CNN on the buttocks and thighs. Note, hypertrichosis of the sacral area. Melanoma developing in a giant CNN is difficult to diagnose early in a setting of such highly abnormal tissue.*

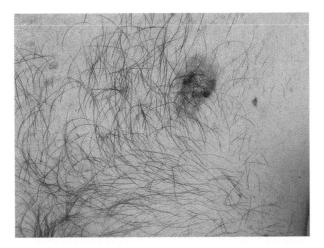

Figure 10-8 Melanoma: arising in small congenital nevus *A nodule with variegation of color (pink, tan, brown, gray) arising in a tan, 2-cm congenital nevomelanocytic nevus on the anterior pectoral region of a 40-year-old white male.*

CUTANEOUS MELANOMA

Melanoma in Situ

The clinical features of this lesion are not clearly presented. The histologic definition of melanoma in situ is used when the atypical melanocytes are confined to the epidermis, the epidermal rete architecture is lost, basilar melanocytic hyperplasia occurs without concentration on rete, melanocytes are distributed throughout the epidermis (pagetoid spread), and continuous cytologic atypia is present. Although some texts describe the clinical lesion as "relatively flat"—an oxymoron—in our experience the lesion is a *macule* with irregular borders and marked variegation of color: brown, dark brown, and black (Figs. 10-9 and 10-10), but without gray or blue, as this occurs only when melanin or melanocytes are located in the dermis. The clinical distinction between melanoma in situ and severely atypical dysplastic nevi may be not be possible. Most life insurance companies at the present time do not regard this lesion as a malignancy, but it definitely is.

SCREENING TECHNIQUE FOR MELANOMA RISK IN NEW PATIENTS

1. *Ask about family history of melanoma or "atypical" nevi (irregular/prominent large moles).* Remember that the term *skin cancer* can be interpreted loosely to mean epithelial cancers rather than melanoma, and the history of melanoma therefore may be difficult or impossible to validate.

2. *Determine the skin phenotype.* Ask only one question: "Do you tan easily?"

   • If "Yes," the person is skin phototype III or IV
   • If "No," the person is skin phototype I or II

   Skin phototypes I and II are considerably more at risk.

3. *Perform a full-body examination to determine the number of moles.* A count of more than 50 moles ≥2 mm in diameter indicates increased risk. (Note, however, that some people at risk may not have any moles, for example, persons with red hair or freckling.) Examine the fingers, toes, plantar and palmar surfaces, and mucocutaneous areas particularly in sub-Saharan Africans, African Americans, Asians, and Native Americans; and examine the scalp.

4. *Perform a full-body examination to determine types of moles.* The types of moles are:

   • *Acquired common moles:* <5 mm in diameter and usually distinctly elevated
   • *Acquired "atypical" moles:* Often large (5 mm in diameter or larger), "flat" in appearance (but actually slightly elevated with side-lighting), light brown, pink to dark (often of variegated color patterns with irregular, indistinct, "fuzzy" borders or "fried egg" appearance)
   • *Congenital melanocytic nevi:* Present in the first 2 weeks of life, verified by birth photograph or by direct or indirect report from patients. Elevated throughout the lesion and often with dark terminal hairs and a "pebbly" surface. Absolute size cannot be used to exclude a lesion as congenital

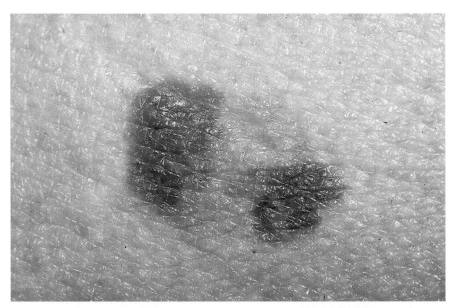

Figure 10-9 Melanoma in situ, superficial spreading type *A 1.3 cm macule on the lateral neck of a 70-year-old white male was first noted five years previously, gradually increasing in size. The central tan area probably represents an original lesion which extends bilaterally. Dermatopathology of the lesions showed a superficial spreading melanoma in situ.*

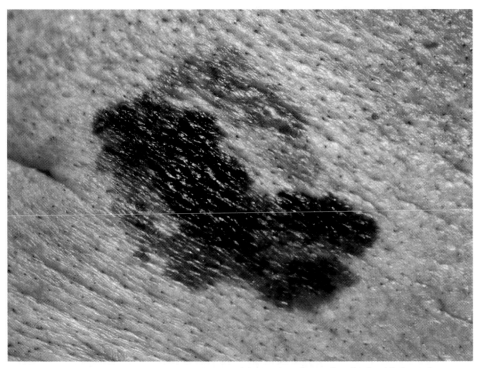

Figure 10-10 Melanoma in situ: lentigo maligna *A large macule on the cheek with irregular borders and striking variegation of melanin pigment (white, tan, brown, dark brown, black).*

I. **Incidence** (United States, 38,300* new cases in 1996) Three percent of all cancers (excluding nonmelanoma skin cancer).

   A. Overall annual crude incidence rates (United States)
      Caucasians   10.4 per 100,000 population per year (1988)

   B. Increasing with time (U.S. whites) (SEER incidence rates, age-adjusted for (U.S. whites), 1970–1992.

      1. 1970   4.5 per 100,000 population per year
      2. 1975   7.3 per 100,000 population per year
      3. 1980   10.0 per 100,000 population per year
      4. 1985   11.8 per 100,000 population per year
      5. 1990   12.9 per 100,000 population per year
      6. 1992   13.6 per 100,000 population per year

II. **Frequency for Type of Melanoma**

   A. Superficial spreading   70%
   B. Nodular   16%
   C. Lentigo maligna melanoma   5%
   D. Unclassified (includes acral lentiginous type)   9%

III. **Mortality** Overall deaths in 1995 (United States, 7300); melanoma represents 1 to 2% of all cancer deaths. In the period 1973 to 1992, there was a 34% increase in the rate of deaths from melanoma; this was the third highest of all cancers. Over this period the percentage change in mortality rates for males exceeded that for females at 47.9 and 16.9%, respectively. In 1992, the death rate from melanoma was 5.9 times higher for whites than for blacks combined (2.5 and .4 per 100,000 population, respectively).

*Estimated [CA Cancer J Clin 46(1); Jan/Feb. 1996].

Superficial Spreading Melanoma

Superficial spreading melanoma (SSM) is one of two major cancers [SSM and nodular melanoma (NM)] that arise in melanocytes of persons with white skin. It arises most frequently on the upper back and occurs as a moderately slow-growing lesion over a period of years. SSM has a distinctive morphology: a uniformly elevated, flattened lesion (plaque). The pigment variegation of SSM is similar to but often less striking than the variety of color present in most lentigo maligna melanomas. The color display is a mixture of brown, dark brown, blue, black, and red, with slate-gray or gray regions in areas of tumor regression.

EPIDEMIOLOGY

Age of Onset   30 to 50 (median, 37) years of age.

Sex   Slightly higher incidence in females.

Race   In world surveys, white-skinned persons overwhelmingly predominate. Only 2% were brown- or black-skinned. Furthermore, brown and black persons have melanomas usually occurring on the extremities; half of brown and black persons have primary melanomas arising on the sole of the foot.

Incidence   SSM constitutes 70% of all melanomas arising in white persons. Melanoma accounts for about 5% of all skin cancers, but new cases increase each year by 7%.

Predisposing and Risk Factors   Four important risk factors, in order of importance, are *presence of precursor lesions* (Clark's dysplastic melanocytic nevus, congenital melanocytic nevus; pages 272 and 278); *family history* of melanoma in parents, children, or siblings; *light skin color* with inability to tan with ease (skin phototypes I and II); and *excessive sun exposure,* especially during preadolescence. Especially increased incidence in young urban professionals, with a frequent pattern of intermittent, intense sun exposure ("weekenders") or winter holidays near the equator.

PATHOGENESIS

In the early stages of growth there is an intraepidermal or "radial growth" phase, during which tumorigenic pigment cells are confined to the epidermis and thus cannot metastasize (called *melanoma in situ*) or "thin" SSM, in which the tumor cells are confined to the epidermis and upper dermis. This "grace period" of the radial growth phase, with potential for cure, is followed by the invasive "vertical growth" phase, in which malignant cells consist of a tumorigenic nodule that invades the dermis with potential for metastasis (Fig. 10-27).

The pathophysiology of SSM is not yet understood. Certainly, in some considerable number of SSM, sunlight exposure is a factor, and both SSM and NM are related to occasional bursts of recreational sun exposure during a susceptible period (<14 years). About 10% of the 47,000 new melanomas each year occur in high-risk families. The rest of the cases may occur sporadically among persons without a specific genetic risk. Persons at high risk inherit the gene in a mutated form of a normal gene that controls melanocytic proliferation.

HISTORY

The usual history of superficial spreading melanoma is a change in a previously existing pigmented lesion (dysplastic nevus, congenital nevomelanocytic nevus, common acquired nevomelanocytic nevus). The patient or close relative may note a gradual darkening in one area of the nevus, and as the dark areas increase there will develop variegation of color with mixes of brown, dark brown, black and the "telltale" blue or blue gray. Also, the borders may become irregular with pseudopods and a notch. With the invasion into the dermis there is the clinical appearance of a papule or nodule.

PHYSICAL EXAMINATION

Diagnosis Made on findings verified by histopathology.

The five cardinal features of SSM are as follows (ABCDE rule):

A, for asymmetry

B, border is irregular and scalloped

C, color is mottled, haphazard display of brown, black, gray, pink

D, diameter is large—greater than a pencil eraser (6 mm)

E, (1) *enlargement,* growth in size, very important sign of evolving melanoma, and
  (2) *elevation* is almost always present with surface distortion, subtle or obvious, and assessed by side-lighting of lesion.

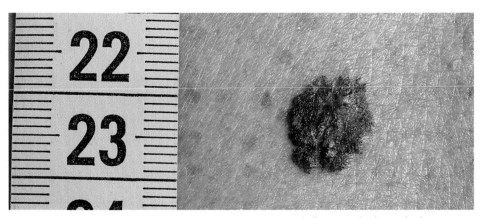

Figure 10-11 Superficial spreading melanoma arising de novo *A flat-topped, elevated, plaque on the trunk with sharply demarcated and irregular margins exhibiting variegation of melanin pigmentation, which ranges from light brown to dark brown and black as well as hues of red. The surface is irregular with a cobblestoned pattern.*

Skin Lesions (Figs. 10-11 to 10-16) Flattened papule, becoming a plaque, and then developing one or more nodules.

Color Dark brown, black, with admixture of pink, gray, and blue-gray hues—with marked variegation and a haphazard pattern. White areas indicate regressed portions.

Size Mean diameter 8 to 12 mm. Early lesions, 5 to 8 mm or smaller; late lesions, 10 to 25 mm.

Shape Asymmetric (one half unlike the other), oval with irregular borders and often with one or more indentations (notches). Sharply defined.

Distribution Isolated, single lesions; multiple primaries are rare. Back (males and females); legs (females, between knees and ankles); anterior trunk and legs in males; relatively fewer lesions on covered areas, e.g., swimsuit, bra.

Wood's Lamp Useful for defining borders.

Epiluminescence Microscopy Increases diagnostic accuracy by 30%.

General Examination
Always search for regional nodes.

LABORATORY EXAMINATIONS

Dermatopathology Malignant melanocytes expand in a pagetoid pattern, e.g., in multiple layers within the epidermis and superficial papillary body of the dermis (radical growth phase). They occur singly and in nests (see Fig. 10-27) and are S-100 and usually also HMB-45 positive. In the vertical growth phase, present clinically as small nodules, they expand further into the reticular dermis and beyond (for microstaging, see Table 10-3).

COURSE AND PROGNOSIS

Left untreated, SSM develops deep invasion (vertical growth) over months to years. Prognosis is summarized in Table 10-4. Melanoma was responsible for about 7300 deaths in 1996—three times the number of deaths from other skin cancers.

MANAGEMENT

Biopsy Total excisional biopsy with narrow margins—optimal biopsy procedure, where possible. Incisional or punch biopsy acceptable when total excisional biopsy cannot be performed or when lesion is large, requiring extensive surgery to remove the entire lesion.

Surgical Treatment See page 302.

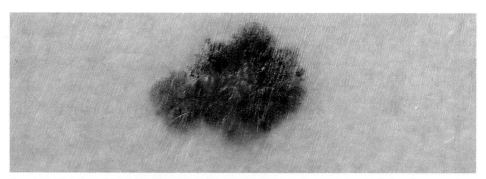

Figure 10-12 Superficial spreading melanoma arising de novo *An asymmetrical, flat plaque with irregular and sharply defined margins. The melanin pigmentation ranges from light brown to pink, dark brown, black, and blue. A dark red-black nodule represents vertical growth and invasion of this SSM.*

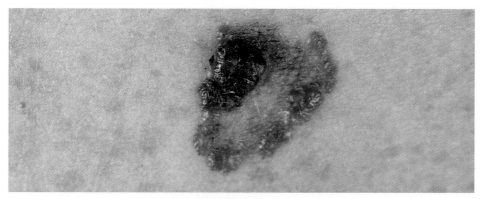

Figure 10-13 Superficial spreading melanoma arising de novo *A lesion resembling a fried egg with a flat portion with color variegation (horizontal growth phase) with a black nodule arising within it (vertical invasive growth phase). The central, whitish-bluish area represents inflammatory regression of the melanoma.*

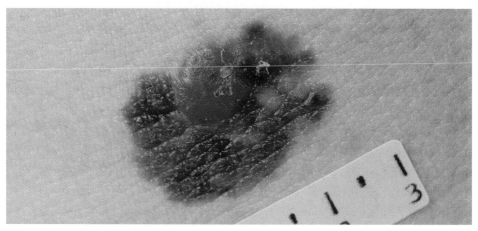

Figure 10-14 Superficial spreading melanoma arising within dysplastic nevus *A macule with a red-brown nodule arising within it: the macular portion (a preexisting dysplastic nevus) shows variegation of melanin pigmentation; the nodule shows slight erosion and crusting and represents the invasive vertical growth phase.*

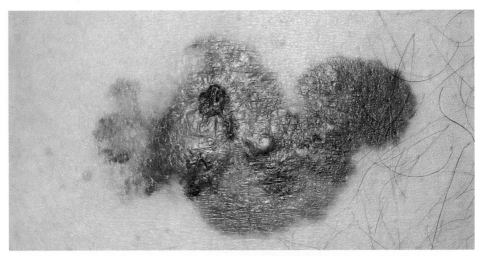

Figure 10-15 Superficial spreading melanoma *A highly characteristic lesion with all features of SSM:* A*symmetry,* B*orders which are highly irregular,* C*olors that are widely variegated,* D*iameter much greater than 1-cm, and* E*levation of the central portion. Note also ulceration in the central portion of the lesion.*

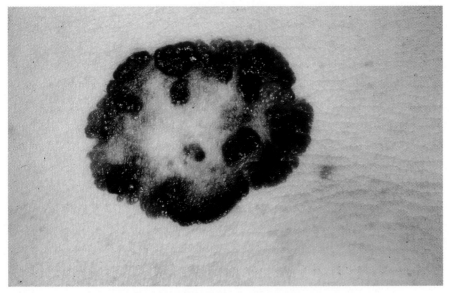

Figure 10-16 Superficial spreading melanoma *An annular lesion with central resolution (regression) having a white scar-like appearance and peripheral extension with black, irregular scalloped borders.*

Nodular Melanoma

Nodular melanoma (NM) is second in frequency (14%) after superficial spreading melanoma (SSM) in most series, occurring largely in middle life in persons with white skin and, as in SSM, on the less commonly exposed areas. The tumor from the beginning is in the "vertical growth" phase and could appropriately be called a *deeply penetrating melanoma* (as opposed to SSM (Fig. 10-28)). NM is uniformly elevated and presents as a thick plaque or an exophytic, polypoid or dome-shaped lesion. The color pattern is usually not variegated, and the lesion is uniformly blue or blue-black or, less commonly, can be very lightly pigmented or nonpigmented (amelanotic melanoma) and confused with a pyogenic granuloma or other nonpigmented tumors. NM is the one type of primary melanoma that arises quite rapidly (4 months to 2 years) from normal skin or from a melanotic nevus as a nodular (vertical) growth without an adjacent epidermal component, as is always present in SSM and LMM.

EPIDEMIOLOGY

Age of Onset   Median age is 50 years.

Sex   Equal incidence in males and females.

Race   NM occurs in all races, but in the Japanese it occurs eight times more frequently (27%) than SSM (3%).

Incidence   NM constitutes 15 to 30% of the melanomas in the United States.

Predisposing Risk Factors   Four important risk factors, in order of importance, are *presence of precursor lesions* (Clark's dysplastic melanocytic nevus, congenital nevomelanocytic nevus); *family history* of melanoma in parents, children, or siblings; *light skin color* with inability to tan with ease; and *excessive sun exposure,* especially during preadolescence. Especially increased incidence in young urban professionals with a frequent pattern of intermittent intense sun exposure ("weekenders" or winter holidays near the equator).

PATHOGENESIS

Both SSM and NM occur in approximately the same sites (upper back in males, lower legs in females), and presumably the same pathogenetic factors are operating in NM as were described in SSM. For the growth pattern of NM, see Figure 10-28. The reason for the high frequency of NM in the Japanese is not known.

HISTORY

This type of melanoma may arise in a preexisting nevus, but more commonly arises *de novo* from normal skin. In contrast to superficial spreading melanoma, the melanoma evolves over a few months. This type of melanoma has relatively rapid growth over several months, which is often noted by the patient, as a new "mole" that was not present before. It appears as a solid blue or blue black lesion or, rarely, it may have the same hue as normal skin color.

PHYSICAL EXAMINATION

Skin Lesions   Uniformly elevated "blueberry-like" nodule (Figs. 10-17 and 10-18) or ulcerated or "thick" plaque; may become polypoid.

Color   Uniformly dark blue, black, or "thundercloud" gray; polypoid lesions may appear pink (amelanotic) with trace of brown.

Size   1 to 3 cm (early lesions) but may grow much larger if undetected.

Shape   Oval or round, usually with smooth, not irregular, borders, as in all other types of melanoma. Sharply defined.

Distribution   Same as SSM. In the Japanese, NM occurs on the extremities (arms and legs).

General Medical Examination   Always search for nodes.

DIFFERENTIAL DIAGNOSIS

Blue/Black Papule/Nodule NM can be confused with *hemangioma* (long history) and *pyogenic granuloma* (short history—weeks) and is sometimes almost indistinguishable from *pigmented basal cell carcinoma* although it is usually softer; it is easy to diagnose this tumor with the dermatoscope. However, a "blueberry-like" nodule of recent origin (6 months to 1 year) should be excised or, if large, an incisional biopsy is mandatory for histologic diagnosis.

PROGNOSIS

Summarized in Table 10-4.

MANAGEMENT

Biopsy Total excisional biopsy with narrow margins—optimal biopsy procedure, where possible. Incisional or punch biopsy acceptable when total excisional biopsy cannot be performed or when lesion is large, requiring extensive surgery to remove the entire lesion.

Surgical Treatment See page 302.

Dermatopathology Malignant melanocytes, which appear as epithelioid, spindle, or small atypical cells, show little lateral (radial) growth within and below the epidermis and invade vertically into the dermis and underlying subcutaneous fat (see Figure 10-28). They are S-100 and usually HMB-45 positive. For microstaging, see Table 10-3.

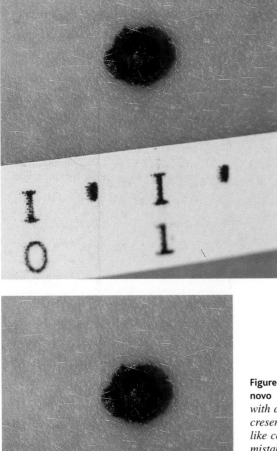

Figure 10-17 Nodular melanoma arising de novo *A 5-mm black papule on the posterior thigh of a 31-year-old female. The lesion had been present for less than one year.*

Figure 10-18 Nodular melanoma arising de novo *An eroded, bleeding, black nodule with an eccentric, gray-black, noneroded, cresent-shaped portion, having a mushroom-like configuration. Such lesions can be mistaken for a vascular lesion such as a pyogenic granuloma and should be excised, and the diagnosis confirmed histologically.*

Lentigo Maligna and Lentigo Maligna Melanoma

Lentigo maligna melanoma is the least common (<5%) of the three principal melanomas of white persons [superficial spreading melanoma (SSM), nodular melanoma (NM), and lentigo maligna melanoma (LMM)] and occurs in older persons on the most sun-exposed areas, the face and forearms. Although there is still some debate about the role of sunlight in the pathogenesis of malignant melanoma, few question the role of sunlight in the pathogenesis of LMM; the tumor was first noted on the faces of women working outdoors in the vineyards of France by Dubreuilh, who called it *melanosis circumscripta praeblastomatosa*. Lentigo maligna (LM) is a *flat* (macular) intraepidermal neoplasm and a melanoma in situ. It is the precursor or evolving lesion of LMM. Focal papular and nodular areas signal invasion into the dermis; the lesion is then called LMM.

EPIDEMIOLOGY

Age of Onset   Median age is 65 for LMM.

Sex   Equal incidence in males and females.

Race   Rare in brown- (e.g., Asians, East Indians) or black-skinned (African Americans) persons. Highest incidence in whites and skin phototypes I, II, and III.

Incidence   5% of primary cutaneous melanomas.

Predisposing Factors   Same factors as in sun-induced nonmelanoma skin cancer (squamous cell carcinoma and basal cell carcinoma): older population, outdoor occupations (farmers, sailors, construction workers).

PATHOGENESIS

In contrast to SSM and NM, which appear to be related to intermittent high-intensity sun exposure and occur on the intermittently exposed areas (back and legs) of young or middle-aged adults, LM and LMM occur on the face, neck, and dorsa of the forearms or hands; furthermore, LM and LMM occur almost always in older persons with evidence of heavily sun-damaged skin (telangiectasia, marked freckling, atrophy, solar keratosis, basal cell carcinoma). The evolution of the lesion is shown in Figure 10-26.

HISTORY

LMM very slowly evolves from LM over a period of several years, sometimes 20 years.

PHYSICAL EXAMINATION

Skin Lesions

Type   *Lentigo Maligna*   Uniformly *flat*, macule (Fig. 10-10).

Lentigo Maligna Melanoma   Flat with focal areas of papules and nodules (Fig. 10-19, center).

Color   *Lentigo Maligna*   Striking variations in hues of brown and black, appears like a "stain," haphazard network of black on a background of brown (Fig. 10-10). The clinical change that indicates the development of LMM is a very dark brown or black pigmentation within the background of LM or appearance of papules or plaques.

Lentigo Maligna Melanoma   Same as LM plus gray areas (indicates focal regression), and blue areas indicate dermal pigment (melanocytes or melanin). Papules or nodules may be blue, black, or pink (Fig. 10-19). Rarely, LMM may be nonpigmented.

Size   *Lentigo Maligna*   3 to 20 cm or larger.

Lentigo Maligna Melanoma   Same as LM.

Shape   *Lentigo Maligna and Lentigo Maligna Melanoma*   Irregular borders, often with a notch, "geographic" shape with inlets and peninsulas. Sharply defined (Fig. 10-10).

Distribution   *Lentigo Maligna and Lentigo Maligna Melanoma*   Single isolated lesion on the sun-exposed areas: forehead, nose, cheeks, neck, forearms, and dorsa of hands; rarely on lower legs.

Other Skin Changes in Areas of Tumor   Sun-induced changes: solar keratosis, freckling, telangiectasia, thinning of the skin, i.e., dermatoheliosis.

General Medical Examination

Check for regional lymphadenopathy.

DIFFERENTIAL DIAGNOSIS

Variegate Tan-Brown Macule/Papule/Nodule
LMM and LM are unique dark flat lesions, with focal elevations (papules and nodules) in LMM. *Seborrheic keratoses* may be dark but are exclusively papules or plaques and have a characteristic stippled surface, often with a verrucous component, i.e., a "warty" surface that, when scratched, exhibits fine scales; also "horn cysts" often can be seen with the dermatoscope. *Solar lentigo,* although macular, does not exhibit the intensity or variegation of brown, dark brown, and black hues seen in LM.

LABORATORY EXAMINATIONS

Dermatopathology LM shows increased numbers of atypical melanocytes distributed in a single layer along the basal layer and above the basement membrane. Atypical melanocytes are usually singly dispersed, but may also aggregate to small nests and extend into the hair-follicles reaching the mid-dermis, even in the preinvasive stage of LM. In LMM, they invade the dermis (vertical growth phase) and expand vertically into the deeper tissues just as in SSM and NM (see Figure 10-26). For microstaging, see Table 10-3.

PROGNOSIS

Summarized in Table 10-3.

MANAGEMENT

See also page 302.
1. Excise with 1-cm or greater margin beyond the clinically visible lesion, provided the flat component does not involve a major organ. Use of Wood's lamp helps in defining borders. ≥2 mm tumor thickness excise with 2 cm margin.
2. Excise down to the fascia. Graft may be needed. Margin width >1 cm is determined by location; a greater margin should be obtained if technically possible.
3. No node dissection recommended unless nodes are clinically palpable. Sentinel node to be done in lesions >1.5 mm in terms of thickness.

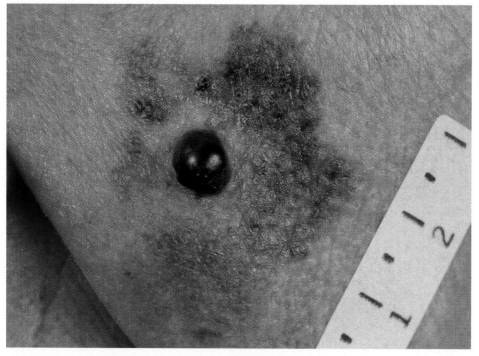

Figure 10-19 Lentigo maligna melanoma *A typical large lentigo maligna (in situ melanoma) on the left cheek with a black nodule of invasive melanoma arising within it.*

Desmoplastic Melanoma

The term *desmoplasia* refers to connective tissue proliferation and, when applied to malignant melanoma, describes different clinical presentations; however, each has a similar microscopic pathology characterized by (1) a dermal fibroblastic component of melanoma with only minimal or absent melanocytic proliferation at the dermal-epidermal junction, (2) nerve-centered superficial malignant melanoma with or without an atypical intraepidermal melanocytic component, or (3) other lesions in which the tumor appears to arise in lentigo maligna or, rarely, in acral lentiginous melanoma or superficial spreading melanoma. Also, desmoplastic melanoma (DM) growth patterns have been noted in recurrent malignant melanoma. The primary tumors occur on the head and neck, most commonly on the face, but may be first noted on the trunk or extremities. DM occurs more frequently in women and in persons with dermatoheliosis ("photoaging"). The diagnosis requires an experienced dermatopathologist; S-100 immunoperoxidase–positive spindle cells need to be identified in the matrix collagen. HMB-45 staining may be negative.

EPIDEMIOLOGY

Age of Onset Median age at diagnosis, 56 years (range, fourth to ninth decades).

Sex More common in women.

Race Skin phototypes I to III.

Incidence Rare.

Etiology Since most, but not all, lesions appear on the sun-damaged skin of the head and neck, ultraviolet radiation exposure has been implicated in the pathogenesis, just as it has in superficial spreading melanoma, lentigo maligna melanoma, and nodular melanoma.

Predisposing and Risk Factors DM occurs most frequently on the head and neck, in a distribution similar to lentigo maligna and lentigo maligna melanoma.

PATHOGENESIS

DM may be a variant of lentigo maligna melanoma in that most lesions occur on the head and neck in patients with sun-damaged skin. DM is more likely to recur locally and metastasize than lentigo maligna melanoma, however.

HISTORY

Duration of Lesion Months to many years. DM is commonly misdiagnosed clinically as a dermatofibroma or neurofibroma because of the absence of color.

Skin Symptoms Asymptomatic. Early and slowly growing lesions are often overlooked by the patient, even though visible on the face and neck.

PHYSICAL EXAMINATION

Skin Lesions

Type *Macule* Early lesions may appear as variegated lentiginous macules, at times with small blue-gray dermal nodules (Fig. 10-20). The lesions actually may arise in lentigo maligna melanoma.

Papule/Nodule May appear as a dermal nodule, with or without any epidermal involvement.

Color Tumors commonly lack any melanin pigmentation. When melanin is principally contained in malignant melanocytes in the dermis, DM may be gray to blue (Fig. 10-20).

Size Because of delay in correct diagnosis, DM may be large.

Palpation Early lesions often cannot be palpated. Older nodular lesions are firm, like a dermal scar or dermatofibroma.

Shape Borders are irregular when epidermal involvement is present, as in lesions arising in lentigo maligna melanoma.

Distribution 85% of DM occurs on the head and neck, and the majority of these on the face, but lesions also occur rarely on the trunk and in acral areas.

DIFFERENTIAL DIAGNOSIS

Blue/Gray Nodule   Basal cell carcinoma, blue nevus, cellular blue nevus, Spitz (spindle cell) nevus, metastatic melanoma to skin, LM, LMM.

LABORATORY EXAMINATIONS

Dermatopathology

A typical junctional melanocytic proliferation, either individual or focal nests, occurs, resembling lentigo maligna. S-100–positive spindle-shaped cells embedded in matrix collagen that widely separates the spindle-cell nuclei. Small aggregates of lymphocytes are commonly seen at the periphery of DM. Neurotropism is characteristic, i.e., fibro-blast-like tumor cells around or within endoneurium of small nerves. DM often has a thickness of 2 mm. Often, DM is seen with a background of severe solar damage to the dermis.

Histologic Differential Diagnosis   Pigmented malignant schwannoma, blue nevus, malignant melanoma arising in a blue nevus, cellular blue nevus, dermatofibroma, neurofibroma, scar, desmoplastic Spitz nevus, lentigo maligna melanoma.

DIAGNOSIS

It is essential to obtain an adequate biopsy; punch biopsies can be misleading.

COURSE AND PROGNOSIS

Diagnosis of DM is often delayed because of the bland clinical appearance and ill-defined margins. There are mixed views about the prognosis of DM. In one series, approximately 50% of patients experienced a local recurrence after primary excision of DM, usually within 3 years of excision; some patients experienced multiple recurrences. Lymph node metastasis occurs less often than local recurrence. In one series, 20% developed metastases, and DM was regarded as a more aggressive tumor than lentigo maligna melanoma.

MANAGEMENT

See Management, page 302.

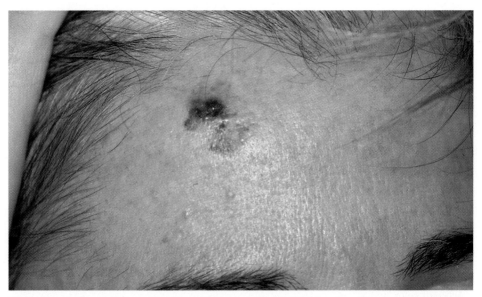

Figure 10-20   Desmoplastic melanoma   *A large nodule with bluish-red and brown portion in an elderly male; lesions often are surrounded by a macular portion resembling lentigo maligna. A nonmelanoma skin cancer had been previously excised from the temple.*

Acral Lentiginous Melanoma

Acral lentiginous melanoma (ALM) is a special presentation of cutaneous melanoma arising on the sole, palm, fingernail or toenail bed. ALM occurs most often in Asians, sub-Saharan Africans, and African Americans, comprising 50 to 70% of the melanomas of the skin found in these populations. It occurs most often in older males (60 years) and often grows slowly over a period of years. The delay in development of the tumor is the reason these tumors are often discovered only when nodules appear or in case of nail involvement, the nail is shed; therefore, the prognosis is poor. The tumor may be misdiagnosed as a verruca plantaris, subungual hematoma, or an onychomycosis of the fingernail or the nail of the large toe. Subungual melanoma most often occurs on the nail bed of the thumb or large toe. The clinical features are less striking than in other melanomas, appearing in the radial growth phase as macules: dark brown, blue-black, or black, with little variegation and often ill-defined.

EPIDEMIOLOGY

Age of Onset Median age is 65.

Sex Male:female ratio 3:1.

Race The best data are on American blacks and Japanese brown-skinned persons, and the incidence of melanoma is about one-seventh that of white persons. ALM is the principal melanoma in the Japanese and in American and sub-Saharan African blacks. ALM accounts for 50 to 70% of melanomas in Japanese.

Incidence 7 to 9% of all melanomas; in whites, 2 to 8%.

Predisposing Factors There are pigmented lesions on the soles of African blacks that are regarded by some as precursor lesions. Subungual melanoma is the most frequent type of ALM in white persons, but trauma has not been proved to be a factor.

PATHOGENESIS

Relatively rare compared to SSM in whites. Probably same incidence in Asians/blacks who have fewer melanomas in general. The pigmented macules that are frequently seen on the soles of African blacks could be comparable with Clark's dysplastic melanocytic nevi.

HISTORY

ALM is slow growing (about 2.5 years from appearance to diagnosis). The tumors occur on the volar surface (palm or sole) and in their radial growth phase may appear as a gradually enlarging "stain"; brown-black or bluish and occupying relatively large areas (8 to 12 cm) of the sole especially. ALM subungual (thumb or great toe) melanoma appears first in the nail bed and involves, over a period of 1 to 2 years, the nail matrix, eponychium, and nail plate. In the vertical growth phase nodules appear; often there are areas of ulceration, and nail deformity may occur.

PHYSICAL EXAMINATION

Skin Lesions

Palm or Sole *Type* Macular lesion in the radial growth phase (Fig. 10-22) with focal papules and nodules developing during the vertical growth phase (Figs. 10-21 and 10-22).

Color Marked variegation of color including brown, black, blue, depigmented pale areas.

Size 3 to 12 cm.

Shape Irregular borders like lentigo maligna melanoma; usually well-defined but not infrequently ill-defined.

Distribution Soles, palms, fingers, and toes.

Subungual *Type* Subungual macule beginning at the nail matrix and extending to involve the nail bed and nail plate (Fig. 10-22). Papules, nodules, and destruction of the nail plate may occur in the vertical growth phase.

Color Dark brown or black pigmentation that may involve the entire nail. Often the nodules or papules are unpigmented. Amelanotic melanoma is often overlooked for weeks to months.

Distribution Thumb or great toe.

DIFFERENTIAL DIAGNOSIS

Variegated Macule/Nodule (Volar) ALM (plantar type) is not infrequently regarded as a "plantar wart" and treated as such. Examination with Wood's lamp may reveal extensive, barely visible pigmentation far beyond what appears to be the borders when viewed with normal light.

Subungual Discoloration ALM (subungual) is usually considered to be traumatic bleeding under the nail; and, in fact, subungual hematomas may persist for over 1 year, but usually the whole pigmented area moves gradually forward. Distinction of ALM from subungual hemorrhage can be made by epiluminescence microscopy (>95%) as the hue of the pigment is purple rather than brown or black, as in a melanoma. With the destruction of the nail plate, the lesions are most often regarded as "fungal infection." When nonpigmented tumor nodules appear, they are misdiagnosed as a pyogenic granuloma.

LABORATORY EXAMINATIONS

Dermatopathology The histologic diagnosis of the radial growth phase of the volar type of ALM may be difficult and may require large incisional biopsies to provide for multiple sections. There is usually an intense lymphocytic inflammation at the dermal-epidermal junction. Characteristic large melanocytes with prominent dendrites along the basal cell layer may extend as large nests into the dermis, as long eccrine ducts. Invasive malignant melanocytes are often spindle shaped, so that ALM frequently has a desmoplastic appearance histologically.

PROGNOSIS

The volar type of ALM can be deceptive in its clinical appearance, and "flat" lesions may be quite deeply invasive. Survival rates (5 years) are less than 50%. The subungual type of ALM has a better 5-year survival rate (80%) than does the volar type. There are so few patients that the data are probably not accurate. Poor prognosis for the volar type of ALM may be related to inordinate delay in the diagnosis.

MANAGEMENT

In considering surgical excision, it is important that the extent of the lesion be ascertained by viewing the lesion with a Wood's lamp and epiluminescence microscopy. The borders of the tumor are indistinct or blurred. There may be a spread of pigment around the nail and onto the nail fold. Subungual ALM and volar type ALM: amputation [toe(s), finger(s)] and volar and plantar ALM wide excision with split skin grafting. Sentinel lymph node procedure necessary in most cases (see Management, page 302).

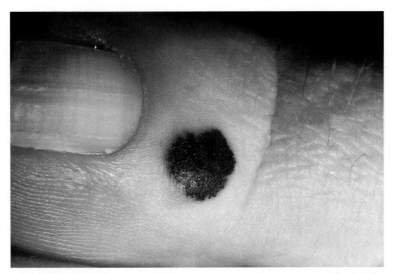

Figure 10-21 Acral lentiginous melanoma arising on the toe *A black nodule with slightly irregular border of a 45-year-old white female of Celtic heritage. The lesion was treated with amputation of the toe at the metatarso-phalangeal joint.*

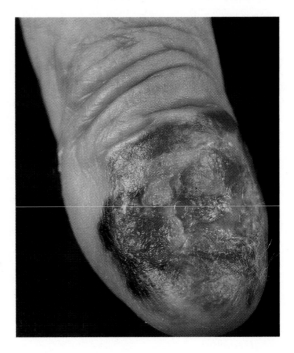

Figure 10-22 Acral lentiginous melanoma *The tumor has replaced the entire nail bed and surrounding skin; the most peripheral parts are macular and resemble a lentigo maligna. The central portion is amelanotic and ulcerated.*

MALIGNANT MELANOMA OF THE MUCOSA

Malignant melanomas arising in the mucosal epithelial lining of the respiratory tract, gastrointestinal and genitourinary tracts are very rare, with an annual incidence of .15% per 100,000 individuals. Major sites of the mucosal melanomas are the vulva and vagina (45%), the head and neck, and the nasal and oral cavity (43%). Mucosal melanomas are so rare that there are no large data bases compared to those for cutaneous melanoma; therefore, pathologic microstaging has not been possible, and the fine tuning of the prognosis that has been useful in cutaneous melanoma (Breslow thickness and Clark levels) has so far not been possible in mucosal melanoma.

Melanomas of the Oral Cavity There is a delay in diagnosis of melanoma of the oral and nasal surfaces. Although melanosis of the mucosa is common in blacks and East Indians, it involves the buccal, mucosal, and gingival bilaterally (see Disorders of Oropharynx, Section 29); when there is a single area of melanosis, a biopsy should be performed to rule out melanoma; this is also true of pigmented nevi in the oral cavity, which should be excised (see Disorders of Oropharynx, Section 29).

Melanomas in the Female Genital Tract These melanomas mostly arise from the labia minora and fewer from the clitoris and the labia majora. Most tumors extend to the vagina at the mucocutaneous border. Vulva melanomas are often flat like lentigo maligna melanoma with large areas of melanoma in situ, and this is important to ascertain in planning excision of all the lesion to prevent recurrence; the Wood's light should be used to outline the periphery of the lesion, as is done in lentigo maligna melanoma (see Disorders of the Genitalia, Perineum, and Anus, Section 30). Vulva melanoma is treated with radical surgery, most often combined with pre operative low-fraction, high-dose irradiation of the whole pelvis.

Anorectal Mucosal Melanoma This melanoma presents with a localized, often polypoid or nodular primary tumor (stage I). The largest experience at the M.D. Anderson Cancer Center recommends the following: for resectable lesions, local resection with negative margins in order to preserve the anal sphincter, followed by adjuvant radiation to the primary site and to the clinically negative inguinal lymph node areas. In more advanced local disease a radical excision is first done followed by adjuvant therapy plus radiation.

Inasmuch as most mucosal melanomas have a high risk of recurrence and metastasis even after complete surgical excision, the tumor should be treated from the beginning with aggressive systemic chemotherapeutic adjuvant therapy.

Table 10-3 Histologic Microstaging of Melanoma

According to Clark	According to Breslow
Level I Melanoma cells confined to epidermis	Thickness of lesion is measured microscopically in mm from granular layer of epidermis down to the deepestpoint of tumor penetration.
Level II Melanoma cells invade dermal papillae	Cutoff points that are relevant for prognosis (see Table 10-4)
Level III Melanoma cells completely occupy papillary layer	≤0.75 mm
Level IV Melanoma cells invade mid-reticular dermis	≤1.5 mm
Level V Melanoma cells invade subcutaneous fat	≥3 mm

METASTATIC MELANOMA

Metastatic melanoma occurs in 15 to 26% of stage I and stage II melanoma. The spread of disease from the primary site usually occurs in a stepwise sequence: local recurrence (Fig. 10-23) (within the scar), if not excised totally. The usual sequence, however, is → regional metastasis (Figs. 10-24 and 10-25) → distant metastasis. It should be noted that distant metastasis can occur skipping the regional lymph nodes.

Sentinel node biopsy can accurately predict the presence of metastatic melanoma within regional lymph nodes with the identification of malignant cells in permanent H&E sections; staining for S-100 protein and HMB-45 are helpful.

Sentinel node localization: When the nodes are not palpable, it is not certain if there are micrometastases; these can be detected by the *sentinel node technique,* which involves a multidisciplinary approach: surgery, nuclear medicine, and pathology. The hypothesis is that the *first* node draining a lymphatic basin, called the *sentinel node,* can predict the presence or absence of metastasis in all the nodes in that basin. Lymphatic mapping (LM) and sentinel lymphadenectomy (SL) are either performed on the same day with a single injection of filtered Tc-99m SC, which is the most useful method for probe-directed LM/SL or, alternatively, one day after lymphoscintigraphy, sentinel node biopsy is performed, guided by a gamma probe and blue dye and the sentinel node is subjected to histopathology and immunohistochemistry. Lymph node dissection is performed only if metastasis is found in the sentinel node. The sentinel node technique is essential in making a decision about the use of adjuvant therapy. In one large recent British report of 247 consecutive patients who had stage I or stage II melanoma, 48 (24%) had metastasis in a sentinel node. Fifteen patients developed recurrence after removal of a tumor-negative sentinel node; six relapsed in the previously mapped basin (false-negative rate 11%). The overall survival rate at 3 years was 93% if the sentinel node was negative and 67% if it was positive. Sentinel node status and Breslow thickness were strong predictors of recurrence and survival. LM is also useful in locating the drainage areas, especially in primary tumors on trunk, which can drain on either side.

Regional nodal metastases within 3 years are related to the thickness of the primary: <.76 mm = 2 to 3%, .76 to 1.49 mm = 25%, 1.5 to 4 mm = 57%, >4 mm = 62%.

Local recurrence (as defined by tumor in the scar) occurs in 1.3%, and the 5-year disease-free survival rate in these patients is 83%. Visceral metastases occur in the lung (18 to 36%), liver (14 to 29%), brain (12 to 20%), and bone (11 to 17%).

Melanoma without a primary tumor is rare, 1 to 6%. *Melanoma may have a late recurrence* (10 or more years). The usual time is 14 years, but there have been "very late" recurrences (more than 15 years) in one series at the Massachusetts General Hospital with 0.072% 20/2766.

Patients with a solitary metastasis confined to the subcutaneous, nonregional lymph nodes or lung are most likely to benefit from surgical intervention.

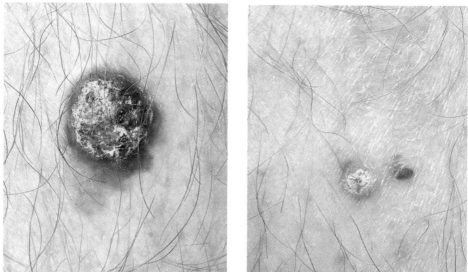

Figure 10-23   Metastatic melanoma: recurring in excision scar   A. *A pigmented lesion on the shin of a 35-year-old male, present for <2 years. The dermatopathology was initially interpreted as a spindle cell (Spitz) nevus. The primary lesion site was not reexcised.* **B.** *Three papules are seen around the excision site scar, one of which is a blue-brown color. The histology from the excised lesion was reviewed and revised as a superficial spreading melanoma.*

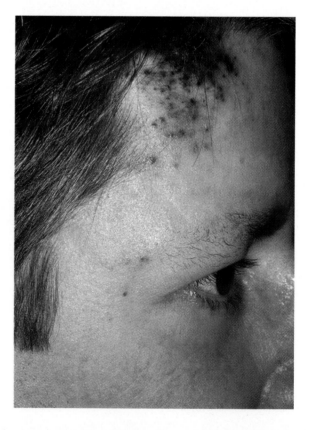

Figure 10-24   Metastatic melanoma: multiple dermal metastases
Multiple blue and blue-gray dermal nodules on the forehead and throughout the scalp of a 45-year-old male. The patient bumped his scalp, resulting in a large ecchymosis $2\frac{1}{2}$ months previously. As the ecchymosis resolved, the dermal nodules became apparent. Cervical lymph nodes were enlarged; needle aspiration demonstrated metastatic melanoma in the nodes as well. The primary melanoma presumably arose in the scalp but was not detected.

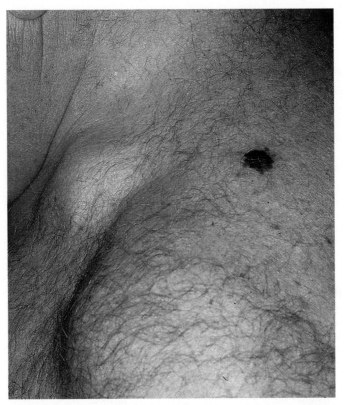

Figure 10-25 Metastatic melanoma: superficial spreading melanoma with supraclavicular lymph node metastasis *A pigmented lesion on the left upper back had been noted by the patient (a 72-year-old male) and physicians for at least 20 years. The patient presented with lymphadenopathy, a metastasis from the previously undiagnosed melanoma.*

Management of Cutaneous Melanoma

For the Examining Physician

1. Histologic diagnosis is necessary in all pigmented lesions with the following three physical characteristics—the hallmarks of atypicality in a pigmented lesion:

   a. Irregularity of the borders: with pseudopods, a notch, or even a "maple leaf" configuration. (Figs. 10-10 and 10-13).

   b. An irregular array of colors: a gradation of red, gray, or blue, admixed with brown or black, displayed in a disorderly, haphazard pigment pattern. *Additional indications:* black nodules with uniform borders, irregularly pigmented lesions with uniform borders.

   c. Increases in size. It is recommended that the ABCDE rule be observed (see below).

2. All congenital melanocytic nevi should be considered for excision, regardless of size. Lesions should be followed with photography until they can be excised some time before puberty. The timing of excision for small congenital lesions depends on the clinical characteristics (light brown, uniform color is a sign of benignancy), on whether general anesthesia is needed, and on the disability that will result from surgery. All giant nevi should be removed if feasible.

3. Any pigmented lesion striking a physician's eye as "out of the ordinary" should be further evaluated (i.e., excision or referral for same).

4. All patients with a history of melanoma should be examined thoroughly for atypical melanocytic nevi (dysplastic nevi) and for the appearance of new primary melanomas. Patients with dysplastic nevi should be followed at 6-month intervals.

Six Signs of Malignant Melanoma

ASYMMETRY in shape—one-half unlike the other half
BORDER is irregular—edges irregularly scalloped
COLOR is mottled—haphazard display of colors; shades of brown, black, gray, red, and white
DIAMETER is usually large—greater than the tip of a pencil eraser (6 mm)
ELEVATION is almost always present—surface distortion is assessed by side-lighting. Melanoma *in situ* and acral lentiginous lesions may be flat
ENLARGEMENT—a history of an increse in the size of lesion is perhaps one of the most important signs of malignant melanoma

A   **ASYMMETRY** in shape—one-half unlike the other half

B   **BORDER** is irregular—edges irregularly scalloped

C   **COLOR** is mottled—haphazard display of colors; shades of brown, black, gray, red, and white

D   **DIAMETER** is usually large—greater than the tip of a pencil eraser (6.0 mm)

E   **ELEVATION** is almost always present—surface distortion is assessed by side-lighting. Melanoma *in situ* and acral lentiginous lesions may be flat
ENLARGEMENT—a history of an increase in the size of lesion is perhaps one of the most important signs of malignant melanoma

5. All blood relatives of patients with melanoma should be examined for dysplastic nevi and early primary melanoma. (The presence of a family history increases the risk 8- to 13-fold for an individual.)

6. All white patients presenting for any problem should be examined for the presence of large melanocytic nevi (>1 cm), for dysplastic nevi, and for nevi on the scalp, mucous membrane, and anogenital area. All black persons should be examined for pigmented lesions of the soles, nail beds, and mucous membranes.

Advice to the Patient

The following advice should be given about pigmented lesions. Seek prompt examination for the following:

All persons with a family history of melanoma

All persons with skin phototypes I and II, especially those with a history in youth of intense or prolonged sun exposure

Any pigmented mole that was present at birth

Any newly appearing mole after puberty

All persons with many (uncountable!) moles >2 mm in diameter and/or with any number of moles >5 mm in diameter

Any changing mole—in size, color, or border

Any mole that itches or is tender for more than 2 weeks

Any mole that is considered "ugly" because of its size, color, pattern, or borders

Persons with skin phototypes I and II should *never* sunbathe. Persons with dysplastic nevi or a melanoma, regardless of skin phototype, should *never* sunbathe or do outdoor work without appropriate clothing. Sunscreens with a sun protection factor (SPF) of >30 should be used in all persons with dysplastic nevi or a previous history of melanoma and in persons with skin phototypes I and II. Avoid exposure to artificial forms of ultraviolet radiation (sunbeds and sunlamps).

GUIDELINES FOR BIOPSY AND SURGICAL TREATMENT OF PATIENTS WITH MELANOMA

I. Biopsy

- Total excisional biopsy with narrow margins—optimal biopsy procedure, where possible.
- Incisional or punch biopsy acceptable when total excisional biopsy cannot be performed on when lesion is large, requiring extensive surgery to remove the entire lesion.
- When sampling the lesion: If raised, remove the most raised area; if flat, remove the darkest area.

II. Melanoma In Situ

- Excise with .5-cm margin.

III. Lentigo Maligna Melanoma

- Excise with a 1-cm margin beyond the clinically visible lesion or biopsy scar—unless the flat component involves a major organ (e.g., the eyelid), in which case lesser margins are acceptable. For lentigo maligna melanoma on areas other than the head and neck, the excision margins are the same as for superficial spreading melanoma, nodular melanoma, and acral melanoma.
- Excise down to the fascia or to the underlying muscle where fascia is absent. Skin flaps of skin grafts may be used for closure.
- No node dissection is recommended unless nodes are clinically palpable and suspicious for tumor.
- See recommendation for sentinel node studies for thickness >1 mm (page 299).

IV. Superficial Spreading Melanoma, Nodular Melanoma, and Acral Melanoma

- Melanoma in situ: excise with a >.5 cm margin from the lesion edge.

THICKNESS <1 MM

- Excise with a 1-cm margin from the lesion edge.
- Excise down to the fascia or to the underlying muscle where fascia is absent. Direct closure without graft is often possible.

- Node dissection is not recommended unless nodes are clinically palpable and suspicious for tumor.

THICKNESS 1 MM TO 4 MM

- Excise 2 cm from the edge of the lesion, except on the face, where narrower margins may be necessary.
- Excise down to the fascia or to the underlying muscle where fascia is absent. Graft may be required.
- The sentinel node procedure for tumors with thickness >1mm with injections of blue dye or, if available, technetium-99 with gamma-probe localization permits a minimally invasive technique for detecting melanoma metastasis in regional nodes (page 299).
- Sentinel node lymphadenectomy can be selectively performed and, therefore, ELND can be done only for those nodal basins with occult tumor cells. Local excision plus elective lymph node dissection results in a significant improvement in disease-free survival and overall survival. (Shen et al. Ann Surg. Oncol 2000: March (2): 114–119).
- If the sentinel node (lymph node closest to the site of the primary melanoma) is positive the regional lymphadenectomy is performed. If the sentinel node is negative, then the patient is spared an ELND.
- If regional node is positive and completely resected with no evidence of distant disease, adjuvant therapy with interferon-alpha-2b is discussed. In this setting, results of recent ECOC Est 1689 trials have demonstrated improvement in median relapse-free survival and 5-year relapse-free survival rates of node-positive, resected patients given high-dose interferon as compared with controls; also results of the Austrian Cooperative Melanoma Group show significantly increased relapse-free 5-year survival rates in node-negative, no ELND treated >1.5 mm primary melanoma patients given low-dose interferon.
- Therapeutic nodal dissection is recommended if nodes are clinically palpable and suspicious for tumor and no evidence of distant disease is present.

- Excise 3 cm from the edge of the lesion, except on the face, where narrower margins may be necessary.
- Excise down to the fascia or to the underlying muscle where fascia is absent. Graft may be required.
- Elective nodal dissection is not recommended.

- Sentinel node procedure recommended (see above).
- Therapeutic nodal dissection is recommended if nodes are clinically suspicious for tumor and no evidence of distant disease is present.

Table 10-4 EIGHT-YEAR SURVIVAL RATES FOR PATIENTS WITH CLINICAL STAGE I MELANOMA IN THE VERTICAL GROWTH PHASE BASED ON SINGLE FACTOR ANALYSIS OF PROGNOSTIC VARIABLES

Variable	Categories	8-Year Survival Rate (%)
Mitotic rate/mm^2	0.0	95.1
	0.1–6.0	79.4
	>6.0	38.2
TILs[a]	Brisk	88.5
	Nonbrisk	75.0
	Absent	59.3
Thickness[b]	<0.76 mm	93.2
	0.76–1.69	85.6
	1.70–3.60	59.8
	>3.60	33.3
Anatomic site	Extremities	87.3
	Head, neck, and trunk	62.4
	Volar or subungual	46.2
Sex	Female	83.8
	Male	56.6
Regression	Absent	77.0
	Present	60.0

[a]Tumor-infiltrating lymphocytes.
[b]Tumor thickness (level of invasion) is the most important single prognostic variable and thus decisive for theraputic decisions.
SOURCE: Modified from Clark WH Jr, et al. Model predicting survival in stage I melanoma based on tumor progression. *J Natl Cancer Inst* 81:1893, 1989.

Table 10-5 AMERICAN JOINT COMMISSION ON CANCER (AJCC) STAGING SYSTEM (1992)

TNM STAGING OF MELANOMA

Primary tumor (pT)

pTX	Primary tumor cannot be assessed.
pTO	No evidence of primary tumor.
pTis	Melanoma in situ (atypical melanocytic hyperplasia, severe melanocytic dysplasia), not an invasive lesion (Clark level I).
pT1	Tumor ≤.75 mm in thickness and invading the papillary dermis (Clark level II).
pT2	Tumor >.75 mm but ≤1.5 mm in thickness and/or invades the papillary-reticular dermal interface (Clark level III).
pT3	Tumor >1.5 mm but ≤4 mm in thickness and/or invades the reticular dermis (Clark level IV).
pT3a	Tumor >1.5 mm but ≤3 mm in thickness.
pT3b	Tumor >3 mm but ≤4 mm in thickness.
pT4	Tumor >4 mm in thickness and/or invades the subcutaneous tissue (Clark level V) and/or satellite(s) within 2 cm of the primary tumor.
pT4a	Tumor >4 mm in thickness and/or invades the subcutaneous tissue.
pT4b	Satellite(s) within 2 cm of the primary tumor.

Regional lymph nodes (N)

NX	Regional lymph nodes cannot be assessed.
N0	No regional lymph node metastasis.
N1	Metastasis ≤3 cm in greatest dimension in any regional lymph node(s).
N2	Metastasis >3 cm in greatest dimension in any regional lymph node(s) and/or intransit metastasis.[a]
N2a	Metastasis >3 cm in greatest dimension in any regional lymph node(s).
N2b	In-transit metastasis.[a]
N2c	Both (N2a and N2b).

Distant Metastasis

MX	Presence of distant metastasis cannot be assessed.
M0	No distant metastasis.
M1	Distant metastasis.
M1a	Metastasis in skin or subcutaneous tissue or lymph node(s) beyond the regional lymph nodes.
M1b	Visceral metastasis.

STAGE GROUPING

Stage I	pT1	N0	M0
	pT2	N0	M0
Stage II	pT3	N0	M0
	pT4	N0	M0
Stage III	Any pT	N1	M0
	Any pT	N2	M0
Stage IV	Any pT	Any N	M1

[a]In-transit metastasis involves skin or subcutaneous tissue more than 2 cm from the primary tumor not beyond the regional lymph nodes.

Table 10-6 WORK-UP OF MELANOMA

- **PRIMARY MELANOMA Stage I or II (no nodes palpated)**
  Chest roentgenogram
  Liver function tests, especially LDH
  Lymphatic mapping and sentinel lymphadenectomy in stage I thickness >1.5 mm.[a]
- **PRIMARY MELANOMA WITH LOCAL-REGIONAL DISEASE**
  Stage III, Satellites and Local Recurrence
  Complete blood count
  Liver function tests, especially LDH
  Chest roentgenogram
  CT scans: abdomen, pelvis (with disease below the waist), neck (with disease in the head and neck)
  Stage IV
  Same as for stage III
  CT scan of the chest
  MRI of the brain
  Bone scan
  GI series (on the basis of symptoms)

[a]Lymphatic mapping and sentinel lymphadenectomy can be cautiously performed in patients who have undergone previous wide local excision if the primary resection margin was no greater than 2 cm and the primary was not in a region of ambiguous drainage. Lymphatic mapping may be inaccurate when melanomas have been resected with large margins, especially if the wound was closed with rotation flaps, and when melanomas are on the head and neck or trunk regions.

Table 10-7 FOLLOW UP PRIMARY MELANOMA

Stage I < 1 mm	Stages I–II	Stage III
Every 3-6 months* for 3 years	Lymph nodes negative	Lymph nodes positive
Review of systems	Every 3-6 months* for 3 years	Every 3-6 months for 3 years
Physical examination	Review of systems	Then 3-12 months for 2 years
Annual examination for life	Physical examination	Annual examination for life
	Liver function (LDH)	Review of systems
	Chest x-ray and CT scans every 6 months	Physical examination
	Annual examination for life	Chest x-ray and CT scans every 6 months
		CBC, liver function (LDH)

*Familial melanoma dysplastic nevus syndrome every 3 months for 3 years, and then every 6 months for 5 years, and then annually for life.

Primary Melanoma of the Skin: Three Major Types

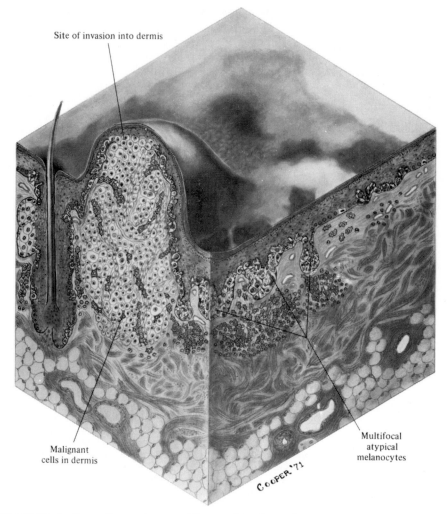

Figure 10-26 Lentigo maligna melanoma *Illustrated is a large, flat, variegated, freckle-like macule (not elevated above the plane of the skin) with irregular borders. These areas show increased numbers of melanocytes, usually atypical and bizarre and distributed in a single layer along the basal layer; at certain places in the dermis, malignant melanocytes have invaded and formed huge nests. At the left is a large nodule that is composed of large epithelioid cells in this illustration; the nodules of all three types of melanoma are indistinguishable from each other.*

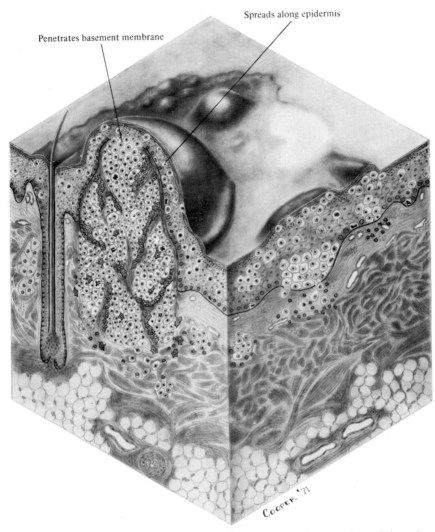

Penetrates basement membrane

Spreads along epidermis

COOPER '71

Figure 10-27   Superficial spreading melanoma   *The border is irregular and elevated throughout its entirety; biopsy of the area surrounding the large nodule shows a pagetoid distribution of large melanocytes throughout the epidermis in multiple layers, occurring singly or in nests, and uniformly atypical. On the left is a large nodule, and scattered throughout the surrounding portion of the nodule are smaller popular and nodular areas. The nodules also may show spindle cells or small malignant melanocytes as in lentigo maligna melanoma and nodular melanoma.*

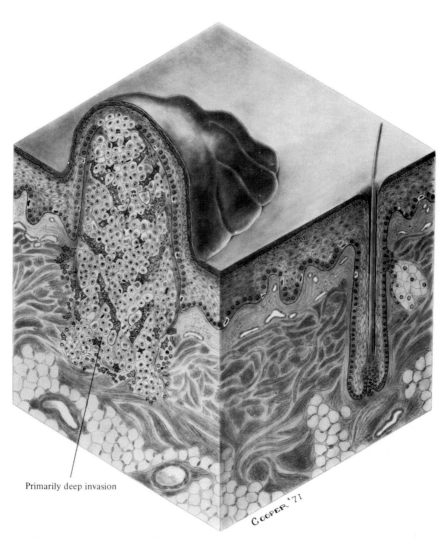

Primarily deep invasion

Figure 10-28   Nodular melanoma   *This arises at the dermal-epidermal junction and extends vertically in the dermis; intraepidermal growth is present only in a small group of tumor cells that conjointly are also invading the underlying dermis. The epidermis lateral to the areas of this invasion does not demonstrate atypical melanocytes. As in lentigo maligna melanoma and superficial spreading melanoma, the tumor may show large epithelioid cells, spindle cells, small malignant melanocytes, or mixtures of all three.*

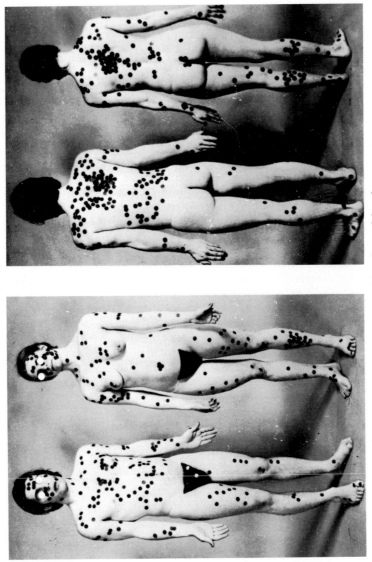

Figure 10-29 *Localization of malignant melanoma in 731 males and females.*

PIGMENTARY DISORDERS

Normal skin color is composed of a mixture of four biochromes, namely, (1) *reduced hemoglobin* (blue), (2) *oxyhemoglobin* (red), (3) *carotenoids* (yellow; exogenous from diet), and (4) *melanin* (brown). However, it is the *total amount of melanin pigment* that is the principal determinant of the skin color. Variations in the amount and distribution of melanin in the skin, furhermore, are the basis of the three principal human skin colors: black, brown, and white. These three basic skin colors are genetically determined and are called *constitutive melanin pigmentation;* also, the normal basic skin color pigmentation can be increased deliberately by exposure to ultraviolet radiation or pituitary hormones, and this is called *inducible melanin pigmentation.*

The basic (*constitutive*) melanin *and inducible* melanin pigmentation determines what is called the *skin phototype* (Table 11-1). Ethnicity is not necessarily a part of the definition, e.g., African "black" ethnic persons can be skin phototype III). An East Indian Caucasian can be skin phototype IV or even V. *The skin phototype is an underutilized marker for skin cancer risk (melanoma and non-melanoma), and it should be recorded at the first patient visit.*

Increase of melanin in the epidermis results in a state known as *hypermelanosis.* This reflects one of two types of changes: (1) An increase in the number of melanocytes in the epidermis producing increased levels of melanin, which is called *melanocytotic hypermelanosis* (an example is *lentigo*); (2) *no* increase of melanocytes but an increase in the production of melanin only, which called *melanotic hypermelanosis* (an example is *melasma*). Hypermelanosis of both types (*melanocytotic* and *melanotic*) can result from three factors: *genetic*; *hormonal* (as in Addison's disease), when it is caused by an increase in circulating pituitary melanotropic hormones; and *ultraviolet radiation* (as in tanning, which is related to exposure to UVB, wavelengths 290 to 320 nm, UVA 2, wavelengths 320 to 340 nm, and also, UVA 1 wavelengths 340 to 400 nm.

VITILIGO

Vitiligo is a major medical problem for brown and black persons that can result in severe difficulties in social adjustment. Therefore, it is important for physicians to be aware of the various options for control of this disease. There are some successful therapeutic approaches, and these should be explained to the patient. The patient with vitiligo should be managed by a dermatologist who has experience and can establish the diagnosis, as there are confusing white spots that mimic vitiligo. Vitiligo is characterized clinically by development of totally white macules, microscopically by complete absence of melanocytes, and medically by an increased association with certain medical diseases, particularly thyroid disease.

EPIDEMIOLOGY

Age of Onset Vitiligo may begin at any age, but in 50% of cases it begins between the ages of 10 and 30 years. A few cases have been reported to be present at birth; onset in old age also occurs but is unusual.

Sex Equal in both sexes. The predominance in women suggested by the literature likely may reflect the greater willingness of women to express concern about cosmetic appearance.

Race Appears in all races. The apparently increased prevalence reported in some countries and among darker-skinned persons results from a dramatic contrast between white vitiligo macules and dark skin and from marked social stigma in countries such as India, where the opportunities for advancement or marriage among affected individuals are even today limited.

Incidence Common. Affects up to 1% of the population. This may be related to the basic skin color in which brown and black color accentuates the contrast and makes it a disfigurement.

Inheritance Vitiligo appears to be an inherited disease. More than 30% of affected individuals have reported vitiligo in a parent, sibling, or child. Vitiligo in identical twins has been reported. As many as four genetic loci may be responsible for vitiligo. The risk of vitiligo for children of affected individuals is unknown but may be less than 10%. Individuals from families with an increased prevalence of thyroid disease, diabetes mellitus, and vitiligo appear to be at increased risk for development of vitiligo.

PATHOGENESIS

Three principal theories have been presented about the mechanism of destruction of melanocytes in vitiligo. The *autoimmune theory* holds that selected melanocytes are destroyed by certain lymphocytes that have somehow been activated internally. The *neurogenic hypothesis* is based on an interaction of the melanocytes and the nerve cells. The *self-destruct hypothesis* suggests that melanocytes are destroyed by toxic substances formed as part of normal melanin biosynthesis. While the immediate mechanism for the evolving white macules involves progressive destruction of selected melanocytes by cytotoxic T cells, other genetically determined cytobiologic changes and cytokines must be involved. Because of differences in the extent and course of segmental and generalized vitiligo, the pathogenesis of these two types must be somewhat different.

HISTORY

Characterizations of the onset of vitiligo suggest that there are both predisposing (genetic) and precipitating (environmental) factors. Many patients attribute onset of their vitiligo to physical trauma, illness, or emotional stress. Onset after the death of a relative or after severe physical injury is often mentioned. Even sunburn reaction may precipitate vitiligo.

Table 11-1 CLASSIFICATION OF SKIN PHOTOTYPES (SPT)

SPT	Basic Skin Color	Response to Sun Exposure
I	Pale white	Do not tan; burn easily
II	White	Tan with difficulty; burn easily
III	White	Tan after initial sunburn
IV	Light brown	Tan easily
V	Brown	Tan easily
VI	Black	Become darker*

Questionnaire for estimating the skin phototype in *white* individuals

Question: "Do you tan easily?"

Three Possible Answers:	Skin Phototype
"No, I burn easily"	I AND II
"I burn first and then tan"	III
"Yes, I tan easily"	IV

NOTE: After excessive solar exposure even SPT VI can have a sunburn.

PHYSICAL EXAMINATION

Skin Lesion

Macules, 5 mm to 5 cm *or more* in diameter (Figs. 11-1 and 11-2). "Chalk" or pale white. Newly developed macules, however, may be "off-white" in color; this represents a transitional phase. The disease progresses by gradual enlargement of the old macules or by development of new ones. Variants are trichrome (three colors) and quadrichrome (white, light brown, dark brown, black). Pigmentation around a hair follicle in a white macule may represent residual pigmentation or return of pigmentation (Fig. 11-3). Confetti-sized hypomelanotic macules also may be observed. Inflammatory vitiligo has an elevated erythematous margin and may be pruritic; this appears to have no special significance. *Convex margins* (as if the pathologic process of depigmentation were flowing into normally pigmented skin). *Round, oval,* or *elongated. Linear* or artifactual macules represent the isomorphic or "Koebner" phenomenon, i.e., the induction of the depigmentation by physical trauma.

Distribution (Figure 11-I) Depigmentation occurs in three general patterns. The *focal* type is characterized by one or several macules in a single site; this may be an early evolutionary stage of one of the other types in some cases. The *segmental* type is characterized by one or several macules in one band on one side of the body; this type is associated rarely with distant vitiligo macules or with further evolution of the disease to generalized vitiligo. The most common type is *generalized* vitiligo, characterized by widespread distribution of depigmented macules, often in a remarkable symmetry (Fig. 11-2). Typical macules occur around the eyes and mouth and on digits, elbows, and knees, as well as on the low back and in genital areas. The *"lip-tip" pattern* involves the skin around the mouth as well as on distal fingers and toes; lips, nipples, and genitalia (tip of the penis) may

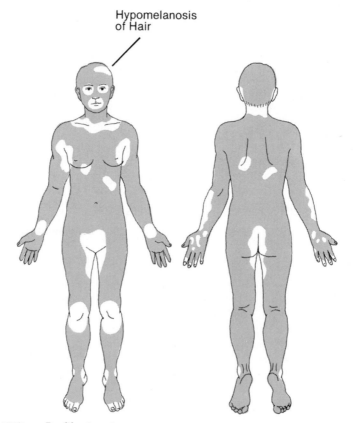

Hypomelanosis of Hair

Figure 11-I   Vitiligo *Predilection sites.*

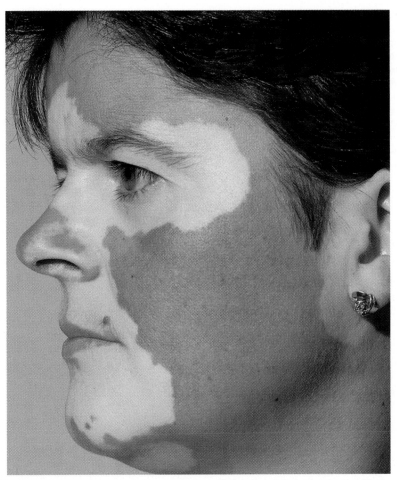

Figure 11-1 Vitiligo: face *Extensive depigmentation of the central face. Involved vitiliginous skin has convex borders, extending into the normal pigmented skin. Note the chalk-white color and sharp margination.*

be involved. Extensive generalized vitiligo may leave only a few normally pigmented areas of skin; this is referred to as *vitiligo universalis* (Fig. 11-4).

Associated Cutaneous Findings White hair and prematurely gray hair, alopecia areata, and halo nevi. In older patients, photoaging as well as solar keratoses may occur in vitiligo macules with history of long exposures to sunlight. Squamous cell carcinoma has rarely been reported, limited to the white macules.

General Examination Vitiligo is not uncommonly associated with thyroid disease (up to 30% of all vitiligo cases: Hashimoto's thyroiditis, Graves' disease), also diabetes melli-

tus—probably less than 5%, pernicious anemia (uncommon, but increased risk), Addison's disease (uncommon), and multiple endocrinopathy syndrome (rare). Ophthalmologic examination may reveal evidence of healed chorioretinitis or iritis (probably less than 10% of all cases). Vision is unaffected. Hearing is normal.

DIFFERENTIAL DIAGNOSIS

Lupus erythematosus (atypical, asymmetric pattern, serologic studies for ANA are positive).
Pityriasis alba (slight scaling, fuzzy margins, off-white color).

Piebaldism (congenital, white forelock, stable, dorsal pigmented stripe on back, distinctive pattern with large hyperpigmented macules in the center of the hypomelanotic areas).

Pityriasis versicolor alba (fine scales with greenish-yellow fluorescence under Wood's lamp, positive KOH; this may be confusing as the depigmentation remains months after infection has ceased).

Chemical leukoderma (history of exposure to certain phenolic germicides, confetti macules). This is a difficult differential diagnosis, as melanocytes are absent as in vitiligo.

Leprosy (endemic areas, off-white color, *anesthetic* macules).

Nevus depigmentosus (stable, congenital, off-white macules, unilateral).

Hypomelanosis of Ito (bilateral, Blaschko's lines, marble cake pattern; 60 to 75% have systemic involvement—CNS, eyes, musculoskeletal system).

Nevus anemicus (does not enhance with Wood's lamp; does not show erythema after rubbing).

Tuberous sclerosis [stable, congenital off-white macules (polygonal, ash-leaf shape, occasional segmental macules, and confetti macules), also facial angiofibromas which come later at 4 years of age].

Leukoderma associated with melanoma (may not be true vitiligo inasmuch as the macules may repigment spontaneously and melanocytes, although reduced, are usually present).

Postinflammatory leukoderma [off-white macules (usually a history of psoriasis or eczema in the same macular area), not so sharply defined].

Mycosis fungoides (may be confusing as only depigmentation may be present and biopsy is necessary).

Vogt-Koyanagi-Harada syndrome (vision problems, photophobia, bilateral dysacousia).

Waardenburg's syndrome (commonest cause of congenital deafness, white macules and white forelock, iris heterochromia).

LABORATORY EXAMINATIONS

Diagnosis usually can be established on clinical grounds alone; however, in certain difficult cases, a skin biopsy may be required (see Dermatopathology, below). Chemical leukoderma (a vitiligo-like process caused by certain known chemicals) can be diagnosed only on clinical grounds and history.

Wood's Lamp Examination   Wood's lamp examination is required to evaluate macules, particularly in lighter skin types, and to identify macules in sun-protected areas in all but the darkest skin types.

Dermatopathology   Established vitiligo macules show normal skin except for an absence of melanocytes. There may be melanocytes at the margins (normal numbers of melanocytes that appear relatively inactive or reduced numbers that are highly activated) and a mild lymphocytic response. These changes are not diagnostic for vitiligo, however—only consistent with it.

Electron Microscopy   Electron microscopy has demonstrated other changes in skin affected by vitiligo; these include changes in keratinocytes: spongiosis, exocytosis, basilar vacuopathy, and necrosis. Extracellular granules and lymphocytes have been seen in the epidermis.

Laboratory Studies T_4, TSH (radioimmunoassay), fasting blood glucose, complete blood count with indices (pernicious anemia), ACTH stimulation test for Addison's disease, if suspected.

DIAGNOSIS

Normally, diagnosis of vitiligo can be made readily on clinical examination of a patient with progressive, acquired, chalk-white, bilateral (ususally symmetric), sharply defined macules in typical sites (periorbital, perioral, neck, penis, perineum, axillae, and points of pressure such as the elbow, malleoli, knees, lumbosacral area).

COURSE AND PROGNOSIS

Vitiligo is a chronic disease. The course is highly variable, but rapid onset followed by a period of stability or slow progression is most characteristic. Up to 30% of patients may report some spontaneous repigmentation in a few areas—particularly areas that are exposed to the sun. Rarely is this sufficient to satisfy the cosmetic burden that the patient feels. Rapidly progressive or "galloping" vitiligo may quickly lead to extensive depigmentation with a total loss of pigment in skin and hair, but not eyes.

Segmental vitiligo is a special subset that usually develops in one unilateral region; usu-

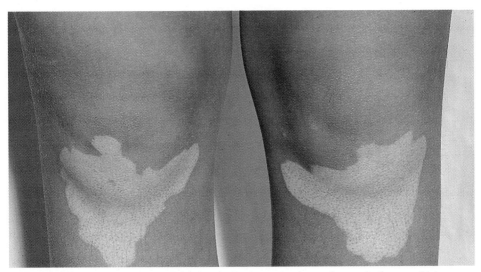

Figure 11-2 Vitiligo: knee *Depigmented, sharply demarcated macules on the knees, which may have arisen after minor trauma (Koebner phenomenon). Apart from the loss of pigment, vitiliginous skin appears normal.*

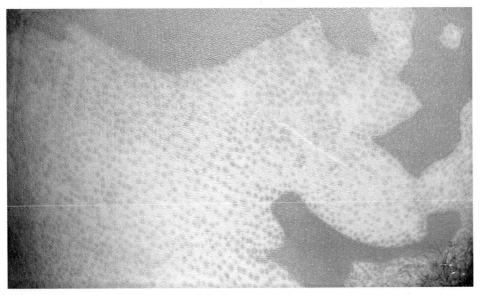

Figure 11-3 Vitiligo repigmentation *A follicular pattern of repigmentation (PUVA therapy) extensively occurring in a large vitiliginous macule. Melanocytes persist in the hair follicle epithelium and serve to repopulate involved skin, spontaneously or with photochemotherapy.*

ally, but not always, does not extend beyond that initial one-sided region; and once present, is very stable.

The treatment of vitiligo-associated disease (i.e., thyroid disease) appears to have no impact on the course of vitiligo.

MANAGEMENT

There is a widespread perception, even among dermatologists, that vitiligo is not treatable with any method. This is regrettable, because affected patients are denied treatments that are available and effective when given by those dermatologists who can establish the diagnosis, select the option for treatment, and be persistent until the cosmetic improvement is acceptable. The duration of the vitiligo has no effect on the success of the repigmentation with PUVA photochemotherapy.

The eight aproaches in the management of vitiligo are as follows:

1. **Sunscreens** The dual objectives of sunscreens are protection of involved skin from acute sunburn reaction and limitation of tanning of normally pigmented skin. Sunscreens with a sun protection factor of more than 30 are reasonable choices to prevent sunburn for most patients. However, since their ability to limit the tanning reaction is inversely proportional to skin phototype, opaque sunscreens should be more effective in limiting the tanning reaction in fairer-skinned individuals. While all skin phototypes have a need for sun protection, sunscreens alone are often perfectly adequate management for those vitiligo patients with skin phototypes I, II, and sometimes III (those who burn and then tan).

2. **Cosmetic Coverup** The objective of coverup with dyes or makeup is to hide the white macules so that the vitiligo is not apparent. Vitadye (ICN) and Dy-o-Derm (Owen Laboratories) both come in one color, are easy to apply, and do not rub off but gradually wash or wear off. So-called self-tanning agents, which contain dihydroxyacetone, are available in a number of formulations; many contain sunscreens that are effective for much less time than the dye is present. Estée Lauder preparations have been found particularly useful by patients. Covermark (Lydia O'Leary) and Dermablend (Flori Roberts) are cos-

metics available to match most skin hues; they do not wash off but do rub off. Other preparations may be found at cosmetic counters.

Repigmentation The objective of repigmentation (Figs. 11-3 and 11-5) is the permanent return of normal melanin pigmentation. This may be achieved for local macules with topical glucocorticoids or topical psoralens and UVA (long-wave ultraviolet light) and for widespread macules with oral psoralens and UVA.

3. **Topical Glucocorticoids** Initial treatment with intermittent (4 weeks on, 2 weeks off) topical Class I glucocorticoid ointments is practical, simple, and safe for single or a few macules. If there is no response in 2 months, it is unlikely to be effective. Physician monitoring every 2 months for signs of early steroid atrophy and telangiectasia is required.

4. **Topical Photochemotherapy** Much more complicated is the use of UVA or sunlight and topical 8-methoxypsoralen (8-MOP; this substance is highly phototoxic and the phototoxicity lasts for 3 days or more. This procedure should be undertaken for small macules only by experienced physicians and well-informed patients. As with oral psoralens, it may require 15 or more treatments to initiate response and 100 or more to finish.

5. **Systemic Photochemotherapy** For more widespread vitiligo, oral PUVA is more practical and carries less risk of severe phototoxicity than topical phototherapy. Oral phototherapy may be done with sunlight and 5-methoxypsoralen (5-MOP) (available in Europe) or with artificial UVA (doctor's office or other approved unit) and 5-MOP, or 8-MOP (Fig. 11-5). Ophthalmologic examination and a blood ANA test are required before starting therapy.

Outdoor PUVA therapy, when available (in summer or in areas with year-round sunlight); treatment may be initiated with 1.2 mg/kg 5-MOP followed 2 h later by 5 min of sunlight (less in the southern regions). Treatments should be twice weekly, though not on two consecutive days, and sunlight exposure should increase by 3 to 5 min per treatment until a sign of response or of slight phototoxicity (i.e., redness) occurs. In some patients, mild phototoxicity is required for response, and in a few it

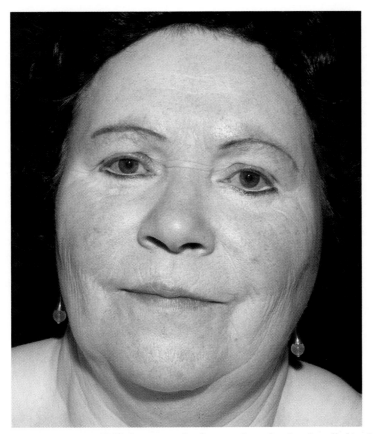

Figure 11-4 Universal vitiligo *Vitiliginous macules have coalesced to involve all skin sites with complete depigmentation of skin and hair in a female. The patient is wearing a black wig, and has darkened the brows with eyebrow pencil and eyelid margins with eye liner.*

causes koebnerization. Individualization of treatment is required. *The unavailability of 5-MOP in the U.S. is a serious problem as trioxsalen is no longer available* and, therefore, there is no safe treatment for vitiligo with sunlight and psoralens; 8-MOP is too phototoxic to use for outdoor vitiligo therapy. The treatment of vitiligo in the United States must be oral 8-MOP plus UVA irradiators. This creates an economic problem for those patients who cannot afford the cost of UVA irradiation.

Indoor PUVA therapy is as effective as is PUVA with sunlight; it can be controlled more rigorously but has the significant disadvantage of additional cost. Either .2 to .4 mg/kg 8-MOP (well absorbed, efficient, potentially very phototoxic, with significant risk of nausea) 1 h before UVA exposure or 1.2 mg/kg 5-MOP (less phototoxic than 8-MOP and no nausea) 2 h be-

fore UVA exposure. Initial UVA exposure should be 1 J/cm^2 and increments (twice weekly, not on two consecutive days) of .5 (8-MOP) to 1 J/cm^2 per treatment until evidence of response or of phototoxicity appears. The latter is the guide to sustaining or increasing the UVA dose until reasonable repigmentation has been established or until progress has started—in the form of tiny macules of pigmentation (Fig. 11-3). When this occurs, it is a good prognostic sign for successful repigmentation.

Oral PUVA photochemotherapy with either 8-MOP or 5-MOP is up to 85% effective in more than 70% of patients with vitiligo of the head, neck, upper arms and legs, and trunk. Distal hands and feet are poorly responsive and, when present alone, are not usually worth treating. Genital areas should be shielded and not treated.

Macules that have totally repigmented usually stay that way in the absence of injury or sunburn (85% likelihood up to 10 years); macules less than fully repigmented will slowly reverse once treatments have been discontinued. Maintenance treatments are not required.

Risks of treatment with PUVA acutely include nausea, gastrointestinal upset, sunburn reaction, hyperpigmentation of the normal skin, and dryness. Chronic effects include photoaging, PUVA lentigines, keratoses (including leukokeratoses), skin cancers (we have seen 1 in more than 30 years of collective experience with more than 4000 patients), and cataracts (we have not observed any).

Standard PUVA precautions should apply; we advise against oral PUVA in children younger than 10 years of age. For children we now use narrow-band UVB 311 nm without oral psoralens and with reasonable success. Treatment is most likely to be successful in highly motivated patients who have reasonable objectives and understand the risks and benefits. While PUVA photochemo-therapy is not a cure, most patients who are responding well to treatment do not at the same time develop new vitiligo macules.

6. **Narrow-band UVB 311 nm** This new light source, which is not available widely, appears to be effective *without* the use of psoralens, but there is new evidence that it is more effective when combined with oral 8-MOP. Comparative studies are in progress to quantify the addition of psoralens to UVB 311 nm and also to compare the responses to PUVA treatment for vitiligo.

7. **Minigrafting** Minigrafting may be a useful technique for refractory and stable segmental vitiligo macules. PUVA may be required after the procedure to unify the color between the graft sites. The demonstrated occurrence of koebnerization in donor sites in generalized vitiligo restricts this procedure to those who have limited cutaneous areas at risk for vitiligo (i.e., segmental vitiligo in which there is no koebnerization of normal skin). "Pebbling" of the grafted site may occur.

Depigmentation The objective of depigmentation is "one" skin color in patients with extensive vitiligo or in those who have failed PUVA, who cannot use PUVA, or who reject the PUVA option.

8. **Bleaching** Monobenzylether of hydroquinone 20% cream (monobenzone 20%)

of *normally pigmented skin* is a permanent, irreversible process. Since application of monobenzone 20% may be associated with satellite depigmentation, this treatment cannot be used selectively to bleach certain areas of normal pigmentation, since there is a real likelihood that new and distant white macules will develop over the months of use. Bleaching with monobenzone 20% normally requires the application twice daily to the body, takes 2 to 3 months to initiate response, and up to 9 to 12 months or more to complete. Erythema, dryness, and itching are possible side effects. Contact dermatitis is observed uncommonly. The success rate is over 90%. Periodically, after sun exposure, an occasional patient will observe focal repigmentation that requires a month or so of local use of monobenzone 20% to reverse; use of a sunscreen containing titanium dioxide or zinc oxide should reduce this risk.

The end-stage color of depigmentation with monobenzone 20% is chalk-white, as in vitiligo macules. Most patients are quite satisfied with the uniformity and the finality of the results. An occasional patient may wish to take 30 to 60 mg β-carotene per day to impart an off-white color to the skin; other than the color change, the only side effect of β-carotene is uncommon of diarrhea.

All those who have bleached are at risk for sunburn from acute solar irradiation. Avoidance of midday sun exposure and use of a sunscreen with a high sun protection factor are urged.

No long-term untoward effects have been reported from the use of monobenzylether of hydroquinone 20% cream. *But note that the depigmentation achieved is permanent;* the patient must understand this fact. With the development of a new therapy that could dramatically change the color, repigmentation will not be successful in patients who have had the melanocytes destroyed. This is especially true for those patients with a long life span such as children or young adults, as research is now being done on pathogenesis and treatment that may alter the type of therapy given, such as cytokines. Depigmented areas may repigment in the exposed areas, and bleaching should be done again.

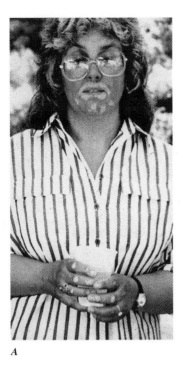

A

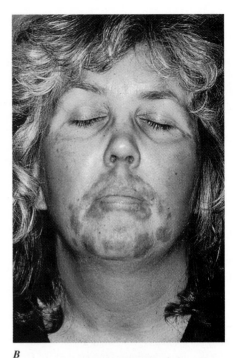

B

Figure 11-5 Vitiligo: repigmentation *The patient is being treated with photochemo-therapy (PUVA).* **A.** *Repigmentation has been uniform except periorally and on the hands, sites that are often resistant to the treatment;* **B.** *Repigmentation may sometimes exceed the color of normal skin "overshoot phenomenon." Here islands of repigmen-tation have created spotted macules in a background of depigmentation, resulting in significant cosmetic disfigurement.* **C.** *However, with further therapy hyperpigmented macules and normal skin blend in color; In a five-year follow-up, there was virtually no loss of pigment in the areas that had been repigmented.*

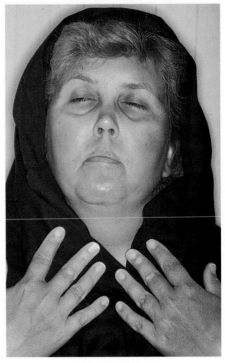

C

ALBINISM

Albinism describes a group of genetic alterations of the melanin pigment system that affect skin, hair follicles, and eyes. It principally involves the synthesis of melanin in these sites, but a normal number of melanocytes is present; also included are some alterations of the pathways of the CNS. Albinism (Table 11-2) can affect the eyes, ocular albinism (X-linked recessive or autosomal recessive), or the eyes and skin, oculocutaneous albinism (OCA). In OCA, the disorder is autosomal recessive, with dilution of normal amounts of skin, hair, and melanin pigment; nystagmus and iris translucency are always present, and there is a reduction of visual acuity, sometimes severe enough to cause severe impairment of vision.

EPIDEMIOLOGY

Age of Onset   Present at birth.

Prevalence   OCA 1:20,000.

Race   Hermansky-Pudlak syndrome (OCA and a platelet disorder) is seen in Hispanics from Puerto Rico, in persons of Dutch origin, and in East Indians from Madras.

CLASSIFICATION (TABLE 11-2)

OCA 1: Type I tyrosinase-negative; OCA1B tyrosinase-positive, with defects in the tyrosinase-melanin pathway catalyzed by tyrosinase. Molecular studies have defined several types of OCA resulting in mutations of the tyrosinase gene, which are the basis of yellow, minimal-pigment, and temperature-sensitive OCA. In OCA2, or P-related OCA, related to the P gene.

Changes that affect the membrane of the pigment organelle, the melanosome, and other organelles, *Chédiak-Higashi syndrome (CHS)*, in which there are prominent hematologic abnormalities (giant granules in the platelets and thrombocytopenia) and repeated bacterial infections resulting from depressed degranulation response and bactericidal functions. Also, *Hermansky-Pudlak syndrome (HPS)*, characterized by a mild to severe bleeding diathesis because of defective platelets; there is a lack of storage of granules or dense bodies, and platelets fail to undergo secondary aggregation when stimulated.

PATHOGENESIS

The defect in melanin synthesis has been shown to result from absence of the activity of the enzyme tyrosinase. Tyrosinase is a copper-containing enzyme that catalyzes the oxidation of tyrosine to dopa and the subsequent dehydrogenation of dopa to dopa-quinone. Recent cloning of complementary DNAs (cDNAs) encoding tyrosinase has made it possible to directly characterize the mutations in the tyrosinase gene responsible for deficient tyrosinase activity in several types of albinism. In type IA, two different missense mutations, one from each parent, result in amino acid substitutions within one of the two copper-binding sites (Table 11-2).

HISTORY

Duration   Present at birth. Patients with albinism early in life need to avoid the sun because of repeated sunburns, especially as toddlers.

Systems Review   HPS: epistaxis, gingival bleeding, excessive bleeding after childbirth or tooth extraction, fibrotic restrictive lung disease.

Family History   There may be no family history of albinism in the autosomal recessive or X-linked recessive types.

Social History   Albinos, excluding CHS and HPS types, live an essentially normal life, except for problems with vision and, in lower latitudes, the development of skin cancers and dermatoheliosis.

PHYSICAL EXAMINATION

General Appearance "Poring" (eyes half closed, squinting) when in sunlight.

Skin Varied, depending on the type: "Snow" white, creamy white, light tan (Table 11-2).

Hair White (tyrosinase-negative), yellow, cream, or light brown (tyrosinase-positive), red, platinum.

Eyes The eye changes are the essential physical finding that define the syndrome of albinism; the skin color and hair color can vary from snow white to brown, but it is the eye findings that permit the diagnosis (Fig. 11-6). Nystagmus, a feature always present, results from hypoplasia of the fovea with reduction of visual acuity and alteration in the formation of the optic nerves; this misrouting of the optic paths is also associated with an alternating strabismus

and diminished stereoacuity. The diagnostic features in the eye that identify albinism are therefore nystagmus and iris translucency (Fig. 11-7), reduction of visual acuity, decreased retinal pigment, foveal hypoplasia, and strabismus.

LABORATORY EXAMINATIONS

Dermatopathology

Light Microscopy Melanocytes are present in the skin and hair bulb in all types of albinism. The dopa reaction of the skin and hair is markedly reduced or absent in the melanocytes of the skin and hair, depending on the type of albinism (tyrosinase-negative or tyrosinase-positive).

Electron Microscopy Melanosomes are present in melanocytes in all types of albinism, but depending on the type of albinism, there is a reduction of the melanization of melanosomes,

Table 11-2 CLASSIFICATION OF ALBINISM

Type	Subtypes	Gene Locus	Includes	Clinical Findings
OCA1	OCA1A	Tyrosinase	Tyrosine-negative OCA	White hair and skin, eyes (pink at birth → blue)
	OCA1B	Tyrosinase	Minimal pigment OCA	White to near-normal skin and hair pigmentation
			Yellow OCA	Yellow (pheomelanin) hair, light red or brown hair
			Temperature-sensitive OCA	May have near-normal pigment but not in axilla
			Autosomal recessive OA (some)	
OCA2	P		Tyrosinase-positive	Yellow hair, skin "creamy" white (Africa)
			Brown OCA	Light brown/tan skin (Africa)
OCA3	TRP1		Autosomal recessive OCA (some)	
			Rufous OCA	Red and red-brown skin and brown eyes (Africa)
HPS	HPS		Hermansky-Pudlak syndrome	Skin/hair as in OCA1A or OACA1B or OCA2, bleeding diathesis (Puerto Rico)
CHS	CHS		Chediak-Higashi syndrome	Silver hair/hypopigmentation/ serious medical problems
OA1	OA1		X-linked OA	Normal pigmentation of skin, any hair

NOTE: OCA, oculocutaneous albinism; TRP1, tyrosine-related protein 1; OA, ocular albinism

SOURCE: Modified from RA King and WS Oetting: Albinism, in IM Freedberg, AZ Eisen, K Wolff, KF Austen, LA Goldsmith, SI Katz, and TB Fitzpatrick (eds): *Fitzpatrick's Dermatology in General Medicine,* 5th ed. New York, McGraw-Hill, 1999.

with many melanosomes being completely un-melanized (stage I) in tyrosinase-negative al-binism. Melanosomes in the albino melanocytes are transferred in a normal manner to the ker-atinocytes. In OA1 (ocular albinism) there are large organelles in the skin and eye called *melanin macroglobules.*

Hematology and General Medical Morpho-logic, chemical, and functional defects of platelets in the HPS; also interstitial pulmonary fibrosis and granulomatous colitis.

Molecular Testing Now available and makes it possible to classify the specific gene alteration in various types of albinism. This, however, is not necessary to diagnose or manage the prob-lem.

DIAGNOSIS

White persons with very fair skin (skin photo-type I), blond hair, and blue eyes may mimic albinos, but they do not have eye changes (iris translucency, nystagmus). Some persons with albinism who have constitutive black or brown skin color may have a dilution of their skin color from black to a light brown and have the ca-pacity to tan; also, some types may have brown irides but still have iris translucency. Therefore, iris translucency and the presence of other eye findings in the fundus are the pathognomonic signs of albinism. The hair and skin color may vary from normal to absent melanin, and the various types are listed in Table 11-2. The spe-cial types of albinism are diagnosed on the ba-sis of clinical presentation of the hair and skin pigmentation as well as hematologic studies (HPS).

SIGNIFICANCE

Albinism is an important disease to recognize early in life in order to begin prophylactic mea-sures to prevent dermatoheliosis and skin can-cer, i.e., protective clothing, sunblocks, and sun avoidance in peak periods during the day (1 to 2 h either side of noon, depending on the lati-tude).

COURSE AND PROGNOSIS

Albinos with tyrosinase-positive OCA form melanin pigment in the hair, skin, and eyes dur-ing early life, the hair becoming cream, yellow, or light brown, and the eye color changing from light gray to blue, hazel, or even brown.

Albinos living in central Africa who are un-protected from the sun develop squamous cell carcinomas early in life, and this significantly shortens their life span; few survive to the age of 40 years because of metastasizing squamous cell carcinoma. Dermatoheliosis and basal cell carcinomas are frequent in albinos living in temperate climates. Melanomas are, curiously, very rare in albinos living in Africa; when they occur, they are usually amelanotic. Melanocytic nevi occur in albinism and also may be ame-lanotic, but they may be pigmented depending on the type of albinism.

MANAGEMENT

Eye Every albino should be under the care of an ophthalmologist.

Skin A lifetime program with a dermatologist beginning in infancy, including the following:

Yearly examination by a dermatologist to detect skin changes: solar keratoses, skin cancers, and dermatoheliosis.

Daily application of topical, potent, broad-spec-trum SPF>30 sunblocks, including lip sun-blocks.

Avoidance of sun exposure in the high solar in-tensity season during the 1 to 2 h either side of noon, depending on the latitude, in the winter also.

Use of topical tretinoin for dermatoheliosis and for its possible prophylactic effect against sun-induced epithelial skin cancers. Treat-nent of solar keratoses to prevent the devel-opment of squamous cell carcinomas which are not infrequent, especially in the third-world countries.

Systemic β-carotene (30 to 60 mg tid) im-parts a more normal color to the skin and may have some protective effect on the development of skin cancers, although this has been proved only in mice.

General It is helpful for albinos to belong to a national volunteer group of albinos in the United States called the *N*ational *O*rganization for *A*lbinism and *H*ypomelanosis (NOAH). (Noah, the builder of the ark in the old Testa-ment, was alleged to be an albino.) This group assists albinos in various ways, especially in dealing with vision problems: obtaining driver's license, etc.

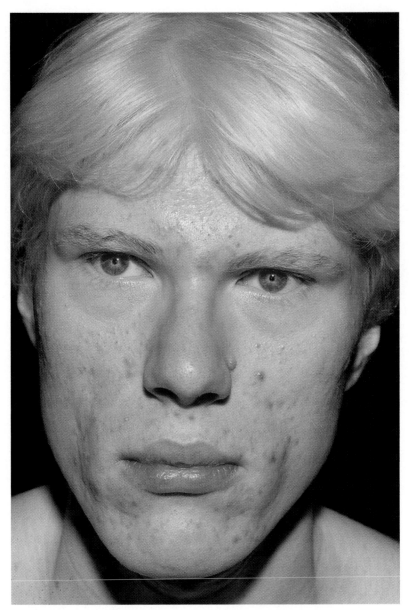

Figure 11-6 Oculocutaneous albinism *White skin and white eyelashes; scalp hair and eyebrows have been darkened with dye. The irises appear translucent. Heme pigment gives the face a pinkish hue; mild papulopustular acne is present. Carotene ingestion colors the central face a yellow-orange hue. The slight divergent strabism is due to nystagmus.*

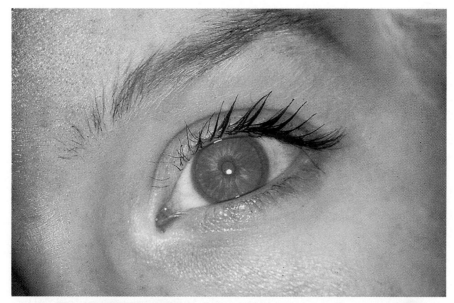

Figure 11-7 Iris translucency with albinism *Iris translucency is a sine qua non in all types of oculocutaneous albinism, even in those patients in which the iris is brown. The iris is rarely pink except in infants, and the diagnosis of albinism depends on the detection of iris translucency. This is best done in a dark room with a flashlight pointed at the sclera. In this photograph the iris translucency appeared because of the strobe light.*

MELASMA

Melasma (Greek: "a black spot") is an acquired light- or dark-brown hyperpigmentation that occurs in the exposed areas, most often on the face, and results from exposure to sunlight; may be associated with pregnancy, with ingestion of contraceptive hormones, or possibly with certain medications such as diphenylhydantoin, or may be idiopathic.
Synonyms: Chloasma (Greek: "a green spot"), mask of pregnancy.

EPIDEMIOLOGY

Age of Onset   Young adults.

Sex   Females>>males; about 10% of patients with melasma are men.

Race   Melasma is more apparent or more frequent in persons with brown or black constitutive skin color (persons from Asia, the Middle East, India, South America).

Incidence   Common, especially among persons with constitutive brown skin color and who are taking contraceptive regimens and who live in sunny areas. During the early clinical trials of estrogen–synthetic progesterone combinations, which were done in the Caribbean in brown-skinned Hispanic women, melasma occurred in 20% of the patients. Melasma has recently been appearing in menopausal women as a result of regimens for prevention of osteoporosis using a combination of estrogens *and* progesterone (medroxyprogesterone, or Provera); melasma did not appear in those women who were given estrogen replacement treatment but without progesterone. Melasma is still occurring in women given the contraceptive agents that are combinations of estrogen-type compounds and progestational agents.

Geography   More apparent or more frequent in sunny areas of the world, especially in the Caribbean and in countries bordering on the Mediterranean.

Precipitating Factors   Sun exposure plus pregnancy or oral contraceptives, diphenylhydantoin; cosmetics probably do not play a role.

PATHOGENESIS

Unknown. Estrogen preparations alone, however, given to postmenopausal women do not cause melasma, despite sun exposure. However, pregnancy causes melasma, and combinations of estrogen and progestational agents, as used for contraception, are the most frequent cause of melasma.

HISTORY

Duration of Lesions   The pigmentation usually evolves quite rapidly over weeks, particularly after exposure to sunlight.

Relationship of Melasma to Other Factors Season (more apparent in summer months in northern latitudes), medications (following or during ingestion of oral contraceptives), menses (during premenstrual period, a darkening of preexisting melasma may sometimes occur), pregnancy.

PHYSICAL EXAMINATION

Skin Lesions   Completely macular hyperpigmentation, the hue and intensity depending largely on the skin phototype of the patient (Fig. 11-8). Light or dark brown or even black. Color is usually uniform but may be splotchy. Most often symmetric.

Shape and Border of Individual Lesions   The pattern follows the areas of exposure, and the lesions have serrated, irregular, and geographic borders.

Distribution   Two-thirds on central part of the face: cheeks (Fig. 11-8), forehead, nose, upper lip, and chin; a smaller percentage on the malar or mandibular areas of the face and occasionally the dorsa of the forearms.

Wood's Lamp Examination   A marked accentuation of the hyperpigmented macules. *This contrast is not accentuated in patients with a normal brown or black skin.* This has been mistakenly interpreted as a "dermal" melasma.

DIFFERENTIAL DIAGNOSIS

Postinflammatory hypermelanotic macules.

LABORATORY EXAMINATIONS

Dermatopathology Increase in production and transfer of melanosomes to the keratinocytes in the epidermis.

Wood's Illumination Allow for dark adaptation.

DIAGNOSIS

Clinical findings.

SIGNIFICANCE

While this is a strictly cosmetic problem, it is very disturbing to both males and females, especially persons with brown skin color and good tanning capacity (skin phototype). For a discussion of how to determine skin phototype (SPT I to VI), see Table 11-1.

COURSE AND PROGNOSIS

Melasma may disappear spontaneously over a period of months after delivery or after cessation of contraceptive hormones. Melasma may or may not return with each subsequent pregnancy.

MANAGEMENT

Topical Two commercially available topical treatments (in the United States) are (1) 3% hydroquinone solution used in combination with topical .025% tretinoin gel and (2) a new combination of 4% hydroquinone and glycolic acid in a cream base; both of these are effective.

Under no circumstances should monobenzylether of hydroquinone or the other ethers of hydroquinone (monomethyl- or monoethyl-) be used in the treatment of melasma because these drugs can lead to a permanent loss of melanocytes with the development of a disfiguring spotty leukoderma. These drugs are limited to the treatment of extensive vitiligo in older persons to depigment the remaining normal pigment and provide one skin color, and eliminate the "harlequin" appearance of subtotal vitiligo.

Prevention It is essential that the patient use, every morning, an *opaque* sunblock containing titanium dioxide and/or zinc oxide; the action spectrum of pigment darkening extends into the visible range, and even the potent (with high SPF) transparent sunscreens are completely ineffective in blocking visible radiation.

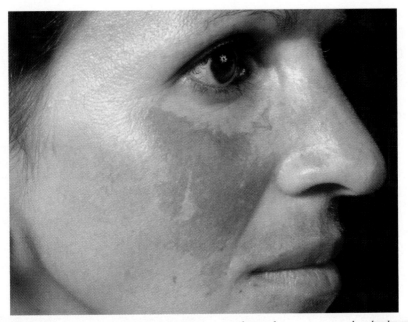

Figure 11-8 Melasma *Well-demarcated, hyperpigmented macules are seen on the cheek, nose, and forehead.*

HYPERPIGMENTATION AND HYPOPIGMENTATION FOLLOWING INFLAMMATION OF THE SKIN

Hyperpigmentation

Postinflammatory epidermal melanin hyperpigmentation is a major problem for patients with skin phototypes IV, V, and VI (Figs. 11-9 and 11-10). This disfiguring pigmentation can develop with acne (Fig. 11-9), psoriasis (Fig. 11-10), atopic dermatitis, contact dermatitis, or lichen planus, or after any type of trauma to the skin. It may persist for weeks to months but does respond to topical hydroquinone, which accelerates its disappearance.

The lesions are characteristically limited to the site of the preceding inflammation and have indistinct, feathered borders. Some drug eruptions may be associated with dermal melanin hyperpigmentation. Dermal melanin hyperpigmentation may also be associated with lichen planus and cutaneous lupus erythematosus. This dermal hyperpigmentation may be persistent, and there is no treatment.

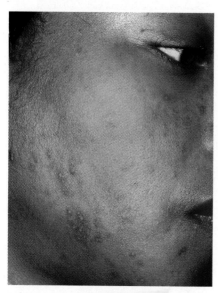

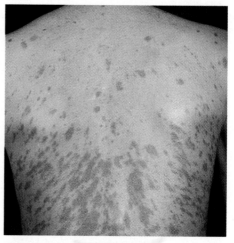

Figure 11-10 Postinflammatory hyperpigmentation *May follow a drug eruption or psoriasis, especially in skin phototypes V and VI as was the case in this middle-age East Indian female. Postinflammatory hyperpigmentation is a major problem in young females with skin phototypes V and VI.*

Figure 11-9 Hypermelanosis with acne *This condition is a major complaint of this 18-year-old African American (skin phototype V). The acne is not the problem now; it is the disfiguring hypermelanosis. This hyperpigmentation can be markedly reduced with topical hydroquinone solution, 3%, applied daily. During the depigmentation, the patient must use an opaque sunblock containing titanium dioxide daily to prevent the pigment darkening that occurs with daily sun exposure.*

PIGMENTARY DISORDERS

Hypopigmentation

Postinflammatory hypomelanosis is always related to loss of melanin. It is a special feature of pityriasis versicolor in which the hypopigmentation may remain for weeks after the active infection has disappeared; this poses a special problem in deciding whether the hypopigmentation is vitiligo or some other type of hypomelanosis. In hypopigmentation associated with pityriasis versicolor (Fig. 11-11) a biopsy of the skin reveals the presence of melanocytes, which are not present in vitiligo. Hypomelanosis is not uncommonly seen in atopic dermatitis, psoriasis (Fig. 11-12), guttate parapsoriasis, pityriasis lichenoides chronica. It may also be present in cutaneous lupus erythematosus, alopecia mucinosa, mycosis fungoides, lichen striatus, and seborrheic dermatitis. Hypomelanosis may follow dermabrasion and chemical peels; and in these conditions there is a "transfer block," in which melanosomes are present in melanocytes but are not transferred to keratinocytes, resulting in hypomelanosis. The lesions are usually not chalk white as in vitiligo but "off" white and have indiscrete margins (Fig. 11-12). A common type of hypopigmentation is associated with pityriasis alba, especially on the face (Fig. 11-13). Hypomelanosis not uncommonly follows intralesional glucocorticoid injections; but when the injections are stopped, a normal pigmentation develops in the areas. Depending on the associated disorder, postinflammatory hypomelanosis may respond to oral PUVA photochemotherapy.

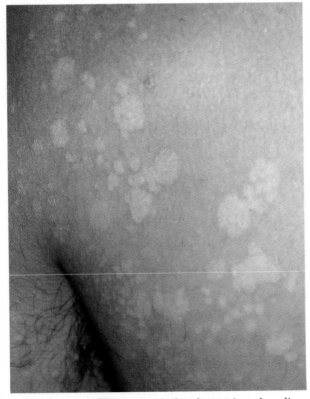

Figure 11-11 **Pityriasis versicolor** *Hypopigmented, sharply marginated, scaling macules on the shoulder area of an individual with brown skin. Gentle abrasion of the surface accentuates the scaling. This type of hypomelanosis can remain long after the eruption has been treated and the primary process is resolved.*

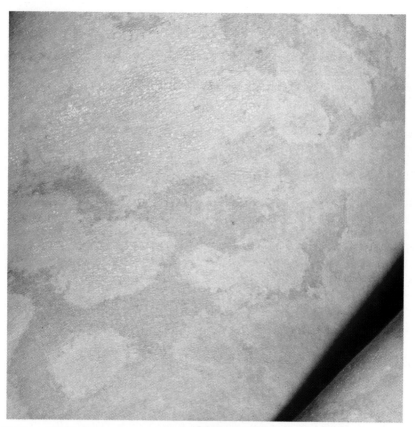

Figure 11-12   Postinflammatory hypomelanosis (psoriasis)   *The hypomelanotic lesions correspond exactly to the antecedent eruption. There is some residual psoriasis within the lesions.*

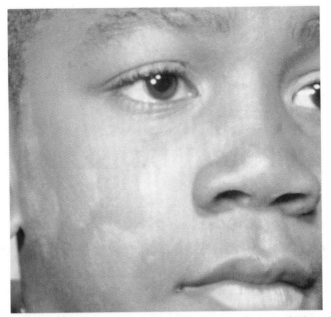

Figure 11-13 Pityriasis alba (PA) *A common disfiguring hypomelanosis, which, as the name indicates, is a white area (alba) with scaling (pityriasis.) It is observed in a large number of children in the summer in temperate climates. It is mostly a cosmetic problem in persons with brown or black skin. Among 200 patients, 90% ranged from 6 to 12 years of age. In young adults, PA quite often occurs on the arms and trunk. Curiously, PA is not often observed after age 30. The lesions are light brown or pale white and occur most often on the face (especially the cheeks); extensive PA can be seen on the upper extremities and trunk. Its pathogenesis is unknown, but some believe it is a form of eczematous dermatitis, but there is no spongosis (the "hallmark" of allergic eczema). On histologic examination, melanocytes are shown to be reduced in number and there are fewer melanosomes, but transfer of melanosomes does occur. Management is satisfactory with low-potency corticosteroids; and if this is not effective, oral PUVA is efficacious. The lesions disappear spontaneously in the winter in temperate climates.*

SKIN SIGNS OF IMMUNE, AUTOIMMUNE, AND RHEUMATIC DISEASES

SYSTEMIC AMYLOIDOSIS

Amyloidosis is an extracellular deposition in various tissues of amyloid fibril proteins and of a protein called *amyloid P component* (*AP*); the identical component of AP is present in the serum and is called *SAP*. These amyloid deposits can affect normal body function. *Acquired systemic amyloidosis* (*AL*), known as *primary amyloidosis*, occurs in patients with B cell or plasma cell dyscrasias and multiple myeloma in whom fragments of monoclonal immunoglobulin light chains form amyloid fibrils. *Secondary amyloidosis* (*AA*) occurs in patients after chronic inflammatory disease, in whom the fibril protein is derived from the circulating acute-phase lipoprotein known as *serum amyloid A*. Clinical features of AL (primary amyloidosis) include a combination of macroglossia and cardiac, renal, hepatic, and GI involvement, as well as carpal tunnel syndrome and *skin lesions*. These occur in 30% of patients; and since they occur early in the disease, they are an important clue to the diagnosis. There are few or no characteristic skin lesions in AA (secondary amyloidosis), which usually affects the liver, spleen, kidneys and adrenals; but there is a certain degree of overlap, and some skin lesions occur. In addition, skin manifestations may also be associated with a number of (rare) heredofamilial syndromes.

AL, Acquired Systemic Amyloidosis, Primary Amyloidosis

EPIDEMIOLOGY

Age of Onset Sixth decade.

Sex Equal incidence.

Precipitating Factors Multiple myeloma in many but not all patients, B cell and plasma cell dyscrasias.

Systemic Symptoms Fatigue, weakness, anorexia, weight loss, malaise. Dyspnea; symptoms related to hepatic, renal and GI involvement; paresthesia related to carpal tunnel syndrome.

PHYSICAL EXAMINATION

Skin Lesions *Purpura* following trauma, "pinch" purpura (Fig. 12-1), occurs on the face and especially around the eyes and in papular and nodular lesions. Smooth, waxy *papules* with (Fig. 12-1) or without purpura, sometimes involving large surface areas. Smooth, waxy *nodules* with or without purpura.

Distribution Around the eyes, central face, extremities, body folds, axillae, umbilicus, anogenital area.

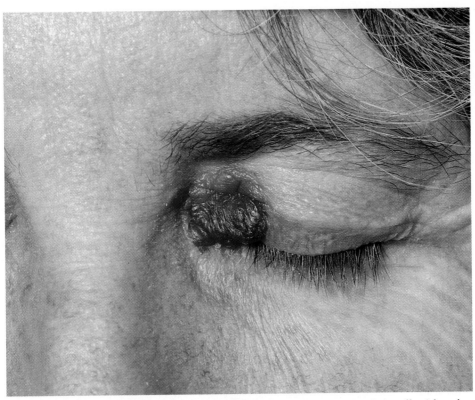

Figure 12-1 **Primary systemic amyloidosis: "pinch purpura"** *The topmost papule is yellowish and nonhemorrhagic; the lower portion is hemorrhagic. So-called "pinch purpura" of the upper eyelid can appear in amyloid nodules after pinching or rubbing the eyelid.*

Mucous Membranes Macroglossia: diffusely enlarged and firm, "woody" (Figure 12-2). This also occurs in AA.

General Examination Kidney—nephrosis; nervous system—peripheral neuropathy, carpal tunnel syndrome; CVS—partial heart block, congestive heart failure; hepatic—hepatomegaly; GI—diarrhea, sometimes hemorrhagic, malabsorptions; lymphadenopathy.

DIFFERENTIAL DIAGNOSIS

Purpura Thrombocytopenic purpura, actinic (Bateman's) purpura, scurvy.

Macroglossia Hypothyroidism.

Papules and Nodules Granuloma annulare, sarcoidosis, lymphomas, xanthomas, necrobiosis lipoidica.

LABORATORY EXAMINATIONS

Hematology Thrombocytosis >500,000/μL may be present.

Urinalysis Proteinuria.

Chemistry Increased serum creatinine; hypercalcemia.

Immunoglobulin Studies Increased IgG. Monoclonal protein in two-thirds of patients with primary or myeloma-associated amyloidoses.

Dermatopathology Accumulation of faintly eosinophilic masses of amyloid in the papillary body near the epidermis, in the papillary and reticular dermis, in sweat glands, around and within blood vessel walls. Use thioflavin and examine the sections for an apple-green birefringence with a simple polarization microscope.

DIAGNOSIS

The combination of purpuric skin lesions, waxy papules, macroglossia, carpal tunnel syndrome, and cardiac symptoms and signs. A tissue diagnosis can be made from the skin biopsy. Scintigraphy after injection of ^{123}I-labeled SAP is now available for estimating the extent of the involvement and can serve as a guide for treatment.

COURSE AND PROGNOSIS

Poor, especially if there is renal involvement. Amyloidosis AL with multiple myeloma has an especially poor prognosis, with 18- to 24-month survival.

MANAGEMENT

Cytotoxic drugs can modify the course of amyloidosis AL associated with multiple myeloma.

AA, Secondary Aymloidosis

There are no characteristic skin lesions in AA, except macroglossia and, occasionally, papules and hemorrhage; hyperpigmentation.

Localized Cutaneous Amyloidosis

Three not uncommon varieties of localized amyloidosis that are unrelated to the systemic amyloidoses are *lichenoid amyloidosis* (discrete, very pruritic, brownish-red papules on the legs); *nodular amyloidosis* (single or multiple, smooth, nodular lesions with or without purpura on limbs, face, or trunk); and *macular amyloidosis* (pruritic, gray-brown, reticulated macular lesions occurring principally on the upper back; the lesions often have a distinctive "ripple" pattern). In lichenoid and macular amyloidosis the amyloid fibrils in skin are keratin-derived. Although these three localized forms of amyloidosis are confined to the skin and unrelated to systemic disease, the skin lesions of nodular amyloidosis are identical to those that occur in amyloidosis AL, where amyloid fibrils derive from immunoglobulin light chain fragments.

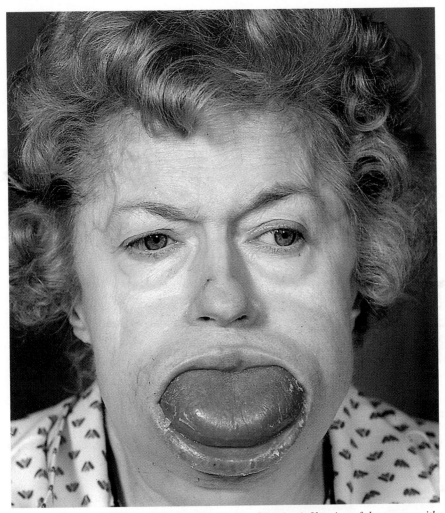

Figure 12-2 Primary systemic amyloidosis: macroglossia *Massive infiltration of the tongue with amyloid has caused immense enlargement; the tongue cannot be retracted completely into the mouth because of its size. (Courtesy of Evan Calkins, MD.)*

URTICARIA AND ANGIOEDEMA

Urticaria is composed of wheals (transient edematous papules and plaques, usually pruritic and due to edema of the papillary body) (Fig. 12-3). Angioedema is a larger edematous area that involves the dermis *and* subcutaneous tissue. Urticaria and/or angioedema may be acute recurrent or chronic recurrent. There are some syndromes with angioedema in which urticarial wheals are rarely present (e.g., hereditary angioedema).

EPIDEMIOLOGY

Incidence

15 to 23% of the population may have had this condition during their lifetime. Chronic urticaria is likely to be present at some time in about 25% of patients with urticaria.

Etiology

Angioedema and urticaria can be classified as IgE-mediated, complement-mediated, anti-FcεRI autoantibody-mediated, related to physical stimuli (cold, sunlight, pressure), or idiosyncratic. The syndrome known as *angioedema-urticaria-eosinophilia syndrome* is related to the action of the eosinophil major basic protein, and *hereditary angioedema* is related to decreased or dysfunctional C1-esterase inhibitor.

Etiologic Types

Immunologic *IgE-Mediated* Often with atopic background. Antigens: food (milk, eggs, wheat, shellfish, nuts), therapeutic agents, drugs (penicillin) (See also Drug-Induced Acute Urticaria, Angioedema, Edema, and Anaphylaxis, Section 18), parasites. **Complement-Mediated** By way of immune complexes activating complement and releasing anaphylatoxins that induce mast cell degranulation. Serum sickness, administration of whole blood, immunoglobulins.

Physical   Urticaria   Dermographism Although 4.2% of the normal population have it, symptomatic dermographism is a nuisance. Linear urticarial lesions occur after stroking or scratching the skin; it itches and fades in 30 min (Fig. 12-4).

Cold Urticaria Usually in children or young adults; urticarial lesions confined to sites exposed to cold. "Ice cube" test establishes diagnosis.

Solar Urticaria Urticaria after solar exposure. Action spectrum 290 to 500 nm; histamine is one of the mediators.

Cholinergic Urticaria Exercise to the point of sweating provokes typical (small, papular) highly pruritic urticarial lesions and establishes diagnosis (Fig. 12-5).

Pressure Angioedema History of swelling induced by pressure (buttock swelling when seated, hand swelling after hammering, foot swelling after walking). No laboratory abnormalities; no fever. Urticaria may occur in addition to angioedema.

Vibratory angioedema May be familial (autosomal dominant) or sporadic. It is believed to result from histamine release from mast cells caused by a "vibrating" stimulus—rubbing a towel across the back produces lesions, but direct pressure (without movements) does not.

Urticaria Due to Mast Cell-Releasing Agents Urticaria/angioedema and even anaphylaxis-like syndromes may occur with radiocontrast media and as a consequence of intolerance to salicylates, azo dyes, and benzoates (See also Drug-Induced Urticaria, Angioedema, Edema, and Anaphylaxis, Section 18).

Urticaria Associated with Vascular/Connective Tissue Autoimmune Disease Urticarial vasculitis is a form of cutaneous vasculitis associated with urticarial skin lesions that persist longer than 12 to 24 h, can be associated with purpura, and can show residual pigmentation due to hemosiderin after involution. There is only slow change of size and configuration. Often associated with hypocomplementemia and renal disease. Urticarial lesions also may be associated with SLE and Sjögren's syndrome, which usually, but not always, represent urticarial vasculitis (page 393).

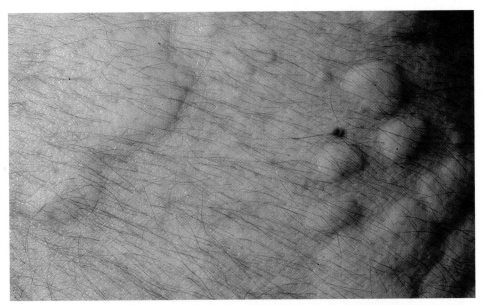

Figure 12-3 Urticaria *Wheals with white-to-light-pink color centrally and peripheral erythema in a close-up view. These are the classic lesions of urticaria. It is characteristic that they are transient and highly pruritic.*

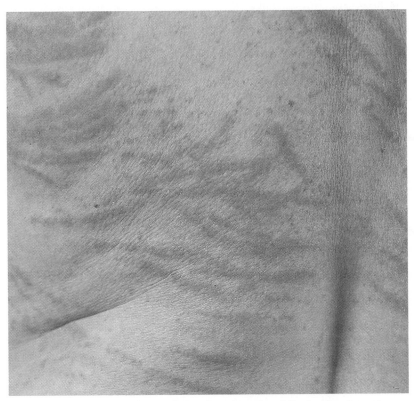

Figure 12-4 Urticaria: dermatographism *Urticaria as it appeared 5 min after the patient scratched himself because of itchiness of his otherwise normal skin. The patient had experienced generalized pruritus for several months with no spontaneously occurring urticaria.*

Hereditary Angioedema (HAE) A serious autosomal dominant disorder; involves angioedema of the face (Fig. 12-6 A and B) and extremities, episodes of laryngeal edema, and acute abdominal pain caused by angioedema of the bowel wall. Urticaria does not usually occur, but there may be an erythema marginatum-like eruption. Laboratory abnormalities involve the complement system: decreased levels of C1-esterase inhibitor (85%) or dysfunctional inhibitor (15%), low C4 value in the presence of normal C1 and C3 levels. Angioedema results from bradykinin formation, since C1-esterase inhibitor is also the major inhibitor of the Hageman factor and kallikrein, the two enzymes required for kinin formation. Episodes can be life threatening.

Angioedema-Urticaria-Eosinophilia Syndrome Severe angioedema, only occasionally with pruritic urticaria, involving the face, neck, extremities, and trunk that lasts for 7 to 10 days. There is fever and marked increase in normal weight (increased by 10 to 18%) owing to fluid retention. No other organs are involved. Laboratory abnormalities include striking leukocytosis (20,000 to 70,000/μL) and eosinophilia (60 to 80% eosinophils), which are related to the severity of attack. There is no family history. Prognosis good.

Clinical Types

Acute Urticaria (<30 Days) Usually large wheals often associated with angioedema (Fig. 12-7), often IgE-dependent with atopic background, related to alimentary agents, parasites, and penicillin. Also, complement-mediated in serum sickness-like reactions (whole blood, immunoglobulins, penicillin). Often accompanied by angioedema. (See also Drug-Induced Acute Urticaria, Angioedema, Edema, and Anaphylaxis, Section 18.)

Chronic Urticaria (>30 Days) Small and large wheals (Fig. 12-8). Rarely IgE-dependent but often due to anti-FcεR autoantibodies; etiology unknown in 80% and therefore considered idiopathic; emotional stress often seems to be an exacerbating factor. Intolerance to salicylates, benzoates. Chronic urticaria affects predominantly adults and is approximately twice as common in women as in men. Up to 40% of patients with chronic urticaria of more than 6 months' duration still have urticaria 10 years later.

PATHOGENESIS

Lesions in acute IgE-mediated urticaria result from antigen-induced release of biologically active molecules from mast cells or basophilic leukocytes sensitized with specific IgE antibodies (type I anaphylactic hypersensitivity). Mediators released increase venular permeability and modulate the release of biologically active molecules from other cell types.

In complement-mediated urticaria, complement is activated by immune complexes; this results in the release of anaphylatoxins, which, in turn, induce mast cell degranulation.

In chronic idiopathic urticaria, histamine derived from mast cells in the skin is considered the major mediator. Other mediators, including eicosanoids and neuropeptides, also may play a part in producing the lesions, but direct measurement of these mediators has not been reported. Intolerance to salicylates and food preservatives and additives, such as benzoic acid and sodium benzoate, as well as several azo dyes, including tartrazine and sunset yellow; is presumably mediated by abnormalities of the arachidonic acid pathway.

In 40% of patients with chronic urticaria an anti-FcεRI autoantibody has been identified and a positive correlation between histamine-releasing activity and disease activity has been demonstrated. Clinically, patients with these autoantibodies are indistinguishable from those without them. These autoantibodies may explain why plasmapheresis, intravenous immunoglobulins, and cyclosporine induce remission of disease activity in these patients. The concept that some chronic urticarias are a manifestation of autoimmune mast cell disease is also supported by the association of chronic urticaria with autoimmune thyroid disease (14%).

In hereditary angioedema, decreased or dysfunctional C1-esterase inhibitor leads to increased kinin formation. The angioedema-urticaria-eosinophilia syndrome may result from the eosinophilia that is markedly elevated in the skin. In this syndrome, the eosinophilia increases and decreases with the angioedema and urticaria; major basic protein is distributed after its release from the eosinophil between the collagen bundles, and mast cells in the dermis show degranulation.

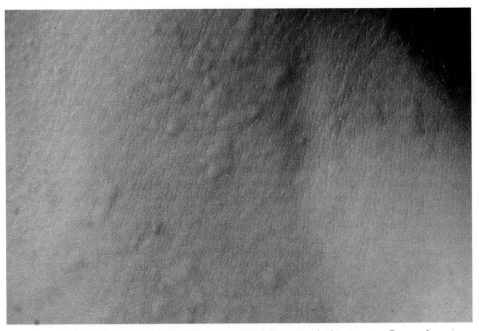

Figure 12-5 Cholinergic urticaria *Small urticarial papules on pink skin (axon reflex erythema) occurring on the neck within 30 min of vigorous exercise.*

HISTORY

Duration of Lesions Hours. Urticarial eruption, pruritus, pain on walking (in foot involvement), flushing, burning, and wheezing (in cholinergic urticaria). Fever in serum sickness and in the angioedema-urticaria-eosinophilia syndrome; in angioedema, hoarseness, stridor, dyspnea. Arthralgia (serum sickness, urticarial vasculitis), abdominal colicky pain in HAE.

PHYSICAL EXAMINATION

Skin Lesions Transient, skin colored-*papules*— many small (1 to 2 mm are typical in cholinergic urticaria), pruritic (Fig. 12-5,). *Wheals*— small (1 cm) to large (8 cm), edematous plaques (Figs. 12-3, 12-7, and 12-8) may be erythematous or white with an erythematous halo, round, oval, arciform, annular, serpiginous due to resolution in one area and progression in another. Lesions are pruritic and transient and the distribution may be localized, regional, or generalized. *Angioedema*—skin-colored, transient enlargement of portion of face (eyelids, lips, tongue) (Figs. 12-6 and 12-7), extremity, or other sites due to subcutaneous edema.

Sites of Predilection Sites of pressure, exposed areas (solar urticaria, cold urticaria), trunk, hands and feet, lips, tongue, ears.

DIFFERENTIAL DIAGNOSIS

Urticarial Wheals Insect bites, adverse drug reactions, urticarial contact dermatitis, urticarial vasculitis.

LABORATORY EXAMINATIONS

For general medical workup, to rule out systemic disease in chronic urticaria (SLE, urticarial vasculitis, Sjögren's syndrome).

Dermatopathology Edema of the dermis or subcutaneous tissue, dilatation of venules but no evidence of vascular damage. Mast cell degranulation. The predominant perivascular inflammatory cell types are activated lymphocytes of the T helper phenotype.

Serology Search for hepatitis-associated antigen, assessment of the complement system, assessment of specific IgE antibodies by RAST, anti-FcεRI autoantibodies.

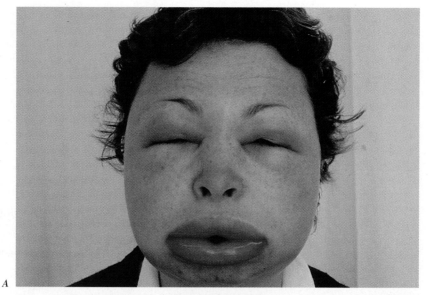

A

Figure 12-6   Hereditary angioedema   A. *Severe edema of the face during an episode leading to grotesque disfigurement.* **B.** *Angioedema will subside within hours. The patient had a positive family history and had multiple similar episodes including colicky abdominal pain.*

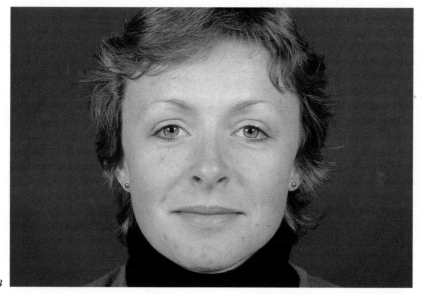

B

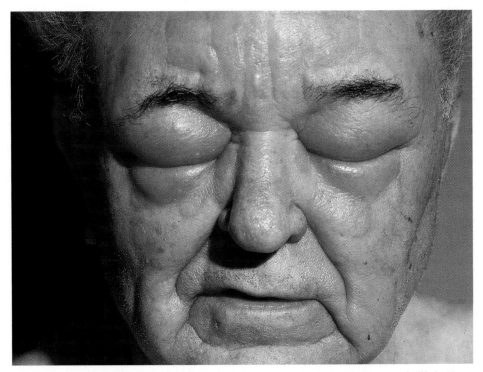

Figure 12-7 Acute urticaria and angioedema *Occurred after the patient had eaten shellfish. He had similar episodes previously, but had never established a link with seafood.*

Hematology The erythrocyte sedimentation rate (ESR) is often elevated in persistent urticaria (urticarial vasculitis), and there may be hypocomplementemia; transient eosinophilia in urticaria from reactions to foods, parasites, and drugs; high levels of eosinophilia in the angioedema-urticaria-eosinophilia syndrome.

Complement Studies Screening for functional C1 inhibitor.

Ultrasonography For early diagnosis of bowel involvement; if abdominal pain is present, this may indicate edema of the bowel.

Parasitology Stool specimen for presence of parasites.

DIAGNOSIS

A detailed history (previous diseases, drugs, foods, parasites, physical exertion, solar exposure) is of utmost importance. Most difficult to evaluate is chronic urticaria. A practical approach to the diagnosis of chronic urticaria is shown in Table 12-1. A careful history of medications including aspirin and nonsteroidal anti-inflammatory drugs should be obtained. If *physical urticaria* is suspected, appropriate challenge testing should be performed. *Cholinergic urticaria* can best be diagnosed by exercise to sweating and intracutaneous injection of acetylcholine or mecholyl, which will produce micropapular whealing. *Solar urticaria* is verified by testing with UVB, UVA, and visible light. *Cold urticaria* is verified by a wheal response to the application to the skin of an ice cube or a test tube containing ice water. If urticarial wheals do not disappear in 24 h or less, urticarial vasculitis should be suspected and a biopsy done. The *angioedema-urticaria-eosinophilia syndrome* has high fever, high leukocytosis (mostly eosinophils), a striking increase in body weight due to retention of water, and a cyclic pattern that may occur and recur over a period of years. *Hereditary angioedema* has a positive family history and is characterized by angioedema of the face and extremities as the result of trauma, abdominal pain, and decreased levels of C4 and C1-esterase inhibitor or a dysfunctional inhibitor.

COURSE AND PROGNOSIS

Half the patients with urticaria alone are free of lesions in 1 year, but 20% have lesions for more than 20 years. Prognosis is good in most syndromes except hereditary angioedema, which may be fatal if untreated.

MANAGEMENT

Prevention Try to prevent attacks by elimination of etiologic chemicals or drugs: aspirin and food additives, especially in chronic recurrent urticaria—rarely successful.

Antihistamines H_1 blockers, e.g., hydroxyzine, terfenadine; or loratadine, cetirizine, fexofenadine. 180 mg/d of fexofenadine or 10 to 20 mg/d of loratadine usually controls most cases of chronic urticaria, but cessation of therapy usually results in a recurrence; if they fail, H_1 and H_2 blockers (cimetidine) and/or mast cell-stabilizing agents (ketotifen). Doxepin, a tricyclic antidepressant with marked H_1 antihistaminic activity, is valuable when severe urticaria is associated with anxiety and depression.

Prednisone Indicated for angioedema-urticaria-eosinophilia syndrome.

Danazol Long-term therapy for hereditary angioedema; whole fresh plasma or C1-esterase inhibitor in the acute attack.

Table 12-1 FEATURES OF COMMON TYPES OF CHRONIC URTICARIA

Type of Urticaria	Age Range of Patients (years)	Principal Clinical Features	Associated Angio-edema	Diagnostic Test
Chronic idiopathic	20–50	Profuse or sparse generalized, pink or pale edematous papules or wheals, often annular with itching	Yes	—
Symptomatic dermographism	20–50	Itchy, linear wheals with a surrounding bright-red flare at sites of scratching or rubbing	No	Light stroking of skin causes an immediate wheal with itching
Other physical urticarias Cold	10–40	Itchy, pale or red wheal or swelling at sites of contact with cold surfaces or fluids	Yes	10-min application of an ice pack causes a wheal within 5 min. of the removal of ice
Pressure	20–50	Large, painful or itchy red swelling at sites of pressure (soles, palms or waist)	No	Application of pressure perpendicular to skin produces persistent red swelling after a latent period of 1–4 h
Solar	20–50	Itchy, pale or red swelling at site of exposure to UV or visible light	Yes	Irradiation by a 2.5-kW solar simulator (290–690 nm) for 30–120s causes wheals in 30 min
Cholinergic	10–50	Itchy, small (<5 mm) monomorphic pale or pink papular wheals on trunk, neck, and limbs	Yes	Exercise or a hot shower elicits an eruption, acute stressful situation

SOURCE: From MW Greaves: Chronic urticaria: A review. *N Engl J Med* 332:1767, 1995.

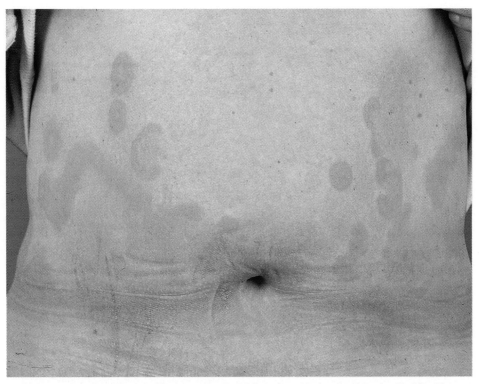

Figure 12-8 Chronic urticaria *Chronic urticaria of 5-yr duration in an otherwise healthy 50-year-old female. Eruptions occur on an almost daily basis and, as they are highly pruritic, greatly impair the patient's quality of life. Although suppressed by antihistamines, there is an immediate recurrence after treatment is stopped. Repeated laboratory and clinical examinations have not revealed an apparent cause.*

BEHÇET'S SYNDROME

Behçet's syndrome (BS) is a perplexing multisystem inflammation which, in the most recent definition of diagnostic criteria, has one basic major feature—recurrent oral aphthous ulcers (AU)—and two of the following features: recurrent genital AU, eye lesions (posterior uveitis), skin lesions (erythema nodosum or pustules). Other manifestations include synovitis, neurologic disorders, and thrombophlebitis.
Synonym: Behçet's disease.

EPIDEMIOLOGY

Age of Onset   Third and fourth decades.

Sex   Males > females.

Prevalence   Highest in Japan (1:10,000), Southeast Asia, the Middle East, southern Europe. Rare in northern Europe, United States.

PATHOGENESIS

Etiology unknown. In the eastern Mediterranean and East Asia, HLA-B5 and HLA-B51 association; in the United States and Europe, no consistent HLA association. The lesions could be the result of an accumulation of neutrophils in the sites of immune complex–mediated vasculitis.

HISTORY

Painful ulcers erupt in a cyclic fashion in the oral cavity and/or genital mucous membranes. Orodynophagia and oral ulcers may persist/recur weeks to months before other symptoms appear.

PHYSICAL EXAMINATION

Skin and Mucous Membranes   *Aphthous Ulcers (AU)*   Punched-out ulcers (3 to >10 mm) with rolled or overhanging borders and necrotic base; (see Fig. 29-4) red rim; occur in crops (2 to 10) on oral mucous membrane (100%), (see Fig. 29-4) vulva, penis, and scrotum; (Figs. 12-9 and 12-10) very painful.

Erythema Nodosum-Like Lesions   Painful inflammatory nodules on the arms and legs (40%) (see Fig. 5-25).

Other   Inflammatory pustules, inflammatory plaques resembling those in Sweet's syndrome (acute febrile neutrophilic dermatosis) (see Fig. 5-29), pyoderma gangrenosum-like lesions, palpable purpuric lesions of necrotizing vasculitis.

Systemic Findings   *Eye*   Posterior uveitis anterior uveitis, retinal vasculitis, vitreitis, hypopyon, secondary cataracts, glaucoma, neovascular lesions.

Musculoskeletal   Nonerosive, asymmetric oligoarthritis.

Neurologic   Onset delayed, occurring in one-quarter of patients. Meningoencephalitis, benign intracranial hypertension, cranial nerve palsies, brainstem lesions, pyramidal/extrapyramidal lesions, psychosis.

Vascular   Aneurysms, arterial occlusions, venous thrombosis, varices; hemoptysis. Coronary vasculitis: myocarditis, coronary arteritis, endocarditis, valvular disease.

GI Tract   AU throughout.

DIFFERENTIAL DIAGNOSIS

Oral and Genital Ulcers   Viral infection (HSV), VZV, hand-foot-and-mouth disease, herpangina, chancre, histoplasmosis, SCC.

LABORATORY EXAMINATIONS

Dermatopathology   Extravasation of erythrocytes, leukocytoclasia. Later: fully-developed leukocytoclastic vasculitis with fibrinoid necrosis of blood vessel walls.

Pathergy Test   Positive pathergy test read by physician at 24 or 48 h, after skin puncture with a sterile needle. Leads to inflammatory pustule.

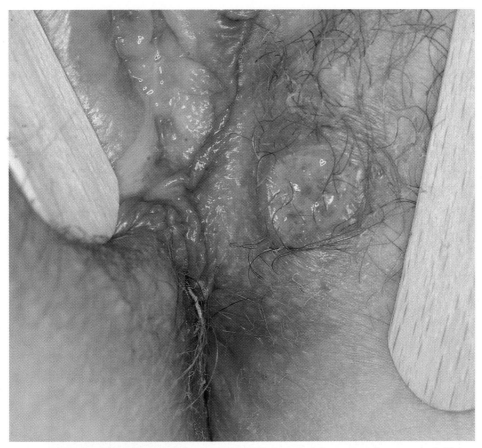

Figure 12-9 Behçet's syndrome: genital ulcers *Multiple large aphthous-type ulcers on the labial and perineal epithelium. In addition, this 25-year-old patient of Turkish extraction had aphthous ulcers in the mouth and previously experienced an episode of uveitis.*

HLA Typing Significant association with HLA-B5 and HLA-B51, particularly in Japanese, Koreans, and Turks, and in the Middle East.

Other Examinations Nonspecific, varying with specific organ system involved.

DIAGNOSIS

Proposed criteria for Behçet's syndrome include the presence of oral AU plus two of the following: recurrent genital AU, eye lesions, skin lesions, or positive pathergy test.

COURSE AND PROGNOSIS

Highly variable course, with recurrences and remissions; the mouth lesions are always present; remissions may last for weeks, months, or years. With CNS involvement, there is a higher mortality rate. In the eastern Mediterranean and East Asia, severe course, one of leading causes of blindness.

MANAGEMENT

Aphthous Ulcers Potent topical glucocorticoids. Intralesional triamcinolone, 3 to 10 mg/ml, injected into ulcer base. Thalidomide, 100 mg PO bid. Colchicine, .6 mg PO 2 to 3 times a day. Dapsone.

Systemic Involvement Prednisone with or without azathioprine, cyclophosphamide, azathioprine alone, chlorambucil, cyclosporine.

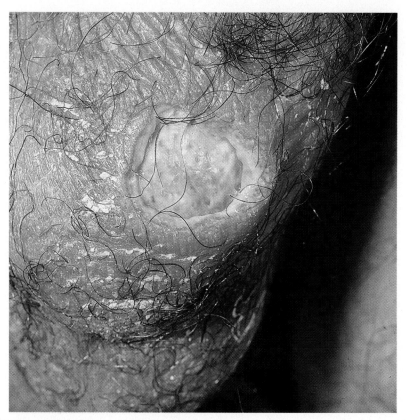

Figure 12-10 Behçet's syndrome *A large, punched-out ulcer on the scrotum of a 40-year-old Korean. The patient also had aphthous ulcers in the mouth and pustules on the thighs and buttocks.*

DERMATOMYOSITIS

Dermatomyositis (DM) is a systemic disease characterized by violaceous (heliotrope) inflammatory changes of the eyelids and periorbital area; erythema of the face, neck, and upper trunk; and flat-topped violaceous papules over the knuckles. It is associated with a polymyositis, interstitial pneumonitis, myocardial involvement, and vasculitis.

EPIDEMIOLOGY

Age of Onset Juvenile. Adults >40 years. Rare; incidence >6 cases per million, but this is based on hospitalized patients and does not include individuals without muscle involvement.

Etiology Unknown. In persons >55 years of age often associated with malignancy. Associated malignant tumors: breast, lung, ovary, stomach, colon, uterus.

Clinical Spectrum Ranges from DM with only cutaneous inflammation (amyopathic DM) to polymyositis with only muscle inflammation. Cutaneous involvement occurs in 30 to 40% of adults and 95% of children with dermatomyositis/polymyositis.

HISTORY

±Photosensitivity. Manifestations in skin disease may precede myositis or vice versa; often, both are detected at the same time. Muscle weakness, difficulty in rising from supine position, climbing stairs, raising arms over head, turning in bed. Dysphagia; burning and pruritus of the scalp.

PHYSICAL EXAMINATION

Skin Lesions Periorbital heliotrope (reddish purple) flush, usually associated with some degree of edema (Fig. 12-11). May extend to involve scalp, upper chest, and arms (Fig. 12-12). Papular dermatitis with varying degrees of violaceous erythema (Fig. 12-12) and scaling on forehead, scalp, cheeks, neck, and upper chest. Flat-topped, violaceous papules (Gottron's papule/sign) (Fig. 12-13) with various degrees of atrophy on the nape of the neck and shoulders and over the knuckles and interphalangeal joints. (Fig. 12-13) *Note:* In lupus, lesions usually occur in the interarticular region of the fingers (see Fig. 12-22). Periungual erythema with telangiectasia, thrombosis of capillary loops, in-

farctions. Lesions over elbows and knuckles may evolve to erosions and ulcers that heal with stellate scarring. Long-lasting lesions may evolve into poikiloderma (mottled discoloration with red, white, and brown). Calcification in subcutaneous/fascial tissues common later in course of juvenile DM, particularly about elbows, trochanteric, and iliac region; may evolve to calcinosis universalis.

Muscle ±Muscle atrophy, ±muscle tenderness. Progressive muscle weakness affecting proximal/limb girdle muscles. Difficulty or inability to rise from sitting or supine position without using arms. Difficulty in raising arms above head and difficulty in climbing stairs.

Occasional involvement of facial/bulbar, pharyngeal, and esophageal muscles. Deep tendon reflexes within normal limits.

DIFFERENTIAL DIAGNOSIS

Lupus erythematosus, mixed connective tissue disease, steroid myopathy, trichinosis, toxoplasmosis.

LABORATORY EXAMINATIONS

Chemistry During acute active phase: elevation of creatine phosphokinase (65%) most specific for muscle disease; also, aldolase (40%), glutamic oxaloacetic transaminase, lactate dehydrogenase.

Autoantibodies ANA in <60%, antibodies to Jo-1 in 30%.

Urine Elevated 24-h creatine excretion (>200 mg/24 h).

Electromyography Increased irritability on insertion of electrodes, spontaneous fibrillations, pseudomyotonic discharges, positive sharp waves: excludes neuromyopathy. With evidence of denervation, suspect coexisting tumor.

MRI MRI of muscles reveals focal lesions.

ECG Evidence of myocarditis; atrial, ventricular irritability; atrioventricular block.

X-Ray of Chest ±Interstitial fibrosis.

X-Ray of Esophagus Reduced peristalsis.

Pathology *Skin* Flattening of epidermis, hydropic degeneration of basal cell layer, edema of upper dermis, scattered inflammatory infiltrate, PAS-positive fibrinoid deposits at dermal-epidermal junction and around upper dermal capillaries, accumulation of acid mucopolysaccharides in dermis.

Muscle Biopsy shoulder/pelvic girdle; one that is weak or tender, i.e., deltoid, supraspinatus, gluteus, quadriceps. Histology—segmental necrosis within muscle fibers with loss of cross-striations; waxy/coagulative type of eosinophilic staining; with or without regenerating fibers; inflammatory cells, histiocytes, macrophages, lymphocytes, plasma cells. Histology of adult DM, polymyositis, and myositis in patients with other connective tissue diseases is indistinguishable. Vasculitis is seen in juvenile DM. MRI-guided needle biopsy of muscle may replace conventional muscle biopsy in the future.

DIAGNOSIS

Proximal muscle weakness with two of three laboratory criteria, i.e., elevated serum "muscle enzyme" levels, characteristic electromyographic changes, diagnostic muscle biopsy.

COURSE AND PROGNOSIS

Patients 50 years of age with dermatomyositis have a higher risk of developing cancer than do patients with polymyositis. With treatment prognosis is relatively good except in patients with malignancy and those with pulmonary involvement. With aggressive immunosuppressive treatment the 8-year survival rate is 70 to 80%. Current recommendation is that patients >50 years of age be investigated for associated malignancy: carcinoma of the breast, ovary, bronchopulmonary, GI tract. Most cancers occur within 2 years of diagnosis. Successful treatment of the neoplasm often followed by improvement/resolution of DM.

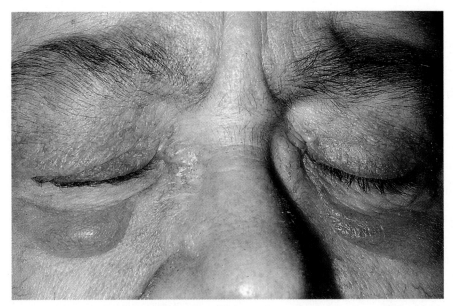

Figure 12-11 Dermatomyositis *Heliotrope (reddish purple) erythema of upper eyelids and edema of the lower lids. This 55-year-old female had experienced severe muscle weakness of the shoulder girdle and presented with a lump in the breast that proved to be carcinoma.*

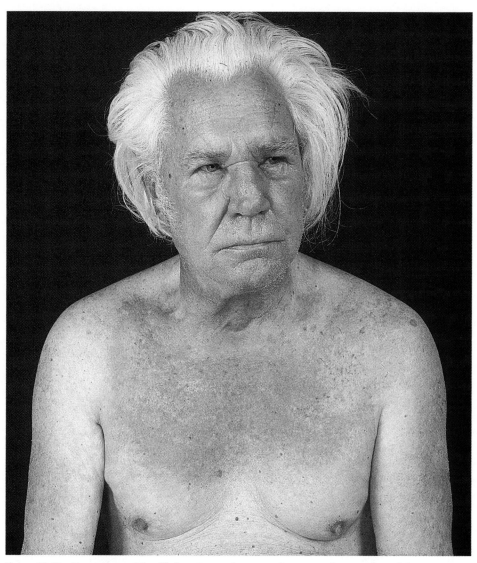

Figure 12-12 Dermatomyositis *Violaceous erythema on the upper chest, neck, and face; periorbital heliotrope (violet color) with edema. The patient could barely lift his arms and couldn't climb stairs.*

MANAGEMENT

Prednisone .5 to 1 mg/kg of body weight per day, increasing to 1.5 mg/kg if lower dose ineffective. Taper when "muscle enzyme" levels approach normal. Best if combined with azathioprine, 2 to 3 mg/kg/d.

Note: Steroid myopathy may occur after 4 to 6 weeks of therapy.

Alternatives Methotrexate, cyclophosphamide are alternatives, and high-dose IV immunoglobulin bolus therapy at monthly intervals spares glucocorticoid doses to achieve or maintain remissions.

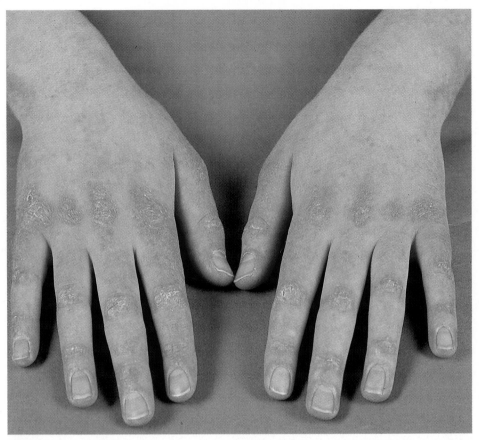

Figure 12-13 Dermatomyositis *Violaceous erythema and Gottron's papules on the dorsum of the hands and fingers, especially over the metacarpophalangeal and interphalangeal joints; the light-protected areas of the forearms are not involved. Periungual erythema and telangiectasis.*

GRAFT-VERSUS-HOST DISEASE

Graft-versus-host disease (GVHD) is an immune disorder caused by the reaction of histoincompatible, immunocompetent donor cells against the tissues of an immunoincompetent host (graft-versus-host reaction, GVHR), characterized by acute cutaneous changes ranging from maculopapular eruption to toxic epidermal necrolysis, diarrhea, and liver dysfunction, as well as chronic changes comprising lichenoid eruptions and sclerodermatous changes.

EPIDEMIOLOGY

Incidence Allogeneic bone marrow transplantation (BMT): 60 to 80% of successful engraftments. Autologous BMT: mild cutaneous GVHD occurs in 8%. Low incidence after blood transfusion in immunosuppressed patients, maternal-fetal transfer in immunodeficiency disease.

Acute GVHD

PATHOGENESIS

GVHR associated with inflammatory reaction mounted by the donor cells against specific host organs—skin, liver, or GI tract. Severity of GVHD related to histocompatibility match between donor and recipient and preparatory regimen used. With successful engraftment, there is replacement of host marrow by immunocompetent donor cells capable of reacting against the "foreign" tissue antigens of the host.

HISTORY

During the first 3 months after BMT (usually between 14 and 21 days): mild pruritus, localized/generalized; pain on pressure, palms/soles. Nausea/vomiting, abdominal pain; watery diarrhea. Jaundice; dark yellow urine.

PHYSICAL EXAMINATION

Skin Lesions Initially, subtle, discrete macules and/or papules on upper trunk, hands/feet, especially palms/soles. Painful. (Figure 12-14); mild edema with violaceous hue, periungual and on pinna. If controlled/resolved, erythema diminishes with subsequent desquamation and postinflammatory hyperpigmentation. If progresses, macules/papules become generalized, confluent, and evolve into erythroderma. Subepidermal bullae, especially over pressure/trauma sites, palms/soles. Positive Nikolski sign. If bullae widespread with rupture/erosion, toxic epidermal necrolysis-like (TEN-like) form of acute cutaneous GVHR (Fig.12-15) (For staging, see Table 12-2).

Mucosa Lichen planus-like lesions in buccal mucosa; erosive stomatitis, oral and ocular sicca-like syndrome; esophagitis/esophageal strictures. Keratoconjunctivitis.

General Findings Fever, jaundice, nausea, vomiting, right upper quadrant pain/tenderness, cramping abdominal pain, diarrhea, serositis, pulmonary insufficiency, dark urine.

DIFFERENTIAL DIAGNOSIS

Exanthematous drug reaction, viral exanthem, TEN, erythroderma.

Table 12-2 CLINICAL STAGING OF ACUTE GVHD (SKIN)

1. Erythematous maculopapular eruption involving <25% of body surface
2. Erythematous maculopapular eruption involving 25 to 50% of body surface
3. 50% of body surface, erythroderma
4. Bulla formation

LABORATORY EXAMINATIONS

Chemistry Elevated SGOT, bilirubin, alkaline phosphatase.

Dermatopathology Basal vacuolization several days before clinically detectable lesions—focal vacuolization of basal cell layer, apoptosis of individual keratinocytes; mild perivenular mononuclear cell infiltrate—increasing vacuolization/cellular necrosis; apposition of lymphocytes to necrotic keratinocytes (satellitosis); vacuoles coalesce to form subepidermal clefts—subepidermal blister formation—endothelial cell swelling. Immunocytochemistry: HLA-DR expression of keratinocytes precedes morphologic changes and thus represents important, early diagnostic sign. (For staging, see Table 12-2.)

DIAGNOSIS

Clinical findings confirmed by skin biopsy.

COURSE AND PROGNOSIS

Mild to moderate GVHD responds well to treatment. Prognosis of TEN-like GVHR grave.

Severe GVHD susceptible to infections—bacterial, fungal, viral (CMV, HSV, VZV). Acute GVHD is primary or associated cause of death in 15 to 70% of BMT recipients.

MANAGEMENT

Topical Glucocorticoids Potent glucocorticoid ointment gives symptomatic relief and adequate control in cases of mild to moderate cutaneous GVHD.

Prednisone 80 to 100 mg/d for mild to moderate cutaneous GVHD.

Cyclosporine Added to prednisone for severe cutaneous disease, ±GI or liver GVHD. Once cutaneous as well as GI and liver manifestations of GVHD have been controlled, cyclosporine and prednisone can be tapered and eventually discontinued.

PUVA Effective for subacute and chronic GVHD (see below). Extracorporeal photopheresis is being evaluated.

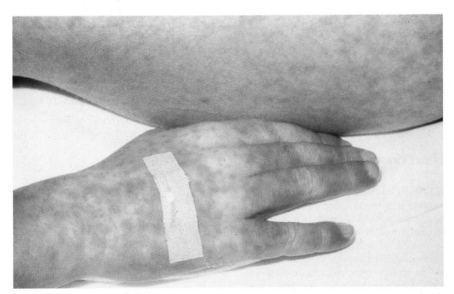

Figure 12-14 Acute graft-versus-host disease *Discrete and confluent, erythematous, blanchable macules and papules involving the hands and the trunk. Note the relative sparing over the wrist and metacarpophalangeal and proximal interphalangeal joints. These relatively mild cutaneous lesions were not associated with intestinal or hepatic involvement.*

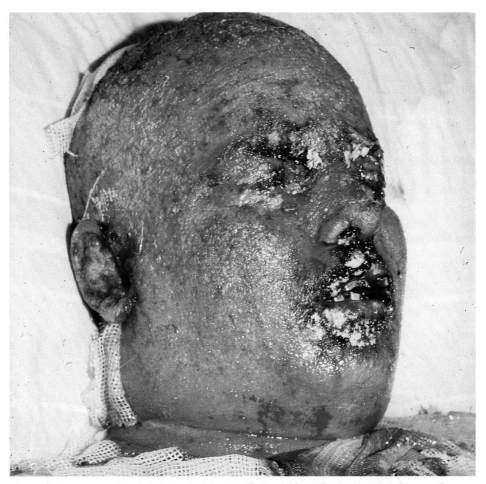

Figure 12-15 Acute graft-versus-host disease *Confluent epidermal necrosis, sloughing, and bleeding resembling toxic epidermal necrolysis, on the face and entire trunk after allogeneic BMT. This is clearly a very severe condition.*

Chronic GVHD

HISTORY

>100 days after BMT. Either evolving from acute GVHD or arising de novo. Acute GVHD is not always followed by chronic GVHD. Clinical classification thus distinguishes between quiescent onset, progressive onset, and de novo chronic cutaneous GVHD. Chronic GVHD occurs in 25% of recipients of marrow from an HLA-identical sibling who survive >100 days.

PHYSICAL EXAMINATION

Skin Lesions Flat-topped (lichen planus-like) papules of violaceous color, initially on distal extremities but later generalized (Fig. 12-16). Confluent areas of dermal sclerosis (Fig. 12-17) with overlying scale resembling scleroderma mainly on trunk, buttocks, hips, and thighs. With more severe disease, severe generalized sclerodermoid changes with necrosis and ulceration on acral and pressure sites. Hair loss; anhidrosis, vitiligo-like hypopigmentation.

General Findings Chronic liver disease, general wasting.

DIFFERENTIAL DIAGNOSIS

Lichen planus, lichenoid drug reaction, scleroderma, poikiloderma.

LABORATORY EXAMINATIONS

Chemistry Elevated transaminases, gamma-GT

Dermatopathology Hyperkeratosis, mild hypergranulosis, mild irregular acanthosis or atrophy, moderate basal vacuolization; rare individual cell necrosis, mild perivascular mononuclear cell infiltrate, melanin incontinence; loss of hair follicles, entrapment of sweat glands; dense dermal sclerosis.

COURSE AND PROGNOSIS

Sclerodermoid GVHD with tight skin/joint contracture may result in impaired mobility, ulcerations. Permanent hair loss; xerostomia, xerophthalmia, corneal ulcers, blindness. Malabsorption. Mild chronic cutaneous GVHD may resolve spontaneously. Chronic GVHD may be associated with recurrent and occasionally fatal bacterial infections.

MANAGEMENT

Topical corticosteroids and PUVA are very effective. Systemic immunosuppression with prednisone, cyclosporine and azathioprine, in various combinations. Thalidomide. Extracorporeal photopheresis is being evaluated.

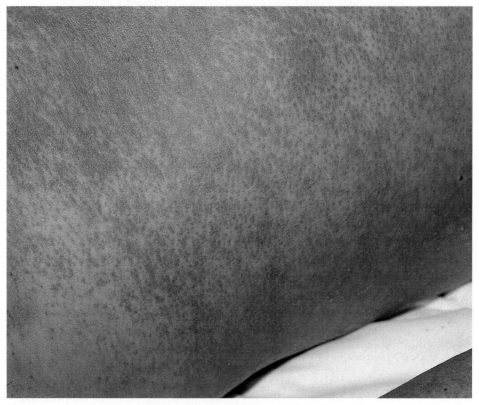

Figure 12-16 Chronic graft-versus-host disease *Violaceous lichen planus-like, perifollicular papules becoming confluent on the trunk, occurring 3 months after allogeneic BMT.*

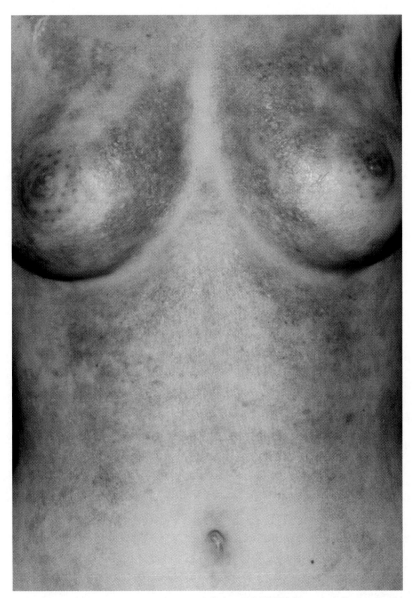

Figure 12-17   Chronic graft-versus-host disease   *A lichenoid GVHR has partially resolved leading to pronounced macular gray-brown follicular hyperpigmentation, confluent on the breasts, upper chest, and anterior abdomen. Sclerosis of the tissue now supervenes, the skin feels bound down on palpation, similar to progressive systemic sclerosis (scleroderma).*

LIVEDO RETICULARIS

Livedo reticularis (LR) is a mottled bluish (livid) discoloration of the skin that occurs in a netlike pattern. It is not a diagnosis in itself but a reaction pattern.

CLASSIFICATION

Idiopathic livedo reticularis (ILR) is a purple/livid discoloration of the skin that occurs in a netlike pattern (diameter of mesh <3 cm). It involves large areas of the lower, sometimes upper extremities and the trunk and disappears after warming. It is a physiologic phenomenon (*synonym:* cutis marmorata).

Secondary (symptomatic) Livedo Reticularis (SLR) is a purple discoloration that occurs in a starburst or lightning-like pattern, netlike but with open (not annular) meshes and is mostly, but not always confined to the lower extremities and buttocks. It is not a diagnosis in itself but a reaction pattern and often indicative of serious systemic disease Table 12-3. Because it differs clinically from ILR and also has a different significance, European dermatologists prefer the term *livedo racemosa.*

Sneddon's Syndrome refers to extensive SLR with hypertension, cerebrovascular accidents, and transient ischemic attacks.

Symptomatic Livedo Reticularis (Livedo Racemosa)

ETIOLOGY

That of associated disorder.

PATHOGENESIS

LR pattern due to vasospasm or obstruction of perpendicular arterioles, perforating dermis from below. Cyanotic periphery of each web of net caused by deoxygenated blood in surrounding horizontally arranged venous plexuses. When factors such as cold cause increased viscosity/low flow rates in superficial venous plexus, further deoxygenation occurs and cyanotic reticular pattern becomes more pronounced. Elevation of limb decreases intensity of color due to increased venous drainage. LR may result from arteriolar disease causing obstruction to inflow and blood hyperviscosity or from obstruction to outflow of blood in venules.

HISTORY

Appearance or worsening with cold exposure. ±Numbness, tingling associated. Worse during winter months.

PHYSICAL EXAMINATION

Skin Lesions Blotchy, arborizing, lightning-like, starburst or mottled pattern of cyanosis. (Figure 12-18), Netlike webs are open (semicircular) and within webs of skin is normal to pallid and feels cool. Symmetric, arms/legs, buttocks; less commonly, body. On exposure to cold, livedo becomes more pronounced but never fades completely on warming. It never ulcerates. *Note:* When associated with *livedoid vasculitis,* ulceration about ankles and forefeet may occur.

General Examination Symptoms of underlying disease (Table 12-3).

DIFFERENTIAL DIAGNOSIS

Idiopathic livedo reticularis Cutis marmorata (transient physiologic mottling of skin that resolves on warming), livedoid vasculitis (segmental hyalinizing vasculitis causing atrophie blanche), erythema ab igne.

LABORATORY EXAMINATIONS

Laboratory Varies with associated disorders.

Dermatopathology Vascular pathology of underlying disease. SLR with livedoid vasculi-

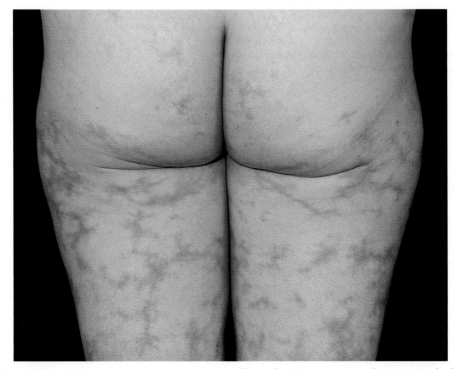

Figure 12-18 Symptomatic livedo reticularis *A netlike, arborizing pattern on the posterior thighs and buttocks defined by violaceous, erythematous streaks resembling lightning. The skin within the erythematous areas is normally pale. This occurred in a patient with labile hypertension and multiple cerebrovascular attacks and was thus pathognomonic for Sneddon's Syndrome.*

Table 12-3 DISORDERS ASSOCIATED WITH SYMPTOMATIC LIVEDO RETICULARIS

Vascular Obstruction	Viscosity Changes	Drugs
Atheroemboli	Thrombocythemia	Amantadine
Arteriosclerosis	Polyglobulinemia	Quinine
Polyarteritis nodosa	Cryoglobulinemia	Quinidine
Cutaneous polyarteritis nodosa	Cold agglutinemia	
Rheumatoid vasculitis	DIC	
Livedoid vasculitis	Lupus erythematosus	
Sneddon's syndrome	Anticardiolipin syndrome	
	Leukemia/lymphoma	

tis: arteriolar intimal proliferation with dilated numerous capillaries, thickening of walls of venules, hyalinization of walls of small arterial vessels, lymphocytic perivascular infiltration. In Sneddon's syndrome: vascular changes as in endarteritis obliterans.

DIAGNOSIS

Clinical diagnosis confirmed by laboratory data supporting diagnosis of associated disorder.

COURSE AND PROGNOSIS

Course/prognosis of SLR depends on that of associated disorder.

MANAGEMENT

Keep from chilling. Pentoxifylline, 400 mg PO tid. and low-dose aspirin may be helpful.
  Treat associated disorder.

Sneddon's Syndrome

A potentially life-threatening disease of unknown etiology occurring more often in females than males and manifesting mainly in skin and the central nervous system.

EPIDEMIOLOGY

Rare but underdiagnosed.

HISTORY

Skin lesions precede neurologic symptoms often by years.

PHYSICAL EXAMINATION

Skin lesions represent classical SLR (livedo racemosa on lower extremities, buttocks, sometimes arms. (Fig. 12-18)
  Neurologic symptoms include headaches, labile hypertension, transient ischemic attacks, transient amnesia, transient aphasia, palsy, and cerebrovascular insult.

LABORATORY EXAMINATIONS

Dermatopathology Endotheliitis → proliferation of subumbilical myofibroblasts → vascular occlusion and fibrosis. Cytotoxic antiendothelial cell antibodies in a small percentage of patients. There may be antiphospholipid antibodies.

MANAGEMENT

Longtime low-dose heparin, aspirin.
  Note: Sneddon's syndrome is not identical with antiphospholipid syndrome although dermatologic manifestations (SLR) may be indistinguishable. Also, it may be associated (in a very small percentage of patients) with livedoid vasculitis—in this case, ulceration may occur around ankles or acrally.

LUPUS ERYTHEMATOSUS

Lupus erythematosus (LE) is the designation of a spectrum of diseases that are linked by distinct clinical findings and distinct patterns of polyclonal B cell immunity. It ranges from life-threatening manifestations of systemic lupus erythematosus (SLE) to the limited and exclusive skin involvement in chronic cutaneous lupus erythematosus (CCLE). More than 85% of patients with LE have skin lesions, which can be classified into LE-specific and -nonspecific. An abbreviated version of Gilliam's classification of LE-specific lesions is given in Table 12-4.

Systemic Lupus Erythematosus

This serious multisystem autoimmune disease is based on polyclonal B cell immunity which involves connective tissue and blood vessels. The clinical manifestations include fever (90%); skin lesions (85%); arthritis; CNS, renal, cardiac, and pulmonary disease. Systemic lupus erythematosus (SLE) may uncommonly develop in patients with chronic cutaneous lupus erythematosus (CCLE); however, lesions of CCLE are common in SLE.

EPIDEMIOLOGY

Age of Onset   30 (females), 40 (males).

Sex   Male:Female ratio 1:8.

Race   More common in blacks.

Other Features   Family history (<5%); an SLE syndrome can be induced by drugs (hydralazine, certain anticonvulsants, and procainamide), but rash is a relatively uncommon feature of drug-induced SLE.

PATHOGENESIS

The tissue injury in the epidermis results from the deposition of immune complexes at the dermal-epidermal junction. Immune complexes selectively generate the assembly of the membrane-attack complex, which mediates membrane injury. CD3+ lymphocytes of the cytotoxic suppressor type.

HISTORY

Lesions present for weeks (acute), months (chronic). Sunlight may cause an exacerbation of SLE (36%). Pruritus, burning of skin lesions. Fatigue (100%), fever (100%), weight loss, and malaise. Arthralgia or arthritis, abdominal pain.

PHYSICAL EXAMINATION

Skin Lesions   Comprise acute cutaneous LE (ACLE) lesions (Table 12-4) in the acute phases of the disease and subacute (SCLE) and chronic cutaneous LE (CCLE) lesions. Whereas ACLE lesions occur only in acute or subacute SLE, SCLE and CCLE lesions are present in subacute and chronic SLE but may also occur in acute SLE. ACLE lesions are typically precipitated by sunlight.

ACLE Lesions

Butterfly Rash   Erythematous, confluent, macular butterfly eruption on the face (Fig. 12-19) sharply defined with fine scaling; erosions (acute flares) and crusts.

Generalized ACLE   Erythematous, discrete, papular or urticarial lesions on the face, on the dorsa of hands, arms, and V of the neck.

Others   Bullae, often hemorrhagic (acute flares).

Papules and scaly *plaques* as in SCLE (Fig. 12-20) and discoid plaques as in CCLE (Fig. 12-21), predominantly in the face and on the arms.

Erythematous, sometimes violaceous, slightly scaling, densely set and confluent *papules* on the dorsa of the finger (usually with sparing of the articular regions (Fig. 12-22)—note difference to dermatomyositis). *Palmar erythema*, mostly on fingertips, *nailfold telangiectasias*.

"Palpable" purpura (vasculitis), lower extremities. (see Fig. 12-31)

Urticarial lesions with purpura (urticarial vasculitis). (see Fig. 12-39)

Scalp   Discoid lesions associated with patchy alopecia. Diffuse alopecia.

Mucous Membranes   Ulcers arising in purpuric necrotic lesions on palate (80%), buccal mucosa, or gums.

Sites of Predilection   Localized or generalized, preferentially in light-exposed sites. Face (80%); scalp (discoid lesions); presternal, shoulders; dorsa of the forearms, hands, fingers, fingertips.

Extracutaneous Multisystem Involvement   Arthralgia or arthritis (80%), renal disease (50%), pericarditis (20%), pneumonitis (20%), gastrointestinal (due to arteritis and sterile peritonitis), hepatomegaly (30%), myopathy (30%), splenomegaly (20%), lymphadenopathy (50%), peripheral neuropathy (14%), CNS disease (10%), seizures or organic brain disease (14%).

LABORATORY EXAMINATIONS

Pathology *Skin*   Atrophy of epidermis, liquefaction degeneration of the dermal-epidermal junction, edema of the dermis, dermal lymphocytic infiltrate, and fibrinoid degeneration of the connective tissue and walls of the blood vessels.

Immunofluorescence of Skin   The lupus band test (direct immunofluorescence demonstrating IgG, IgM, C3) shows granular or globular deposits of immune reactants in a bandlike pattern along the dermal-epidermal junction. This is positive in lesional skin in 90% and in the clinically normal skin (sun-exposed, 70 to 80%; non-sun-exposed, 50%); in the latter case, indicative of renal disease and hypocomplementemia.

Table 12-4   ABBREVIATED GILLIAM CLASSIFICATION OF SKIN LESIONS ASSOCIATED WITH LE

I. LE-specific skin disease (cutaneous LE[a] [CLE])
   A. Acute cutaneous LE [ACLE]
      1. Localized ACLE (malar rash; butterfly rash)
      2. Generalized ACLE (macolupapular lupus rash, malar rash, photosensitive lupus dermatitis)
   B. Subacute cutaneous LE [SCLE]
      1. Annular SCLE
      2. Papulosquamous SCLE (disseminated DLE, subacute disseminated LE, maculopapular photosensitive LE)
   C. Chronic cutaneous LE (CCLE)
      1. Classic discoid LE [DLE]
         a. Localized DLE
         b. Generalized DLE
      2. Hypertrophic/verrucous DLE
      3. Lupus profundus
      4. Mucosal DLE
         a. Oral DLE
         b. Conjunctival DLE
      5. Lupus tumidus (urticarial plaque of LE)
      6. Chilblains LE (chilblains lupus)
      7. Lichenoid DLE (LE/lichen planus overlap)
II. LE-nonspecific skin disease
   These range from necrotizing and urticarial vasculitis to livedo reticularis, Raynaud's phenomenon, dermal mucinosis, and bullous lesions in LE

[a] Alternative or synonymous terms are listed in parentheses; abbreviations are indicated in brackets.
SOURCE: Reprinted and modified from RD Sontheimer with permission from Stockton Journals, Macmillan Press, Ltd.

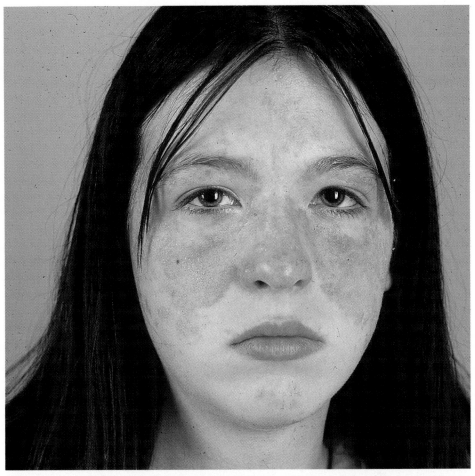

Figure 12-19 Acute systemic lupus erythematosus *Bright red, sharply defined erythema with slight edema and minimal scaling in a "butterfly pattern" on the face. This is the typical "malar rash." Note also that the patient is female and young.*

Other Organs The fundamental lesion is fibrinoid degeneration of connective tissue and walls of the blood vessels associated with an inflammatory infiltrate of lymphocytes and plasma cells.

Serology ANA positive (>95%); peripheral pattern of nuclear fluorescence. Anti-double-stranded DNA antibodies, anti-Sm antibodies and rRNP antibodies are specific for SLE; low levels of complement (especially with renal involvement). Anticardiolipin autoantibodies (lupus anticoagulant) are present in a specific subset (anticardiolipin syndrome); SS-A(Ro) autoantibodies have a low specificity for SLE but are specific in the subset of subacute cutaneous lupus erythematosus (SCLE) (see below).

Hematology Anemia [normocytic, normochromic, or rarely, hemolytic Coombs-positive, leukopenia (>4000/μL)], lymphopenia, thrombocytopenia, elevated ESR (a good guide to activity of the disease).

Urinalysis Persistent proteinuria, casts.

DIAGNOSIS

Made on the basis of clinical findings, histopathology, lupus band test, and serology within the framework of the revised American Rheumatism Association (ARA) criteria for classification of SLE (Table 12-5).

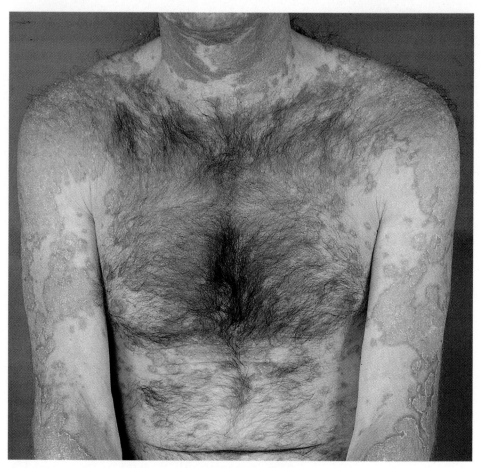

Figure 12-20 Subacute cutaneous lupus erythematosus *Widely scattered, erythematous-to-violaceous, scaling, well-demarcated plaques on the trunk, neck, and arms, mimicking the clinical appearance of psoriasis vulgaris.*

SKIN SIGNS OF IMMUNE, AUTOIMMUNE, AND RHEUMATIC DISEASES

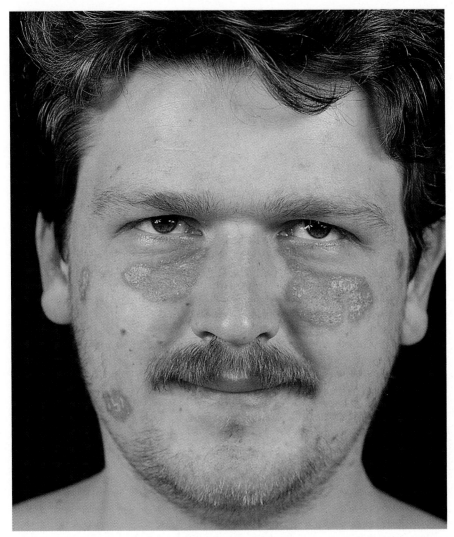

Figure 12-21 Chronic cutaneous lupus erythematosus *Well-demarcated, erythematous, hyperkeratotic plaques with atrophy, follicular plugging, and adherent scale on both cheeks. This is the classic presentation of chronic discoid LE.*

Table 12-5 1982 REVISED ARA CRITERIA FOR CLASSIFICATION OF SYSTEMIC LUPUS ERYTHEMATOSUS[a]

Criterion	Definition
1. Malar rash	Fixed erythema, flat or raised, over the malar eminences, tending to spare the nasolabial folds.
2. Discoid rash	Erythematous raised patches with adherent keratotic scaling and follicular plugging; atrophic scarring may occur in older lesions.
3. Photosensitivity	Skin rashes as a result of unusual reaction to sunlight, by patient history or physician observation.
4. Oral ulcers	Oral or nasopharyngeal ulceration, usually painless, observed by a physician.
5. Arthritis	Nonerosive arthritis involving two or more peripheral joints, characterized by tenderness, swelling, or effusion.
6. Serositis	a. Pleuritis—convincing history of pleuritic pain or rub heard by a physician or evidence of pleural effusion *or* b. Pericarditis—documented by ECG or rub or evidence of pericardial effusion.
7. Renal disorder	a. Persistent proteinuria—.5g/d or >3+ if quantitation not performed *or* b. Cellular casts—may be red cell, hemoglobin, granular, tubular, or mixed.
8. Neurologic disorder	a. Seizures—in the absence of offending drugs or known metabolic derangements, e.g., uremia, ketoacidosis, or electrolyte im-balance *or* b. Psychosis—in the absence of offending drugs or known metabolic derangements, e.g., uremia, ketoacidosis, or electro- lyte imbalance.
9. Hematologic disorder	a. Hemolytic anemia—with reticulocytosis *or* b. Leukopenia—<4000/μL total on two or more occasions *or* c. Lymphopenia—<1500/μL on two or more occasions *or* d. Thrombocytopenia—<100,000/μL in the absence of offending drugs.
10. Immunologic disorder	a. Anti-DNA—antibody to native DNA in abnormal titer *or* b. Anti-Sm—presence of antibody to Sm nuclear antigen *or* c. Positive finding of antiphospholipid antibodies based on (1) an abnormal serum level of IgG or IgM anticardiolipin antibodies, (2) a positive test result for lupus anticoagulant using a standard method, or (3) a false-positive serologic test for syphilis known to be positive for at least 6 months and confirmed by negative *Treponema pallidum* immobilization or fluorescent treponemal antibody absorption test.
11. Antinuclear antibody	An abnormal titer of antinuclear antibody by immunofluorescence of an equivalent assay at any point in time and in the absence of drugs known to be associated with "drug-induced lupus" syndrome.

[a] The proposed classification is based on 11 criteria. For the purpose of identifying patients in clinical studies, a person shall be said to have SLE if any 4 or more of the 11 criteria are present, serially or simultaneously, during any interval of observation.

SOURCE: Reprinted from Tan EM et al., *Arthritis Rheumatism*, 25:1271–1277, 1982. Used by permission of the American College of Rheumatology.

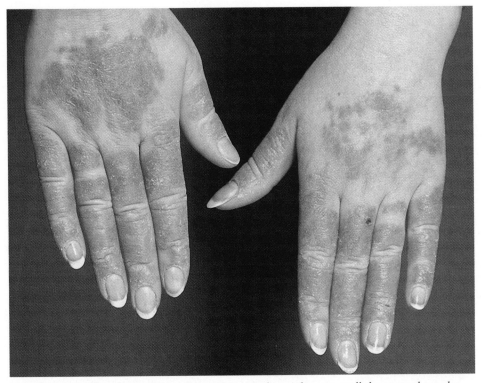

Figure 12-22 Acute systemic lupus erythematosus *Red-to-violaceous, well-demarcated papules and plaques on the dorsa of the fingers and hands, characteristically sparing the skin overlying the joints. This is an important differential diagnostic sign when considering dermatomyositis, which characteristically involves these sites.*

PROGNOSIS

Five-year survival is 93%.

MANAGEMENT

General Measures Rest, avoidance of sun exposure.

Indications for Prednisone (60 mg/d in divided doses): (1) CNS involvement, (2) renal involvement, (3) severely ill patients without CNS involvement, (4) hemolytic crisis.

Concomitant Immunosuppressive Drugs Azathioprine or cyclophosphamide, depending on organ involvement and activity of disease. In renal disease cyclophosphamide IV bolus therapy.

Antimalarials Hydroxychloroquine is useful for treatment of the skin lesions in subacute and chronic SLE, but does not reduce the need for prednisone. Observe precautions in the use of hydroxychloroquine.

Cutaneous Lupus Erythematosus

Subacute Cutaneous Lupus Erythematosus (SCLE)

Skin lesions of subacute cutaneous lupus erythematosus (SCLE) are annular or psoriasiform. (Fig. 12-20) There is no follicular plugging, no scarring, and little atrophy, all of which are frequently noted in CCLE. Patients with SCLE may have a few of the criteria of SLE as defined by the American Rheumatism Association, including photosensitivity, arthralgias, serositis, renal disease, and serologic abnormalities; (Table 12-5); practically all have anti-Ro (SS-A) and most have anti-La (SS-B) antibodies. The serious criteria of SLE are uncommon: severe vasculitis, severe CNS disease, or progressive renal disease. Nonetheless, most patients have a mild form of SLE so that SCLE is not a purely cutaneous disease. The clinical skin lesions are the distinctive feature of SCLE.

EPIDEMIOLOGY

Age of Onset   Young and middle-aged.

Race   Uncommon in blacks or Hispanics.

Sex   Females > males.

Incidence   About 10% of the LE population.

Precipitating Factors   Sunlight exposure.

HISTORY

Rather sudden onset with annular or psoriasiform plaques erupting on the upper trunk, arms, dorsa of the hands, usually after exposure to sunlight; mild fatigue, malaise; some arthralgia, fever of unknown origin.

PHYSICAL EXAMINATION

Skin Lesions   *Two Types*   *Psoriasiform* Papulosquamous, sharply defined, with slight delicate scaling (Fig. 12-20), evolving into bright red confluent plaques that are oval, arciform, or polycyclic, just as in psoriasis.
  Annular   Bright red annular lesions with central regression and little scaling. In both there may be telangiectasia, but there is no follicular plugging and less induration than in CCLE. Lesions resolve with slight atrophy (no scarring) and hypopigmentation.

Other Lesions   Periungual telangiectasia, diffuse nonscarring alopecia.

Distribution   Scattered, disseminated in light-exposed areas: shoulders, extensor surface of the arms, dorsal surface of the hands, upper back, V-neck area of the upper chest.

DIFFERENTIAL DIAGNOSIS

Scaly Red Plaques   Dermatomyositis, secondary syphilis, psoriasis, seborrheic dermatitis, tinea corporis.

LABORATORY EXAMINATIONS

Dermatopathology   Liquefaction degeneration of the basal layer and edema of the upper dermis that can sometimes lead to cleft formation. Colloid bodies in the epidermis and at the junction. 60% have immune deposits in dermal-epidermal junction.

UV Testing   Most patients have a lower than normal UVB MED. Typical SCLE lesions may develop in UVB test sites.

Serology   ANA present in 60 to 80%. Antibodies to Ro(SS-A) antigen in more than 80%, to La(SS-B) in 30 to 50%; high levels of circulating immune complexes.

Other Laboratory Tests   Patients with SCLE, particularly those with manifest systemic involvement, may have a number of laboratory abnormalities, including anemia, leukopenia, lymphopenia, hematuria, proteinuria, and depressed complement levels.

DIAGNOSIS

Clinical findings confirmed by histology and immunopathology. The extensive involvement is far more than is ever seen in CCLE, and the distinctive eruption is a marker for SCLE.

COURSE AND PROGNOSIS

A better prognosis than for SLE in general. Some patients may have renal (and CNS) involvement and thus have a guarded prognosis. The skin lesions can disappear completely, but occasionally, a vitiligo-like leukoderma remains for some months. Women with Ro(SS-A)–positive SCLE may give birth to babies with neonatal lupus and congenital heart block.

MANAGEMENT

Topical Anti-inflammatory glucocorticoids are only partially helpful.

Systemic Systemic treatment is usually required. Thalidomide (100 to 300 mg/d) is very effective for skin lesions but not for systemic involvement. Hydroxychloroquine, 400 mg/d; if this does not control the skin lesions, quinacrine hydrochloride, 100 mg/d, can be added. The bizarre yellow skin color caused by quinacrine can be somewhat modified by β-carotene, 60 mg tid.

Chronic Cutaneous Lupus Erythematosus (CCLE)

This chronic, indolent skin disease is characterized by sharply marginated, scaly, infiltrated, and later atrophic red ("discoid") plaques, usually occurring on habitually exposed areas. (Fig. 12-21) This disorder, in most cases, is purely cutaneous without systemic involvement. However, CCLE lesions may occur in SLE. CCLE may manifest as chronic discoid LE (CDLE) or LE panniculitis.

Classic Chronic Discoid LE (CDLE)

EPIDEMIOLOGY

Age of Onset 20 to 45 years.

Sex Females > males.

Race Possibly more severe in blacks.

HISTORY

Can be precipitated by sunlight but to a lesser extent than ACLE or SCLE. Lesions last for months to years. Usually no symptoms, sometimes slightly pruritic or smarting. No general symptoms.

PHYSICAL EXAMINATION

Skin Lesions Bright red papules evolving into plaques, sharply marginated, with adherent scaling (Fig. 12-21). Scales are difficult to remove and show spines on the undersurface (magnifying lens) resembling carpet tacks. Plaques are round or oval, annular or polycyclic, with irregular borders and expand in the periphery and regress in the center, resulting in depression of lesions, atrophy, and eventually scarring. (Fig. 12-23) Follicular plugging (closely set and often in clusters) and dilated follicles may persist in atrophic and scarred lesions but eventually disappear so that smooth, whitish scarred lesions result that are partially surrounded by a still active inflammatory and raised border. (Fig. 12-23) While active lesions are bright red, "burned out" lesions may be pink or white (hypomelanosis) macules and scars, but scarred lesions may also show hyperpigmentation, especially in persons with brown or black skin. (Fig. 12-23)

Distribution and Sites of Predilection CDLE may be localized or generalized, occurring predominantly on the face and scalp; otherwise: dorsa of forearms, hands, fingers, toes, and less frequently, the trunk.

Scalp Scarring alopecia with residual inflammation and follicular plugging. (Fig. 12-23)

Mucous Membranes Less than 5% of patients have lip involvement (hyperkeratosis, hypermelanotic scarring, erythema) and atrophic erythematous or whitish areas with or without ulceration on the buccal mucosa, tongue, and palate.

DIFFERENTIAL DIAGNOSIS

The discoid lesions of CDLE may closely mimic *actinic keratosis. Plaque psoriasis* and scaling discoid LE without atrophy and scarring may be difficult to distinguish, especially on the dorsa of the hands; histopathology permits distinction. *Polymorphous light eruption* LE (PMLE) may pose a problem. PMLE disappears in the winter in northern latitudes, does not develop atrophy or follicular plugging, and does not occur in unexposed areas—mouth, hairy scalp. *Lichen planus* can be confusing, but the biopsy is distinctive. *Lupus vulgaris* and *tinea facialis.*

LABORATORY EXAMINATIONS

Dermatopathology Hyperkeratosis, atrophy of the epidermis, follicular plugging, liquefaction degeneration of the basal cell layer. In the dermis there is edema, dilatation of small blood vessels, and perifollicular and periappendageal lymphocytic inflammatory infiltrate. Strong PAS reaction of the subepidermal, thickened basement zone.

Immunofluorescence Positive in active lesions at least 6 weeks old. Granular deposits of IgG, >IgM at the dermal-epidermal junction. This is known as the *lupus band test* (LBT) and is positive in 90% of active lesions not recently treated with topical glucocorticoids but negative in burned-out (scarred) lesions and in the normal skin, both sun-exposed and nonexposed. SLE, in contrast, has a positive LBT in lesional as well as in normal sun-exposed (70 to 80%) and nonexposed (50%) skin.

Serology Low incidence of ANA in a titer >1:16.

Hematology Occasionally leukopenia (<4500/μL).

DIAGNOSIS

Clinical findings confirmed by histology.

COURSE AND PROGNOSIS

Only 1 to 5% may develop SLE; with localized lesions, complete remission occurs in 50%; with generalized lesions, remissions are less frequent (<10%). *Note again:* CCLE lesions may be the presenting cutaneous sign of SLE.

MANAGEMENT

Prevention Topical sunscreens (SPF 30) routinely.

Local Glucocorticoids Topical fluorinated glucocorticoids (with caution). Intralesional triamcinolone acetonide, 3 to 5 mg/ml, for small lesions.

Antimalarial Hydroxychloroquine, ≤6.5 mg/kg of body weight per day. If hydroxychloroquine is ineffective, add quinacrine, 100 mg tid. Monitor for side effects.

Retinoid Hyperkeratotic CDLE lesions respond well to systemic etretinate (1 mg/kg of body weight).

Chronic Lupus Panniculitis

Chronic lupus panniculitis is a form of CCLE in which there are firm, circumscribed subcutaneous nodules on the face, scalp, breast, upper arms, thighs, and buttocks. Most but not all patients also have typical lesions of DLE. Usually a form of cutaneous lupus, but may occur in SLE. *Synonym:* Lupus erythematosus profundus.

HISTORY

May precede or follow the onset of discoid lesions by several years. Nodules are either tender, asymptomatic, and sometimes painful.

PHYSICAL EXAMINATION

Skin Lesions Deep-seated nodules or platelike infiltrations with or without grossly visible epidermal changes or change of color; lesions

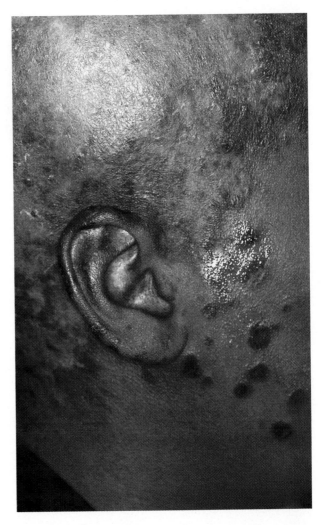

Figure 12-23 Chronic cutaneous lupus erythematosus
Widespread involvement of the scalp has led to complete hair loss with residual erythema, atrophy, and scarring. Sharp demarcation of the confluent lesions in the periphery and the raised border indicate that these lesions originally were CDLE plaques, as can still be seen on the cheek. Note the intense lesional hyperpigmentation that can occur in blacks.

evolve into deep depressions. (Fig. 12-24) Plaques or nodules are indolent and firm, sometimes tender or painful, and are better felt than seen; the overlying skin may be normal or exhibit typical lesions of CDLE.

Ulcers may develop in the plaques or nodules, and in this case there may be scarring.

Distribution Scalp, face, upper arms, (Fig. 12-24) trunk (especially the breasts), thighs, and buttocks.

Systems Review In one series, 35% of the patients had mild SLE.

DIFFERENTIAL DIAGNOSIS

Morphea, erythema nodosum, sarcoid, miscellaneous types of panniculitis.

LABORATORY EXAMINATIONS

Dermatopathology Subcutaneous layer. Necrobiosis with fibrinoid deposits, dense lymphocytic infiltrates; later, hyalinization of the fat lobules; there may be considerable mucinous deposits and also rarely vasculitis.

Other In patients with SLE there are typical hematologic and serologic abnormalities.

MANAGEMENT

Systemic Same as for CCLE, discoid type.

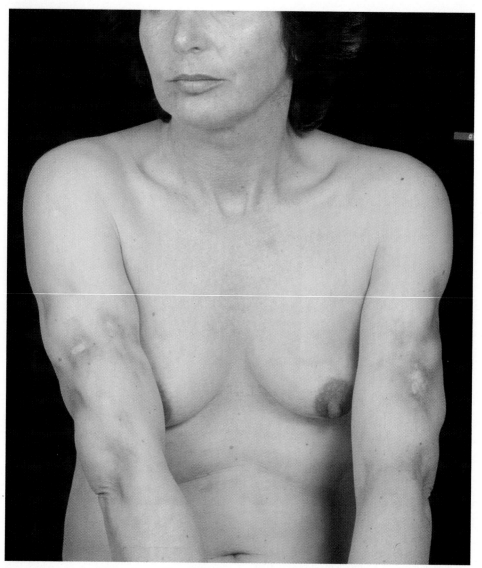

Figure 12-24   Lupus panniculitis   *Chronic panniculitis with atrophy of the subcutaneous tissue, resulting in large sunken areas of overlying skin, representing resolving lesions. Where erythema is still visible, palpation reveals firm subcutaneous nodules and plaques. Also, some lesions reveal scarring in the center.*

SCLERODERMA

Scleroderma is a multisystem disorder characterized by inflammatory, vascular, and sclerotic changes of the skin and various internal organs, especially the lungs, heart, and GI tract.
Synonyms: Progressive systemic sclerosis, systemic sclerosis, systemic scleroderma.

EPIDEMIOLOGY

Age of Onset 30 to 50 years.

Sex Female:male ratio 4:1.

Etiology Unknown.

CLASSIFICATION

Systemic scleroderma can be divided into two subsets: *limited systemic scleroderma* (lSSc) and *diffuse systemic scleroderma* (dSSc). lSSc comprises 60% of scleroderma patients; patients are usually female, older than those with dSSc, and have a long history of Raynaud's phenomenon with skin involvement limited to hands, feet, face, and forearms (acrosclerosis) and a high incidence of anticentromeric antibodies. lSSc includes the CREST syndrome, and systemic involvement may not appear for years; patients usually die of other causes. dSSc patients have a relatively rapid onset and diffuse involvement, not only of hands and feet but also of the trunk and face, synovitis, tendosynovitis, and early onset of internal involvement. Anticentromere antibodies are uncommon, but Scl-70 (antitopoisomerase I) antibodies are present in 33%.

Clinical Variant CREST syndrome, i.e., *C*alcinosis cutis + *R*aynaud's phenomenon + *E*sophageal dysfunction + *S*clerodactyly + *T*elangiectasia.

HISTORY

Raynaud's phenomenon with digital pain, coldness, rubor with pain and tingling. Pain/stiffness of fingers, knees. Migratory polyarthritis. Heartburn, dysphagia, especially with solid foods. Constipation, diarrhea, abdominal bloating, malabsorption, weight loss. Exertional dyspnea, dry cough.

PHYSICAL EXAMINATION

Skin *Hands/Feet Early:* Raynaud's phenomenon with triphasic color changes, i.e., pallor, cyanosis, rubor (Fig. 12-25). Precedes sclerosis by months and years. Nonpitting edema of hands/feet. Painful ulcerations at fingertips ("rat bite necrosis") (Fig. 12-26), knuckles; heal with pitted scars. *Late:* sclerodactyly with tapering of fingers (madonna fingers) with waxy, shiny, hardened skin, which is tightly bound down and does not permit folding or wrinkling; (Fig. 12-25); leathery crepitation over joints, flexion contractures; periungual telangiectasia, nails grow claw-like over shortened distal phalanges. Bony resorption and ulceration results in loss of distal phalanges (Fig. 12-25).

As sclerosis proceeds proximally, there is loss of sweat glands with anhidrosis and thinning and complete loss of hair on distal extremities.

Face Early: periorbital edema. *Late:* edema and fibrosis result in loss of normal facial lines, masklike (patients look younger than they are) (Fig. 12-27), thinning of lips, microstomia, radial perioral furrowing, small sharp nose. Telangiectasia and diffuse hyperpigmentation.

Trunk In dSSc the chest and proximal upper and lower extremities are involved early. Tense, stiff, and waxy appearing skin that cannot be folded (Fig. 12-27). Impairment of respiratory movement of chest wall and of joint mobility.

Other Changes *Cutaneous Calcification* Occurs on finger tips or over bony prominences or any sclerodermatous site; may ulcerate and extrude white paste.

Color Changes Hyperpigmentation that may be generalized and on the extremities may be accompanied by perifollicular hypopigmentation.

Mucous Membranes Sclerosis of sublingual ligament; uncommonly, painful induration of gums, tongue.

Distribution of Lesions *Early:* in lSSc early involvement is seen on fingers, hands, and face, and in many patients scleroderma remains confined to these regions. *Late:* the distal upper and lower extremities may be involved and occasionally the trunk. In dSSc sclerosis of the extremities and the trunk may start soon or soon after or concomitant with acral involvement.

CREST Syndrome

Matlike telangiectasia, especially the face (Fig. 12-28), upper trunk, and hands; also in the entire GI tract. Calcinosis over bony prominences, finger tips, elbows, and trochanteric regions.

PATHOGENESIS

Pathogenesis unknown. Primary event might be endothelial cell injury in blood vessels, the cause of which is unknown. Early in course, target organ edema occurs, followed by fibrosis; cutaneous capillaries are reduced in number; remainder dilate and proliferate, becoming visible telangiectasia. Fibrosis due to overproduction of collagen by fibroblasts.

GENERAL EXAMINATION

Esophagus Dysphagia, diminished peristalsis, reflux esophagitis.

Gastrointestinal System Small intestine involvement may produce constipation, diarrhea, bloating, and malabsorption.

Lung Pulmonary fibrosis and alveolitis. Reduction of pulmonary function due to restricted movement of chest wall.

Heart Cardiac conduction defects, heart failure, pericarditis.

Kidney Renal involvement occurs in 45%. Slowly progressive uremia, malignant hypertension.

Musculoskeletal System Carpal tunnel syndrome. Muscle weakness.

DIFFERENTIAL DIAGNOSIS

Diffuse Sclerosis Mixed connective tissue disease, eosinophilic fasciitis, scleromyxedema, morphea, porphyria cutanea tarda, chronic graft-versus-host disease, lichen sclerosus et atrophicus, polyvinyl chloride exposure, adverse drug reaction (pentazocine, bleomycin).

LABORATORY EXAMINATIONS

Dermatopathology *Early:* mild cellular infiltrate around dermal blood vessels, eccrine coils, and at the dermal subcutaneous interphase. *Late:* epidermis shows disappearance of rete ridges, increased eosinophilia, broadening and homogenization of collagen bundles, obliteration and decrease of interbundle spaces, thickening of dermis with replacement of upper or total subcutaneous fat by hyalinized collagen. Paucity of blood vessels, thickening/hyalinization of vessel walls.

Autoantibodies Patients with dSSc have circulating autoantibodies by ANA testing. Autoantibodies react with centromere proteins or DNA topoisomerase I; fewer patients have antinucleolar antibodies. Anticentromeric autoantibodies occur in 21% of dSSc and 71% of CREST patients, DNA topoisomerase I (Scl-70) antibodies in 33% of dSSc and 18% of CREST patients.

DIAGNOSIS

Clinical findings confirmed by dermatopathology.

COURSE AND PROGNOSIS

Course characterized by slow, relentless progression of skin and/or visceral sclerosis; however, the 10-year survival rate is >50%. Renal disease is the leading cause of death; also, cardiac and pulmonary involvement. Spontaneous remissions do occur. lSSc, which includes the CREST syndrome, progresses more slowly and has a more favorable prognosis; some cases do develop visceral involvement.

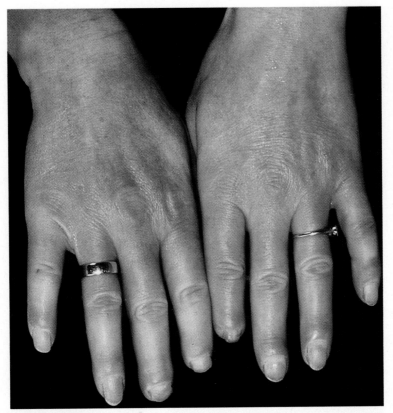

Figure 12-25 Scleroderma: Raynaud's phenomenon and acrosclerosis *Hands and fingers are edematous (nonpitting) with both erythema and vasoconstriction (blue and white); skin is shiny, bound down; hair is absent due to sclerosis. Distal fingers are tapered and the phalanges on some fingers shortened (index fingers), which is associated with bony resorption. Nail dystrophy.*

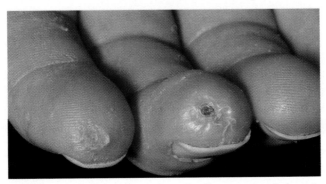

Figure 12-26 Scleroderma: acrosclerosis *Typical "rat bite" necroses and ulcerations of fingertips.*

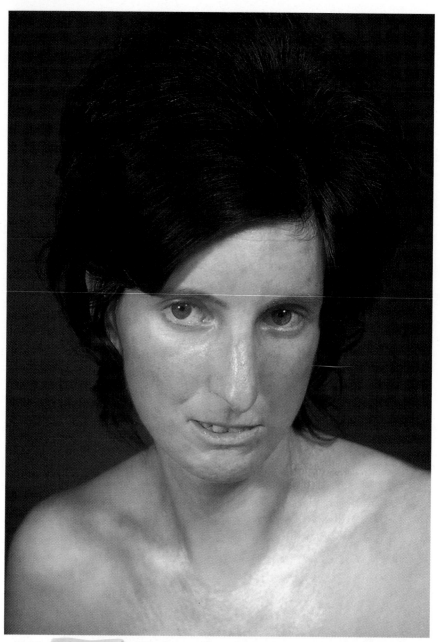

Figure 12-27 **Scleroderma** *Masklike facies with stretched, shiny skin and loss of normal facial lines giving a younger appearance than actual age; the hair and eyebrows are dyed black. Thining of the lips and perioral sclerosis result in small mouth, which is asymmetric, creating a snarling appearance. Sclerosis and multiple telangiectases are also present on the shoulders and chest.*

SKIN SIGNS OF IMMUNE, AUTOIMMUNE, AND RHEUMATIC DISEASES

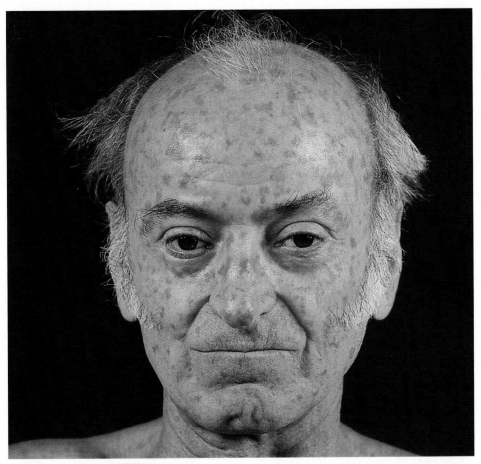

Figure 12-28   Scleroderma: CREST syndrome   *Numerous macular or matlike telangiectases without other findings of scleroderma on the face. Complete features include **c**alcinosis cutis, **R**aynaud's phenomenon, **e**sophageal dysmotility, **s**clerosis, and **t**elangiectasias.*

| **MANAGEMENT**

Symptomatic   Systemic glucocorticoids may be of benefit for limited periods early in the disease. All other systemic treatments (EDTA, aminocaproic acid, D-penicillamine, *para*-aminobenzoate, colchicine, immunosuppressive drugs) have not been shown to be of lasting benefit. Presently, interferon-γ is being tested clinically, as is photopheresis.

Scleroderma-Like Conditions

A scleroderma-like condition, as is seen in systemic sclerosis, occurs in persons exposed to polyvinyl chloride. Bleomycin also produces pulmonary fibrosis and Raynaud's phenomenon. Cutaneous changes indistinguishable from dSSc-like sclerosis of skin, accompanied by myalgia, pulmonitis, myocarditis, neuropathy, and encephalopathy are related to the ingestion of certain lots of l-tryptophan (*arthralgia-myalgia syndrome*); the *toxic oil syndrome* that occurred in an epidemic in Spain in 1981 affecting 25,000 people was due to the consumption of denatured grape seed oil. After an acute phase, with rash, fever, pulmonitis, and myalgia, the syndrome progresses to a condition with neuromuscular abnormalities and scleroderma-like skin lesions.

RAYNAUD'S DISEASE/RAYNAUD'S PHENOMENON

Raynaud's phenomenon (RP) is digital ischemia that occurs on exposure to cold and/or as a result of emotional stress. The various causes of RP include *rheumatic disorders* [systemic scleroderma (85%), SLE (35%), dermatomyositis (30%), Sjögren's syndrome, rheumatoid arthritis, polyarteritis nodosa], *diseases with abnormal blood proteins* (cryoproteins, cold agglutinins, macroglobulins), *drugs* (β-adrenergic blockers, nicotine), *arterial diseases* (arteriosclerosis obliterans, thromboangiitis obliterans), and *carpal tunnel syndrome*. When no etiology is found for RP, the term Raynaud's disease (RD) is used. It is primarily RD that is summarized below.

EPIDEMIOLOGY

Age of Onset Young adults or at menopause.

Sex Female >> male.

Incidence As high as 20% in young women.

Occupation May occur in persons using vibratory tools (chain saw users), meat cutters, typists, and pianists.

Precipitating Factors Cold, mental stress, certain occupations (see above), smoking.

PATHOGENESIS

The vasomotor tone is regulated by the sympathetic nervous system. The centers for vasomotor tone are located in the brain, the spinal cord, and the peripheral nerves. Vasodilatation occurs only on withdrawal of the sympathetic activity. It is conjectured that there may be a "local fault" in which blood vessels are abnormally sensitive to cold.

HISTORY

Numbness and/or pain worse in winter in temperate climates, in the cold (meat cutters); previous treatment (drugs), occupation (using vibratory tools) have to be explored. Careful review is important to detect diseases in which RP is associated: arthralgia, fatigue, dysphagia, muscle weakness, etc.

PHYSICAL EXAMINATION

Skin

Types of Skin Changes *The Episodic Attack* There is blanching or cyanosis of the fingers or toes, extending from the tip to various levels of the digits. The finger distal to the line of ischemia is white or blue and cold (Fig. 12-29); the proximal skin is pink and warm. When the digits are rewarmed, the blanching may be replaced by cyanosis because of slow blood flow; at the end of the attack, the normal color or a red color reflects the reactive hyperemic phase. To recapitulate, the sequence of color changes is white → blue → red. Rarely, the tip of the nose, earlobes, or the tongue may be involved. Blanching may occur in one or two digits or in all the digits; often the thumb is spared. The feet are involved in only 40%.

Repeated or Persistent Vascular Vasospasm Patients with RP often have a persistent vasospasm rather than episodic attacks. Skin changes include trophic changes with development of taut, atrophic skin and shortening of the terminal phalanges—this is called *sclerodactyly*. Acrogangrene is rare in RD (<1%). In RP associated with scleroderma, painful ulcers and fissures develop (Fig. 12-30); sequestration of the terminal phalanges or the development of gangrene may lead to autoamputation of the fingertips.

Nails

Pterygium, clubbing.

DIFFERENTIAL DIAGNOSIS

See Table 12-6.

SKIN SIGNS OF IMMUNE, AUTOIMMUNE, AND RHEUMATIC DISEASES

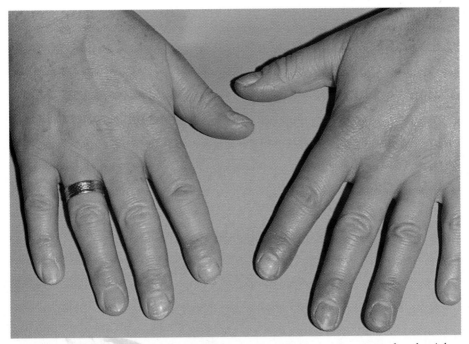

Figure 12-29 Raynaud's disease *The left hand exhibits a distal cyanosis compared to the right hand; it is seen especially well in the nail beds. Unilateral episodes such as this one may occur after contact with a cold object.*

Table 12-6 CAUSES OF RAYNAUD'S PHENOMENON

Connective tissue disease
  Scleroderma
  Systemic lupus erythematosus
  Dermatomyositis and polymyositis
  Mixed connective tissue disease
  Rheumatoid arthritis
  Polyarteritis and vasculitis
  Sjögren syndrome
Obstructive arterial disease
  Arteriosclerosis obliterans
  Thromboangiitis obliterans
  Arterial embolism
  Thoracic outlet syndrome
Neurogenic disorders
  Carpal tunnel syndrome
  Reflex sympathetic dystrophy
  Hemiplegia
  Poliomyelitis
  Multiple sclerosis
  Syringomyelia
Drugs
  β-adrenergic blockers
  Ergot preparations
  Methysergide
  Bleomycin and vinblastine
  Clonidine
  Bromocriptine
  Cyclosporine
Trauma
  Vibratory tools
  Hypothenar hammer syndrome
  Pianists, typists
  Meat cutters
Hematologic causes
  Cryoproteins
  Cold agglutinins
  Macroglobulins
  Polycythemia
Miscellaneous
  Hypothyroidism
  Vinyl chloride disease
  Neoplasms
  Vasculitis and hepatitis B antigenemia
  Arteriovenous fistula
  Intraarterial injections

SOURCE: TD Coffman: Cutaneous changes in peripheral vascular disease, in Fitzpatrick et al. (eds): *Dermatology in General Medicine*, 4th ed. New York, McGraw-Hill, 1993; chapter 167.

LABORATORY EXAMINATIONS

Serology ANA and other tests to rule out scleroderma, lupus erythematosus, immunoproteins.

DIAGNOSIS

The vascular changes in RP are characteristic; when no other disease is discovered (see above), the diagnosis is RD.

COURSE AND PROGNOSIS

RP may disappear spontaneously; it progresses in about 1 of 3 patients.

MANAGEMENT

Prevention Education regarding the use of loose-fitting clothing, and avoiding cold and pressure on the fingers. Giving up smoking is mandatory.

Systemic Therapy Drug therapy such as reserpine and nifedipine should be used only in patients who have severe RD.

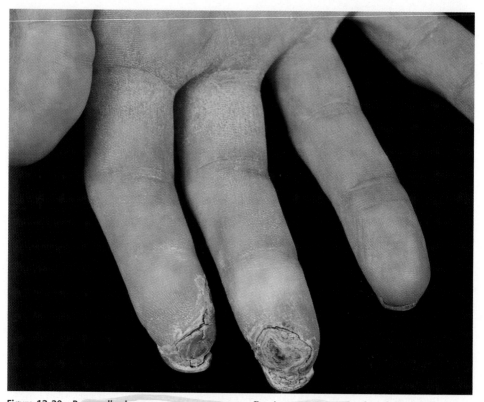

Figure 12-30 Raynaud's phenomenon: acrogangrene *Persistent vasospasm of medium-sized arterioles can sometimes lead to gangrene of the terminal digits as illustrated in this patient with scleroderma.*

VASCULITIS

Hypersensitivity Vasculitis

Hypersensitivity vasculitis (HV) encompasses a heterogeneous group of vasculitides associated with hypersensitivity to antigens from infectious agents, drugs, or other exogenous or endogenous sources, characterized pathologically by involvement of postcapillary venules and inflammation and fibrinoid necrosis. Clinically, skin involvement is characteristic, manifested by "palpable purpura." Systemic vascular involvement occurs, chiefly in the kidney, muscles, joints, GI tract, and peripheral nerves. Schönlein-Henoch purpura is a type of HV associated with IgA.

Synonyms: Allergic cutaneous vasculitis, necrotizing vasculitis.

CLASSIFICATION

Exogenous Stimuli Proved or Suspected

Infectious diseases Hepatitis B virus, hepatitis C virus, group A hemolytic streptococcus, *Staphylococcus aureus, Mycobacterium leprae.*

Drugs Sulfonamides, penicillin, serum, others.

Endogenous Antigens Likely Involved   Vasculitis associated with:

Neoplasms Lymphoproliferative disorders, carcinoma of kidney.
Connective tissue diseases SLE, rheumatoid arthritis, Sjögren's syndrome.
Other underlying diseases Cryoglobulinemia, paraproteinemia, hypergammaglobulinemia.
Congenital deficiencies of the complement system.

EPIDEMIOLOGY

Age of Onset   All ages.

Sex   Equal incidence in males and females.

Etiology   Idiopathic 50%.

PATHOGENESIS

The most frequently postulated mechanism for the production of necrotizing vasculitis is the deposition in tissues of circulating immune complexes. Initial alterations in venular permeability, which may facilitate the deposition of complexes at such sites, may be due to the release of vasoactive amines from platelets, basophils, and/or mast cells. Immune complexes may activate the complement system or may interact directly with Fc receptors on endothelial cell membranes. When the complement system is activated, the generation of anaphylatoxins C3a and C5a can degranulate mast cells. Also, C5a can attract neutrophils that could release lysosomal enzymes during phagocytosis of complexes and subsequently damage vascular tissue.

HISTORY

A new drug taken during the few weeks before the onset of HV is a likely etiologic agent, as may be a streptococcal infection, a known vascular/connective tissue disease, or paraproteinemia. Onset and course: acute (days, as in drug-induced or idiopathic), subacute (weeks, especially urticarial types), chronic (recurrent over years). Symptoms are pruritus, burning pain; there may be no symptoms. Fever, malaise; symptoms of peripheral neuritis, abdominal pain (bowel ischemia), arthralgia, myalgia, kidney involvement (microhematuria), CNS involvement.

PHYSICAL EXAMINATION

Skin Lesions   The hallmark is *palpable purpura*. This term describes the palpable petechiae that present as bright red, well-demarcated macules and papules with a central, dot-like hemorrhage (Fig. 12-31) (petechiae due to coagulation defects or thrombocytopenia are strictly macular and, therefore, not palpable). Lesions are scattered, discrete or confluent, and are primarily localized to the lower third of legs and the ankles (Fig. 12-31), but may spread to the buttocks and arms. Stasis factor aggravates or precipitates lesions. Purpuric lesions do not blanch (with a glass slide). Red initially, they turn purple and even black in the center. In the case of massive inflammation, purpuric papules convert to hemorrhagic blisters, become necrotic, and even ulcerate (Fig. 12-32).

DIFFERENTIAL DIAGNOSIS

Thrombocytopenic purpura, rash such as exanthematous drug eruption in setting of thrombocytopenia, disseminated intravascular coagulation (DIC) with purpura fulminans, septic vasculitis (rickettsial spotted fevers), septic emboli (infective endocarditis), bacteremia [disseminated gonococcal infection, meningococcemia (acute/chronic)], other noninfectious vasculitides.

LABORATORY EXAMINATIONS

Hematology   Rule out thrombocytopenic purpura.

ESR   Elevated.

Serology   Serum complement is reduced or normal in some patients, depending on associated disorders.

Urinalysis   RBC casts, albuminuria.

Others   Depending on underlying disease.

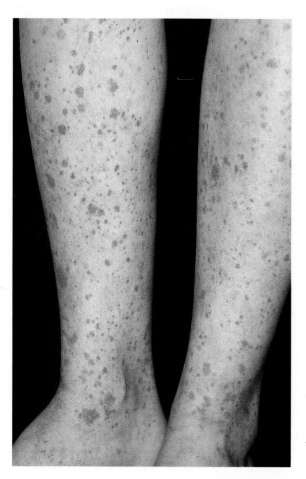

Figure 12-31   Hypersensitivity vasculitis   *Multiple sites of cutaneous vasculitis present clinically as "palpable purpura" on the lower extremities. Although appearing to the eye as macules, the lesions can be palpated, and this contrasts with petechiae, for instance, in thrombocytopenic purpura. The lesions shown here do not blanch with a glass slide, indicating hemorrhage.*

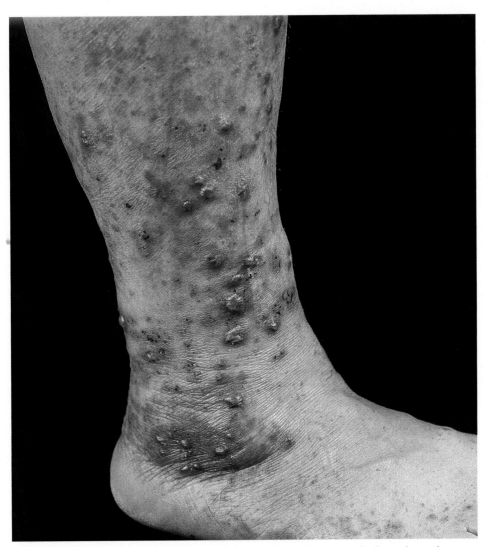

Figure 12-32 Hypersensitivity vasculitis *A limited number of lesions on the lower leg and forefoot with palpable purpura and hemorrhagic bullae. These lesions may progress to necrosis and ulceration.*

Dermatopathology *Necrotizing vasculitis.* Deposition of eosinophilic material (fibrinoid) in the walls of postcapillary venules in the upper dermis, and perivenular and intramural inflammatory infiltrate consisting predominantly of neutrophils. Extravasated RBC and fragmented neutrophils ("nuclear dust"). Frank necrosis of vessel walls. Intramural C3 and immunoglobulin deposition is seen with immunofluorescent techniques.

DIAGNOSIS

Based on clinical appearance and histopathology.

COURSE AND PROGNOSIS

Depends on underlying disease. In the idiopathic variant, multiple episodes can occur over the course of years. Usually self-limited, but irreversible damage to kidneys can occur.

MANAGEMENT

Antibiotics Antibiotics for patients in whom vasculitis follows bacterial infection.

Prednisone For patients with moderate to severe disease.

Cytotoxic Immunosuppressives Cyclophosphamide, azathioprine are used, usually in combination with prednisone.

Schönlein-Henoch Purpura

This is a specific subtype of hypersensitivity vasculitis that occurs mainly in children but also affects adults. There is a history of upper respiratory tract infection (75%), involving group A streptocuocci. The disorder consists of palpable purpura accompanied by bowel angina (diffuse abdominal pain that is worse after meals) or bowel ischemia, usually including bloody diarrhea, kidney involvement (hematuria and red cell casts), and arthritis. Histopathologically, there is necrotizing vasculitis and the immunoreactants deposited in skin are IgA. Long-term morbidity may result from progressive renal disease (5%).

Polyarteritis Nodosa

Polyarteritis nodosa (PAN) is a multisystem, necrotizing vasculitis of small- and medium-sized muscular arteries characterized by its involvement of the renal and visceral arteries. There is a form of PAN that is restricted to skin (*cutaneous* PAN).
Synonyms: Periarteritis nodosa, panarteritis nodosa.

EPIDEMIOLOGY

Age of Onset Mean age 45 years.

Sex Male:female ratio 2.5:1.

Etiology Unknown.

Clinical Variants *Cutaneous PAN* is a rare variant with symptomatic vasculitis limited to skin and at times peripheral nerves.

PATHOGENESIS

Necrotizing inflammation of small- and medium-sized muscular arteries; may spread circumferentially to involve adjacent veins. Lesions segmental, tend to involve bifurcations of arteries. About 30% of cases associated with hepatitis B antigenemia, i.e., immune complex formation.

HISTORY

Chronic Disease Syndrome GI involvement: nausea, vomiting, abdominal pain, hemorrhage, perforation, infarction. CVS: congestive heart failure, pericarditis, conduction system defects, myocardial infarction. Paresthesias, numbness.

Cutaneous PAN Pain in nodules, ulcers, involved extremities; aching during flares and physical activity. Myalgia. Neuralgia, numbness, mild paresthesia.

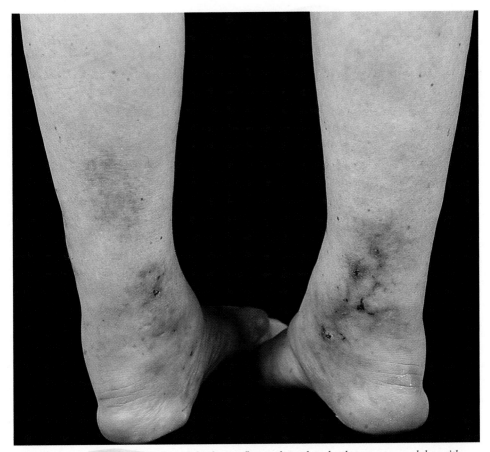

Figure 12-33 Polyarteritis nodosa *Multiple, confluent, dermal and subcutaneous nodules with ulceration (note starburst pattern of lesions) occurring on the medial aspect of the lower legs; lesions represent cutaneous infarctions. Scar on the left posterior calf represents a previous site of cutaneous polyarteritis nodosa ulceration.*

PHYSICAL EXAMINATION

Skin Lesions Occur in 15% of cases. Subcutaneous inflammatory, bright red to bluish nodules (.5 to 2 cm) that follow the course of involved arteries. Violaceous, become confluent to form painful subcutaneous plaques (Fig. 12-33), and accompanied by livedo reticularis; "starburst" livedo is pathognomonic and marks a cluster of nodular lesions (Fig. 12-33). Ulcers may follow ischemia of nodules. They usually occur on the lower extremities, usually bilaterally. Lower legs, thighs. Other areas: arms, trunk, head, neck, buttocks. Livedo reticularis may extend to trunk. Duration—days

to months. Resolves with residual violaceous or postinflammatory hyperpigmentation. Skin lesions in systemic and cutaneous PAN are identical.

GENERAL EXAMINATION

Cardiovascular Elevated blood pressure.

Neurologic CNS: cerebrovascular accident. Peripheral nerves: mixed motor/sensory involvement with mononeuritis multiplex pattern.

Muscles Diffuse myalgias (excluding shoulder and hip girdle), lower extremities.

Eye Hypertensive changes, ocular vasculitis, retinal artery aneurysm, optic disc edema/atrophy.

Kidney BUN ↑, keratinin clearance ↓.

TESTES Pain and tenderness.

DIFFERENTIAL DIAGNOSIS

Other vasculitides and panniculitides.

LABORATORY EXAMINATIONS

Dermatopathology *Best yield: biopsy of nodular skin lesion (deep wedge biopsy).* Polymorphonuclear neutrophils infiltrate all layers of muscular vessel wall and perivascular areas; later, mononuclear cells. Fibrinoid necrosis of vessel wall with compromise of lumen, thrombosis, infarction of tissues supplied by involved vessel, with or without hemorrhage. Skin pathology is identical in systemic and cutaneous PAN.

CBC Commonly neutrophilic leukocytosis; rarely, eosinophilia; anemia of chronic disease. ± Elevated ESR.

Serology Antineutrophil cytoplasmic autoantibodies (p-ANCA) in serum. Hepatitis B surface antigenemia in 30% of cases.

Chemistry Elevated creatinine, BUN.

Arteriography Aneurysms in small- and medium-sized muscular arteries of kidney/hepatic/visceral vasculature.

COURSE AND PROGNOSIS

Untreated, very high morbidity and mortality rates characterized by fulminant deterioration or by relentless progression associated with intermittent acute exacerbations. Death from renal failure, bowel infarction and perforation, cardiovascular complications, intractable hypertension. Lesions may heal with scarring and further occlusion or aneurysmal dilatations. Effective treatment reduces morbidity and mortality rates. *Cutaneous PAN:* chronic relapsing benign course.

MANAGEMENT

Systemic PAN *Combined Therapy* Prednisone, 1 mg/kg of body weight per day, and cyclophosphamide, 2 mg/kg/d.

Cutaneous PAN Nonsteroidal anti-inflammatory agents, prednisone.

Wegener's Granulomatosis

Wegener's granulomatosis (WG) is a systemic vasculitis, defined by a clinical triad of manifestations that includes involvement of the upper airways, lungs, and kidneys and by a pathologic triad consisting of necrotizing granulomas in the upper respiratory tract and lungs, vasculitis involving both arteries and veins, and glomerulitis.

EPIDEMIOLOGY

Age of Onset Mean age 40 years, but occurs at any age.

Sex Male: female ratio 1.3: 1.

Race Rare in blacks.

Etiology Unknown.

Clinical Variants Variants limited to kidneys; i.e., glomerulitis occurs in 15% of cases. Limited to respiratory tract.

PATHOGENESIS

Immunopathogenesis unclear. Possibly an aberrant hypersensitivity response to an exogenous or endogenous antigen that enters through or resides in upper airways. Clinical symptomatology caused by necrotizing vasculitis of small arteries and veins. Pulmonary involvement: multiple, bilateral, nodular infiltrates. Similar infiltrates in paranasal sinuses, nasopharynx.

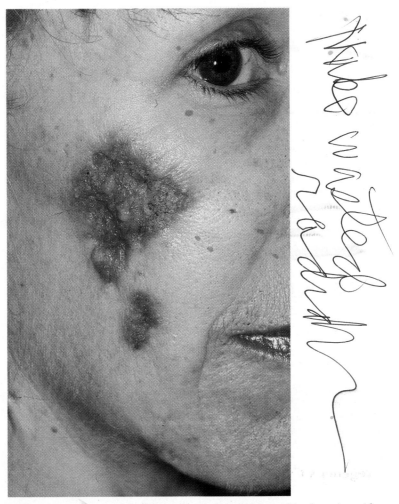

Figure 12-34   Wegener's granulomatosis *A pyoderma gangrenosum-like irregular ulceration with jagged and undermined borders is often the first manifestation of Wegener's gramulomatosis.*

HISTORY

Chronic disease syndrome. Fever. Paranasal sinus pain, purulent or bloody nasal discharge. Cough, hemoptysis, dyspnea, chest discomfort.

PHYSICAL EXAMINATION

Skin Lesions Overall in 50% of patients, but in only 13% of patients at initial presentation. *Ulcers with jagged, undermined borders* most typical; resemble pyoderma gangrenosum (Fig. 12-34). *Papules, vesicles, palpable purpura* as in hypersensitivity (necrotizing) vasculitis (Fig. 12-35), subcutaneous nodules, plaques, noduloulcerative lesions as in PAN. Most common on lower extremities. Also, face, trunk, upper limbs.

Mucous Membranes Oral ulcerations (Fig. 12-36). Often first symptom. ±Nasal mucosal ulceration, crusting, blood clots; nasal septal perforation; saddle-nose deformity. Eustachian tube occlusion with serous otitis media; ±pain. External auditory canal: pain, erythema, swelling. Marked gingival hyperplasia.

Eye 65%. Mild conjunctivitis, episcleritis, scleritis, granulomatous sclerouveitis, ciliary vessel vasculitis, retroorbital mass lesion with proptosis.

Nervous System Cranial neuritis, mononeuritis multiplex, cerebral vasculitis.

Renal Disease 85%. Signs of renal failure in advanced WG.

DIFFERENTIAL DIAGNOSIS

Cutaneous Necrosis + Respiratory Tract Disease Other vasculitides, Goodpasture's syndrome, tumors of the upper airway/lung, infectious/noninfectious granulomatous diseases (especially blastomycosis), midline granuloma, angiocentric lymphoma, allergic granulomatosis.

LABORATORY EXAMINATIONS

Hematology Mild anemia. Leukocytosis. ±Thrombocytosis.

ESR Markedly elevated.

Chemistry Impaired renal function.

Urinalysis Proteinuria, hematuria, RBC casts.

Serology Antineutrophil cytoplasmic autoantibodies (ANCA) are seromarkers for WG. Two ANCA patterns occur in ethanol-fixed neutrophils: cytoplasmic pattern (c-ANCA) and perinuclear pattern (p-ANCA). A 29-kDa protease (PR-3) is the major antigen for c-ANCA; myeloperoxidase, that for p-ANCA. c-ANCA has been associated predominantly with WG and is considered specific for this condition; p-ANCA with microscopic polyarteritis, PAN, other vasculitides, idiopathic necrotizing and crescentic glomerulonephritis. Titers correlate with disease activity. Hypergammaglobulinemia, particularly IgA class.

Pathology All involved tissues including skin: necrotizing vasculitis of small arteries/veins with intra- or extravascular granuloma formation. Kidneys: focal/segmental glomerulonephritis.

Imaging *Paranasal sinuses* Opacification, with or without sclerosis. *Chest:* pulmonary infiltrates, nodules, consolidation, cavitation; upper lobes.

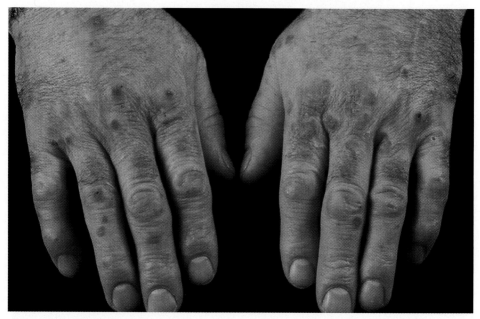

Figure 12-35 Wegener's granulomatosis *A limited number of erythematous, purpuric, non-blanchable papules and nodules on the dorsa of fingers and hands; a few lesions have central areas of infarction. These lesions are very similar to those of hypersensitivity vasculitis and also occur on the lower legs.*

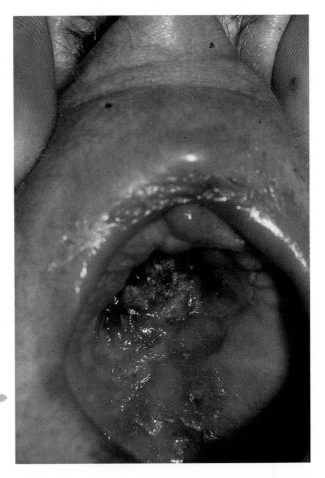

Figure 12-36 Wegener's granulomatosis *A large ulcer on the palate covered by a dense, adherent, necrotic mass; similar lesions occur in the sinuses and tracheobronchial tree.*

DIAGNOSIS

Disease triad of necrotizing granulomatous vasculitis of upper and lower respiratory tract associated with glomerulonephritis and c-ANCA.

COURSE AND PROGNOSIS

Untreated, usually fatal because of rapidly progressive renal failure. With combination cyclophosphamide plus prednisone therapy, long-term remission is achieved in 90% of cases.

MANAGEMENT

Treatment of Choice Cyclophosphamide plus prednisone.

Cyclophosphamide 2 mg/kg of body weight per day. Dose should be adjusted to keep leukocyte count >5000/μL (neutrophil count> 1500/μL) to avoid infections associated with neutropenia. Therapy should be continued for 1 year after complete remission, then tapered and discontinued. *Alternative drug:* azathioprine in similar doses if cyclophosphamide is not tolerated.

Prednisone 1 mg/kg of body weight per day for 1 month, and then changed to alternate-day doses which are tapered and then discontinued after 6 months of therapy.

Trimethoprimsulfamethoxazole as adjunctive therapy and/or prevention of upper airway bacterial infections that promote disease flare.

Giant Cell Arteritis

Giant cell arteritis is a systemic granulomatous vasculitis of medium- and large-sized arteries, most notably the temporal artery and other branches of the carotid artery, characterized by headaches, fatigue, fever, anemia, and high ESR, in elderly patients.

Synonyms: Temporal arteritis, cranial arteritis.

EPIDEMIOLOGY

Age of Onset   Elderly, usually >55 years.

Sex   Females>males.

Etiology   Unknown. Probably via cell-mediated immunity.

Clinical Variants   Temporal arteritis is a characteristic regional expression of giant cell arteritis affecting the temporal and other cranial arteries, which may or may not be accompanied by clinical symptoms of systemic involvement. Association with polymyalgia rheumatica.

HISTORY

Fatigue. Fever. Chronic disease syndrome. Headache usually bilateral. Scalp pain. Claudication of jaw/tongue while talking/chewing. Eye involvement: transient impairment of vision, ischemic optic neuritis, retrobulbar neuritis, persistent blindness. Systemic vasculitis: claudication of extremities, stroke, myocardial infarction, aortic aneurysms/dissections, visceral organ infarction. Polymyalgia rheumatica syndrome: stiffness, aching, pain in the muscles of the neck, shoulders, lower back, hips, thighs.

PATHOGENESIS

Systemic vasculitis of multiple medium- and large-sized arteries. Symptoms secondary to ischemia.

PHYSICAL EXAMINATION

Skin Lesions   Superficial temporal arteries are swollen, prominent, tortuous, ±nodular thickenings (Fig. 12-37). Tender. Initially, involved artery pulsates; later, occluded with loss of pulsation. ±Erythema of overlying skin. Gangrene, i.e., skin infarction of the area supplied by affected artery in the temporal/parietal scalp with sharp, irregular borders; ulceration with exposure of bone (Fig. 12-38). Scars at sites of old ulcerations. Postinflammatory hyperpigmentation over involved artery.

General Examination   Findings in other organ systems related to tissue ischemia/infarction.

DIFFERENTIAL DIAGNOSIS

Gangrenous zoster of the scalp, caustic necrosis due to acids, third-degree burns.

LABORATORY EXAMINATIONS

CBC   Normochromic/slightly hypochromic anemia.

ESR   Markedly elevated.

Temporal Artery Biopsy   Biopsy tender nodule of involved artery with or without overlying affected skin after Doppler flow examination. Lesions focal; section serially. Panarteritis with inflammatory mononuclear cell infiltrates within the vessel wall with frequent giant cell granuloma formation. Intimal proliferation with vascular occlusion, fragmentation of internal elastic lamina, extensive necrosis of intima and media.

DIAGNOSIS

Clinical appearance verified by biopsy of temporal artery.

COURSE AND PROGNOSIS

Untreated, can result in blindness secondary to ischemic optic neuritis. Excellent response to glucocorticoid therapy. Remission after several years.

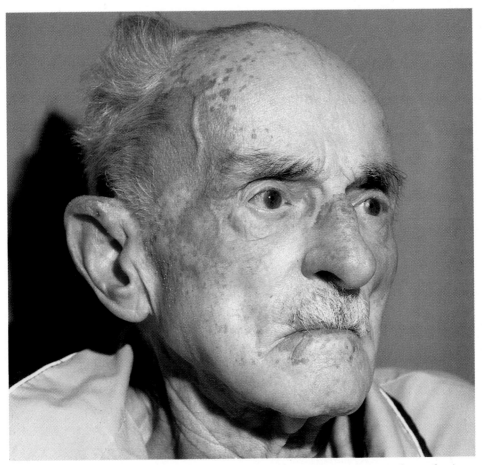

Figure 12-37 Giant cell arteritis *The superficial temporal artery is prominent, and on palpation is tender and pulseless in an elderly male who has excruciating headaches and progressive impairment of vision. An incidental finding is extensive vitiligo with islands of repigmentation.*

MANAGEMENT

Prednisone Initially, 40 to 60 mg/d; taper when symptoms abate; continue 7.5 to 10 mg/d for 1 to 2 years.

Methotrexate Observations indicate that low-dose (15 to 20 mg) methotrexate, once a week, may have a considerable glucocorticoid-sparing effect in giant cell arteritis.

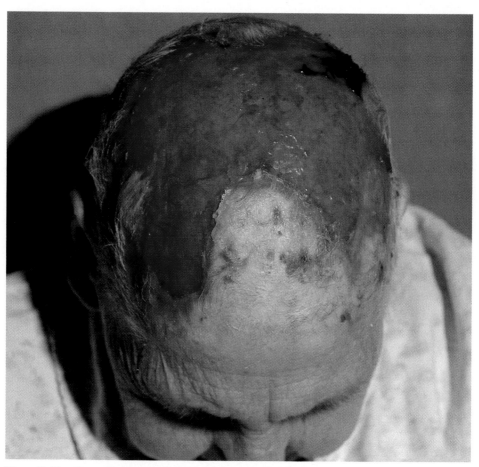

Figure 12-38 Giant cell arteritis *Extensive bilateral infarction and ulceration of the scalp of an elderly female secondary to vascular occlusion of temporal arteries.*

Urticarial Vasculitis

Urticarial vasculitis is a multisystem disease characterized by cutaneous lesions resembling urticaria, except that wheals persist more than 24 h, generally up to 3 to 4 days. Fever, arthralgia, elevated sedimentation rate, and histologic findings of a leukocytoclastic vasculitis are also present. The syndrome is often accompanied by various degrees of extracutaneous involvement. May be cutaneous manifestations of SLE.

Synonym: Urticaria perstans.

EPIDEMIOLOGY

Age of Onset   Majority 30 to 50 years.

Sex   Female:male ratio 3:1.

Etiology   In patients with serum sickness; in collagen vascular diseases, in particular, lupus erythematosus; with certain infections (e.g., hepatitis B); and idiopathic.

Incidence   <5% of patients with urticaria.

PATHOGENESIS

Thought to be an immune complex disease, similar to hypersensitivity vasculitis. Deposition of antigen-antibody complexes in cutaneous blood vessel walls leads to complement activation, resulting in neutrophil chemotaxis; collagenase and elastase released from neutrophils cause vessel wall and cell destruction.

HISTORY

Lesions may be associated with itching, burning, stinging sensation, pain, tenderness. Fever (10 to 15%). Arthralgias with or without arthritis in one or more joints (ankles, knees, elbows, wrists, small joints of fingers). Nausea, abdominal pain. Cough, dyspnea, chest pain, hemoptysis. Pseudotumor cerebri. Cold sensitivity. Renal involvement: diffuse glomerulonephritis.

PHYSICAL EXAMINATION

Skin Lesions   Urticaria-like (i.e., edematous), raised, occasionally indurated, erythematous, circumscribed wheals (Fig. 12-39); occasionally with angioedema. Eruption occurs in transient crops, usually lasting more than 24 h and up to 3 to 4 days, changing shape slowly, often reveal purpura on blanching (glass slide), and resolve with a yellowish-green color and hyperpigmentation.

General Examination   Extracutaneous manifestations: joints (70%), GI tract (20 to 30%), CNS (>10%), ocular system (>10%), kidneys (10 to 20%), lymphadenopathy (5%).

DIFFERENTIAL DIAGNOSIS

Urticaria, serum sickness, other vasculitides, SLE, urticaria in acute hepatitis B infection.

LABORATORY EXAMINATION

Dermatopathology   Biopsy of early lesions may show inflammation of dermal venules primarily with neutrophils without necrotizing vasculitis. Later, frank leukocytoclastic vasculitis. In some patients there is no histologic evidence of leukocytoclastic vasculitis, and these lesions are most often related to circulating immune complex (Gell and Coombs type III) immunologic reactions that occur 1 to 2 weeks after exposure to antigens such as heterologous serum or certain infectious agents or drugs.

Urinalysis   10% of patients—microhematuria, proteinuria.

ESR   Elevated.

Serologic Findings   Hypocomplementemia (70%); circulating immune complexes.

DIAGNOSIS

Clinical suspicion confirmed by skin biopsy.

Disease Associations   SLE and other collagen vascular autoimmune disease.

COURSE AND PROGNOSIS

Most often this syndrome has a chronic (months to years) but benign course. Episodes recur over periods ranging from months to years. Renal disease occurs only in hypocomplementemic patients.

MANAGEMENT

Rule out vascular/connective tissue disease.

First Line H_1 and H_2 blockers [doxepin (10 mg bid to 25 mg tid) plus cimetidine (300 mg tid)/ranitidine (150 mg bid)] *plus* a nonsteroidal anti-inflammatory agent [indomethacin (75 to 200 mg/d)/ibuprofen (1600 to 2400 mg/d)/naprosyn (500 to 1000 mg/d)]

Second Line   Colchicine, .6 mg bid or tid *or* dapsone, 50 to 150 mg/d.

Third Line   Prednisone.

Fourth Line   Cytotoxic immunosuppressive agents (azathioprine, cyclophosphamide).

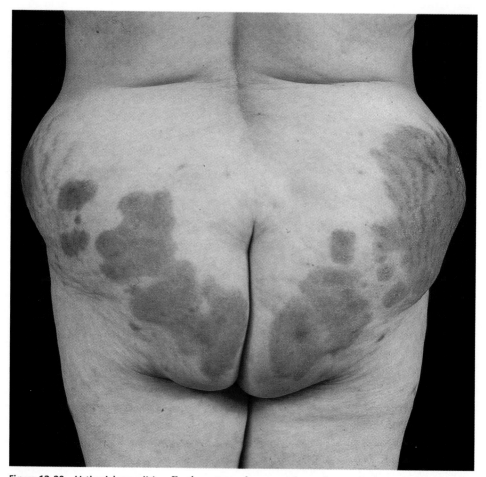

Figure 12-39   Urticarial vasculitis   *Erythematous plaques and papules on the buttocks do not blanch on diascopy (compression of the lesional skin with glass). In contrast to the lesions of urticaria, which usually resolve within 24 h, those of urticarial vasculitis persist for up to 3 days before resolving with residual hyperpigmentation (hemosiderin deposition). Urticarial lesions change shape in a short time, while those of urticarial vasculitis change slowly.*

Nodular Vasculitis

Nodular vasculitis is a form of lobular panniculitis associated with subcutaneous blood vessel vasculitis with subsequent ischemic changes that produce lipocyte injury, necrosis, inflammation, and granulation. An immune complex–mediated vascular injury has been hypothesized, but in most cases there is no direct evidence to support an immunologic mechanism. Synonyms are *erythema induratum* and *Bazin's disease,* but these terms are now reserved for those cases of nodular vasculitis that are associated with *Mycobacterium tuberculosis.*

EPIDEMIOLOGY

Age of Onset   Middle-aged to older persons.

Sex   Usually females.

Etiology   Immune complex–mediated vascular injury due to bacterial antigens has been implicated. Immunoglobulins, complement, and bacterial antigens have been found by immunofluorescence and in some cases mycobacterial DNA sequences by PCR. Bacterial cultures are invariably negative.

Dermatopathology   Tuberculoid granulomas, foreign body giant cell reaction, and necrosis of fat lobules. Medium-sized vessel vasculitis, predominantly venular but sometimes arterial, in the septal areas. Fibrinoid necrosis or a granulomatous chronic inflammatory infiltrate invades between the fat cells, gradually replacing adipose tissue and leading to fibrosis.

HISTORY

Chronic, recurrent, often bilateral, subcutaneous nodules and plaques with ulceration of the legs. Usually asymptomatic but may be tender. Often in middle-aged females with stubby column-like legs who work in the cold.

PHYSICAL EXAMINATION

Skin Lesions   Erythematous tender or asymptomatic subcutaneous nodules or plaques (Fig. 12-40) on the calves, rarely on shins and thighs. Lesions become bluish red in color, are firm, and fluctuate before ulcerating (Fig. 12-40). Ulcers drain serous/oily fluid, are ragged, punched-out, and have violaceous or brown margins. They persist for prolonged periods before healing with atrophic scars.

Associated Findings   Follicular perniosis, livedo, varicose veins, and a cool, edematous skin.

General Examination   Patients are usually healthy.

DIFFERENTIAL DIAGNOSIS

Red Nodules on Legs   Erythema nodosum, other forms of panniculitis, cutaneous panarteritis nodosa. *Note:* Erythema nodosum is hot, very tender, and never ulcerates.

LABORATORY EXAMINATIONS

Skin Testing   Patients with an association with mycobacterial infection are highly sensitive to tuberculin and purified protein derivative (PPD); and, therefore, skin testing to mycobacterial antigens should be performed. In such patients, mycobacterial DNA sequences can be found by PCR.

DIAGNOSIS

By clinical findings and biopsy.

COURSE AND PROGNOSIS

Chronic recurrent, scarring.

MANAGEMENT

Antituberculous therapy in those cases where a mycobacterial etiology is proved. In other cases, bed rest, tetracyclines, and potassium iodide have proved effective. Systemic glucocorticoids are sometimes necessary for remission. In some cases dapsone is effective.

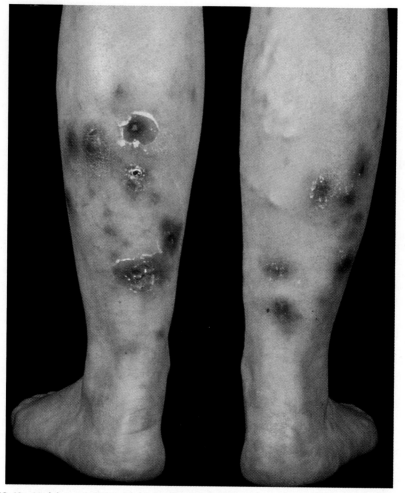

Figure 12-40 Nodular vasculitis *Multiple, deep-seated, brown to bluish nodules, particularly on the posterior aspects of both lower legs. The lesions, which are relatively asymptomatic, may undergo necrosis forming slowly healing ulcers. Varicose veins are also seen on the right calf.*

KAWASAKI'S DISEASE

Kawasaki's disease (KD) is an acute febrile illness of infants and children, characterized by cutaneous and mucosal erythema and edema with subsequent desquamation, cervical lymphadenitis, and complicated by coronary artery aneurysms (20%).
Synonym: Mucocutaneous lymph node syndrome.

EPIDEMIOLOGY

Age of Onset   Peak incidence at 1 year, mean 2.6 years, uncommon after 8 years. Most cases of KD in adults probably represent toxic shock syndrome.

Sex   Male predominance, 1.5:1.

Race   USA> Japanese> African Americans> white children.

Etiology   Idiopathic.

Season   Winter and spring.

Geography   First reported in Japan, 1961; United States, 1971. Epidemics.

Clinical Phases

Phase I: Acute Febrile Period   Abrupt onset of fever, lasting approximately 12 days, followed (usually within 1 to 3 days) by most of the other principal features.

Phase II: Subacute Phase   Lasts approximately until day 30 of illness; fever, thrombocytosis, desquamation, arthritis, arthralgia, carditis; highest risk for sudden death.

Phase III: Convalescent Period   Begins within 8 to 10 weeks after onset of illness; begins when all signs of illness have disappeared and ends when ESR returns to normal; very low mortality rate during this period.

PATHOGENESIS

Generalized vasculitis. Endarteritis of vasavasorum involves adventitia/intima of proximal coronary arteries with ectasia, aneurysm formation, vessel obstruction, and distal embolization with subsequent myocardial infarction. Other vessels: brachiocephalic, celiac, renal, iliofemoral arteries. Increased activated helper T cells and monocytes, elevated serum-soluble interleukin (IL)-2 receptor levels, elevated levels of spontaneous IL-1 production by peripheral blood mononuclear cells, anti-endothelial antibodies, and increased cytokine-inducible activation antigens on the vascular endothelium occur in KD. T cell response is driven by a conventional antigen.

HISTORY

Prodrome   Usually none.

Symptoms   Fever, sudden onset. Constitutional symptoms of diarrhea, arthralgia, arthritis, meatitis, tympanitis, photophobia.

PHYSICAL EXAMINATION

Skin Lesions

Phase I   Lesions appear 1 to 3 days after onset of fever. Duration 12 days average. Nearly all mucocutaneous abnormalities occur during this phase.

Exanthem   Erythema usually first noted on palms/soles, spreading to involve trunk and extremities within 2 days. First lesions: erythematous macules; lesions enlarge and become more numerous (Fig. 12-41). Type: urticaria-like lesions most common; morbilliform pattern second most common; scarlatiniform and erythema multiforme-like in <5% of cases. Confluent macules to plaque-type erythema on perineum, which persist after other findings have resolved. Edema of hands/feet: deeply erythematous to violaceous; brawny swelling with fusiform fingers. Palpation: lesions may be tender.

Mucous Membranes   Bulbar conjunctivae: bilateral vascular dilatation (conjunctival injection); noted 2 days after onset of fever; duration, 1 to 3 weeks (throughout the febrile course). Lips: red, dry, fissured, hemorrhagic crusts; duration, 1 to 3 weeks. Oropharynx: diffuse erythema. Tongue: "strawberry" tongue (erythema and protuberance of papillae of tongue).

Phase II Desquamation highly characteristic; follows resolution of exanthem (Fig. 12-42). Begins on tips of fingers and toes at junction of nails and skin; desquamating sheets of palmar/plantar epidermis are progressively shed.

Phase III Beau's lines (transverse furrows on nail surface) may be seen. Possible telogen effluvium.

General Findings Meningeal irritation. Pneumonia. Lymphadenopathy, usually cervical node: ≥1.5 cm, slightly tender, firm. Arthritis/arthralgias, knees, hips, elbows. Pericardial tamponade, dysrhythmias, rubs, congestive heart failure, left ventricular dysfunction.

DIFFERENTIAL DIAGNOSIS

Juvenile rheumatoid arthritis, infectious mononucleosis, viral exanthems, leptospirosis, Rocky Mountain spotted fever, toxic shock syndrome, staphylococcal scalded-skin syndrome, erythema multiforme, serum sickness, systemic lupus erythematosus, Reiter's syndrome.

LABORATORY EXAMINATIONS

Chemistry Abnormal liver function tests.

Hematology Leukocytosis ($>$18,000/μL).

Phase II Thrombocytosis after the tenth day of illness. Elevated ESR.

Phase III ESR returns to normal.

Urinalysis Pyuria.

Dermatopathology Arteritis involving small and medium-sized vessels with swelling of endothelial cells in postcapillary venules, dilatation of small blood vessels, lymphocytic/monocytic perivascular infiltrate in arteries/arterioles of dermis.

Electrocardiography Prolongation of PR and QT intervals; ST-segment and T-wave changes.

Echocardiography Coronary aneurysms.

Cardiac Angiography Coronary aneurysms in 25% of cases.

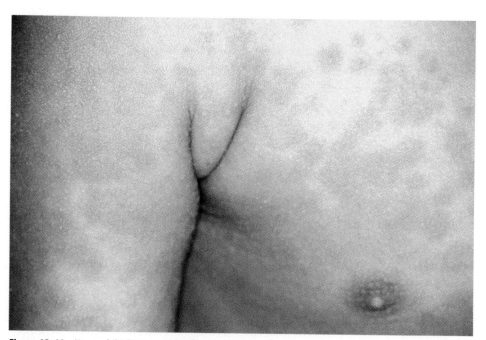

Figure 12-41 Kawasaki's disease *Blotchy erytema on the trunk of a child; bulbar conjunctivitis, lymphadenopathy and strawberry tongue were also present.*

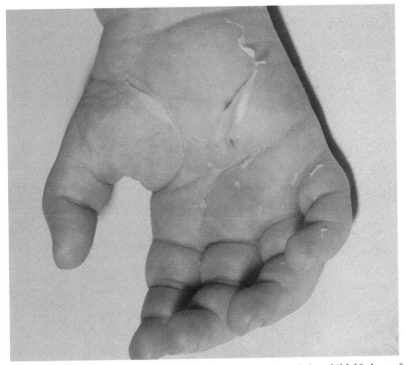

Figure 12-42 Kawasaki's disease *Shedding of the skin on the palm of this child 10 days after the acute illness.*

Diagnosis Diagnostic criteria: fever spiking to >39.4°C, lasting ≥5 days without other cause, associated with four of five criteria: (1) bilateral conjunctival injection; (2) at last one of following mucous membrane changes: injected/fissured lips, injected pharynx, "strawberry" tongue; (3) at least one of the following extremity changes: erythema of palms/soles, edema of hands/feet, generalized/periungual desquamation; (4) diffuse scarlatiniform erythroderma, deeply erythematous maculopapular rash, iris lesions; and (5) cervical lymphadenopathy (at least one lymph node ≥1.5 cm in diameter).

COURSE AND PROGNOSIS

Clinical course triphasic. Uneventful recovery occurs in majority. Cardiovascular system complications in 20%. Coronary artery aneurysms occur within 2 to 8 weeks, associated with myocarditis, myocardial ischemia/infarction, pericarditis, peripheral vascular occlusion, small bowel obstruction, stroke. Case fatality rate, .5 to 2.8% of cases, and is associated with coronary artery aneurysms.

MANAGEMENT

Diagnosis should be made early and attention directed at prevention of the cardiovascular complications.

Hospitalization Recommended during the phase I illness, monitoring for cardiac and vascular complications.

Systemic Therapy

Intravenous Immunoglobulin 2 g/kg as a single infusion over 10 h together with aspirin.

Aspirin 100 mg/kg/d until fever resolves or until day 14 of illness, followed by 5 to 10 mg/kg/d until ESR and platelet count have returned to normal.

Glucocorticoids Contraindicated. Associated with a higher rate of coronary aneurysms.

REITER'S SYNDROME

Reiter's syndrome (RS) is defined by an episode of peripheral arthritis of more than 1 month's duration occurring in association with urethritis and/or cervicitis and frequently accompanied by keratoderma blennorrhagicum, circinate balanitis, conjunctivitis, and stomatitis. The classic triad is arthritis, urethritis, and conjunctivitis.

EPIDEMIOLOGY

Age of Onset 22 years (median) in postvenereal type.

Sex 90% of patients are males (postvenereal type).

Race Most common in Caucasians from northern Europe; rare in Asians and African blacks.

Genetic Diathesis HLA-B27 occurs in up to 75% of Caucasians with RS but in only 8% of healthy Caucasians. Patients who are HLA-B27–negative have a milder course, with significantly less sacroiliitis, uveitis, and carditis.

Associated Disorders Incidence of RS may be increased in HIV-infected individuals.

Etiology Unknown.

PATHOGENESIS

RS appears linked to two factors: *genetic factors*, i.e., HLA-B27 in up to 75% of affected Caucasians (8% incidence in unaffected Caucasians) and *enteric pathogens* such as *Salmonella enteritidis, S. typhimurium, S. heidelberg; Yersinia enterocolitica, Y. pseudotuberculosis; Campylobacter fetus; Shigella flexneri*. Two patterns are observed: the *epidemic form*, which follows venereal exposure, the most common type in the United States and the United Kingdom; and the *postdysenteric form*, the most common type of RS in continental Europe and North Africa.

HISTORY

Onset 1 to 4 weeks after infection: enterocolitis (shigellosis or other enteric pathogen infection); nongonococcal urethritis (*Chlamydia* or *Ureaplasma urealyticum*). Urethritis and/or conjunctivitis usually first to appear, followed by arthritis.

Symptoms consist of malaise, fever, dysuria, urethral discharge. Eyes: red, slightly sensitive. Arthritis: tendon/fascia inflammation results in pain over ischial tuberosities, iliac crest, long bones, ribs; heel pain at site of attachment of plantar aponeurosis and/or Achilles tendon; back pain; joint pains.

PHYSICAL EXAMINATION

Skin Lesions Resemble those of psoriasis, especially on palms/soles, glans penis, mouth. *Keratoderma blennorrhagicum* (KDB): brownish-red papules or macules, sometimes topped by vesicles that enlarge; centers of lesions become pustular and/or hyperkeratotic, crusted (Fig. 12-43), i.e., resembling mollusk shells, mainly on palms and soles. Scaling erythematous, psoriasiform plaques on scalp, elbows, and buttocks. Erosive patches resembling pustular psoriasis may occur, especially on shaft of penis, scrotum. *Circinate balanitis* (Fig. 12-44): shallow erosions with serpiginous, micropustular borders if uncircumcised; crusted and/or hyperkeratotic plaques if circumcised, i.e., psoriasiform.

Nails Small subungual pustules; extensive involvement may result in onycholysis and extensive subungual hyperkeratosis with erythema surrounding the nail.

Mucous Membranes *Urethra* Sterile serous or mucopurulent discharge.

Mouth Erosive lesions on tongue or hard palate resembling migratory glossitis.

Eyes Conjunctivitis, mild, evanescent, bilateral; anterior uveitis.

Systemic Findings Arthritis: oligoarticular, involving up to six joints, asymmetric; most commonly knees, ankles, small joints of feet; diffuse swelling of fingers and toes.

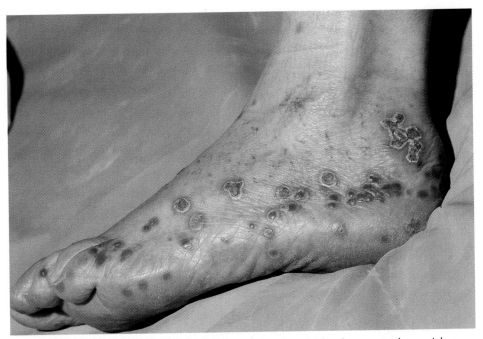

Figure 12-43   Reiter's syndrome: keratoderma blennorrhagicum   *Red-to-brown papules, vesicles, and pustules with central erosion and characteristic crusting and peripheral scaling on the dorsilateral and plantar foot.*

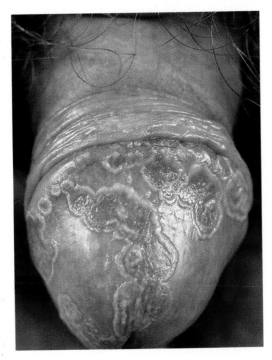

Figure 12-44   Reiter's syndrome: balanitis circinata   *Moist, well-demarcated erosions with a slightly raised micropustular circinate border on the glans penis.*

DIFFERENTIAL DIAGNOSIS

Arthritis Plus Skin Lesions   Psoriasis vulgaris with psoriatic arthritis, disseminating gonococcal infection, SLE, ankylosing spondylitis, rheumatoid arthritis, gout, Behçet's disease.

LABORATORY EXAMINATIONS

Hematology   Nonspecific findings: anemia, leukocytosis, thrombocytosis, elevated ESR.

Culture   Urethral culture negative for gonococcus.

Serology   ANA, rheumatoid factor negative. Rule out HIV infection.

Dermatopathology   Spongiosis, vesiculation; later, psoriasiform epidermal hyperplasia, spongiform pustules, parakeratosis. Perivascular neutrophilic infiltrate in superficial dermis; edema.

DIAGNOSIS

Clinical findings; ruling out other spondylo- and reactive arthropathies.

COURSE AND PROGNOSIS

Only 30% of RS patients develop complete triad of arthritis, urethritis, conjunctivitis; 40% have only one manifestation, i.e., incomplete RS. Majority have self-limited course, with resolution in 3 to 12 months. RS may relapse over many years in 30%. Chronic deforming arthritis in 10 to 20%.

MANAGEMENT

Prior Infection   Role of antibiotic therapy unproven in altering course of postvenereal RS.

Cutaneous Manifestations   Similar to management of psoriasis (see Psoriasis and Ichthyosiform Dermatoses, Section 3). Balanitis: low-potency glucocorticoids. Palmar/plantar: potent glucocorticoid preparations, which are more effective under plastic occlusion. Extensive or refractory disease: phototherapy and PUVA.

Prevention of Articular Inflammation/Joint Deformity   Rest, nonsteroidal anti-inflammatory agents. Occasionally, phenylbutazone is indicated. In HIV-infected individuals, zidovudine may ameliorate RS.

Methotrexate, Etretinate   Effective in treatment of arthritis and cutaneous manifestations.

SARCOIDOSIS

Sarcoidosis is a chronic granulomatous inflammation affecting diverse organs, but it presents primarily as skin lesions, eye lesions, bilateral hilar lymphadenopathy, and pulmonary infiltration.

EPIDEMIOLOGY

Age of Onset   Under 40 years (range 12 to 70 years).

Sex   Equal incidence in males and females.

Race   All races. In the United States and South Africa, much more frequent in blacks. The disease occurs worldwide; frequent in Scandinavia.

Other Factors   Etiology unknown. The disease can occur in families.

HISTORY

Onset of lesions: days (presenting as acute erythema nodosum) or months (presenting as asymptomatic sarcoidal papules or plaques on skin or pulmonary infiltrate discovered on routine chest radiography). Constitutional symptoms such as fever, fatigue, weight loss, arrhythmia.

PHYSICAL EXAMINATION

Skin Lesions   Brownish, purple infiltrated plaques that may be annular, polycyclic, serpiginous, and occur mainly on extremities, buttocks, and trunk. (Fig. 12-45) Central clearing with slight atrophy may occur. Multiple scattered maculopapular or papular lesions, .5 to 1 cm, yellowish brown, or purple occur mainly on the face (Fig. 12-46) and extremities. Occasionally, nodules, firm, purple or brown, may arise on the face, trunk, or extremities; and diffuse, violaceous, soft doughy infiltrations may occur on the nose, cheeks, or earlobes (*lupus pernio*). (Fig. 12-47) Sarcoidosis tends to infiltrate old scars, which then exhibit translucent purple-red or yellowish papules or nodules. *Note:* On blanching with glass slide, all cutaneous lesions of sarcoidosis reveal "apple jelly" yellowish brown color. On the scalp sarcoidosis may cause scarring alopecia with brownish sarcoidal infiltrates still present in the scarred tissue.

Systems Review   Enlarged parotids, pulmonary infiltrates, cardiac dyspnea, neuropathy, uveitis, kidney stones. In acute bilateral hilar sarcoidosis, particularly in young women, the first clinical manifestations of sarcoidosis may be erythema nodosum and arthritis. This combination is called *Sjögren syndrome*. The *Heerford syndrome* describes patients with fever, parotid enlargement, uveitis, and facial nerve palsy.

LABORATORY EXAMINATIONS

Dermatopathology   Large islands of epithelioid cells with a few giant cells and lymphocytes (so-called naked tubercles). Asteroid bodies in large histiocytes; occasionally fibrinoid necrosis.

Skin Tests   Intracutaneous tests for recall antigens usually but not always negative.

Imaging   Systemic involvement is verified radiologically by gallium scan and transbronchial, liver, or lymph node biopsy. In 90% of patients: hilar lymphadenopathy, pulmonary infiltrate.

Blood Chemistry   Increased level of serum angiotensin-converting enzyme (ACE), hypergammaglobulinemia, hypercalcemia.

DIAGNOSIS

Tissue biopsy of skin or lymph nodes is the best criterion for diagnosis of sarcoidosis.

Systemic Sarcoidosis

Systemic glucocorticoids for active ocular disease, active pulmonary disease, cardiac arrhythmia, CNS involvement, or hypercalcemia.

Cutaneous Sarcoidosis

Glucocorticoids *Local* Intralesional triamcinolone, 3 mg/mL, effective for small lesions.

Systemic Glucocorticoids for widespread or disfiguring involvement.

Hydroxychloroquine 100 mg bid for widespread or disfiguring lesions refractory to intralesional triamcinolone. Only sometimes effective.

Methotrexate Low-dose for widespread skin and systemic involvement. Not always effective.

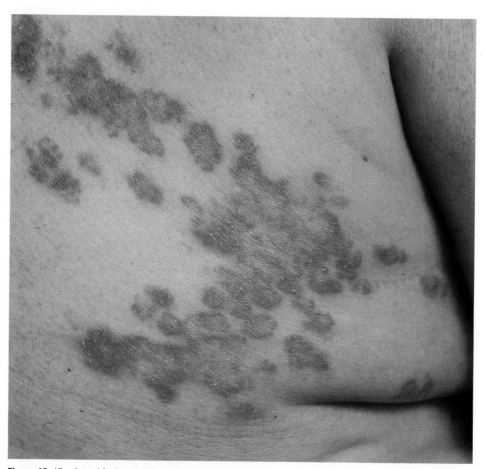

Figure 12-45 Sarcoidosis: granulomatous lesions *Multiple, circinate, confluent, firm, brownish-red, infiltrated plaques that show a tendency to resolve in the center. Thus, the annular appearance. The lesions are diascopy positive, i.e., an "apple-jelly" tan-pink color remains in lesions after compression with glass.*

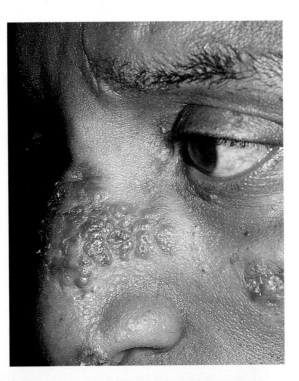

Figure 12-46 Sarcoidosis
Brownish-to-purple papules coalescing to irregular plaques, occurring on the face of this man who also had massive pulmonary involvement. Blanching with a glass slide reveals "apple-jelly" color in the lesions.

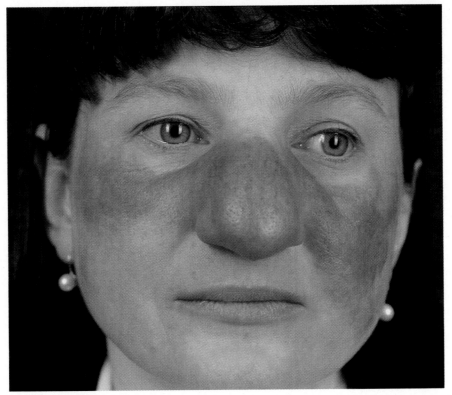

Figure 12-47 Sarcoidosis *This is the classic appearance of "lupus pernio" with violaceous, soft, doughy infiltrations on cheeks and nose, which is thus grossly enlarged.*

GENETIC, METABOLIC, ENDOCRINE, AND NUTRITIONAL DISEASES

DISEASES IN PREGNANCY

Pruritic Urticarial Papules and Plaques of Pregnancy

Pruritic urticarial papules and plaques of pregnancy (PUPPP) is a distinct pruritic eruption of pregnancy that usually begins in the third trimester, most often in primigravidae. There is no increased risk of fetal morbidity or mortality.

Synonyms: Polymorphic eruption of pregnancy, toxemic rash of pregnancy, late-onset prurigo of pregnancy.

EPIDEMIOLOGY

Age of Onset   Average age 27 years.

Etiology   Unknown. The development of striae has been theorized to be a trigger for PUPPP. A relationship with maternal and fetal weight gain has been proposed but challenged.

Incidence   Estimated to be 1:120 to 240 pregnancies.

Risk Factors   76% of patients are primigravidae. Some cases have been associated with polyhydramnios.

PATHOGENESIS

Not understood. There is little evidence to suggest that PUPPP is an autoimmune disease. This reaction may represent a maternal response to paternal antigens expressed in the fetal placenta. No HLA subtypes appear to be predisposed when patients are compared with North American controls.

HISTORY

Average time of onset is 36 weeks of gestation, usually 1 to 2 weeks before delivery. *Symptoms and signs can start in the postpartum period.* Pruritus develops on the abdomen, often in the striae distensae, and is severe enough to disrupt sleep. The skin lesions evolve over 1 to 2 weeks and taper off over 7 to 10 days.

PHYSICAL EXAMINATION

Skin Lesions   Erythematous papules, 1 to 3 mm (Fig. 13-1), quickly coalescing into urticarial plaques (Fig. 13-2) with polycyclic shape and arrangement; blanched halos around the periphery of lesions. Vesicles, 2 mm, may occur in the plaques, but bullae are absent. Target lesions are observed in 19%. Although pruritus is the chief symptom, excoriations are infrequent.

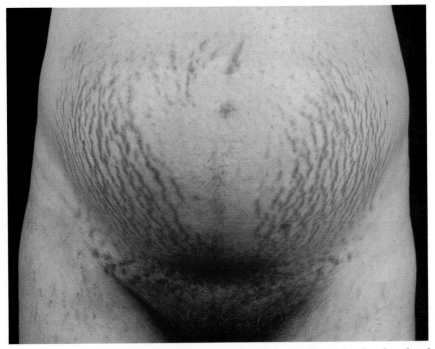

Figure 13-1 Pruritic urticarial papules and plaques of pregnancy *Small papules distributed and confluent within striae distensae on the abdomen in a pregnant woman (35 weeks of gestation). Note sparing of periumbilical skin. Lesions were extremely pruritic, causing sleepless nights and great stress.*

Distribution 50% of the women affected have papules and plaques in the striae distensae (Fig. 13-1); the abdomen, buttocks, thighs (Fig. 13-2), upper inner arms, and lower back also may be affected. The face, breasts, palms, and soles are rarely involved. The periumbilical area is usually spared (Fig. 13-1).

Mucous Membranes No lesions.

DIFFERENTIAL DIAGNOSIS

Pruritic Abdominal Rash in Late Pregnancy Herpes gestationis, adverse cutaneous drug reaction, allergic contact dermatitis, metabolic pruritus, atopic dermatitis.

LABORATORY EXAMINATIONS

Laboratory Findings Moderately elevated leukocyte count and erythrocyte sedimentation rate (ESR) consistent with third-trimester pregnancy. Normal human chorionic gonadotropin, estrogen, and progesterone. No circulating com-

plement-binding herpes gestationis (HG) factor. (See Herpes Gestationis, page 409).

Histology Superficial or mid-dermal, loosely arranged perivascular lymphohistiocytic infiltrate with rare eosinophils, dermal edema. Focal parakeratosis, spongiosis, microvesiculation, or exocytosis. Overall, the histologic findings are nondiagnostic.

Direct Immunofluorescence No consistent findings of immunoreactants in lesional or perilesional skin.

DIAGNOSIS

Clinical; immunofluorescence studies may be needed to differentiate PUPPP from herpes gestationis (HG), especially if there are papulovesicular lesions. HG has to be excluded because it has been claimed that it may be associated with increased risk of fetal morbidity and mortality. It often starts in the periumbilical areas, and the striae are not prominently involved. HG always has C3 deposition at the basement membrane zone and is associated with HLA-B8, -DR3.

COURSE AND PROGNOSIS

The majority of women studied do not have a recurrence in the postpartum period or with subsequent pregnancies or with the use of oral contraceptives. A recurrence is usually much milder than the original episode. The symptoms usually resolve within 10 days of delivery.

In one large series, there were no premature or postmature infants or spontaneous abortions; one stillborn (one of a set of twins) was reported. No consistent congenital abnormalities have been observed.

MANAGEMENT

Tropical High-potency topical steroids may relieve the pruritus within 24 to 72 h. Application of topical steroids often can be tapered off after 1 week of therapy. Baths and emollients may be helpful as supportive measures.

Systemic Oral prednisone in doses of 10 to 40 mg/d has been used for severe cases; often the symptoms are relieved in 24 h. Oral antihistamines are generally ineffective.

Delivery The symptoms can be so severe and exhausting for the pregnant woman that early delivery may be a consideration; often, however, the patient is better within several days.

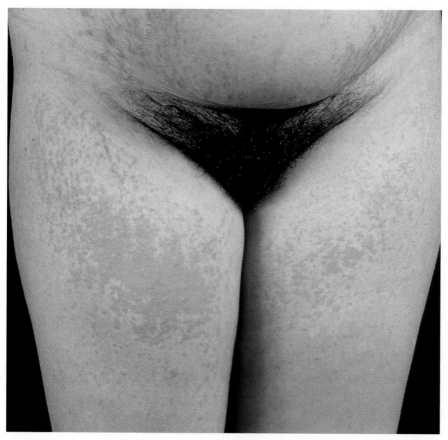

Figure 13-2 Pruritic urticarial papules and plaques of pregnancy *Papular lesions characteristically also occur on the thighs, where they coalesce to urticarial plaques. Note that excoriations are absent despite the often excrutiating pruritus.*

Herpes Gestationis

Herpes gestationis (HG)[1] is a pruritic polymorphic inflammatory dermatosis of pregnancy and the postpartum period. It is an autoimmune process with circulating complement-fixing IgG antibodies in the serum. It creates severe discomfort for the affected, but it is debated whether fetal prognosis is impaired.

EPIDEMIOLOGY

Age of Onset   Usually between the fourth and seventh months of pregnancy but has been reported also during the first trimester and in the postpartum period. Postpartum exacerbations are common. HG may or may not recur in subsequent pregnancies and is exacerbated by the use of estrogen- or progesterone-containing medications (e.g., contraceptives).

Sex   Pregnant women.

Race   All races.

Incidence   Estimated to be 1:10,000 deliveries.

PATHOGENESIS

Etiology unknown. The C3 deposition at the basement membrane and HG factor suggest an immunologic mechanism similar to that in bullous pemphigoid. It is postulated that IgG antibodies arise in response to antigenic stimulus peculiar to pregnancy, perhaps in the amnion. These antibodies have specificity for a 180-kDa antigen, a hemidesmosomal peptide. Antibodies deposited on the basement membrane zone activate the complement cascade, which in turn generates an inflammatory response.

Relationship between HG and bullous pemphigoid is unresolved. This relationship is suggested by the morphologic similarity of lesions, similar immunopathology, and the fact that the HG antigen is very closely related to, if not identical with, the 180-kDa bullous pemphigoid antigen.

Hormonal factors undoubtedly play an important role. Onset in pregnancy or thereafter, postpartum flares, and exacerbations with hormone-producing tumors or contraceptives.

[1]HG is a morphologic term because of the grouping of vesicular lesions. HG is unrelated to any known viral infection.

HISTORY

Extremely pruritic eruption that causes great anxiety, particularly in primigravidae. Family history is noncontributory.

PHYSICAL EXAMINATION

Skin Lesions   Papulovesicular eruption, mainly on the abdomen and lateral sides of the trunk but also involving other areas, including palms, soles, chest, back, and face. Lesions vary from erythematous, edematous papules to urticarial lesions (Fig. 13-3) and large, tense bullae that evolve into erosions and crusts. Grouping of lesions is pronounced, hence the name *herpes gestationis*. Milder cases present with only a few erythematous papules or isolated edematous urticarial plaques.

Mucous Membranes   Spared.

Hair and Nails   Spared.

Systemic Review   Negative.

DIFFERENTIAL DIAGNOSIS

Pruritic Eruption in Pregnancy   Pruritic urticarial papules and plaques of pregnancy that usually occur late in pregnancy are also severely pruritic, generally are not vesicular, and have no immunoreactants at the epidermal-dermal junction. Other papular eruptions in pregnancy: erythema multiforme, dermatitis herpetiformis, bullous pemphigoid, adverse cutaneous drug reaction, atopic dermatitis.

LABORATORY EXAMINATIONS

Dermatopathology   Lymphohistiocytic infiltrates with eosinophils and occasional neutrophils around superficial and deep dermal-vascular plexus. Edema of the dermal papillae and epidermis with vesicular lesions showing subepidermal blister formation in a bulbous teardrop shape, liquefaction degeneration of basal cells of variable degree, and characteristic foci of basal cell necrosis over the tips of the dermal papillae, spongiosis.

Immunopathology Heavy homogeneous linear deposition of C3 along basement membrane zone in peribullous and urticarial lesions and perilesional normal-appearing skin. Concomitant deposition of IgG in 30 to 40% of patients that is IgG1. Occasional IgA and IgM and, rarely, properdin factor B, or C1q and C4. Immunofluorescence findings persist for months and up to a year after lesions have resolved.

A serum complement-fixing factor, termed *HG factor*, is an avidly complement-fixing IgG1 antibody, (which often escapes detection by routine indirect immunofluorescence because of low concentration) in all patients. This factor binds to amniotic epithelial basement membrane.

Immunogenetic Studies Marked increase in HLA-B8, HLA-DR3, and HLA-DR4.

DIAGNOSIS

Clinical setting confirmed by histology and immunofluorescence.

Fetal Involvement

One study reveals significant fetal death and premature deliveries in a larger series of HG patients, whereas other studies suggest that there is no increase in fetal mortality. Children born of affected mothers usually have no skin lesions; but in some reports babies have been described with urticarial, vesicular, and bullous lesions that resolve spontaneously. C3 deposition has been noted in clinically normal as well as affected infant skin, and HG factor has been detected in the sera of some infants born to affected mothers.

MANAGEMENT

Systemic glucocorticoids given orally in doses equivalent to 20 to 40 mg of prednisone. Exacerbation during remission may require higher doses. Prednisone is gradually tapered during the postpartum period. A few patients do not require systemic prednisone and can be controlled with antihistamines and topical steroids.

Infants born to affected mothers who have received high doses of prednisone should be examined carefully by a neonatologist for adrenal insufficiency. Cutaneous lesions in infants are transient and do not require therapy.

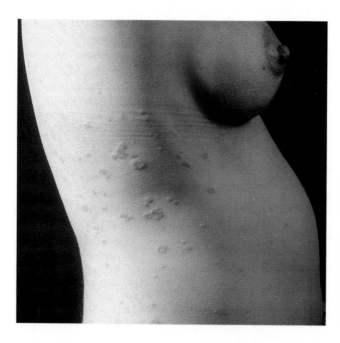

Figure 13-3 Herpes gestationis *Very pruritic papules and urticarial plaques in a pregnant woman at 28 weeks of gestation. Although herpes gestationis is a blistering disease, it often presents initially as shown here. Note also that, in contrast to PUPPP (Fig. 13-1), the abdomen and thus the striae are spared.*

DIABETES MELLITUS

CLASSIFICATION OF DIABETES MELLITUS (DM)

Primary
  Insulin-dependent DM (IDDM, type 1)   Non-insulin-dependent DM (NIDDM, type 2): non-obese NIDDM, obese NIDDM, maturity-onset DM of the young (MODY)

Secondary
  Pancreatic disease, hormonal abnormalities, drug-, chemical-induced, insulin receptor abnormalities, genetic syndromes

SKIN DISEASES ASSOCIATED WITH DIABETES MELLITUS

ACANTHOSIS NIGRICANS AND LIPODYSTROPHY
Associated with insulin resistance in DM. Insulin-like epidermal growth factors may cause epidermal hyperplasia.

ADVERSE CUTANEOUS DRUG REACTIONS (Section 18)
Insulin: local reactions—lipodystrophy with decreased adipose tissue at sites of subcutaneous injection; Arthus-like reaction with urticarial lesion at site of injection.
Systemic insulin allergy: Urticaria, serum sickness-like reactions.
Oral hypoglycemic agents: Exanthematous eruptions, urticaria, erythema multiforme, photosensitivity.

CALCIPHYLAXIS

CUTANEOUS PERFORATING DISORDERS
Rare conditions in which horny plugs perforate into the dermis or dermal debris is eliminated through epidermis.

DIABETIC BULLAE (*Bullosis diabeticorum*)

DIABETIC DERMOPATHY
Circumscribed, atrophic, slightly depressed, brownish lesions on the anterior lower legs. The pathogenic significance of diabetic angiopathy remains to be established but is often accompanied by microangiopathy.

ERUPTIVE XANTHOMAS

GRANULOMA ANNULARE

INFECTIONS (Sections 20 and 21)
Poorly controlled DM associated with increased incidence of primary (furuncles, carbuncles) and secondary *Staphylococcus aureus* infections (paronychia, wound/ulcer infection, cellulitis (*S. aureus*, group A streptococcus), erythrasma, dermatophytoses (tinea pedis, onychomycosis), candidiasis (mucosal and cutaneous), mucormycosis with necrotizing nasopharyngeal infections.

NECROBIOSIS LIPOIDICA

PERIPHERAL NEUROPATHY (Diabetic foot)

PERIPHERAL VASCULAR DISEASE (Section 14)
Small-vessel vasculopathy (microangiopathy): Involves arterioles, venules, and capillaries. Characterized by basement membrane thickening and endothelial cell proliferation. Presents clinically as acral erysipelas-like erythema, ±ulceration.
Large-vessel vasculopathy: Incidence greatly increased in DM. Ischemia is most often symptomatic on lower legs and feet with gangrene and ulceration. Predisposes to infections.

SCLEREDEMA
Synonym: Scleredema adultorum of Buschke. Need not be associated with DM. Onset correlates with duration of DM and with presence of microangiopathy. Skin findings: poorly demarcated scleroderma-like induration of the skin and subcutaneous tissue of the upper back, neck, proximal extremities. Rapid onset and progression.

XANTHOMAS
Disseminated, varied, associated with DM. Occurs in setting of grossly uncontrolled DM and very high serum triglycerides.

Diabetic Bullae

Large, intact bullae arise spontaneously on the lower legs, feet, dorsa of the hands and fingers on noninflamed bases (Fig. 13-4). When ruptured, oozing bright red erosions result but heal after several weeks. Localization on dorsa of hand and fingers suggests porphyria cutanea tarda, but abnormalities of porphyrin metabolism are not found. Neither trauma nor an immunologic mechanism has been implicated. Histologically, bullae show intra- or subepidermal clefting without acantholysis. The 46-year-old diabetic male shown in Figure 13-4 had his great toe amputated because of gangrene. One year after surgery he started to develop bullae in the pretibial areas and dorsum of the foot as shown in the illustration.

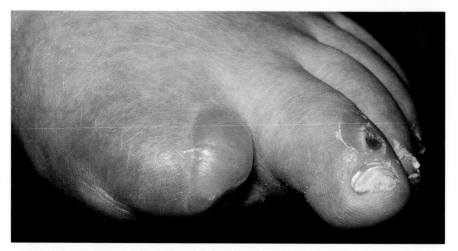

Figure 13-4 Diabetic bulla *A large, intact bulla is seen on the stump of the amputated great toe and a crusted erosion on the second toe. The patient has many of the vascular complications of diabetes mellitus, i.e., renal failure with renal transplantation, blindness secondary to retinopathy, and artherosclerosis obliterans resulting in amputation of the great toe. Diabetic bullae have occurred previously on his lower legs.*

Diabetic Foot and Diabetic Neuropathy

Peripheral neuropathy is responsible for the "diabetic foot." Others factors are angiopathy, atherosclerosis, infection. Diabetic neuropathy is combined motor and sensory. Motor neuropathy leads to weakness and muscle wasting distally. Autonomic neuropathy accompanies sensory neuropathy and leads to anhidrosis, which may not be confined to the distal extremities. Sensory neuropathy predisposes to neurotropic ulcers over bony prominences of feet, usually on the great toe and sole as shown here (Fig. 13-5). Ulcers are surrounded by a ring of callus and may extend to interlying joint and bone, leading to osteomyelitis.

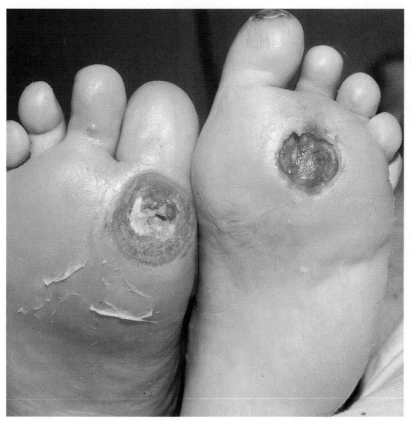

Figure 13-5 Diabetic, neuropathic ulcers on the soles *Two large ulcers overlying the first right and second left metacarpophalangeal joints. The patient, a 56-year-old male with diabetes mellitus of 20 years' duration, has significant sensory neuropathy of the feet and lower legs as well as peripheral vascular disease.*

Diabetic Dermopathy

Circumscribed, atrophic, slightly depressed lesions on the anterior lower legs that are asymptomatic (Fig. 13-6). They arise in crops and gradually resolve, but new lesions appear. The pathogenic significance of diabetic angiopathy remains to be established, but it is often accompanied by micro-angiopathy.

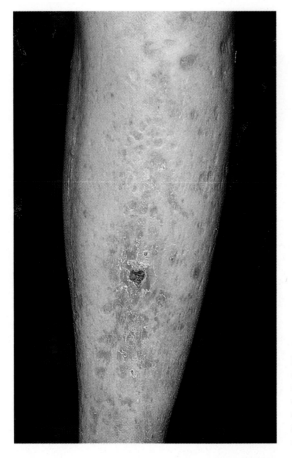

Figure 13-6   Diabetic dermopathy   *A crusted erosion at the site of traumatic injury and many old pink depressed areas are seen on the anterior leg of a 56-year-old male with diabetes mellitus. The other leg had identical findings.*

Necrobiosis Lipoidica

Necrobiosis lipoidica (NL) is a cutaneous disorder often, but not always, associated with diabetes mellitus. The lesions are distinctive, sharply circumscribed, multicolored plaques occurring on the anterior and lateral surfaces of the lower legs.

Synonym: Necrobiosis lipoidica diabeticorum.

EPIDEMIOLOGY

Age of Onset Young adults, early middle age, but not uncommon in juvenile diabetics.

Sex Female:male ratio 3:1 in both diabetic and nondiabetic forms.

Incidence <1% of diabetic individuals.

Etiology Unknown.

Precipitating Factors A history of preceding trauma to the site can be a factor in the initial development of the lesions; for this reason, NL is often present on the shins and over the bony areas of the feet.

PATHOGENESIS

The arteriolar changes in the areas of necrobiosis of the collagen have been thought by some to be precipitated by aggregation of platelets. The granulomatous inflammatory reaction is believed to be due to alterations in the collagen. The severity of NL is not related to the severity of the diabetes mellitus. Furthermore, control of the diabetes has no effect on the course of NL.

HISTORY

NL occurs often in the setting of long-standing juvenile-onset diabetes. Slowly evolving and enlarging over months, persisting for years. Cosmetic disfigurement but pain in lesions that develop ulcers.

Relationship to DM One-third of patients have clinical DM; one-third have abnormal glucose tolerance only; one-third have normal glucose tolerance.

PHYSICAL EXAMINATION

Skin Lesions Lesion starts as brownish-red or skin-colored papule that slowly evolves into well-demarcated waxy plaques of variable size (Fig. 13-7). The sharply defined and slightly elevated border retains a brownish-red color, whereas the center becomes depressed and acquires a yellow-orange hue. Through the shiny and atrophic epidermis multiple telangiectasias of variable size are seen. Larger lesions formed by centrifugal enlargement or merging of smaller lesions acquire a serpiginous or polycyclic configuration. Ulceration commonly occurs within the plaques (Fig. 13-8), and healed ulcers result in depressed scars. Burned-out lesions appear as tan areas with telangiectasia.

Distribution Usually 1 to 3 lesions; >80% occur on the shin; at times symmetric. Less commonly, on feet, arms, trunk, or face and scalp; rarely may be generalized.

DIFFERENTIAL DIAGNOSIS

Sarcoidosis, granuloma annulare (not infrequently coexists with NL), xanthoma.

LABORATORY EXAMINATIONS

Dermatopathology Sclerotic collagen and obliteration of the bundle pattern, necrobiosis of connective tissue, and concomitant granulomatous infiltration in lower dermis. Fat-containing foam cells are often present, imparting the yellow color to the clinical lesion. Dermal blood vessels show microangiopathy with endothelial thickening and focal deposits of PAS-positive material.

Immunofluorescence Presence of immunoglobulins and complement (C3) in the walls of the small blood vessels.

Chemistry Abnormal glucose tolerance test.

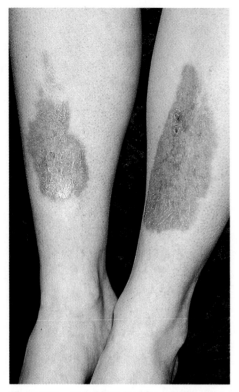

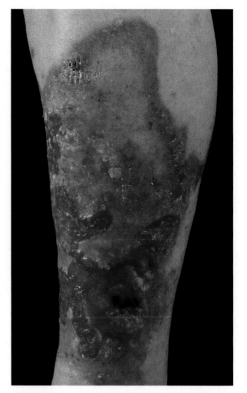

Figure 13-7 Necrobiosis lipoidica, diabeticorum: early *Large, symmetric plaques with active yellow-orange to tan-pink, well-demarcated, raised, firm borders in the pretibial regions of a 25-year-old diabetic female. The central parts of the lesions are depressed with atrophic changes of epidermal thinning and telangiectasias against yellow background.*

Figure 13-8 Necrobiosis lipoidica, late with ulceration *A very extensive plaque of necrobiosis lipoidica on the lower leg of a diabetic female. The lower portion has undergone necrosis with extensive, deep ulceration. These lesions can become very painful.*

DIAGNOSIS

The lesions are so distinctive that biopsy confirmation is not necessary; biopsy may be required in early stages to rule out granuloma annulare.

COURSE AND PROGNOSIS

The lesions are indolent and can enlarge to involve large areas of the skin surface unless treated. The lesions are unsightly, and patients are often upset about the cosmetic appearance. Ulcerated areas within NL are painful but usually can be healed over time.

MANAGEMENT

Glucocorticoids

Topical The application of potent glucocorticoids under occlusion is helpful in some cases; however, ulcerations may occur when NL is occluded.

Intralesional Intralesional triamcinolone, 5 mg/mL, into active lesions or lesion margins usually arrests extension of plaques of NL. This is the best treatment, with 3 to 5 mg/mL triamcinolone suspension.

Ulceration Most ulcerations within NL lesions heal with local wound care; if not, excision of entire lesion with grafting may be required.

Calciphylaxis

Calciphylaxis is characterized by progressive cutaneous necrosis associated with small- and medium-sized vessel calcification occurring in the setting of end-stage renal disease, diabetes mellitus, and hyperparathyroidism. Cutaneous involvement presents as initial painful geographic areas of ischemia that progress to gangrene and ulceration of the subcutaneous fat, dermis, and epidermis; secondary infection and sepsis are common.

Synonym: Widespread systemic calcification.

EPIDEMIOLOGY

Age of Onset   Middle to old age.

Sex   Equal.

Risk Factors   End-stage renal disease, diabetes mellitus, advanced HIV disease.

PATHOGENESIS

The pathogenesis is poorly understood. In animal models, calciphylaxis is described as a condition of induced systemic hypersensitivity in which tissues respond to appropriate challenging agents with calcium deposition. Calciphylaxis is associated with chronic renal failure, secondary hyperparathyroidism, and an elevated calcium phosphate end product. Implicated "challenging agents" include glucocorticoids, albumin infusions, intramuscular tobramycin, iron dextran complex, calcium heparinate, immunosuppressive agents, and vitamin D.

HISTORY

Even early infarctive lesions are exquisitely tender.

Systems Review   Occurs in end-stage renal disease. Most patients are diabetic. Onset often closely follows initiation of hemo- or peritoneal dialysis.

PHYSICAL EXAMINATION

Skin Lesions   Initially preinfarctive ischemic plaques occur, appearing as mottling or having a livedo reticularis pattern, dusky red to violaceous (Fig. 13-9). Bullae may form over ischemic tissue. As epidermis/dermis eventually becomes necrotic, central infarcted sites are black, resulting in tightly adherent black, leathery slough Fig. 13-9. Lesions gradually enlarge over weeks to months; and, when debrided, deep ulcers reaching down to the fascia result. Ischemic skin frequently becomes secondarily infected; infection can remain localized or become invasive, causing cellulitis and bacteremia.

Large areas of induration can be defined on palpation as platelike subcutaneous masses that extend beyond infarcted or ulcerated areas. Even early lesions are extremely tender, unless advanced sensory neuropathy coexists.

Distribution   Distal extremities, most commonly on the lateral and posterior calves; abdomen, buttocks; fingers; glans penis.

DIFFERENTIAL DIAGNOSIS

Panniculitis, vasculitides, necrobiosis lipoidica with ulceration, dystrophic calcinosis cutis, metastatic calcification (calcium deposited in dermis and not the subcutaneous fat), scleroderma, atheroembolization, atherosclerosis obliterans, disseminated intravascular coagulation (purpura fulminans), pyoderma gangrenosum, warfarin necrosis, heparin necrosis. *Vibrio vulnificus* cellulitis, other necrotizing cellulitides.

LABORATORY EXAMINATIONS

Chemistry   Azotemia. Calcium $\times$ phosphate ion product usually elevated.

Parathormone (PTH)   Levels usually elevated.

Cultures   Rule out secondary infection.

Dermatopathology   Incisional biopsy shows calcification of the media of small- and medium-sized blood vessels in the dermis and subcutaneous tissue. Intraluminal fibrin thrombi are present. Ischemia results in intralobular or septal fat necrosis, accompanied by a sparse lymphohistiocytic infiltrate.

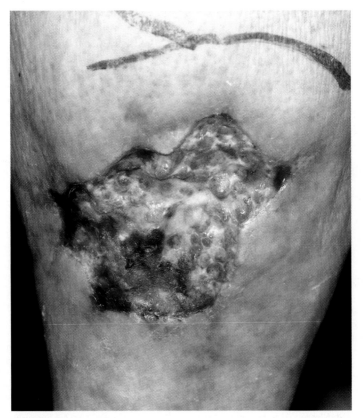

Figure 13-9 Calciphylaxis *A very large ulceration of the right calf, surrounded by a mottled violaceous zone of ischemia, in a diabetic female with renal failure. The areas outlined in blue demarcated subcutaneous induration corresponding to sites of early calciphylaxis. The ulcer is sharply demarcated with eschar in a portion and extending into the subcutaneous fat; the lesion was extremely painful and, secondarily infected with* Xanthomonas maltophilia. *The reticulated and mottled surrounding skin is ischemic and may become necrotic.*

Imaging Radiographs of affected extremities show calcium deposition outlining small and large vessels. Microcalcification of calciphylaxis is difficult to visualize.

DIAGNOSIS

Made on history of renal failure, clinical findings, elevated PTH level, elevated calcium × phosphate ion product, and histologic features.

COURSE AND PROGNOSIS

The course in most patients tends to be slowly progressive despite all therapeutic interventions. Pain is a constant feature, associated with ischemia and secondary infection. In advanced disease, gangrene of fingers, toes, and penis may result in autoamputation. Local infection and sepsis are common complications. Overall, the prognosis is poor, and the mortality rate is very high.

MANAGEMENT

Calciphylaxis is best managed by early diagnosis, treatment of renal failure, partial parathyroidectomy when indicated, aggressive debridement of necrotic tissue, and avoidance of precipitating factors such as systemic glucocorticoids.

GENETIC, METABOLIC, ENDOCRINE, AND NUTRITIONAL DISEASES

HEREDITARY HEMORRHAGIC TELANGIECTASIA

Synonym: **OSLER-WEBER-RENDU SYNDROME**

Hereditary hemorrhagic telangiectasia is an autosomal dominant condition affecting blood vessels, especially in the mucous membranes of the mouth and the GI tract. The disease is frequently heralded by recurrent epistaxis that appears often in childhood. The diagnostic lesions are small, pulsating, macular and papular, usually punctate, telangiectases (Fig. 13-10) on the lips, face, palms/soles, fingers/toes, nail beds, tongue, conjunctivae, nasopharynx, and throughout the GI and genitourinary tracts. In the 18-year-old male, shown in the illustration, there had been repeated epistaxis, but the telangiectasias had gone unnoticed until the patient was evaluated for anemia. Careful history then revealed that the patient's father had a minor form of the same condition. Pulmonary A-V fistulas may occur. Chronic blood loss results in anemia. Electrocautery and pulse dye laser are used to destroy cutaneous and accessible mucosal lesions. Estrogens have been used to treat recalcitrant bleeding.

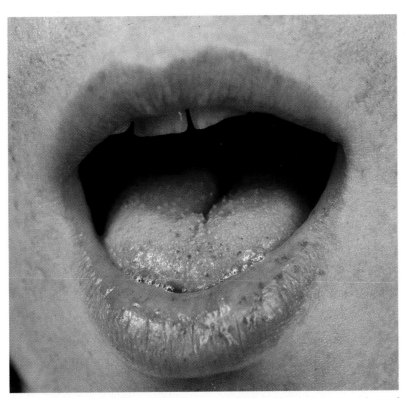

Figure 13-10   Hereditary hemorrhagic telangiectasia   *Multiple 1–2-mm, discrete, red macular and papular telangiectases on the lower lip and tongue.*

CUSHING'S SYNDROME AND HYPERCORTICISM

Cushing's syndrome (CS) is characterized by truncal obesity, moon face, acne, abdominal striae, hypertension, decreased carbohydrate tolerance, protein catabolism, psychiatric disturbances, and amenorrhea and hirsutism in females associated with excess adrenocorticosteroid of endogenous or exogenous source. Cushing's disease refers to CS associated with pituitary adrenocorticotropic hormone (ACTH)-producing adenoma. CS medicamentosum refers to CS caused by exogenous administration of glucocorticoids.

A plethoric obese person with a "classic" habitus that results from the redistribution of fat: moon facies Fig. 13-11, "buffalo" hump, truncal obesity, and thin arms. Purple striae, mostly on the abdomen and trunk; atrophic skin with easy bruising and telangiectasia; facial hypertrichosis with pigmented hairs and often increased lanugo hairs on the face and arms; androgenetic alopecia in females. Acne of recent onset (without comedones) or flaring of existing acne. General symptoms consist of fatigue and muscle weakness, hypertension, personality changes, amenorrhea in females, polyuria, and polydipsia. Work-up includes determination of blood glucose, serum potassium, and free cortisol in 24-h urine. Abnormal dexamethasone suppression test with failure to suppress endogenous cortisol secretion when dexamethasone is administered. Elevated ACTH. CT scan of the abdomen and the pituitary. Assessment of osteoporosis. Management consists of elimination of exogenous glucocorticoids or the detection and correction of underlying endogenous cause.

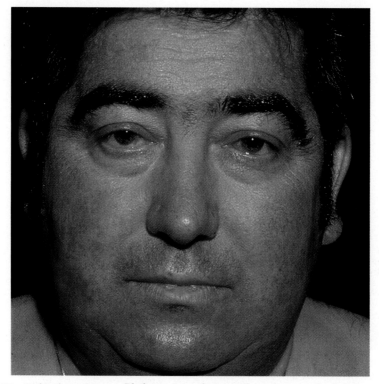

Figure 13-11   Cushing's syndrome   *Plethoric moon facies with erythema and telangiectases of cheek and forehead; the face, neck, and supraclavicular areas show increased deposition of fat.*

GRAVES' DISEASE AND HYPERTHYROIDISM

Graves' disease (GD) is a disorder with three major manifestations: hyperthyroidism with diffuse goiter, ophthalmopathy, and dermopathy. The manifestations often do not occur together, may not occur at all, and run courses that are independent of each other.

Dermopathy (pretibial myxedema) Early lesions: bilateral, asymmetric, firm, non-pitting nodules and plaques that are pink, skin-colored, or purple (Fig. 13-12, right). Late lesions: confluence of early lesions, which symmetrically involve the pretibial regions and may, in extreme cases, result in grotesque involvement of entire lower legs and dorsa of feet; smooth surface with orange peel-like appearance, later becomes verrucous (Fig. 13-12, right).

Fingers show acropachy, which represents diaphyseal proliferation of the periosteum and clubbing (Fig. 13-12, left); a special type of onycholysis (Plummer's nail) (Section 28) is also seen in which the free edge of the nail becomes undulated and curves upward.

Ophthalmopathy of GD has two components, spastic (stare, lid lag, lid retraction) and mechanical (proptosis (Fig. 13-12, top), oph-thalmoplegia, congestive oculopathy, chemosis, conjuctivitis, periorbital swelling, and potential complications of corneal ulceration, optic neuritis, optic atrophy). Exophthalmic ophthalmoplegia: ocular muscle weakness with inward gaze, convergence, strabismus, diplopia.

Thryoid Diffuse toxic goiter, asymmetric, lobular. Asymmetric and lobular thyroid enlargement, often with the presence of a bruit.

MANAGEMENT

Thyrotoxicosis Antithyroid agents block thyroid hormone synthesis. Ablation of thyroid tissue, surgically or by radioactive iodine.

Ophthalmopathy Symptomatic treatment in mild cases. Severe cases: prednisone 100 to 120 mg/d initially, tapering to 5 mg/d. Orbital radiation. Orbital decompression.

Dermopathy Topical glucocorticoid preparations under plastic occlusion for several months are usually effective. Low-dose oral glucocorticoids (prednisone, 5 mg/d).

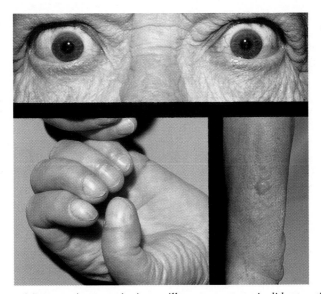

Figure 13-12 Graves' disease *A composite image illustrates: proptosis, lid retraction; thyroid acropachy (osteoarthropathy) with clubbing; and the pink- and skin-colored papules, plaques in the pretibial region.*

HYPOTHYROIDISM AND MYXEDEMA

Myxedema results from insufficient production of thyroid hormones and can be caused by multiple disturbances, characterized by accumulation of water-binding mucopolysaccharides in the dermis, resulting in thickening of facial features and doughy induration of the skin. Cretinism denotes hypothyroidism dating from birth, resulting from developmental abnormalities. Hypothyroidism may be *thyroprivic* (e.g., congenital, primary idiopathic, postablative); *goitrous* (e.g., heritable biosynthetic defects, maternally transmitted, iodine deficiency, drug-induced or chronic thyroiditis); *trophoprivic* (e.g., pituitary); or *hypothalamic* [e.g., infection (encephalitis), neoplasm].

Early symptoms of **myxedema** are slow in developing, are nonspecific, and are often overlooked: fatigue, lethargy, cold intolerance, constipation, stiffness and cramping of muscles, carpal tunnel syndrome, menorrhagia. *Later*: intellectual and motor activity slow, appetite declines, weight increases, and voice becomes deeper.

There is a dull, expressionless facies (Fig. 13-13), with puffiness of eyelids. The nose is broadened, and the lips are thick. Skin appears swollen, cool, waxy, rough, dry, coarse, and pale due to increased concentration of water and mucopolysaccharides and vasoconstriction; increased skin creases (Figure 13-13). Palms and soles are yellow-orange due to carotenemia, palmoplantar keratoderma.

The hair is dry, coarse, and brittle. There is thinning of hair due to slow growth in the scalp, beard (Fig. 13-13), and sexual areas. Eyebrows: alopecia of the lateral one-third. The nails are brittle, and grow slowly. The tongue is large, smooth, red, and clumsy.

Workup Includes thyroid function tests, TSH, scintigraphic imaging and serum cholesterol ($\uparrow$).

Management By replacement therapy.

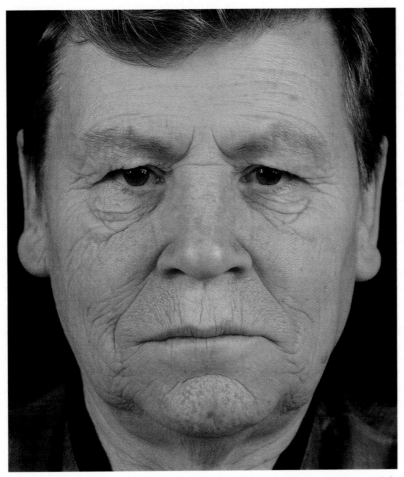

Figure 13-13 Myxedema *Dry, pale skin; thinning of the lateral eyebrows; puffiness of the face and eyelids; increased number of skin creases; dull, expressionless, beardless facies.*

ADDISON'S DISEASE

Addison's disease is a syndrome resulting from adrenocortical insufficiency caused by infections (e.g., tuberculosis) and is characterized as an autoimmune disease. The disease is insidious and is characterized by progressive generalized brown hyperpigmentation, slowly progressive weakness, fatigue, anorexia, nausea, and, frequently, GI symptoms (vomiting and diarrhea). The patients state that their summer tan did not fade during the winter, or that friends comment that they are "getting darker." Weakness is a prominent symptom, occurring first after stress and then progressing to chronic weakness, fatigue, and weight loss.

Suggestive laboratory changes include a low-serum sodium, a high-serum potassium, and elevation of the blood urea nitrogen. The diagnosis is confirmed by specific tests of adrenal insufficiency. Nausea, vomiting, and diarrhea are frequent complaints. There may be orthostatic hypotension with dizziness and syncope.

The patient may appear completely normal except for a generalized brown hyperpigmentation. There is increased brown melanin hyperpigmentation in those areas where pigmentation normally occurs. It is therefore the *change* in the intensity of the pigmentation in these areas or *the development of new areas* of pigmentation, e.g., gingival or buccal mucous membrane, that is significant. The intensity of the pigmentation is related to skin phototype; but even light-skinned persons (SPT I and II) can develop marked pigmentation where they have increased blood levels of melanotropins. Pigmentation occurs in areas that are *normally* hyperpigmented: around the eyes, gingival and buccal mucous membrane, tongue, nipples, creases of the palms, over bony prominences (Fig. 13-14), in the linea nigra (abdomen), axillae, and anogenital areas in males and females. Pigmentation also develops in new scars following surgery.

The differential diagnosis includes hemochromatosis, porphyria cutanea tarda, chronic renal failure, hepatic cirrhosis, functioning benign endocrine tumors, such as chromophobe adenomas that produce ACTH and associated peptides [i.e., Nelson's syndrome, metastatic cancers (especially lung), carcinoid, Whipple's intestinal lipodystrophy, vitamin B_{12} deficiency, chemotherapy (doxorubicin, busulfan, bleomycin, systemic 5-fluorouracil), and systemic scleroderma] in the early stages before the induration is detectable. The diagnosis may be subtle since the problem may not present with a change in skin pigmentation but with only abdominal symptoms (i.e., weakness, weight loss, vague abdominal pain, and diarrhea). If the diagnosis is abnormal, generalized pigmentation can be docu-

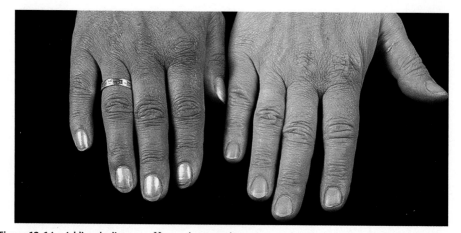

Figure 13-14 Addison's disease *Hyperpigmentation representing an accentuation of normal pigmentation on the hand of a patient with Addison's disease (left). For comparison, the hand of a normal individual, matched for ethnic pigmentation, is shown on the right.*

mented and the patient will have GI complaints. The laboratory diagnosis may be impossible in the early phases of the disease. A screening test used for diagnosis is: plasma cortisol 30 to 60 min after 250 μg cosyntropin intramuscularly or intravenously. Diffused, increased brown melanin hyperpigmentation of recent onset must always be thoroughly investigated and diagnosed since the treatment of Addison's disease can be lifesaving. Adrenal crises, in fact, can be fatal and may be precipitated by trauma (auto accidents, surgery) or severe illness. This disease should be managed by an endocrinologist. Hormone replacement is given using hydrocortisone 20 to 30 mg/d with two-thirds of the dose taken in the morning $\pm$ .05 to .1 mg fludrocortisone for the mineralocorticoid component of the adrenal hormones.

GENERALIZED PRURITUS WITHOUT DIAGNOSTIC SKIN LESIONS

Persistent severe pruritus, like pain, is a dominating factor in existence; from day to day it takes over one's life. Intense pruritus may, in fact, be more maddening for the patient than pain because there is no effective medication to control the pruritus; pain usually can be controlled with analgesics. The physician, therefore, feels somewhat helpless in the management of these unfortunate patients. Pruritus leads to sleepless nights; a state of permanent fatigue ensues that precludes work and confounds family relationships. The approach to the patient with generalized pruritus without identifiable skin lesions is to consider this symptom in the same manner as a patient with factitious (i.e., not based on organic disease) dermatosis—*generalized pruritus and factitious dermatosis are both diagnoses of exclusion:* all organic causes must be excluded within reasonable limits.

The differential diagnosis of generalized pruritus is presented in Table 13-1, the workup of these patients is presented in Table 13-2, and pruritus ani is presented in Table 13-3. The appearance of a typical patient is shown in Figure 13-15.

Table 13-1 DIFFERENTIAL DIAGNOSIS OF PRURITUS

Metabolic and Endocrine Conditions	Malignant Neoplasms	Drug Ingestion	Infestations
Hyperthyroidism	Lymphoma and	Subclinical drug	Scabies[1]
Diabetes mellitus	leukemia	sensitivities:	Pediculosis corporis
Hypothyroidism	Other cancer (rare)	Aspirin, alcohol,	Hookworm
Chronic	Multiple myeloma	dextran, polymyxin	(ancylostomiasis)
renal failure		B, morphine, codeine,	Onchocerciasis
		scopolamine, D-	Ascariasis
		tubocurarine	

Hematologic Disease	Hepatic Disease	Psychogenic States	Miscellaneous Conditions
Polycythemia vera	Obstructive biliary	Transitory:	Dry skin (xerosis)
Paraproteinemia from	disease	Periods of emotional	"Senile" pruritus[2]
iron deficiency	Pregnancy (intrahepatic	stress	Pregnancy-related
	cholestasis)	Persistent:	disorders
		Delusions of parasitosis	Fiberglas exposure
		Psychogenic pruritus	Various primary skin
		Neurotic excoriations	diseases

[1]Diagnostic lesions may or may not present.

[2]Unexplained intense pruritus in patients over 70 years without obvious "dry skin" and with no apparent emotional stress.

Table 13-2 APPROACH TO THE DIAGNOSIS OF GENERALIZED PRURITUS WITHOUT DIAGNOSTIC SKIN LESIONS

It is critical to recognize that nonspecific skin changes can be induced by rubbing and scratching. The false conclusion that a dermatologic cause for itching is necessarily present just because a rash can be seen is a trap that must be avoided.

The approach to the patient with persistent generalized pruritus begins with careful examination of the skin, followed by additional attention to the general history, review of systems, general physical examination, and investigations as outlined below.

Initial Visit

1. Detailed history of pruritus:
   - Are there any skin lesions that precede the itching?
   - Severity: Does the itching keep the patient awake?
2. History of constitutional symptoms, weight loss, fatigue, fever, malaise
3. Has there been a recent emotional stress situation?
4. History of oral or parenteral medication that can be a cause of generalized pruritus without a rash
5. Examine carefully for subtle primary skin disorders as a cause of the pruritus; xerosis or asteatosis, scabies, pediculosis (nits?)
6. General physical examination including *all* the lymph nodes; rectal examination and stool guaiac in adult patients (depending on the individual clinical situation, may be deferred to second or later visit)
7. If pruritus has been present for more than 2 weeks, obtain additional data (see nos. 1 – 4 below)
8. If dry skin or winter itch is a reasonable possible explanation, give the patient bath oil, followed by an emollient ointment. No soap; the bath is therapeutic, not for cleansing the skin; shower to clean.
9. Check for dermographism.
10. Follow-up appointment in 2 weeks

Subsequent Visit(s)

If no relief from symptomatic treatment given on the first visit, proceed as follows:
1. Refer patient to a dermatologist.
2. Obtain chest roentgenogram.
3. Detailed review of systems.
4. Laboratory tests: complete blood tests including erythrocyte sedimentation rate, fasting blood sugar, renal function tests, liver function tests, hepatitis antigens, thyroid tests, stool for parasites.
5. If the diagnosis has not been established at this point, the patient should be referred to an internist for complete workup including pelvic examination and Pap smear.

SOURCE: Bernhard JD, ed. *Itch Mechanisms and Management of Pruritis.* New York, McGraw-Hill, 1994, pp. 211–215.

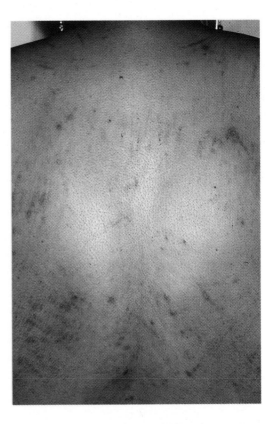

Figure 13-15 Pruritus without diagnostic skin lesions *This patient had multiple scratch marks due to compulsive scratching because of severe pruritus. There were no other, and in particular, no diagnostic lesions. Work up revealed biliary cirrhosis without jaundice.*

Table 13-3 PRURITUS ANI

Many patients, in desperation, become resigned to accepting pruritus ani as part of their lives and endure the embarrassment and the sleepless nights.

Pruritus ani is pruritus of the anal skin without evidence of a primary dermatologic disorder sometimes seen in this region, *viz,* dermatophytosis, candidiasis, psoriasis, or seborrheic dermatitis. Pinworms are a rare cause and are seen usually only in children. The major factor in the pathogenesis of pruritus ani is irritation from the presence of fecal soiling on the anal skin; this is most often the result of incomplete cleansing of the area after defecation but also results in some persons from the weakness of the anal sphincter, which allows for fecal soiling when the rectum is distended by the arrival of feces or with flatus. The vicious cycle is irritation → itching → rubbing with the development of lichenificiation → more pruritus. When lichenificiation is present, control begins with a *very limited* course of potent topical corticosteroids to reduce lichenification. The main thrust of the management, however, must be directed at two provoking factors:

1. *Paroxysmal compulsive rubbing and scratching of the anal sphincter and skin around it.* Anxiety and stress appear to contribute to the itching. The "fits" of rubbing or scratching occur most often after defecation and at night, when the patient is often awakened by the itching. These bouts of pruritus can be somewhat relieved by menthol-camphor lotions.
2. *Poor anal hygiene.* Strict, "squeaky" clean and cleansing with cotton pledgets soaked in witch hazel is ideal. Whenever possible, a shower or tub bath is the best method of cleansing; a more convenient method is with a bidet. After cleansing the area, liberal application of talcum powder helps absorb the fecal soiling that can occur during the day; ointments and oily lotions may actually aggravate the pruritus.

SCURVY

Scurvy is an acute or chronic disease of infancy and of middle and old age caused by dietary deficiency of ascorbic acid (vitamin C). The disorder is characterized principally by anemia, hemorrhagic manifestations in the skin (ecchymoses and perifollicular hemorrhage) and in the musculoskeletal system (hemorrhage into periosteum and muscles), and changes in the gums (loosening of teeth, bleeding gums).
Synonym: Vitamin C deficiency.

EPIDEMIOLOGY AND ETIOLOGY

Age of Onset   6 to 12 months; middle to old age.

Etiology *Infancy/Childhood*   Diet consisting of only processed milk with no added citrus fruit or vegetables. Result of parental neglect.

Adulthood   Edentulous persons who live alone, cook for themselves, and do not eat salads and uncooked vegetables. Affected individuals often have other dietary deficiencies as well.

Precipitating Factors
Pregnancy, lactation, and thyrotoxicosis increase requirements of ascorbic acid; alcoholism.

PATHOGENESIS

Humans are unable to synthesize ascorbic acid and require it as an essential dietary vitamin. Total-body pool of vitamin C varies from 1.5 to 3 g. First symptoms of depletion (i.e., petechial hemorrhages and ecchymoses) occur when pool size is $< .5$ g.

The best-understood function of vitamin C is in synthesis of collagen. Deficiency leads to impairment of peptidyl hydroxylation of procollagen, reduction in collagen formation, and secretion with associated capillary fragility.

HISTORY

With no vitamin C intake, symptoms of scurvy occur after 1 to 3 months. Lassitude, weakness, arthralgia, and myalgia.

PHYSICAL EXAMINATION

Skin Lesions   Petechiae, follicular hyperkeratosis with perifollicular hemorrhage, especially on the lower legs (Fig. 13-16). Hair becomes fragmented and buried in these perifollicular hyperkeratotic papules (corkscrew hairs); extensive ecchymoses (Fig. 13-17), which can be generalized. Nails: Splinter hemorrhages.

Mouth   Gingiva: swollen, purple, spongy, and bleeds easily; findings occur in more advanced scurvy. Loosening and loss of teeth.

Musculoskeletal   Hemorrhage into periosteum of long bones and into joints causes painful swellings and, in children, epiphyseal separation. Sternum may sink inward: scorbutic rosary (elevation at rib margins).
Retrobulbar, subarachnoid, intracerebral hemorrhage can cause death.

DIFFERENTIAL DIAGNOSIS

Thrombocytopenia, senile purpura, coagulopathy, anticoagulant drug therapy (warfarin, heparin), cryoglobulinemia, vasculitis.

Gingival Hypertrophy
Poor dental hygiene, drug-induced gingival hyperplasia, leukemia, pregnancy.

LABORATORY EXAMINATIONS

Hematology   Normocytic, normochromic anemia resulting from bleeding into tissues. Folate deficiency is also common, resulting in macrocytic anemia. Positive capillary fragility test.

Chemistry   Platelet ascorbic acid level usually $<25\%$ of normal value, serum ascorbic acid level $\downarrow$.

Imaging   X-ray findings diagnostic.

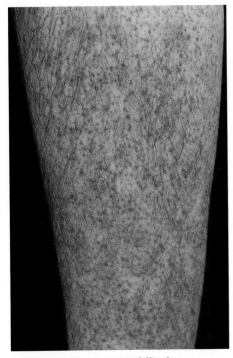

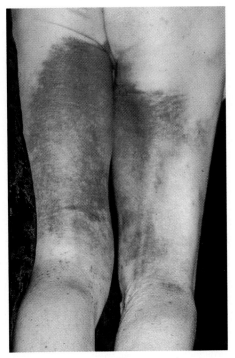

Figure 13-16 Scurvy *Perifollicular hemorrhage on the leg. The follicles are often plugged by keratin (perifollicular hyperkeratosis). This eruption occurred in a 46-year-old alcoholic, homeless male, who also had bleeding gums and loose teeth.*

Figure 13-17 Scurvy *These extensive ecchymoses occurred in an edentulous 65-year-old male who lived alone and whose food intake consisted mainly of biscuits soaked in water.*

DIAGNOSIS

Clinical findings confirmed by low ascorbic acid level.

COURSE AND PROGNOSIS

Unless treated, scurvy is fatal. On treatment, spontaneous bleeding ceases within 24 h, muscle and bone pain fade quickly, bleeding from gums stops in 2 to 3 days.

MANAGEMENT

In suspected cases, blood should be obtained for ascorbic acid level and therapy begun immediately.

Ascorbic Acid 100 mg 3 to 5 times daily until 4 g is given; then 100 mg/d is curative in days to weeks.

ZINC DEFICIENCY AND ACRODERMATITIS ENTEROPATHICA

Acrodermatitis enteropathica (AE) is a genetic disorder of zinc absorption, presenting in infancy, characterized by a triad of acral dermatitis (face, hands, feet, anogenital area), alopecia, and diarrhea; nearly identical clinical findings occur in other individuals with acquired zinc deficiency (AZD) due either to dietary deficiency or failure of intestinal absorption.

EPIDEMIOLOGY

Age of Onset *AE:* in infants bottle-fed with bovine milk, days to few weeks. In breast-fed infants, soon after weaning. *AZD:* older individuals.

Etiology *AE:* autosomal recessive trait resulting in failure to absorb zinc. *AZD:* secondary to reduced dietary intake of zinc, malabsorption (regional enteritis, after intestinal bypass surgery for obesity), chronic alcoholism, increased urinary loss (nephrotic syndrome), hypoalbuminemic states, penicillamine therapy, high catabolic states (trauma, burns, surgery), hemolytic anemias; adolescents who eat dirt, prolonged parenteral nutrition without supplemental zinc.

PATHOGENESIS

In AE, patients do not absorb enough zinc from the diet. The specific ligand involved in basic transport mechanisms for zinc that might be abnormal in AE is not known. The defect appears to be somewhere in the early stages of zinc nutriture, where zinc is presented to the intestinal brush border. This defect can be overcome by increased zinc supply in the diet. It is not known how zinc deficiency leads to skin and other lesions.

HISTORY

AE usually starts when infant is weaned and placed on cow's milk. *AZD* concomitant with dietary change or underlying illness.

PHYSICAL EXAMINATION

Skin Findings Patches and plaques of dry, scaly, sharply marginated and brightly red, eczematous dermatitis evolving into vesiculobullous, pustular, erosive, and crusted lesions (Figs. 13-18, 13-19A). Initially occur in the perioral and anogenital areas. Later, scalp, hands and feet, flexural regions, trunk. Fingertips glistening, erythematous, with fissures and secondary paronychia. Perlèche. Lesions become secondarily infected with *Candida albicans, Staphylococcus aureus.* Impaired wound healing.

Hair and Nails Diffuse alopecia, graying of hair. Paronychia, nail ridging, loss of nails.

Mucous Membranes Red, glossy tongue; superficial aphthous-like erosions; secondary oral candidiasis.

General Examination Photophobia, irritable, depressed mood. Children with AE whine and cry constantly. Failure of growth.

DIFFERENTIAL DIAGNOSIS

Atopic dermatitis, seborrheic dermatitis, psoriasis, mucocutaneous candidiasis, glucagonoma syndrome.

LABORATORY EXAMINATIONS

CBC Anemia.

Chemistry Low serum/plasma zinc levels.

Urine Reduced urinary zinc excretion.

Dermatopathology Psoriasiform dermatitis with large, pale keratinocytes in the upper epidermis; prominent parakeratosis. There may be intraepidermal clefts with acantholysis and blisters. Sparse, superficial, perivascular lymphohistiocytic infiltrate and tortuous capillaries in the papillary dermis.

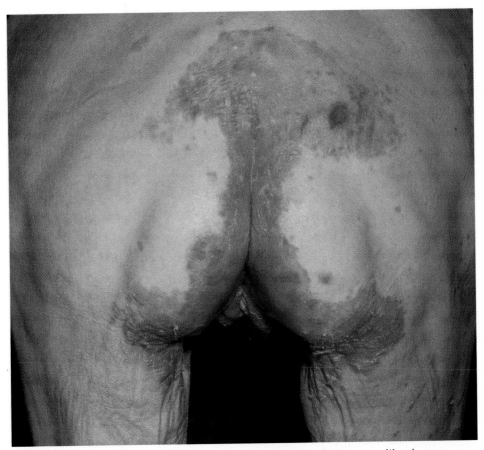

Figure 13-18   Zinc deficiency   *Well-demarcated, psoriasiform and eczematous-like plaques overlying the sacrum, intergluteal cleft, buttocks, and hip in a 60-year-old alcoholic female whose diet had consisted of pickles and cheap wine. She also had a similar eruption around the mouth, perleche, atrophic glossitis, and had glistening, shiny, oozing fingertips.*

DIAGNOSIS

Clinical diagnosis confirmed by zinc blood levels and histopathology.

COURSE AND PROGNOSIS

Before it was known that AE is due to deficient zinc uptake from the diet, it was usually fatal in infancy or early childhood. Patients failed to thrive and suffered from severe candidal and bacterial infections. After zinc replacement, severely infected and erosive skin lesions heal within 1 to 2 weeks (Fig. 13-19b), diarrhea ceases, and irritability and depression of mood improve within 24 h.

MANAGEMENT

Dietary or IV supplementation with zinc salts in 2 to 3 times the required daily amount restores normal zinc status in days to weeks.

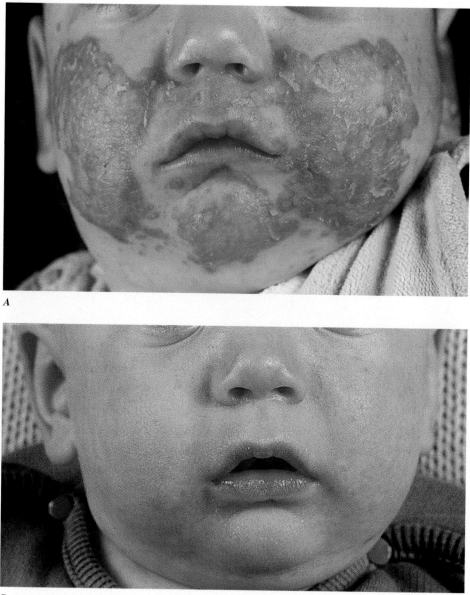

Figure 13-19 Acrodermatitis enteropathica A. *Sharply demarcated, symmetric, partially erosive, scaly, and crusted plaques on the face of an infant after weaning. Similar lesions were also found in the perigenital and perianal regions and on the fingertips. The child was highly irritable, whining, and crying and had diarrhea.* **B.** *Within 24 h after zinc replacement, the irritability and diarrhea ceased and the infant's mood improved; and after 10 days the perianal and perigenital lesions had healed.*

PELLAGRA

Pellagra is related to niacin deficiency. Niacinamide is an important constituent of coenzyme I (NAD) and coenzyme II (NADP), which function in oxidation-reduction reactions as a hydrogen ion donor and acceptor, respectively. The essential amino acid tryptophan is converted in the body to niacin. Pellagra may arise from a diet deficient in niacin or tryptophan, or both. A predominantly maize-based diet is usually implicated, but only when the maize is steamed or cooked. Pellagra is characterized by "3Ds": *d*ermatitis, *d*iarrhea and *d*ementia. Skin changes are determined by exposure to sunlight and pressure. The disorder begins with a symmetric itching and smarting erythema on the dorsa of the hands, neck, and face. Vesicles and bullae may erupt and break, so that crusting occurs and lesions become scaly (Fig. 13-20). Later, skin becomes indurated, lichenified, rough, covered by dark scales and crusts; there are cracks and fissures and a sharp demarcation from normal skin (Fig. 13-20). The distribution is striking: dorsa of hands and fingers ("gauntlet" of pellagra), band-like around the neck ("Casal's necklace"), dorsa of feet up to malleoli with sparing of the heel, and butterfly region of the face.

Diagnosis is verified by detection of decreased levels of urinary metabolites. Oral administration of 100 to 300 mg niacinamide plus other vitamins of the B complex lead to complete resolution.

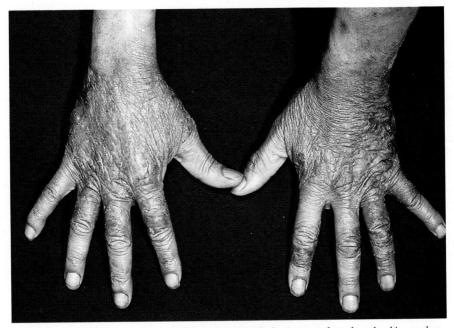

Figure 13-20   "Gauntlet" of pellagra   *Indurated, lichenified, pigmented, and scaly skin on the dorsa of the hands in a patient with niacin deficiency.*

PSEUDOXANTHOMA ELASTICUM

Pseudoxanthoma elasticum (PXE) is a serious hereditary disorder of connective tissue that involves the elastic tissue in the skin, blood vessels, and eyes. The principal skin manifestations are a distinctive *peau d'orange* surface pattern resulting from closely grouped clusters of yellow (chamois-colored) papules in a reticular pattern on the neck, axillae, and other body folds. The effects on the vascular system include gastrointestinal (GI) hemorrhage, hypertension occurring in young persons and resulting from involvement of renal arteries, and claudication. Ocular manifestations ("angioid" streaks and retinal hemorrhages) can lead to blindness.

EPIDEMIOLOGY

Age of Onset   20 to 30 years.

Incidence   1:40,000 to 1:160,000.

Inheritance   Autosomal recessive (most common) and autosomal dominant.

PATHOGENESIS

Biochemical defect is not known. Abnormalities of both collagen and elastic tissues result in fragmented and calcified elastic fibers in skin, eyes, arteries.

HISTORY

Asymptomatic skin lesions, usually present by age 30 but may go undetected until old age. There may be symptoms relating to multisystem involvement. Decreased visual acuity in a young person. Coronary artery disease: angina pectoris, myocardial infarction. Peripheral vascular disease: claudication, such as cardiac disease, hematemesis and melena, symptoms associated with hypertension. History of miscarriages.

PHYSICAL EXAMINATION

Skin Lesions   Yellow, chamois-colored papules, coalescing to form larger plaques on the sides of neck (Fig. 13-21), axillae, groin, abdomen, and thighs. Papules are arranged in a reticulated or linear pattern with furrows between individual plaques (Fig. 13-21). Skin of involved sites becomes redundant, lax, soft, and may hang in folds.

Mucous Membranes   Yellow papules may be present on the soft palate, labial mucosa, rectum, and vagina.

Eyes   Angioid streaks (Fig. 13-22), which are slate-gray, wider than blood vessels, and extend across the fundus, radiating from the optic disc (streaks represent rupture of Bruch's membrane secondary to elastic fiber defect). Macular degeneration. Retinal hemorrhages. Diminished visual acuity; blindness. Alteration of retinal pigmentation.

General Examination   Decreased or absent peripheral pulses. Hypertension. Mitral valve prolapse.

DIFFERENTIAL DIAGNOSIS

Lax Yellow Plaque(s)   Cutis laxa, Ehlers-Danlos syndrome, xanthomatosis.

Angioid Streaks   Sickle cell anemia, Paget's disease of bone, hyperphosphatemia.

LABORATORY EXAMINATIONS

Dermatopathology   Biopsy of scar can detect characteristic changes of PXE *before typical skin changes are apparent.* Swelling and irregular clumping and basophilic staining of elastic fibers in reticular dermis; with von Kossa stain, elastic fibers appear curled and "chopped up" with calcium deposition.

Imaging   X-ray: extensive calcification of the peripheral arteries of the lower extremities. Arteriography of symptomatic vessels.

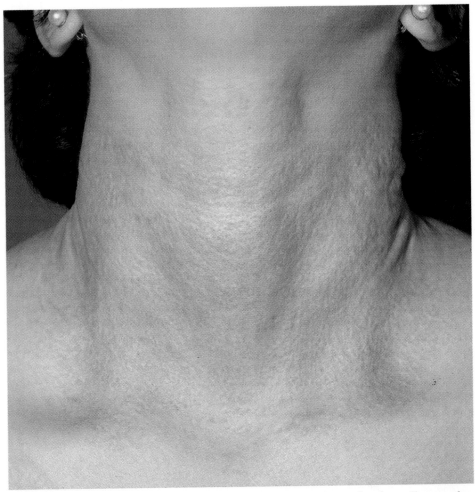

Figure 13-21   Pseudoxanthoma elasticum   *Multiple, confluent, chamois-colored or yellow papules (pseudoxanthomatous) created a large, circumferential, pebbled plaque on the neck in a 32-year-old woman. Changes in the connective tissue in this condition lead to excessive folds on the lateral neck.*

DIAGNOSIS

By the skin lesions, which are distinctive, confirmed by biopsy. Angioid streaks are also characteristic.

COURSE AND PROGNOSIS

The course is inexorably progressive. Gastric artery hemorrhage occurs commonly, resulting in hematemesis. Peripheral vascular disease presents as premature cerebrovascular accidents, atherosclerosis obliterans, or bowel angina. Pregnancies are complicated by miscarriage, cardiovascular complications. Life span is often shortened due to myocardial infarction or massive GI hemorrhage.

MANAGEMENT

Genetic counseling. Evaluate family members for PXE. Obstetrician should be aware of PXE diagnosis and follow patient carefully. Regular reevaluation by primary care physician is mandatory. For symptomatic involvement by various systems, patient should be referred to dermatologist, ophthalmologist, gastroenterologist, cardiologist, neurologist. Surgery can correct some disfiguring cutaneous changes.

Eye   Laser surgery for retinal hemorrhages.

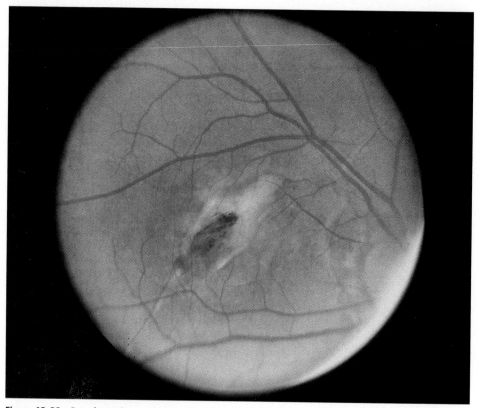

Figure 13-22   Pseudoxanthoma elasticum: angioid streak in retina   *Yellowish streaks wider than blood vessels extend across the fundus in a distribution more or less radial from the optic disk.*

TUBEROUS SCLEROSIS

Tuberous sclerosis is an autosomal dominant disease arising from a genetically programmed hyperplasia of ectodermal and mesodermal cells and manifested by a variety of lesions in the skin, CNS (hamartomas), heart, kidney, and other organs. The principal early manifestations are the triad of seizures, mental retardation, and congenital white spots (macules). Facial angiofibromata are pathognomonic but do not appear until the third or fourth year.

EPIDEMIOLOGY

Incidence   In institutions, 1:100 to 1:300; in general population, 1:20,000 to 1:100,000.

Age of Onset   Infancy.

Sex   Equal incidence.

Race   All races.

Heredity   Autosomal dominant. The genes for tuberous sclerosis have been mapped to chromosomes 16p13 and 9q34.

PATHOGENESIS

Genetic alterations of ectodermal and mesodermal cells with hyperplasia, with a disturbance in embryonic cellular differentiation.

HISTORY

White macules are present at birth or appear in infancy (80% occur by 1 year of age, 100% appear by 2 years); >20% of angiofibromata are present at 1 year of age, 50% occur by 3 years. Seizures (infantile spasms) occur in 86%; the earlier the onset of seizures, the worse the mental retardation. Mental retardation (49%).

PHYSICAL EXAMINATION

Skin Lesions   (96% incidence).

Hypomelanotic Macules   Present at birth in >80% of patients—"off-white"; one or many, usually more than three. Polygonal or "thumbprint," .5 to 2 cm; lance ovate or "ash-leaf" spots (Fig. 13-23), 3 to 4 cm (up to 12 cm); tiny white macules or "*confetti*," 1 to 2 mm (Fig. 13-24). White macules occur on trunk (56%), lower extremities (32%), upper extremities (7%), head and neck (5%).

Papules/Nodules   .1 to .5 cm, dome-shaped and smooth, exhibiting red or skin color (Fig. 13-25). Occur in the center of the face. They are firm and disseminated but may coalesce; termed adenoma sebaceum but represent angiofibromas (present in 70%).

Plaques   Represent connective tissue nevi ("shagreen" patch), present in 40%; skin colored; occur on the back and buttocks.

Periungual Papules or Nodules   Ungual fibromas (Koenen's tumors) present in 22%, arise late in childhood and have the same pathology (angiofibroma) as the facial papules. (see Fig. 28-20)

SPECIAL EXAMINATIONS

Illumination   (allow for dark adaptation) Wood's lamp examination should always be used to detect white macules with a decreased melanin pigmentation, particularily in light-skinned persons in whom white spots shine up with Wood's light.

Hair   Depigmented tufts of hair present at birth.

Associated Systems   CNS (tumors producing seizures), eye (gray or yellow retinal plaques, 50%), heart (benign rhabdomyomas), hamartomas of mixed-cell type (kidney, liver, thyroid, testes, and GI system)

DIFFERENTIAL DIAGNOSIS

Features   Associated with multiple endocrine neoplasia, Type 1.

White Spots   Focal vitiligo, nevus anemicus, tinea versicolor, nevus depigmentosus, postinflammatory hypomelanosis.

Angiofibromas   Tricholemmoma, syringoma, skin-colored papules on the face, dermal nevi. *Note:* angiofibromata of the face (Fig. 13-25) have been mistaken for and treated as acne vulgaris.

Periungual Fibromas Verruca vulgaris.

LABORATORY EXAMINATIONS

Dermatopathology *White Macules* Decreased number of melanocytes, decreased melanosome size, decreased melanin in melanocytes and keratinocytes.

Angiofibromata Proliferation of fibroblasts, increased collagen, angioneogenesis, capillary dilatation, absence of elastic tissue.

Brain "Tubers" are gliomas.

IMAGING

Skull X-Ray Multiple calcific densities.

CT Scan Ventricular deformity and tumor deposits along the striothalamic borders.

MRI Subependymal nodules.

Electroencephalography Abnormal.

Renal Ultrasound Reveals renal hamartoma.

DIAGNOSIS

The diagnosis may be difficult or impossible in an infant or child if one or two white macules are the only cutaneous finding. More than five is highly suggestive. Even when typical white "ash-leaf" or "thumbprint" macules (Fig. 13-23) are present, it is necessary to confirm the diagnosis. Confetti spots (Fig. 13-24) are virtually pathognomonic. A pediatric neurologist can then evaluate the patient with a study of the family members and by obtaining various types of imaging as well as electroencephalography. Mental retardation and seizures may be absent.

COURSE AND PROGNOSIS

A serious autosomal disorder that causes major problems in behavior, because of mental retardation, and in therapy, to control the serious seizure problem present in many patients.

In severe cases, 30% die before the fifth year of life, and 50 to 75% die before reaching adult age. Malignant gliomas are not uncommon. Genetic counseling is imperative.

MANAGEMENT

Prevention Counseling.

Treatment Laser surgery for angiofibromas.

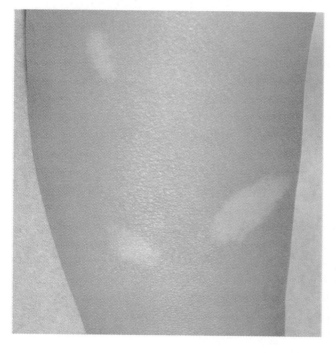

Figure 13-23 Tuberous sclerosis: ash-leaflet hypopigmented macules *Three well-demarcated, elongated (ash-leaflet shaped), hypomelanotic macules on the lower leg of a child with tan skin.*

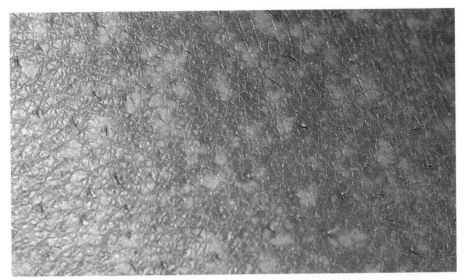

Figure 13-24 Tuberous sclerosis: "confetti" macules *Multiple, discrete, small, confetti-like, hypopigmented macules of variable size on the leg. These lesions are pathognomonic.*

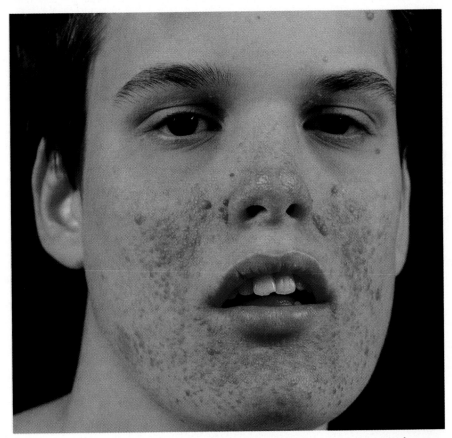

Figure 13-25 Tuberous sclerosis: angiofibromata *Confluent, small, angiomatous (erythematous, glistening) papules on the lower half of the face. These lesions were not present during the first few years of life; appeared only after the age of 4 years.*

NEUROFIBROMATOSIS

Neurofibromatosis (NF) is an autosomal dominant trait manifested by changes in the skin, nervous system, bones, and endocrine glands. These changes include a variety of congenital abnormalities, tumors, and hamartomas. Two major forms of NF are recognized: (1) classic von Recklinghausen's NF, termed *NF1* and first described in 1882; and (2) central, or acoustic NF, termed *NF2*. Both types have café-au-lait macules and neurofibromas, but only NF2 has *bilateral* acoustic neuromas (unilateral acoustic neuromas are a variable feature of NF1). An important diagnostic sign present only in NF1 is pigmented hamartomas of the iris (Lisch nodules).

EPIDEMIOLOGY

Incidence   *NF1:* 1:4000; *NF2:* 1:50,000.

Race   All races.

Sex   Males slightly more than females.

Heredity   Autosomal dominant; the gene for NF1 is on chromosome 17 (q 1.2) and that for NF2 is on chromosome 22.

PATHOGENESIS

Action of an abnormal gene on cellular elements derived from the neural crest: melanocytes, Schwann cells, endoneurial fibroblasts.

HISTORY

Café-au-lait (CAL) macules are not usually present at birth but appear during the first 3 years; neurofibromata appear during late adolescence. Neurofibromata may be tender to firm; pressure causes pain. Clinical manifestations in various organs are related to pathology: hypertensive headaches (pheochromocytomas), pathologic fractures (bone cysts), mental retardation, brain tumor (astrocytoma), short stature, precocious puberty (early menses, clitoral hypertrophy).

PHYSICAL EXAMINATION

Appearance of Patient   Patients not uncommonly consult physician only because of the physical disfigurement.

Skin Lesions   *CAL macules*   Light- or dark-brown *uniform* melanin pigmentation with sharp margination. Lesions vary in size from multiple "freckle-like" tiny macules <2 mm (Fig. 13-26), to very large brown macules >20-cm (Fig. 13-27). The common size, however, is 2 to 5 cm. Tiny freckle-like lesions in the axillae are highly characteristic ("axillary freckling") (Fig. 13-26). CAL macules also vary in number, from a few to hundreds. A few CAL macules (three or less) may be present in 10 to 20% of the normal population.

Papules/Nodules   (Neurofibromas)   Skin-colored, pink, or brown (Fig. 13-27); flat, dome-shaped or pedunculated; soft or firm; "buttonhole sign"—invagination with the tip of the index finger is pathognomonic.

Plexiform Neuromas   Drooping, soft, doughy (Fig. 13-27); may be massive, involving entire extremity, the head, or a portion of the trunk.

Distribution   Randomly distributed (Figure 13.27) but may be localized to one region (segmental NF1). The segmental type may be heritable or a localized hamartoma.

Other Physical Findings   *Eyes*   Pigmented hamartomas of the iris (Lisch nodules) begin to appear at age 5 and are present in 20% of children with NF before age 6; they can be found in 95% of patients with NF1 after age 6 but are not present in NF2. Lisch nodules are visible only with slit-lamp examination and appear as "glassy," transparent, dome-shaped, yellow-to-brown papules up to 2 mm. They do not correlate with the severity of the disease.

Musculoskeletal   Cervicothoracic kyphoscoliosis, segmental hypertrophy.

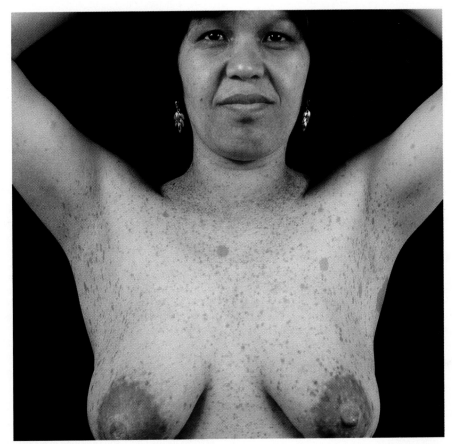

Figure 13-26   von Recklinghausen's disease (NF1)   *Several larger (>1 cm) café-au-lait macules on the upper chest and multiple small macules in the axillae (axillary "freckling") in a brown-skinned female. Myriads of early, small, pink-tan neurofibromata on the chest, breasts, and neck.*

Adrenal Pheochromocytoma Elevated blood pressure and episodic flushing.

Peripheral Nervous System Elephantiasis neuromatosa (gross disfigurement from neurofibromatosis of the nerve trunks).

Central Nervous System Optic glioma, acoustic neuroma (rare in NF1 and unilateral, but bilateral in NF2), astrocytoma, meningioma, neurofibroma.

DIFFERENTIAL DIAGNOSIS

Brown CAL-Type Macules Albright's syndrome (polyostotic fibroma, dysplasia, and precocious puberty), normal (present in 10 to 20% of population).

LABORATORY EXAMINATIONS

Dermatopathology More than 10 *melanin macroglobules* per 5 high-power fields in "split" dopa preparations. The melanin macroglobules also can be seen in routine H&E sections. They do not occur in Albright's syndrome.

Wood's Lamp Examination In white persons with pale skin, the CAL macules are more easily visualized with Wood's lamp examination.

DIAGNOSIS

Two of the following criteria:

1. Multiple CAL macules—more than six lesions with a diameter of 1.5 cm in adults and more than five lesions with a diameter of .5 cm or more in children younger than 5 years.
2. Multiple freckles in the axillary and inguinal regions

3. Based on clinical and histologic grounds, two or more neurofibromas of any type, or one plexiform neurofibroma
4. Sphenoid wing dysplasia or congenital bowing or thinning of long bone cortex, with or without pseudoarthrosis
5. Bilateral optic nerve gliomas
6. Two or more Lisch nodules on slit-lamp examination
7. First-degree relative (parent, sibling, or child) with NF1 by the preceding criteria

COURSE AND PROGNOSIS

It is important to establish the diagnosis in order to do genetic counseling and to follow patients for development of malignancy. Also, neurofibromatosis support groups help with social adjustment in severely affected persons.

There is variable involvement of the organs affected over time, from only a few pigmented macules to marked disfigurement with thousands of nodules, segmental hypertrophy, and plexiform neuromas. The mortality rate is higher than in the normal population, principally because of the development of neurofibrosarcoma during adult life. Other serious complications are relatively infrequent.

MANAGEMENT

An orthopedic physician should manage the two major bone problems: kyphoscoliosis and tibial bowing. A plastic surgeon can do reconstructive surgery on the facial asymmetry. The language disorders and learning disabilities should be evaluated by a psychologist. Close follow-up annually should be mandatory to detect sarcomas that may arise within plexiform neuromas. Surgical removal of pheochromocytoma.

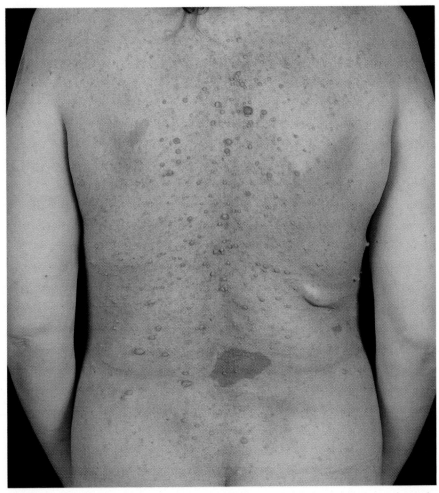

Figure 13-27 von Recklinghausen's disease (NF1) *Skin-colored and pink-tan, soft papules and nodules on the back are neurofibromata; the lesions first appeared during late childhood. Three large café-au-lait macules on the back and right arm. The large, soft, ill-defined, subcutaneous nodule on the right lower back and on the right posterior axillary line are plexiform neuromas.*

XANTHOMAS

Cutaneous xanthomas are yellow-brown, pinkish, or orange macules, papules, plaques, nodules, or infiltrations in tendons. They are characterized histologically by accumulations of xanthoma cells—macrophages containing droplets of lipids. A xanthoma may be a symptom of a general metabolic disease, a generalized histiocytosis, or a local cell dysfunction. The classification is based on this principle: (1) xanthomas due to hyperlipidemia and (2) normolipidemic xanthomas. The cause of xanthomas in the first group may be a primary hyperlipidemia, mostly genetically determined (Table 13-4), or secondary hyperlipidemia, associated with certain internal diseases such as biliary cirrhosis, diabetes mellitus, chronic renal failure, alcoholism, hyperthyroidism, and monoclonal gammopathy, or with intake of certain drugs such as beta-blockers and estrogens.

Some of the xanthomas are associated with high plasma low-density lipoprotein (LDL)–cholesterol levels, and therefore with a serious risk of atheromatosis and myocardial infarction. For that reason laboratory investigation of plasma lipid levels is always necessary. As a first step, cholesterol and triglycerides should be determined after overnight fasting. The second step is plasma electrophoresis, which separates high-density lipoprotein (HDL), very-low density lipoprotein (VLDL), chylomicrons, and VLDL remnants. Apoproteins are lipid-free protein components of plasma lipoproteins. They are able to solubilize cholesterol esters and triglycerides for transport.

In some cases an apoprotein deficiency is present. Table 13-5 shows correlations of clinical xanthoma type and lipoprotein disturbances.

Table 13-4   CLASSIFICATION OF GENETIC HYPERLIPIDEMIAS

Frederickson Type	Classification	Lipid Profile
I	Familial lipoprotein lipase deficiency (hyperchylomicronemia, hypertriglyceridemia) (FLD)	TG++, C normal, CM++, HDL −/normal
IIa	Familial hypercholesterolemia (FH)	TG normal, C+, LDL+
IIb	Familial combined hyperlipidemia (FCL)	TG+, C+, LDL+, VLDL+
III	Familial dysbetalipidemia (remnant particle disease) (FD)	TG+, C+, IDL+, CM remnants +
IV	Familial hypertriglyceridemia (FLT)	TG+, C normal/+, VLDL++ VLDL++
V	Familial combined hypertriglyceridemia (FHT)	TG+, C+, VLDL++, CM++

NOTE: TG = triglycerides, C = cholesterol, CM = chylomicrons, HDL = high-density lipoproteins, LDL = low-density lipoproteins, VLDL = very-low-density lipoproteins, IDL = intermediate-density lipoproteins, + = raised, − = lowered.

Table 13-5   RELATION OF XANTHOMA TYPE TO LIPOPROTEIN DISTURBANCES

Xanthelasma palpebrarum	Normolipemic (~50%) or FH, FD
Xanthoma tendineum	FH (type IIa)
Xanthoma tuberosum	FD, FHT, FH (if homozygous) (type III, V, IIa)
Xanthoma eruptivum (or tuberoeruptivum)	FD, FHT, FLD (rare)
Xanthochromia and xanthoma striatum palmare	FD (type III)
Xanthoma planum (generalized)	Patients often develop a monoclonal gammopathy associated with myeloma (type III), macroglobulinema, or lymphoma, and with normal plasma lipid levels. Less commonly, FHT may be present.

Xanthelasma

Synonyms: Xanthelasma palpebrarum, periocular xanthoma.

EPIDEMIOLOGY

Age of Onset   Over 50 years; when in children or young adults, it is associated with familial hypercholetserolemia (FH) or familial dysbetalipidemia (FD).

Sex   Either.

Incidence   Most common of all xanthomas.

SIGNIFICANCE

May be an isolated finding unrelated to hyperlipidemia, but sometimes there is an elevation of LDL. A markedly increased LDL is a sign of FH or FD.

HISTORY

Duration of Lesions   Months, with slow enlargement from tiny spot.

Skin Symptoms   None.

PHYSICAL EXAMINATION

Skin Lesions   Soft, polygonal yellow-orange papules and plaques localized to upper eyelids (Fig. 13-28) and around inner canthus.

LABORATORY EXAMINATIONS

Cholesterol estimation in plasma; if enhanced, screening for type of hyperlipidemia.

COURSE AND PROGNOSIS

If due to hyperlipidemia, complication with atherosclerotic cardiovascular disease may be expected.

In approximately 50% of these patients, no metabolic disturbances are found. In others, xanthelasma is a sign of familial hyperlidemia (FH or FD). When total lipids and total cholesterol content of the serum are within normal limits, no further lipid analysis is necessary.

MANAGEMENT

Laser, excision, electrodesiccation, or topical application of trichloroacetic acid. Recurrences are not uncommon.

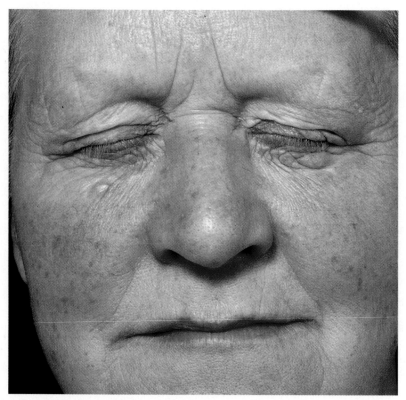

Figure 13-28   Xanthelasma   *Multiple, longitudinal, creamy-orange, slightly elevated dermal papules on the eyelids of a normolipemic individual.*

Xanthoma Tendineum

These subcutaneous tumors are yellow or skin-colored and move with the extensor tendons (Fig. 13-29). They are a symptom of familial hypercholesterolemia (FH) that presents as a type IIa hyperlipidemia. This condition is autosomal recessive with a different phenotype in the heterozygote and homozygote. In the homozygote, the xanthomata appear in early childhood and the cardiovascular complications in early adolescence; the elevation of the LDL content of the plasma is extreme. These patients rarely attain ages above 20 years.
Synonym: Tendinous xanthoma.

MANAGEMENT

A diet low in cholesterol and saturated fats, supplemented by cholestyramine or statins. In extreme cases, measures such as portacaval shunt or liver transplantation have to be considered.

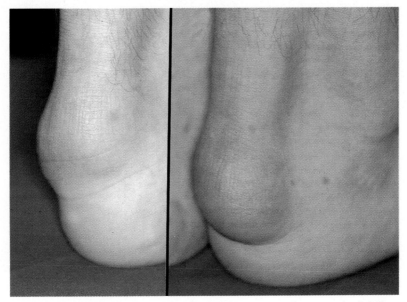

Figure 13-29 Tendinous xanthomas *Large subcutaneous tumors adherent to the Achilles tendons.*

Xanthoma Tuberosum

This condition comprises yellowish nodules (Fig. 13-30) located especially on the elbows and knees by confluence of concomitant eruptive xanthomas. They are to be found in patients with FD, familial combined hypertriglyceridemia (FHT), and familial lipoprotein lipase deficiency (FLD). In homozygous patients with FH, the tuberous xanthomas are flatter and skin-colored. They are not accompanied by eruptive xanthomas.

Synonym: Tuberous xanthoma.

MANAGEMENT

Treatment of the underlying condition.

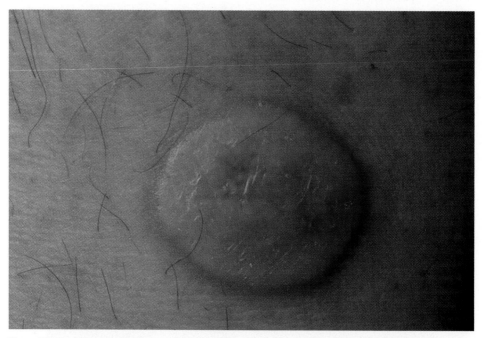

Figure 13-30   Tuberous xanthoma   *Flat-topped, yellow, firm tumor with an erythematous margin.*

Eruptive Xanthoma

These discrete inflammatory-type papules "erupt" suddenly and in showers, appearing typically on the buttocks.

ETIOLOGY

A sign of FHT, FD, the very rare FLD, and diabetes out of control.

HISTORY

Lesions appear suddenly.

PHYSICAL EXAMINATION

Skin Lesions Dome-shaped papules, discrete. Nodules represents confluent papules. Initially red, then yellow center with red halo. Lesions may be scattered discrete in a localized region (e.g. elbows (Fig. 13-31), buttocks or appear as "tight" clusters that become confluent to form "tuberoeruptive" xanthomas.

Distribution

Papules: buttocks, elbows, knees, back, or anywhere else.
"Tuberoeruptive" lesions: mostly on elbows.

MANAGEMENT

React very favorably to a low-calorie and low-fat diet.

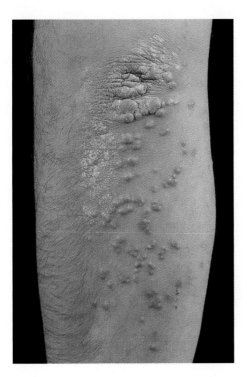

Figure 13-31   Papular eruptive xanthomas   *Multiple, discrete, red-to-yellow papules becoming confluent on the elbow of an individual with uncontrolled diabetes mellitus; lesions were present on both elbows and buttocks.*

Xanthoma Striatum Palmare (XSP)

This condition is characterized by yellow-orange, flat or elevated infiltrations of the volar creases of palms and fingers (Fig. 13-32). Pathognomonic for FD (type III). Next to XSP, FD also presents with tuberous xanthoma (Fig. 13-30), and xanthelasma palpebrarum (Fig. 13-28).

Patients with FD are prone to atherosclerotic cardiovascular disease, especially ischemia of the legs and coronary vessels.

MANAGEMENT

Patients with FD react very favorably to a diet low in fats and carbohydrates. If necessary, this may be supplemented with statins, fibrates, or nicotinic acid.

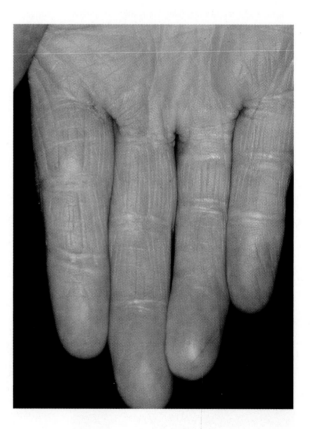

Figure 13-32 Xanthoma striatum palmare *The palmar creases are yellow, often a subtle lesion noticeable only upon close examination.*

NORMOLIPEMIC PLANE XANTHOMA

Xanthoma planum is a normolipemic xanthoma that consists of diffuse orange-yellow pigmentation of the skin (Fig. 13-33). There is a recognizable border. These lesions can be idiopathic or secondary to leukemia, but the most common association is with multiple myeloma. The lesions may precede the onset of multiple myeloma by many years.

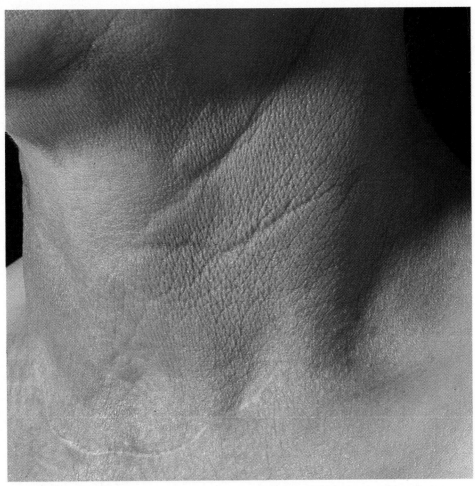

Figure 13-33 Plane xanthoma *Yellowish-reddish, slightly elevated plaques on the neck, noticeable mainly because of the accentuation of the skin texture in a normolipemic patient with lymphoma. Plane xanthomas occur most commonly on the upper trunk and neck and also occur in individuals with myeloma.*

SKIN SIGNS OF VASCULAR INSUFFICIENCY

ATHEROSCLEROSIS, ATHEROEMBOLIZATION, AND ARTERIAL INSUFFICIENCY

Atherosclerosis obliterans (ASO), especially of the lower extremities, is associated with a spectrum of cutaneous findings, ranging from slowly progressive ischemic changes to the sudden appearance of ischemic lesions following atheroembolization. Atheroembolism is the phenomenon of dislodgement of atheromatous debris from an affected artery or aneurysm with centrifugal microembolization and resultant ischemic and infarctive cutaneous lesions.

EPIDEMIOLOGY

Age of Onset   Middle-aged to elderly.

Sex   Males > females.

Incidence   Atherosclerosis is the cause of 90% of arterial disease in developed countries, affecting 5% of men older than 50 years; 10% (20% of diabetics) of all men with atherosclerosis develop critical limb ischemia.

Risk Factors for Atherosclerosis   Cigarette smoking, hyperlipidemia, low high density lipoprotein (HDL), high cholesterol, high low density lipoprotein (LDL), hypertension, diabetes mellitus, hyperinsulinemia, abdominal obesity, family history of premature ischemic heart disease, personal history of cerebrovascular disease or occlusive peripheral vascular disease.

Diabetes Mellitus and Lower Leg Ischemia   Gangrene of lower extremities is estimated to be from 8 to 150 times more frequent in diabetic than in nondiabetic individuals, most often occurring in those who smoke.

PATHOGENESIS

Atherosclerosis is the most common cause of arterial insufficiency and may be generalized or localized to the coronary arteries, aortic arch vessels to the head and neck, or those supplying the lower extremities, i.e., femoral, popliteal, anterior and posterior tibial arteries. Atheromatous narrowing of arteries supplying the upper extremities is much less common. Atheromatous deposits and thromboses occur commonly in the femoral artery in Hunter's canal and in the popliteal artery just above the knee joint. The posterior tibial artery is most often occluded where it rounds the internal malleolus, the anterior tibial artery where it is superficial and becomes the dorsalis pedis artery. Atheromatous material in the abdominal or iliac arteries also can diminish blood flow to the lower extremities as well as break off and embolize (atheroembolization) downstream to the lower extremities. Detection of atherosclerosis is often delayed until an ischemic event occurs, related to critical decrease in blood flow.

In addition to large-vessel arterial obstruction, individuals with diabetes mellitus often have microvasculopathy associated with endothelial cell proliferation and basement membrane thickening of arterioles, venules, and capillaries.

Atheroembolism   Multiple small deposits of fibrin, platelet, and cholesterol debris embolize from proximal atherosclerotic lesions or

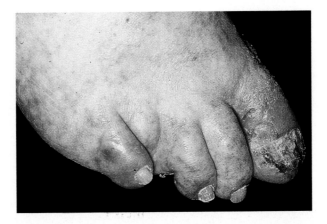

Figure 14-1 Atherosclerosis obliterans with ischemic skin changes *The great toe shows ischemic and preinfarctive changes and early ulceration. The forefoot is white; and there is mottled, livedoid erythema distally and livid erythema on the tips of the toes. The fourth digit had been amputated previously because of gangrene. In this 68-year-old diabetic woman, the iliac artery was occluded.*

aneurysmal sites. Occurs spontaneously or after intravascular surgery or procedures such as arteriography, fibrinolysis, or anticoagulation. Emboli tend to lodge in small vessels of skin and muscle and usually do not occlude large vessels.

HISTORY

Symptoms *Atherosclerosis of Lower Extremity Arteries* Early symptom is usually pain on exercise, i.e., *intermittent claudication.* With progressive arterial insufficiency, pain and/or paresthesias at rest occur in leg and/or foot, especially at night.

Atheroembolism Often occurs after an intraarterial procedure. Acute pain and tenderness at site of embolization. "Blue toe," "purple toe" syndrome: peripheral ischemia, livedo reticularis of sudden onset.

Individuals with arterial insufficiency of the lower extremities often have symptoms of ischemic heart disease (coronary artery disease or arteriosclerotic heart disease), atherosclerosis obliterans, diabetes mellitus. An episode of cutaneous atheroembolization may be accompanied by embolization to kidney, pancreas, muscle, etc.

PHYSICAL EXAMINATION

Atherosclerosis/Arterial Insufficiency

Skin Lesions General findings associated with ischemia include pallor, cyanosis, livedoid vascular pattern (Fig. 14-1) loss of hair on affected limb. Earliest infarctive changes (Fig. 14-1) include well-demarcated maplike areas of epidermal necrosis. Later, dry black gangrene may occur over the infarcted skin (purple cyanosis → white pallor → black gangrene) (Fig. 14-2). With shedding of slough, well-demarcated ulcers with underlying structures such as tendons can be seen. Microangiopathy in diabetic patients may present as acral erysipelas-like erythema (Fig. 14-1).

Palpation Pulse of large vessels usually diminished or absent. In diabetics with mainly microangiopathy, gangrene may occur in the setting of adequate pulses. Temperature of foot: cool to cold.

Pain Early infarctive lesions painful on palpation; ischemic ulcers are painful; in diabetics with neuropathy and ischemic ulcers, pain may be minimal or absent.

Distribution Ischemic ulcers may first appear between toes at sites of pressure and beginning on fissures on plantar heel. Dry gangrene of feet, starting at the toes or at pressure sites (Fig. 14-2).

General Examination Buerger's sign: with significant reduction in arterial blood flow, limb elevation causes pallor (best noted on plantar foot); dependency causes delayed and exaggerated hyperemia. Auscultation over stenotic arteries reveals bruits.

Atheroembolization

Skin Lesions Violaceous livedo reticularis on legs, feet, but also as high up as buttocks (Fig. 14-3A). Ischemic changes with poor return of color after compression of skin. "Blue toe" (Fig. 14-3B): indurated, painful plaques often fol-

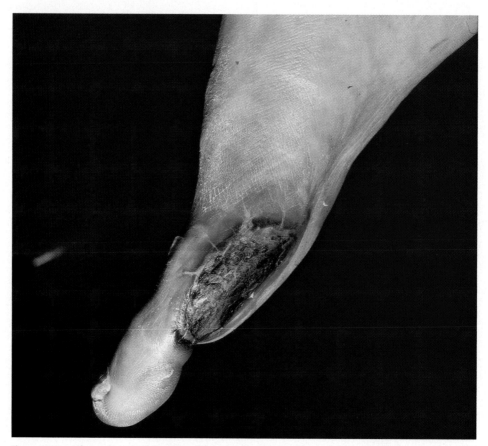

Figure 14-2 **Atherosclerosis obliterans** *There is distal ischemia and dry gangrene on the base of the great toe with purple cyanosis of the forefoot.*

lowing livedo reticularis on calves and thighs that may undergo necrosis (Fig. 14-4), become black and crusted, and ulcerate. Cyanosis and gangrene of digits.

General Examination *Pulses* Distal pulses may remain intact.

DIFFERENTIAL DIAGNOSIS

Intermittent Claudication Pseudoxanthoma elasticum, Buerger's disease (thromboangiitis obliterans), arthritis, gout.

Painful Foot Gout, interdigital neuroma, onychomycosis with ingrowing great toenails, flat feet, calcanean bursitis, plantar fasciitis.

Ischemic and Infarctive Lesions of Leg/Foot Vasculitis, chilblains, Raynaud's phenomenon

(vasospasm), disseminated intravascular coagulation (purpura fulminans), cryoglobulinemia, hyperviscosity syndrome (macroglobulinemia), septic embolization (infective endocarditis), nonseptic embolization (ventricular mural thrombus with myocardial infarction, atrial thrombus with atrial fibrillation), aneurysms (dissecting, thrombosed), drug-induced necrosis (warfarin, heparin), ergot poisoning, intraarterial injection, livedo reticularis syndromes, external compression (popliteal entrapment, cervical rib).

LABORATORY EXAMINATIONS

Hematology Rule out anemia, polycythemia.

Lipid Studies Hypercholesterolemia (>240 mg/dL), often associated with rise in low-

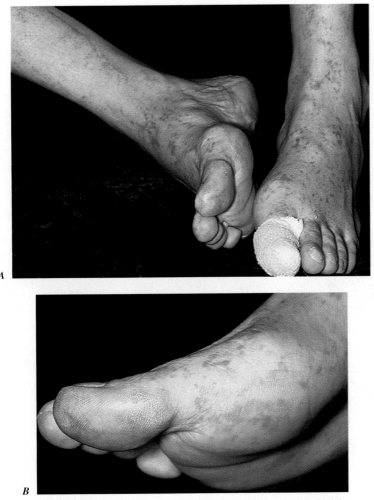

Figure 14-3 Atheroembolism after angiography A. *A mottled, violaceous, vascular pattern on the feet and ankles. The findings were noted after intravascular catheterization and angiography in an individual with ASO. The dressing on the great toe protects an ischemic ulcer.* B. *Close-up of the mottled, violaceous, vascular pattern on the foot and the "blue toe."*

density lipoprotein (LDL). Hypertriglyceridemia (250 mg/dL), often associated with rise in very-low-density lipoproteins (VLDL) and remnants of their catabolism (mainly intermediate-density lipoprotein, IDL).

Dermatopathology of Atheroembolism Deep skin and muscle biopsy specimen shows arterioles occluded by multinucleated foreign-body giant cells and fibrosis surrounding biconvex, needle-shaped clefts corresponding to the cholesterol crystal microemboli.

Doppler Studies Show reduced or interrupted blood flow.

Digital Plethysmography With exercise can unmask significant atherosclerotic involvement of lower extremity arteries.

X-Ray Calcification can be demonstrated intramurally; often the calcification represents medial sclerosis that may be present in the absence of significant atherosclerosis.

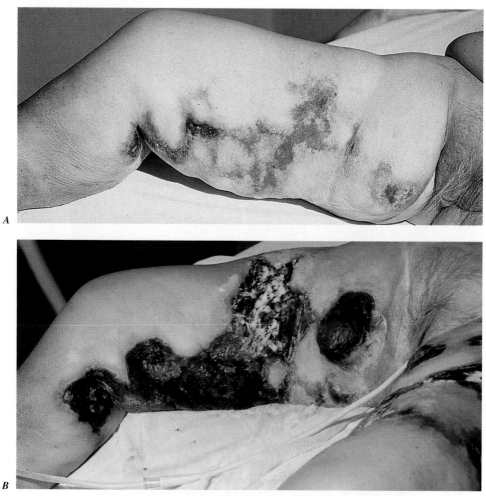

Figure 14-4 Atheroembolism with cutaneous infarction A. *Violaceous plaques and cutaneous infarctions with a linear arrangement on the medial thigh of a 73-year-old woman with atherosclerosis, heart failure, and diabetes. B. Within 48 h the initial changes progressed to become far more extensive with large areas of infarction.*

Arteriography Atherosclerosis is best visualized by angiography. With atheroembolization, ulceration of atheromatous plaques seen in abdominal aorta or more distally.

DIAGNOSIS

Clinical suspicion confirmed by arteriography and deep skin biopsy (atheroembolism).

COURSE AND PROGNOSIS

Arterial insufficiency can be a slowly progressive disease or punctuated by episodes of complete occlusion or embolism. Approximately 5% per year of individuals with intermittent claudication progress to pain at rest or gangrene. A much higher percentage die from other complications of atherosclerosis such as ischemic heart disease.

Poor tissue perfusion makes infection more likely, with interdigital tinea pedis, leg/foot ulcers, or small breaks and fissures in the skin. Chronic lymphedema, prior saphenous venous harvesting, and prior episodes of cellulitis increase the likelihood of cellulitis.

Atherosclerosis of coronary and carotid arteries usually determines survival of patient; involvement of lower extremity arteries often causes significant morbidity and is commonly associated with coronary artery involvement as well. Balloon angioplasty, endarterectomy, and bypass procedure have improved prognosis of patients with atherosclerosis. Amputation rates have been lowered from 80% to less than 40% by aggressive vascular surgery.

Atheroembolism May be a single episode if atheroembolization follows intraarterial procedure. May be recurrent if spontaneous and associated with significant tissue necrosis.

MANAGEMENT

Prevention Goal of management is prevention of atherosclerosis rather than treatment of ischemic complications.

Diet First step in management of primary hyperlipidemia: Reduce intake of saturated fats and cholesterol as well as calories.

Exercise Useful adjunct to diet. Walking increases new collateral vessels in ischemic muscle.

Hypertension Reduce elevated blood pressure.

Cigarette Smoking Discontinue.

Blood Correct anemia or polycythemia.

Positioning of Ischemic Foot As low as possible without edema.

Drug Therapy Recommended for adults with LDL cholesterol >190 mg/dL or >160 mg/dL in the presence of two or more risk factors after an adequate trial of at least 3 months of diet therapy alone. Initiation of drug therapy usually commits patients to lifelong treatment. Drugs act primarily by lowering LDL cholesterol and include bile acid-binding resins, nicotinic acid, and HMG-CoA reductase inhibitors.

Intermittent Claudication

Medical Management Encourage walking to create new collateral vessels.

Surgical Management Endarterectomy or bypass for aortic iliac occlusions and for extensive femoral popliteal disease.

Ischemia/Infarction of Foot/Leg

Surgical Management Distal bypass surgery of three crural arteries.

Atheroembolization Response to surgical revascularization or thrombolytic therapy often poor.

Medical Management Heparin and warfarin. Analgesics.

Surgical Management Debridement of necrotic tissue locally or amputation if indicated. Remove or bypass atherosclerotic vessel or aneurysm. Amputation of leg/foot: indicated when medical and surgical management has failed.

THROMBOPHLEBITIS AND DEEP VENOUS THROMBOSIS

Superficial phlebitis is an inflammatory thrombosis of a superficial normal vein, usually due to infection or trauma from needles and catheters, or of a varicose vein usually in the context of the chronic venous insufficiency (CVI) syndrome. Deep venous thrombosis is due to thrombotic obstruction of a vein with or without an inflammatory response and occurs due to slow blood flow, hypercoagulability, or changes in the venous walls. The most common causes are shown in Table 14-1

ETIOLOGY AND PATHOGENESIS

The thrombus originates in an area of low venous flow. An occlusion of a vein by thrombus imposes a block to venous return which leads to increased venous pressure and edema in the distal limb. An inflammatory response to the thrombus causes pain and tenderness. If the venous pressure is too high, arterial limb flow may rarely be compromised and ischemia of the distal limb may occur. The thrombus in the vein often has a free-floating tail, which may break off to produce a pulmonary embolus. Organization of the thrombus in the vein destroys the venous walls, and this leads to post-phlebitic syndrome.

HISTORY

Patients complain of pain or aching in the involved limb or notice limb swelling. Some patients may have no symptoms. Pulmonary embolus may be the first indication of deep venous thrombosis.

CLINICAL MANIFESTATIONS

Superficial thrombophlebitis is diagnosed by the characteristic induration of a superficial vein with redness and increased heat (Fig. 14-5). Deep venous thrombosis presents with a swollen, warm, tender limb (Fig. 14-6) with prominent distended collateral veins. Pitting edema may occur but is not always present, and a tender cord may be felt where the vein is thrombosed. With iliofemoral thrombophlebitis the limb is swollen from the foot to the inguinal region and tenderness is not present in the limb, but collateral veins may form from the thigh to the abdominal wall. Two types are recognized: the limb may be very pale (phlegmasia alba dolens) or may be cyanotic with cold digits if

Table 14-1 PREDISPOSING FACTORS IN DEEP VENOUS THROMBOSIS[a]

COMMON FACTORS

Major surgery	Oral contraceptives
Fractures	Malignancies
Congestive heart failure	Venous varicosities
Acute myocardial infarction	Previous history of venous thrombosis
Stroke	Leiden factor 5 mutation
Pregnancy and postpartum	Severe pulmonary insufficiency
Spinal cord injuries	Prolonged immobilization
Shock	

LESS COMMON FACTORS

Sickle cell anemia	Antithrombin III deficiency
Homocystinuria	Antiphospholipid antibodies
Protein C or S deficiency	Ulcerative colitis

[a]SOURCE: TD Coffman: Cutaneous changes in peripheral vascular disease, in IM Freedberg, AZ Eisen, K Wolff, KF Austen, LA Goldsmith, SI Katz, TB Fitzpatrick (eds): *Fitzpatrick's Dermatology in General Medicine,* 5th ed. New York, McGraw-Hill, 1999, p. 1954.

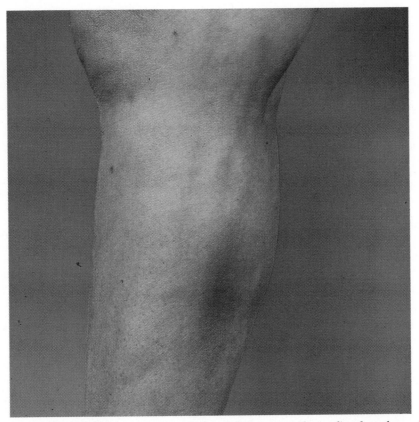

Figure 14-5 Superficial phlebitis *A linear painful erythematous cord extending from the popliteal fossa to the mid-calf in a 35-year-old man who had moderate varicosities. Phlebitis occurred after a 15-h flight.*

the arterial inflow is compromised (phlegmasia cerulea dolens). In thrombosis of calf veins the calf and foot are swollen and warm, and there is deep tenderness of the calf often without a palpable cord (Fig. 14-6).

Migratory phlebitis describes an excessive inflammatory induration of superficial veins that migrates within a defined region of the body. *Mondor's disease* is an inflamed, subcutaneous vein from the breast to the axillary region that during healing leads to a shortening of the venous cord that puckers the skin. Migratory phlebitis may be associated with thromboangiitis obliterans and malignancies, but Mondor's disease has no special associations.

LABORATORY EXAMINATIONS

Venous imaging by bimodal duplex ultrasound and Doppler examination reveals an absence of flow or of the normal respiratory venous flow variations in proximal venous occlusions. For thrombophlebitis of the calf veins, intravenous [^{125}I]fibrinogen or a venogram gives a definite diagnosis.

DIFFERENTIAL DIAGNOSIS

Lymphedema, cellulitis, erysipelas, superficial phlebitis, lymphangitis. An uncommon differential diagnosis is rupture of the plantar muscle, which produces pain, swelling, and ecchymotic areas in the dependent ankle area.

MANAGEMENT

The treatment of deep venous thrombosis is anticoagulation. IV heparin is given at a loading dose of 5000 U and approximately 1000 U/h thereafter. The partial thromboplastin time (PTT) should be 1.5 to 2 times normal. Low-molecular-weight heparin is also effective, and warfarin can be started orally at the same time and should overlap heparin for 5 days until the necessary factors for blood clotting are depressed. Patients should be treated for 3 months with anticoagulation. Elastic stockings and compression are mandatory and should be worn for at least three months, and ambulation should be started as soon as symptoms subside.

SKIN SIGNS OF VASCULAR INSUFFICIENCY

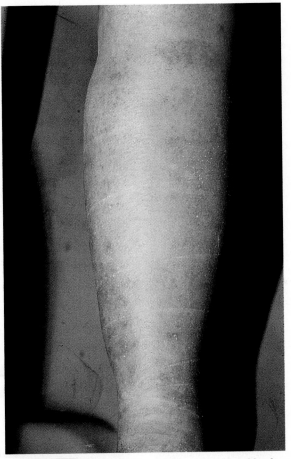

Figure 14-6 Deep venous thrombosis *The leg is swollen, pale, with a blotchy cyanotic discoloration, and is painful. The episode occurred after abdominal surgery.*

CHRONIC VENOUS INSUFFICIENCY

Chronic venous insufficiency (CVI) results from failure of return of venous blood and increased capillary pressure; the resultant changes include edema, stasis dermatitis, hyperpigmentation, fibrosis of the skin and subcutaneous tissue (lipodermatosclerosis) of the leg, and ulceration.

EPIDEMIOLOGY

Age of Onset   Varicose veins: peak incidence of onset 30 to 40 years.

Sex   Varicose veins are three times more common in women than in men.

Etiology   CVI is most commonly associated with varicose veins and the postphlebitic syndrome. Varicose veins are an inherited characteristic.

Aggravating Factors   Varicose veins: pregnancy, increased blood volume, increased cardiac output, increased venocaval pressure, effect of progesterone on smooth muscle of vein wall.

PATHOGENESIS

The valves of the deep veins of the calf are damaged and incompetent at restricting backflow of blood. The communicating veins that connect deep and superficial calf veins are damaged, which also causes CVI in that blood flows from deep veins to superficial venous plexus. Fibrin is deposited in the extravascular space and undergoes organization, resulting in sclerosis and obliteration of lymphatics and microvasculature. Perivascular fibrosis results in diminished nutrition of the epidermis, which breaks down with ulcer formation.

This cycle repeats itself: initial event → aggravation of venous stasis and varicose vein dilatation → lipodermatosclerosis → new thrombosis → stasis dermatitis → ulceration.

HISTORY

Prior episode(s) of superficial phlebitis and deep vein thrombosis. Risk factors for deep leg vein thrombosis include antepartum/postpartum state, minor leg injuries, pelvic lower abdominal operations, medical illnesses, prolonged recumbency.

CVI commonly associated with heaviness or aching of leg, which is aggravated by standing (dependency) and relieved by walking. Lipodermatosclerosis may limit movement of ankle and cause pain and limitation of movement, which in turn increases stasis. History of leg edema aggravated by dependency (end of the day, standing), summer season. Shoes feel tight in the evening. Night cramps. Atrophie blanche may occur at sites of trauma.

PHYSICAL EXAMINATION

Varicose Veins   A simple staging system for CVI is shown in Table 14-2. Superficial leg veins are enlarged, tortuous, with incompetent valves; best evaluated with the patient standing (Fig. 14-7). "Blow-out" at sites of incompetent communicating veins, tourniquet test (see below).

Edema   Dependent; improved or resolved in the morning after a night in the horizontal position.

Eczematous (stasis) Dermatitis   Occurs in setting of CVI about the lower legs and ankles (Fig. 14-8). It is a classic eczematous dermatitis with inflammatory papules, scaly and crusted erosions; in addition, there is stippled pigmentation, dermal sclerosis, and excoriations due to scratching. It must be distinguished from contact dermatitis secondary to topical agents, with which it is often combined. In addition, there

Table 14-2   STAGING OF CVI (ACCORDING TO WIDMER)

Stage	Characteristics
I	Edema, subfascial congestion, ankle flare (phlebectasia around ankle)
II	Lipodermatosclerosis, pigmentation, stasis dermatitis, atrophie blanche
III	All of the above and ulcers, scars

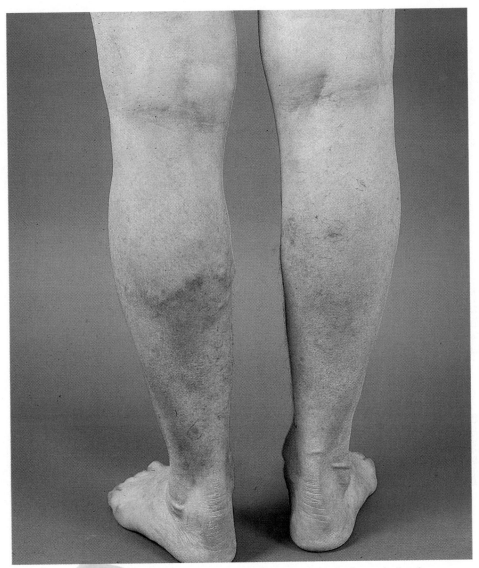

Figure 14-7   Varicose veins   *There are meandering irregular varicose veins on both calves, left>right, with superficial phlebectasia.*

may be concomitant irritant dermatitis due to secretion from stasis ulcer and bacterial colonization. If extensive, may be associated with generalized eczematous dermatitis, i.e., "id" reaction or autosensitization.

Pigmentation Stippled with recent and old hemorrhages (Fig. 14-9).

Atrophie blanche Ivory-white depressed plaques (Fig. 14-9) on the ankle and/or foot; stippled pigmentation; hemosiderin-pigmented border, usually within stasis dermatitis.

Ulceration Occurs in 30% of cases; very painful "hyperalgesic micro-ulcer" in area of atrophie blanche (Fig 14-9); larger superficial or deep ulcers, sharply defined with deep margin, necrotic base surrounded by atrophie blanche, stasis dermatitis, and lipodermatosclerosis (Fig. 14-10).

Lipodermatosclerosis Inflammation, induration, pigmentation of lower third of leg creating "champagne bottle" or "piano leg" appearance with edema above and below the sclerotic region (Fig. 14-10). "Groove sign" created by varicose veins meandering through sclerotic tissue. A verrucous epidermal change can occur overlying the sclerosis, referred to as elephantiasis nostras verrucosa. In long-standing sclerosis, calcification can occur.

Distribution Edema: dorsa of feet, ankles, legs. Pigmentation: over varices, at ankles, around the legs. *Ulcers:* usually medially and above ankles (Fig. 14-10).

DIFFERENTIAL DIAGNOSIS

Varicose Veins Post-thrombotic syndrome, Klippel-Trenaunay-Weber syndrome, Parkes-Weber syndrome (congenital arteriovenous fistulas).

Deep Vein Phlebitis Superficial thrombophlebitis, muscle trauma, hematoma.

Edema Right-sided heart failure, hypoalbuminemia, Kaposi's sarcoma, pretibial myxedema (Graves' disease), iliac vein compression.

Pigmentation Progressive pigmentary purpura, minocycline pigmentation.

Stasis Dermatitis Nummular eczema, atopic dermatitis, asteatotic eczema, allergic contact dermatitis, irritant dermatitis.

Leg Ulcer (page 468)

LABORATORY EXAMINATIONS

Cultures Rule out secondary bacterial infection.

Doppler Studies Evaluate arterial flow in patients with poor peripheral pulses.

Phlebography Contrast medium is injected into veins to detect incompetent veins and venous occlusion.

Color-Coded Duplex Sonography Detects incompetent veins. Venous occlusion due to thrombus.

Arteriography Rule out significant arterial insufficiency.

Imaging X-ray may (10% of chronic cases) show subcutaneous calcification, i.e., postphlebitic subcutaneous calcinosis. Bony changes include periostitis underlying ulceration, osteoporosis as a result of disuse, fibrous ankylosis of ankle. Osteomyelitis.

Tourniquet Test A tourniquet is applied to the leg that has been elevated to empty the veins; when the patient stands up and the tourniquet is released, there is instant filling of a varicose vein due to absent or ill-functioning valves.

Dermatopathology *Early:* small venules and lymphatic spaces appear dilated; edema of extracellular space with swelling and separation of collagen bundles. *Subsequently:* capillaries dilated, congested with tuft formation and tortuosity of venules; deposition of fibrin. *Endothelial cell hypertrophy:* may be associated with venous thrombosis; angioendotheliomatous proliferation mimicking Kaposi's sarcoma. In all stages, extravasation of red blood cells (RBCs) that break down forming hemosiderin, which is taken up by macrophages. Lymphatic vessels become encased in a fibrotic stroma, i.e., dermatoliposclerosis. Calcification of fat and fibrous tissue may occur.

DIAGNOSIS

Usually made on history, clinical findings, and Doppler sonography.

MANAGEMENT

Prerequisite Compression dressings or stockings.

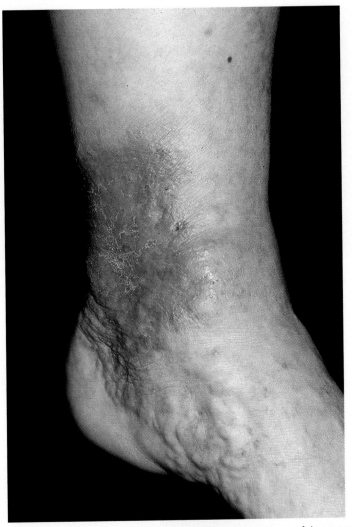

Figure 14-8 Stasis dermatitis in CVI *A patch of eczematous dermatitis overlying venous varicosities on the medial ankle in a 59-year-old woman. The lesion is scaly, itching, and there are small scars from previous ulcerations.*

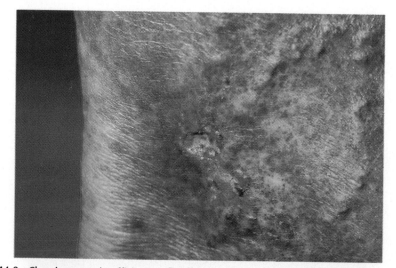

Figure 14-9   Chronic venous insufficiency   *Small varicose veins meandering through an area of diffuse and mottled pigmentation due to hemosiderin and ivory-white patches of atrophie blanche and a small ulcer with a necrotic base. Such lesions are both itchy and painful.*

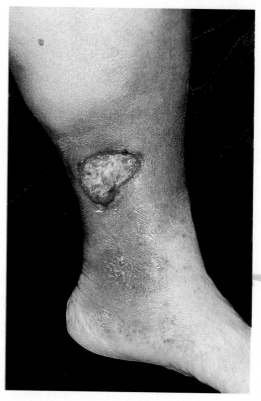

Figure 14-10   Chronic venous insufficiency and lipodermatosclerosis   *The ankle is relatively thin and the upper calf edematous, creating a "champagne bottle" or "piano leg" appearance. An ulcer with a necrotic base is present proximal to the ankle within an area of pronounced lipodermatosclerosis, and stasis dermatitis is seen over the malleolus. The patient had a history of deep vein thrombosis and pulmonary embolism.*

Atrophie Blanche Avoid trauma to area involved. Intralesional triamcinolone into painful lesions. Compression.

Varicose Veins *Injection Sclerotherapy* A sclerosing agent such as tetradecyl sulfate is injected into varicosities, followed by prolonged compression. Used mainly to treat minor branch varicosities not associated with saphenous incompetence and new branch vein varicosities developing after surgery. Recurrence is very common within 5 years.

Vascular Surgery Incompetent perforating veins are identified, ligated, and cut, followed by stripping long and/or short saphenous veins out of the main trunk. Residual perforating veins are the main cause of recurrences after surgery. In patients with combined arterial and CVI, bypass or angioplasty may prove beneficial.

LEG ULCERS

Leg ulcers occur relatively commonly in late middle and old age, arising in association with chronic venous insufficiency, chronic arterial insufficiency, or peripheral sensory neuropathy; in some patients, a combination of these factors. Leg ulcers are associated with significant long-term morbidity and often do not heal unless the underlying problem(s) is corrected.

EPIDEMIOLOGY

Age of Onset Venous ulcers: middle-aged and elderly. Arterial ulcer: >45 years.

Sex Venous ulcers: females>males.

Etiology In developed countries, most common causes include chronic venous insufficiency (80% of cases), arterial insufficiency (5 to 10%), neuropathy, diabetes mellitus; in many cases, several of these factors are in play.

Prevalence >600,000 cases in the United States. The incidence of deep vein thrombosis appears to be decreasing. Arterial insufficiency is becoming more common in an aging population.

Risk Factors Venous ulcers: minor injury, malnutrition, sedentary lifestyle.

Inheritance Half of patients have a family history of leg ulcers (presumably related to inheritance of valvular defects).

PATHOGENESIS

Venous Ulcers (See also Chronic Venous Insufficiency.) In half of patients venous ulcers are associated with prior venous thrombosis and in the other half with incompetence of superficial or communicating veins. Calf muscle pump dysfunction may occur because of deep venous insufficiency or obstruction, perforator incompetence, superficial venous insufficiency, arterial fistulas, neuromuscular dysfunction; commonly, a combination of these factors is in play. High venous pressure associated with capillary tortuosity and increased capillary permeability to large molecules results in deposition of a pericapillary fibrin layer. This layer is a barrier to diffusion of oxygen and other nutrients, resulting in ischemia and necrosis. Factors precipitating epidermal necrosis include minor trauma (scratch, knock) or contact dermatitis.

Arterial Ulcers See Atherosclerosis (page 452).

Neuropathic Ulcers Foot ulcers in diabetic patients are usually associated with both sensory neuropathy and ischemia, often complicated by infection. Pressure over prominences of foot leads progressively to callosity formation, autolysis, and finally ulceration. (See also Section 13.)

HISTORY

Venous Ulcers Lower leg. Aching and swelling of legs that are exacerbated by dependency and relieved by elevation of leg. Stasis dermatitis associated with pruritus and weeping. Varicose veins, thrombosis, lipodermatosclerosis.

Arterial Ulcers Lower leg, toes. Intermittent claudication and pain, even at rest, as disease progresses. Characteristically, painful at night and often quite severe; may be worse when legs elevated, improving on dependency. Risk factors: cigarette smoking, diabetes mellitus.

Neuropathic Ulcers Soles, toes, heel. Most commonly associated with diabetes of many years' duration. Early symptoms of neuropathy include paresthesia, pain, anesthesia of leg and foot. Patients are often unaware of prior trauma that commonly precedes ulcerations of heel, plantar metatarsal area, or great toe.

Systems Review See Atherosclerosis, Atheroembolization, and Arterial Insufficiency (page 452) and Chronic Venous Insufficiency (page 462).

PHYSICAL EXAMINATION

Ulcers Associated with Chronic Venous Insufficiency

Venous ulcers arise in the setting of varicose veins, edema, induration, and/or lipodermatosclerosis. Varicose veins are best evaluated with the patient standing.

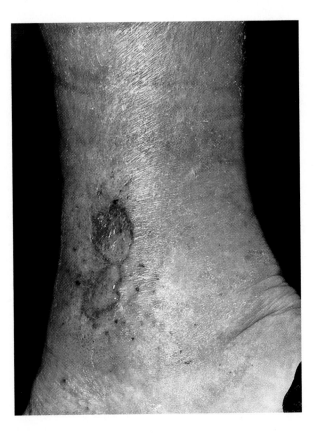

Figure 14-11 Venous insufficiency
*Two coalescing ulcers with a
necrotic base in an area of
atrophie blanche, lipodermatosclerosis, and stasis dermatitis.
Scratch marks indicate itchiness
of surrounding skin, while the
ulcers are painful.*

Skin Lesions *Eczematous (stasis) Dermatitis.*
(Figs. 14-8 and 14-11) *Lipodermatosclerosis*:
induration and fibrosis of dermis and subcutaneous tissue; (Fig. 14-10); may precede venous
ulceration (Figs. 14-10 and 14-11). Chronic
lymphedema may be associated with epidermal
hyperplasia, termed *elephantiasis nostras verrucosa*.

Venous Ulcers Painful, sometimes not. Ulceration preceded by ischemia that presents as
a red or blue-red patch or atrophie blanche
(Fig. 14-9). Minor trauma to this site often precipitates ulceration. Ulcers are usually punched
out with irregular shaggy brown to brown-red
borders (Figs. 14-10 and 14-11) which are hard
due to lipodermatosclerosis. Cellulitis may
complicate stasis dermatitis or venous ulcers;
repeated episodes cause additional damage to
lymphatic drainage, thus compounding chronic
lymphedema, lipodermatosclerosis, and pigmentation. Immobility of ankle joint results in
fibrous or bony ankylosis. Arterial pulses palpable (unless there is also arterial insufficiency).

Distribution Ulcers commonly develop on the
medial lower aspect of the calf (Fig. 14-10), especially over malleolus (lateral as well as medial), in the area supplied by incompetent perforating veins (Fig. 14-11). Stasis ulcers also
can develop in the most dependent parts of a
pendulous abdominal panniculus in a massively
obese individual.

Ulcers Associated with Chronic Arterial Insufficiency

Skin Lesions Ulcer(s) are painful. Punched
out, with sharply demarcated borders (Fig.
14-12). A tissue slough is often present at the
base, under which tendons can be seen. Exudation minimal. Associated findings of ischemia:
loss of hair on feet and lower legs; shiny atrophic skin. Stasis pigmentation and lipodermatosclerosis are absent. Pulses diminished or
absent.

Distribution Occur over sites of pressure or
trauma: bony prominences (pretibial) (Fig 14-12),
supramalleolar distal points such as toes.

Ulcers Associated with Hypertension (Martorell's Ulcer)

Skin Lesions Ulcer(s): punched out, sharply demarcated borders, with surrounding halo of erythema, very painful, often crusted (Fig. 14-13). Pain relieved by placing leg in dependent position.

Distribution Anterior external aspect of leg between middle and lower third of limb.

Neuropathic and Diabetic Ulcers (see Diabetes Mellitus, Section 13)

The typical diabetic neuropathic foot is numb, warm, and dry, with palpable pulses.

Skin Lesions Ulcers commonly surrounded by thick callus. Base: dry, gray or black (see Fig. 13-5). Other findings include Charcot's arthropathy and neuropathic edema. Initially, change is loss of sensation of light touch of great toe and then foot; subsequently, ankle jerk reflex is lost; then joint position sense.

Distribution Ulcers occur at points of high-pressure loading, especially on the soles, metatarsal head, great toe, heel or at sites of deformity.

General Findings

Cardiovascular System Cardiac function and peripheral pulses should be evaluated in all patients with leg ulcers. Measure systolic blood pressure at ankle.

Nervous System Neurologic findings should be evaluated in all patients with leg ulcers.

DIFFERENTIAL DIAGNOSIS

First Line Squamous cell carcinoma (*Note:* squamous cell carcinoma can arise in long-standing venous ulcer), basal cell carcinoma, gumma, ecthyma, injection drug user (skin popping), pressure ulcer (ski boot), necrobiosis lipoidica.

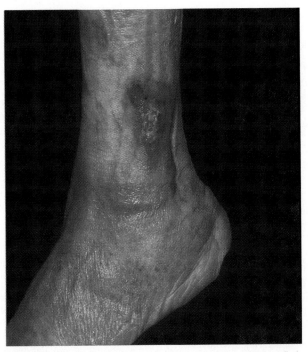

Figure 14-12   Chronic arterial insufficiency with a sharply defined, "punched out" ulcer with irregular outlines.   *The extremity was pulseless, and there was massive ischemia on the toes.*

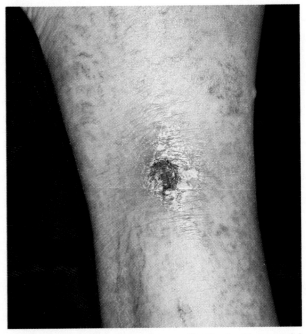

Figure 14-13   Ulcer associated with hypertension (Martorell's Ulcer)   *Very painful, crusted ulcer on the anterior external aspect of the lower leg in a patient with uncontrolled hypertension.*

Second Line Vasculitis (polyarteritis nodosa), erythema induratum, calciphylaxis, other infection [Buruli ulcer, *Mycobacterium marinum* infection, leprosy, invasive fungal infection, chronic herpes simplex ulcer (HSV)], extravasation of intravenous fluid, sickle cell anemia, polycythemia vera, pyoderma gangrenosum, necrobiosis lipoidica with ulceration, factitia.

LABORATORY EXAMINATIONS

Hematology, Chemistry, Serology According to suspected cause.

Patch Testing Rule out associated allergic contact dermatitis when leg ulcers are associated with surrounding eczematous dermatitis to commonly used topical agents such as neomycin, parabens, lanolin, nitrofurazone, bacitracin, or formaldehyde.

Vascular Blood Flow Studies Measure systolic blood pressure at ankle. Doppler sonography, color-coded duplex sonography, photoplethysmography, phlebography; arteriography.

Imaging Rule out underlying osteomyelitis by x-ray examination. When indicated, additional studies such as CT scan, bone scan, gallium scan, or bone biopsy can be performed. Charcot's arthropathy occurs in diabetics, involving the metatarsotarsal joints.

Dermatopathology Biopsy of ulcer margin indicated if ulcer(s) not improved after 3 months of therapy. Rule out vasculitis or inflammatory/infectious etiology (gumma); rule out underlying malignancy or malignant transformation (squamous cell carcinoma).

DIAGNOSIS

History and clinical findings confirmed by appropriate laboratory examinations.

COURSE AND PROGNOSIS

With correction of underlying causes, ulcers heal with initial formation of pink granulation tissue at the base, which is reepithelialized by epithelium from residual skin appendages or surrounding epidermis.

Infection Ulcers provide an easy portal of entry for infection, which should be suspected if pain appears or increases in intensity. Infection can occur relatively superficially in ulcer base or be more invasive with cellulitis and possible lymphangitis or bacteremia.

Eczematous Dermatitis Can be either stasis dermatitis, irritant dermatitis, or allergic contact dermatitis to one of many medicaments used in topical treatments.

Neoplasia Ulcers can heal with a pseudoepitheliomatous epidermal hyperplasia within the scar, mimicking squamous cell carcinoma. Squamous cell carcinoma and, less commonly, basal cell carcinoma can, however, arise at sites of chronic (years) ulceration.

Venous Ulcers Heal with adequate management. Invariably recur, usually on multiple occasions, unless underlying causes are corrected.

Arterial Ulcers Do not heal unless arterial blood flow is corrected. Diabetic patients are particularly predisposed to ulcers and frequently have several etiologic factors in play, i.e., peripheral vascular disease, neuropathy, infection, and impaired healing.

Neurotrophic Ulcers Rule out underlying osteomyelitis in patients with prolonged purulent drainage from ulcers.

MANAGEMENT

In general, factors such as anemia and malnutrition should be corrected to facilitate healing. Control hypertension. Weight reduction in the obese. Exercise; mobilize patient. Correct edema caused by cardiac, renal, or hepatic dysfunction. Secondary infection should be treated with effective antibiotics.

Venous Ulcers Ulceration tends to be recurrent unless underlying risk factors are corrected, i.e., corrective surgery and/or elastic stockings worn on a daily basis; beware of excess compression in patients with underlying arterial occlusion. Leg elevation. Unna boot; replace weekly. Intermittent pneumatic compression.

Treat Underlying Eczematous Dermatitis
Whether atopic, stasis, or allergic contact eczematous dermatitis, should be treated initially with moist dressings for the acute exudative phase and subsequently with moderate to potent glucocorticoid ointment for a limited time. Hydrated petrolatum for xerosis.

Debridement Moist saline dressings, changed frequently. Surgical debridement to remove necrotic tissue.

Systemic Antimicrobial Agents Treat secondarily infected ulcer or complications of lymphangitis or cellulitis.

Skin Grafting Large ulcers with healthy granulation tissue in the base can be grafted by pinch or split-thickness methods. The patient's own epidermis can be cultured in vitro and used for grafting.

Arterial Ulcers ***Symptomatic*** Analgesics for ischemic pain.

Increase Local Blood Flow Stop smoking. Control hypertension, diabetes. Exercise to increase collateral circulation. Elevate head of bed. Keep legs and feet warm.

Debridement Moist saline dressings, changed frequently. Surgery is usually contraindicated.

Systemic Antimicrobial Agents Treat secondarily infected ulcer or complications of lymphangitis or cellulitis.

Arterial Reconstruction Endarterectomy to remove localized atheromatous plaques; reconstruction/bypass of occluded areas. Consider in patients with pain at rest or failure of ulcer to heal.

Neuropathic Ulcers ***Prevention*** Distribute weight off pressure points with special shoes.

Treatment Debride callus around ulcer margin. Total-contact plaster casting removes pressure from ulcer site.

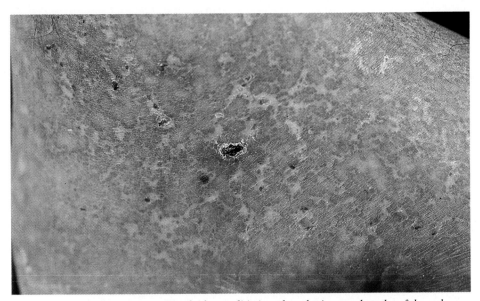

Figure 14-14 Livedoid vasculitis *Livedoid vasculitis is a thrombotic vasculopathy of dermal vessels confined to the lower extremities and starting mostly in the ankle region. It is characterized by a triad of livedo reticularis, atrophie blanche, and very painful, small punched-out ulcers that have a very poor tendency for healing. It is a reaction pattern of the skin that often recurs in winter or summer (livedo reticularis with winter and summer ulcerations) and is histologically characterized by fibrin thrombi in small- and medium-sized dermal veins and arteries with wedge-shaped necrosis and hyalinization of the vessel walls (segmental hyalinizing vasculitis). Livedoid vasculitis may be idiopathic or may be associated with Sneddon's syndrome, anti-phospholipid antibody syndrome or conditions of hypercoagulability or hyperviscosity. Treatment consists of bed rest, analgesics, low-dose heparin, and platelet aggregation inhibitors. Larger ulcers will have to be excised and grafted.*

PRESSURE ULCERS

Pressure ulcers develop at body-support interfaces over bony prominences as a result of external compression of the skin, shear forces, and friction, which produce ischemic tissue necrosis. Pressure ulcers occur in patients who are obtunded mentally or have diminished sensation (as in spinal cord disease) in the affected region. Secondary infection results in localized cellulitis, which can extend locally into bone or muscle or into the bloodstream with resultant bacteremia and sepsis.

Synonyms: Pressure sore, bed sore, decubitus ulcer.

EPIDEMIOLOGY

Age of Onset Any age. Risk factors for pressure ulcers are more common in the elderly. In many individuals, risk factors persist for the life of the patient. The greatest prevalence of pressure ulcers is in elderly, chronically bedridden patients.

Sex Equally prevalent in both sexes.

Prevalence Acute care hospital setting, 3 to 14%; long-term care settings, 15 to 25%; home-care settings, 7 to 12%; spinal cord units, 20 to 30%.

PATHOGENESIS

External compression of the dermis and hypodermis leads to ischemic tissue damage and necrosis. Risk factors for developing pressure ulcers: inadequate nursing care, diminished sensation/immobility (obtunded mental status, spinal cord disease), hypotension, fecal or urinary incontinence, presence of fracture, hypoalbuminemia, and poor nutritional status. The mean skin capillary pressure is approximately 25 mmHg. External compression with pressures <30 mmHg occludes the blood vessels so that the surrounding tissues become anoxic. Amount of damage is proportional to extent and duration of pressure. Healthy individuals can tolerate higher pressures. Repositioning the patient every 1 or 2 h prevents the interface skin over a bony prominence from becoming ischemic, with subsequent ulcer formation. Secondary bacterial infection can enlarge the ulcer rapidly, extend to underlying structures (as in osteomyelitis), and invade the bloodstream, with bacteremia and septicemia. Infection also impairs or prevents healing.

HISTORY

Ulcers often develop within the first 2 weeks of acute hospitalization and more rapidly if the patient experiences significant immobilization. Painful unless there is altered sensorium.

PHYSICAL EXAMINATION

Skin Lesions *Clinical Categories of Pressure Ulcers* Early change: localized erythema that blanches on pressure.

Stage I: Nonblanching erythema of intact skin
Stage II: Necrosis, superficial or partial-thickness involving the epidermis and/or dermis. Bullae → necrosis of dermis (black) → shallow ulcer.
Stage III: Deep necrosis, crateriform ulceration with full-thickness skin loss (Fig. 14-15); damage or necrosis can extend down to, but not through, fascia.
Stage IV: Full-thickness ulceration with extensive damage/necrosis (Fig. 14-16) to muscle, bone, or supporting structures. May enlarge to many centimeters. May or may not be tender. Borders may be undetermined.

Well-established pressure ulcers are widest at the base and taper to a cone shape at the level of skin. Ulcers with devitalized tissue at the base (eschar) have a higher chance of secondary infection. Purulent exudate and erythema surrounding the ulcer suggest infection. Foul odor suggests anaerobic infection.

Distribution Occur over bony prominences: sacrum (60%) (Fig. 14-16) > ischial tuberosities, greater trochanter (Fig. 14-15), heel > elbow, knee, ankle, occiput.

General Examination Fever, chills, or increased pain of ulcer suggests possible cellulitis or osteomyelitis.

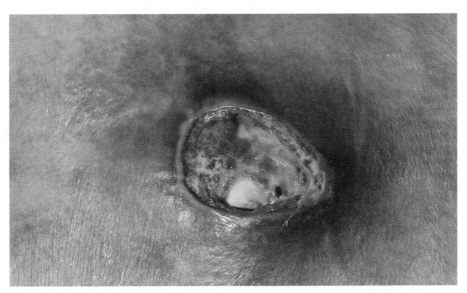

Figure 14-15 Pressure ulcer, stage III *Well-demarcated crateriform ulcer with full thickness skin loss extending down to fascia over greater trochanteric region.*

DIFFERENTIAL DIAGNOSIS

Infectious ulcer (actinomycotic infection, deep fungal infection, chronic herpetic ulcer), thermal burn, malignant ulcer (cutaneous lymphoma, basal cell or squamous cell carcinoma), pyoderma gangrenosum, rectocutaneous fistula.

LABORATORY EXAMINATIONS

Hematologic Studies Elevated white blood cell count and erythrocyte sedimentation rate suggest infection (osteomyelitis or bacteremia).

Wound Culture *Bacterial Culture* Infection must be differentiated from colonization. Culture of the ulcer base detects only surface bacteria. Optimal culture technique: Deep portion of punch biopsy specimen obtained from the ulcer base is minced and cultured for aerobic and anaerobic bacteria. Most infections are polymicrobial and difficult to diagnose. Commonly cultured pathogens include: *Staphylococcus aureus*, methicillin-resistant *S. aureus*, group A streptococcus, enterococcus, *Proteus mirabilis*, *Pseudomonas aeruginosa*, *Haemophilus influenzae* (scalp ulcers), anaerobes, *Bacillus fragilis*.

Viral Culture Rule out chronic herpes simplex virus ulcer.

Blood Culture Bacteremia often follows manipulation of ulcer (within 1 to 20 min of beginning the debridement); resolves within 30 to 60 min. Anaerobes are commonly present; frequently polymicrobial.

Pathology

Skin Biopsy Epidermal necrosis with eccrine duct and gland necrosis. Variable infiltrate of neutrophils and mononuclear cells around necrotic eccrine glands. Deep ulcers show wedge-shaped infarcts of the subcutaneous tissue, obstruction of the capillaries with microthrombi, and endothelial cell swelling followed by endothelial cell necrosis and secondary inflammation.

Bone Biopsy Essential for diagnosing continuous osteomyelitis; specimen is examined histologically and microbiologically.

Imaging It is difficult to distinguish osteomyelitis from chronic pressure-related changes by radiogram or scan.

DIAGNOSIS

Usually made clinically. Complications are assessed with data on cultures, biopsies, and imaging. Osteomyelitis occurs in nonhealing pressure ulcers; combination of elevated ery-

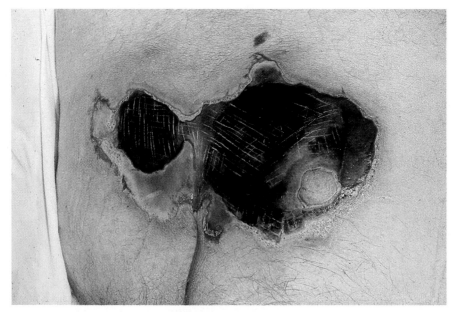

Figure 14-16 Pressure ulcer, stage IV *Huge black necrosis over sacral area in a patient who had been bedridden after a stroke. Debridement of necrotic tissue revealed involvement of fascia and bone.*

throcyte sedimentation rate, leukocytosis, and x-ray examination leads to diagnosis with 90% sensitivity and specificity.

COURSE AND PROGNOSIS

If pressure is relieved, some changes are reversible; intermittent periods of pressure relief increase resistance to compression. Osteomyelitis occurs in nonhealing pressure ulcers (32 to 81%). Septicemia is associated with a high mortality rate. Overall, patients with pressure ulcers have a fourfold risk of prolonged hospitalization and of dying when compared with patients without ulcers. With proper treatment, stages I and II ulcers heal in 1 to 2 weeks and stages III and IV ulcers heal in 6 to 12 weeks. Manipulation of pressure ulcers can cause bacteremia.

MANAGEMENT

Prophylaxis in At-Risk Patients Reposition patient every 2 h (more often if possible); massage areas prone to pressure ulcers while chang-

ing position of patient; inspect for areas of skin breakdown over pressure points.

- Use interface air mattress to reduce compression.
- Minimize friction and shear forces by using proper positioning, transferring, and turning techniques.
- Clean with mild cleansing agents, keeping skin free of urine and feces.
- Minimize skin exposure to excessive moisture from incontinence, perspiration, or wound drainage.
- Maintain head of the bed at a relatively low angle of elevation (<30 degrees).
- Evaluate and correct nutritional status; consider supplements of vitamin C and zinc.
- Mobilize patients as soon as possible.

Stages I and II Ulcers Topical antibiotics (not neomycin) under moist sterile gauze may be sufficient for early erosions. Normal saline wet-to-dry dressings may be needed for debridement. If ulcer does not heal by 30% within 2 weeks, consider hydrogels or hydrocolloid dressings.

Stages III and IV Ulcers Surgical management includes: debridement of necrotic tissue, bony prominence removal, flaps and skin grafts.

Infectious Complications *Continuous Osteomyelitis* Prolonged course of antimicrobial agent depending on sensitivities, with or without surgical debridement of necrotic bone.

Transient Bacteremia Treatment is usually not indicated.

Sepsis Marked by elevated temperature, chills, hypotension, and tachycardia and/or tachypnea. Massive antibiotic treatment according to antibiogram.

SKIN SIGNS OF SYSTEMIC CANCERS

MUCOCUTANEOUS SIGNS OF SYSTEMIC CANCERS

Mucocutaneous findings may suggest systemic cancers in several ways: associations of heritable mucocutaneous disorders with systemic cancers; by action at a distance, i.e., paraneoplastic syndromes; or spread to skin or mucosal sites by direct, lymphatic, or hematogenous extension (cutaneous metastasis).

CLASSIFICATION

Heritable Disorders

Cowden's syndrome, Peutz-Jeghers syndrome, Muir-Torre syndrome, Gardner's syndrome, von Recklinghausen's disease.

Paraneoplastic Syndromes

Association With Underlying Cancer Malignant acanthosis nigricans, tripe palms, Bazex's syndrome, carcinoid syndrome, erythema gyratum repens, hypertrichosis lanuginosa, ectopic ACTH syndrome, glucagonoma syndrome, neutrophilic dermatoses (Sweet's syndrome, pyoderma gangrenosum), paraneoplastic pemphigus, dermatomyositis, pruritus, palmar keratoses, migratory phlebitis (Trousseau's syndrome).

Possible Association with Underlying Cancer Arsenical keratoses, acquired ichthyosis, vasculitis.

Cutaneous Metastases

Direct Extension Paget's disease, extramammary Paget's disease.

Metastasis Persistent tumor, lymphatic extension, hematogenous spread.

METASTATIC CANCER TO THE SKIN

Metastatic cancer to the skin is characterized by solitary or multiple dermal or subcutaneous nodules, occurring as metastatic cells from a distant noncontiguous primary malignant neoplasm, that are transported to and deposited in the skin or subcutaneous tissue by hematogenous or lymphatic routes or across the peritoneal cavity.

EPIDEMIOLOGY

Age of Onset   Any age, but usually older.

Sex   Frequency of primary tumors varies with sex.

Females   Breast (69%), large intestine (9%), melanoma (5%), lung (4%), ovary (4%), sarcoma (2%), uterine cervix (2%), pancreas (2%), squamous cell carcinoma (SCC) of oral cavity (1%), bladder (1%).

Males   Lung (24%), large intestine (19%), melanoma (13%), SCC of oral cavity (12%), kidney (6%), stomach (6%), urinary bladder (2%), salivary glands (2%), breast (2%), 1% each in prostate, thyroid, liver, SCC of skin.

Incidence   .7 to 9% of all patients with cancer.

PATHOGENESIS

Includes detachment of cancer cells from primary tumor, invasion, intravasation into blood or lymphatic vessel, circulation, stasis within vessel, extravasation, invasion into tissue, proliferation at metastatic site. The growth of metastases depends on proliferation of metastatic cells, cytokine and growth factor release from cancer and stromal cells, angiogenesis, and immune reactions. Three patterns of metastases are observed: mechanical tumor stasis (anatomic proximity and lymphatic draining), site-specific (selective attachment of tumor cells to specific organ), nonselective (independent of mechanical or organ-specific factors).

HISTORY

Prior history of primary internal cancer or may be first sign of visceral cancer. In one series, underlying cancer had been undiagnosed in 60% of patients with lung cancer, in 53% with renal cancer, in 40% with ovarian cancer. Of patients with cutaneous metastases, skin lesion(s) was presenting sign in 37% of men but in only 6% of women.

History of cancer chemotherapy.

PHYSICAL EXAMINATION

Skin Lesions   Nodule (Figs. 15-1A and 15-1B), raised plaque, thickened fibrotic area. First detected when <5 mm. Fibrotic area may resemble morphea; occurring on scalp, may produce alopecia. Initially, epidermis is intact (Fig. 15-1A), stretched over nodule; in time, surface may become ulcerated or hyperkeratotic (Fig. 15-2). May appear inflammatory, i.e., pink to red (Figs. 15-1B, 15-2, and 15-3). Metastatic melanoma to dermis: blue to gray to black nodules (Fig. 15-4). Firm to indurated. May be solitary, few, or multiple.

Distribution   Lung cancer to trunk, scalp. Hypernephroma to scalp, operative scar.

Patterns of Cutaneous Involvement

Breast

Inflammatory metastatic carcinoma: erythematous patch or plaque with an active spreading border (carcinoma erysipeloides) (Fig. 15-3). Most often with breast cancer that may spread within lymphatics to skin of involved breast, resulting in inflammatory plaques resembling erysipelas. Breast most common primary, but occurs with others as well (pancreas, parotid, tonsils, colon, stomach, rectum, melanoma, pelvic organs, ovary, uterus, prostate, lung).

Telangiectatic metastatic carcinoma (carcinoma telangiectaticum): Breast cancer appearing as pinpoint telangiectases with dilated capillaries where it is associated with carcinoma erysipeloides. Violaceous papulovesicles resembling lymphangioma circumscriptum (Fig. 15-3).

En cuirasse metastatic carcinoma: diffuse morphea-like induration of skin. Begins as

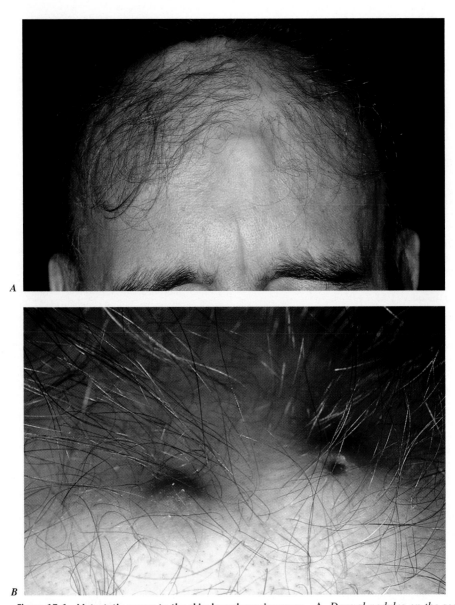

Figure 15-1 Metastatic cancer to the skin: bronchogenic cancer A. *Dermal nodules on the scalp of a patient undergoing chemotherapy for metastatic lung cancer; the nodules were only apparent following loss of hair during chemotherapy. The anterior nodule is asymptomatic, noninflamed.* B. *Close-up of posterior lesions: erythematous nodules; crust at a biopsy site.*

scattered, firm, lenticular papulonodules overlying erythematous or red-blue smooth cutaneous surface. Papulonodules coalesce into sclerodermoid plaque with no associated inflammation. Usually local extension of breast cancer occurring in the presternal re-

gion, which resembles a metal breastplate of a cuirassier. Also occurs with primary of lung, GI tract, kidney.

Breast carcinoma of inframammary crease: cutaneous exophytic nodule resembling primary SCC or basal cell carcinoma of skin.

SKIN SIGNS OF SYSTEMIC CANCERS

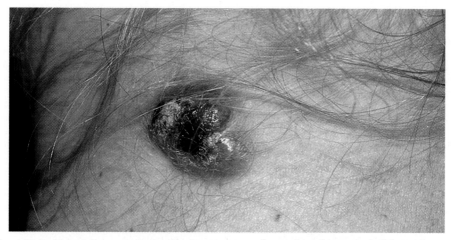

Figure 15-2 Metastatic cancer to the skin: breast cancer *Large, hyperkeratotic nodule on the posterior neck in a 40-year-old woman with metastatic breast cancer, present for 6 months; became ulcerated; similar but smaller lesions were present on the scalp and back.*

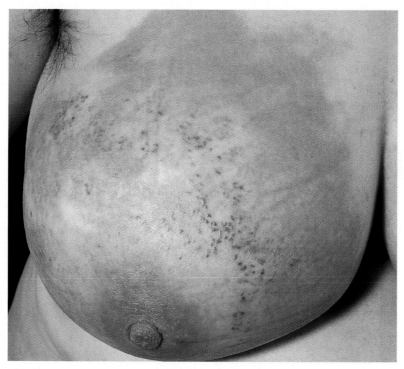

Figure 15-3 Metastatic cancer to the skin: inflammatory breast cancer (carcinoma erysipelatoides) *The breast is enlarged with an inflammatory, erythematous plaque resembling cellulitis or erysipelas on most of the surface; the cancer has spread via the cutaneous lymphatics. In addition, the breast is studded with numerous small, papular, erythematous telangiectases (telangiectatic carcinoma).*

Nodular metastatic carcinoma: multiple firm papulonodules or nodules. Usually multiple, may be solitary. May have keratotic core resembling keratoacanthoma (Fig. 15-2).

Paget's disease: sharply demarcated plaque or patch of erythema and scaling occurring on nipple or areola associated with underlying breast cancer (see Fig. 15-5).

Alopecia neoplastica: occurs via *hematogenous spread.* On scalp, areas of hair loss resembling alopecia areata; well-demarcated, red-pink, smooth surface.

Large Intestines   Often presents on skin of abdomen or perineal regions; also, scalp or face. Most originate in rectum. May present with metastatic inflammatory carcinoma (like carcinoma erysipeloides) of inguinal region, supraclavicular area, or face and neck. Less commonly, sessile or pedunculated nodules on buttocks, grouped vascular nodules of groin or scrotum, or facial tumor. Rarely, cutaneous fistula after appendectomy or resembling hidradenitis suppurativa.

Lung Carcinoma   May produce a large number of metastatic nodules in a short period. Most commonly, reddish nodule(s) (Fig. 15-1*B*) on scalp. Trunk: symmetric; along direction of intercostal vessels, may be zosteriform; in scar (thoracotomy site or needle aspiration tract).

Hypernephroma   Can produce solitary lesion; also widespread. Usually appear vascular, ±pulsatile, ±pedunculated; can resemble pyogenic granuloma. Most common on head (scalp) and neck; also trunk and extremities.

Malignant Melanoma   May spread from primary cutaneous site to distant cutaneous site by lymphatic vessels. Primary sites also can be noncutaneous: eye, cervix, oral cavity. Cutaneous metastases of unknown primary also occur. Nodules, single or multiple (Fig. 15-4). Usually deeply pigmented; amelanotic variants occur.

Carcinoma of Bladder, Ovary   Can spread contiguously to abdominal and inguinal skin similarly to breast cancer, as described above, and look like erysipelas.

Miscellaneous Patterns   With dilation of lymphatics and superficial hemorrhage, may resemble lymphangioma. With lymph stasis and dermal edema, resembles pigskin or orange peel. May metastasize hematogenously to scalp, forming many subcutaneous nodules with "bag of marbles" feel to scalp.

Sister Mary Joseph nodule is metastatic carcinoma to umbilicus from intraabdominal carcinoma, most commonly stomach, colon, ovary, pancreas; however, primary may be in breast. Easier to detect by palpation than by visual detection. Can be firm to indurated nodules, ±fissuring, ±ulceration, ±vascular appearance, ±discharge. In 15% may be initial presentation of primary malignancy (differential diagnosis: endometriosis of skin).

DIFFERENTIAL DIAGNOSIS

"Blueberry Muffin Baby"   Neuroblastoma, congenital leukemia.

Multiple Cylindroma-like Lesions: (Smooth Nodules on Scalp)*   Prostate adenocarcinoma, lung cancer, breast cancer.

Epidermal Inclusion or Pilar Cyst-like Lesions   Cancer of prostate, colon, breast.

Kaposi's Sarcoma-like Lesions   Cancer of kidney.

Pyogenic Granuloma-like Lesions   Amelanotic melanoma, renal cancer.

Alopecia Areata-like Lesions   Breast cancer.

Lymphangioma-like Lesions   Cancer of breast, lung, cervix, ovary.

Morphea-like lesions   Cancer of breast, stomach, lung, mixed tumors, lacrimal gland.

LABORATORY EXAMINATIONS

Dermatopathology   Carcinomatous deposits tend to spread in dermal lymphatic vessels, with resultant "Indian file" appearance of strands of cells. At times, cell differentiation sufficient to predict primary site; however, many times cells anaplastic. ±Dilatation of lymphatics secondary to carcinomatous lymphatic obstruction. Hypernephroma produces marked vascular proliferation.

Imaging   Look for primary tumor.

---

*Cylindromas are rare adnexal tumors of the scalp mimicking marbles tucked under the skin.

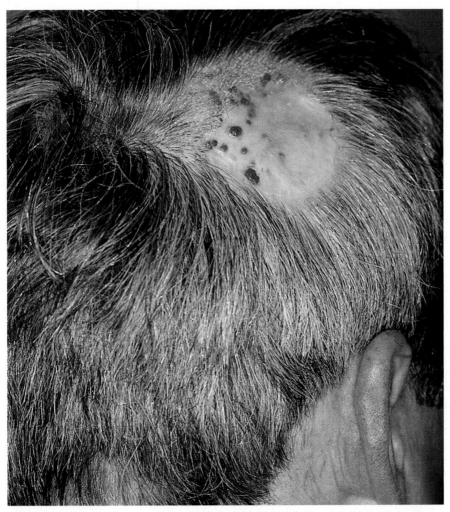

Figure 15-4 Recurrent melanoma *The primary melanoma had been excised from the scalp 2 years previously and the excision site grafted. The first recurrences were noted 6 months previously; the site was reexcised and a regional lymph node dissection performed. Melanoma recurring as red-purple dermal papules are seen at the grafted site and on the neck, along the surgical scar.*

DIAGNOSIS

Clinical history of internal cancer suggests diagnosis, confirmed by skin biopsy.

COURSE AND PROGNOSIS

In individuals with known cancer, cutaneous metastases are indicative of a poor prognosis. Average survival after detection of cutaneous metastasis only 3 months except for contiguous spread of breast cancer, which may last for years. With Paget's disease of breasts, prognosis better if no tumor palpable or no adenopathy.

MANAGEMENT

With solitary or few lesions and if patient not terminal, excision may be indicated.

PAGET'S DISEASE

Mammary Paget's Disease

Mammary Paget's disease (MPD) is a malignant neoplasm that unilaterally involves the nipple or areola and simulates a chronic eczematous dermatitis; it is associated with underlying intraductal carcinoma of the breast.

EPIDEMIOLOGY

Age of Onset 56 years (mean).

Sex Females, with rare examples in males.

Incidence 1 to 4% of all breast cancers.

HISTORY

Insidious onset over several months or years, may be asymptomatic. Pruritus, pain, burning. Discharge, bleeding, ulceration, nipple invagination.

PHYSICAL EXAMINATION

Skin Lesions Red, scaling plaque, rather sharply marginated, oval with irregular borders. When scale is removed, the surface is moist and oozing (Fig. 15-5). Lesions range in size from .3 to 15 cm. In early stages there is no induration of the plaque; but later, induration and infiltration develop, and nodules may be palpated in breast. At initial presentation an underlying breast mass is palpable in less than half of patients.

Distribution Single lesion localized to one nipple and areola. May uncommonly occur bilaterally. May also develop in ectopic breast tissue in females and males.

Regional Lymph Nodes Lymph node metastases occur more often when MPD is associated with an underlying palpable mass.

DIFFERENTIAL DIAGNOSIS

Red Areolar/Periareolar Plaque Eczematous dermatitis, psoriasis, benign ductal papilloma, nipple-areola retention hyperkeratosis, impetigo, pityriasis versicolor, SCC *in situ*, familial pemphigus.

Eczematous dermatitis of the nipples is usually bilateral; it is without any induration and responds rapidly to topical glucocorticoids. Nevertheless, be suspicious of Paget's disease if "eczema" persists for longer than 3 weeks.

LABORATORY AND SPECIAL EXAMINATIONS

Dermatopathology Neoplastic cells in epidermis. Typical large rounded cells with a large nucleus and without "intercellular bridges" (Paget's cells) that stain much lighter than surrounding keratinocytes.

Mammography Define underlying intraductal carcinoma.

DIAGNOSIS

Clinical findings confirmed by biopsy findings.

COURSE AND PROGNOSIS

When breast mass is not palpable, 92% of patients survive 5 years; 82%, 10 years. When breast mass is palpable, 38% survive 5 years; 22%, 10 years. Prognosis worse when there is lymphadenopathy.

MANAGEMENT

Surgery, radiotherapy, and/or chemotherapy as in any other breast carcinomas. Lymph node dissection if regional nodes are palpable.

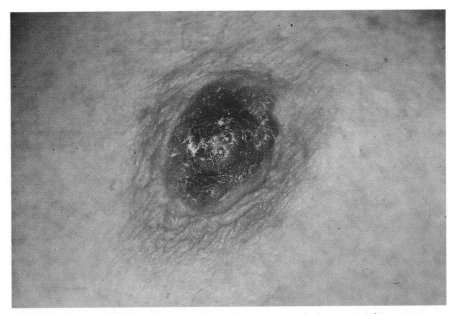

Figure 15-5 Mammary Paget's disease *A sharply demarcated red plaque mimicking eczema on the nipple. The plaque is slightly indurated and there is slight scaling; any red, eczema-like lesion on the nipple and areola that does not respond to topical corticosteroids should be biopsied.*

Extramammary Paget's Disease

Extramammary Paget's disease (EPD) is a neoplasm of the anogenital and axillary skin, histologically and clinically similar to Paget's disease of the breast, and often represents an intraepidermal extension of a primary adenocarcinoma of underlying apocrine glands or of the lower gastrointestinal, urinary, or female genital tracts.

EPIDEMIOLOGY

Age of Onset   >40 years.

Sex   Women >men.

CLASSIFICATION

- Unassociated with underlying cancer.
- Associated with underlying cancer, adjacent apocrine cancer, or eccrine gland carcinoma.
- Associated with another type of cancer, usually of gastrointestinal (GI) or genitourinary (GU) tract.

PATHOGENESIS

The histogenesis of EPD is not uniform. Paget cells in the epidermis may occur as an in situ upward extension of an in situ adenocarcinoma in deeper glands (25%). Alternatively, EPD may have a multifocal primary origin in the epidermis and its related appendages. The primary tumor and Paget cells are usually mucus-secreting. Primary tumors in the anorectum can arise within the rectal mucosa or intramuscular glands.

HISTORY

Insidious onset, slow spread, +itching.

PHYSICAL EXAMINATION

Skin Lesions   Erythematous plaque, +scaling, +erosion (Fig. 15-6), +crusting, +exudation; eczematous-appearing lesions. Borders sharply defined (Fig. 15-6), geographic configuration.

Distribution   Most commonly anogenital region (vulva, scrotum, penis, perianal, perineal skin) (Fig. 15-6) also, axilla, external ear canal, eyelids, umbilicus, pubic area. Rarely, more than one site involved simultaneously.

General Examination   Rectum, urethra, cervix should be examined for primary adenocarcinoma.

Rectal Examination, Proctoscopy, Sigmoidoscopy, Barium Enema   For perineal/perianal EPD, searching for underlying carcinoma.

Cystoscopy, Intravenous Pyelogram   For genital EPD, searching for underlying carcinoma.

Pelvic Examination   For vulvar EPD, searching for underlying carcinoma.

DIFFERENTIAL DIAGNOSIS

Red Plaque   Eczematous dermatitis, lichen simplex chronicus, lichen sclerosus et atrophicus, lichen planus, inverse pattern psoriasis, intertriginous, *Candida* intertrigo, SCC in situ (erythroplasia of Queyrat), human papillomavirus–induced SCC in situ, (amelanotic) superficial spreading melanoma.

LABORATORY EXAMINATIONS

Dermatopathology

Characteristic Paget cells are dispersed between keratinocytes, occur in clusters, extend down into adnexal structures (hair follicles, eccrine ducts). Adnexal adenocarcinoma is often found when carefully searched for. Dermis shows chronic inflammatory reaction. Paget cells are characterized by clear, abundant cytoplasm and do not form intercellular bridges with adjacent keratinocytes. Both the cells and their nuclei are rounded; nuclei are vesicular or hyperchromatic. Cytoplasm PAS-positive, diastase-resistant, supporting glandular origin.

DIAGNOSIS

Clinical suspicion confirmed by skin biopsy.

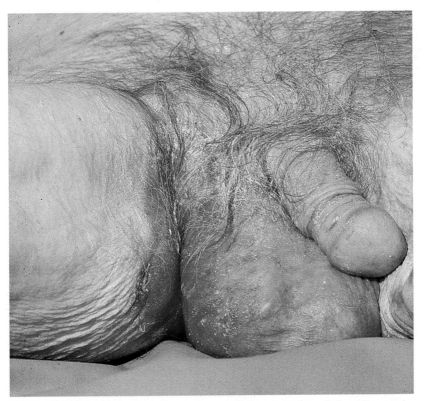

Figure 15-6 Extramammary Paget's disease *Moist, well-demarcated, eroded, oozing, erythematous plaque on the scrotum and inguinal fold in an older male. The lesion is commonly mistaken for* Candida *intertrigo and, unsuccessfully treated as such.*

COURSE AND PROGNOSIS

EPD remains in situ in the epidermis and adnexal epithelium in >65% of cases. Prognosis related to existence of underlying adenocarcinoma. When no underlying neoplasm is present, there is a high recurrence rate, even after apparently adequate excision; this is due to the multifocal origin in the epidermis and adnexal structures.

MANAGEMENT

EPD is usually much larger than is apparent clinically. Surgical excision must be controlled histologically (Mohs' microscopic surgery). If Paget cells are in dermis and regional lymph nodes are palpable, lymph node dissection may improve prognosis.

COWDEN'S SYNDROME (MULTIPLE HAMARTOMA SYNDROME)

Cowden's syndrome (named after the propositus) is a rare, autosomal dominant heritable cancer syndrome with variable expressivity in a number of systems in the form of multiple hamartomatous neoplasms of ectodermal, mesodermal, and endodermal origin. There is a special susceptibility for breast and thyroid cancers; and the skin lesions, which are special adnexal tumors (tricholemmomas), are important markers because they portend the onset of breast and thyroid cancers.

CLINICAL MANIFESTATION

Skin lesions, which may appear first in childhood but develop over time, consist of *tricholemmomas,* skin-colored, pink (Fig. 15-7), or brown papules having the appearance of flat warts on the central area of the face, perioral areas, lips near the angles of the mouth, and the ears; *translucent punctate keratoses* of the palms and soles; and *hyperkeratotic, flat-topped papules* on the dorsa of the hands and forearms. Mucous membrane lesions are characteristic: *papules* of the gingival, labial (Fig. 15-7), and palatal surfaces; they are whiter than the surrounding mucosa and often coalesce, giving a "cobblestone" appearance. *Papillomas* of the buccal mucosa and the tongue.

Systems Review In addition to breast cancer (20%), which is often bilateral, and thyroid cancer (8%), there are various internal hamartomas:

Breasts—fibrocystic disease, fibroadenomas, adenocarcinoma, gynecomastia in males; *Thyroid*—goiter, adenomas, thyroglossal duct cysts, follicular adenocarcinoma; *GI tract*—hamartomatous polyps throughout tract but increased in large bowel, adenocarcinoma arising in polyp; *Female genital tract*—ovarian cysts, menstrual abnormalities; *Musculoskeletal*—craniomegaly, kyphoscoliosis, "adenoid" facies, high-arched palate; *CNS*—mental retardation, seizures, neuromas, ganglioneuromas, and meningiomas of the ear canal.

SIGNIFICANCE

It is important to establish the diagnosis of Cowden's syndrome so that these patients can be followed carefully to detect breast and thyroid cancers.

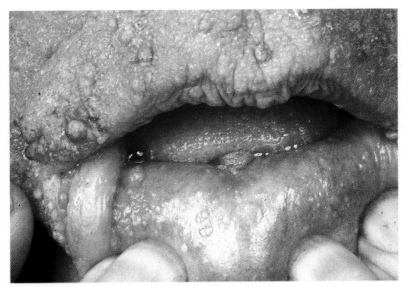

Figure 15-7 Cowden's syndrome: tricholemmomas *Multiple skin-colored warty papules on the face, as well as on the mucosa of the lower lip.*

GLUCAGONOMA SYNDROME

Glucagonoma syndrome is a rare but well-described clinical entity caused by excessive production of glucagon in an α cell tumor of the pancreas, characterized by superficial migratory necrolytic erythema (MNE) with erosions that crust and heal with hyperpigmentation, a beefy-red tongue, and angular cheilitis.

EPIDEMIOLOGY

Age of Onset   Middle-aged to elderly.

Etiology   Most cases associated with glucagonoma, but pathogenesis of MNE is not known. There exists MNE without glucagonoma.

PATHOGENESIS

Most cases are associated with glucagon production by a pancreatic glucagonoma. Pathogenesis of cutaneous findings is unknown; may be related to nutritional deficiency. Isolated cases have been reported of MNE associated with advanced hepatic cirrhosis and a bronchial carcinoma.

HISTORY

Rash unresponsive to conventional therapy. Weight loss, abdominal pain, diabetes.

PHYSICAL EXAMINATION

Skin Lesions   Inflammatory red plaques (Fig. 15-8) of gyrate, circinate, arcuate, annular shape, enlarge with central clearing, resulting in geographic areas that become confluent (Fig. 15-9). Borders show vesiculation to bulla formation, crusting, and scaling (Figs. 15-8 and 15-9). Lesions involve perioral and perigenital regions and flexures and intertriginal areas. Fingertips red, shining, erosive.

Mucous Membranes   Glossitis, angular cheilitis (Fig. 15-8), blepharitis.

General Examination   Wasting, malnutrition.

DIFFERENFTIAL DIAGNOSIS

Moist Red Plaque(s)   Acrodermatitis enteropathica, zinc deficiency, pustular psoriasis, mucocutaneous candidiasis, Hailey-Hailey disease (familial pemphigus).

LABORATORY EXAMINATIONS

Chemistry   Fasting plasma glucagon level to >1000 ng/L (normal 50 to 250 ng/L) makes the diagnosis. Hyperglycemia, reduced glucose tolerance. Associated findings: severe malabsorption, gross hypoaminoacidemia, low serum zinc.

Dermatopathology   Early skin lesions show bandlike upper epidermal necrosis with retention of pyknotic nuclei and pale keratinocyte cytoplasm (electron microscopy shows vacuolar degeneration and lysis of organelles).

CT Scan, Angiography   Locates tumor within pancreas.

DIAGNOSIS

Clinical findings confirmed by skin biopsy and serum glucagon levels.

COURSE AND PROGNOSIS

Depends on the aggressiveness of the glucagonoma. Hepatic metastases have occurred in 75% of patients at the time of diagnosis. If these are slow-growing, patients may have prolonged survival, even with metastatic disease.

MANAGEMENT

MNE   Responds poorly to all types of therapy. Some cases have responded partially to zinc replacement. MNE resolves after tumor excision.

Surgery   Surgical excision of glucagonoma achieves cure in only 30% of cases because of persistent metastases (usually liver). Surgery also reduces tumor masses and associated symptoms.

Chemotherapy   Poor response.

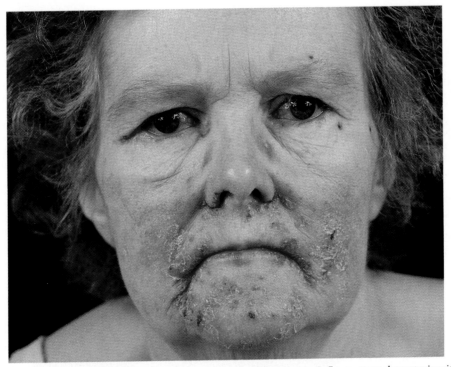

Figure 15-8   Glucagonoma syndrome: migratory necrolytic erythema   *Inflammatory dermatosis with angular cheilitis, inflammatory, scaly, erosive and crusted plaques and fissures around the nose, mouth, and medial aspects of the eyes.*

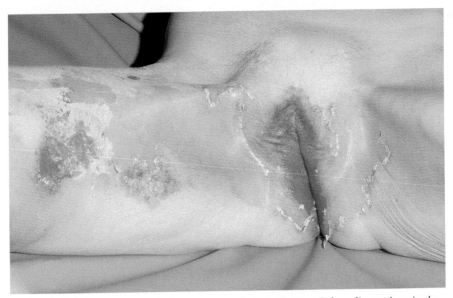

Figure 15-9   Glucagonoma syndrome: migratory necrolytic erythema   *Polycyclic erosions in the anogenital gluteal and sacral regions. Sharply defined with necrotic flaccid epidermis still covering part of these erosions.*

GLUCAGONOMA SYNDROME

PEUTZ-JEGHERS SYNDROME

Peutz-Jeghers syndrome (PJS) is a familial (autosomal dominant, spontaneous mutation in 40%) polyposis characterized by many small, pigmented brown macules (lentigines) on the lips, oral mucous membranes (brown to bluish black), and also on the bridge of nose, palms, soles. There are usually, but not always, multiple hamartomatous polyps in the small bowel, as well as in the large bowel and stomach, that cause abdominal symptoms such as pain, GI bleeding, anemia. Whereas pigmented macules are congenital or develop in infancy and early childhood, polyps come on in late childhood or before age 30. Macules on the lips may disappear over time, but not the pigmentation of the mouth; and therefore the mouth pigmentation is the sine qua non for the diagnosis (Fig. 15-10). The lentigines occur in some patients who never have abdominal lesions. Adenocarcinoma may develop in polyps and there is an increased incidence of breast, ovarian, and pancreatic cancer.

There is a normal life expectancy unless carcinoma develops in the GI tract. Malignant neoplasms may be more frequent in the Japanese with this syndrome, and prophylactic colectomy has been recommended for these patients.

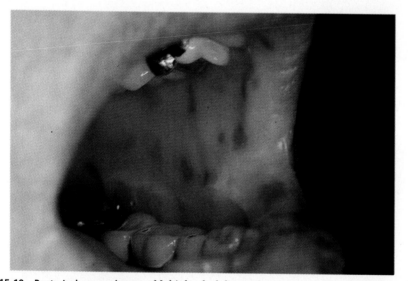

Figure 15-10   Peutz-Jeghers syndrome   *Multiple, dark-brown lentigines on the vermilion border of the lip and the buccal mucosa. This patient had GI bleeding due to hamartomatous polyps in the small bowel.*

SKIN SIGNS OF SYSTEMIC CANCERS

MALIGNANT ACANTHOSIS NIGRICANS

Like other forms of acanthosis nigricans (AN), malignant AN starts as a diffuse, velvety thickening and hyperpigmentation chiefly on the neck, axillae and other body folds, as well as the perioral and periorbital, umbilical, mamillary, and genital areas, giving the skin a dirty appearance (Fig. 15-11). Hyperpigmentation and hyperkeratosis soon lead to a rugose, mamillated, and papillomatous surface (Fig. 15-11); verrucous growths also involve the vermilion border of the lips (Fig. 15-12); and the knuckles and the palms show maximal accentuation of the palmar ridges (tripe hands) (Fig. 15-13). On the oral mucous membranes there is a velvety texture with delicate furrows, and there are warty papillomatous thickenings periorally.

Malignant AN differs from other forms of AN primarily because of (1) the more pronounced velvety hyperkeratosis and hyperpigmentation, (2) the pronounced mucosal involvement and involvement of the mucocutaneous junction, (3) tripe hands, and (4) weight loss and wasting due to the underlying malignancy.

AN may precede by 5 years other symptoms of a malignancy, usually adenocarcinoma of the GI or GU tract, bronchocarcinoma, or, less commonly, lymphoma. Malignant AN is a truly paraneoplastic disease, and a search for underlying malignancies is imperative. Removal of malignancy is followed by regression of AN.

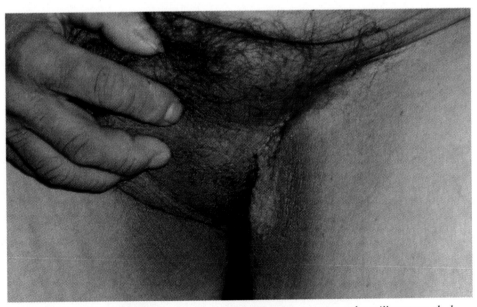

Figure 15-11   Acanthosis nigricans   *Poorly defined, velvety, verrucous and papillomatous, dark-chocolate-brown plaques on the medial thighs and scrotum. Similar changes were also present in the axillae and neck and the vermilion border of the lips was covered with velvety, raspberry-like growths.*

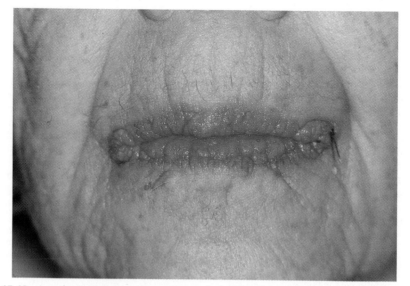

Figure 15-12   Acanthosis nigricans   *Verrucous and mamillated growths on the vermilion border of the lips in a patient with carcinoma of the stomach. The gastric cancer was suspected because of these raspberry-like growths, acanthosis nigricans of the major skin folds, and weight loss.*

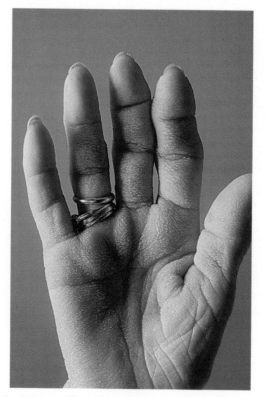

Figure 15-13   Acanthosis nigricans   *The palmar ridges of the palm show maximal accentuation, thus resembling the mucosa of the stomach of a ruminant (tripe palm).*

PARANEOPLASTIC PEMPHIGUS (PNP)

Mucous membranes primarily and most severely involved. Lesions combine features of pemphigus vulgaris (page 94) and erythema multiforme (page 136), clinically, histologically, and immunopathologically. Most prominent clinical findings consist of severe oral and conjunctival erosions (Fig. 15-14) in a patient with an underlying neoplasm, usually a lymphoma. PNP sera immunoprecipitate from human keratinocyte extracts a complex of five polypeptides that are not yet fully characterized but include bullous pemphigoid antigen I, desmoplakin I, and another desmosomal plaque protein. Autoantibodies of PNP cause blistering in neonatal mice. Treatment is directed toward elimination or suppression of malignancy but may also require systemic glucocorticoids.

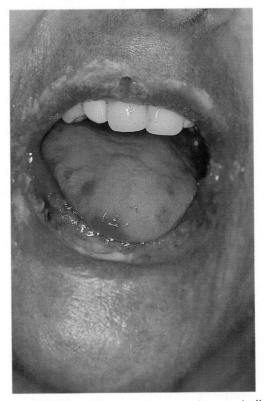

Figure 15-14 Paraneoplastic pemphigus *Severe erosions covering practically the entire mucosa of the oral cavity with partial sparing of the dorsum of the tongue. Lesions are extremely painful interfering with adequate food intake. This patient had non-Hodgkin's lymphoma as underlying malignancy.*

SKIN SIGNS OF HEMATOLOGIC DISEASES

THROMBOCYTOPENIC PURPURA

Thrombocytopenic purpura (TP) is characterized by cutaneous hemorrhages occurring in association with a reduced platelet count; hemorrhages are clinically usually small (petechiae) but at times larger (ecchymoses) and occur at sites of minor trauma/pressure (platelet count $<40,000/\mu L$) or spontaneously (platelet count $<10,000/\mu L$).

EPIDEMIOLOGY

Age of Onset Acute idiopathic thrombocytopenic purpura (ITP)—children; drug-induced and autoimmune TP—adults.

Sex Both sexes; HIV-associated thrombocytopenic purpura—homosexual men.

Etiology *Decreased Platelet Production* Direct injury to bone marrow, drugs (cytosine arabinoside, daunorubicin, cyclophosphamide, busulfan, methotrexate, 6-mercaptopurine, vinca alkaloids, thiazide diuretics, ethanol, estrogens), replacement of bone marrow, aplastic anemia, vitamin deficiencies, Wiskott-Aldrich syndrome.

Splenic Sequestration Splenomegaly, hypothermia.

Increased Platelet Destruction *Immunologic:* autoimmune TP, drug hypersensitivity (sulfonamides, quinine, quinidine, carbamazepine, digitoxin, methyldopa), after transfusion. *Nonimmunologic:* infection, prosthetic heart valves, disseminated intravascular coagulation (generalized stimulus; localized stimulus, Kasabach-Merritt syndrome), thrombotic thrombocytopenic purpura.

PATHOGENESIS

Platelet plugs by themselves effectively stop bleeding from capillaries and small blood vessels but are incapable of stopping hemorrhage from larger vessels. Platelet defects therefore produce problems with small-vessel hemostasis, small hemorrhages in the skin or in the CNS.

HISTORY

Usually sudden appearance of asymptomatic hemorrhagic skin and/or mucosal lesions.

PHYSICAL EXAMINATION

Skin Lesions *Petechiae*—small (pinpoint to pinhead), red, nonblanching macules that are not palpable and turn brown as they get older; later acquiring a yellowish-green tinge (Fig. 16-1). *Ecchymoses*—black-and-blue spots; larger area of hemorrhage. *Vibices*—linear hemorrhages, (Fig. 16-1) due to trauma or pressure. Most common on legs and upper trunk, but may be anywhere.

Mucous Membranes *Petechiae*—most often on palate (Fig. 16-2), gingival bleeding.

General Examination Possible CNS hemorrhage, anemia.

DIFFERENTIAL DIAGNOSIS

Nonhemorrhagic Blanching Vascular Lesions Telangiectasia/erythema, spider nevi, Osler's disease.

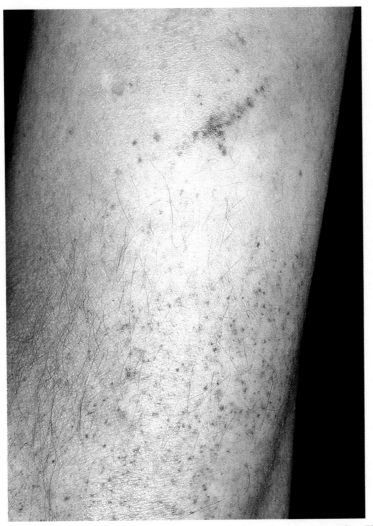

Figure 16-1 Thrombocytopenic purpura *Myriads of petechiae on the upper arm of an HIV-infected 25-year-old male were the presenting manifestation of (vibices) his disease. A linear arrangement of petechiae with an ecchymosis at the site of minor trauma.*

True Hemorrhagic Lesions Bateman's (actinic or senile) purpura, purpura of scurvy, progressive pigmentary purpura (Schamberg's disease), purpura following severe Valsalva maneuver (coughing, vomiting/retching), traumatic purpura, factitial or iatrogenic purpura, Gardner-Diamond syndrome (autoerythrocyte sensitization syndrome), *palpable nonblanching purpura-vasculitis.*

LABORATORY EXAMINATIONS

Hematology Thrombocytopenia.

Bone Marrow Aspiration Defines state of platelet production.

Serology Rule out HIV disease.

Lesional Skin Biopsy May be contraindicated due to postoperative hemorrhage; however, usually can be controlled by suturing biopsied site.

DIAGNOSIS

Clinical suspicion confirmed by platelet count.

COURSE AND PROGNOSIS

Varies with the etiology.

MANAGEMENT

Identify underlying cause and correct, if possible. If platelet count is very low ($<$10,000/μL), bed rest to reduce risk of hemorrhage.

Oral Glucocorticoids, High-Dose Immunoglobulins

Platelet Transfusions If platelet count $<$10,000/μL, platelet transfusion may be indicated.

Chronic ITP Splenectomy may be indicated.

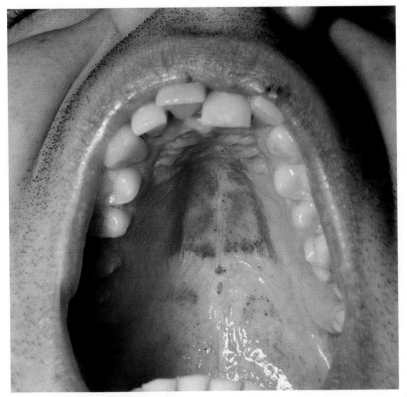

Figure 16-2   Thrombocytopenic purpura   *May first manifest on the oral mucosa or conjunctiva. Here multiple petechial hemorrhages are seen on the palate.*

DISSEMINATED INTRAVASCULAR COAGULATION

Disseminated intravascular coagulation (DIC) is a widespread blood clotting disorder occurring within blood vessels, associated with a wide range of clinical circumstances (bacterial sepsis, obstetric complications, disseminated malignancy, massive trauma), and manifested by purpura fulminans (cutaneous infarctions and/or acral gangrene) or bleeding from multiple sites. The spectrum of clinical symptoms associated with DIC ranges from relatively mild and subclinical to explosive and life-threatening.

Synonyms: Purpura fulminans, consumption coagulopathy, defibrination syndrome, coagulation-fibrinolytic syndrome.

EPIDEMIOLOGY

Age of Onset All ages, occurs in children.

Etiology Events that Initiate DIC *Massive Tissue Destruction* Tumor products, crushing trauma, extensive surgery, severe intracranial damage; retained contraception products, placental abruption, amniotic fluid embolism; certain snake bites; hemolytic transfusion reaction; acute promyelocytic leukemia; burn injuries.

Extensive Destruction of Endothelial Surfaces, Exposure to Foreign Surfaces Vasculitis in Rocky Mountain spotted fever, meningococcemia, or occasionally gram-negative septicemia, group A streptococcal infection, heat stroke, malignant hyperthermia; extensive pump oxygenation (repair of aortic aneurysm); eclampsia, preeclampsia; giant hemangioma (Kasabach-Merritt syndrome); immune complexes; postvaricella purpura gangrenosa.

Events that Complicate and Propagate DIC Shock, complement pathway activation.

PATHOGENESIS

Uncontrolled activation of coagulation results in thrombosis and consumption of platelets/clotting factors II, V, VIII. Secondary fibrinolysis. If the activation occurs slowly, excess activated products produced, predisposing to vascular infarctions/venous thrombosis. If the onset is acute, hemorrhage surrounding wound sites and IV lines/catheters or bleeding into deep tissues is usually seen.

HISTORY

Hours to days; rapid evolution. Usually complication developing during convalescence from etiologic circumstances. Fever, chills associated with onset of hemorrhagic lesions.

PHYSICAL EXAMINATION

Skin Lesions

Infarction (purpura fulminans) (Fig. 16-3): massive ecchymoses with sharp, irregular ("geographic") borders with deep purple color and erythematous halo, ±evolution to hemorrhagic bullae and blue to black gangrene (Fig. 16-4); multiple lesions are often symmetric; distal extremities, areas of pressure; lips, ears, nose, trunk; peripheral acrocyanosis followed by gangrene on hands (Fig. 16-5), feet, tip of nose, with subsequent autoamputation if patient survives.

Hemorrhage from multiple cutaneous sites, i.e., surgical incisions, venipuncture or catheter sites.

Mucous Membranes Hemorrhage from gingiva.

General Examination High fever, tachycardia, ±shock. Multitude of findings depending on the associated medical/surgical problem.

DIFFERENTIAL DIAGNOSIS

Large Cutaneous Infarctions Necrosis after initiation of warfarin therapy, heparin necrosis, calciphylaxis, atheroembolization.

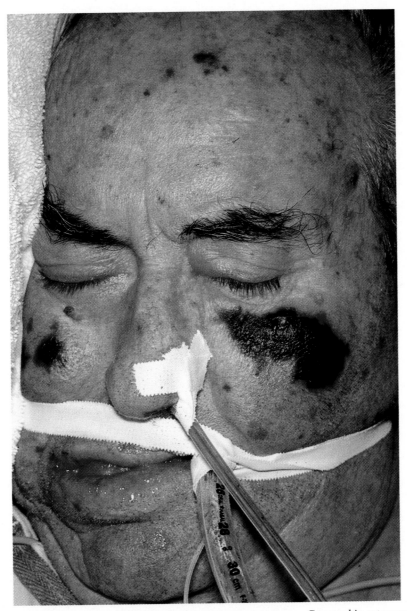

Figure 16-3 **Disseminated intravascular coagulation: purpura fulminans** *Geographic cutaneous infarctions on the cheeks with smaller lesions on the forehead; lesions were also present on the hands, elbows, thighs, and feet. The patient was a diabetic with* Staphylococcus aureus *sepsis and died within 24 h after onset of the purpuric lesions.*

LABORATORY EXAMINATIONS

Dermatopathology Occlusion of arterioles with fibrin thrombi. Dense PMN infiltrate around infarct and massive hemorrhage.

Hematologic Studies CBC Schistocytes (fragmented RBCs), arising from RBC entrapment and damage within fibrin thrombi, seen on blood smear; platelet count low. Leukocytosis.

Coagulation Studies Reduced plasma fibrinogen; elevated fibrin degradation products; prolonged PT, PTT, and thrombin time.

DIAGNOSIS

Clinical suspicion confirmed by coagulation studies.

COURSE AND PROGNOSIS

Mortality rate is high. Surviving patients require skin grafts or amputation for gangrenous tissue. Common complications: severe bleeding, thrombosis, tissue ischemia/necrosis, hemolysis, organ failure.

MANAGEMENT

Correct reversible cause. Vigorous antibiotic therapy for infections. Control bleeding or thrombosis: heparin, pentoxyphyllin. Prevent recurrence in chronic DIC.

SKIN SIGNS OF HEMATOLOGIC DISEASES

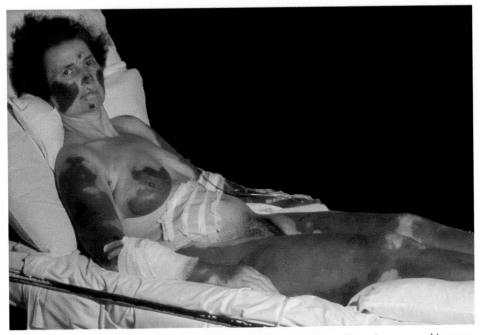

Figure 16-4   Disseminated intravascular coagulation: purpura fulminans   *Extensive geographic areas of cutaneous infarction with hemorrhage involving the face, breast, and extremities; although the patient looked alert, she died within several days. This catastrophic event followed sepsis after abdominal surgery.*

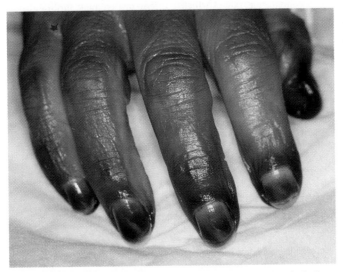

Figure 16-5   Disseminated intravascular coagulation   *Gangrene of the distal phalanges in meningococcal sepsis, which progressed to involve the full lengths of the fingers and necessitated amputation after the patient's recovery.*

DISSEMINATED INTRAVASCULAR COAGULATION

CRYOGLOBULINEMIA

Cryoglobulinemia (CG) is the presence of serum immunoglobulin (precipitates at low temperature and redissolves at 37°C) complexed with other immunoglobulins or proteins. Associated clinical findings include purpura in cold-exposed sites, Raynaud's phenomenon, cold urticaria, acral hemorrhagic necrosis, bleeding disorders, vasculitis, arthralgia, neurologic manifestations, hepatosplenomegaly, and glomerulonephritis.

EPIDEMIOLOGY

Age of Onset, Sex Those of associated disorders.

Etiology That of associated disorders.

CLASSIFICATION OF CRYOGLOBULINEMIA AND ASSOCIATED DISEASES

Type I Cryoglobulins Monoclonal immunoglobulins (IgM, IgG, IgA, light chains). Cutaneous, vasomotor symptoms such as acral gangrene; renal/neurologic problems. *Associated diseases:* plasma cell dyscrasias such as multiple myeloma, Waldenström's macroglobulinemia, lymphoproliferative disorders such as chronic lymphocytic leukemia.

Type II Cryoglobulins Mixed cryoglobulins: two immunoglobulin components, one of which is monoclonal (usually IgG, less often IgM) and one polyclonal; components interact and cryoprecipitate. Cutaneous, vasomotor symptoms, palpable purpura, Raynaud's phenomenon; renal/neurologic problems. *Associated diseases:* multiple myeloma, Waldenström's macroglobulinemia, chronic lymphocytic leukemia; rheumatoid arthritis, systemic lupus erythematosus, Sjögren's syndrome.

Type III Cryoglobulins Polyclonal immunoglobulins that form cryoprecipitate with polyclonal IgG or a nonimmunoglobulin serum component occasionally mixed with complement and lipoproteins. Probably represents immune complex disease in which the complexes form cryoprecipitates; palpable purpura, Raynaud's phenomenon; renal/neurologic problems. *Associated diseases:* Autoimmune diseases; connective tissue diseases; wide variety of infectious diseases, i.e., hepatitis B, hepatitis C, Epstein-Barr virus infection, cytomegalovirus infection, subacute bacterial endocarditis, leprosy, syphilis, β-hemolytic streptococcal infections.

PATHOGENESIS

Precipitation of cryoglobulins (when present in large amounts) causes vessel occlusion, also associated with hyperviscosity (type I); immune complex deposition followed by complement activation and inflammation; platelet aggregation/consumption of clotting factors by cryoglobulins, causing coagulation disorder; small vessel thromboses and vasculitis produced by immune complexes (types II and III).

HISTORY

Cold sensitivity, <50% of cases. Chills, fever, dyspnea, diarrhea may occur following cold exposure. Purpura also may follow long periods of standing or sitting. Due to other organ system involvement, arthralgia, renal symptoms, neurologic symptoms, abdominal pain, arterial thrombosis.

PHYSICAL EXAMINATION

Skin Lesions

Noninflammatory purpura (usually type I): occurs at cold-exposed sites, e.g., helix (Fig. 16-6), tip of nose. *Palpable purpura* (usually types II and III) as in hypersensitivity vasculitis, occurring in crops on lower extremities with extension to thighs, abdomen, precipitated by standing up; less commonly by cold. *Livedo reticularis* mostly on lower and upper extremities. *Acrocyanosis* and *Raynaud's phenomenon*, with or without severe resultant gangrene of fingertips and toes (usually types I or II) (Fig. 16-7). *Urticaria* induced by cold, associated with purpura.

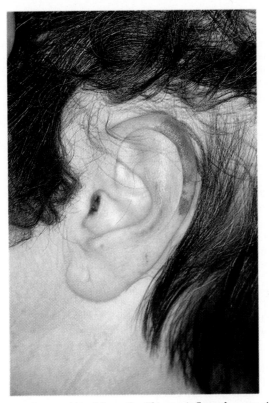

Figure 16-6 Cryoglobulinemia: monoclonal (type I)   *This noninflamed, purpuric lesion on the helix appeared on the first cold day in the fall.*

General Examination Related to underlying diseases. Renal involvement: 30 to 60% of individuals with essential mixed CG (type II) develop renal disease with hypertension, edema, or renal failure. Neurologic involvement: peripheral sensorimotor polyneuropathy, presenting as paresthesias or foot drop. Arthritis. Hepatosplenomegaly.

DIFFERENTIAL DIAGNOSIS

Cold agglutinins, cryofibrinogenemia.

LABORATORY EXAMINATIONS

Cryoglobulins Blood drawn into warmed syringe, RBC removed via warmed centrifuge. Plasma refrigerated in a Wintrobe tube at 4°C for 24 to 72 h; then centrifuged and cryocrit determined.

Type I Usually high (75 mg/mL).

Type II Often very high; typical monoclonal spike not always present on immunoelectrophoresis.

Type III Usually low (<1 mg/mL). Polyclonal immunoglobulin complexes or polyclonal immunoglobulin–nonimmunoglobulin cryoprecipitates; IgM-IgG cryoglobulins most frequent. C1q may be present in cryoprecipitates.

Bone Marrow Aspiration Diagnose myeloproliferative states.

Other Renal involvement: urinalysis shows proteinuria, hematuria, pyuria, red cell casts. Hepatic involvement: increased alkaline phosphatase.

Serology IgG monoclonal rheumatoid factors present in 10% of cases of type I CG, ANA; antigens of, and antibodies to hepatitis B virus (HBV) and hepatitis C virus (HCV).

Dermatopathology *Type 1* (monoclonal): Dermal vessels contain intraluminal amorphous eosinophilic material, mainly precipitated cryoglobulin; inflammatory infiltrate usually absent. *Types II and III*: leukocytoclastic vasculitis, with or without intraluminal cryoprecipitate.

DIAGNOSIS

Clinical suspicion confirmed by detection of cryoglobulins.

COURSE AND PROGNOSIS

Cyclic eruptions usually induced by cold or fluctuations of activity of underlying disease. Prognosis depends on underlying disease; often guarded.

MANAGEMENT

Treatment based on severity of symptoms and morbidity and mortality of underlying disease.

NSAIDs For mild dermatologic and articular symptoms.

Glucocorticoids For severe visceral involvement.

Cytotoxic Agents (cyclophosphamide, melphalan, chlorambucil) For renal disease; often combined with prednisone.

Plasmapheresis at 37°C For rapidly progressive disease.

Cryofiltration For patients refractory to other therapies.

Interferon α For patients with hepatitis C-associated CG.

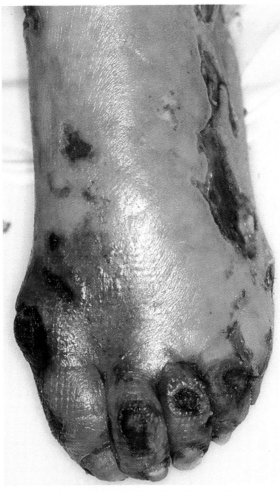

Figure 16-7   Cryoglobulinemia: mixed (type II)   *Associated Raynaud's phenomenon and arterial occlusion have resulted in extensive necroses, hemorrhage, and ulcerations on the skin of the foot.*

LANGERHANS CELL HISTIOCYTOSIS

Langerhans cell histiocytosis (LCH) is an idiopathic group of disorders characterized histologically by proliferation and infiltration of tissue by Langerhans cell–type histiocytes that fuse into multinucleated giant cells and form granulomas with eosinophils. LCH is characterized clinically by cutaneous findings that range from soft tissue swelling to eczema-like and seborrheic dermatitis–like changes and ulceration and by lytic bony lesions.

Synonyms: Type II histiocytosis, eosinophilic granuloma, Hand-Schüller-Christian disease, Letterer-Siwe syndrome (LSS).

CLASSIFICATION

The disorders of xanthohistiocytic proliferation involving histiocytes, foam cells, and mixed inflammatory cells are divided into Langerhans cell histiocytosis (LCH, formerly, histiocytosis X) and non-Langerhans cell histiocytoses (nonhistiocytosis X). A simplified classification of LCH is presented in Table 16-1.

EPIDEMIOLOGY

Age of Onset *Unifocal LCH* Most commonly, childhood and early adulthood.

Multifocal LCH Most commonly, childhood.

LSS More commonly, first few years; also, adult form.

Sex Males>females.

Etiology Unknown.

Incidence Rare, .5 per 100,000 children in the United States (estimate).

PATHOGENESIS

The stimulus for the proliferation of Langerhans cells is unknown.

HISTORY

Unifocal LCH Systemic symptoms uncommon. Pain and/or swelling over underlying bony lesion. Disruption of teeth with mandibular disease, fracture, otitis media due to mastoid involvement; recalcitrant ulcer on oral mucosa or genital region. Often, lesions are asymptomatic and diagnosed on radiographs for unrelated disorders.

Multifocal LCH Erosive skin lesions are exudative, pruritic, or painful, with poor response to local treatments. Moist scalp and intertriginous lesions may have offensive odor. Associated disorders include otitis media caused by destruction of temporal and mastoid bones, proptosis due to orbital masses, loose teeth with infiltration of maxilla or mandible, anterior and/or pituitary dysfunction with involvement of sella turcica associated with growth retardation. Diabetes insipidus occurs secondary to hypothalamic or pituitary involvement. Triad of lytic skull lesions, proptosis, and diabetes insipidus: Hand-Schüller-Christian disease. Lung involvement associated with chronic cough, pneumothorax.

LSS Child is systemically ill with a course that resembles a systemic infection or malignancy. Hepatomegaly, petechiae, and purpura, generalized skin eruption.

PHYSICAL EXAMINATION

Skin Lesions *Unifocal LCH*

1. Swelling over bony lesion, over long (e.g., humerus) or flat bone (e.g., rib, mastoid), tender.
2. Cutaneous/subcutaneous nodule, yellowish, may be tender and break down, occurring anywhere.
3. Sharply marginated ulcer, usually in genital and perigenital regions or oral mucous membrane (gingiva, hard palate). Necrotic base, draining, tender (Fig. 16-8).

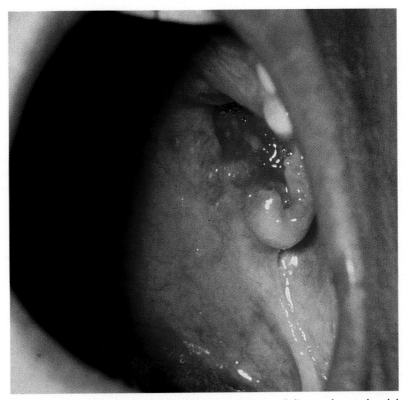

Figure 16-8 Langerhans cell histiocytosis: eosinophilic granuloma *Solitary, ulcerated nodule with loss of teeth on the gingival ridge near the palate, associated with involvement of the maxillary bone. Lesion was asymptomatic and only when the molars were lost did the patient consult a physician.*

Table 16-1 CLASSIFICATION OF LCH

Unifocal LCH Most commonly manifested by a single osteolytic bony lesion. Skin and soft tissue lesions not so uncommon (known as *eosinophilic granuloma*).

Multifocal LCH Similar to unifocal LCH; however, bony lesions are multiple and interfere with function of neighboring structures. Multifocal LCH involves bones, skin (second most frequently involved organ), soft tissue, lymph nodes, lungs, and pituitary glands (known as *Hand-Schüller-Christian disease*).

Letterer-Siwe Syndrome (LSS) The most aggressive of multifocal LCH forms, with skin involvement and infiltration of various organs causing organomegaly, thrombocytopenia. Guarded prognosis.

Multifocal LCH

As in unifocal LCH; in addition, regionally localized (head) or generalized (trunk) eruptions. Papulosquamous, seborrheic dermatitis-like (scaly, oily), eczematous dermatitis-like lesions (Fig. 16-9); sometimes vesicular; or purpuric (Fig. 16-10) Turn necrotic and may become heavily crusted. Removal of crusts leaves small, shallow punched-out ulcers (Fig. 16-10). Intertriginous lesions coalesce (Fig. 16-11), may be erosive and exudative, become secondarily infected and ulcerate (Fig. 16-11). Mandibular and maxillary bone involvement may result in loss of teeth (Fig. 16-8). Ulceration of vulva (Fig. 16-11).

LSS

Skin lesions as in multifocal LCH but more widespread, disseminated (Fig. 16-10).

Distribution *Tumorous swelling*: calvarium, sphenoid bone, sella turcica, mandible, long bones of upper extremities. *Papulosquamous eruptions* on scalp (Fig. 16-9), face, and trunk, particularly abdomen and buttocks (Fig. 16-10). *Erosions* and ulcers occur in groin, axillae, anogenital region (Fig. 16-11), retroauricularregion, neck. *Ulcers*: vulva, gingiva.

General Findings

Multifocal LCH Bony lesions occur in calvarium, sphenoid bone, sella turcica, mandible, long bones of upper extremities, and vertebrae. Associated findings of pituitary involvement.

LSS Hepatosplenomegaly, lymphadenopathy, involvement of lungs and other organs, bone marrow; thrombocytopenia.

DIFFERENTIAL DIAGNOSIS

Unifocal LCH Rule out other causes of lytic bony lesion.

Multifocal LCH Infectious and neoplastic disorders.

LSS Infectious and neoplastic disorders.

LABORATORY EXAMINATIONS

Radiographic Findings

Unifocal LCH Single osteolytic lesion in a long or flat bone (in children, calvarium, femur; in adults, rib).

Multifocal LCH Osteolytic lesions in calvarium, sphenoid bone, sella turcica, mandible, vertebrae, and/or long bones of upper extremities. Chest: diffuse micronodular and interstitial infiltrate in midzones and bases of lungs with sparing of costophrenic angles; later, honeycomb appearance, pneumothorax. Extent of osseous involvement established by bone scanning.

LSS Scans show organomegaly.

Histopathology Constant histologic feature of LCH is proliferation of Langerhans cells with abundant pale eosinophilic cytoplasm and indistinct cell borders; a folded, indented, kidney-shaped nucleus with finely dispersed chromatin; and small, inconspicuous nucleoli. For diagnostic purposes, Langerhans cells in LCH have to be recognized by morphologic, ultrastructural (Birbeck granules), histochemical, and immunohistochemical markers (Table 16-2).

DIAGNOSIS

Confirmation of diagnosis by biopsy (skin, bone, or soft tissue/internal organs). Since skin is the organ most frequently involved after bone, skin biopsies have great diagnostic significance (see Histopathology, above).

COURSE AND PROGNOSIS

Unifocal LCH Benign course with excellent prognosis for spontaneous resolution.

Multifocal LCH Spontaneous remissions possible. Prognosis poorer at extremes of age and with extrapulmonary involvement.

Table 16-2 DIAGNOSIS IN LCH

Presumptive diagnosis
   Clinical + histopathologic
Diagnosis (two or more criteria)
   ATPase+
   S-100 protein+
   α-D-mannosidase+
   Peanut agglutinin+
Definite diagnosis
   CD1a+
   Birbeck granules+

          SKIN SIGNS OF HEMATOLOGIC DISEASES

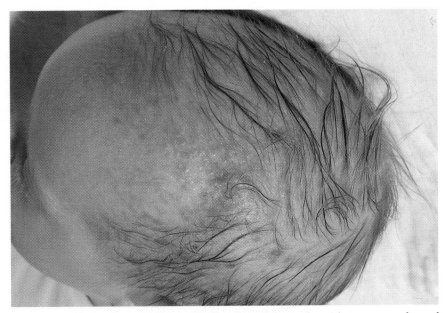

Figure 16-9 Langerhans cell histiocytosis *Small, yellow-pink papules with a greasy scale on the scalp in this infant. These were the only lesions at first presentation and were mistaken for infantile seborrheic dermatitis. Only after lesions proved refractory to topical treatment and additional purpuric and crusted lesions appeared on the trunk, was a biopsy performed and the correct diagnosis established.*

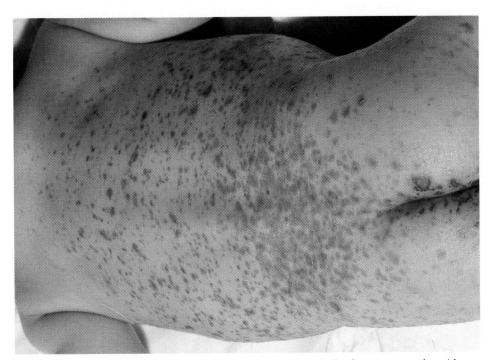

Figure 16-10 Langerhans cell histiocytosis: Letterer-Siwe syndrome *Erythematous papules with purpura, crusting, and ulceration becoming confluent on the trunk and the intergluteal fold of a young child.*

LSS Commonly fulminant and fatal. Spontaneous remissions uncommon. Current scoring systems for evaluation of prognosis are based on number of organs involved, presence or absence of organ dysfunction, and age. The worst prognosis is in the very young with multifocal LCH and organ dysfunction.

MANAGEMENT

Unifocal LCH Curettage with or without bony chip packing. Low-dose (300 to 600 rad) radiotherapy. Extraosseous soft tissue lesions: surgical excision or low-dose radiotherapy.

Multifocal LCH Diabetes insipidus and growth retardation treated with vasopressin and human growth hormone. Low-dose radiotherapy to bony lesions. Systemic treatment with glucocorticoids or vinblastine, mercaptopurine, and methotrexate, given as single agents or in combination, also with epipodophyllotoxin (etoposide). Topical glucocorticoids for discrete cutaneous lesions. Cutaneous lesions respond best to PUVA or topical nitrogen mustard but also to thalidomide.

LSS Only a few controlled studies of chemotherapy exist. The use of vinblastine results in complete or partial remission in 55%; combination chemotherapy in 70%. PUVA is effective in cutaneous lesions.

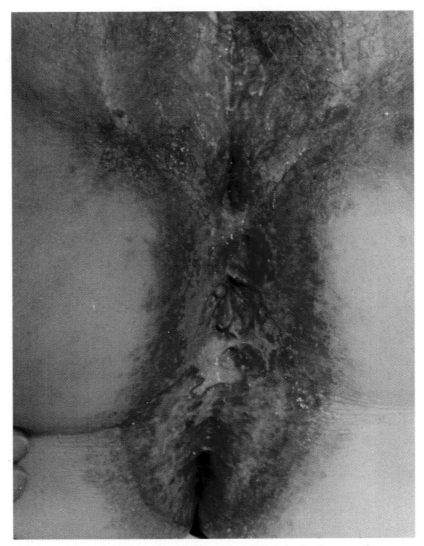

Figure 16-11   Langerhans cell histiocytosis: Letterer-Siwe syndrome   *Confluent erythematous papules with hemorrhage, necrosis, scaling, and ulceration in the anogenital and perineal region in a 65-year-old female.*

MASTOCYTOSIS SYNDROMES

Mastocytosis is associated with an abnormal accumulation of mast cells in the skin and at various systemic sites, which, because of pharmacologically active substances, is manifested clinically by local cutaneous and systemic symptoms. A consensus-based classification that divides mastocytosis into four categories is given in Table 16-3.

A classification of cutaneous mastocytosis is shown in Table 16-4.

Most patients with mastocytosis have only skin involvement, and most of these have no systemic symptoms (flushing, vomiting, syncope, etc.). However, up to half of patients with systemic mastocytosis may not have any skin findings.

EPIDEMIOLOGY

Age of Onset MC and UP: onset between birth and 2 years of age (55%), but mastocytosis can occur at any age; infancy-onset UP rarely associated with systemic mastocytosis.

Sex Slight male: female predominance.

Prevalence Unknown.

PATHOGENESIS

Mast cells contain several pharmacologically active substances that are associated with the clinical findings in mastocytosis: histamine (urticaria, GI symptoms), prostaglandin D_2 (flush, cardiovascular symptoms, GI symptoms), heparin (bleeding into lesion at biopsy site), neutral protease/acid hydrolases (patchy hepatic fibrosis, bone lesions).

HISTORY

Stroking lesion causes it to itch and to wheal (Darier's sign). Various drugs are capable of causing mast cell degranulation and release of pharmacologically active substances that exacerbate skin lesions (whealing, itching) and cause flushing: alcohol, dextran, polymyxin B, morphine, codeine. Flushing episode can also be elicited by heat or cold and may be accompanied by headache, nausea, vomiting, diarrhea, dyspnea/wheezing, syncope. Systemic involvement may lead to symptoms of malabsorption; portal hypertension. Bone pain. Neuropsychiatric symptoms (malaise, irritability).

PHYSICAL EXAMINATION

Skin Lesions *Mastocytoma* **(MC)** Macular to papular to nodular lesions (Fig. 16-12), yellow to tan-pink, which become erythematous and raised (urticate) when stroked due to degranulation of mast cells (Darier's sign); in some patients, lesions become bullous. Often solitary; may be multiple, but few.

Urticaria pigmentosa **(UP)** Tan macules to slightly raised tan to brown papules/nodules (Fig. 16-13). Disseminated, few or .100 with widespread symmetric distribution. Darier's sign (whealing) after rubbing, (Fig. 16-13), in infants may become bullous. Bright-red diffuse flushing occurring spontaneously, after rubbing of skin, after ingestion of alcohol or mast cell–degranulating agents.

Telangiectasia macularis eruptiva perstans **(TMEP)** Freckle-like, brownish macules (Fig.

Table 16-3 CONSENSUS REVISED CLASSIFICATION OF MASTOCYTOSIS

I. Indolent
   A Syncope
   B Cutaneous disease
   C Ulcer disease
   D Malabsorption
   E Bone marrow mast cell aggregates
   F Skeletal disease
   G Hepatosplenomegaly
   H Lymphadenopathy
II. Hematologic disorder
   Myelodysplastic
III. Aggressive
   Lymphadenopathic mastocytosis
IV. Mastocytic leukemia

SOURCE: From DO Metcalfe, J Invest Dermatol 96:64s, 1991.

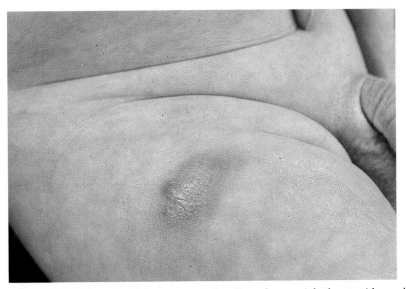

Figure 16-12 Mastocytosis: solitary mastocytoma *A solitary, brown-pink plaque with poorly demarcated borders on the thigh of a young child; the lesion was tan and flat prior to stroking (positive Darier's sign). When stroked very vigorously, a blister developed.*

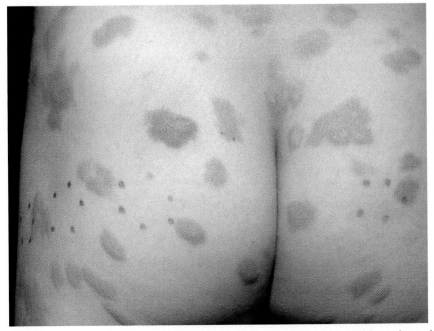

Figure 16-13 Mastocytosis: generalized urticaria pigmentosa *Multiple, flat-topped papules and small plaques of brownish color on the buttocks of a child. Lesions are asymptomatic. Rubbing a lesion has resulted in urtication and an axon flare, a positive Darier's sign.*

16-14) with fine telangiectasia in long-standing lesions. Hundreds of lesions, trunk >extremities; lesions may be confluent. Urticate with gentle stroking. Dermatographism.

Diffuse cutaneous mastocytosis (**DCM**) Yellowish, thickened appearance of large areas of skin; "doughy." Smooth with scattered elevation, resembling leather, "pseudoxanthomatous mastocytosis" (compare with pseudoxanthoma elasticum), skin folds exaggerated, especially in axilla/groin. Large bullae may occur after trauma or spontaneously. DCM may present as erythroderma (Fig. 16-15).

Dermatopathology Accumulation of normal-looking mast cells in dermis. Mast cell infiltrates may be sparse (spindle-shaped mast cells) or densely aggregated (cuboidal shape) and have a perivascular or nodular distribution. Pigmentation due to increased melanin in basal layer.

Systemic Symptoms Flushing, accompanied by wheezing, asthmatic attacks, nausea, vomiting, diarrhea, syncope.

Bone pain/spontaneous fractures with osteolytic lesions.

Neuropsychiatric symptoms, malaise, irritability.

Malabsorption, weight loss.

DIFFERENTIAL DIAGNOSIS

Mastocytoma Juvenile xanthogranuloma, Spitz nevus.

Flushing Carcinoid syndrome.

UP, DCM, TMEP Histiocytosis X, secondary syphilis, papular sarcoid, generalized eruptive histiocytoma, non-histiocytosis X of childhood.

LABORATORY EXAMINATIONS

CBC Systemic mastocytosis: anemia, leukocytosis, eosinophilia.

Blood Tryptase levels↑, coagulation parameters.

Urine Patients with extensive cutaneous involvement may have increased 24-h urinary histamine excretion.

Bone Scan and Imaging Define bone involvement (lytic bone lesions, osteoporosis, or osteosclerosis) and small bowel involvement. Small bowel "follow-through" to detect lesions in the small intestine.

Bone Marrow Smear and/or biopsy for morphology and mast cell markers.

DIAGNOSIS

Clinical suspicion, positive Darier's sign, confirmed by skin biopsy.

COURSE AND PROGNOSIS

Most cases of solitary mastocytoma and generalized UP in children resolve spontaneously. Adults with onset of UP or TMEP with extensive cutaneous involvement have a higher risk for development of systemic mastocytosis than do infants, in whom systemic mastocytosis is rare. In young children, acute and extensive degranulation may be life-threatening (shock).

MANAGEMENT

Avoidance of drugs that may cause mast cell degranulation and histamine release: alcohol, dextran, polymyxin B, morphine, codeine, scopolamine, D-tubocurarine, nonsteroidal anti-inflammatory agents.

Antihistamines, both H_1 and H_2, either alone or with ketotifen. Disodium cromoglycate, 200 mg qid, may ameliorate pruritus, flushing, diarrhea, abdominal pain, and disorders of cognitive function. PUVA treatment is effective for skin lesions, but recurrence is common.

Table 16-4 CLASSIFICATION OF CUTANEOUS MASTOCYTOSIS

Generalized	Urticaria pigmentosa (UP)
	Telangiectasia macularis eruptiva perstans (TMEP)
	Diffuse cutaneous mastocytosis (DCM)
Localized	Mastocytoma (MC) (solitary or a few)

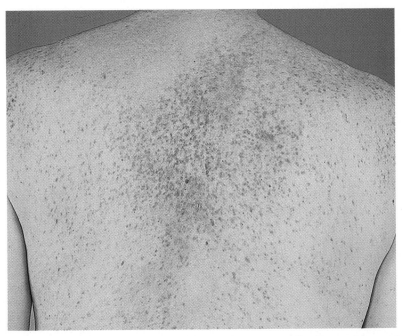

Figure 16-14 Mastocytosis: telangiectasia macularis eruptiva perstans *Small, tan-pink macules and telangiectases on the back.*

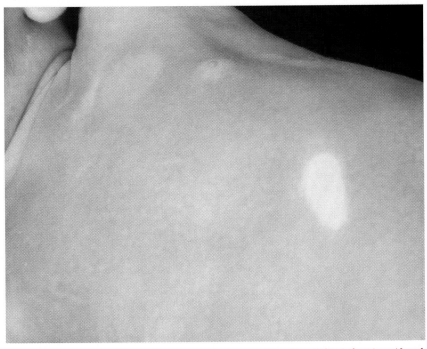

Figure 16-15 Mastocytosis: diffuse cutaneous mastocytosis *The skin of this infant is uniformly erythrodermous secondary to infiltrating mast cells with several spared, white areas of normal skin. In this child there were systemic symptoms associated with the flare of this erythroderma: syncope, wheezing and diarrhea.*

LEUKEMIA CUTIS

Leukemia cutis (LC) is a localized or disseminated skin infiltration by leukemic cells. It is usually a sign of dissemination of systemic disease or relapse of existing leukemia.

EPIDEMIOLOGY

Age of Onset Any age; more common in persons older than 50 years, depends on type of leukemia.

Sex No predilection, but a slightly higher number of cases involving men have been reported.

Incidence Uncommon overall; reported incidence varies from <5 to 50%, depending on the type of leukemia.

Associated Diseases Both acute and chronic leukemias, including the leukemic phase of non-Hodgkin's lymphoma and hairy cell leukemias. Most commonly occurs with acute monocytic leukemia M5 and acute myelomonocytic leukemia M4.

HISTORY

Most commonly after or concurrent with diagnosis of hematologic malignancy; occasionally precedes the symptoms of systemic leukemia.

PHYSICAL EXAMINATION

Skin Lesions Pattern of presentation of LC is variable and may have features that overlap with other (inflammatory) eruptions. Most common lesions are small (2 to 5 mm) papules (Fig. 16-16), nodules (Fig. 16-17), or plaques. LC lesions are usually somewhat more pink, violaceous, or darker than normal skin, always palpable, indurated, firm or guttate psoriasiform or lymphomatoid papulosis-like lesions, but usually not tender. Localized or disseminated (Fig. 16-16); usually on trunk, extremities (Fig. 16-17), and face but may occur at any site. May be hemorrhagic when associated with thrombocytopenia or ulcerate (Fig. 16-18). Erythroderma may (rarely) occur. Leukemic gingival infiltration (hypertrophy) occurs with acute monocytic leukemia. Similar lesional morphologies occur with different types of leukemia (Fig. 16-18), or, a specific type of leukemia may present with a variety of morphologies.

Inflammatory disorders occurring in patients with leukemia are modified by the participation of leukemic cells in the infiltrate, resulting in unusual presentation of such disorder, e.g., psoriasis with hemorrhage or erosions/ulcerations.

Associated Reaction Patterns Sweet's syndrome; bullous pyoderma gangrenosum lesions; urticaria; palpable purpura (necrotizing vasculitis).

General Examination Systemic signs associated with hematologic malignancy. Not infrequently, cutaneous manifestation may be the initial presenting symptom and may contribute importantly to the diagnosis.

DIFFERENTIAL DIAGNOSIS

The differential diagnosis is large because of the broad clinical manifestations of LC and the many nonspecific inflammatory reactions that are common in leukemic patients. It is most important to differentiate LC from a wide variety of disseminated infections occurring in the immunocompromised, neutropenic host, including bacterial sepsis (*Staphylococcus aureus, Pseudomonas aeruginosa*), fungemia (*Candida, Aspergillus*), and disseminated viral infections (herpes simplex virus, varicella-zoster virus). Inflammatory disorders that must be ruled out include neutrophilic dermatoses (Sweet's syndrome, pyoderma gangrenosum), adverse cutaneous drug reactions, transfusion-associated graft-versus-host disease, vasculitis, and erythema multiforme.

LABORATORY EXAMINATIONS

Hematology Leukemic cells are usually visible in the smear of peripheral blood, but they are absent in aleukemic leukemia.

Bone Marrow Aspirate Confirms the diagnosis and defines the type.

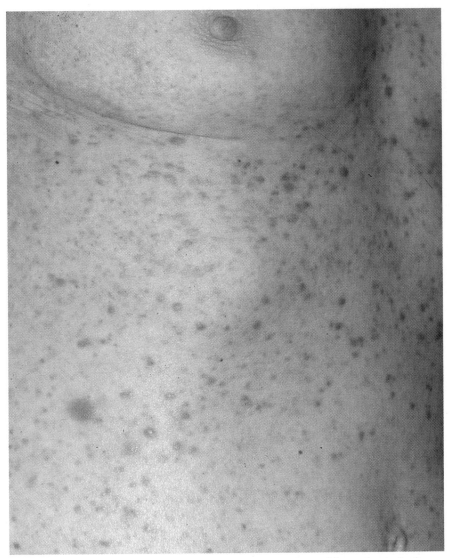

Figure 16-16　Leukemia cutis　*Hundreds of tan-pink papules and a nodule on the trunk of a female with acute myelogenous leukemia arose during a one-week interval. Per se these lesions are "nonspecific" and do not present a diagnosis; but when such an eruption is seen, one should perform a peripheral blood count and a biopsy.*

Dermatopathology Dermis, subcutaneous large perivascular, periadnexal, or diffuse. Leukemic cells. Touch preparation from a skin biopsy along with the clinical findings may be sufficient to suggest a rapid diagnosis of LC.

Immunophenotyping Conforms with type of leukemia.

DIAGNOSIS

Hematologic studies with complete analysis of bone marrow aspirate and peripheral blood smear and cutaneous histology and immunophenotyping are needed to make the diagnosis. If cutaneous findings precede any systemic disease, careful assessment of peripheral blood smears and bone marrow biopsies must be made.

COURSE AND PROGNOSIS

The prognosis for the LC is directly related to the prognosis for the systemic disease.

MANAGEMENT

Therapy is usually directed at the leukemia itself. However, systemic chemotherapy sufficient for bone marrow remission may not treat the cutaneous lesions effectively. Thus, a combination of systemic chemotherapy and local electron-beam therapy or PUVA may be necessary for chemotherapy-resistant LC lesions.

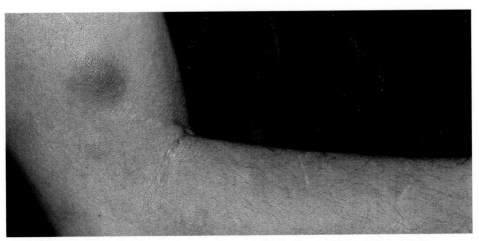

Figure 16-17 Leukemia cutis *A large, dark-brown nodule and a smaller papule on the upper arm of a male with acute myelogenous leukemia; six similar nodules were also present on the trunk.*

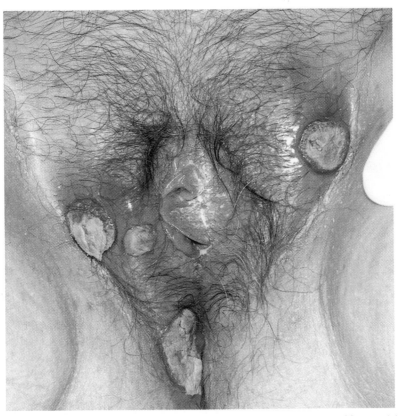

Figure 16-18 Leukemia cutis: chloroma *Large, ulcerated, green-hued tumors (chloromas) in the inguinal and perineal regions of a female with acute myelogenous leukemia; similar lesions were also present in the axillae and on the tongue.*

CUTANEOUS LYMPHOMAS AND SARCOMA

LYMPHOMATOID PAPULOSIS

Lymphomatoid papulosis is an asymptomatic, chronic, self-healing, polymorphous eruption characterized by recurrent crops of lesions that regress spontaneously, with histologic features of lymphocytic atypia. It is a low-grade, self-limited T cell lymphoma with a low but real risk of progression to more malignant forms of lymphoma.

EPIDEMIOLOGY

Incidence   1.2 to 1.9 cases per million.

Age of Onset   Childhood to elderly; average age 40 years.

Sex   Both sexes.

Inheritance   None; occurs sporadically.

Etiology   Unknown

PATHOGENESIS

Unknown; considered to be a low-grade lymphoma controlled by host mechanisms without systemic involvement. Antigens shared with and occasional progression to Hodgkin's disease or cutaneous T cell lymphoma suggest a low-grade lymphoma, perhaps induced by chronic antigenic stimulation. Lymphomatoid papulosis may begin as a chronic, reactive, polyclonal lymphoproliferative phenomenon that sporadically overwhelms host immune defenses and evolves into a clonal, antigen-independent, true lymphoid malignancy. Belongs in the spectrum of primary cutaneous Ki-1+ lymphoproliferative disorders, including pseudo-Hodgkin's disease of the skin, regressing atypical histiocytosis, Hodgkin's lymphoma, and Ki-1+ large cell lymphoma.

HISTORY

Usually asymptomatic; occasionally, lesions are pruritic, tender, or painful. Negative history of weight loss, anorexia, fever, sweating. If these are present, pursue workup for systemic lymphoma.

PHYSICAL EXAMINATION

Skin Finding   Erythematous to red-brown. Papules (Fig. 17-1) and nodules, 2 to 5 mm in diameter, which are initially smooth and hemorrhagic, later hyperkeratotic, with central, black necrosis, crusting (Fig. 17-1), and ulceration. Few to hundreds of lesions, arranged at random and often grouped, appear in crops of recurrent, self-healing eruptions primarily on trunk and extremities; rarely, oral and genital mucosa. Lesions may resolve spontaneously at any point in their evolution, and only those that progress to necrosis or ulceration produce atrophic hyper- or hypopigmented scarring. Individual lesions evolve over a 2- to 8-week period.

Other Organ Systems   Uninvolved.

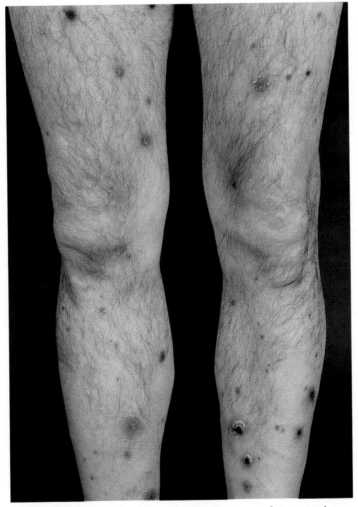

Figure 17-1 Lymphomatoid papulosis *Crops of reddish-brown papules appear in waves involving the entire body. Lesions are asymptomatic, become hyperkeratotic, crusted and necrotic in the center. Since lesions arise asynchronously, all stages in this evolution are present simultaneously.*

DIFFERENTIAL DIAGNOSIS

Multiple Papules/Nodules in Various Stages of Development *Pityriasis lichenoides et varioliformis acuta (Mucha-Habermann disease)*—clinically similar without histologic atypia. *Lymphoma cutis, Hodgkin's or non-Hodgkin's type*—clinically progressive, histologically malignant. *Large-cell anaplastic T cell lymphoma, regressing atypical histiocytosis;* papular mycosis fungoides; also histiocytosis X, papular drug eruption, papular urticaria, scabies.

LABORATORY EXAMINATIONS

Dermatopathology Superficial or deep, perivascular or interstitial mixed-cell infiltrate, wedge-shaped, sometimes interstitial. Epidermis: focal spongiosis, mild exocytosis, necrotic keratinocytes, necrosis, or ulceration. Frequent extravasated erythrocytes. Small-vessel lymphocytic vasculitis in 10% of cases. Cytologically, atypical cells may comprise 50% of infiltrate. *Type A:* large, atypical histiocytic-looking lymphocytes with abundant cytoplasm, convoluted nucleus with occasional binucleation, multipolar mitosis, and Reed-Sternberg-like cells. *Type B:* smaller, atypical lymphocytes with cerebriform nuclei, epidermotropism, and occasional mitosis.

Immunohistochemistry Predominantly activated, interleukin-2 receptor–positive, HLA-DR–positive, Ki-1 (CD30)–positive T helper cells (CD4). Southern blot hybridization: clonal T cell population in 50%.

Other Negative workup for systemic involvement.

DIAGNOSIS

Based on typical histology and immunohistochemistry, lack of systemic involvement by history and physical examination. May necessitate periodic biopsy to rule out blastic transformation, especially with tumor formation. No reliable histologic, immunohistochemical, or genotypic test available for prediction of risk of progression to lymphoma.

COURSE AND PROGNOSIS

Chronic atypical eruption of low but real malignant potential may prove emotionally and diagnostically challenging for physician and patient alike.

May remit in 3 weeks or continue for decades. Patients may experience periods without lesions or have continuous, repetitive outbreaks. In 10 to 20% of patients, lymphomatoid papulosis is preceded by, associated with, or followed by another type of lymphoma: mycosis fungoides, Hodgkin's disease, or CD30+ large cell lymphoma. May persist despite systemic chemotherapy for concurrent lymphoma.

MANAGEMENT

No treatments have proved consistently effective, as is evidenced by the multiple reported therapies. Topical agents include glucocorticoids and carmustine (BCNU). Electron-beam irradiation has been employed as well. PUVA may control the disease but does not affect the long-term prognosis. Tetracyclines, sulfones, systemic glucocorticoids, and even acyclovir have been reported as effective by some researchers. A wide spectrum of systemic agents has been used, including retinoids, methotrexate, chlorambucil, cyclophosphamide, cyclosporine, and interferon-α2b, none with lasting effect.

KAPOSI'S SARCOMA

Kaposi's sarcoma (KS) is a multisystem vascular neoplasia characterized by mucocutaneous violaceous lesions and edema as well as involvement of nearly any organ. Many individuals with KS are in some degree immunocompromised, especially those with HIV disease.

Synonym: Multiple idiopathic hemorrhagic sarcoma.

EPIDEMIOLOGY

Etiopathogenesis DNA of human herpesvirus type 8 (HHV-8), has been identified in tissue samples of all variants of KS. There is seroepidemiologic evidence that this virus is somehow involved in the pathogenesis.

Age of Onset

Classic KS Peak incidence after the sixth decade.

African-Endemic KS Two distinct age groups: young adults, mean age 35; and young children, mean age 3 years.

HIV-Associated KS Young adults.

Sex

Much more common in males in all variants, but HIV-associated KS occurs almost exclusively in homosexual males; rarely women may have HIV-associated KS when they acquire HIV infection via heterosexual exposure from a bisexual male.

Incidence

Classic KS Not so uncommon in eastern and southern Europe. Rare in the United States in people of Eastern or Ashkenazi Jewish extraction. Increasing incidence in Sweden before onset of HIV pandemic.

African-Endemic KS 9 to 12.8% of all malignancies in Zaire.

Iatrogenic Immunosuppression–Associated KS Rare.

HIV-Associated KS In HIV-infected individuals, the risk for KS is 20,000 times that of the general population, 300 times that of other immunosuppressed individuals. Early in the HIV epidemic in the United States and Europe, 50% of homosexual men at the time of initial diagnosis of AIDS had KS; currently, the incidence is 18% in this risk group.

Clinical Variants of KS

Classic or European KS Occurs in elderly males of eastern European heritage (Mediterranean and Ashkenazi Jewish). Predominantly arises on the legs; also occurs in lymph nodes and abdominal viscera, slowly progressive.

African-Endemic KS (Non-HIV-Associated) Four clinical patterns are recognized:

Nodular Type Runs a rather benign course with a mean duration of 5 to 8 years and resembles classic KS.

Florid or Vegetating Type Characterized by more aggressive biologic behavior. Is also nodular but may extend deeply into the subcutis, muscle, and bone.

Infiltrative Type Shows an even more aggressive course with florid mucocutaneous and visceral involvement.

Lymphadenopathic Type Predominantly affects children and young adults. Frequently confined to lymph nodes and viscera, but occasionally also involves the skin and mucous membrane.

Iatrogenic Immunosuppression–Associated KS Occurs in recipients of renal transplants and individuals with cancer treated with cytotoxic chemotherapy. Resolves on cessation of immunosuppression.

HIV-Associated KS Associated with HIV infection, rapid progression, extensive systemic involvement.

Risk Factors

African-Endemic KS No evidence of underlying immunodeficiency.

Iatrogenic Immunosuppression–Associated KS Most commonly in solid-organ transplant recipients as well as individuals treated chronically with immunosuppressive drugs. Arises on average 16.5 months after transplantation.

HIV-Associated KS At the time of initial presentation, one in six HIV-infected individuals with KS have CD4+ T cell counts of ≥500/μL.

PATHOGENESIS

KS cells likely are derived from the endothelium of the blood/lymphatic microvasculature. Not a true malignancy but rather a widespread cellular proliferation in response to angiogenic substances. KS lesions produce factors that promote their own growth as well as the growth of other cells, but it is not known how HHV-8 induces/promotes proliferation of endothelial cells.

HISTORY

Mucocutaneous lesions are usually asymptomatic but are associated with significant cosmetic stigma. At times lesions may ulcerate and bleed easily. Large lesions on palms or soles may impede function. Lesions on the lower extremities that are tumorous, ulcerated, or associated with significant edema often give rise to moderate to severe pain. Urethral or anal canal lesions can be associated with obstruction. GI involvement rarely causes symptoms. Pulmonary KS can cause bronchospasm, intractable coughing, progressive respiratory failure, shortness of breath.

PHYSICAL EXAMINATION

Skin Lesions KS most often begins as an ecchymotic-like macule (Fig. 17-2). Macules evolve into papules (Fig. 17-3), plaques, nodules, and tumors that are violaceous, red, pink, or tan (Figs. 17-2 and 17-3) and become purple-brownish (Fig. 17-4 and 17-5) with a greenish hemosiderin halo as they age. Almost all KS lesions are palpable, feeling firm to hard even when they are in a macular stage. Often oval initially, and on the trunk often arranged parallel to skin tension lines (Fig. 17-6). Lesions may initially occur at sites of trauma, usually in the acral regions. In time, individual lesions may enlarge and become confluent, forming tumor masses. Secondary changes to larger nodules and tumors include erosion, ulceration, crusting, and hyperkeratosis.

Lymphedema usually occurs on the lower extremities (Fig. 17-4) and results from confluent masses of lesions due to deeper involvement of lymphatics and lymph nodes. Distal edema may initially be unilateral but later becomes symmetric and involves not only the lower legs but also the genitalia and/or face. Areas of tense edema have a peau d'orange appearance. Long-standing confluent lesions associated with edema of a limb can evolve to fibrosis, contracture, and atrophy with subsequent loss of function of the extremity.

Distribution Wide-spread or localized. In classic KS, lesions almost always occur on the feet and legs or the hands and slowly spread centripedally (Figs. 17-2 and 17-3). Tip of nose (Fig. 17-5), periorbital areas, ears, and scalp as well as penis and legs may also be involved, but involvement of the trunk is rare. In HIV-associated KS there is early involvement of the face (Fig. 17-5) and wide-spread distribution on the trunk (Fig. 17-6).

Mucous Membranes Oral lesions are the first manifestation of KS in 22% of cases; often a marker for CD4+ T cell counts of <200/μL. Very common (50% of individuals) on hard palate, appearing first as a violaceous stain, which evolves into papules and nodules with a cobblestone appearance. Lesions also arise on soft palate, uvula, pharynx, gingiva, and tongue. Conjunctival lesions uncommon.

General Examination KS lesions of the viscera, though common, are often asymptomatic. This is particularly true for classic KS. At autopsy of HIV-infected individuals with mucocutaneous KS, 75% have visceral involvement (bowel, liver, spleen, lungs).

Lymph Nodes In HIV-associated KS, lymph nodes involved in half of cases, and in African-lymphadenopathic KS, in all.

Urogenital Tract Prostate, seminal vesicles, testes, bladder, penis, scrotum.

Lung Pulmonary infiltrates, particularly in HIV-associated KS.

GI Tract GI hemorrhage, rectal obstruction, protein-losing enteropathy can occur.

Other Heart, brain, kidney, adrenal glands.

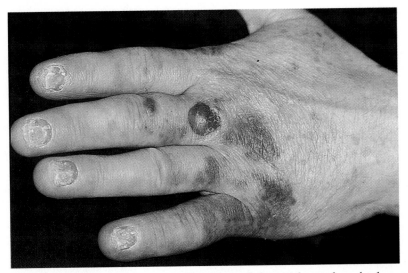

Figure 17-2 Classic Kaposi's sarcoma *An ecchymotic purple-brownish macule and a 1-cm nodule on the dorsum of the hand of a 65-year-old male of Ashkenazi Jewish extraction. The lesion was originally mistaken for a bruise as were similar lesions on the feet and on the other hand. The appearance of brownish nodules together with additional macules prompted a referral of this otherwise completely healthy patient to a dermatologist who diagnosed Kaposi's sarcoma, which was verified by biopsy. Note also onychomycosis.*

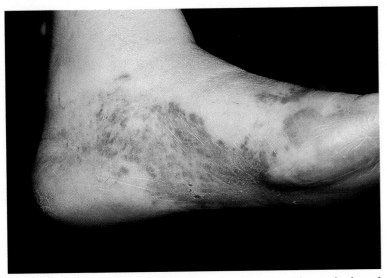

Figure 17-3 Classic Kaposi's sarcoma *Multiple purplish confluent papules on the foot of a 60-year-old Greek patient. Since lesions were asymptomatic, they first went unnoticed and were later ignored. Only when similar lesions arose proximally on the lower leg and also on the other foot, did the patient seek medical advice.*

DIFFERENTIAL DIAGNOSIS

Single Pigmented Lesion Dermatofibroma (sclerosing hemangioma), pyogenic granuloma, hemangioma, bacillary (epithelioid) angiomatosis, melanocytic nevus, ecchymosis, granuloma annulare, insect bite reactions, stasis dermatitis.

LABORATORY EXAMINATIONS

Skin Biopsy The diagnosis of KS should be confirmed histologically in all patients.

Dermatopathology Discrete intradermal nodule with vascular channels lined by atypical endothelial cells among a network of reticulin fibers and extravasated erythrocytes with hemosiderin deposition. Three histologic stages are described:

Patch stage: In the reticular dermis, proliferation of small, irregular, and jagged endothelial-lined spaces surrounding normal dermal vessels and adnexal structures; variable, inflammatory lymphocytic infiltrate (±plasma cells). Promontory sign: a normal vessel or adnexal structure protruding into an ectatic space.

Plaque stage: Spindle cells expand throughout dermal collagen bundles forming irregular, cleftlike, angulated vascular channels that contain variable numbers of RBCs. Hemosiderin deposits; eosinophilic hyaline globules. Peripheral perivascular inflammatory infiltrate.

Nodular stage: Spindle cells in sheets and fascicles with mild to moderate cytologic atypia, single-cell necrosis, trapped RBCs within an extensive network of slitlike vascular spaces.

Culture Rule out secondary infections in ulcerated/crusted lesions.

Chest X-Ray Difficult to distinguish pulmonary KS from *Pneumocystis carinii* pneumonia. In KS, pulmonary nodules and pleural effusions more common.

DIAGNOSIS

Confirmed on lesional skin biopsy.

COURSE AND PROGNOSIS

Classic KS Average survival, 10 to 15 years; usually die of unrelated causes. Secondary malignancies arise in >35% of cases.

African-Endemic KS Mean survival in young adults, 5 to 8 years; young children, 2 to 3 years.

Iatrogenic Immunosuppression–Associated KS Course may be chronic or rapidly progressive; KS usually resolves after immunosuppressive drugs are discontinued.

HIV-Associated KS HIV-infected individuals with high CD4+ T cell counts can have stable or slowly progressive disease for many years. Rapid progression of KS can occur after decline of CD4+ T cell counts to low values, prolonged systemic glucocorticoid therapy, or illness such as *P. carinii* pneumonia. KS of the bowel and/or lungs is the cause of death in 10 to 20% of patients. Patients with only a few lesions, present for several months, without history of opportunistic infections, and CD4+ T cell counts >200/μL tend to respond better to therapy and probably have a better overall prognosis. Immunosuppression caused by prednisone or methotrexate may precipitate appearance of KS, which may regress when these agents are withheld. At time of initial diagnosis, 40% of KS patients have GI involvement; 80% at autopsy. Reduced survival rate in patients with GI involvement. Pulmonary KS has high short-term mortality rate, i.e., median survival <6 months.

MANAGEMENT

The goal of therapy for KS is to control symptoms of the disease, not cure. A number of local and systemic therapeutic modalities are effective in controlling symptoms. Classic KS responds well to radiotherapy of involved sites. African-endemic KS, when symptomatic, responds best to systemic chemotherapy. Immunosuppressive drug–associated KS regresses or resolves when drug dosages are reduced or discontinued. HIV-associated KS usually responds to a variety of local therapies; for extensive mucocutaneous involvement or visceral involvement, chemotherapy is indicated.

Local therapy is usually directed at individual lesions that are cosmetically disturbing (e.g., on the face), bulky, bleeding, cause functional disturbance on the palms or soles, or cause lymphatic obstruction and lymphedema.

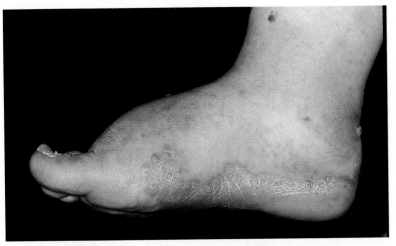

Figure 17-4 Classic Kaposi's sarcoma *Brownish confluent plaques on the sole have become hyperkeratotic and pea-sized purplish nodules have arisen on the lower leg. Involvement of lymphatics has led to pronounced edema of the forefoot, which indicates that the disease process is further advanced than in the patient shown in Figure 17-3.*

Limited Intervention

Radiotherapy Indicated for tumorous lesions, confluent lesions with a large surface area, large lesions on distal extremity, large oropharyngeal lesions. Dosing: 8 Gy in a single fraction for small lesions, 800 to 3000 rads in single or divided dose.

Cryosurgery A cryospray device should be used. Indicated for deeply pigmented, protruding nodules. Best results with two freeze-thaw cycles. Pain is moderate during freeze cycle. Treated lesions heal with crust formation. KS often persists in deeper portions of lesion. Violaceous lesion is replaced with a white scar. Secondary infection is uncommon.

Laser Surgery Pulsed-dye laser effective for small superficial lesion.

Electrosurgery Effective for ulcerated, bleeding nodular lesion; must use a smoke evacuator in conjunction.

Excisional Surgery Effective for selected small lesions. Not a realistic approach to the patient with many lesions.

Intralesional Cytotoxic Chemotherapy

Vinblastine .1 mg (.5 mL of a .2 mg/mL solution) injected per square centimeter of lesion; for refractory lesions, incremental doses of up to .2 mg/cm^2 can be given. Most effective for small, early, papular lesions. Larger nodular lesions respond more slowly. The maximal total vinblastine dose injected should not exceed 2 mg per clinic visit. Some lesions heal with blister formation, crusting and scarring. Inadvertent injection near a cutaneous sensory nerve can result in a neutric pain that can last up to a month.

Vincristine and Bleomycin Have also been used for intralesional therapy.

Aggressive Intervention

Single-Agent Chemotherapy

Adriamycin, 20 mg/m^2.
Vinblastine, IV bolus .1 mg/kg weekly.
Lipid formulations of daunorubicin and doxirubicin (Daunosome and Doxol) are effective and less toxic than older formulations.
Etoposide (VP16), given orally.
Paclitaxel (Taxol), given intravenously every 3 weeks.

Combination Chemotherapy

Vincristine (2 mg) + bleomycin (15 units/m^2) + adriamycin (20 mg/m^2) is given every other week in patients with relatively advanced KS. Interferon α (15 million units/d) + zidovudine (600 mg/d).

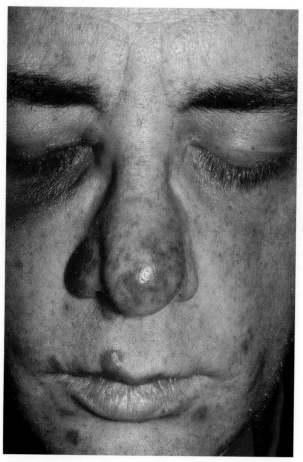

Figure 17-5 HIV-associated Kaposi's sarcoma *Multiple bruise-like purplish and brownish macules, papules and nodules are present not only on the face but also on the trunk and the extremities of this 29-year-old male homosexual with AIDS. Note also swelling of the nose. Early involvement of the face is typical for HIV-associated KS.*

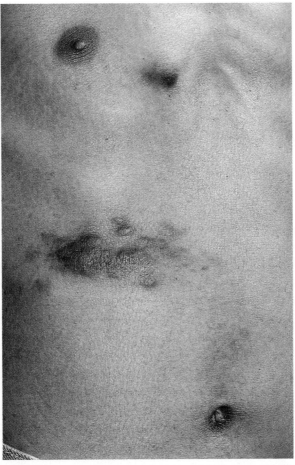

Figure 17-6 HIV-associated Kaposi's sarcoma *Multiple purplish plaques and nodules on the trunk of a homosexual AIDS patient. The patient had CD4+ T cell counts <200/μL and marked mucous membrane involvement, Pneumocystis carinii and Candida.*

ADULT T CELL LEUKEMIA/LYMPHOMA

Adult T cell leukemia/lymphoma (ATLL) is a neoplasm of CD4+ T cells, caused by human T cell lymphotrophic virus I (HTLV-I), manifested by skin infiltrates, hypercalcemia, visceral involvement, lytic bone lesions, and abnormal lymphocytes on the peripheral smears.

EPIDEMIOLOGY

Age of Onset   Average age, 35 to 55 years.

Sex   Males >females.

Race   Japanese, blacks.

Etiology   HTLV-I, a human retrovirus. Malignant cells are activated CD4+ T cells with an increased expression of the α chain of the interleukin-2 receptor. Infection by the virus usually does not cause disease, which suggests that other environmental factors are involved. Immortalization of some infected CD4+ T cells, increased mitotic activity, genetic instability, and impairment of cellular immunity can all occur after infection with HTLV-I. These events may increase the probability of additional genetic changes which, by chance, may lead to the development of leukemia in some people (≤5%). Most of these effects have been attributed to the HTLV-I–encoded protein tax.

Transmission   Sexual intercourse; perinatally; exposure to blood or blood products (same as HIV). Leukemia develops 20 to 40 years after infection.

Geography   Southwestern Japan (Kyushu), Africa, Caribbean Islands, southeastern United States.

Classification   Four main categories. In the relatively indolent smoldering and chronic forms, the median survival is 2 years or more. In the acute and lymphomatous forms, it ranges from 4 to 6 months.

HISTORY

Fever, weight loss, abdominal pain, diarrhea, pleural effusion, ascites, cough, sputum.

PHYSICAL EXAMINATION

Skin Findings   Lesions occur in 50% of patients with ATLL. Single to multiple erythematous, violaceous, brown papules (Fig. 17-7), ±purpura; firm nodules (Fig. 17-8); papulosquamous lesions, large plaques, ±ulceration; trunk>face>extremities; generalized erythroderma; poikiloderma; diffuse alopecia.

General Examination *Abdomen*   Hepatomegaly (50%), splenomegaly (25%).

Lymph Nodes   Lymphadenopathy (75%) sparing mediastinal lymph nodes.

DIFFERENTIAL DIAGNOSIS

Multiple Cutaneous Nodules   Cutaneous T cell lymphoma (mycosis fungoides), Sézary's syndrome.

LABORATORY EXAMINATIONS

Hematology   WBC ranges from normal to 500,000/μL. Peripheral blood smear—polylobulated lymphocytic nuclei, resembling Sézary cells.

Dermatopathology   Perivascular and/or diffuse infiltrates with large abnormal lymphocytes in the upper to middle dermis; epidermis often spared. Alternatively, dense intradermal infiltration and Pautrier's microabscesses, composed of many large abnormal lymphocytes, ±giant cells.

Chemistry   Hypercalcemia: 25% at time of diagnosis of ATLL; >50% during clinical course. Hypercalcemia felt to be due to osteoclastic bone resorption.

Serology   Seropositive (ELISA, Western blot) to HTLV-I; in IV drug users, up to 30% have dual retroviral infection with both HTLV-I and HIV.

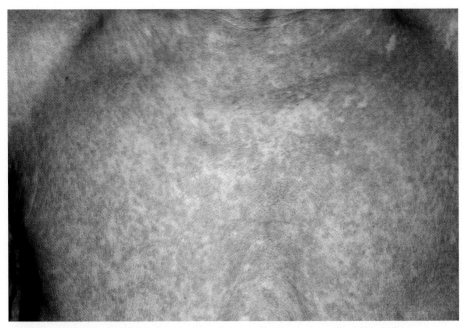

Figure 17-7 Adult T cell leukemia/lymphoma *A generalized eruption of small, confluent violaceous papules with a predilection for the trunk. The patient had fever, weight loss, abdominal pain, massive leukocytosis with Sézary cells in smear, lymphadenopathy, hepatosplenomegaly and hypercalcemia.*

DIAGNOSIS

Characteristic clinical findings, seropositivity to HTLV-I, confirmation of integration of HTLV-I proviral DNA in the cellular DNA of the ATLL cells.

COURSE AND PROGNOSIS

Course may be smoldering or chronic for prolonged period (abnormal lymphocytosis, skin infiltrates, modest bone marrow involvement) or massive lymphoma. Mean survival with acute crisis in hypercalcemic patients 12.5 weeks (range 2 weeks to 1 year); if normocal-

cemic, 50 weeks. Cause of death: opportunistic infections, disseminated intravascular coagulation.

MANAGEMENT

Various regimens of cytotoxic chemotherapy; the rates of complete response are <30%, and responses lack durability. The acute and lymphomatous forms resist conventional cytotoxic chemotherapy. Excellent results have been obtained with the combination of oral zidovudine and subcutaneous interferon-α. Obtain HTLV-I serology of family members, sexual partners. If seropositive, should not donate blood.

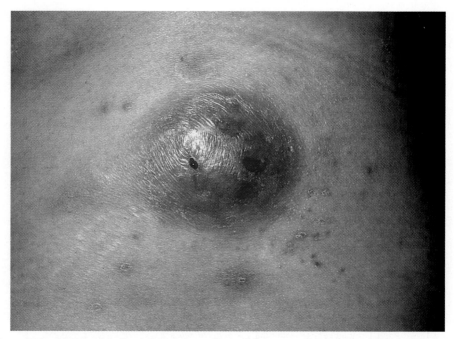

Figure 17-8   Adult T cell leukemia/lymphoma   *Firm, violaceous to brownish nodules as shown here are another cutaneous manifestation of ATLL. These nodules may ulcerate.*

CUTANEOUS T CELL LYMPHOMA

Cutaneous T cell lymphoma (CTCL) is a term that applies to T cell lymphoma first manifested in the skin, but since the neoplastic process involves the entire lymphoreticular system, the lymph nodes and internal organs become involved in the course of the disease. CTCL is a malignancy of helper T cells (CD4+).
Synonym: Mycosis fungoides.

EPIDEMIOLOGY

Age of Onset 50 years (range 5 to 70 years).

Sex Male: female ratio 2:1.

Incidence Uncommon but not rare.

Etiology Unknown. Human T cell lymphotrophic virus (HTLV) in some patients.

HISTORY

For months to years, often preceded by various diagnoses such as psoriasis, nummular dermatitis, and "large plaque" parapsoriasis. Symptoms: pruritus, often intractable, but may be none.

PHYSICAL FINDINGS

Skin Findings Randomly distributed, scaling or nonscaling plaques in different shades of red. Well or ill-defined; at first superficial, much like eczema or psoriasis or mimicking dermatophytosis ("mycosis"), (Fig. 17-9), and later becoming thicker. Round, oval, but often also arciform, annular, and of bizarre configuration (Fig. 17-10). Lesions are randomly distributed but in early stages often spare exposed areas.

Later lesions consist of nodules (Fig. 17-11) and tumors with or without ulceration (Figs. 17-11 and 17-12). Extensive infiltration can cause leonine facies (Fig. 17-13). Confluence may lead to erythroderma (see Section 6). There is palmoplantar keratoderma and there may be hair loss. Poikiloderma may be present from the onset or develop later.

General Examination Lymphadenopathy.

Sézary's Syndrome This is a leukemic form of CTCL consisting of (1) erythroderma, (2) lymphadenopathy, (3) elevated WBC ($>20,000/\mu$L) with a high proportion of so-called Sézary cells, (4) hair loss, and (5) pruritus. (See page 542.)

DIFFERENTIAL DIAGNOSIS

Scaling Plaques (Fig. 17-9) High index of suspicion is needed in patients with atypical or refractory "psoriasis," "eczema," and poikiloderma atrophicans vasculare. Repeated biopsies are necessary. CTCL often mimics psoriasis in being a scaly plaque and disappearing with exposure to sunlight.

LABORATORY EXAMINATIONS

Dermatopathology Repeated and multiple biopsies often are necessary to finally establish the diagnosis. Bandlike and patchy infiltrate in upper dermis of atypical lymphocytes (mycosis cells) extending to skin appendages. Mycosis cells (Lutzner cells): T cells with hyperchromatic, irregularly shaped (cerebriform) nuclei. Mitoses vary from rare to frequent. Abnormal T cells can be identified by electron microscopy (and by experienced investigators by light microscopy): typically convoluted nucleus. Microabscesses in the epidermis containing mycosis cells (Pautrier's microabscesses).

Monoclonal antibody techniques: Mycosis cells are activated CD4+ T cells; T cell receptor rearrangement studies: monoclonal.

Hematology Eosinophilia, 6 to 12%, can increase to 50%. Buffy coat: abnormal circulating T cells (Sézary type) and increased WBC ($20,000/\mu$L). Bone marrow examination is not helpful in early stages.

Chemistry Lactic dehydrogenase isoenzymes 1, 2, and 3 increased in erythrodermic stage.

Chest X-Ray Search for hilar lymphadenopathy.

Imaging In stage I and stage II disease, diagnostic imaging (CT, gallium scintigraphy, liver-spleen scan, and lymphangiography) does not provide more information than biopsies of lymph nodes.

CT Scan With more advanced disease, to search for retroperitoneal nodes in patients with extensive skin involvement, lymphadenopathy, or tumors in the skin.

Liver-Spleen Scan To identify any focal areas.

DIAGNOSIS

In the early stages, the diagnosis of CTCL is a problem. Clinical lesions may be typical, but histologic confirmation may not be possible for years despite repeated biopsies. One-micrometer thick sections may be helpful. For early diagnosis, cytophotometry (estimation of aneuploidy and polyploidy) and estimation of the indentation of pathologic cells (nucleocontour index) are helpful. Fresh tissue should be sent for immunophenotyping of infiltrating T cells by use of monoclonal antibodies and T cell receptor rearrangement studies. Lymphadenopathy and the detection of abnormal circulating T cells in the blood appear to correlate well with *internal* organ involvement. See TNM classification and staging, Tables 17-1 and 17-2.

COURSE AND PROGNOSIS

Unpredictable; CTCL (pre-CTCL) may be present for years. Course varies with the source of the patients studied. At the NIH there was a median survival time of 5 years from the time of the histologic diagnosis, while in Europe a less malignant course is seen (survival time, up to 10 to 15 years). This, however, may be due to patient selection. Prognosis is much worse when (1) tumors are present (mean survival, 2.5 years), (2) there is lymphadenopathy (mean survival, 3 years), (3) >10% of the skin surface is involved with pretumor-stage CTCL, and (4) there is a generalized erythroderma. Patients younger than 50 years have twice the survival rate of patients older than 60 years.

MANAGEMENT

In the pre-CTCL stage, in which the histologic diagnosis is only compatible, but not confirmed, PUVA photochemotherapy is the most effective treatment. For histologically proven plaque-stage disease with no lymphadenopathy and no abnormal circulating T cells, PUVA photochemotherapy is also the method of choice. Also used at this stage are topical chemotherapy with nitrogen mustard in an ointment base (10 mg/dL) and total body electron-beam therapy, singly or in combination. Isolated tumors

---

Table 17-1 TNM CLASSIFICATION OF CTCL (MYCOSIS FUNGOIDES)

T: Skin	T_0 Clinically and/or histologically suspicious lesions
	T_1 Limited plaques, papules, or eczematous patches covering less than 10% of the skin surface
	T_2 Generalized plaques, papules, or erythematous patches covering more than 10% of the skin surface
	T_3 Tumors (1 or more)
	T_4 Generalized erythroderma
N: Lymph nodes	N_0 No clinically abnormal peripheral nodes, pathology negative for MF
	N_1 Clinically abnormal peripheral lymph nodes, pathology negative for MF
	N_2 No clinically abnormal peripheral lymph nodes, pathology positive for MF
	N_3 Clinically abnormal peripheral lymph nodes, pathology positive for MF
B: Blood	B_0 Less than 5% atypical circulating lymphocytes
	B_1 Greater than 5% atypical circulating lymphoctyes (Sézary's)
M: Visceral organs	M_0 No visceral organ involvement
	M_1 Histologically proven visceral involvement

NOTE: MF, mycosis fungoides.

CUTANEOUS LYMPHOMAS AND SARCOMA

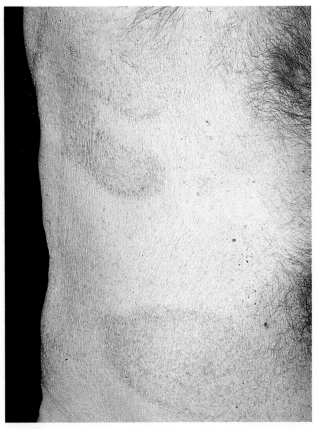

Figure 17-9 Cutaneous T cell lymphoma/mycosis fungoides *In early stages lesions consist of randomly distributed, well- or ill-defined plaques. They may be scaly and appear in various shades of red. They mimick eczema, psoriasis or dermatophytosis.*

that may develop should be treated with local x-ray or electron-beam therapy. For extensive plaque stage with multiple tumors or in patients with lymphadenopathy or abnormal circulating T cells, electron-beam plus chemotherapy is probably the best combination for now; randomized, controlled studies of various combinations are in progress. Also, extracorporeal PUVA photochemotherapy is being evaluated in patients with Sézary's syndrome.

Table 17-2 STAGING SYSTEM FOR CTCL

Stage	T	N	M
IA	T_1	N_0	M_0
IB	T_2	N_0	M_0
IIA	T_{1-2}	N_1	M_0
IIB	T_3	N_{0-1}	M_0
III	T_4	N_{0-1}	M_0
IVA	T_{1-4}	N_{2-3}	M_0
IVB	T_{1-4}	N_{0-3}	M_1

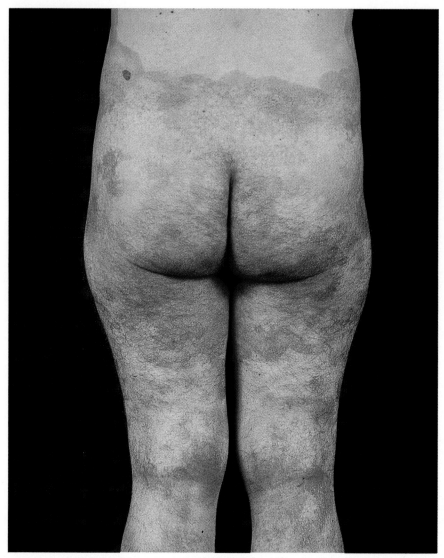

Figure 17-10   Cutaneous T cell lymphoma/mycosis fungoides   *More advanced stages show confluence of plaques with bizarre configuration and areas of poikiloderma. This patient had been treated unsuccessfully for psoriasis for two years before a biopsy and the correct diagnosis was made.*

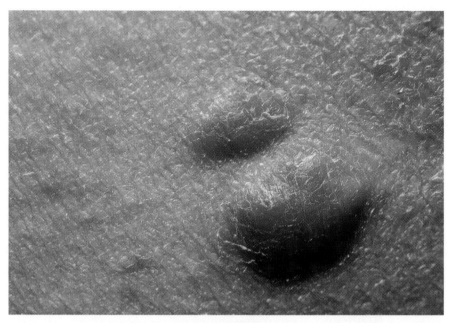

Figure 17-11 Cutaneous T cell lymphoma/mycosis fungoides *Early nodular stage with reddish-brownish smooth or scaly nodules within an eczema-like plaque.*

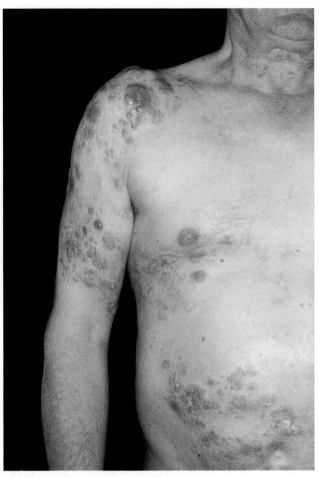

Figure 17-12   Cutaneous T cell lymphoma/mycosis fungoides: tumor stage   *Scaly and crusted eczema-like plaques seen on the abdomen have turned papular and nodular on the shoulder and arm. This patient was staged IIB (T_3 N_1 M_0).*

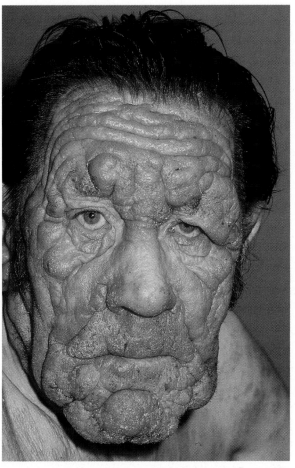

Figure 17-13 Cutaneous T cell lymphoma/mycosis fungoides: leonine facies *In this 50-year-old patient the disease had started with extremely pruritic, generalized eczema-like plaques on the trunk that had been treated as eczema over a course of four years. Massive nodular infiltration of the face occurred only recently leading to a leonine facies.*

SÉZARY'S SYNDROME

Sézary's syndrome is a rare special variant of cutaneous T cell lymphoma (CTCL) (mycosis fungoides) characterized by universal erythroderma, peripheral lymphadenopathy, and cellular infiltrates of atypical lymphocytes (Sézary cells) in the skin and in the blood. The disease may arise de novo or, less commonly, result from extension of a preexisting circumscribed CTCL. It usually occurs in patients older than 60 years and more commonly in males than in females.

Patients appear sick, shivering, and scared and there is generalized scaling erythroderma with considerable thickening of the skin. Because of the bright red color, the syndrome has been called the "red man syndrome" (see Section 6). There is diffuse hyperkeratosis of palms and soles, diffuse hair loss which can lead to baldness, and generalized lymphadenopathy.

DIFFERENTIAL DIAGNOSIS

Any exfoliative dermatitis can mimic Sézary's syndrome (see Section 6). Adult T cell leukemia/lymphoma.

LABORATORY EXAMINATIONS

Dermatopathology Like CTCL. The lymph nodes may contain nonspecific inflammatory cells (dermatopathic lymphadenopathy), or there can be a complete replacement of the nodal pattern by Sézary cells. The cell infiltrates in the viscera in CTCL are the same as are present in the skin. However, Sézary cells are not absolutely specific for Sézary syndrome, since these atypical lymphocytes can occur in nonspecific exfoliative dermatitis. Immunophenotyping: CD4 + T cells; T cell–receptor rearrangement: monoclonal process.

Hematology There may be a moderate leukocytosis or a normal WBC. The buffy coat contains from 15 to 30% atypical lymphocytes (Sézary cells).

DIAGNOSIS

The three features are erythroderma, generalized lymphadenopathy, and presence of increased numbers of atypical lymphocytes in the buffy coat.

COURSE AND PROGNOSIS

Without treatment, the course is progressive, and patients die from opportunistic infections.

MANAGEMENT

As in CTCL, plus appropriate supportive measures required for erythroderma. (See Cutaneous T Cell Lymphoma, pages 535–541.

CUTANEOUS B CELL LYMPHOMA

A clonal proliferation of B lymphocytes can be confined to the skin or more often is associated with systemic B cell lymphoma. Rare. Occurs in individuals older than 50 years and consists of crops of asymptomatic nodules and plaques, red to plum color (Fig. 17-14) with a smooth surface, firm, nontender, cutaneous or subcutaneous (Figs. 17-14 and 17-15). Dermatopathology shows dense nodular or diffuse monomorphous infiltrates of lymphocytes usually separated from the epidermis by a zone of normal collagen. B cell–specific monoclonal antibody studies facilitate differentiation of cutaneous B cell lymphoma from pseudolymphoma and cutaneous T cell lymphoma and permit more accurate classification of the cell type. Most cases react with CD19, 20, 22, and 28. Genetyping studies confirm diagnosis with immunoglobulin gene rearrangement.

Patients should be investigated thoroughly for nodal and extracutaneous disease; if found, bone marrow, lymph node, and peripheral blood studies will show morphologic cytochemical and immunologic features similar to those of the cutaneous infiltrates. Management consists of x-ray therapy to localized lesions and chemotherapy for systemic disease.

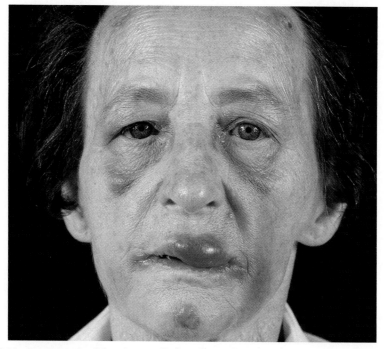

Figure 17-14   Cutaneous B cell lymphoma   *Red to plum color, smooth, firm nodules on the face of a 62-year-old female with systemic B cell lymphoma (leukemia). Nodules erupted suddenly and were accompanied by diffuse hemorrhage due to thrombocytopenia.*

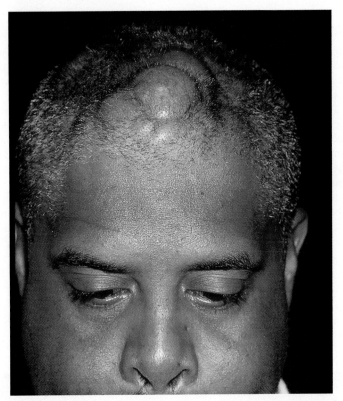

Figure 17-15   Cutaneous B cell lymphoma   *Smooth, cutaneous and subcutaneous nodules. Nontenderness and firmness were the first symptoms of B cell lymphoma (leukemia).*

DERMATOFIBROSARCOMA PROTUBERANS

A rare, recurring, and locally aggressive tumor that usually presents as indurated plaque with firm smooth protuberant nodules, varying from flesh color to reddish-brown, (Fig. 17-16), and often measuring several centimeters in diameter. Initially often presenting as atrophic, depressed, scar-like lesion, it develops into nodular masses, firm and irregular. Most commonly occurs on the trunk. The tumor histologically shows cartwheel-like arrangements of fibroblasts, seen as short fascicles running at right angles to one another. The tumor may be monomorphous—often mimicking scarred tissue—but mitosis may be present. Immunohistochemistry nearly always shows CD34 positivity.

A wide local excision with at least a 2-cm free margin is the treatment of choice, but recurrences are common. Locally aggressive metastases are extremely rare but do occur.

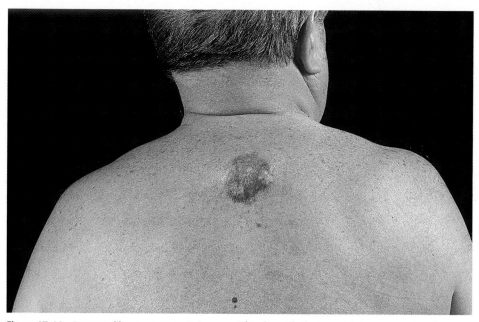

Figure 17-16   Dermatofibrosarcoma protuberans   *This firm, flesh- to reddish-brown colored nodular plaque started as a firm papule and was completely asymptomatic. The patient consulted a physician for cosmetic reasons only. Excision with 3 cm margins and split-skin grafting resulted in a cure.*

ADVERSE CUTANEOUS DRUG REACTIONS

Adverse cutaneous drug reactions (ACDRs) are common in hospitalized patients (2 to 3% experience ACDRs) as well as in ambulatory patients. Complications of drug therapy, overall, are the most common adverse event for hospitalized individuals, accounting for 19% of such events. ACDRs in an ambulatory practice occur frequently, many commonly used drugs having reaction rates of greater than 1%. Most reactions are mild, accompanied by pruritus, and resolve promptly after the offending drug is discontinued. However, severe, life-threatening ACDRs do occur and are unpredictable. Drug eruptions can mimic virtually all the morphologic expressions in dermatology and must be the first consideration in the differential diagnosis of a suddenly appearing symmetric eruption. Drug eruptions are caused by immunologic or nonimmunologic mechanisms and are provoked by systemic or topical administration of a drug. The majority are based on a hypersensitivity mechanism and may be of types I, II, III, or IV.

CLASSIFICATION

Immunologically Mediated ACDR   See Table 18-1.

Nonimmunologic Drug Eruptions

Idiosyncrasy Sensu Strictiori   Reactions due to hereditary enzyme deficiencies.

Cumulation   Reactions are dose dependent, based on the total amount of drug ingested: pigmentation due to gold, amiodarone, or minocycline.

Reactions due to Combination of a Drug with Ultraviolet Irradiation (Photosensitivity)   Reactions may have a toxic or immunologic (allergic) pathogenesis.

Irritancy/Toxicity of a Topically Applied Drug 5-fluorouracil, imiquimod.

Individual Idiosyncrasy to a Topical or Systemic Drug

Mechanisms Not Yet Known

GUIDELINES FOR ASSESSMENT OF POSSIBLE ACDRs[1]

- Exclude alternative causes, especially infections, in that many infections (especially viral) are difficult to distinguish clinically from the adverse effects of drugs used to treat infections.
- Examine interval between introduction of a drug and onset of the reaction.
- Note any improvement after drug withdrawal.
- Determine whether similar reactions have been associated with the same compound.
- Note any reaction on readministration of the drug.

FINDINGS INDICATING POSSIBLE LIFE-THREATENING ACDR[1]

Cutaneous

Confluent erythema
Facial edema or central facial involvement
Skin pain

[1] Source: From Roujeau JC, Stern RS: Severe adverse cutaneous reactions to drugs. N Engl J Med 331:1272, 1994.

Palpable purpura
Skin necrosis
Blisters of epidermal detachment
Positive Nikolsky's sign (epidermis separates readily from dermis with lateral pressure)
Mucous membrane erosions
Urticaria
Swelling of the tongue

General

High fever (temperature >40°C)
Enlarged lymph nodes
Arthralgias or arthritis
Shortness of breath, wheezing, hypotension

TYPES OF CLINICAL REACTIONS

Exanthematous Reactions (See also Section 23). Most common type of ACDR. Can occur with nearly any drug. Initial reaction usually occurs <14 days after drug therapy initiated; recurs shortly after rechallenge with sensitizing agent.

Urticaria/Angioedema (See also Section 12) Second most common type of ACDR after exanthematous reaction. May occur with/without angioedema. Onset: usually within 36 h after initial exposure; within minutes after rechallenge. Aspirin and NSAIDs are common causes; also codeine, penicillin, blood transfusion. Drugs that release mast cell mediator(s) (and thus cause urticaria): opiates, codeine, amphetamine, polymyxin B, atropine, hydralazine, pentamidine, quinine, radiocontrast media. Drugs that may cause urticaria/angioedema by pharmacologic mechanisms: cyclooxygenase inhibitors (aspirin, indomethacin); ACE inhibitors (captopril, enalapril).

Angioedema (alone) Uncommon. Characterized by edema of deep dermis, subcutaneous and submucosal areas.

Anaphylaxis and Anaphylactoid Reactions (See also Section 12) The most serious type of adverse drug reaction: occurs within minutes or hours after administration of drug; may be systemic life-threatening reaction. Most commonly caused by radiographic contrast media, antibiotics, extracts of allergens; more common with parenteral than oral administration. Intermittent administration may predispose to anaphylaxis.

Serum Sickness Onset: 5 to 21 days after initial exposure. Minor form: fever, urticaria, arthralgia. Major (complete) form: fever, urticaria, angioedema, arthralgia, arthritis, lymphadenopathy, eosinophilia, ±nephritis, ±endocarditis. Implicated drugs include IV IgG immunoglobulin (IVIG), antibiotics, and bovine serum albumin (used for oocyte retrieval during in vitro fertilization).

Erythema Multiforme (See also Section 5) Majority of cases considered to be associated with reactivated HSV infection.

Stevens-Johnson Syndrome (SJS) (See also Section 5) A moderate mucocutaneous and systemic reaction. With more severe mucocutaneous and systemic involvement, clinical findings merge into toxic epidermal necrolysis.

Toxic Epidermal Necrolysis (TEN) (See also Section 5). A severe, life-threatening mucocutaneous and systemic reaction.

Fixed Drug Eruptions Appears 30 min to 8 h after readministration in sensitized individuals. Lesions often solitary, recurring at same site; may be multiple. More numerous lesions occur after repeated administration; multiple bullous lesions can mimic those of TEN.

Lichenoid Eruptions (See also Section 5) May be extensive, occurring weeks to months after initiation of drug therapy; may progress to exfoliative dermatitis. Adnexal involvement may result in alopecia, anhidrosis. Resolution after discontinuation slow, 1 to 4 months; up to 24 months after gold. May be photodistributed or bullous. Oral involvement occurs with some drugs.

Photosensitivity (See also Section 8) Classified as phototoxic (occurring in all individuals if dosing high enough, only at sites of light exposure), photoallergic (may be eczematous or lichenoid), or photocontact reactions. Some drugs cause both phototoxic and photoallergic reactions.

Photoonycholysis (See Section 28)

Porphyria, Pseudoporphyria, and Photosensitivity (See also Section 8) Porphyria cutanea tarda (PCT) may be precipitated by drugs in sun-exposed sites. Pseudo-PCT with bulla formation can also be a drug-induced reaction.

Purpura (Petechia, Ecchymosis) Drug-induced (allergic or cytotoxic) thrombocytopenia results in petechiae/ecchymoses if platelet counts are <30,000/μL. Hemorrhage into a morbilliform ACDR occurs not uncommonly on the legs. The use of oral, inhalation, and topical glucocorticoids is associated with ecchymoses, usually on the extremities in areas of dermatoheliosis. Progressive pigmented purpura has also been reported to associated with drug therapy.

Acneform Eruptions Folliculocentric pustules, usually without comedones. Drugs: glucocorticoids (parenteral, topical), ACTH, anabolic steroids, oral contraceptives, halogens (iodides, bromides), isoniazid, danazol, lithium, azathioprine.

Pustular Eruptions Toxic pustuloderma, acute generalized exanthematous pustulosis. Must be differentiated from pustular psoriasis; eosinophil in the infiltrate suggests ACDR. Drugs: ampicillin, amoxicillin, macrolides, tetracyclines.

Pityriasis Rosea-Like (Pityriasiform) Reactions Caused by gold therapy, captopril, and other drugs.

Psoriasiform Reactions (See also Section 3) Drugs reported to exacerbate psoriasis: antimalarials; β-blockers; lithium salts; nonsteroidal anti-inflammatory drugs (NSAIDs) (ibuprofen, indomethacin); miscellaneous (captopril, cimetidine, clonidine, gemfibrozil, interferon, methyldopa, penicillamine, trazadone).

Eczematous Eruptions Systemic administration of a drug to an individual who has been previously sensitized to the drug by topical application can provoke a widespread eczematous dermatitis (systemic contact-type dermatitis medicamentosa) or urticaria. Systemically administered drugs that reactivate allergic contact dermatitis to related topical agents (systemic drug/topical agent): ethylenediamine antihistamines, aminophylline/aminophylline suppositories, ethylenediamine HC1; procaine/benzocaine; iodides, iodinated organic compounds, radiographic contrast media/iodine; streptomycin, kanamycin, paramomycin, gentamicin/neomycin sulfate; nitroglycerine tablets/nitroglycerin ointment; disulfuram/thiuram.

Exfoliative Dermatitis and Erythroderma (See also Section 6) This widespread or generalized reaction may follow an exanthematous ACDR or begin with erythema and exudation in body folds and progress to become generalized. In individuals previously sensitized by topical administration of a drug, systemic administration of the sensitizing agent (or closely related compound) may cause a generalized eczematous dermatitis. The most commonly implicated drugs are sulfonamides, antimalarials, phenytoin, and penicillin.

Erythema Nodosum Reported with sulfonamides, other antimicrobial agents, analgesics, oral contraceptives, G-CSF, all-*trans*-retinoic acid.

Lupus Erythematosus (LE)-Like Syndrome 5% of cases of systemic LE are drug-induced. Cutaneous manifestations, including photosensitivity, urticaria, erythema multiforme-like lesions, Raynaud's phenomenon, are not common, however.

Dermatomyositis-Like Reactions Reported with penicillamine, NSAIDs, carbamazepine.

Scleroderma-Like Reactions Reported with penicillamine, bleomycin, bromocriptine, sodium valproate, 5-hydroxytryptophan, acetanilide contaminating rapeseed cooking oil.

Bullous Eruptions Differential diagnosis: fixed drug eruption, drug-induced vasculitis, SJS, TEN, porphyria, pseudoporphyria, drug-induced pemphigus, drug-induced pemphigoid, drug-induced linear IgA disease, bulla over pressure areas in sedated patients.

Pseudolymphoma Anticonvulsant drugs (phenytoin, carbamazepine), allopurinol, antidepressants, phenothiazines, benzodiazepam, antihistamines, β-blockers, lipid-lowering agents, cyclosporine, D-penicillamine.

Cutaneous Necrosis Drugs can cause cutaneous necrosis when given orally or at sites of injection. Warfarin-induced cutaneous necrosis is a rare reaction with onset between the third and fifth days of anticoagulation therapy with the warfarin derivatives and indandione compounds, manifested by sharply demarcated, purpuric cutaneous infarction. Risk factors: higher initial dosing, obesity, female sex; individuals with hereditary deficiency of protein C, a natural anticoagulant protein; protein S or antithrombin III deficiency. Idiosyncratic reaction. In individuals with hereditary deficiency of protein C, a natural anticoagulant protein, warfarin greatly depresses protein C levels before decreasing other vitamin K-dependent coagulation factors, inducing a transient hypercoagulable state and thrombus formation. Lesions vary with severity of reaction: petechiae to ecchymoses to tender hemorrhagic infarcts to extensive necrosis. *Early:* large indurated dermal plaque(s). *Later:* quickly evolve to well-demar-

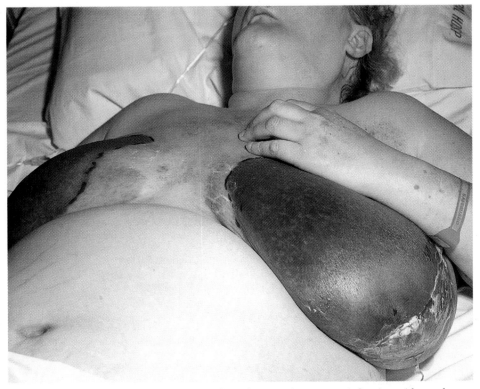

Figure 18-1 Cutaneous necrosis: warfarin *Bilateral areas of cutaneous infarction with purple-to-black coloration of the breast surrounded by an area of erythema, occurred on the fifth day of warfarin therapy.*

cated, deep purple to black, geographic areas of necrosis (Fig. 18-1). Hemorrhagic bullae, large erosions may complicate infarcts. Later, deep tissue sloughing and ulceration if lesions are not debrided and grafted. Often single; may present as two lesions, one on either breast. Distribution: areas of abundant subcutaneous fat: breasts, buttocks, abdomen, thighs, calves; acral areas are spared. Histology: epidermal necrosis, thrombosis, and occlusion of most blood vessels, scanty inflammatory response. Coagulation studies: usually within normal limits. Differential diagnosis: Purpura fulminans (disseminated intravascular coagulation), hematoma/ecchymosis in overly anticoagulated patient, necrotizing soft tissue infection, vasculitis, rare necrosis after vasopressin treatment, brown recluse spider bite. Depending on severity of reaction, lesions may subside, heal by granulation, or require surgical intervention. If area of necrosis is large in an elderly, debilitated patient, may be life-threatening. If warfarin is inadvertently readministered, reaction recurs.

Cutaneous necrosis can occur at sites of injection of several drugs. Heparin can cause cutaneous necrosis, usually at the site of subcutaneous injection (Fig. 18-2). Interferon-α can cause necrosis and ulceration at injections sites, often in the lower abdominal panniculus (Fig. 18-3). Extravasation of chemotheraeutic drugs such as doxorubicin can be followed by skin necrosis with ulceration.

Drug-Induced Pigmentation (See also Section 11) Associated with post-inflammatory hyperpigmentation, increased melanin synthesis, increased lipofuscin synthesis, or cutaneous deposition of drug-related material.

Drug-Induced Alopecia (See Section 27)

Drug-Induced Hypertrichosis (See Section 27)

Drug-Induced Nail Changes (See Section 28)

LABORATORY EXAMINATIONS

Hematology Eosinophil count >1000/μL. Lymphocytosis with atypical lymphocytes.

Chemistry Abnormal results of liver function tests.

DIAGNOSIS

Usually made on clinical findings. Lesional skin biopsy is helpful in defining the type of reaction pattern occuring but does not help in identifying the offending drug. Skin tests and radioallergosorbent tests are helpful in diagnosing IgE-mediated type I hypersensitivity reactions, more specifically to penicillins.

MANAGEMENT

In most cases, the implicated or suspected drug should be discontinued. In some, such as with morbilliform eruptions, the offending drug can be continued, and the eruption may resolve. In cases of urticaria/angioedema or early SJS/TEN, the ACDR can be life-threatening, and the drug should be discontinued.

Table 18-1 IMMUNOLOGICALLY MEDIATED ADVERSE CUTANEOUS DRUG REACTIONS

Type of Reaction	Pathogenesis	Example of Causative Drug(s)	Clinical Pattern
Type I	IgE-mediated; immediate-type immunologic reactions	Penicillin	Urticaria/angioedema of skin/mucosa, edema of other organs, and fall in blood pressure (anaphylactic shock). Occur more commonly if drug (antigen) is administered intravenously than by mouth.
Type II	Drug + cytotoxic antibodies cause lysis of cells such as platelets or leukocytes	Penicillin, cephalosporins, sulfonamides, rifampin	
	Drug + antibodies (immune complexes) cause lysis or phagocytosis	Quinine, quinidine, salicylamide, isoniazid, chlorpromazine, sulfonamides, sulfonylureas	
Type III	IgG or IgM antibodies formed to drug; immune complexes deposited in small vessel activate complement and recruitment of granulocytes		Vasculitis; urticaria-like lesions; Stevens-Johnson syndrome; toxic epidermal necrolysis ?Fixed drug eruption Arthritis, nephritis, alveolitis, hemolytic anemia, thrombocytopenia, agranulocytosis Onset of reaction: 5–7 days between introduction of drug and appearance of reaction
Type IV	Cell-mediated immune reaction. Sensitized lymphocytes react with drug, liberating cytokines, which trigger cutaneous inflammatory response response	Sulfamethoxazole	Morbilliform (exanthematous) reactions; photoallergic reactions ?Fixed drug eruption ?Bullous eruption ?Lichenoid Stevens-Johnson syndrome; toxic epidermal necrolysis

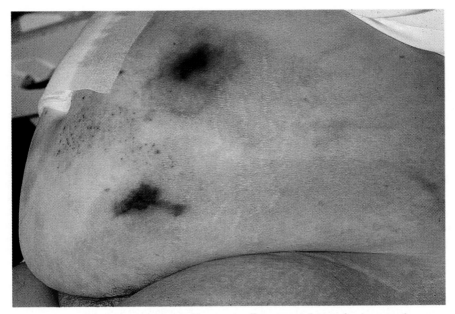

Figure 18-2   Cutaneous necrosis: heparin   *Two areas of cutaneous hemorrhagic necrosis with surrounding erythema on the abdomen occurring postoperatively in a female treated with heparin.*

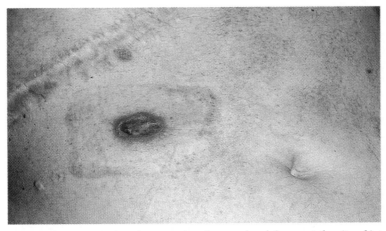

Figure 18-3   Cutaneous necrosis: interferon-α   *An ulcer on the abdomen at the site of interferon injection. The patient has had liver transplantation and acquired hepatitis C virus infection during the procedure.*

EXANTHEMATOUS DRUG REACTIONS

An exanthematous drug reaction (eruption) is an adverse hypersensitivity reaction to an ingested or parenterally administered drug characterized by a cutaneous eruption that mimics a measles-like viral exanthem; systemic involvement is minimal.
Synonyms: Morbilliform drug reaction, maculopapular drug reaction.

EPIDEMIOLOGY

Age of Onset Less common in the very young.

Incidence Most common type of cutaneous drug reaction.

Etiology *Drugs with a high probability of reaction* (3 to 5%): penicillin and related antibiotics, carbamazepine, allopurinol, gold salts (10 to 20%). *Medium probability:* sulfonamides (bacteriostatic, antidiabetic, diuretic), NSAIDs, hydantoin derivatives, isoniazid, chloramphenicol, erythromycin, streptomycin. *Low probability* (≤1%): barbiturates, benzodiazepines, phenothiazines, tetracyclines.

PATHOGENESIS

Exact mechanism unknown. Probably delayed hypersensitivity. Rash with Epstein-Barr virus (EBV) and cytomegalovirus (CMV) mononucleosis probably not allergic.

HISTORY

Mononucleosis Up to 100% of patients with primary EBV or CMV infection (infectious mononucleosis syndrome) given ampicillin or amoxicillin develop an exanthematous drug eruption.

HIV Infection 50 to 60% of HIV-infected patients who receive sulfa drugs (i.e., trimethoprim-sulfamethoxazole) develop eruption. With immune restitution with highly-active antiretroviral therapy (HAART), previously tolerant individuals may develop ACDR as CD4+ cell count rises.

Drug History Increased incidence of reactions in patients on allopurinol given ampicillin/amoxicillin.

Prior Drug Sensitization Patients with prior history of exanthematous drug eruption will most likely develop a similar reaction if rechallenged with same drug. About 10% of patients sensitive to penicillins who are given cephalosporins will exhibit cross-drug sensitivity and develop eruption. Patients sensitized to one sulfa-based drug (bacteriostatic, antidiabetic, diuretic) may cross-react with another category of the drug in 20% of cases.

Onset *Early Reaction* In previously sensitized patient, eruption starts within 2 or 3 days after readministration of drug.

Late Reaction Sensitization occurs during administration or after completing course of drug; peak incidence at ninth day after administration. However, ACDR may occur at any time between the first day and 3 weeks after the beginning of treatment. Reaction to penicillin can begin 2 or more weeks after drug is discontinued.

Skin Symptoms Usually quite pruritic, disturbs sleep. Painful skin lesions, suggest more serious ACDR such as toxic epidermal necrolysis.

Systems Review ±.Fever chills.

PHYSICAL EXAMINATION

Skin Lesions Macules and/or papules, a few millimeters to 1 cm in size (Fig. 18-4). Purpura may be seen in lesions of lower legs. In individuals with thrombocytopenia, exanthematous eruptions can mimic vasculitis because of intralesional hemorrhage. *May progress to generalized exfoliative dermatitis, especially if drug not discontinued.* Scaling and/or desquamation may occur with healing; also, erythema multiforme-like.

Color Bright or "drug" red. Resolving lesions have hues of tan and purple. In time, lesions become confluent forming large macules, polycyclic/gyrate erythema, reticular eruptions, sheet-like erythema, erythroderma.

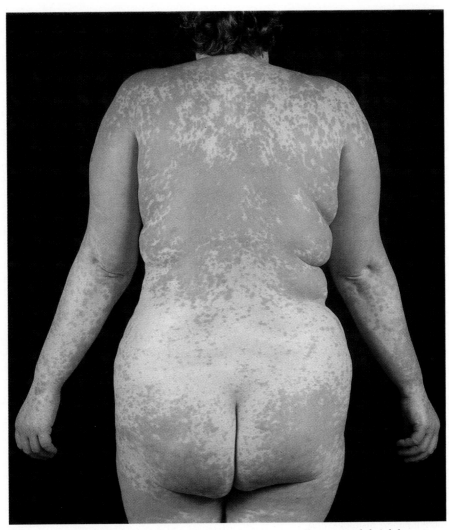

Figure 18-4   Exanthematous drug eruption: ampicillin   *Symmetrically arranged, brightly erythematous macules and papules, discrete in some areas and confluent in others on the back and extremities.*

Distribution Symmetric (Fig.18-4). Almost always on trunk and extremities. Confluent lesions in intertriginous areas, i.e., axilla, groin, inframammary area. Palms and soles variably involved. In children, may be limited to face and extremities. Eruption may be accentuated in striae. May spare face, nipple, periareolar area, surgical scar. Reactions to ampicillin usually appear initially on the elbows, knees, and trunk, extending symmetrically to most areas of the body.

Mucous Membranes Enanthem on buccal mucosa.

Reactions to Specific Drugs *Ampicillin, Amoxicillin* Up to 100% of patients with EBV or CMV mononucleosis syndrome given ampicillin, amoxicillin developed drug eruptions.

NSAIDs Incidence: 1 to 3%. Site: trunk, pressure areas. Onset: 1 to 2 weeks after beginning therapy.

Barbiturates Morphology: macular or maculopapular; scarlatiniform. Site: face, trunk. Onset: few days after initiation of therapy. Cross-reactivity with other barbiturates: not universal.

Nitrofurantoin Associated findings: fever, peripheral eosinophilia, pulmonary edema, chest pain, dyspnea. Onset: 2 weeks after initiation of therapy; within hours if previously sensitized.

Hydantoin Derivatives Morphology: macular or confluent erythema. Site: begins on face, spreads to trunk and extremities (see Section 18). Onset: 2 weeks after initiation of therapy. Associated findings: fever, peripheral eosinophilia; facial edema; lymphadenopathy (can mimic lymphoma histologically).

Isoniazid Morphology: morbilliform; may evolve to exfoliative dermatitis. Associated findings: fever; hepatitis.

Benzodiazepines Incidence: very low. Onset: few days after initiation of therapy. Rechallenge: frequently rash does not occur.

Phenothiazines Site: begins on face, spreads to trunk (mainly back) and extremities. Onset: between second and third weeks after initiation of therapy. Associated findings: periorbital edema. Rechallenge: rash may not occur. Cross-reactivity: common.

Carbamazepine Morphology: diffuse erythema; severe erythroderma may follow. Site: begins on face, spreads rapidly to all areas; may occur in photodistribution. Onset: 2 weeks after initiation of therapy. Associated findings: facial edema. Early findings of SJS/TEN mimic those of exanthematous reactions.

Sulfonamides Incidence: common in up to 50 to 60% of HIV-infected patients. Morphology: morbilliform, erythema multiforme-like.

Allopurinol Incidence: 5%. Morphology: morbilliform. Begins on face, spreads rapidly to all areas; may occur in photodistribution Onset: 2 to 3 weeks after initiation of therapy. Associated findings: facial edema; systemic vasculitis, especially involving kidneys. Rash may fade in spite of continued administration.

Gold Salts Incidence: 10 to 20% of patients; dose-related. Morphology: diffuse erythema; exfoliative dermatitis, lichenoid, hemorrhagic, bullous, or pityriasis rosea-like eruptions may follow.

General Examination Drug fever. Findings associated with the indication for drug administration.

DIFFERENTIAL DIAGNOSIS

Exanthematous Eruption Viral exanthem (often begins on face, progresses to trunk; may be accompanied by conjunctivitis, lymphadenopathy, fever), secondary syphilis, atypical pityriasis rosea, early widespread allergic contact dermatitis.

LABORATORY EXAMINATIONS

Hemogram Peripheral eosinophilia.

Dermatopathology Perivascular lymphocytes and eosinophils.

DIAGNOSIS

Clinical diagnosis, at times confirmed by histologic findings, correlated with history of drug administration.

COURSE

After discontinuation of drug, rash usually fades; however, it may worsen for a few days. The eruption may begin after the drug has been discontinued. Occasionally fades even though drug is continued. Eruption usually recurs with rechallenge, although not always. In some cases of exanthematous ampicillin reactions, readministration of the drug does not cause the eruption. Duration of ampicillin eruption after discontinuation of drug: 3 to 5 days. If drug is continued, exfoliative dermatitis may develop. Of more concern, a morbilliform eruption may be the initial presentation of a more serious eruption, i.e., SJS, TEN, hypersensitivity syndrome, or serum sickness.

MANAGEMENT

The definitive step in management is to identify the offending drug and discontinue it.

Indications for Discontinuation of Drug Urticaria (concern for anaphylaxis), facial edema, blisters, mucosal involvement, ulcers, palpable or extensive purpura, fever, lymphadenopathy.

Symptomatic Treatment Oral antihistamine to alleviate pruritus.

Glucocorticoids *Potent Topical Glucocorticoid Preparation* May help speed resolution of eruption, especially if secondary changes of eczematous dermatitis have occurred due to scratching.

Oral or IV Glucocorticoids Provides symptomatic relief. If offending drug cannot be substituted or omitted, systemic glucocorticoids can be administered to treat the ACDR; also, to induce more rapid remission.

Prevention The patient must be aware of his or her specific drug hypersensitivity and that other drugs of the same class can cross-react. Although an exanthematous drug eruption may not recur if the drug is given again, readministration is best avoided by using a different agent. Wearing a medical alert bracelet is advised.

DRUG-INDUCED ACUTE URTICARIA, ANGIOEDEMA, EDEMA, AND ANAPHYLAXIS

Drug-induced urticaria and angioedema occur due to a variety of mechanisms and are characterized clinically by transient wheals and larger edematous areas that involve the dermis and subcutaneous tissue (angioedema). In some cases, cutaneous urticaria/angioedema is associated with systemic anaphylaxis, which is manifested by respiratory distress, vascular collapse, and/or shock.

Synonym: Angioneurotic edema.

EPIDEMIOLOGY

Classification of Pathogenesis of Reactions

Immune-Mediated (Allergic) Urticaria/Angioedema *IgE-Mediated* Antibiotics (especially penicillins), radiographic contrast agents.

Complement-Mediated By way of immune complexes activating complement and releasing anaphylatoxins that induce mast cell degranulation. Serum sickness, administration of whole blood, immunoglobulins.

Immune Complex–Mediated Reactions resemble serum sickness, penicillin.

Nonallergic Urticaria (Anaphylactoid Reactions) *Analgesics/Anti-inflammatory Drugs (NSAIDs)* Drugs inhibit or block cyclooxygenase enzyme in prostaglandin synthesis. Also associated with rhinosinusitis and asthma.

Radiographic Contrast Media Most reactions are nonallergic; rarely, allergic.

Angiotensin-Converting Enzyme (ACE) Inhibitors In .1 to .2% of patients, ACE inhibitors induce a rapid swelling in the nose, throat, mouth, glottis, larynx, lips, and/or tongue. May be due to inhibition of kinin metabolism. Not dose-related; nearly always develops within the first week of therapy, usually within the first few hours after the initial dose. Individuals undergoing hemodialysis with high-flux dialysis membranes (increases bradykinin production) at much higher risk (up to 35%).

Calcium-Channel Blockers Nifedipine produces peripheral edema in 10 to 30% of treated patients. The edema is localized to the lower legs and feet and probably occurs secondary to vasodilation of dependent arterioles and small blood vessels rather than to generalized fluid retention.

Drugs Releasing Histamine See below.

Drugs Causing Urticaria/Angioedema/Anaphylaxis

Antibiotics and Chemotherapeutic Agents Penicillins: ampicillin, amoxicillin, dicloxacillin, mezlocillin, penicillin G, penicillin V, ticarcillin. Cephalosporins, including third generation. Sulfonamides and derivatives.

CVS Drugs Amiodarone, procainamide.

Immunotherapeutics, Vaccines Antilymphocyte serum, levamisole, horse serum.

Cytostatic Agents L-Asparaginase, bleomycin, cisplatin, daunorubicin, 5-fluorouracil, procarbazine, thiotepa.

ACE Inhibitors Captopril, enalopril, lininopril.

Calcium-Channel Blockers Nifedipine, diltiazem, verapamil.

Drugs Releasing Histamine Centrally acting drugs (morphine, meperidine, atropine, codeine, papaverine, propanidid, alfaxalone); muscle relaxants (D-tubocurarine, succinylcholine); sympathomimetics (amphetamine, tyramine); hypotensive agents (hydralazine, tolazoline, trimethaphan camsylate); antimicrobial agents (pentamidine, propamidine, stilbamidine, quinine, vancomycin); others (radiographic contrast media).

Incidence Angioedema occurs in 1 per 10,000 courses of penicillin and leads to death in 1 to 5 per 100,000 courses. Angioedema associated with ACE inhibitors occurs in 2 to 10 per 10,000 new users.

PATHOGENESIS

IgE-mediated urticaria: Lesions result from antigen-induced release of biologically active molecules (leukotrienes, prostaglandins) from mast cells or basophilic leukocytes sensitized with specific IgE antibodies (type I, anaphylactic hypersensitivity). Mediators released increase venular permeability, modulate the release of biologically active materials from other cell types. In sensitized individuals, a very small amount of drug can trigger a serious reaction. Parenteral administration of the drug in a sensitized individual is much more likely to trigger anaphylaxis than oral administration. Urticaria can be immediate or accelerated, depending on whether IgE molecules are present before drug exposure or are formed during exposure. In complement-mediated urticaria, complement is activated by immune complexes, leading to the release of anaphylatoxins, which, in turn, induce mast cell degranulation. Intolerance to salicylates is presumably mediated by abnormalities of the arachidonic acid pathway.

HISTORY

Time from Initial Drug Exposure to Appearance of Urticaria *IgE-Mediated* Initial sensitization, usually 7 to 14 days; urticaria may occur while the drug is still being administered or after it is discontinued. In previously sensitized individuals, usually within minutes or hours.

Immune Complex–Mediated Initial sensitization, usually 7 to 10 days, but as long as 28 days; in previously sensitized individuals, symptoms appear 12 to 36 h after drug re-administered.

Analgesics/Anti-Inflammatory Drugs Occurs after administration of drug by 20 to 30 min (up to 4 h).

Prior Drug Exposure *Radiographic Contrast Media* 25 to 35% probability of repeat reaction in individuals with history of prior reaction to contrast media.

Duration of Lesions Hours.

Skin Symptoms Pruritus, burning of palms/soles, auditory canal. With airway edema, difficulty breathing.

Constitutional Symptoms IgE-mediated: flushing, sudden fatigue, yawning, headache, weakness, dizziness; numbness of tongue, sneezing, bronchospasm, substernal pressure, palpitations; nausea, vomiting, crampy abdominal pain, diarrhea.

Systems Review Arthralgia.

PHYSICAL EXAMINATION

Skin Lesions

Urticaria Large wheals (Fig. 18-5) that appear and resolve within a few hours, spontaneously or with therapy; reappear. Pink with larger lesions having white central area surrounded by an erythematous halo. Oval, arciform, annular, polycyclic, serpiginous, and bizarre patterns. Target and iris lesions occur. Initial part of lesion resolves as the newer portions advance centrifugally, at times merging with other lesions. Transient, hours.

Distribution Localized, regional, or generalized.

Angioedema Extensive tissue swelling with involvement of deep dermal and subcutaneous tissues. Often pronounced on face with skin-colored enlargement of portion of face (eyelids, lips, tongue) (Fig. 18-5).

Distribution Genitalia, or any site; upper airway with possible obstruction of breathing.

General Findings *IgE-Mediated Reactions* Hypotension. Bronchospasm, laryngeal edema.

DIFFERENTIAL DIAGNOSIS

Acute Edematous Red Pruritic Plaque(s) Allergic contact dermatitis (poison ivy, poison oak dermatitis), cellulitis, insect bite(s).

LABORATORY EXAMINATIONS

Dermatopathology Edema of the dermis or subcutaneous tissue, dilation of venules, mild perivascular infiltrate, mast cell degranulation.

Complement Levels Decreased in serum sickness.

Ultrasonography For early diagnosis of bowel involvement; presence of abdominal pain may indicate edema of the bowel.

DIAGNOSIS

Clinical diagnosis, at times confirmed by histologic findings.

COURSE AND PROGNOSIS

Drug-induced urticaria/angioedema usually resolves within hours to days to weeks after the causative drug is withdrawn.

MANAGEMENT

The offending drug should be identified and withdrawn as soon as possible.

Prevention *Previously Sensitized Individuals* The patient should carry information listing drug sensitivities (wallet card, bracelet).

Radiographic Contrast Media Avoid use of contrast media known to have caused prior reaction. If not possible, pretreat patient with antihistamine and prednisone (1 mg/kg) 30 to 60 min before contrast media exposure.

Treatment of Acute Severe Urticaria/Anaphylaxis *Epinephrine* .3 to .5 mL of a 1:1000 dilution subcutaneously, repeated in 15 to 20 min. Maintain airway. Intravenous access.

Antihistamines H_1 blockers or H_2 blockers or combination.

Systemic Glucocorticoids *Intravenous* Hydrocortisone or methylprednisolone for severe symptoms.

Oral Prednisone, 70 mg, tapering by 10 or 5 mg daily over 1 to 2 weeks, is usually adequate.

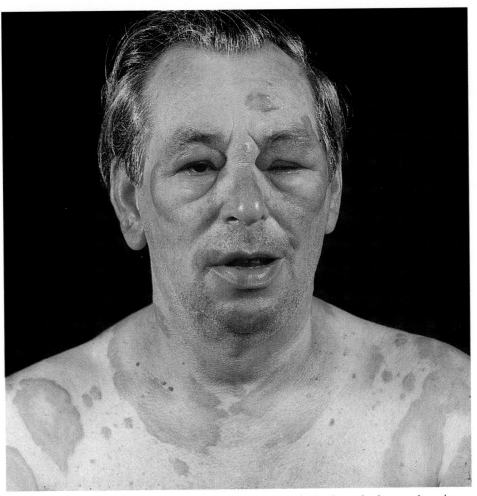

Figure 18-5 **Drug-induced urticaria: penicillin** *Large, urticarial wheals on the face, neck, and trunk with angioedema in the periorbital region.*

FIXED DRUG ERUPTION

A fixed drug eruption (FDE) is an adverse cutaneous reaction to an ingested drug, characterized by the formation of a solitary, but at times multiple, plaque, bulla, or erosion; if the patient is rechallenged with the offending drug, the FDE occurs repeatedly at the identical skin site (i.e., fixed) within hours of ingestion.

EPIDEMIOLOGY

Most Commonly Implicated Agents

Antimicrobial agents
   Tetracyclines (tetracycline, minocycline)
   Sulfonamides, including "nonabsorbable" drugs; cross-reactions with antidiabetic and diuretic sulfa drug may occur.
   Metronidazole
   Nystatin
Anti-inflammatory agents
   Salicylates
   NSAIDs
   Phenylbutazone
   Phenacetin
Psychoactive agents
   Barbiturates, including Fiorinal
   Quaalude, Doriden
Oral contraceptives
Quinine (including quinine in tonic water), quinidine
Phenolphthalein
Many other commonly used drugs
Food coloring: in food or medications

PATHOGENESIS

Unknown.

HISTORY

Drug History Patients frequently give a history of identical lesion(s) occurring at the identical location. FDEs may be associated with a headache for which the patient takes a barbiturate containing analgesic, with constipation for which the patient takes a phenolphthalein-containing laxative, or with a cold for which the patient takes an over-the-counter medication containing a yellow dye. The offending "drug" in food dye-induced FDE may be difficult to identify, i.e., yellow dye in Galliano liqueur or phenolphthalein in maraschino cherries; quinine in tonic water.

Skin Symptoms Usually asymptomatic. May be pruritic or burning. Painful when eroded. Patients note a residual area of postinflammatory hyperpigmentation between attacks.

Time to Onset of Lesion(s) Occur from 30 min to 8 h after ingestion of drug in previously sensitized individual.

Duration of Lesion(s) Lesions persist if drug is continued. Resolve days to few weeks after drug is discontinued.

PHYSICAL EXAMINATION

Skin Lesions The characteristic early lesion is a sharply demarcated macule (Fig. 18-6), round or oval in shape, occurring within hours after ingestion of the offending drug. Initially, erythema, then dusky red to violaceous. After healing, dark brown with violet hue postinflammatory hyperpigmentation. Most commonly, lesions are solitary, but they may be multiple (Fig. 18-7) with random distribution; numerous lesions may simulate toxic epidermal necrolysis (Fig. 18-7). Size varies from a few millimeters up to 10 to 20 cm in diameter. Within a few hours the lesion becomes edematous, thus forming a plaque, which may evolve to become a bulla and then an erosion. Eroded lesions, especially on genital or oral mucosa, are quite painful (Fig. 18-6).

Distribution Genital skin is most commonly involved site, but any site may be involved; perioral, periorbital. Occur in conjunctivae, oropharynx; may simulate herpes simplex, conjunctivitis, or urethritis.

DIFFERENTIAL DIAGNOSIS

Solitary Genital Erosion Recurrent herpetic lesion.

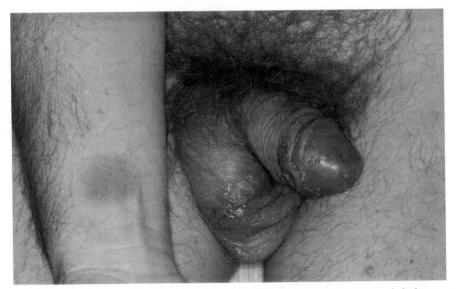

Figure 18-6 Fixed drug eruption: phenolphthalein   *A violet plaque on the wrist, eroded plaques on the glans penis and scrotum, associated with extensive intraoral erosions. This was the fourth such episode and followed ingestion of a phenolphthalein-containing laxative.*

Multiple Erosions Stevens-Johnson syndrome, toxic epidermal necrolysis.

Oral Erosion(s) Aphthous stomatitis, primary herpetic gingivostomatitis, erythema multiforme.

LABORATORY EXAMINATIONS

Dermatopathology Similar to findings in erythema multiforme: individual keratinocyte necrosis, basal vacuolization, dermal edema, perivascular and interstitial lymphohistiocytic infiltrate, at times with eosinophils. Subepidermal vesicles and bullae with overlying epidermal necrosis. Between outbreaks, the site of FDE shows marked pigmentary incontinence with melanin in macrophages in upper dermis.

Patch Test Suspected drug can be placed as a patch test at a previously involved site; an inflammatory response occurs in 30% of cases.

DIAGNOSIS

Made on clinical grounds. Readministration of the drug confirms diagnosis but should be avoided.

COURSE AND PROGNOSIS

FDE resolves within a few weeks of withdrawing the drug. Recurs within hours after ingestion of a single dose of the drug.

MANAGEMENT

Treatment of Lesion(s) Identify and withhold the offending drug. A newly erupted lesion of FDE presents as an inflammatory plaque, with or without erosion. Noneroded lesions can be treated with a potent topical glucocorticoid ointment or intralesional triamcinolone. Eroded cutaneous lesions can be treated with bacitracin or Silvadene ointment and a dressing until the site is reepithelialized. Postinflammatory hyperpigmentation (dermal melanin) may persist at the site of an FDE for months or years and does not respond to hydroquinone therapy.

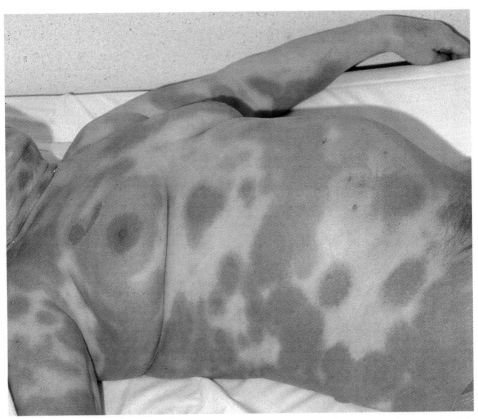

Figure 18-7   Generalized fixed drug eruption: tetracycline   *Multiple, confluent, violaceous-red, oval erythematous areas, some of which later became bullous. The eruption may be difficult to distinguish from toxic epidermal necrolysis.*

DRUG HYPERSENSITIVITY SYNDROME

Hypersensitivity syndrome is an idiosyncratic adverse drug reaction that begins acutely in the first 2 months after initiation of drug and is characterized by fever, severe disease with characteristic infiltrated papules and facial edema or an exfoliative dermatitis, lymphadenopathy, hematologic abnormalities (eosinophilia, atypical lymphocytes), and organ involvement (hepatitis, carditis, interstitial nephritis, or interstitial pneumonitis). The mortality rate is 10% if unrecognized and untreated. Lesional biopsy specimens show a lymphocytic infiltrate, at times mimicking a cutaneous lymphoma.

Synonym: Drug rash with eosinophilia and systemic symptoms (DRESS).

EPIDEMIOLOGY

Race Reactions to antiepileptic drugs may be higher in black individuals.

Etiology Most commonly: antiepileptic drugs (phenytoin, carbamazepine, phenobarbital; cross-sensitivity among these three drugs is common) and sulfonamides (antimicrobial agents, dapsone, sulfasalazine). Less commonly: allopurinol, gold salts, sorbinil, minocycline, zalcitabine, calcium channel blockers, ranitidine, thalidomide, mexiletine.

PATHOGENESIS

Some patients have a genetically determined inability to detoxify the toxic arene oxide metabolic products of anticonvulsant agents. Slow *N*-acetylation of sulfonamide and increased susceptibility of leukocytes to toxic hydroxylamine metabolites are associated with higher risk of hypersensitivity syndrome.

HISTORY

Onset 2 to 6 weeks after drug is initially used, and later than most other serious skin reactions.

Prodrome Fever, rash.

Systems Review Fever.

PHYSICAL EXAMINATION

Skin Lesions *Early:* morbilliform eruption (Fig. 18-8) on face, upper trunk, upper extremities; cannot be distinguished from exanthematous drug eruption. May progress to generalized exfoliative dermatitis/erythroderma, especially if drug is not discontinued. Eruption become infiltrated and indurated with edematous follicular accentuation. Facial edema (especially periorbially) is characteristic. Dermal edema may result in blister formation. Sterile folliculocentric as well as non-follicular pustules may occur. Eruption may become purpuric on legs. Scaling and/or desquamation may occur with healing.

Distribution Symmetric. Almost always on trunk and extremities. Lesions may become confluent and generalized.

Mucous Membranes Cheilitis, erosions, erythematous pharynx, enlarged tonsils.

General Examination Elevated temperature (drug fever).

Lymph Nodes Lymphadenopathy frequent ±tender; usually due to benign lymphoid hyperplasia.

Other Involvement of liver, heart, lungs, joints, muscles, thyroid, brain also occurs.

DIFFERENTIAL DIAGNOSIS

Early That of morbilliform eruptions. Can mimic early measles or rubella.

Later Serum sickness, drug-induced vasculitis, Henoch-Schönlein purpura, cryoglobulin-associated vasculitis, vasculitis associated with infection and collagen vascular diseases.

Rash Plus Lymphadenopathy Rubella, primary EBV or CMV mononucleosis syndrome.

LABORATORY EXAMINATIONS

Hemogram Peripheral eosinophilia (30% of cases). Leukocytosis. Mononucleosis-like atypical lymphocytes.

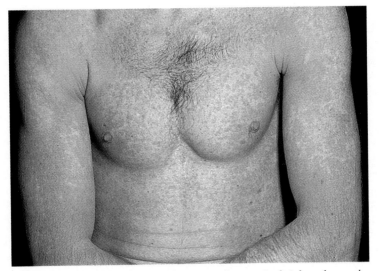

Figure 18-8 Drug hypersensitivity syndrome: phenytoin *Symmetric, bright red, exanthematous eruption, confluent in some sites: the patient had associated lymphadenopathy.*

Chemistries Hepatitis.

Histology *Skin* Lymphocytic infiltrate, dense and diffuse or superficial and perivascular. ±Eosinophils or dermal edema. In some cases, band-like infiltrate of atypical lymphocytes with epidermotrophism simulating cutaneous T cell lymphoma.

Lymph Nodes Benign lymphoid hyperplasia. Uncommonly atypical lymphoid hyperplasia, pseudolymphoma.

Liver Eosinophilic infiltrate or granulomas.

Kidney Interstitial nephritis.

DIAGNOSIS

Proposed Diagnostic Criteria (1) Cutaneous drug eruption. (2) Hematologic abnormalities (eosinophilia ≥1500/μL or presence of atypical lymphocytes). (3) Systemic involvement (adenopathies ≥2 cm in diameter or hepatitis (SGOT ≥2N) or interstitial nephritis or interstitial pneumonitis or carditis). Diagnosis is confirmed if three criteria are present.

COURSE AND PROGNOSIS

Rash and hepatitis may persist for weeks after drug is discontinued. In patients treated with systemic glucocorticoids, rash and hepatitis may recur as glucocorticoids are tapered. Lymphadenopathy usually resolves when drug is withdrawn; however, rare progression to lymphoma has been reported. Rarely, patients die from systemic hypersensitivity such as with eosinophilic myocarditis. Clinical findings recur if drug is given again.

MANAGEMENT

Identify and discontinue the offending drug.

Symptomatic Treatment Oral antihistamine to alleviate pruritus.

Glucocorticoids *Topical* High-potency topical glucocorticoids applied bid are usually helpful in relieving cutaneous symptoms of pruritus but do not alter systemic hypersensitivity.

Systemic Prednisone (.5 mg/kg per day) usually results in rapid improvement of symptoms and laboratory parameters.

Future Drug Therapy Cross-sensitivity between various aromatic antiepileptic drugs occurs, making it difficult to select alternative anticonvulsant therapy.

Prevention The individual must be aware of his or her specific drug hypersensitivity and that other drugs of the same class can cross-react. These drugs must never be readministered. Patient should wear a medical alert bracelet.

DRUG-INDUCED PIGMENTATION

Drug-induced alterations in pigmentation are relatively common, resulting from a variety of endogenous and exogenous pigments, and can be of significant cosmetic concern to the patient.

CAUSATIVE DRUGS

The following drugs are capable of inducing hyperpigmentation of skin and/or mucosa:

Antiarrhythmic: amiodarone
Antimalarial: chloroquine, hydroxychloroquine, quinacrine, quinine
Antimicrobial: minocycline, clofazimine, zidovudine
Antiseizure: hydantoins
Cytostatic: bleomycin, cyclophosphamide, doxorubicin, daunorubicin, busulfan, 5-fluorouracil, dactinomycin
Heavy metals: silver, gold, mercury
Hormones: adrenocorticotropic hormone (ACTH), estrogen/progesterone
Psychiatric: chlorpromazine

PATHOGENESIS

Increase in melanin ACTH, phenytoin, estrogen/progesterone.

Increase in hemosiderin Minocycline.

Increase in exogenous pigment Minocycline (metabolite of minocycline).

PHYSICAL EXAMINATION

Skin Findings

Amiodarone

>75% of patients after 40-g cumulative dose after >4 months of therapy. More common in skin phototypes I and II. Lipofuscin-type pigment deposited in macrophages and endothelial cells. Low-grade or minimal photosensitivity; limited to the light-exposed areas in a small proportion (8%) of patients. Dusky-red erythema and, later, blue-gray dermal melanosis (ceruloderma) (Fig. 18-9) in exposed areas (face and hands); "phototoxic"-type erythema (rare).

Other adverse effects of amiodarone Pulmonary fibrosis, pneumonitis, hepatotoxicity, thyroid disturbances, neuropathy, and myopathy.

Course The low-grade photosensitivity disappears 12 to 24 months after drug is discontinued; the long period results from the gradual elimination of the photoactive drug from the lysosomal membranes. The pigmentation also disappeared after 33 months in one patient who was followed carefully (Fig. 18-9).

Minocycline

Onset delayed, usually after total dose of >50 g, but may occur after a small dose. Not melanin but an iron containing brown pigment, located in the dermal macrophages; stippled or diffuse. Blue-gray or slate-gray pigmentation (Fig. 18-10).

Distribution Extensor legs, ankles, dorsa of feet, face, especially around eyes; sites of trauma or inflammation such as acne scars, contusions, abrasions; hard palate, teeth; nails.

Internal sites Bones, cartilage, thyroid ("black thyroid").

Course Discoloration gradually disappears over a period of months after drug is discontinued.

Clofazimine

Reddish brown (range, pink to black).

Distribution Light-exposed areas; conjunctivae; accompanied by red sweat, urine, feces. Subcutaneous fat is orange.

Zidovudine

Brown.

Distribution Brown macules on lips or oral mucosa; longitudinal brown bands in nails.

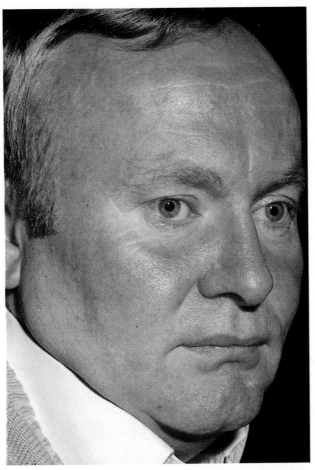

Figure 18-9 Drug-induced pigmentation: amiodarone *A striking slate-gray pigmentation in a photodistribution of the face. The blue color (ceruloderma) is due to the deposition of melanin and lipofuscin contained in macrophages and endothelial cells in the dermis. The pigmentation is reversible, but it may take up to a year or more to complete resolution. In this patient it took 33 months for the ceruloderma to disappear.*

Antimalarials (Chloroquine, Hydroxychloroquine, Quinacrine)

Occurs in 25% of individuals who take the drug for >4 months. Brownish, gray-brown, and/or blue-black, due to melanin, hemosiderin, as well as quinacrine-containing complexes; quinacrine: yellow, yellow-green.

Distribution Over shins; face, nape of neck; hard palate (sharp line of demarcation at soft palate); under finger- and toenails; also may occur in cornea and retina; quinacrine: skin and sclerae (resembling icterus); yellow-green fluorescence of nail bed with Wood's lamp.

Course Discoloration disappears within a few months after drug discontinued; quinacrine dyschromia can fade after 2 to 6 months even though drug is continued.

Phenytoin

Dose High over a long period of time (>1 year).

Discoloration Spotty, resembling melasma, in light-exposed areas. Melanin pigmentation.

Bleomycin

Mechanism unknown. Tan to brown to black.

Distribution Increase in epidermal melanin at sites of minor inflammation, i.e., parallel linear streaks at sites of dermatographism induced by excoriation ("flagellate" pigmentation), most commonly on the back, elbows, small joints, nails.

Cyclophosphamide (Cytoxan)

Brown discoloration.

Arrangement Diffuse or discrete macules.

Distribution Elbows; palms with Addisonian-like pigmentation and macules.

Busulfan (Myleran)

Occurs in 5% of treated patients. Addisonian-like pigmentation.

Distribution Face, axillae, chest, abdomen, oral mucous membranes.

ACTH

Addisonian pigmentation of skin and oral mucosa. First 13 amino acids of ACTH are identical to α-melanocyte–stimulating hormone (MSH).

Estrogens/Progesterone

Caused by endogenous and exogenous estrogen combined with progesterone, i.e., during pregnancy or with oral contraceptive therapy. Sunlight causes marked darkening of pigmentation. Tan/brown (melasma or chloasma).

Distribution Face, especially forehead, cheeks, and perioral area; also occurs on linea alba, nipples/areolae, vulva.

Course Discoloration may persist despite discontinuation of drug.

Chlorpromazine and Other Phenothiazines

Occurs after long-term (>6 months), high-dose (>500 mg/d) therapy. Phototoxic reaction. Slate-gray, blue-gray, or brownish.

Distribution Areas exposed to light, i.e., chin and cheeks.

Course After discontinuation of drug, discoloration usually fades slowly.

Silver (Argyria or Argyrosis)

Source Silver nitrate nose drops; silver sulfadiazine applied as an ointment (Silvadene).

Pigment Silver sulfide (silver nitrate converted into silver sulfide by light, as in photographic film). Blue-gray discoloration.

Site Primarily areas exposed to light, i.e., face, dorsa of hands, nails, conjunctiva; also diffuse.

Gold (Chrysiasis)

Source Organic colloidal gold preparations used in therapy of rheumatoid arthritis. 5 to 25% of all treated patients and is dose-dependent.

Dose In high-dose therapy, appears in a short time; with lower dose, occurs after months. Blue-gray to purple discoloration.

Distribution Light-exposed areas; sclerae.

Course Persists long after drug is discontinued.

Iron

Source IM iron injections; multiple blood transfusions. Brown or blue-gray discoloration.

Distribution Generalized; also, local deposits at site of injection.

Carotene

Source Ingestion of large quantities of β-carotene–containing vegetables; β-carotene tablets (Lumitene). Yellow-orange discoloration.

Distribution Most apparent on palms and soles.

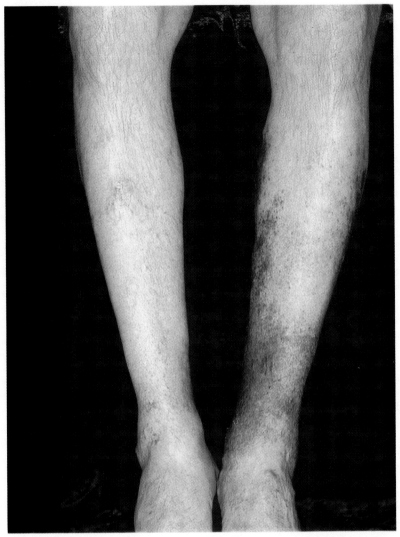

Figure 18-10 Drug-induced pigmentation: minocycline *Stippled, blue-gray macular pigmentation on the lower legs. The patient had taken minocycline for years for rosacea. The pigmentation was much more pronounced on the left leg, associated with varicose veins, chronic venous insufficiency, and chronic edema. A melon-sized inguinal hernia was also present with striking pigmentation of the enlarged scrotum.*

CUTANEOUS SIGNS OF INJECTING DRUG USE

Injecting drug users often develop cutaneous stigmata as a result of their habit, whether injecting subcutanenously or intravascularly. Cutaneous lesions range from foreign body response to injected material, infections, and scars.

Cutaneous Injection Reactions

Cutaneous Injury   Multiple punctures at sites of cutaneous injection, often linear over veins (Fig. 18-11).

Foreign Body Granuloma   Subcutaneous injection of adulterants (talc, sugar, starch, baking soda, flour, cotton fibers, glass, etc.) can elicit a foreign body response ±granuloma (Fig. 18-12).

Intravascular Injection Reactions

Venous Injury   Intravenous injection can result in thrombosis, thrombophlebitis, septic phlebitis. Chronic edema of the upper extremity is common.

Arterial Injury   Chronic intraarterial injection can result in injection site pain, cyanosis, erythema, sensory and motor deficits, and vascular compromise (vascular insufficiency/gangrene).

Infections

Transmission of Infectious Agents   Injecting drug use can result in transmission of HIV, hepatitis B virus (HBV), hepatitis C virus (HCV) with subsequent life-threatening systemic infections.

Injection Site Infections   Local infections include cellulitis (Fig. 18-12), abscess formation, lymphangitis, septic phlebitis/thrombophlebitis. The most common organisms are those from the drug users, i.e.; *Staphylcoccus aureus* and group A streptococcus. Less common microbes: enteric organism, anaerobes, *Clostridium botulinum,* oral flora, fungi (*Candida albicans*), and polymicrobial infections.

Systemic Infections   Intravenous injection of microbes can result in infection of vascular endothelium, most commonly heart valve with infectious endocarditis.

Scars

Linear Scars   Multiple cutaneous punctures result in linear scarring along the course of veins, i.e., "needle tracks" (Fig. 18-11). These are found on the forearms, dorsum of the hands, wrists, antecubital/popliteal fossae, penis.

Atrophic Punched-Out Scars   Result from subcutaneous injections (i.e., "skin popping") after an inflammatory (sterile or infected) response to injected material.

Tattoos   Carbon on needles (after flame sterilization) can result in inadvertent tattooing and pigmented linear scars.

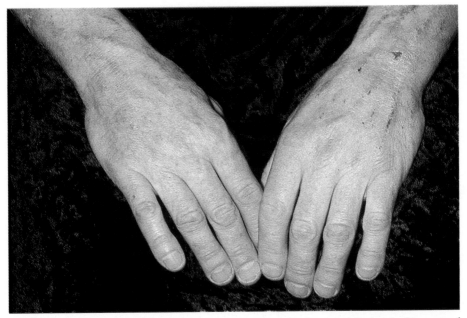

Figure 18-11   Injecting drug use: injection tracks over veins on the dorsum of the hand   *Linear tracks with punctures, fibrosis, and crusts were created by daily injections into the superficial veins.*

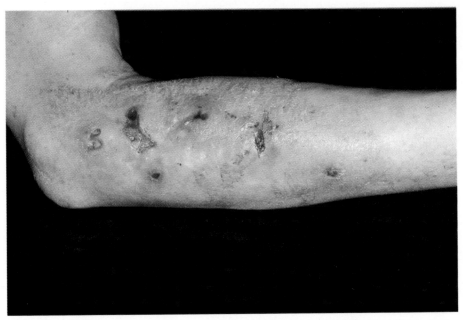

Figure 18-12   Injecting drug use: cellulitis and foreign body response at injection site   *The patient injected into the subcutaneous tissue as well as veins of the forearm, resulting in foreign body response and* S. aureus *cellulitis with associated bacteremia and infectious endocarditis.*

DISORDERS OF PSYCHIATRIC ETIOLOGY

Classification of Disorders of Psychiatric Etiology

Compulsive habits
  Neurotic excoriations
Delusions
  Delusions of parasitosis
  Dysmorphic syndrome
Factitious syndromes

NEUROTIC EXCORIATIONS

Neurotic excoriations are not an uncommon problem occurring in females more than in males and in the third to fifth decades. They may relate the onset to a specific event or to chronic stress; they deny picking and scratching. The clinical lesions are an admixture of several types of lesions, principally excoriations, all produced by habitual picking of the skin with the fingernails (Figs. 19-1 through 19-3); most often on the upper back (Fig. 19-2), face (most common) (Fig. 19-1), and extremities. There may be depigmented (Fig. 19-2) atrophic (scars) macules, or hyperpigmented macules. *The lesions are located only on sites that the hands can reach, thus sparing the center of the back;* the face. The diagnosis can be deceptive and what prima facie appears to be neurotic excoriations could be a serious cause of pruritus. Psychiatric guidance may be necessary if the problem is not solved, as it can be very disfiguring on the face and disruptive to the patient and the family. The course is prolonged, unless life adjustments are made. Pimozide (Orap) has been helpful but must be used with caution and with the advice and guidance of a psychopharmacologist. Also, antidepressant drugs may be used.

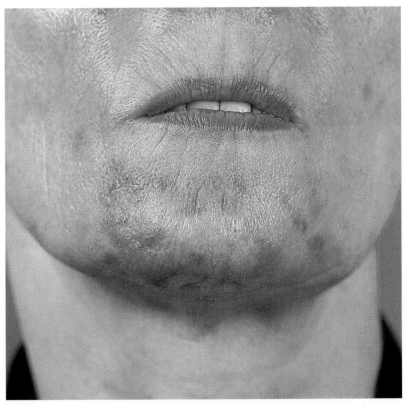

Figure 19-1 **"Neurotic" excoriations: chin** *Multiple erythematous and pigmented macules and a few crusted erosions on the chin of a 45-year-old woman with mild facial acne. No primary lesions are seen. The patient, who is moderately depressed, has mild acneform lesions, which she compulsively picks with her fingernail.*

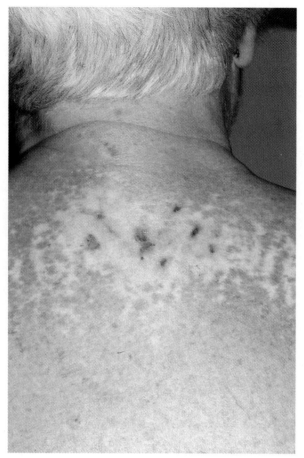

Figure 19-2 "Neurotic" excoriations: upper back *Excoriations of the upper mid-back and linear areas of postinflammatory depigmentation in a 66-year-old diabetic female. Lesions have been present for at least 10 years but resolved for one month with intralesional triamcinolone and cloth tape occlusion. Once the protection was removed, the patient resumed excoriating the site.*

DISORDERS OF PSYCHIATRIC ETIOLOGY

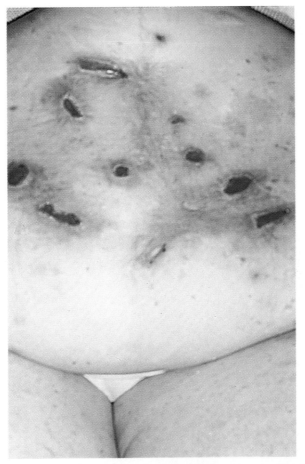

Figure 19-3 "Neurotic" excoriations: abdomen *Large linear ulcerations on the abdomen of a severely depressed 51-year-old diabetic female. The lesions had been present for several years, worsening after the death of her husband. The ulcers were secondarily infected with* Staphylococcus aureus. *The lesions resolved with occlusion of the site but recurred whenever she had access to the skin. She was unable to control her compulsive behavior of picking at the site with her fingernails.*

DELUSIONS OF PARASITOSIS

This rare generalized disorder, which occurs in adults and is present for months or years, is associated with pain or paresthesia and is characterized by the presence of numerous skin lesions, mostly excoriations, which the patient truly believes are the result of a parasitic infestation (Fig. 19-4). The onset of the initial pruritus or paresthesia may be related to xerosis or, in fact, to a previously treated infestation. It is important to rule out other causes of pruritus. This problem is serious; patients truly suffer and are opposed to seeking psychiatric help (Fig. 19-5). Patients may sell their houses to move away from the offending parasite.

The patient should see a psychiatrist for at least one visit and for recommendations of drug therapy: pimozide plus an antidepressant. Treatment is often difficult.

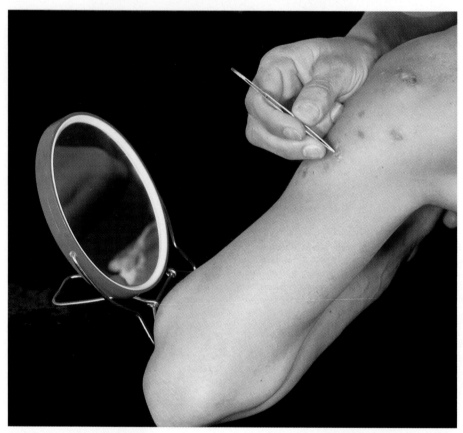

Figure 19-4   Delusions of parasitosis   *Usually patients collect small pieces of debris from their skin by scratching with their nails or an instrument and submit them to the doctor for examination for parasites. Occasionally this can progress to an aggressive behavior such as depicted in this case where the patient posed to demonstrate how she removes the "parasites" from her skin with a mirror and tweezers. "Objects" are then meticulously collected on a piece of paper that is submitted for examination. In the majority of cases, patients are not dissuaded from their monosymptomatic delusion.*

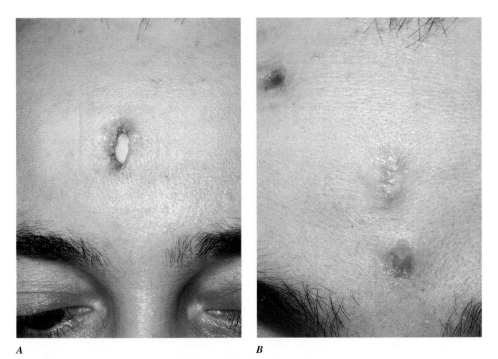

A   B

Figure 19-5 Delusions of parasitosis A. *A sharply marginated ulcer on the forehead extending to the skull in a 32-year-old male. The patient saw fat lobules, considered them as parasites and picked them out with a needle. Similar lesions were also present on the neck. The ulcer had recently been excised by a plastic surgeon; however, the patient resumed picking at the site shortly after the procedure.* **B.** *The ulcer was occluded for two weeks preventing manipulation; the ulcer healed completely but new excoriations are seen. The patient was a successful business man; he refused psychiatric consultation.*

FACTITIOUS SYNDROMES (MUNCHAUSEN'S SYNDROME)

The term *factitial* means "artificial," and in this condition there is a self-induced dermatologic lesion(s) (1) for which the patient claims no responsibility, or (2) it is determined that the patient is deliberately mutilating the skin. It occurs in young adults, more female than male. The history is vague ("hollow" history) of the evolution of the lesions. The lesions may be present for weeks to months to years (Fig. 19-6).

Patient may be normal looking and act normal in every respect, although frequently there is a strange affect and bizarre personality. The skin lesions consist of scars, ulcers, sphacelus (dense adherent necrotic membrane) (Fig. 19-6). The shape of the lesions may be linear, bizarre shapes, geometric patterns, single or multiple, and rarely occurring on the face. It is important to rule out chronic infections, granulomas, and vasculitis. The diagnosis can be difficult, but the nature of the lesions (bizarre shapes) may immediately suggest an artificial etiology. It is important to rule out every possible cause and perform a biopsy before assigning the diagnosis of *dermatosis artefacta*, both for the benefit of the patient and because the physician may be at risk for malpractice if he or she fails to diagnose a true pathologic process. This makes the task difficult. There is often serious personality and/or psychosocial stress.

The condition demands the utmost tact on the part of the physician, who can avert a serious outcome (i.e., suicide) by attempting to gain enough empathy with the patient to ascertain the cause. This varies with the nature of the psychiatric problem. The condition may persist for years in a patient who has selected his or her skin as the target organ of his or her conflicts. Consultation and even management with a psychiatrist are mandatory in most patients.

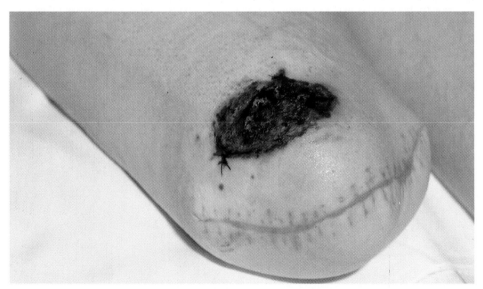

Figure 19-6 Factitious syndrome *This sharply demarcated necrosis was self-inflicted by the covert application of potassium hydroxide incorporated into soap and applied to the skin with a tightly fitting bandage. Similar ulcers had previously been present first on the toes and later on the lower extremities and had led to successive steps of amputation.*

DYSMORPHIC SYNDROME (DS)

Patients with dysmorphic syndrome (dysmorphia, Greek: "ugly") regard their image as distorted in the eyes of the public; this becomes almost an obsession. The patient with DS does not consult a psychiatrist, but a dermatologist or plastic surgeon. The typical patient with DS is a single, female, young adult who is an anxious and unhappy person. Common dermatologic complaints are facial (wrinkles, acne, scars, hypertrichosis, dry lips), scalp (incipient baldness, increased hair growth), genital [normal sebaceous glands on the penis, red scrotum (males), red vulva, vaginal odor], hyperhidrosis, and bromhidrosis. Management is a problem. One strategy is for the dermatologist to agree with the patient that there is a problem and thus establish rapport; in a few visits the complaint can be explored and further discussed. If the patient and physician do not agree that the complaint is a vastly exaggerated skin or hair change, then the patient should be referred to a psychiatrist; this latter plan is usually not accepted, in which case the problem may persist indefinitely.

BACTERIAL INFECTIONS INVOLVING THE SKIN

SUPERFICIAL CUTANEOUS INFECTIONS

Three superficial bacterial "infections" of the stratum corneum and hair follicle occur, associated with overgrowth of normal flora at sites of occlusion and high surface humidity: erythrasma, pitted keratolysis, and trichomycosis. Trichomycosis, a misnomer in that the causative agents are *Corynebacteria* and not fungi, presents as adherent granular nodules of hairs in the axillae (trichomycosis axillaris) or pubic area; the underlying skin is normal. Intertrigo is a nonspecific inflammation of naturally opposed skin, the diagnosis being made after specific infectious causes such as erythrasma or candidiasis are ruled out.

Erythrasma

Erythrasma (Greek: "red spot") is a chronic bacterial infection caused by *Corynebacterium minutissimum* affecting the intertriginous areas of the toes, groins, and axillae, which mimics epidermal dermatophyte infections.

EPIDEMIOLOGY

Age of Onset Adults.

Etiology *C. minutissimum,* gram-positive rod (diphtheroid), part of normal skin flora, which causes superficial infection under certain conditions.

Predisposing Factors Humid cutaneous microclimate: warm and/or humid climate or season; occlusive clothing/shoes; obesity. Prolonged occlusion of skin, maceration. Diabetes.

HISTORY

Symptoms Usually asymptomatic. Occasionally, burning sensation, pruritus. Duration: weeks to months to years.

PHYSICAL EXAMINATION

Skin Lesions Macule, sharply marginated (Fig. 20-1). Scaling at sites not continuously occluded. In web spaces of feet, may be macerated (Fig. 20-2), eroded, or fissured. Often symmetric or in multiple web spaces. Red or brownish red; postinflammatory hyperpigmentation in more heavily melanized individuals. If pruritic, secondary changes of excoriation, lichenification.

Sites of Predilection Toe webspaces (Fig. 20-2) >> groin folds (thigh in contact with scrotum) (Fig. 20-1)> axillae; also, intertriginous skin under panniculus, intergluteal, inframammary.

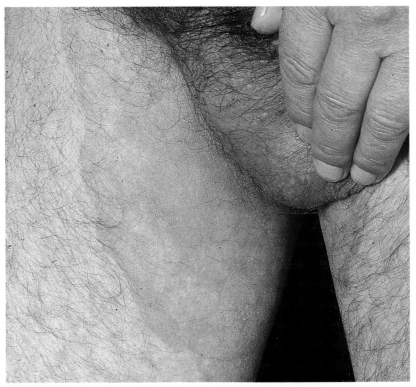

Figure 20-1 Erythrasma: groins *Sharply marginated, brownish-red, slightly scaling macular patch on the inguinal area (infectious intertrigo) appears bright coral-red when examined with a Woods lamp. KOH preparation was negative for hyphae.*

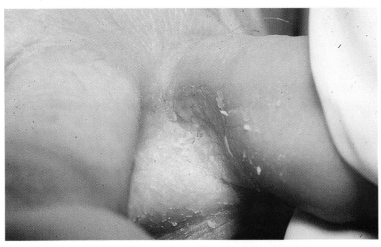

Figure 20-2 Erythrasma: webspace *This macerated interdigital webspace (infectious intertrigo) appeared bright coral-red when examined with a Wood's lamp; KOH preparation was negative for hyphae. The webspace is the most common site for erythrasma in temperate climates. In some cases, interdigital tinea pedis and/or pseudomonal intertrigo may also be present.*

DIFFERENTIAL DIAGNOSIS

Well-Demarcated Intertriginous Plaque Dermatophytosis, intertriginous candidiasis, pityriasis versicolor, pitted keratolysis, inverse-pattern psoriasis, seborrheic dermatitis, acanthosis nigricans.

LABORATORY EXAMINATIONS

Wood's Lamp The diagnosis is made by demonstration of the characteristic coral-red fluorescence (attributed to coproporphyrin III). May not be present if patient has bathed recently.

Direct Microscopy Negative for fungal forms on KOH preparation of scales. In the web spaces of the feet, concomitant interdigital tinea pedis may also be present. Gram or Giemsa stains may show fine bacterial filaments.

Bacterial Culture Heavy growth of *Corynebacterium*. Rules out *Staphylococcus aureus,* group A streptococcus, and *Candida* infection. In some cases, concomitant *Pseudomonas aeruginosa* web space infection (feet) is also present.

DIAGNOSIS

Clinical findings, absence of fungi on direct microscopy, positive Wood's lamp examination.

COURSE

Relapses occur if predisposing causes are not corrected. Secondary prophylaxis usually indicated.

MANAGEMENT

Prevention Wash with benzoyl peroxide (bar or wash). Wear less occlusive clothing. Use powder such as Zeasorb AF powder.

Topical Therapy Benzoyl peroxide (2.5%) gel daily after showering for 7 days. Topical erythromycin solution bid for 7 days. Topical antifungal agents such as clotrimazole, miconazole, or econazole.

Systemic Antibiotic Therapy Erythromycin or tetracycline, 250 mg qid for 14 days.

Pitted Keratolysis

Pitted keratolysis (PK) presents as defects in the thickly keratinized skin of the plantar foot with sculpted pits of variable depth, depending on the thickness of the stratum corneum, usually associated with pedal hyperhidrosis, caused by *Micrococcus sedentarius.*

EPIDEMIOLOGY

Etiology *M. sedentarius.*

Age of Onset Young adults.

Sex Males > females.

Predisposing Factors Hyperhidrosis of the feet; occlusive footwear.

HISTORY

Skin Symptoms Usually asymptomatic. Foot odor. Uncommonly, itching, burning, tenderness. Often mistaken for tinea pedis.

PHYSICAL EXAMINATION

Skin Lesions Pits in stratum corneum, 1 to 8 mm in diameter (Fig. 20-3). Pits can remain discrete or, more often, become confluent, forming large areas of eroded stratum corneum. Involved areas are white when stratum corneum is fully hydrated. Symmetric or asymmetric involvement of both feet.

Distribution: Toe webs; all or heel of foot in contact with shoe.

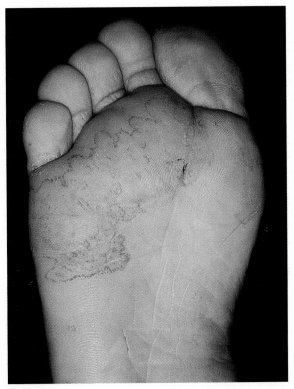

Figure 20-3 Pitted keratolysis *The stratum corneum of the anterior plantar foot shows a large erosion with well-dermarcated scalloped margins, formed by the confluence of multiple, confluent erosions (defects in the stratum corneum or "pits").*

DIFFERENTIAL DIAGNOSIS

Erosion in Multiple Webspaces of Feet Interdigital tinea pedis, *Candida* intertrigo, erythrasma, *Pseudomonas* web space infection.

LABORATORY EXAMINATIONS

Direct Microscopy KOH preparation negative for hyphae.

Wood's Lamp Examination Negative for bright coral-red fluorescence (erythrasma).

Culture In some cases, rules out *Staphylococcus aureus,* group A streptococcus, or *Pseudomonas aeruginosa* infection.

DIAGNOSIS

Clinical diagnosis ruling out other causes.

COURSE AND PROGNOSIS

Persists and recurs until the underlying predisposing factors are corrected. Secondary prophylaxis usually indicated.

MANAGEMENT

Prevention Wash affected site with lather from benzoyl peroxide bar or wash. Reduce moisture in shoes with agents such as aluminum chloride or Zeasorb AF powder. Wear less occlusive footwear.

Topical therapy Daily applications of agents such as benzoyl peroxide gel or topical antibiotics such as erythromycin are usually effective.

Intertriginous Infections and Intertrigo

Intertrigo (Latin: *inter* between, *trigo* rubbing) is a nonspecific inflammation of opposed skin, occurring in the submammary region, axillae, groins, and gluteal folds. With increased moisture and maceration, the stratum corneum becomes eroded. The problem is more common in obese individuals who have more skin with more folds. Intertriginous infections caused by bacteria (groups A and B streptococcus, *Corynebacterium minitissimum, Pseudomonas aeruginosa*) and fungi (dermatophytes, *Candida,* and *Malassezia furfur*) must be ruled out. Dermatoses such as psoriasis vulgaris (inverse pattern), seborrheic dermatitis, and atopic dermatitis also occur in body folds, presenting as erythema or erythematous plaques.

Intertrigo is diagnosed in the presence of erythema ± symptoms or pruritus, tenderness, or increased sensitivity, excluding infectious causes. For acutely symptomatic intertrigo, moist dressings and/or Castellani's paint give immediate symptomatic relief. Powders with antibacterial/antifungal activity are helpful for preventing recurrence. In some cases, zinc oxide ointment reduces friction at involved sites. Topical corticosteroid preparations should be avoided because of the risk of cutaneous atrophy at these naturally occluded sites. Weight reduction is ideal but often not possible.

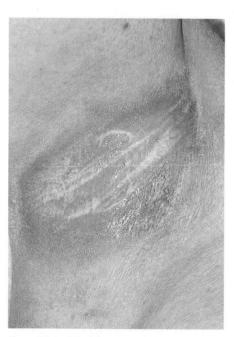

Figure 20-4   Intertrigo: group A streptococcus
A painful erythematous plaque with purulent exudate in the axilla of an HIV-infected woman. (See page 590 for treatment.)

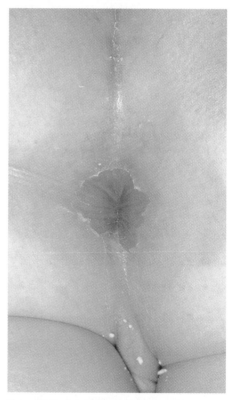

Figure 20-5   Intertrigo: group A streptococcus
Well-dermarcated erythema and erosion in the perineum of an 8-year-old boy associated with pruritus and tenderness; several classmates at school had GAS pharyngitis. (See page 590 for treatment.)

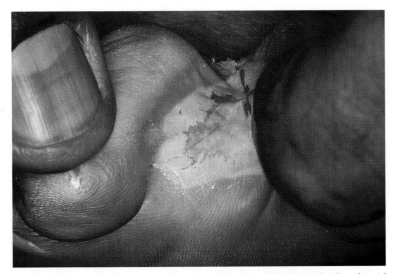

Figure 20-6   Intertrigo: *C. albicans* *Maceration of a webspace of the foot of a female with diabetes. KOH preparation showed yeast with pseudomycelial forms;* C. albicans *was isolated on culture.*

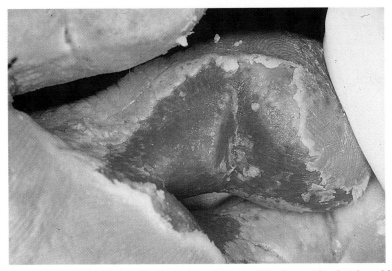

Figure 20-7   Intertrigo: *P. aeruginosa* *Erosion of a webspace of the foot with a bright red base and surrounding erythema. Tinea pedis (interdigital and moccasin-patterns) and hyperhidrosis were also present, which facilitated growth of* Pseudomonas.

PYODERMAS

PATHOGENESIS

Normal skin is heavily colonized by bacterial flora, which are more numerous and diverse in occluded sites. The most common are various nonpathogenic gram-positive bacteria such as *Staphylococcus epidermidis* (coagulase-negative).

- *Staphylococcus aureus* is not one of the normal flora of the skin; it does, however, colonize the nares, perineum, and/or axillae in approximately 20% of individuals. *S. aureus* can be isolated from involved skin in 90% of individuals with atopic dermatitis and from nonlesional skin in 70%.

- Group A β-hemolytic streptococcus (GAS) (*Streptococcus pyogenes*) usually colonizes the skin first and then the nasopharynx. An intact stratum corneum is the most important defense against invasion of pathogenic bacteria. Group B and group G β-hemolytic streptococci (GBS, GGS) colonize the perineum of some individuals and may cause superficial and invasive infections.

Carriers of *S. aureus* and/or GAS are at increased risk for pyodermas, (impetigo/ecthyma; furuncles, carbuncles, abscesses; folliculitis) and soft-tissue infections (erysipelas, cellulitis; gangrenous cellulitis). Frequent hand washing reduces the risk of person-to-person transmission of cutaneous pathogens.

Impetigo and Ecthyma

Staphylococcus aureus and *Streptococcus pyogenes* can cause superficial infections of the epidermis (impetigo) or extending into the dermis (ecthyma), characterized by crusted erosions or ulcers. The infections may arise as primary infections in minor superficial breaks in the skin or as secondary infections of preexisting dermatoses (impetiginization or secondary infection).

EPIDEMIOLOGY

Age of Onset Primary infections more common in children. Secondary infections, any age. Bullous impetigo: children, young adults.

Etiology In the 2000s, *S. aureus* most commonly; also, group A β-hemolytic *Streptococcus pyogenes* (GAS); or mixed *S. aureus* and GAS. Bullous impetigo: 80% caused by phage 2 staphylococci (60% of these of type 71), which produce exotoxins and which also cause staphylococcal scalded-skin syndrome.

Predisposing Factors Colonization of the skin by *S. aureus* and GAS is promoted by warm ambient temperature, high humidity, presence of skin disease (especially atopic dermatitis), age of patient, prior antibiotic therapy, poor hygiene, crowded living conditions, and neglected minor trauma. Topical glucocorticoids have little effect on the microflora of the skin, except in those with atopic dermatitis; topical glucocorticoids applied to atopic dermatitis usually reduce the density of *S. aureus*. Impetiginiza-

tion or secondary infection also occurs in lesions of eczema and scabies. Ecthyma: lesion of neglect—develops in excoriations; insect bites; minor trauma in diabetics, elderly patients, soldiers, and alcoholics.

Portals of Entry of Infection

Primary Impetigo Arises at minor breaks in the skin.

Secondary Impetigo (Impetiginization) Arises in a variety of underlying dermatoses and traumatic breaks in the integrity of the epidermis.

Underlying Dermatoses Inflammatory dermatoses: atopic dermatitis, contact dermatitis, stasis dermatitis, psoriasis vulgaris, chronic cutaneous lupus erythematosus, pyoderma gangrenosum. Bullous disease: pemphigus vulgaris, bullous pemphigoid, sunburn, porphyria cutanea tarda. Ulcers: pressure, stasis. Chronic lymphedema. Umbilical stump. Herpes simplex, varicella, herpes zoster. Dermatophytosis: tinea pedis, tinea capitis.

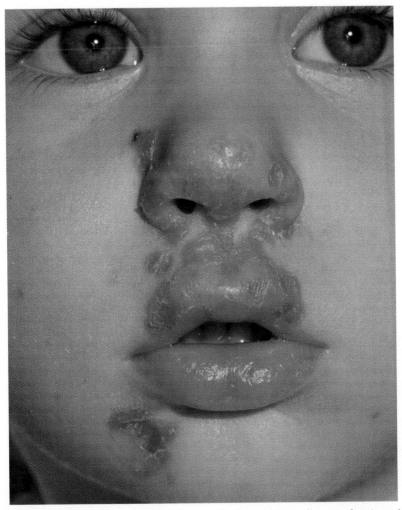

Figure 20-8 Impetigo: group A streptococcus (GAS) *Crusted (golden-yellow, stuck-on) erosions becoming confluent on the nose, cheek, lips, and chin; clinical lesions are preceded by oropharyngeal colonization with GAS.*

Trauma Surgical wounds; abrasion; laceration; puncture; bites: human, animal, insect; burns.

HISTORY

Duration of Lesions Impetigo: days to weeks. Ecthyma: weeks to months.

Symptoms Impetigo: variable pruritus, especially associated with atopic dermatitis. Ecthyma:pain, tenderness.

PHYSICAL EXAMINATION

Skin Lesions

Nonbullous Impetigo

Transient superficial small vesicles or pustules rupture, resulting in erosions, which in turn become surmounted by a crust (Fig. 20-8). Golden-yellow crusts are often seen in impetigo but are not pathognomonic (Fig. 20-9). 1- to 3-cm lesions; central healing often apparent if lesions present for several weeks.

Arrangement Scattered, discrete lesions; without therapy, lesions may become confluent; satellite lesions occur by autoinoculation.

Bullous Impetigo

Vesicles (Fig. 20-10) and bullae (Fig. 20-11) containing clear yellow or slightly turbid fluid without surrounding erythema, arising on normal-appearing skin. With rupture, bullous lesions decompress. If roof of bulla is removed, shallow moist *erosion* forms.

Distribution More common in intertriginous sites.

Ecthyma

Ulceration with a thick adherent crust (Fig. 20-12). Lesions may be tender, indurated.

Distribution More common on distal extremities.

Miscellaneous Physical Findings At times, lymphangitis and/or regional lymphadenopathy.

DIFFERENTIAL DIAGNOSIS

Erosion ± Crust/Scale-Crust Excoriation, perioral dermatitis, seborrheic dermatitis, allergic contact dermatitis, herpes simplex, epidermal dermatophytosis, scabies.

Intact Bulla(e) Allergic contact dermatitis, herpes simplex, herpes zoster, bacterial folliculitis, thermal burns, bullous pemphigoid, dermatitis herpetiformis, porphyria cutanea tarda (dorsa of hands).

Ulcer ± Crust/Scale-Crust Chronic herpetic ulcers, excoriated insect bites, neurotic excoriations, cutaneous diphtheria, porphyria cutanea tarda (dorsa of hands), venous (stasis) and atherosclerotic ulcers (legs).

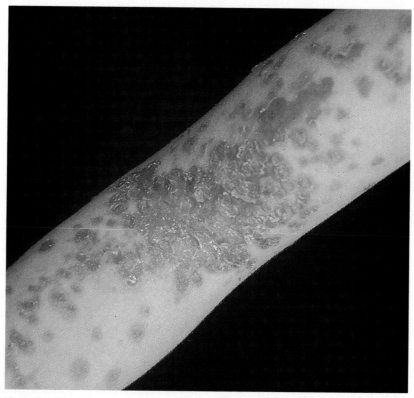

Figure 20-9 Impetigo: *S. aureus* *Crusted erosions on the arm of a child. The confluence of lesions in the antecubital fossae suggests there was prior atopic dermatitis at the site that became secondarily infected.*

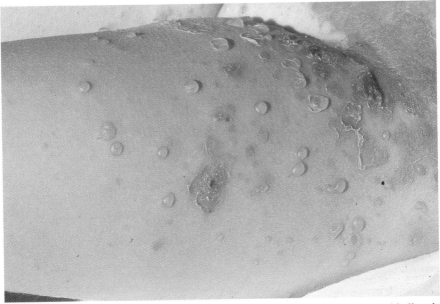

Figure 20-10 Bullous impetigo: *S. aureus* *Scattered, discrete, thin-walled vesicles and bullae that easily rupture and form erosions on the thigh of a child.*

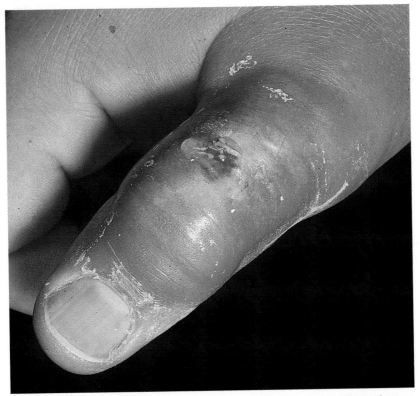

Figure 20-11 Bullous impetigo: *S. aureus* *A large, single bulla with surrounding erythema and edema on the thumb of a child; the bulla has ruptured only in the center and clear serum exudes from it. Due to the thick stratum corneum on hands and feet, an impetigo blister may remain intact for days, which facilitates spread of infection to deeper layers of tissue.*

LABORATORY EXAMINATIONS

Gram's Stain Gram-positive cocci, in chains or clusters, within neutrophils.

Culture *S. aureus,* commonly; GAS (especially from older lesions). Failure of oral antibiotic may be indication of infection by methicillin-resistant *S. aureus.*

Dermatopathology Impetigo: vesicle formation (very early lesion) in the subcorneal or granular region, acantholytic cells, spongiosis, dermal perivascular infiltrate of lymphocytes and neutrophils; gram-positive cocci in blister fluid and within neutrophils.

DIAGNOSIS

Clinical findings confirmed by Gram's stain or culture.

COURSE AND PROGNOSIS

Untreated, lesions of impetigo progress for several weeks, in some cases forming ecthyma. Untreated or neglected impetigo can progress to ecthyma. With adequate treatment, prompt resolution. Lesions can progress to invasive infection with lymphangitis, suppurative lymphadenitis, cellulitis or erysipelas, bacteremia, septicemia. Nonsuppurative complications of GAS infection include guttate psoriasis, scarlet fever, and glomerulonephritis. Recurrence may occur because of failure to eradicate organism or reinfection from a family member. Ecthyma often heals with scar. Recurrent *S. aureus* or GAS infections can occur by recolonization from a family member or a family dog.

MANAGEMENT

Prevention Benzoyl peroxide wash (soap bar). Check family members for signs of impetigo. Between 20 and 25% of individuals are nasal carriers of *S. aureus.*

Topical treatment Mupirocin (pseudomonic acid) ointment is highly effective in eliminating both GAS and *S. aureus,* including methicillin-resistant *S. aureus,* from the nares and cutaneous lesions. Apply three times daily to involved skin and to nares for 7–10 days.

SYSTEMIC ANTIMICROBIAL TREATMENT

Organism	Drug of choice/dose	Alternative Drugs
Group A streptococcus	Penicillin VK: 250 mg qid for 10 days Benzathine penicillin: 600,000 units IM in children 6 years or younger, 1.2 million units if 7 years or older, if compliance is a problem	Erythromycin: 250–500 mg (adults) qid for 10 days Cephalexin: 250–500 mg (adults) qid for 10 days
S. aureus	Dicloxacillin: 250–500 mg (adults) qid for 10 days	Cephalexin: 250–500 mg (adults) qid for 10 days; 40–50 mg/kg/d (children) for 10 days Amoxicillin plus clavulanic acid (β-lactamase inhibitor): 20 mg/kg per day tid for 10 days Clarithromycin: 250–500 mg bid for 10 days
GAS and *S. aureus* in penicillin-allergic patients if organism is sensitive	Erythromycin ethylsuccinate: 1–2 g/d (adults) in four divided doses for 10 days; 40 mg/kg/d (children) qid for 10 days	Azithromycin: 250 mg qd for 5–7 days Clindamycin: 150–300 mg (adults) qid for 10 days; 15 mg/kg/d (children) qid for 10 days
Methicillin-resistant *S. aureus*	Minocycline: 100 mg bid for 10 days	Trimethoprim-sulfamethoxazole: 160 mg trimethoprim + 800 mg sulfamethoxazole bid Ciprofloxacin: 500 mg bid for 7 days

BACTERIAL INFECTIONS INVOLVING THE SKIN

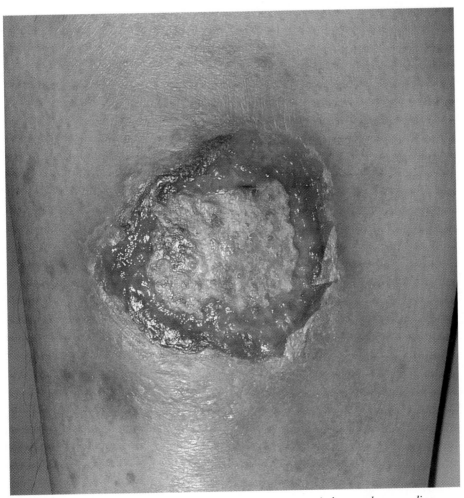

Figure 20-12   Ecthyma   *A large, circumscribed ulcer with a necrotic base and surrounding erythema in the pretibial region. Ecthyma develops on the skin as a result of poor hygiene, minor skin trauma, and crowded living conditions. Most commonly occurs in homeless people or soldiers in combat.*

Infectious Folliculitis

Infectious folliculitis is an infection of the upper portion of the hair follicle, characterized by a follicular papule, pustule, erosion, or crust at the follicular infundibulum; the involvement can extend deeper to the entire length of the follicle (sycosis).

EPIDEMIOLOGY

Regions of the Pilosebaceous and Apocrine Apparatus *Infundibulum:* superior region extending down to the junction of the sebaceous duct with the follicle. *Isthmus:* mid-region between the sebaceous duct and the erector pili muscle protuberance. *Inferior region:* lower region below the erector pili muscle protuberance.

Race *S. aureus* folliculitis on the legs of males: Indians, West Africans. Pseudofolliculitis and keloidal folliculitis in black men can be complicated by *S. aureus* infection.

Predisposing Factors Shaving hairy regions such as the beard area, axillae, or legs facilitates follicular infection. Extraction of hair such as plucking or waxing. Occlusion of hair-bearing areas facilitates growth of microbes: clothing, plastic film, adhesive plaster, position (sitting occludes buttocks, lying in bed occludes back), prosthesis, natural occlusion in intertriginous sites (axillae, inframammary, anogenital). Topical climate with high temperatures and high relative humidity. Topical glucocorticoid preparations. Systemic antibiotic promotes growth of gram-negative bacteria. Diabetes mellitus. Immunosuppression.

HISTORY

Symptoms Duration: days; *S. aureus* and dermatophytic folliculitis can be chronic. Usually nontender or slightly tender; may be pruritic. Uncommonly, tender regional lymphadenitis.

PHYSICAL EXAMINATION

Skin Lesions

Papule or pustule confined to the ostium of the hair follicle, at times surrounded by an erythematous halo. Rupture of pustule leads to superficial erosions or crusts. Scattered discrete or more frequently grouped and clustered. Usually, only a small percentage of follicles in a region is infected. Superficial infection heals without scarring, but in darkly pigmented individuals, postinflammatory hypo- and hyperpigmentation. Extension of infection can progress to abscess or furuncle formation. In chronic folliculitis, a full range of lesions is noted. Pseudofolliculitis barbae caused by penetration of the skin by sharp tips of shaved hairs frequently complicated by *S. aureus* secondary infection.

Distribution *Face* *S. aureus*. Gram-negative folliculitis: resembles or may coexist with acne vulgaris.

Beard Area *S. aureus* folliculitis: folliculitis (sycosis) barbae, most commonly of shaved beard area. Dermatophytic folliculitis: tinea barbae; papulopustules may coalesce to deeply infiltrated kerion. *C. albicans.* Herpes simplex virus. Molluscum contagiosum. Demodicidosis resembles rosacea.

Scalp *S. aureus.* Dermatophytic.

Neck *S. aureus* in shaved area and nape of neck, occipital scalp, especially in diabetics. Pseudofolliculitis in shaved area. Keloidal folliculitis in nape of neck; follicular keloids to large nodular–tumorous keloidal masses.

Legs In western nations, occurs in women who shave legs. In India, a chronic folliculitis occurs in young men, lasting for years. Pustular dermatitis atrophicans of the legs reported commonly from West Africa, usually affecting the shins, sometimes the thighs and forearms.

Trunk *S. aureus* in axillae, especially in those who shave. *P. aeruginosa* ("hot tub") folliculitis. *Pityrosporum* folliculitis. *Candida* folliculitis on the back of hospitalized patients with fever who lie in supine position.

Buttocks Common site for *S. aureus* folliculitis. Dermatophytic.

Variants

S. Aureus **Folliculitis** Can be either superficial folliculitis (infundibular) (follicular impetigo of Bockhart) (Fig. 20-13) or deep (sycosis) (extension beneath infundibulum) with abscess formation (Fig. 20-14). In the shaved beard area,

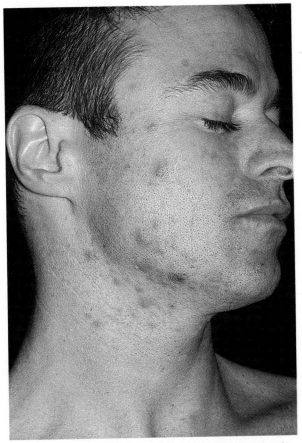

Figure 20-13 Infectious folliculitis, superficial: *S. aureus* *Numerous superficial erythematous papules and crusts of hair follicles in the beard area. The condition was chronic, aggravated by shaving. S. aureus was isolated on culture of the beard area and nares.*

CLASSIFICATION OF INFECTIOUS FOLLICULITIS BY ETIOLOGY

Infectious Agent	Organism
Bacterial	*S. aureus:* superficial (Bockhart's impetigo); deep (sycosis); may progress to furuncle (boil) or carbuncle formation
	Pseudomonas aeruginosa (hot-tub) folliculitis
	Gram-negative folliculitis
Fungal	Dermatophytic folliculitis: tinea capitis, tinea barbae, Majocchi's granuloma
	Pityrosporum folliculitis
	Candida folliculitis
Viral	Herpes simplex virus
	Molluscum contagiosum
Syphilitic	Secondary syphilis, acneform
Infestation	Demodicidosis

also known as sycosis vulgaris or barber's itch. In severe cases (lupoid sycosis), the pilosebaceous units may be destroyed and replaced by fibrous scar tissue.

Gram-Negative Folliculitis   Occurs in individuals with acne vulgaris treated with oral antibiotics. "Acne" typically worsens, having been in good control. Characterized by small follicular pustules and/or larger abscesses on the cheeks.

Hot Tub Folliculitis   Occurs on the trunk following immersion in spa water (Fig. 20-15).

Dermatophytic Folliculitis   Infection begins in the perifollicular stratum corneum and spreads into follicular ostia and hair shafts. (See Section 21.)

Tinea capitis: "gray patch" (alopecia associated with scaling of the scalp) and "black dot" (slight scaling and brittle hair breaking off at skin surface) and kerion (characterized by alopecia and an inflammatory boggy plaque);

follicular involvement may not be apparent due to the more extensive involvement of the skin. Favus is characterized by suppurative and granulomatous folliculitis associated with scarring. In Majocchi's or dermatophytic granuloma, scattered papules and nodules, usually associated with tinea cruris or tinea corporis (Fig. 20-16). (See Section 21.)

***Pityrosporum* Folliculitis**   More common in subtropical and tropical climates. Pruritic, monomorphic eruption characterized by follicular papules and pustules on the trunk, most often on the back (Fig. 20-17), upper arms, and less often on the neck and face; excoriated papules. Absence of comedones differentiates it from acne vulgaris. (See Section 21.)

Candida Albicans   Occurs in sites of occluded skin such as the back of a hospitalized febrile patient or under plastic dressing, especially if topical glucocorticoid preparations are used. Large follicular pustules. (See Section 21.)

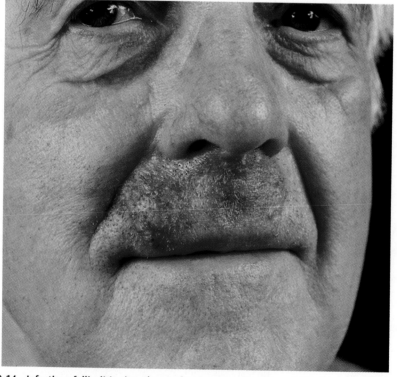

Figure 20-14   Infectious folliculitis, deep (sycosis): *S. aureus*   *Confluent follicular pustules forming a tender, thick, erythematous plaque on the moustache area. The differential diagnosis includes tinea barbae with kerion formation.*

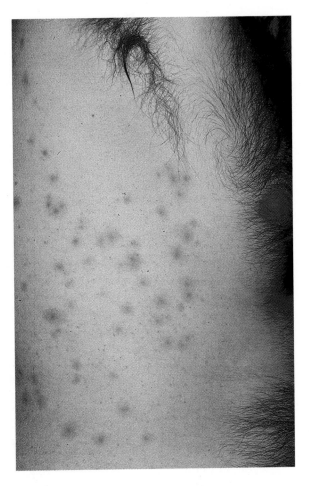

Figure 20-15 Infectious folliculitis: *P. aeruginosa* or "hot tub" *Multiple follicular pustules are present on the trunk, appearing 3 days after bathing in a hot tub.* P. aeruginosa *was isolated on culture from a lesion. The lesions resolved spontaneously within a week.*

Herpetic Folliculitis Occurs predominantly in the beard area (viral sycosis) in men. Characterized by follicular vesicles and later crusts (Fig. 20-18).

Molluscum Sycosis Presents as umbilicated skin-colored papules in a follicular and perifollicular distribution over the beard area.

Syphilitic Folliculitis Manifested by dull red papules; may be arranged in oval groups (corymbiform syphilis). Nonscarring alopecia of the scalp and beard.

Demodicidosis Clinical presentation: perifollicular scaling (pityriasis folliculorum or rosacea-like erythematous follicular papules and pustules with a background of erythema on the face.

DIFFERENTIAL DIAGNOSIS

Follicular Inflammatory Disorders Acneform disorders (acne vulgaris, rosacea, perioral dermatitis), HIV-associated eosinophilic folliculitis, chemical irritants (chloracne), adverse cutaneous drug reactions (halogens, corticosteroids, lithium), perforating folliculitis, follicular atopic dermatitis, keratosis pilaris, keratosis pilaris atrophicans, lichen planopilaris, pityriasis rubra pilaris, vitamin A deficiency, vitamin C deficiency, chronic cutaneous lupus erythematosus, keloidal folliculitis, pseudofolliculitis barbae.

Regional Differential Diagnosis *Face:* tinea barbae, acne, rosacea, perioral dermatitis, keratosis pilaris, pseudofolliculitis barbae (ingrowing hairs), miliaria. *Scalp:* acne necrotica. *Trunk:* acne vulgaris, pustular miliaria, transient acantholytic disease (Grover's disease), scurvy. *Extremities:* keratosis pilaris, scurvy. *Axillae and groins:* hidradenitis suppurativa.

LABORATORY FINDINGS

Direct Microscopy *Gram's Stain* *S. aureus:* gram-positive cocci in grape-like clusters within polymorphonuclear leukocytes and extracellular. Also visualizes fungi.

KOH Preparation Dermatophytes: hyphae. *P. ovale:* multiple yeast forms of *Pityrosporum.* *Candida:* mycelial forms.

Culture *Bacterial:* S. aureus, P. aeruginosa; gram-negative folliculitis: *Proteus, Klebsiella, E. coli.* In cases of chronic relapsing folliculitis, culture nares and perianal region for *S. aureus* carriage. *Fungal:* dermatophytes; *C. albicans.* Viral: herpes simplex virus.

Dermatopathology In the evaluation of a biopsy specimen of a follicular lesion, infectious folliculitis must be differentiated from noninfectious inflammatory follicular and perifollicular disorders. The following features should be evaluated: Are microorganisms present? Is the inflammatory infiltrate predominantly follicular or perifollicular? What region of the pilosebaceous structure is involved? Is the inflammatory process acute suppurative (neutrophilic), chronic lymphocytic, or granulomatous (foreign body response to keratin subsequent to rupture of follicle)? Is any portion of the pilosebaceous structure destroyed?

DIAGNOSIS

Clinical findings confirmed by laboratory findings.

COURSE AND PROGNOSIS

S. aureus folliculitis can progress to deeper follicular and perifollicular infection with furuncle (abscess) formation. Infection of multiple contiguous follicles results in a carbuncle. Many types of infectious folliculitis tend to recur or become chronic unless the predisposing conditions are corrected.

MANAGEMENT

Prophylaxis *Correct underlying predisposing condition.* Washing with antibacterial soap or benzoyl peroxide preparation.

Antimicrobial Therapy *Bacterial Folliculitis* See Table 20-1.
Gram-negative Folliculitis: associated with systemic antibiotic therapy of acne vulgaris. Discontinue current antibiotics. Wash with benzoyl peroxide. In some cases, ampicillin (250 mg qid) or sulfamethoxazole-trimethoprim qid. Isotretinoin.

Fungal Folliculitis Various topical antifungal agents. For dermatophytic folliculitis: terbinafine, 250 mg PO for 14 days, or itraconazole, 100 mg bid for 14 days. For *Candida* folliculitis: fluconazole or itraconazole, 100 mg bid for 14 days.

Herpetic Folliculitis See HSV infections (Section 23).

Demodicidosis Permethrin cream.

Pseudofolliculitis Barbae Rule out secondary *S. aureus* infection. Discontinue shaving. Use beard clipper instead of safety razor. Destruction of hair follicle: electrolysis; laser hair removal.

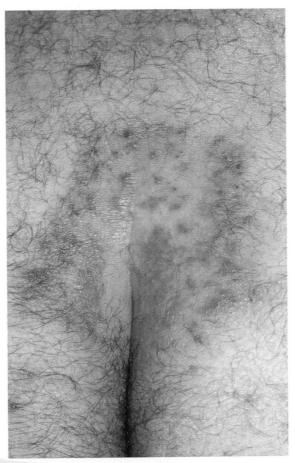

Figure 20-16 Infectious folliculitis: dermatophytic *Multiple follicular papules on the sacral area; similar eruptions were present on the thighs. The patient was an HIV-infected male, who had been treated with topical glucocorticoids and antifungal agents without response. The lesions resolved with oral terbinafine therapy.*

Table 20-1 ORAL ANTIMICROBIAL AGENTS FOR BACTERIAL INFECTIONS

Antimicrobial Agent	Dosing (PO Unless Indicated), Usually For 7 to 14 Days
Natural penicillins	
Penicillin V	250–500 mg tid/qid for 10 days
Penicillin G	600,000–1.2 million U IM qd for 7 days
Benzathine penicillin G	600,000 U IM in children ≤6 years, 1.2 million units if ≥7 years, if compliance is a problem
Penicillinase-resistant penicillins	
Cloxacillin	250–500 mg (adults) qid for 10 days
Dicloxacillin	250–500 mg (adults) qid for 10 days
Nafcillin	1.0–2.0 g IV q4h
Oxacillin	1.0–2.0 g IV q4h
Aminopenicillins	
Amoxicillin	500 mg tid or 875 mg q12h
Amoxicillin plus clavulanic acid (β-lactamase inhibitor)	875/125 mg bid; 20 mg/kg/d tid for 10 days
Ampicillin	250–500 mg qid for 7–10 days
Cephalosporins	
Cephalexin	250–500 mg (adults) qid for 10 days; 40–50 mg/kg/d (children) for 10 days
Cephradine	250–500 mg (adults) qid for 10 days; 40–50 mg/kg/d (children) for 10 days
Cefaclor	250–500 mg q8h
Cefprozil	250–500 mg q12l
Cefuroxime axetil	125–500 mg q12h
Cefixime	200–400 mg q12–24h
Erythromycin group	
Erythromycin ethylsuccinate	250–500 mg (adults) qid for 10 days; 40 mg/kg/d (children) qid for 10 days
Clarithromycin	500 mg bid for 10 days
Azithromycin	Azithromycin: 500 mg on day 1, then 250 mg qd days 2–5
Clindamycin	150–300 mg (adults) qid for 10 days; 15 mg/kg/d (children) qid for 10 days
Tetracylines	
Minocycline	100 mg bid for 10 days
Doxycycline	100 mg bid
Tetracycline	250–500 mg qid
Miscellaneous agents	
Trimethoprim-sulfamethoxazole	160 mg TMP + 800 mg SMZ bid
Metronidazole	500 mg qid
Ciprofloxacin	500 mg bid for 7 days

Figure 20-17 Infectious folliculitis:
Pityrosporum ovale *Multiple,
discrete, follicular papulopustules
on the back, mimicking acne
vulgaris. Lesional biopsy showed
yeast forms of* P. ovale (Mallezzia
furfur). *The lesions resolved after
treatment with oral itraconazole.*

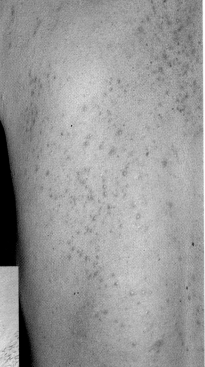

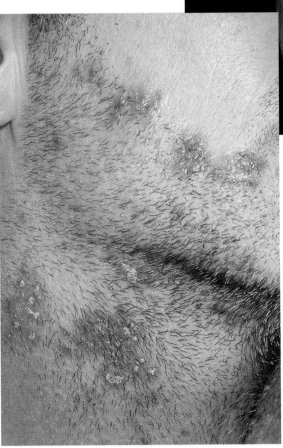

**Figure 20-18 Infectious folliculitis:
herpes simplex virus** *Discrete and
grouped pustules and erosions in
the beard area of an otherwise
healthy 40-year-old male. HSV was
isolated on culture. The initial
diagnosis was* S. aureus *folliculitis;
however, no pathogens were
isolated on bacterial culture. There
was no response to dicloxacillin,
but lesions resolved with oral
acyclovir.*

Abscess, Furuncle, and Carbuncle

An *abscess* is a circumscribed collection of pus appearing as an acute or chronic localized inflammation, associated with tissue destruction. A *furuncle* is an acute, deep-seated, red, hot, tender nodule or abscess that evolves from a staphylococcal folliculitis. A *carbuncle* is a deeper infection comprised of interconnecting abscesses usually arising in several contiguous hair follicles.

EPIDEMIOLOGY

Age of Onset Children, adolescents, and young adults.

Sex More common in boys.

Etiology *Staphylococcus aureus*. Much less commonly, other organisms. Abscesses can be sterile, a response to a foreign body, such as a ruptured inclusion cyst. Dental abscesses can point anywhere on the face, even at sites distant from their origin. Sterile or infected abscesses can occur at injection sites.

Predisposing Factors

- Chronic *S. aureus* carrier state (nares, axillae, perineum, bowel)
- Diabetes mellitus
- Obesity
- Poor hygiene
- Bactericidal defects (e.g., chronic granulomatous disease)
- Chemotactic defects
- Hyper-IgE syndrome (Job's syndrome)

PATHOGENESIS

Folliculitis, furuncles, and carbuncles represent a continuum of severity of staphylococcal infection. These cutaneous infections arise in chronic *S. aureus* carriers. Control/eradication of carrier state treats/prevents folliculitis, furuncle, and carbuncle formation.

HISTORY

Duration of Lesions Days to weeks to months.

Skin Symptoms Throbbing pain and invariably exquisite tenderness.

Constitutional Symptoms Carbuncles may be accompanied by low-grade fever and malaise.

PHYSICAL EXAMINATION

Skin Lesions Lesions are red, hot, and painful/tender.

Abscess May arise in any organ or structure. Abscesses that present on the skin arise in the dermis, subcutaneous fat, muscle, or a variety of deeper structures. Initially, a tender red nodule forms. In time (days to weeks), pus collects within a central space (Fig. 20-19). A well-formed abscess is characterized by fluctuance of the central portion of the lesion. Occur at any cutaneous site. At sites of trauma (Fig. 20-19). Upper trunk for abscesses in ruptured inclusion cysts. Single or multiple.

Furuncle Initially, a firm tender nodule, up to 1 to 2 cm in diameter (Fig. 20-20) with a central necrotic plug. In many individuals, furuncles occur in setting of staphylococcal folliculitis in beard area or neck. Nodule becomes fluctuant with abscess formation below necrotic plug often topped by a central pustule. After rupture or drainage of pustule and discharge of necrotic plug, a nodule with cavitation remains. A variable zone of cellulitis may surround the furuncle. Arise in any hair-bearing region: beard area, posterior neck and occipital scalp, axillae, buttocks. Single or multiple (Fig. 20-21).

Carbuncle Evolution is similar to that of furuncle. Comprised of several to multiple, adjacent, coalescing furuncles (Fig. 20-22). Characterized by multiple loculated dermal and subcutaneous abscesses, superficial pustules, necrotic plugs, and sieve-like openings draining pus.

DIFFERENTIAL DIAGNOSIS

Painful Dermal/Subcutaneous Nodule Ruptured epidermoid or pilar cyst, hidradenitis suppurativa (axillae, groin, vulva), necrotizing lymphangitis.

BACTERIAL INFECTIONS INVOLVING THE SKIN

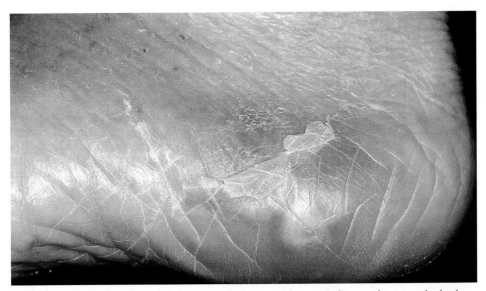

Figure 20-19   Abscess: *S. aureus* *A very tender abscess with surrounding erythema on the heel. The patient was a diabetic with neuropathy and had a sewing needle lodge in the soft tissue, which provided the portal of entry.*

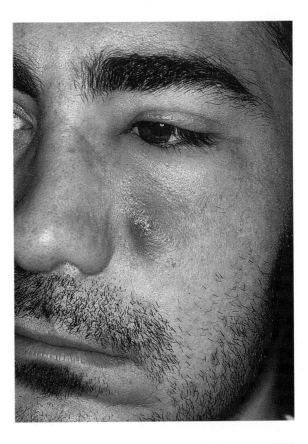

Figure 20-20   Furuncle: *S. aureus*
A painful abscess with associated facial edema in an otherwise healthy 25-year-old male. The patient felt systemically ill. The infection resolved with oral dicloxacillin.

PYODERMAS

LABORATORY EXAMINATIONS

Gram's Strain Gram-positive cocci within PMN leukocytes and in extracellular space.

Bacterial Culture *Pus* Culture of pus isolates *S. aureus*. Sensitivities to antimicrobial agents may determine management.

Hematology Culture if patient is febrile ±constitutional symptoms before beginning treatment.

Antibiotic Sensitivities Identifies methicillin-resistant *S. aureus* and need for changing usual antibiotic therapy.

Dermatopathology Pyogenic infection arising in hair follicle and extending into deep dermis and subcutaneous tissue (furuncle) and with loculated abscesses (carbuncle).

DIAGNOSIS

Clinical findings confirmed by findings on Gram's stain and culture.

COURSE AND PROGNOSIS

Most cases resolve with incision and drainage and systemic antibiotic treatment. At times, however, furunculosis is complicated by bacteremia and possible hematogenous seeding of heart valves, joints, spine, long bones, and viscera (especially kidneys). *S. aureus* can hematogenously disseminate via venous drainage to cavernous sinus with resultant cavernous venous thromboses and meningitis. Some individuals are subject to recurrent furunculosis, particularly diabetics. The incidence of infection caused by methicillin-resistant *S. aureus* is increasing.

MANAGEMENT

The treatment of an abscess, furuncle, or carbuncle is incision and drainage, and systemic antimicrobial therapy.

Prevention Individuals subject to repeated furuncle/carbuncle formation can reduce *S. aureus* carriage by use of an antibacterial soap while bathing. Mupirocin ointment is effective for eliminating nasal carriage.

Surgery Incision and drainage are often adequate for treatment of abscesses, furuncles, or carbuncles. Scissors or scalpel blade can be used to drain loculated pus in carbuncles; if this is not done, resolution of pain and infection can be delayed despite systemic antibiotic therapy. Dental abscesses are often associated with devitalized tooth pulp, which must be removed or the tooth extracted. All foreign matter must be removed: comedone, keratinaceous debride, foreign body.

Adjunctive Therapy Application of heat to the lesion promotes localization/consolidation and aids early spontaneous drainage.

Systemic Antimicrobial Treatment In healthy individuals, incision and drainage are often adequate therapy. Systemic antibiotics speed resolution in healthy individuals and are mandatory in any individual at risk for bacteremia (e.g., immunosuppressed patients). See Table 20-1.

Recurrent Furunculosis Usually related to persistent *S. aureus* in the nares, perineum, and body folds.

Topical Therapy Shower with providone-iodine soap or benzoyl peroxide (bar or wash). Apply mupirocin ointment daily to the inside of nares and other sites of *S. aureus* carriage.

Systemic Therapy Appropriate antibiotic treatment is continued until all lesions have resolved. Secondary prophylaxis may be given once a day for many months.

Carrier State Rifampin: 600 mg PO for 7 to 10 days for eradication of carrier state.

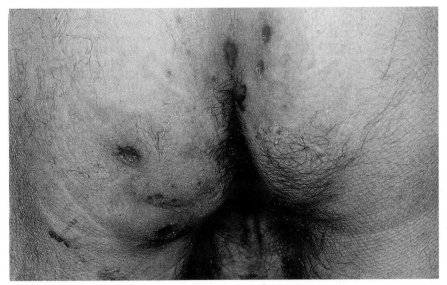

Figure 20-21 Furuncles, multiple: *S. aureus* *Multiple, painful ulcerated nodules on the buttocks of a 20-year-old male who had experienced a recent episode of severe ulcerative colitis.*

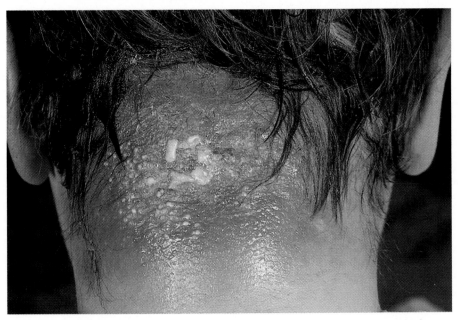

Figure 20-22 Carbuncle: *S. aureus* *A very large, inflammatory plaque studded with multiple pustules, some of which have ruptured, draining pus, on the nape of the neck. This very painful area is surrounded by erythema and edema (cellulitis), extends down to fascia, and has formed from a confluence of many furuncles.*

CLASSIFICATION/DEFINITIONS OF SOFT TISSUE INFECTIONS

Soft tissue infections (STIs), or cellulitides, are characterized by an acute, diffuse, spreading, edematous, suppurative inflammation of the dermis and subcutaneous tissues, often associated with systemic symptoms of malaise, fever, and chills. Non-necrotizing STIs are treated with antibiotics, drainage of abscesses, and supportive measures. Necrotizing STIs are often life-threatening and require, in addition, extensive surgical debridement. See Table 20-2.

Erysipelas A distinct type of superficial cutaneous cellulitis with marked dermal lymphatic vessel involvement presenting as a painful, bright-red, raised, edematous, indurated plaque with advancing raised borders, sharply marginated from the surrounding normal skin. Usually caused by group A β-hemolytic streptococcus (group A streptococcus; very uncommonly group C or G streptococcus) and rarely due to *S. aureus*. Group B streptococci can cause erysipelas in the newborn. Most common cause of virulent soft tissue infection in a healthy host sometimes without evident portal of entry.

Sites of predilection: face, lower legs, areas of preexisting lymphedema, umbilical stump.

Cellulitis Has many of the features of erysipelas but extends into the subcutaneous tissues. Cellulitis is differentiated from erysipelas by two physical findings: cellulitis lesions are not raised, and demarcation from uninvolved skin is indistinct. The tissue feels hard on palpation and is extremely painful. In some cases, even with antibiotic therapy, the overlying epidermis undergoes bulla formation or necrosis, resulting in extensive areas of epidermal sloughing and superficial erosion. In other cases, with or without therapy, infection may localize in the soft tissue, with dermal and subcutaneous abscess formation or necrotizing fasciitis. *S. aureus* and group A streptococci are by far the most common etiologic agents, but occasionally other bacteria are implicated (e.g., group B streptococci in the newborn, pneumococcus, a variety of gram-negative bacilli, and *Cryptococcus*).

Lymphangitis Inflammation of the lymphatic vessels, usually beginning on acral sites such as hands or feet; presents as erythematous streaking on the volar or dorsal aspect of the arm proximal to a finger or hand infection. Several subtypes of necrotizing fasciitis are recognized. Correct diagnosis is imperative in understanding pathogenesis and deciding on the appropriate antimicrobial and surgical therapies.

Gangrenous Cellulitis Characterized by necrosis of the dermis, subcutaneous fat (hypodermis), fascia, or muscle. Classified as necrotizing fasciitis, clostridial soft tissue infections, and progressive bacterial synergistic gangrene.

Necrotizing Soft Tissue Infection (NSTI) Differ from other variants because of significant tissue necrosis, lack of response to antimicrobial treatment alone, and need for surgical debridement of devitalized tissues. Starts with erythema and painful induration of underlying soft tissues; rapid development of black eschar which transforms into liquefied black and malodorous necrotic mass. Divided into three categories: necrotizing cellulitis, necrotizing fasciitis, myonecrosis. In that presence of fascial necrosis can be determined only by surgical exploration and histopathologic examination of involved tissue, necrotizing cellulitis cannot be differentiated from necrotizing fasciitis on clinical grounds alone. NSTI in the genital area is called Fournier's gangrene.

Ecthyma Gangrenosum An NSTI, most commonly caused by *Pseudomonas aeruginosa*, characterized by a cutaneous infarction progressing to large ulcerated gangrenous lesions. Occurs most commonly in the setting of profound prolonged neutropenia and is often followed by *P. aeruginosa* bacteremia. Patients are often immunocompromised.

Table 20-2   ETIOLOGY OF SOFT TISSUE INFECTIONS (STIs)

Type of Infection	Most Common Cause(s)	Uncommon Causes
Erysipelas	Group A streptococcus (GAS)	Group B, C, and G streptococci (GBS, GCS, GGS) *S. aureus*
Cellulitis	*S. aureus,* GAS	GBS, GCS, GGS *Erysipelothrix rhusiopathiae* Pneumococcus *Haemophilus influenzae* (children) *Escherichia coli* *Campylobacter jejuni* *Moraxella* *Serratia, Proteus,* other Enterobacteriaceae *Cryptococcus neoformans* *Legionella pneumophila, L. micdadei* *Bacillus anthracis* (anthrax) *Aeromonas hydrophila* *Vibrio vilnificus, V. alginolyticus*

Cellulitis in children
  Facial/periorbital cellulitis
  Perianal cellulitis
	S. aureus, GAS
	H. influenzae (young children)
	GAS
		GBS (neonates)
		Neisseria meningitidis
		S. aureus

Cellulitis secondary to bacteremia	*P. aeruginosa*	*V. vulnificus* *Streptococcus pneumoniae* GAS, GBS
Crepitant cellulitis	*Clostridia* spp. (*C. perfringens, C. septicum*)	*Bacteroides* spp. Peptostreptococci *E. coli, Klebsiella*
Cellulitis associated with water exposure	*E. rhusiopathiae* (erysipeloid) *V. vulnificus* *Aeromonas hydrophila* *Mycobacterium marinum* (nodular lymphangitis) *M. fortuitum* complex	Seal finger (etiology unknown)

Gangrenous cellulitis
  (infectious gangrene)
  Necrotizing fasciitis (NF)
    Streptococcal gangrene
    Nonstreptococcal NF
	
	GAS
	Mixed infection with one or more anaerobes (*Peptostreptococcus* or *Bacteroides*) *plus* at least one facultative species (non-group A streptococci; members of the Enterobacteriaceae such as *Enterobacter* or *Proteus*)
		
		GBS, GCS, GGS
		Bacillus cereus (granulocytic patients)

Synergistic necrotizing cellulitis[a] (necrotizing cutaneous myositis, synergistic nonclostridial anaerobic myonecrosis)	Polymicrobial with aerobic and anaerobic organisms that originate in the intestine. One-third of patients have positive blood cultures, usually a coliform, *Bacteroides,* or *Peptostreptococcus*	
Aerobes	Coliforms: *E. coli, Proteus, Klebsiella*	
Anaerobes	*Bacteroides, Peptostreptococcus, Clostridium, Fusobacterium*	

(Continued)

Table 20-2 ETIOLOGY OF SOFT TISSUE INFECTIONS (STIs) *(Cont.'d)*

Type of Infection	Most Common Cause(s)	Uncommon Causes
Fournier's gangrene	Similar to nonstreptococcal NF	
Clostridial STI	*C. perfringens*	
	Other histotoxic clostridial spp.	
Anaerobic cellulitis		
Anaerobic myonecrosis (GAS gangrene)		
Spontaneous, nontraumatic anaerobic myonecrosis	*C. septicum* (bacteremic)	
Nonclostridial anaerobic cellulitis	Various *Bacteroides* spp.	
	Peptostreptococci	
	Peptococci	
Progressive bacterial synergistic gangrene (Meleney's gangrene)	Mixed bacterial infection	
Ulcer base	*S. aureus*	*Proteus* spp.
		Other gram-negative bacilli
Advancing margin	Microaerophilic or anaerobic streptococci	
Gangrenous cellulitis in the immunosuppressed individual	*P. aeruginosa* (ecthyma gangrenosum)	Mucoraceae (*Mucor, Rhizopus, Absidia*) *Bacillus* spp.

*Essentially the same as nonstreptococcal NF but with some involvement of adjacent skeletal muscle.

Erysipelas and Cellulitis

Erysipelas and cellulitis are acute, spreading infections of dermal and subcutaneous tissues, characterized by a red, hot, tender area of skin, often at the site of bacterial entry, caused most frequently by group A β-hemolytic streptococci (erysipelas) or *Staphylococcus aureus*.

EPIDEMIOLOGY

Age of Onset Any age. Children <3 years; older individuals.

Etiology Commonly in adults: *S. aureus,* group A β-hemolytic *Streptococcus pyogenes* (GAS); in children: *Haemophilus influenzae* type b (Hib), GAS, *S. aureus.*
Less commonly caused by the following: *H. influenzae,* group B streptococci (GBS), pneumococci, *Erysipelothrix rhusiopathiae.* In patients with diabetes or impaired immunity: *Escherichia coli, Proteus mirabilis, Acinetobacter, Enterobacter, Pseudomonas aeruginosa, Pasteurella multocida, Vibrio vulnificus; Mycobacterium fortuitum* complex; *Cryptococcus neoformans.* In children, uncommonly caused by pneumococci, *Neisseria meningitidis* group B (periorbital).

Portals of Entry Cellulitis can arise via a portal of entry through any mucocutaneous site or, less commonly, spread hematogenously to soft tissue. Bloodborne pathogens causing cellulitis include *S. pneumoniae, V. vulnificus,* and *C. neoformans.*

Underlying Dermatoses

- Bullous disease: pemphigus vulgaris, bullous pemphigoid, sunburn, porphyria cutanea tarda
- Chronic lymphedema
- Dermatophytosis: tinea pedis, tinea capitis, tinea barbae
- Viral infections: herpes simplex, varicella, herpes zoster
- Inflammatory dermatoses: atopic dermatitis, contact dermatitis, stasis dermatitis, psoriasis, chronic cutaneous lupus erythematosus, pyoderma gangrenosum

- Superficial pyoderma: impetigo, folliculitis, furunculosis, carbuncle, ecthyma
- Ulcers: pressure, chronic venous insufficiency, ischemic, neuropathic
- Umbilical stump

Trauma

- Abrasion
- Bites: human, animal, insect
- Burns
- Laceration
- Puncture

Surgical Wound

- Surgical incisions
- Venous access devices

Mucosal Infection

- Oropharynx, nasal mucosa
- Middle ear

Risk Factors Drug and alcohol abuse, cancer and cancer chemotherapy, chronic lymphedema (postmastectomy, postcoronary artery grafting, previous episode of cellulitis), cirrhosis, diabetes mellitus, iatrogenic immunosuppression (neutropenia), immunodeficiency syndromes, malnutrition, neutropenia, renal failure, systemic atherosclerosis.

PATHOGENESIS

After entry, infection spreads to tissue spaces and cleavage planes as hyaluronidases break down polysaccharide ground substances, fibrinolysins digest fibrin barriers, lecithinases destroy cell membranes. Local tissue devitalization, e.g., trauma, is usually required to allow for significant anaerobic bacterial infection. The number of infecting organisms is usually small, suggesting that cellulitis may be more of a reaction to bacterial superantigens than to overwhelming tissue infection.

HISTORY

Incubation Period Few days.

Prodrome Occurs less often than commonly thought. Malaise, anorexia; fever, chills can develop rapidly, before cellulitis is apparent clinically. Higher fever (38.5°C) and chills usually associated with GAS.

Previous Treatment Prior episode(s) of cellulitis in an area of lymphedema.

Drugs Ingesting drug use.

Immune Status Immunocompromised patients susceptible to infection with bacteria of low pathogenicity.

History Local pain and tenderness. Necrotizing infections associated with more local pain and systemic symptoms.

PHYSICAL EXAMINATION

Skin Lesions

Portals of Entry Breaks in skin, ulcers, chronic dermatosis. Red, hot, edematous and shiny plaque, and very tender area of skin of varying size (Fig. 20-23); borders usually sharply defined, irregular, and slightly elevated; bluish purple color with *H. influenzae*. Vesicles, bullae, erosions, abscesses, hemorrhage, and necrosis may form in plaque. Lymphangitis.

Distribution *Adults* Lower leg; most common site, following interdigital tinea. Arm: in young male, consider IV drug use; in female; postmastectomy. Trunk: operative wound site. Face: following rhinitis, conjunctivitis (Fig. 20-23).

Children Cheek, periorbital area, head, neck most common: usually *H. influenzae* (Fig. 20-24). Extremities: *S. aureus,* group A streptococci.

Lymph Nodes Can be enlarged and tender, regionally.

Variants in Infecting Organism

S. aureus Often a portal of entry is apparent; usually a focal infection (Figs. 20-25 and 20-26). Most common pathogen in injection drug user. Toxin syndromes (scalded-skin syndrome, toxic shock syndrome) may occur. Endocarditis may follow bacteremia.

Group A Streptococcus Incidence of invasive GAS infections is increasing. The morbidity and mortality rates are significant: 37% of patients have necrotizing fasciitis and 25% meet the criteria for streptococcal toxic shock syndrome; mortality rate reported to be 21%.

Group B Streptococcus Colonizes anogenital region. Causes anogenital cellulitis, which may extend into pelvic tissues. Following childbirth, known as *puerperal sepsis*.

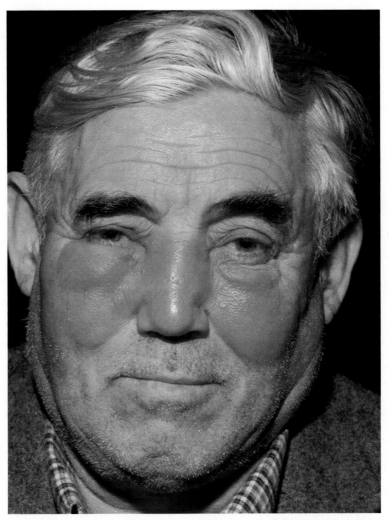

Figure 20-23 Erysipelas: group A streptococcus *Painful, shiny, erythematous, edematous plaques involving eyelids, cheeks, and the nose of an elderly febrile male. On palpation the skin is hot and tender. Portal of entry was conjunctivitis.*

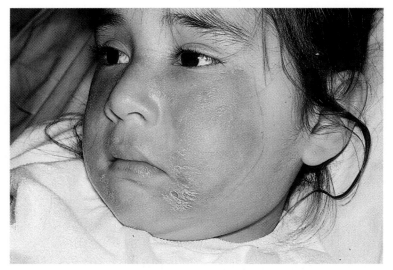

Figure 20-24   Cellulitis: *H. influenzae* *Erythema and edema of the cheek of a young child, associated with fever and malaise.* H. influenzae *was isolated on culture of the nasopharynx. (Courtesy of Sandy Tsao, MD).*

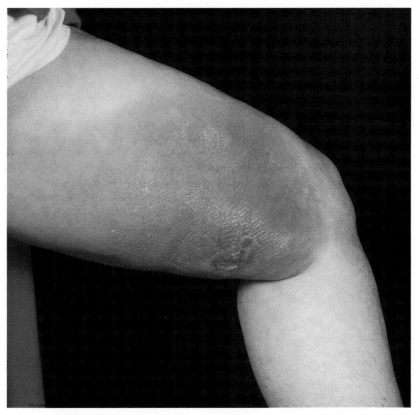

Figure 20-25   Cellulitis: *S. aureus* *Portal of entry of infection is seen on the lateral thigh with necrosis of skin; the infection has extended mainly proximally from this site.*

S. pneumoniae (Pneumococcus) Occurs more commonly in individuals with systemic lupus erythematosus, complement deficiency, HIV disease, glucocorticoid therapy, drug or alcohol abuse. Infected sites show bulla formation, brawny erythema, violaceous hue.

E. rhusiopathiae: erysipeloid Painful, swollen plaque with sharply defined irregular raised border occuring at the site of inoculation, i.e., finger or hand (Fig. 20-27), spreading to wrist and forearm. Color: purplish-red acutely; brownish with resolution. Enlarges peripherally with central fading. Usually no systemic symptoms. Uncommonly, associated with bacteremia and aortic valvulitis. Occurs in individuals who handle game. A typical example would be someone who becomes injured when boning fish.

P. aeruginosa Ecthyma gangrenosum begins as erythematous macule (cutaneous ischemic lesion) that quickly evolves to a bluish or gunmetal gray plaque with an erythematous halo (infarction) (Fig. 20-28 A and B). The epidermis overlying the ischemic area forms a bulla. Epidermis eventually sloughs, forming an ulcer. *Distribution:* most commonly in the axilla, groin, perineum. Usually occurs as solitary lesion but may occur as a few lesions. Lesions associated with *Pseudomonas* septicemia: "rose" spot-like lesions (erythematous macules and/or papules on trunk as in typhoid fever, occur with *Pseudomonas* infection of GI tract, i.e., diarrhea, headache, high fever); painful clustered vesicular to bullous lesions; multiple painful nodules representing small embolic lesions. (See page 652.)

H. influenzae Occurs mainly in children younger than 2 years. Cheek, periorbital area, head, neck most common sites (Fig. 20-24). Clinically, swelling, characteristic violaceous erythema hue. Use of Hib vaccine has dramatically reduced incidence.

V. vulnificus Underlying disorders: cirrhosis, diabetes, immunosuppression. Follows ingestion of raw/undercooked seafood, gastroenteritis, bacteremia with seeding of skin; also exposure of skin to sea water. Characterized by bulla formation, necrotizing vasculitis (Fig. 20-29). Usually on the extremities; often bilateral.

A. hydrophila Exposure to fresh water; preexisting wound. Lower leg. Necrotizing soft tissue infections (NSTI).

Capnocytophaga Canimorsus Immunosuppression or asplenia; exposure to a dog.

P. multocida Follows cat bite.

Clostridium Spp. Associated with trauma, contamination by soil or feces, malignant intestinal tumor. Infection may be characterized by gas, marked systemic toxicity.

M. chelonei–M. fortuitum Complex History of recent surgery, injection, penetrating wound. Low-grade cellulitis. Systemic findings lacking.

C. neoformans Patient always immunocompromised. Red, hot, tender, edematous plaque on extremity. Rarely multiple noncontiguous sites.

General Findings

Fever, signs of sepsis.

DIFFERENTIAL DIAGNOSIS

Erysipelas/Cellulitis Deep vein thrombosis/thrombophlebitis, stasis dermatitis, early contact dermatitis, giant urticaria, fixed drug eruption, erythema nodosum, erythema migrans (Lyme borreliosis), prevesicular herpes zoster, eosinophilic cellulitis, erysipelas-like lesion of familial Mediterranean fever.

Necrotizing Soft Tissue Infections Vasculitis, embolism with infarction of skin, peripheral vascular disease, purpura fulminans, calciphylaxis, warfarin necrosis, traumatic injury, cryoglobulinemia, fixed drug eruption, pyoderma gangrenosum, brown recluse spider bite.

LABORATORY STUDIES

Direct Microscopy *Smears* Gram's stain of exudate, pus, bulla fluid, aspirate, or touch preparation may show bacteria. GAS: chains of gram-positive cocci. *S. aureus:* clusters of gram-positive cocci. Clostridia: gram-negative rods, few neutrophils.

"Touch" Preparation Lesional skin biopsy specimen touched to microscope slide. Potassium hydroxide applied; examined for yeast and mycelial forms of fungus; detects *Candida, Cryptococcus, Mucor.* Gram's stain: detects bacteria.

Cultures Primary lesion, aspirate or biopsy of leading edge of inflammation. Yield of blood cultures very low, in the range of 2%, highest in GAS infections. Fungal and mycobacterial

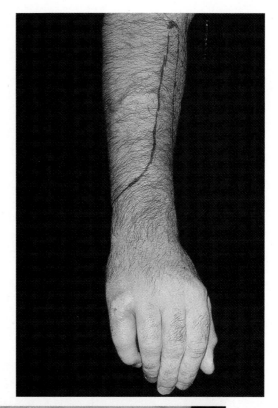

Figure 20-26 Cellulitis originating in furuncle: *S. aureus* *Furuncle on the dorsum of the little finger with proximal extension with cellulitis and lymphangitis in a 40-year-old HIV-infected male. The infection was recurrent, associated with bacteremia, and required inpatient intravenous antibiotic therapy.*

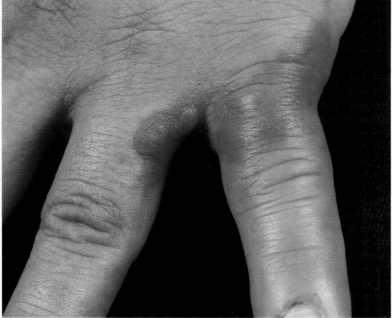

Figure 20-27 Erysipeloid *A well-demarcated, violaceous, cellulitic plaque (without epidermal changes of scale or vesiculation) on the dorsum of the hand and fingers; the site was somewhat painful, tender, and warm.*

CLASSIFICATION/DEFINITIONS OF SOFT TISSUE INFECTIONS

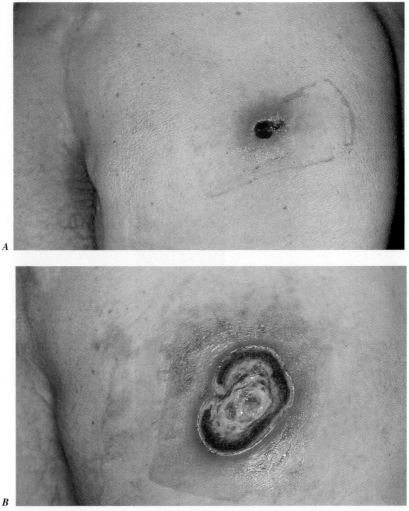

Figure 20-28   Ecthyma gangrenosum: *P. aeruginosa*   A. *An extremely painful, infarcted area with surrounding erythema present for 5 days on the buttock of a neutropenic HIV-infected male. This primary cutaneous infection was associated with bacteremia.* **B.** *Two weeks later, the lesion had progressed to a large ulceration. The patient died three months later of P. aeruginosa pneumonitis.*

cultures indicated in atypical case. Needle aspiration may be helpful. Culture of lesional biopsy specimen.

Hematology   WBC and ESR may be elevated.

Dermatopathology   Helpful in ruling out noninfectious inflammatory dermatoses. In NSTI, vasculitis without thrombosis, paucity of neutrophils at site of infection; bacilli found in media and adventitia, but usually not in intima, of vessel. Helpful with cryptococcal cellulitis.

Immunofluorescent staining with polyclonal and monoclonal antibodies to organisms such as GAS may demonstrate GAS in the reticular dermis.

Imaging   MRI may be helpful in diagnosis of severe acute infectious cellulitis, distinguishing pyomyositis, necrotizing fasciitis, and infectious cellulitis with or without subcutaneous abscess formation. X-ray examination of involved sites helpful in identifying soft tissue gas and extensive soft tissue involvement.

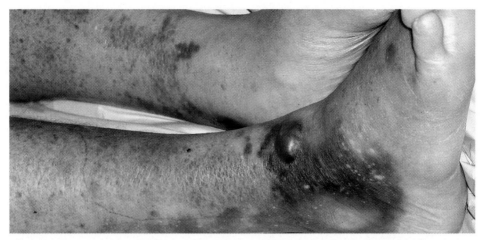

Figure 20-29 Cellulitis: *V. vulnificus* *Bilateral hemorrhagic plaques and bullae on the legs, ankles, and feet of an older diabetic with cirrhosis. Unlike other types of cellulitis in which microorganisms enter the skin locally, that which is caused by* V. vulnificus *usually follows a primary enteritis with bacteremia and dissemination to the skin.*

DIAGNOSIS

Clinical diagnosis. Confirmed by culture in only 25% of cases in immunocompetent patients. Suspicion of necrotizing fasciitis requires immediate deep biopsy and frozen-section histopathology.

COURSE AND PROGNOSIS

When occurring as a local infection in the absence of bacteremia, prognosis is much more favorable. Dissemination of infection (lymphatics, hematogenously) with metastatic sites of infection occurs if treatment is delayed. Abnormal or synthetic heart valve may be colonized and infected. In preantibiotic era, mortality rate was very high. In immuncompromised patients, prognosis, depends on prompt restoration of altered immunity, usually on correction of neutropenia. Without surgical debridement, necrotizing fasciitis is fatal. If neutropenia exists, prognosis depends on recovery of neutrophil count.

MANAGEMENT

Prophylaxis

Individuals with prior episodes of cellulitis Especially in sites of chronic lymphedema: support stockings, antiseptics to skin, chronic secondary antimicrobial prophylaxis (penicillin G, dicloxacillin, or erythromycin, 500 mg/d).

Status postsaphenous vein harvest Especially with tinea pedis: Wash with benzoyl peroxide bar daily, followed by application of topical antifungal cream.

Pneumococcus Immunize those at risk.

HIb Chemoprophylaxis for household contacts <4 years of age if unimmunized.

***Vibrio* spp.** Diabetics, alcoholics, cirrhotics should avoid eating undercooked seafood.

Supportive Rest, immobilization, elevation, moist heat, analgesia

Surgical Intervention Drain abscesses. Debride necrotic tissue. With felon, surgical drainage is required for later lesions to interrupt the cycle of inflammatory-ischemic events.

Antimicrobial Therapy See Table 20-1.

Gangrenous Cellulitis

Gangrenous cellulitis (infectious gangrene) is characterized by rapid progression of infection with extensive necrosis of subcutaneous tissues and overlying skin. Several clinical types of gangrenous cellulitis occur dependent on the causative organism, the anatomic location of the infection, and predisposing conditions (Table 20-3). Several subtypes of necrotizing fasciitis are recognized. Correct diagnosis is imperative in understanding pathogenesis and deciding on the appropriate antimicrobial and surgical therapies.

TYPES OF GANGRENOUS CELLULITIS

Streptococcal Gangrene Caused by group A streptococcus (GAS) (rarely, groups B, C, or G); a similar-appearing NF is caused by other bacterial species (usually a mixture of anaerobic and facultative organisms). Rare entity, with a high mortality rate, usually developing at the site of an injury (minor trauma, laceration, needle puncture, or surgical incision) on an extremity, but can occur in postoperative abdominal incisions. In some cases, there is no obvious portal of entry. GBS have caused a similar process postpartum secondary to infected episiotomy incisions and in adult diabetics unrelated to obstetric complications. GBS gangrene represents a cellulitis that has progressed rapidly to gangrene of the subcutaneous tissue, with subsequent necrosis of the overlying skin. Although streptococcal gangrene may be associated with underlying diseases (diabetes, myxedema), most cases occur in otherwise healthy persons, often in children and the elderly.

Initially, findings of acute cellulitis (local redness, edema, heat, and pain in the involved area), typically on an extremity. Fever and other constitutional symptoms are prominent as the inflammatory process extends rapidly over the next few days. Characteristic findings appear within 36 to 72 h after onset: the involved area becomes dusky blue in color; vesicles or bullae containing initially yellowish, then red-black fluid appear. Infection spreads rapidly along fascial planes resulting in extensive necrotic sloughs. Bullae rupture, and extensive, sharply demarcated cutaneous gangrene develops. At this point the area may be numb, and the black necrotic eschar with surrounding irregular border of erythema resembles a third-degree burn. The eschar sloughs off by the end of 1 week to 10 days. Peripheral areas of involvement develop about the initial site of infection. Metastatic abscesses may occur as a consequence of bacteremia, resembling purpura fulminans but then evolving to dark-colored blebs containing streptococci. Secondary thrombophlebitis is common, but lymphangiitis and lymphadenitis are not.

Necrotizing Fasciitis Other Than That due to Group A Streptococcus Caused by a mixed infection in which one or more anaerobes (e.g., *Peptostreptococcus, Bacteroides*) are involved along with at least one facultative species (non-group A streptococci; members of the Enterobacteriaceae such as *Enterobacter, Proteus,* etc.). Antecedent injury to soft tissues, abdominal surgery, perirectal abscess, decubitus ulcer, and intestinal perforation are common predisposing events. Diabetes mellitus, alcoholism, or parenteral drug abuse are additional contributing factors. The onset is usually acute, and the course is rapidly progressive with high fever and prominent toxicity. Most commonly occurs on the lower extremities, abdominal wall, perineum (Fig. 20-30), and about operative wounds. It is important to recognize that this infection may present in the thigh (dissection along the psoas muscle) or abdominal wall from an intestinal source (occult diverticulitis, rectosigmoid neoplasm). The involved area is swollen, red, warm, painful, and tender. The process is more extensive than the extent of the overlying skin changes would suggest. Within several days the skin color becomes purple, bullae develop, and frank cutaneous gangrene ensues. At this stage the involved area is no longer tender; it has become anesthetic due to occlusion of small blood vessels and destruction of superficial nerves in the subcutaneous tissues. Crepitus is often present, particularly in patients with diabetes mellitus.

Ecthyma gangrenosum (EG) is a primary skin infection, presenting as NF, most commonly caused by *Pseudomonas aeruginosa,* characterized by a cutaneous infarction progressing to large ulcerated gangrenous lesions (Fig. 20-28).

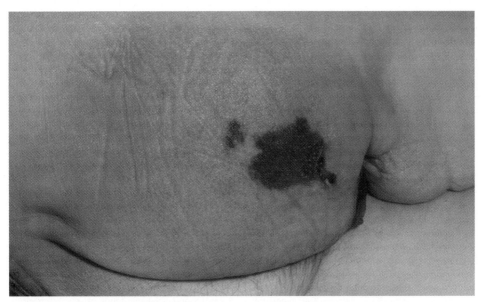

Figure 20-30   Necrotizing fasciitis   *Erythematous, edematous plaque involving the entire buttock with rapidly progressive area of necrosis.*

Table 20-3   CLASSIFICATION OF GANGRENOUS CELLULITIS (INFECTIOUS GANGRENE)

Necrotizing Fasciitis (NF)

- Streptococcal gangrene
- Necrotizing fasciitis other than streptococcal gangrene
- Synergistic necrotizing cellulitis (necrotizing cutaneous myositis, synergistic nonclostridial anaerobic myonecrosis)
- Fournier's gangrene

Clostridial soft tissue infections

- Anaerobic cellulitis
- Anaerobic myonecrosis (gas gangrene)
- Spontaneous, nontraumatic anaerobic myonecrosis

Progressive bacterial synergistic gangrene
Gangrenous cellulitis in the immunosuppressed individual
Localized areas of skin necrosis complicating conventional cellulitis

EG occurs most commonly in the setting of profound prolonged neutropenia and is often followed by *P. aeruginosa* bacteremia.

Synergistic Necrotizing Cellulitis Necrotizing cutaneous myositis, synergistic nonclostridial anaerobic myonecrosis. Highly lethal polymicrobial infection, characterized by extensive necrosis of skin and muscle as well as fascia and subcutaneous tissue with progressive undermining along fascial planes. May be rather indolent initially, presenting over 7 to 10 days with mild symptoms. Individuals are often afebrile or have only low-grade fever, lacking systemic toxicity in the early stages. The lower extremities, perineum, and abdominal wall are common sites.

The initial skin lesion is a small area of necrosis or reddish-brown blister with extreme local tenderness; the superficial appearance belies the widespread destruction of the deeper tissues. Skin sinuses (with surrounding areas of gangrene) are formed, draining foul-smelling brownish ("dishwater") pus. Between the draining tracts the skin appears uninvolved, even though extensive necrosis of underlying fascia, muscle, and subcutaneous tissues has occured. Extensive gangrene of the superficial tissues and fat can be visualized by direct inspection through skin incisions, associated with gelatinous necrosis of fascia and muscle. Gas can be palpated in the tissues in 25% of patients.

Fournier's Gangrene Streptococcal scrotal gangrene, perineal phlegmon. Variant of NF involving the scrotum and penis. Caused by the same mixture of facultative and anaerobic organisms causing NF other than that due to GAS. In rare cases GAS has been implicated. Average age at onset is 50 to 60 years. Most men have underlying disease including diabetes mellitus, ischiorectal abscess, perineal fistual, erysipelas of the perineum, bowel disease (rectal carcinoma, diverticulitis), scrotal trauma, prior urogenital surgery (especially involving the periurethral glands), pressure ulcers of the scrotum and perineum (alcoholics sitting in a drunken stupor), and dissection of pancreatic secretions through the retroperitoneum and into the scrotum. Onset can be insidious, with a discrete area of necrosis on the scrotum, progressing rapidly to advanced skin necrosis over 1 to 2 days. Pain, swelling, and crepitus in the scrotum are marked. Foul smelling drainage occurs, and purplish discoloration of the scrotum progresses to frank gangrene. The infection tends to be superficial, limited to skin and subcutaneous tissue, extending to the base of the scrotum, but may spread to the penis, perineum, and abdominal wall along fascial planes. The testes, glans penis, and spermatic cord usually are spared as they have a separate blood supply. If the process invades the abdominal panniculus of an obese patient, especially one with diabetes mellitus, progression can be extraordinarily rapid.

Clostridial Soft Tissue Infections Classified as *anaerobic cellulitis,* which involves the subcutaneous tissue, and *clostridial or anaerobic myonecrosis (gas gangrene),* occuring in the setting of muscle injury and contamination with soil or other foreign material containing spores of *Clostridium perfringens* or other histotoxic clostridial species. *C. perfringens* is an obligate anaerobe usually present in large numbers as normal flora in human feces and thus can endogenously contaminate skin surfaces. In spite of clostridial contamination of major traumatic open wounds, the incidence of gas gangrene is only 1 to 2%.

Nonclostridial Anaerobic Cellulitis Very similar to clostridial anaerobic cellulitis. The infection is caused by a variety of nonspore-forming anaerobic bacteria (*Bacteroides* spp., peptostreptococcus, *Prevotella* spp.) either alone or mixed with facultative species (Enterobacteriaceae, various streptococci, staphylococci).

Progressive Bacterial Synergistic Gangrene (Meleney's Gangrene) Progressive bacterial synergistic gangrene usually starts in the first or second postoperative week with local redness, tenderness, and swelling. Early infection shows a local tender area of erythema and swelling, which subsequently forms a small, painful, superficial ulcer that gradually enlarges. In established infections, three zones of involvement are characteristic: central area of necrosis (ulceration); middle zone of violaceous, tender edematous tissue; and outer zone of bright erythema. Local pain and tenderness are nearly always present; fever and systemic toxicity, however, are usually absent. Untreated, the ulceration progressively enlarges, ultimately resulting in enormous ulcerations. Meleney's ulcer has the features of progressive bacterial synergistic gangrene (Meleney's gangrene) with associated burrowing necrotic tracts through tissue planes emerging at distant skin sites.

Gangrenous Cellulitis in the Immunosuppressed Individual Caused by the usual agents as well as those not pathogenic in immunocompetent individuals. *P. aeruginosa* primarily infects skin in persons with prolonged neutropenia. Infection begins at sites where skin integrity is lost, or in normal appearing skin, especially in intertriginous areas. Infection causes a septic vasculitis with resultant infarction of skin; the necrotizing infection is referred to as ecthyma gangrenosum. Cutaneous mucormycosis can occur at a site of cutaneous injury in an individual with or without underlying immunocompromise.

DIFFERENTIAL DIAGNOSES OF GANGRENOUS CELLULITIS

Factitial ulcers, pyoderma gangrenosum, purpura fulminans (disseminated intravascular coagulation) calciphylaxis, ischemic necrosis (atherosclerosis obliterans, thromboembolism), fixed drug eruption, warfarin necrosis, heparin necrosis, pressure ulcer, amebic (*Entamoeba histolytica*) skin gangrene after bowel surgery, brown recluse spider bite.

MANAGEMENT

Surgical Debridement Requires early and complete surgical debridement of necrotic tissue in combination with high-dose antimicrobial agents.

Antimicrobial Therapy (See Table 20-1.)

Acute Lymphangitis

Acute lymphangitis is an inflammatory process involving the subcutaneous lymphatic channels. It is due most often to group A streptococcus (GAS) but occasionally may be caused by *Staphylococcus aureus;* rarely, soft tissue infections with other organisms, such as *Pasteurella multocida,* or herpes simplex virus may be associated with acute lymphangitis.

HISTORY

Portal of entry is commonly a wound on an extremity, an infected blister, or a *S. aureus* paronychia. The systemic manifestations of infection may occur either before any evidence of infection is present at the site of inoculation or after the initial lesion has subsided. The patient may notice pain over an area of redness proximal to the original break in the skin. Systemic symptoms are often more prominent than one might expect from the degree of local pain and erythema.

PHYSICAL EXAMINATION

Skin Findings   Red linear streaks, which may be a few millimeters to several centimeters in width, extend from the local lesion toward the regional lymph nodes (Fig. 20-31), which are usually enlarged and tender. Characteristically irregular and tender and may be mistaken for linear excoriations or phytoallergic contact dermatitis (poison ivy or oak). Occasionally, breakdown of overlying skin and ulceration occur in the course of bacterial lymphangitis, but this is rare in the antibiotic era.

DIFFERENTIAL DIAGNOSIS

Linear Lesions on Upper Extremities   Subacute or chronic sporotrichoid syndrome caused by organisms such as *Sporothrix schenckii.*

Linear Lesions on Lower Extremities   Superficial thrombophlebitis.

LABORATORY FINDINGS

Hemogram   WBC may be elevated with a marked increase in polymorphonuclear cells.

Culture   Isolate *S. aureus* or GAS from portal of entry.

DIAGNOSIS

The combination of a peripheral lesion with proximal red linear streaks leading toward regional lymph nodes is diagnostic of lymphangitis.

COURSE AND PROGNOSIS

The frequent development of bacteremia with metastatic infection in various organs makes this a potentially serious disease. The infection responds readily to penicillin therapy if instituted promptly.

MANAGEMENT

See Table 20-1.

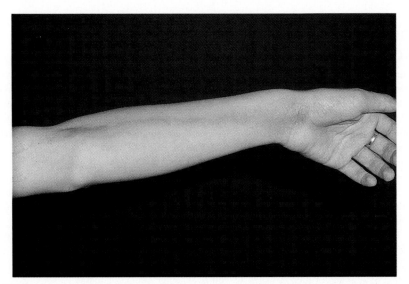

Figure 20-31   Acute lymphangitis   *A tender linear streak extending from the wrist to the upper arm; the infection spreads from the portal of entry within the superficial lymphatic vessels.*

GRAM-POSITIVE INFECTIONS ASSOCIATED WITH TOXIN PRODUCTION

Staphylococcus aureus and group A streptococcus (GAS) produce toxins that have systemic as well as mucocutaneous effects, causing staphylococcal scalded-skin syndrome (SSSS), toxic shock syndrome (TSS), and scarlet fever (SF). Two staphylococcal exotoxins (epidermolytic toxins A and B [ET-A, ET-B]), are responsible for the pathogenic changes of the SSSS. These toxins bind directly to the desmosomal protein desmoglein-1, which results in interdesmosomal splitting and causes blistering and denudation by disruption of the epidermal granular cell layer. These epidermolytic toxins display limited homology to staphylococcal enterotoxins and TSS toxin 1 (TSST-1). TSS is associated with production of TSST-1, enterotoxin B, and enterotoxin C_1. Certain strains of GAS produce a pyrogenic exotoxin, i.e., erythrogenic toxin, which causes scarlet fever and is involved in the pathogenesis of toxin shocklike syndrome (TSLS).

Local production of toxin by *S. aureus* can result in bullous impetigo at the site of infection. Usually, the site of *S. aureus* or GAS infection (may be minimally symptomatic) and toxin production is a distant locus; toxin production and dissemination result in erythema of skin and/or mucosal sites as well as systemic symptomatology.

Staphylococcal Scalded-Skin Syndrome

Staphylococcal scalded-skin syndrome (SSSS) is a toxin-mediated epidermolytic disease characterized by erythema, widespread detachment of the superficial layers of the epidermis, resembling scalding, and occurring mainly in newborns and infants younger than 2 years. Severity ranges from a localized form, bullous impetigo, to a generalized form with extensive epidermolysis and desquamation. The clinical spectrum of SSSS includes (1) bullous impetigo, (2) bullous impetigo with generalization, (3) scarlatiniform syndrome, (4) generalized scalded-skin syndrome.
Synonym: Ritter's disease.

EPIDEMIOLOGY

Age of Onset   Most common in neonates during first 3 months of life. Infants and young children. Rare in adults.

Etiology   *Staphylococcus aureus* of phage group II, mostly type 71, which elaborate two distinct exotoxins, epidermolytic or exfoliative toxins A and B. Site of toxin production: purulent conjunctivitis, otitis media omphalitis, occult nasopharyngeal infection; bullous impetigo.

PATHOGENESIS

In newborns and infants, *S. aureus* colonizes nose, conjunctivae, or umbilical stump with or without causing clinically apparent infection, producing an exotoxin that is transported hematogenously to the skin. In bullous impetigo exotoxin is produced in impetigo lesion. Specific antistaphylococcal antibody, metabolic differences, or greater ability to localize, metabolize, and excrete in individuals older than 10 years probably accounts for decreased incidence of SSSS with older age. At times purulent conjunctivitis, otitis media, or occult nasopharyngeal infection occurs at site of toxin production. The exfoliative toxin causes acantholysis and intraepidermal cleavage within the stratum granulosum. The few cases of SSSS reported in adults were associated with immunodeficiency or renal insufficiency. Local effects of the toxin result in bullous impetigo, but with absorption of the toxin, a mild scarlatiniform rash accompanying the bullous lesions may appear. Conversely, local effects of the toxin may be absent, with systemic absorption resulting in a staphylococcal scarlet fever syndrome. More

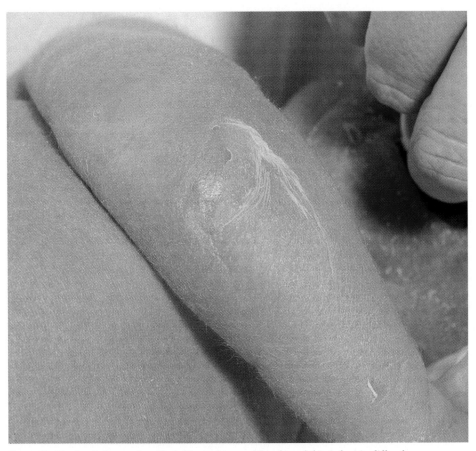

Figure 20-32 Staphylococcal scalded-skin syndrome *The skin of this infant is diffusely erythematous; gentle pressure to the skin of the arm has sheared off the epidermis, which folds like tissue paper.*

extensive epidermal damage is characterized by sloughing of superficial epidermis in SSSS. Healing spontaneously occurs in 5 to 7 days.

HISTORY

Skin Symptoms SSSS: early erythematous areas are very tender.

PHYSICAL EXAMINATION

Skin Lesions *Localized Form* See Bullous Impetigo (page 588), intact flaccid purulent bullae, clustered. Rupture of the bullae results in moist red and/or crusted erosive lesions. Lesions often are clustered in an intertriginous area.

Generalized Form Exotoxin-induced changes: micromacular scarlatiniform rash (staphylococcal scarlet fever syndrome) or diffuse, ill-defined erythema (Fig. 20-32) and a fine, stippled, sandpaper appearance occur initially. In 24 h, erythema deepens in color and involved skin becomes tender. Initially periorificially on face, neck, axillae, groins; becoming more widespread in 24 to 48 h. Initial erythema and later sloughing of superficial layers of epidermis are most pronounced periorificially on face and in flexural areas on neck, axillae, groins, antecubital area, back (pressure points). Condition becomes generalized, resembling scalding. With epidermolysis, epidermis appears wrinkled and can be removed by gentle pressure (skin resembles wet tissue paper) (Nikolsky's sign) (Fig. 20-32). In some infants, flaccid bullae occur. Unroofed epidermis forms erosions with red, moist base. Desquamation occurs with healing (Fig. 20-33).

Mucous Membranes   Uninvolved in SSSS.

General Examination   Possible low-grade fever. Irritable child.

DIFFERENTIAL DIAGNOSIS

Drug-induced toxic epidermal necrolysis, toxic shock syndrome, Kawasaki's syndrome, eczema herpeticum.

LABORATORY EXAMINATIONS

Direct Microscopy *Gram's Stain*   Bullous impetigo: pus in bullae, clumps of gram-positive cocci within PMN SSSS: gram-positive cocci only at colonized site, not in areas of epidermolysis.

Bacterial Culture   Bullous impetigo: *S. aureus* isolated from involved site. SSSS: *S. aureus* only at site of infection (i.e., site of toxin production)—umbilical stump, ala nasi, nasopharynx, conjunctivae, external ear canal, stool. *S. aureus* is not recovered from sites of sloughing skin or bullae.

Dermatopathology   Intraepidermal cleavage with splitting occurring beneath and within stratum granulosum.

DIAGNOSIS

Clinical findings confirmed by bacterial cultures.

COURSE AND PROGNOSIS

In late phases of SSSS, and in an accelerated manner, after adequate antibiotic treatment, the superficially denuded areas heal in 3 to 5 days associated with generalized desquamation in large sheets of skin (Fig. 20-33); there is no scarring. Death can occur in neonates with extensive disease.

MANAGEMENT

General Care   Hospitalization is recommended for neonates and young children, especially if skin sloughing is extensive and parental compliance questionable. Discharge home when significant improvement is apparent. If case is mild and home care reliable, children can be treated with oral antibiotic.

Topical Therapy   Baths or compresses for debridement of necrotic superficial epidermis. Topical antimicrobial agents for impetigo lesions: mupirocin ointment, bacitracin, or silver sulfadiazine ointment. Avoid triple antibiotic ointment containing neomycin, which is a frequent allergen that causes contact dermatitis.

Systemic Antimicrobial Therapy   See Table 20-1.

Adjunctive Therapy   Replace significant water and electrolyte loss intravenously in severe cases.

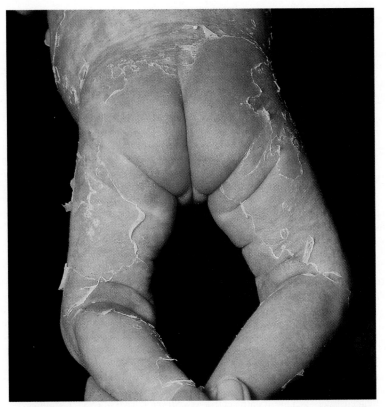

Figure 20-33 Staphylococcal scalded-skin syndrome *In this infant, painful, tender, diffuse erythema was followed by generalized epidermal desquamation.* S. aureus *had colonized the nares with perioral impetigo, the site of exotoxin production.*

Toxic Shock Syndrome

Toxic shock syndrome (TSS) is an acute toxin-mediated illness caused by toxin-producing *Staphylococcus aureus,* characterized by rapid onset of fever, hypotension, generalized skin and mucosal erythema, and multisystem failure, occurring in menstrual (MTSS) and nonmenstrual (NMTSS) patterns. Rarely, group A streptococcus (GAS) produces streptococcal toxic shock-like syndrome (TSLS).

EPIDEMIOLOGY

Age of Onset   MTSS: 23 years (mean age); NMTSS: 27 years (mean age).

Sex   Prior to 1984, more than 99% of cases were in females; after 1984, 55% in females.

Race   In the United States, 97% of MTSS in whites; 87% of NMTSS in whites.

Risk Factors   *MTSS*   Use of vaginal tampon of high absorbency.

Etiology   *S. aureus* producing TSS toxin 1 (TSST-1); other factors. Severe GAS infections also can cause TSLS.

NMTSS   Nonsurgical wounds (burns, skin ulcers, cutaneous and ocular injuries), surgical wounds, nasal packs, postpartum infections, vaginal nonmenstrual origin (contraceptive sponge, contraceptive diaphragm). Influenza.

Streptococcal TSLS   Diabetes mellitus, peripheral vascular disease.

Underlying Disorders   NMTSS can occur secondary to a wide variety of primary *S. aureus* infections as well as secondary infection of underlying dermatoses.

PATHOGENESIS

S. aureus multiplies in foreign body or minor wound infection, elaborating the TSST-1, which is absorbed and causes the clinical changes. TSST-1 causes decreased vasomotor tone and leakage of intravascular fluid. Rapid onset of hypotension followed by tissue ischemia and multisystem organ failure.

HISTORY

Incubation Period   Shorter in NMTSS. After surgical procedure, <4 days.

Symptoms   Recurrent symptoms in MTSS in untreated cases; tampon use. Sudden onset of fever, hypotension. Tingling sensation, hands and feet. Maculopapular eruption, pruritic. Generalized myalgias, muscle tenderness and weakness; headache, confusion, disorientation, seizures; profuse diarrhea; dyspnea.

PHYSICAL EXAMINATION

Skin Lesions   Generalized scarlatiniform erythroderma, most intense around infected area. Macular eruption (see Scarlet Fever). Petechiae, bullae, uncommonly. Edema, extensive generalized nonpitting; most marked on face, hands, feet (Fig. 20-34). Subsequent desquamation of palms, soles.

NMTSS   Look for cutaneous site of infection.

Streptococcal TSS   Cellulitis, necrotizing fasciitis, puerperal sepsis, varicella in children, and rarely asymptomatic streptococcal pharyngitis.

Mucous membranes   Look for forgotten or retained vaginal tampon. Intense erythema and injection of bulbar conjunctivae and mucous membranes of mouth, tongue, pharynx, vagina, tympanic membranes. Strawberry tongue. Subconjunctival hemorrhages. Ulcerations of mouth, vagina, esophagus, bladder.

General Findings   Fever, hypotension, multiorgan system failure. Renal and CNS complications more common in NMTSS.

DIFFERENTIAL DIAGNOSIS

Toxin-Mediated Infections   Staphylococcal scalded-skin syndrome, scarlet fever, GAS TSLS, Kawasaki's disease.

Localized Infections with Abdominal Pain and Shock   Urinary tract infection, pelvic inflammatory disease, septic abortion, gastroenteritis.

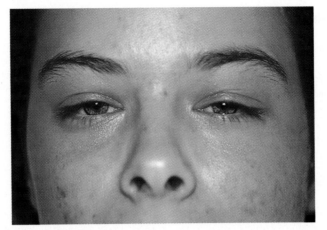

Figure 20-34 Toxic shock syndrome (TSS) *Erythema of the bulbar conjunctivae associated with facial erythema and edema in a female with menstrual TSS.*

Multisystem Infection Septic shock with localized infection (meningococcus, gonococcus, pneumococcus, *Hemophilus influenzae* (type B), leptospirosis, measles, Rocky Mountain spotted fever, tick-borne typhus, viral syndrome (adenoviruses, enteroviruses), Legionnaires' disease, toxoplasmosis.

Multisystem Illness, Possibly of Infectious Etiology Kawasaki's syndrome.

Noninfectious Diseases Systemic lupus erythematosus, acute rheumatic fever, adverse cutaneous drug reactions (Stevens-Johnson syndrome, toxic epidermal necrolysis), juvenile rheumatoid arthritis.

LABORATORY STUDIES

Direct Microscopy *Gram's Stain* Vaginal, wound exudate: many leukocytes and gram-positive cocci in clusters.

Culture Vaginal, wound exudate, foreign body: TSST-1–producing *S. aureus.* Streptococcal TSS: GAS recovered from blood or primary site of infection.

Biopsy Confluent epidermal necrosis, vacuolar alteration of dermal-epidermal junction, subepidermal vesiculation, little or no inflammatory infiltrate in dermis.

DIAGNOSIS

TSS clinical case definition (per CDC):

Fever Temperature ≥38.9°C.

Rash Diffuse macular erythroderma.

Desquamation 1 to 2 weeks after onset of illness, particularly of palms, soles, fingers, toes.

Hypotension Systolic blood pressure ≤90 mmHg for adults. For children, >5th percentile by age 16 or younger. Orthostatic syncope or orthostatic dizziness.

Involvement of Three or More Specific Organ Systems

COURSE AND PROGNOSIS

Diagnosis of NMTSS is often delayed because of the wide variety of clinical settings and associated symptomatology. Complications: refractory hypotension, adult respiratory distress syndrome, cardiomyopathy, arrhythmias, encephalopathy, acute renal failure, metabolic acidosis, liver necrosis, disseminated intravascular coagulation. Recurrence of untreated MTSS is high. Antibiotic therapy and discontinuance of tampons significantly reduce risk. Recurrences after NMTSS are rare. The mortality rate of NMTSS is higher than that of MTSS. Streptococcal TSS: associated with mortality rate of 25 to 50%.

MANAGEMENT

Usually patients are managed best in intensive care facility.

Local Infection Remove potentially foreign bodies. Drain and irrigate infected sites.

Systemic Antimicrobial Therapy IV anti-staphylococcal antibiotic.

Adjunctive Therapy Aggressive monitoring and management of specific organ system failure (i.e., management of fluid, electrolyte, metabolic, and nutritional needs). Methylprednisolone for severe cases.

Scarlet Fever

Scarlet fever (SF) is an acute infection of the tonsils, skin, or other sites by an erythrogenic exotoxin-producing strain of group A streptococcus (GAS), associated with a characteristic toxigenic exanthem.

EPIDEMIOLOGY

Age of Onset Children.
Etiology Usually group A β-hemolytic *Streptococcus pyogenes* (GAS). Uncommonly, exotoxin-producing *Staphylococcus aureus*.

PATHOGENESIS

Erythrogenic toxin production depends on the presence of a temperate bacteriophage. Patients with prior exposure to the erythrogenic toxin have antitoxin immunity and neutralize the toxin. The SF syndrome therefore does not develop in these patients. Since several erythrogenic strains of GAS cause infection, it is theoretically possible to have a second episode of SF. Strain of *S. aureus* can synthesize an erythrogenic exotoxin, producing a scarlatiniform exanthem.

HISTORY

Incubation Period Rash appears 1 to 3 days after onset of infection.

Exposure Household member(s) may be a streptococcal carrier.

PHYSICAL EXAMINATION

Skin Lesions *Site of GAS Infection* Pharyngitis; tonsillitis. Infected surgical or other wound. Impetiginous skin lesion.

Exanthem Finely punctate erythema is first noted on the upper part of the trunk (Fig. 20-35); may be accentuated in skin folds such as neck, axillae, groin, antecubital and popliteal fossae (Pastia's lines). Palms/soles usually spared. Face becomes flushed but with a perioral pallor. Initial punctate lesions become confluently erythematous, i.e., scarlatiniform. Linear petechiae (Pastia's sign) occur in body folds. Intensity of the exanthem varies from mild to moderate erythema confined to the trunk due to an extensive purpuric eruption.

Petechiae Scattered petechiae occur (Rumpel-Leede test for capillary fragility positive).

Desquamation Exanthem fades within 4 to 5 days and is followed by brawny desquamation on the body and extremities and by sheetlike exfoliation on the palms and soles. In subclinical or mild infections, exanthem and pharyngitis may pass unnoticed. In this case patient may seek medical advice only when exfoliation on the palms and soles is noted.

Mucous Membranes *Site of GAS Infection* Acute follicular or membranous tonsillitis. May be asymptomatic or mild and go undetected.

Enanthem Pharynx beefy red. Tongue initially is white with scattered red, swollen papillae (white strawberry tongue) (Fig. 20-36). By the fourth or fifth day, the hyperkeratotic membrane is sloughed, and the lingular mucosa appears bright red (red strawberry tongue) (Fig. 20-36). Punctate erythema and petechiae may occur in the palate.

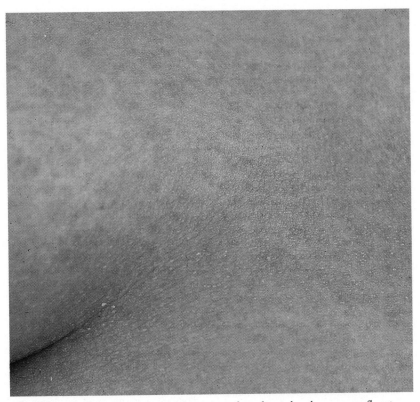

Figure 20-35   Scarlet fever: exanthem   *Finely punctated erythema has become confluent (scarlatiniform); petechiae can occur and have a linear configuration within the exanthem in body folds (Pastia's line).*

General Examination Patient may appear acutely ill with high fever, headache, nausea, vomiting. Anterior cervical lymphadenitis associated with pharyngitis/tonsillitis.

Variant Streptococcal toxic shock-like syndrome (TSLS): toxemia, organ failure, and a scarlatiniform rash associated with GAS cellulitis.

DIFFERENTIAL DIAGNOSIS

Generalized Exanthem Staphylococcal scarlet fever (pharyngitis, tonsillitis, strawberry tongue, and palatal enanthem not seen), staphylococcal or streptococcal toxic shock syndrome, Kawasaki's syndrome, viral exanthem, drug eruption.

LABORATORY STUDIES

Direct Microscopy *Gram's Stain* Gram-positive cocci in chain (GAS) or clusters (*S. aureus*) identified in smear from infected wound or impetiginized skin lesion.

Rapid Direct Antigen Tests (DATs) Used to detect GAS antigens in throat swab specimens.

Culture Isolate GAS or *S. aureus* on culture of specimen from throat or wound.

Serology Serologic tests detect immune responses to extracellular products (streptolysin O, hyaluronidase, DNase B, NADase, and strep-tokinase) and cellular components (M protein, group A antigen) of GAS. Useful in demonstrating antecedent streptococcal infection in individuals who lack documentation of recent GAS infection but who present with nonsuppurative sequelae (rheumatic fever, glomerulonephritis).

DIAGNOSIS

Clinical findings confirmed by detecting streptococcal antigen in a rapid test and/or culturing GAS from throat or wound.

COURSE AND PROGNOSIS

Production of erythrogenic toxin does not alter the course of the GAS infection. In some cases, GAS may enter the bloodstream with resultant high fever and marked systemic toxicity (toxic scarlet fever) and consequent metastatic foci of infection. Suppurative complications of GAS infection include peritonsillar cellulitis, peritonsillar abscess, retropharyngeal abscess; otitis media, acute sinusitis; suppurative cervical lymphadenitis.

Nonsuppurative sequelae of streptococcal infections, i.e., acute rheumatic fever, acute glomerulonephritis, and erythema nodosum, may follow if the infection goes untreated. The incidence of acute rheumatic fever had markedly decreased during the past two decades but is currently on the rise.

MANAGEMENT

Symptomatic therapy	Aspirin or acetaminophen for fever and/or pain.
Systemic antimicrobial therapy	Penicillin is the drug of choice because of its
Goal is to eradicate GAS throat carriage	efficacy in prevention of rheumatic fever.
to prevent Penicillin G benzathine	rheumatic fever
	1.2 million units IM (adults); 600,000 units IM
	(children <60 lbs).
Penicillin V	250 mg PO qid for 10 days.
For penicillin-allergic patients:	
Erythromycin estolate	20 to 40 mg/kg/d.
Erythromycin ethylsuccinate	40 mg/kg/d.
Azithromycin	See Table 20-1.
Clarithromycin	See Table 20-1.
Cephalosporin (for those who cannot	See Table 20-1.
tolerate oral erythromycin)	
Follow-Up	Reculture of throat recommended for
	individuals with history of rheumatic fever or if
	a family member has history of rheumatic
	fever.

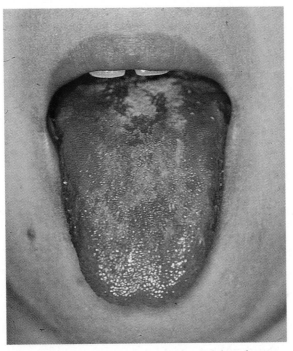

Figure 20-36   Scarlet fever: white and red strawberry tongue   *Bright red tongue with prominent papillae on the fifth day after onset of group A streptococcal pharyngitis in a child. The white patches at the back of the tongue represent residua of the initial white strawberry tongue.*

INFECTIVE ENDOCARDITIS, SEPSIS, AND SEPTIC SHOCK

Infective endocarditis (IE), sepsis, and septic shock are very serious systemic infections with high associated morbidity and mortality rates. Clinical findings often are acute in onset and relatively nonspecific in nature. Cutaneous findings, however, may be extremely helpful in making the correct diagnosis. Early recognition of clinical findings, diagnosis, and initiation of therapy increase the likelihood of a positive outcome.

Infective Endocarditis

Infective endocarditis (IE) is a microbial infection, implanted on a heart valve or on the mural endocardium after bacteremia or fungemia. It is characterized by fever, valvular destruction, and peripheral embolization. Acute IE is most commonly caused by *Staphylococcus aureus,* occurs on normal valves, is rapidly destructive, produces metastatic foci, and is fatal in <6 weeks unless treated. Subacute EI is usually caused by *Streptococcus viridans,* occurs on damaged valves, does not produce metastatic foci, and takes >6 weeks (up to one year) to be fatal.

EPIDEMIOLOGY

Classification by Duration/Onset *Acute Bacterial Endocarditis (ABE)* Caused by more invasive organisms, most commonly *S. aureus*. Can attack normal valve or mural endocardium. Other microorganisms: *Streptococcus pneumoniae* (alcoholics with pneumonia), group A streptococcus (GAS), *Neisseria gonorrhoeae, Salmonella, Pseudomonas aeruginosa* [intravenous drug users (IVDUs)].

Subacute Bacterial Endocarditis (SBE) Defined as duration >6 weeks. Caused by a variety of less virulent bacteria. Commonly, bacteria are members of the indigenous flora. Characteristically, infection is on deformed valves. Agents: streptococci of oral cavity, GI and GU tracts; *Haemophilus* organisms, *S. epidermidis*.

Etiology Most common is bacterial: (1) *S. viridans*, enterococci, and other streptococci account for about 50%; (2) *S. aureus, S. epidermidis,* 20%; (3) no causative agent can be isolated in 15 to 20%; (4) remainder uncommon bacterial and fungal organisms. Staphylococcal, fungal, gram-negative bacterial agents common in IVDUs, as well as polymicrobial IE. *S. aureus* most common cause with a normal valve. Also, fungi (*Candida albicans*), *Rickettsia, Chlamydia*.

Transmission Circumstances that result in transient bacteremia: dental procedures, IVU, various infections, induced abortions, intrauterine contraceptive devices, temporary transvenous pacemakers, prolonged IV infusions, endoscopic procedures. Estimated risk for IE in IVDUs in the United States: 2 to 5% per year.

Risk factors *Underlying Heart Disease* (1) Acquired heart disease—70% (rheumatic valvular disease, calcific stenosis, "floppy" mitral or aortic valves, prolapsing mitral valve leaflet, i.e., "click-murmur" syndrome, idiopathic hypertrophic subaortic stenosis, calcified mitral annulus; (2) congenital heart disease (interventricular septal defect, patent ductus arteriosus, pulmonic valve in tetralogy of Fallot).

Prosthetic Material Prosthetic heart valves, xenografts, intracardiac "patches," vascular prostheses.

IVDU Increasingly common risk factor for IE.

Classification by Valvular Status/IVDU *Native Valve Endocarditis* More common in males; most patients older than 50 years. Streptococci, enterococci, staphylococci cause most cases. Streptococci cause 55% of cases (in non-IVDU): *S. viridans* (75%), normal inhabitants of oropharynx; *S. bovis* in persons older than 60 years (one-third of patients have premalignant or malignant GI lesion); GAS (attacks normal

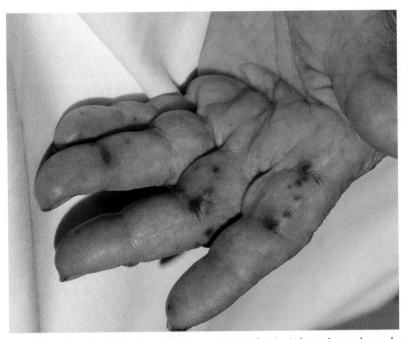

Figure 20-37 Infective endocarditis: Janeway lesions *Hemorrhagic, infarcted macules and papules on the volar fingers in a patient with* S. aureus *endocarditis.*

or damaged valve with rapid destruction); enterococci (6% of cases) (more common in male, average age 60 years). Staphylococci cause 30% of cases *(S. aureus* 5 to 10 times more common than *S. epidermidis).*

IVDU Most common in young males. Increasingly common risk factor for IE. Skin is most common source of infecting microbes. *S. aureus* accounts for 50% of cases; streptococci/enterococci, 20%; fungi (mainly *Candida),* 6%; gram-negative bacilli (usually *Pseudomonas* species), 6%. Tricuspid valve infection is common.

Prosthetic Valve Endocarditis Accounts for 10 to 20% of cases. More common in male older than 60 years; occurs in 1 to 2% of these patients during first year after surgery. Aortic valve >>mitral valve prostheses. Infection usually occurs on suture line. Half of early-onset endocarditis caused by staphylococci: *S. epidermidis > S. aureus.*

PATHOGENESIS

Characteristic lesions of IE are vegetations on valves or elsewhere on endocardium. Usually arises secondary to colonization by microbes of sterile vegetations composed of platelets/fibrin. Sterile vegetations represent nonbacterial thrombotic endocarditis; these form over areas of trauma to endothelium (intracardiac foreign bodies), in areas of turbulence (deformed valves), over scars, or in setting of wasting disease (e.g., malignancy with marantic endocarditis). Vegetations of IE then result from deposition of platelets/fibrin over bacteria, which forms a "protective site" into which phagocytic cells penetrate poorly. Clinical features result from vegetations and immune reaction to infection. With fungal IE, vegetations may be large, occluding valve orifice and forming large peripheral emboli. *S. aureus* can cause rapid valve destruction; healing forms scar, with resulting valvular stenosis or regurgitation. Abscesses may form in myocardium. Other complications include conduction abnormalities, fistulas, or rupture of chordae, papillary muscle, or ventricular septum. Vegetations can embolize to heart, brain, kidney, spleen, liver, extremities, lung, with resultant infarcts and abscesses. Circulating immune complexes may result in glomerulonephritis, arthritis, or various mucocutaneous manifestations of vasculitis.

HISTORY

SBE Fever, sweats, weakness, myalgias, arthalgias, malaise fatigability, anorexia, chilly sensations cough. Recent history of dental extraction or scaling, cystoscopy, rectal surgery, tonsillectomy. Fever, weitht loss, cerebrovascular accident, arthralgia, arthritis, diffuse myalgias.

ABE Onset abrupt with high fever and rigors, rapid downhill course.

IVDU Occurs in .2 to 2% of users annually. Right-sided IE more common than left-sided. *S. aureus* in >50%; 5% polymicrobial. Septic emboli common.

PHYSICAL EXAMINATION

Consider IE in any patient with fever and heart murmur.

Skin Lesions (Table 20-4)

Types *Janeway Lesions Nonpainful,* small, erythematous or hemorrhagic macules or nodules of palms (Fig. 20-3) or soles. More common in ABE but occur in SBE.

Osler's Nodes Tender to painful, purplish, split pea-sized, subcutaneous nodules in the pulp of the fingers and/or toes and thenar and hypothenar eminences (Fig. 20-38). Transient, disappearing within several days (5% of patients). In ABE, associated with minute infective emboli; aspiration may reveal the causative organism, i.e., *S. aureus.* In SBE, associated with immune complexes and small-vessel arteritis of skin.

Subungual Splinter Hemorrhages Linear in the *middle* of the nail bed (IE). (see Section 28). Distal hemorrhages are traumatic.

Petechial Lesions Small, nonblanching, reddish-brown macules. Occur on extremities, upper chest, mucous membranes [conjunctivae (Fig. 20-39), palate]. Occur in crops. Fade after a few days. 20 to 40%.

Clubbing of Fingers Occurs after prolonged course of untreated SBE (15%).

Gangrene of Extremities Secondary to embolization.

Pustular Petechiae, Purulent Purpura With *S. aureus* (Fig. 20-40).

General Examination

Heart SBE, 90% have murmurs; ABE, only two-thirds have murmur, which may change, heart failure.

Eye Petechial and flame-shaped hemorrhages in retina, cotton-wool exudates in fundus, Roth's spots (oval or boat-shaped white areas in the retina that are surrounded by a zone of hemorrhage), endophthalmitis.

Joints Septic arthritis with ABE.

Thromboembolic Phenomena Significant embolic episodes occur in one-third of patients, resulting in stroke, seizures, monocular blindness, mesenteric artery occlusion with abdominal pain, ileus, melena, splenic infarction, pulmonary infarction, gangrene of extremities, mycotic aneurysms.

DIFFERENTIAL DIAGNOSIS

ABE Meningococcemia, disseminated intravascular coagulation.

SBE Acute rheumatic fever, marantic endocarditis, collagen vascular diseases (SLE with cardiac involvement, systemic vasculitis), dysproteinemia, atrial myxoma, organizing left atrial thrombus, atheromatous embolism, cytomegalovirus infection after cardiac surgery (postperfusion syndrome).

LABORATORY EXAMINATIONS

See Table 20-5.

Dermatopathology Osler's node in subacute IE shows aseptic necrotizing vasculitis.

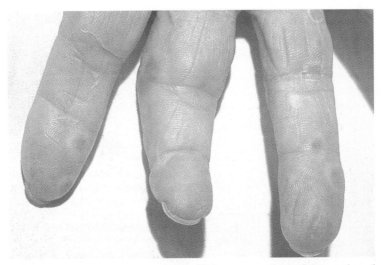

Figure 20-38 Infective endocarditis: Osler's nodes *Violaceous, tender nodules on the volar fingers associated with minute infective emboli or immune complex deposition.*

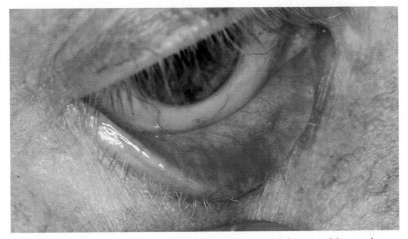

Figure 20-39 Infective endocarditis: subconjunctival hemorrhage *Submucosal hemorrhage of the lower eyelid in an elderly diabetic with enterococcal endocarditis; splinter hemorrhages in the midportion of the nail bed and Janeway lesions were also present.*

Table 20-4 CUTANEOUS MANIFESTATIONS AND CHARACTERISTICS OF INFECTIVE ENDOCARDITIS

Cutaneous Manifestations	Palpation	Morphologic Findings
Osler's node	Tender	Erythematous papules and nodules with white centers; may necrose
Janeway lesions	Nontender	Hemorrhagic papules
Splinter hemorrhages	Nontender	Subungual hemorrhagic streaks

Imaging Echo-Doppler study demonstrates vegetations, acute severe mitral or aortic regurgitation. Evidence of septic pulmonary emboli suggests tricuspid valve IE. Systemic embolization can occur from aortic or mitral valve.

DIAGNOSIS

Clinical diagnosis of IE is made in the following manner:
I. *Definite IE:* 2 major criteria *or* 1 major + 3 minor criteria *or* 5 minor criteria.
  A. Major criteria.
    1. Isolation of *S. viridans, S. bovis,* HACEK-group organisms, or (in the absence of a primary focus) community-acquired *S. aureus* or enterococcus from two separate blood cultures or isolation of a microorganism consistent with endocarditis in (1) blood culture 12 h apart or (2) all of three or most of four or more blood cultures, with first and last at least 1 h apart.
    2. Evidence of endocardial involvement on echocardiography: oscillating intracardiac mass or abscess or new partial dehiscence of prosthetic valve *or* new valvular regurgitation.
  B. Minor criteria.
    1. Predisposing lesion or IVDU.
    2. Fever of 38.0°C.
    3. Major arterial emboli, septic pulmonary infarcts, mycotic aneurysm, intracranial hemorrhage, conjunctival hemorrhages, Janeway lesions.
    4. Glomerulonephritis, Osler's nodes, Roth's spots, rheumatoid factor.

5. Positive blood cultures not meeting the major criterion (excluding single cultures positive for organisms that do not typically cause endocarditis) or serologic evidence of active infection with an organism that causes endocarditis.
6. Echocardiogram consistent with endocarditis but not meeting the major criterion.
II. *Possible IE:* Findings that fall short of "definite" but do not fall into the "rejected" category
III. *Rejected:* Alternative diagnosis or resolution of syndrome or no evidence of IE at surgery or autopsy with 4 days of antibiotic therapy

COURSE AND PROGNOSIS

Varies with the underlying cardiac disease and baseline health of the patient, as well as with the complications that occur. Complications; congestive heart failure, stroke, other systemic embolizations, septic pulmonary embolization. Aortic valve involvement has higher risk of death or need for surgery.

MANAGEMENT

Cure of IE requires eradication of all microbes from vegetation(s). Microbicidal drug regimens must produce high enough concentrations for long enough duration to sterilize vegetation(s).

Antimicrobial Therapy Appropriate IV antibiotic therapy, depending on the sensitivity of the infecting organism.

Surgery Most common indication, congestive heart failure. Valve replacement.

Table 20-5 FREQUENCY OF OCCURRENCE OF LABORATORY MANIFESTATIONS OF INFECTIVE ENDOCARDITIS

Manifestation	% of Cases
Anemia	70–90
Leukocytosis	20–30
Proteinuria	50–65
Microscopic hematuria	30–50
Elevated serum creatinine level	10–20
Elevated ESR	>90
Rheumatoid factor	50
Circulating immune complexes	65–100
Decreased serum complement level	5–40

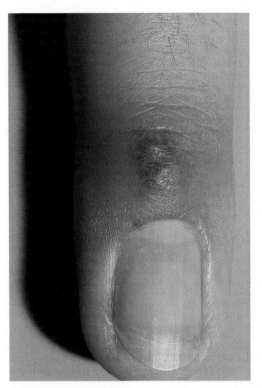

Figure 20-40   Septic vasculitis associated with bacteremia   *Dermal nodule with hemorrhage and necrosis on the dorsum of a finger. This type of lesion occurs with bacteremia (e.g.,* S. aureus*) and fungemia (e.g.,* Candida tropicalis*).*

Sepsis and Septic Shock

Sepsis and septic shock vary in presentation with multiple factors, host response, and the invading microbes. Fever or hypothermias, tachypnea, and tachycardia often herald onset of sepsis, the inflammatory response to microbial invasion.When counterregulatory control mechanisms are overwhelmed, often as the microbes move from a local site to invade the bloodstream, homeostasis may fail, and dysfunction of major organs may supervene (severe sepsis). Further failure of counterregulatory mechanisms leads to septic shock, which is characterized by hypotension as well as organ dysfunction. As sepsis progresses to septic shock, the risk of dying increases substantially. Early sepsis is usually reversible, whereas patients with septic shock often succumb despite aggressive therapy.

EPIDEMIOLOGY

Age of Onset For *Neisseria meningitidis* (NM), highest incidence in children aged 6 months to 3 years (peak, 6 to 12 months); lowest in persons older than 20 years.

Incidence in the United States, 300,000 to 500,000 cases annually with 100,000 deaths. Two-thirds of cases occur in patients hospitalized for other illnesses. Increasing incidence in the United States attributable to aging population, with increasing longevity of patients with chronic diseases.

Etiology Can be a response to any class of microorganisms. Microbial invasion of bloodstream is not essential for development of sepsis; local or systemic spread of microbial signal molecules or toxins can also elicit the reponse. Blood cultures yield bacteria or fungi in 20 to 40% of cases of severe sepsis; 40 to 70% of cases of septic shock. In cases with negative blood cultures, the etiologic agent can be established by culture/microscopic examination of infected material from a local site.

Globally, NM, meningococcus, is a common cause of sepsis and septic shock. NM is a gram-negative, encapsulated coccus. 13 serovars; however, serotypes A, B, C, 29E, W-135 cause 99% of infections. Confined to humans; natural habitat is nasopharynx. Nasopharyngeal carrier rate: in nonepidemic periods, 10%; in closed populations, up to 60 to 80%. Carriage persists for few months. Invasive infection usually occurs within first few days of carriage, before development of protective antibodies.

Risk Groups Influenza A virus infection. Absence of spleen or functional asplenia. Alcoholism. Complement deficiency, especially impaired alternative pathway activation.

Transmission For NM, person-to-person through inhalation of droplets of aerosolized infected nasopharyngeal secretions; direct or indirect oral contact.

Season For NM, highest incidence in midwinter, early spring; lowest in midsummer.

Geography For NM, worldwide. Occurs in epidemics or sporadically. Major outbreaks reported in Africa, China, South America.

Risk Factors Widespread use of antimicrobial agents, glucocorticoids, indwelling catheters, mechanical devices, mechanical ventilation.

Gram-negative Bacillary Bacteremia Diabetes mellitus, lymphoproliferative disease, cirrhosis, burns, invasive procedures or devices, treatment with drugs that cause neutropenia.

Gram-positive Bacteremia Vascular catheterization, presence of indwelling mechanical devices, burns, IVDU.

Fungemia Immunosuppressed patients with neutropenia, often after broad-spectrum antimicrobial therapy.

PATHOGENESIS

Septic response triggered when microorganisms spread from skin or GI tract into contiguous tissues. Localized infection may then lead to bacteremia or fungemia. Microbes can also be introduced into bloodstream directly from such routes as venous access lines. In some cases, however, no primary site of infection is apparent. Septic response occurs when invading microbes have circumvented host's innate and acquired immune defenses. Lipopolysaccharide (LPS) (endotoxin) is the most potent gram-negative bacterial signal molecule. Septic response involves complex interaction among microbial

BACTERIAL INFECTIONS INVOLVING THE SKIN

signal molecules, leukocytes, humoral mediators, and vascular endothelium. Many of the characteristics of sepsis (fever, tachycardia, tachypnea, leukocytosis, myalgias, somnolence) are produced by release of tumor necrosis factor α. Intravenous fibrin deposition, thrombosis, and disseminated intravascular coagulation (DIC) are important features of septic response. C5a and other products of complement activation may promote neutrophil reactions such as chemotaxis, aggregation, degranulation, and oxygen-radical production. The underlying mechanism of tissue damage is widespread vascular endothelial injury, with fluid extravasation and microthrombosis that decrease oxygen and substrate utilization by affected tissues. Nitric oxide is a mediator of septic shock.

For NM, primary focus is usually a subclinical nasopharynx infection. Shortly after adherence to nasopharyngeal mucosa, encapsulated NM are transported through nonciliated epithelial cells in large, membrane-bound vacuoles. Within 24 h NM are observed in submucosa in close proximity to local immune cells and blood vessels. NM gain access to circulation; invading NM may either be killed or multiply and initiate bacteremic stage. Hematogenous dissemination seeds the skin and meninges. Signs/symptoms of systemic disease appear concurrently with meningococcemia, preceding symptoms of meningitis by 24 to 48 h. Edema, infarction of overlying skin, and extravasation of RBC are responsible for the characteristic macular, papular, petechial, hemorrhagic, and bullous lesions. Similar vascular lesions occur in the meninges and in other tissues. Systemic meningococcal infection is primarily a bacteremic disease; NM exhibits marked trophism for meninges and skin, and to a lesser degree for synovia, serosal surfaces, and adrenal glands. NM replicate at a rapid rate; within hours, patient may deteriorate from good health to irreversible shock, marked hemorrhagic diathesis, and death. In chronic meningococcemia, usually during periodic fevers, rash, and joint manifestations, NM can be isolated from the blood; unusual host-parasite relationship is central to this persistent infection.

HISTORY

Symptoms *Acute Meningococcemia* In most cases, nasopharyngeal infection is subclinical; mild URI symptoms occasionally develop. Spiking fever, chills, arthralgia, myalgia.

Stupor, hemorrhagic lesions, hypotension may be evident within a few hours of onset of symptoms in fulminant meningococcemia.

Chronic Meningococcemia Intermittent fever, rash, myalgia, arthralgia, headache, anorexia.

PHYSICAL EXAMINATION

Skin Lesions

Nonspecific Cutaneous Findings Often subtle. Acrocyanosis, ischemic necrosis of peripheral tissues, most commonly digits, associated with hypotension, DIC.

Specific Skin Lesions *Petechiae* Cutaneous/oropharyngeal suggest meningococcal infection; less commonly *Haemophilus influenzae*. In patient with tick bite living in endemic area, Rocky Mountain spotted fever.

Ecthyma Gangrenosum See Figure 20-28. *Pseudomonas aeruginosa* most commonly; also *Aeromonas hydrophila*.

Hemorrhagic Bullous Lesions *Vibrio vulnificus* in patient (diabetes mellitus, liver disease) with history of eating raw oysters (Fig. 20-29) *Capnocytophaga canimorsus* or *C. cynodegmi* following dog bite.

S. aureus (Fig. 20-40).

Generalized Erythema *S. aureus,* group A streptococcus (GAS) with toxic shock syndrome.

Acute Meningococcemia *Early Exanthem* Occurs soon after onset of disease in 75% of cases; pink, 2- to 10-mm macules/papules, sparsely distributed on trunk/lower extremities as well as face, palate, conjunctivae (Fig. 20-41).

Later Lesions Petechiae appear in center of macules. Lesions become hemorrhagic within hours. In severe cases, petechiae may become confluent and develop into hemorrhagic bullae with extensive ulcerations. *Fulminant*: purpura, ecchymoses and confluent, often bizarre-shaped grayish to black necrosis (purpura fulminans) associated with DIC in fulminant disease (Fig. 20-42).

Fulminant Meningococcemia Associated with shock, hypotension, peripheral vasoconstriction with cold cyanotic extremities. Peripheral gangrene may occur, requiring amputation in those who survive.

Complications Intercurrent infections, CNS damage. Patients who recover may have necrosis of skin, distal extremities, tips of ears/nose.

Chronic Meningococcemia Intermittent appearance of lesions. Macular and papular lesions, usually distributed about one or more painful joints or pressure points. Petechiae, which may evolve to vesicles or pustules. Minute hemorrhage with paler areola. Purpuric areas with pale blue-gray centers; hemorrhagic tender nodules.

General Examination

Fever (may be absent in neonates, elderly patients, persons with uremia, alcoholism).

Skin / Soft Tissue Infection as Source of Sepsis Cellulitis, pustules, bullae, hemorrhagic lesions. Hematogenously disseminated toxins can result in diffuse cutaneous reactions such as erythema.

GI Manifestations Nausea, vomiting, diarrhea, ileus; stress ulcer. Liver; cholestatic jaundice; hepatocellular/canalicular dysfunction. Prolonged hypotension: acute hepatic injury; ischemic bowel necrosis.

Acute Meningococcemia High fever, tachypnea, tachycardia, mild hypotension. Patient appears acutely ill with marked prostration.

Meningitis 50 to 88% of patients with meningococcemia develop meningitis. Signs of meningeal irritation, altered consciousness. Agitated, maniacal behavior. Signs of increased intracranial pressure.

Fulminant Meningococcemia More rapid progression and overwhelming character. Occurs in 10 to 20% of cases of meningococcal disease; characterized by development of shock, DIC, and multiple-organ failure.

Less Common Manifestations Arthritis (5 to 10%), pneumonia, sinusitis, otitis media, conjunctivitis, endophthalmitis, endocarditis, pericarditis, urethritis, endometritis.

Chronic Meningococcemia Intermittent fever, arthritis/arthralgia.

DIFFERENTIAL DIAGNOSIS

Acute Meningococcemia and Meningitis Acute bacteremia and endocarditis, acute "hypersensitivity" vasculitis, enteroviral infections, Rocky Mountain spotted fever, toxic shock syndrome.

Chronic Meningococcemia Subacute bacterial endocarditis, acute rheumatic fever, Henoch-Schönlein purpura, rat-bite fever, erythema multiforme, gonococcemia.

LABORATORY EXAMINATIONS

Direct Microscopy Examine skin/mucosal surfaces. Gram stain of material from primary site of infection or from infected cutaneous lesions. In overwhelming infection (pneumococcal sepsis in splenectomized patient or fulminant meningococcemia), microorganisms can be seen in buffy coat. In meningococcemia, scrapings from nodular lesions show gram-negative diplococci.

Hematology Leukocytosis with left shift, thrombocytopenia; later leukopenia. Neutrophils contain toxic granules, Döhle bodies, cytoplasmic vacuoles.

Clotting Studies Prolonged thrombin time, decreased fibrinogen, presence of D-dimers.

Chemistry Hyperbilirubinemia, increased creatinine.

Cultures *Blood* Obtain at least two blood samples (from different venipuncture sites) for culture. Gram-negative bacteremia is low-grade; multiple blood cultures or prolonged incubation of cultures may be necessary. *S. aureus* grows rapidly and is most easily detectable. Negative blood cultures may reflect prior antibiotic administration, slow-growing or fastidious organisms, or absence of microbial invasion of bloodstream. Acute meningococcemia, NM in nearly 100%; meningitis, one-third positive.

Skin/Soft Tissue Obtain cultures from sites of possible cutaneous infection.

CSF Culture Acute meningococcemia, usually positive.

Culture of Lesional Skin Biopsy Specimen Up to 85%.

DIAGNOSIS

Definitive etiologic diagnosis requires isolation of microorganism from blood or local site of infection.

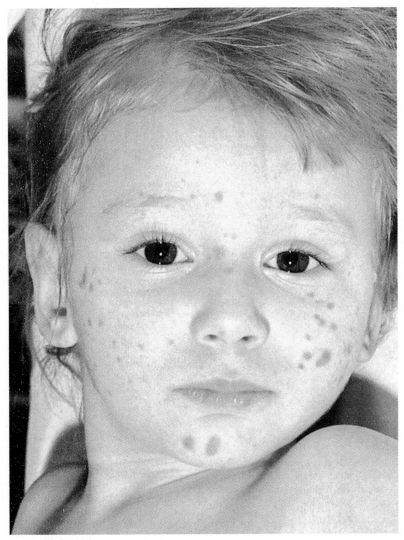

Figure 20-41 Acute meningococcemia *Discrete, pink-to-purple macules and papules as well as purpura on the face of this young child. These lesions represent early disseminated intravascular coagulation with its cutaneous manifestation, purpura fulminans.*

COURSE AND PROGNOSIS

Ventilation-perfusion mismatching produces a fall in arterial P_{O_2} early in course, which may progress to adult respiratory distress syndrome (ARDS). Severe decrease in systemic vascular resistance results in generalized maldistribution of blood flow, functional hypovolemia, diffuse capillary leakage of intravascular components. Cardiac output may intially be elevated; subsequent cardiac dysfunction common. Renal failure occurs due to hypotension and capillary injury. Platelet counts low in patients with DIC; low counts reflect diffuse endothelial injury. Approximately 25 to 35% of patients with severe sepsis and 40 to 45% of those with septic shock die within 30 days; others die within the ensuing 5 months.

Acute Meningococcemia   Untreated, ends fatally. Adequately treated, recovery rate for meningitis or meningococcemia is >90%. Mortality rate for fulminant meningococcemia remains very high. Prognosis is poor when purpura/ecchymoses are present at time of diagnosis.

Chronic Meningococcemia   Untreated, may recur over a few weeks to 8 months; average duration 6 to 8 weeks; may evolve into acute meningococcemia, meningitis, endocarditis; 100% cure with antibiotics.

MANAGEMENT

Requires urgent measures to treat local infection, provide hemodynamic and respiratory support, and eliminate offending organism. Outcome depends on underlying disease.

Immunization for Meningococcus   <20% of NM isolates from associated disease belong to serogroups for which vaccines are available: A, C, W-135, Y.

Prophylaxis of Contacts of Primary Cases of Meningococcemia *Rifampin*   600 mg bid in adults; 10 mg/kg/d as two equal portions in children 1 to 12 years; 5 mg/kg/d as two equal portions for newborns for 2 days.

Minocycline   100 mg bid for 5 days in adults.

Ciprofloxacin   Also effective.

Prevention   Reduce number of invasive procedures, limit use of indwelling vascular and bladder catheters, reduce incidence and duration of profound neutropenia (<500 neutrophils/mL), aggressively treat localized nosocomial infections.

Surgery   Removal or drainage of focal source of infection is essential.

Antimicrobial Therapy   In the absence of an obvious source of infection, antimicrobial regimen differs in the following types of patients: immuncompetent adult, neutropenic patient, splenectomized patient, injecting drug user, HIV-infected patient.

Any febrile patient with a petechial rash should be considered to have NM infection; blood culture should be obtained; treatment begun without awaiting confirmation.

Acute Meningococcemia

Penicillin G   300,000 U/kg/ IV up to 24 million U/d. Alternatives: ceftriaxone, cefotaxime.

Ampicillin   IV for 10 days.

Chloramphenicol   In penicillin-allergic individuals.

Antibiotic Therapy of Sepsis Due to Other Microbes   Depends on the sensitivity of the infecting organism (Tables 20-1 and 20-8).

Hemodynamic, Respiratory, Metabolic Support   Primary goal is to restore adequate oxygen and substrate delivery to tissues. Adequate fluids should be infused to treat intravascular volume depletion. Adrenal insufficiency should be considered in patients with refractory hypotension, fulminant meningococcemia, prior glucocorticoid use, disseminated tuberculosis, HIV disease. Ventilator therapy is indicated for progressive hypoxia, hypercapnia, neurologic deterioration, respiratory muscle failure.

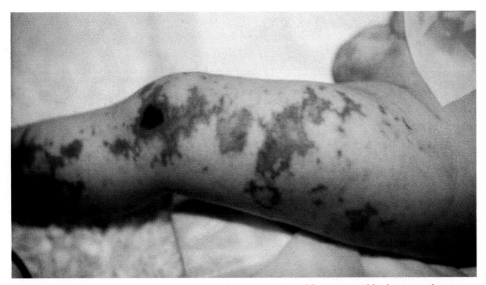

Figure 20-42   Acute meningococcemia: purpura fulminans   *Maplike, gray-to-black areas of cutaneous infarction of the leg in a child with* NM *meningitis and disseminated intravascular coagulation with purpura fulminans.*

GRAM-NEGATIVE INFECTIONS

Bartonella Infections

Bartonella species are tiny gram-negative bacilli that can invade mammalian cells such as endothelial cells and erythrocytes. Clinical syndromes caused by *Bartonella* (Table 20-6) include cat-scratch disease (CSD), bacillary angiomatosis, endocarditis, Oroya fever, and verruga peruana; manifestations vary with the immune status of the host.

Verruga peruana and Oroya fever are caused by *B. bacillliformis,* which is transmitted by the bite of the sandfly *Phlebotomus* in Andean valleys. The initial presentation is of a severe febrile illness associated with profound anemia with significant morbidity and mortality. Verruga peruana, which appears after convalescence from acute Oroya fever, presents as red-purple cutaneous lesions, tiny to sessile to large, pedunculated, and nodular; these lesions resemble the angiomatous lesions of bacillary angiomatosis or Kaposi's sarcoma.

Trench fever is caused by *B. quintana* and *B. henselae,* presenting as a febrile systemic illness with prolonged bacteremia. There are no cutaneous manifestations.

Table 20-6   CLINICAL SYNDROME CAUSED BY *BARTONELLA* SPECIES

Clinical Syndrome	Causative *Bartonella*
Oroya fever	*B. bacilliformis*
Verruga peruana	*B. bacilliformis*
Trench fever	*B. quintana, B. henselae*
Endocarditis (*Bartonella* bacteremic syndrome)	*B. quintana, B. henselae, B. elizabethae*
Cat-scratch disease	*B. henselae*
Cutaneous bacillary angiomatosis	*B. quintana, B. henselae*
Peliosis hepatis (liver involvement)	*B. quintana, B. henselae*
Parenchymal bacillary peliosis (liver and spleen involvement)	*B. quintana, B. henselae*

Cat-Scratch Disease

Cat-scratch disease (CSD) is a benign, self-limited zoonotic infection characterized by a primary skin or conjunctival lesion after cat scratches or contact with a cat and subsequent acute to subacute tender regional lymphadenopathy, as well as systemic symptoms that may be debilitating. *Synonyms:* Cat-scratch fever, benign lymphoreticulosis, nonbacterial regional lymphadenitis.

EPIDEMIOLOGY

Age of Onset Most patients <21 years in the United States.

Sex Males>females.

Incidence 20,000 cases annually in the United States, of whom 2000 are hospitalized.

Etiology *Bartonella henselae, B. quintana.*

Transmission History of cat contact in 90% of cases; of these individuals, 75% have history of scratch, bite, or lick. Blood cultures of kittens frequently are positive for *B. henselae*. Adult cats are blood culture–negative but are *B. henselae*–seropositive. Familial cases may occur shortly after addition of a kitten to the household. Fleas transmit infection between cats. Whether flea bite can transmit infection to humans is unknown.

Season Late fall, winter, or early spring in cooler climates; July and August in warmer climates. Worldwide.

PATHOGENESIS

B. henselae causes granulomatous inflammation in healthy individuals (CSD) and angiogenesis in immuncompromised persons.

HISTORY

Incubation Period Primary lesion at bite/scratch site: 1 to 8 weeks (average, 2 weeks). Regional lymphadenopathy: 5 to 50 days after primary lesion appears. A local primary lesion occurs in about half of patients.

Prodrome Mild fever and malaise occur in less than half the patients. Chills, general aching, and nausea are infrequently present.

PHYSICAL EXAMINATION

Skin Lesions *Primary* Innocuous-looking, small (1.5 cm) papule, vesicle, or pustule at the inoculation site; may ulcerate; skin color pink to red; firm, at times tender. Residual linear cat scratch. Associated regional lymphadenitis (Fig. 20-43). Primary lesion on exposed skin of head, neck, extremities. Uncommonly: urticaria, transient maculopapular eruption, vesiculopapular lesions, erythema nodosum.

Mucous Membranes If portal of entry is the conjunctiva, 3-to 5-mm whitish-yellow granulation on palpebral conjunctiva associated with tender preauricular and/or cervical lymphadenopathy (oculoglandular syndrome of Parinaud).

General Examination Most patients do not have fever. Systemic symptoms common. Regional lymphadenopathy (Fig. 20-43) evident within a few days to a few weeks after the primary lesion, which has usually resolved by the time lymphadenopathy occurs. Nodes are usually solitary, moderately tender, freely movable. Involved lymph nodes: epitrochlear, axillary, pectoral, cervical. Nodes may suppurate. Generalized lymphadenopathy or involvement of the lymph nodes of more than one region is unusual. Less common: encephalitis, pneumonitis, thrombocytopenia, osteomyelitis, hepatitis, abscesses in liver or spleen.

DIFFERENTIAL DIAGNOSIS

Regional Lymphadenopathy, Distal Cutaneous Lesion Suppurative bacterial lymphadenitis, atypical mycobacteria, sporotrichosis, tularemia, toxoplasmosis, infectious mononucleosis, tumors, sarcoidosis, lymphogranuloma venereum, coccidioidomycosis.

Other Cat-Associated Infections *Pasteurella multocida* bite infection, *Capnocytophaga* (DF-2) spp. bite infection, sporotrichosis, *Microsporum canis* dermatophytosis, *Toxocara cata* (larva migrans), *Dirofilaria repens* subcutaneous nodules.

LABORATORY EXAMINATIONS

Hematology WBC usually normal; ESR commonly elevated.

Dermatopathology Primary lesion: middermal, small areas of frank necrosis surrounded by necrobiosis and palisaded histiocytes; multinucleated giant cells and eosinophils also may be seen. Demonstration of small, pleomorphic bacilli in Warthin-Starry–stained sections of primary skin lesion, conjunctiva, or lymph nodes. Lymph nodes: granulomatous inflammation with stellate necrosis without angiomatosis.

Culture Isolation of *B. henselae* from lymph node aspirates is seldom possible, perhaps because the strains of *Bartonella* causing CSD are more fastidious than those that cause bacteremia or because the lymph node aspirates contain few viable bacteria.

Serology Antibodies to *B. henselae* usually positive ≥1:64.

Polymerase Chain Reaction (PCR) *B. henselae* DNA detected in aspirates of pus from involved lymph nodes in 96% of cases.

DIAGNOSIS

Suggested by regional lymphadenopathy developing over a 2- to 3-week period in an individual with cat contact and a primary lesion at the site of contact and confirmed by identification of *B. henselae* from tissue or serodiagnosis.

COURSE AND PROGNOSIS

Self-limiting, usually within 1 to 2 months. Uncommonly, prolonged morbidity with persistent high fever, suppurative lymphadenitis, severe systemic symptoms. Uncommonly, cat-scratch encephalopathy occurs. Antibiotic therapy has not been very effective in altering the course of the infection.

MANAGEMENT

Symptomatic in most cases.

Antimicrobial Therapy In comparison with bacillary angiomatosis, which is also caused by *B. henselae,* specific antimicrobial therapies have not proved effective in treatment of CSD. Ciprofloxacin, doxycycline, erythromycin may be effective.

Surgery Occasionally, surgical drainage of suppurative node is indicated.

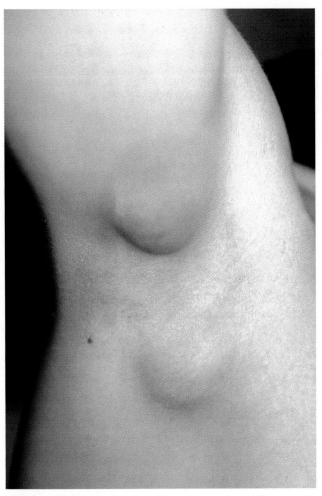

Figure 20-43 Bartonellosis: cat-scratch disease *Acute, very tender, axillary lymphadenopathy in a child; cat scratches were present on the dorsum of the ipsilateral hand. (Courtesy of Howard Heller, M.D.)*

Bacillary Angiomatosis

Bacillary angiomatosis (BA) is a systemic infection caused by *Bartonella* species, occurring nearly exclusively in HIV-infected individuals, characterized by cutaneous vascular tumors resembling Kaposi's sarcoma and symptomatic multisystemic infection, most commonly involving the liver (peliosis hepatis) and/or spleen (parenchymal bacillary peliosis).

EPIDEMIOLOGY

Etiology *B. henselae* and *B. quintana*. In immunocompetent individuals, *B. henselae* is also the agent of cat-scratch disease. Incidence has markedly diminished in HIV disease in past decade.

Reservoir *B. henselae* frequently causes asymptomatic bacteremia in kittens, which has been documented by isolation of the organism by blood cultures or anti-*B. henselae* antibodies. The reservoir for *B. quintana* is unknown.

Transmission (See also Cat-Scratch Disease) Presumably enters percutaneously through minor breaks in the epidermis (scratches or bites). The role of the cat flea in transmission to humans is unclear. Reservoir of *B. quintana* is not known; probably transmitted by ectoparasites (mites, lice).

Risk Factors BA occurs almost exclusively in HIV-infected individuals with advanced immunodeficiency. Uncommonly, in individuals who are immunocompetent, immunocompromised for other reasons, or organ-transplant recipients.

PATHOGENESIS

Bartonella spp. cause vascular proliferation (angiogenesis): *B. bacilliformis,* verruga peruana; *B. henselae* and *B. quintana,* BA.

HISTORY

Incubation Period Unknown, but probably days to weeks.

History Owning or having been scratched by a kitten. Patients with localized infection may be free of systemic symptoms. Those with more widespread disseminated infection have fever, malaise, weight loss.

Cutaneous BA Lesions may be painful, in contrast with Kaposi's sarcoma lesions, which are not painful.

Disseminated BA Skin lesions usually absent. Presents with nausea, vomiting, diarrhea, fever, chills. Bony lesions may cause focal bone pain.

PHYSICAL EXAMINATION

Skin Lesions Papules or nodules resembling angiomas (red, bright red, violaceous, or skin-colored) (Fig. 20-44); up to 2 to 3 cm in diameter; usually situated in dermis with thinning or erosion of overlying epidermis surrounded by a collarette of scale. Pyogenic granuloma– like lesions (Fig. 20-44). Subcutaneous nodules, 1 to 2 cm in diameter, resembling cysts. Uncommonly, abscess formation. Papules/nodules range from solitary lesions to >100 and, rarely, >1000. Firm, nonblanching. Lesions may be nontender or painful, a finding not seen in nodular lesions of Kaposi's sarcoma. Any site, but palms and soles are usually spared. Occasionally, lesions occur at the site of a cat scratch. A solitary lesion presenting as a dactylitis.

Mucous Membranes Angioma-like lesions of lips and oral mucosa. Laryngeal involvement with obstruction.

Systemic Findings Infection may spread hematogenously or via lymphatics to become systemic, commonly involving the liver and spleen (hepatosplenomegaly, liver abscesses, necrotizing splenitis, hepatic/splenic necrotizing granulomata). Lesions also may occur in the heart (cardiac lesions, endocarditis), bone marrow, lymph nodes, muscles, and soft tissues, CNS (brain abscess, aseptic meningitis, encephalopathy).

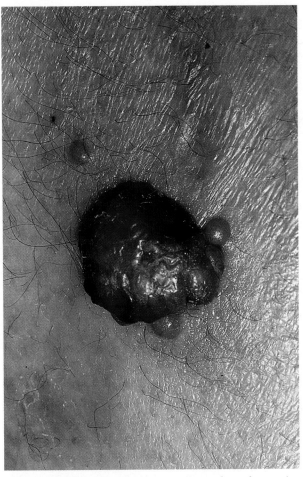

Figure 20-44 Bartonellosis: bacillary angiomatosis *3- to 5-mm cherry hemangioma-like papules and a larger pyogenic granuloma-like nodule on the shin of a male with advanced HIV disease. Subcutaneous nodular lesions were also present.*

DIFFERENTIAL DIAGNOSIS

Multiple Cutaneous Angiomatous Papules/ Nodules Kaposi's sarcoma, pyogenic granuloma, epithelioid (histiocytoid) angioma, cherry angioma, sclerosing hemangioma, disseminated cryptococcosis.

LABORATORY EXAMINATIONS

Histopathology *Dermatopathology* Lobular vascular proliferations composed of plump "epithelioid" endothelia. Neutrophils scattered throughout the lesion, especially around eosinophilic granular aggregates, which are masses of bacteria (visualized by Warthin-Starry staining or electron microscopy).

Liver Biopsy Associated with higher morbidity and mortality rates in that the lesions are vascular tumors. Dilated capillaries or multiple blood-filled cavernous spaces; myxoid stroma containing an admixture of inflammatory cells and granular clumps (*Bartonella*).

Culture *Bartonella* can be isolated from lesional skin biopsy specimens, blood, or other infected tissues on endothelial-cell monolayer.

PCR Detects *Bartonella* DNA in tissue.

Chemistry Bacillary peliosis hepatis associated with elevated γ-glutamyltransferase, alkaline phosphatase.

Serology Anti-*Bartonella* antibodies detected by indirect fluorescent-antibody testing (detected by the Centers for Disease Control and Prevention). Also, enzyme immunoassay for detection of IgG antibodies to *B. henselae*.

Imaging Lesions can be visualized by conventional radiographs and nuclear imaging. Lesions regress with appropriate therapy. CT scan shows hepatomegaly, ±splenomegaly.

DIAGNOSIS

Clinical findings confirmed by demonstration of *Bartonella* bacilli on silver stain of lesional biopsy specimen or culture or antibody studies.

COURSE AND PROGNOSIS

Course variable. In some individuals, lesions regress spontaneously. Untreated systemic infection causes significant morbidity and mortality. With effective antimicrobial therapy, lesions resolve within 1 to 2 weeks. As with other infections occurring in HIV disease, relapse may occur and require lifelong secondary prophylaxis. Azithromycin given for *Mycobacterium avium* complex (MAC) prophylaxis seems to prevent BA. BA does not occur in HIV-infected individuals treated with (and responding to) highly active antiretroviral therapy (HAART).

MANAGEMENT

Prevention HIV-infected individuals should avoid contact with cats, especially kittens, to minimize the risk for acquiring BA, as well as toxoplasmosis.

Antimicrobial Therapy Given for 8 to 12 weeks. A Jarisch-Herxheimer type reaction may occur shortly after beginning therapy.

- Erythromycin 500 mg PO qid *or*
- Doxycycline 100 mg PO bid *or*
- Ciprofloxacin 750 mg PO bid *or*
- Azithromycin 500 mg PO qd

Secondary Prophylaxis Lifelong maintenance if relapses occur.

Tularemia

Tularemia is an acute infection transmitted by handling flesh of infected animals, by the bite of insect vectors, by inoculation of conjunctiva, by ingestion of infected food, or by inhalation; it manifests as four patterns: ulceroglandular, oculoglandular, typhoidal, pulmonary.
Synonyms: rabbit fever, deerfly fever.

EPIDEMIOLOGY

Age of Onset/Sex   Young males.

Etiology   *Francisella tularensis,* a pleomorphic gram-negative coccobacillus.

Occupation   Rabbit hunters, butchers, cooks, agricultural workers, trappers, campers, sheep herders and shearers, mink ranchers, muskrat farmers, laboratory technicians.

Transmission   (1) Small abrasion or puncture wound, bites of infected deerflies/ticks; (2) conjunctival inoculation; (3) ingestion of infected meat; (4) inhalation. Animal reservoir—rabbits, foxes, squirrels, skunks, muskrats, voles, beavers. Insect vectors—ticks (*Ixodes, Dermacentor*), body lice, deerfly.

Season   Greatest frequency in summer (tick season) and rabbit-hunting season.

Geography   Throughout northern hemisphere. United States: midwest in summer; east of Mississippi in winter.

Clinical Syndromes   Ulceroglandular, glandular, pulmonary, oropharyngeal, oculoglandular, typhoidal.

PATHOGENESIS

After inoculation, *F. tularensis* reproduces and spreads through lymphatic channels to lymph nodes and bloodstream.

HISTORY

Incubation Period   2 to 10 days.

Symptoms   Prodrome: headache, malaise, myalgia, high fever. About 48 h after inoculation, pruritic papule develops at the site of trauma or insect bite followed by enlargement of regional lymph nodes.

PHYSICAL EXAMINATION

Skin Lesions   At inoculation site: erythematous tender papule evolving to a vesicopustule, enlarging to crusted ulcer with raised, sharply demarcated margins (96 h) (Fig. 20-45). Depressed center that is often covered by a black eschar (chancriform). Primary lesion on finger/hand at site of trauma/insect bite; groin/axilla after tick bite. After bacteremia, exanthem (trunk and extremities) with macules, papules, petechiae; erythema multiforme; erythema nodosum.

Mucous Membranes   In oculoglandular tularemia, F. tularensis is inoculated into conjunctiva, causing a purulent conjunctivitis with pain, edema, congestion. Small yellow nodules occur on conjunctivae and ulcerate.

General Findings   Fever to 41°C.

Regional Lymph Nodes   As the ulcer develops, nodes enlarge and become tender (chancriform syndrome) (Fig. 20-45). If untreated, become suppurating buboes. Lung consolidation, splenomegaly, generalized lymphadenopathy, hepatomegaly may occur.

Variants   "Typhoidal" form occurs with ingestion of *F. tularensis*, resulting in ulcerative or exudative pharyngotonsillitis with cervical lymphadenopathy. Tularemic pneumonia occurs after bacteremia or inhalation of *F. tularensis.*

DIFFERENTIAL DIAGNOSIS

Inoculation Site   Furuncle, paronychia, ecthyma, anthrax, *Pasteurella multocida* infection, sporotrichosis, *Mycobacterium marinum* infection.

Tender Regional Adenopathy   Herpes simplex virus lymphadenitis, plague, cat-scratch disease, melioidosis or glanders, lymphogranuloma venereum.

LABORATORY EXAMINATIONS

Cultures   Routine culture media do not support the growth of *F. tularensis* from clinical specimens.

Serology   Diagnosis usually confirmed by demonstrating a fourfold rise in acute and convalescent *F. tularensis* antibody titers.

DIAGNOSIS

Clinical diagnosis in a patient with chancriform syndrome with appropriate animal exposure or insect exposure and systemic manifestations. Disease in pneumonic presentation has "flulike" symptomatology and is fatal if unrecognized.

COURSE AND PROGNOSIS

Untreated, mortality rate for ulceroglandular form, 5% typhoidal and pulmonary forms, 30%.

MANAGEMENT

Prevention   Avoid contact with wild rabbits. In tick-infested areas, wear tight wristbands and pants tucked into boots to prevent tick attachment. Inspect for ticks at day's end. Vaccine in development. Wear rubber gloves when handling or processing wild rabbits.

Drug of Choice   Streptomycin, 1 to 2 g/d for 7 to 10 afebrile days, is most effective at cure and prevention of relapse.

Alternatives   Gentamycin, tetracycline, chloramphenicol effect lower cure rate and higher relapse rates.

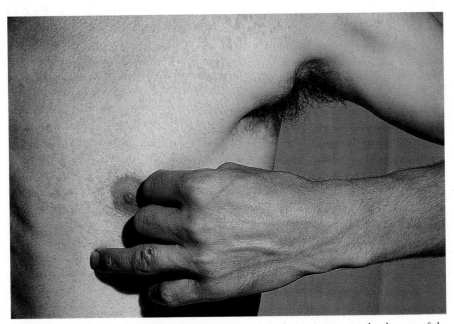

Figure 20-45 Tularemia *A crusted ulcer at the site of inoculation is seen on the dorsum of the left ring finger with associated axillary lymph node enlargement (chancriform syndrome). The infection occurred after the patient killed and skinned a rabbit.*

Cutaneous *Pseudomonas Aeruginosa* Infections ~~not related to~~

Pseudomonas aeruginosa exists in moist environments associated with hospitals. Hospitalized compromised individuals become colonized with the organism. Local invasion can follow colonization of any mucocutaneous site with local infection and/or hematogenous dissemination. Ecthyma gangrenosum (EG) is the necrotizing soft-tissue infection that occurs after local tissue invasion or bacteremic seeding, associated with blood vessel invasion, septic vasculitis, vascular occlusion, and infarction of tissue.

EPIDEMIOLOGY

Etiology *P. aeruginosa* is a small, aerobic gram-negative bacillus; motile by a single polar flagellum. Half of all clinical isolates produce blue-green pigment pyocyanin.

Ecology *P. aeruginosa* is widespread in nature, inhabiting water, soil, plants, and animals, preferring moist environments. Carriage rate is low in healthy individuals. Colonizes skin, external ear, upper respiratory tract, and/or large bowel in those who are naturally or iatrogenically compromised, have received antimicrobial therapy, and/or been exposed to a hospital environment.

Transmission Most infections are hospital acquired. Pseudomonal carriage increases with length of hospital stay and antibiotic administration. Transmitted to patients via hands of hospital personnel or via fomites. Entry sites for bacteremia at breaks in mucocutaneous barriers: sites of trauma, foreign bodies (IV or urinary catheter), aspiration/aerosolization into respiratory tract, decubitus or skin ulcers, thermal burns.

Risk Factors for Invasive Infection Hospitalization; immunocompromise; granulocytopenia; use of cancer chemotherapy, glucocorticoids, antibiotics (recently); catheters (IV, urethral); cancer; debilitation; mucosal ulceration.

PATHOGENESIS

P. aeruginosa rarely causes disease in the healthy host. Infections occur when normal cutaneous or mucosal barriers have been breached or bypassed (e.g., burn injury, penetrating trauma, surgery, endotracheal intubation, urinary bladder catheterization, IV drug abuse); when immunologic defense mechanisms compromised (e.g., by chemotherapy-induced neutropenia, hypogammaglobulinemia, extremes of age, diabetes mellitus, cystic fibrosis, cancer, HIV disease); when protective function of normal bacterial flora has been disrupted by broad-spectrum antimicrobial therapy; and/or when patient has been exposed to reservoirs associated with hospital environment. Infections caused by *P. aeruginosa* begin with superficial colonization of cutaneous or mucosal surfaces and progress to localized bacterial invasion and damage of underlying tissue. Infection may remain anatomically localized or may spread by direct extension to contiguous structures. Blood vessel and bloodstream invasion, dissemination, systemic inflammatory-response syndrome (SIRS) (sepsis syndrome), multiple-organ dysfunction, and, ultimately, death may follow localized infection. The organism and/or its products may cause tissue injury at primary and secondary sites of infection; release of systemically acting toxins or inflammatory mediators of infected host may contribute directly or indirectly to SIRS.

HISTORY

Symptoms Local pain; high fever, chills.

PHYSICAL FINDINGS

Nail Colonization *P. aeruginosa* grows on the undersurface of onycholytic nails, e.g., psoriasis, onychomycosis; the debrided inner surface of the nail plate has a surface green discoloration that can easily be abraded off.

Folliculitis *P. aeruginosa* can infect multiple hair follicles in healthy indivuals after aqueous exposure in hot tubs ("hot-tub folliculitis") or physiotherapy pools, presenting as multiple follicular pustules on the trunk (Fig. 20-15). The infection is self-limited. In immunocompromised host, may progress to EG.

Toe Webspace Infection Intertrigo of toe webspaces. Webspace(s) macerated, moist with green color (Fig. 20-7); usually in the setting of hyperhidrosis, ±macerated interdigital tinea pedis, ±erythrasma, ±keratoderma.

Primary and Secondary Pyoderma *P. aeruginosa* can cause primary infection of hair follicles or small breaks in skin, or secondary infections of sites of trauma, burn injury, inflammatory dermatoses, ulcers. With deeper invasion, necrotizing infection (due to blood vessel invasion and occlusion) occur, i.e., EG. These pyodermas have a typical blue-green exudate and characteristic fruity odor. In thermal burn injury, black, dark brown, or violaceous discoloration of burn eschar may occur.

External Otitis "Swimmer's ear." Moist environment of external auditory canal provides medium for superficial infection, presenting as pruritus, pain, discharge; usually self-limited. Malignant external otitis occurs in elderly diabetics most commonly; may progress to deeper invasive infection.

Ecthyma Gangrenosum Begins as erythematous macule (cutaneous ischemic lesion that quickly evolves to an infarction) (Fig. 20-28). The epidermis overlying the ischemic area may form a bulla or slough with formation of erosion/ulcer. EG usually occurs as solitary lesion but may occur as a few lesions. EG can occur as a complication of primary or secondary pyoderma or of bacteremia. Initially erythematous, progressing to hemorrhagic bluish (so-called gunmetal gray). Fully evolved EG: blackish central necrosis with erythematous halo. Lesions usually tender, but may be painless. Most common sites: axillae, groin, perianal; may occur anywhere, including lip and tongue.

Bacteremia Common primary sites of infection: skin, soft tissues, urinary tract, GI tract, lungs, intravascular foci. EG develops in small minority of patients. Also, multiple subcutaneous nodules.

Endocarditis Left-sided infections present with embolic phenomena: large emboli, ecthyma gangrenosum, Janeway lesions, Osler's nodes (Figs. 20-37 and 20-38).

Gastrointestinal Infection "Rose" spotlike lesions: erythematous macules and/or papules on trunk as in typhoid fever; occur with *Pseudomonas* infection of GI tract, i.e., diarrhea, headache, high fever (Shanghai fever).

General Examination Bacteremia may be associated with SIRS; fever, tachypnea, tachycardia, prostration, hypotension.

DIFFERENTIAL DIAGNOSIS

Ischemic/Infarcted Plaque(s) Other conditions that produce skin lesions by direct involvement of blood vessels such as vasculitis, cryoglobulinemia, fixed drug eruption, pyoderma gangrenosum.

LABORATORY EXAMINATIONS

Cultures In most cases, *P. aeruginosa* can be cultured from both blood and ecthymatous skin lesions. However, EG can remain a localized cutaneous infection, not accompanied by systemic infection; in this case, only culture of exudate or biopsy specimen from the lesion is positive for *P. aeruginosa*.

Dermatopathology Vasculitis without thrombosis. Paucity of neutrophils at site of infection. Bacilli found in media and adventitia, but usually not in intima, of vessel.

DIAGNOSIS

Clinical suspicion confirmed by blood and skin exudate/biopsy specimen culture.

COURSE AND PROGNOSIS

The heterogeneity of infections accounts for substantial differences in short-term and long-term prognosis. Prognosis depends on prompt restoration of altered immunity, usually on correction of neutropenia. When occurring as a local infection in the absence of bacteremia, prognosis is much more favorable.

MANAGEMENT

Correct Predisposing Factors White cell transfusion or G-CSF for granulocytopenia.

Antimicrobial Therapy Antibiotic and dosage are adjusted according to sensitivities and results of cultures.

Surgery After control of infection, areas of infarction should be debrided.

MYCOBACTERIAL INFECTIONS

Mycobacteria are rod-shaped or coccobacilli identified by the property of acid-fastness, a characteristic associated with the composition of their cell walls. They cause infections in select populations globally. Although *Mycobacterium leprae* can be cultured in vivo in mice and armadillos, it causes disease in humans exclusively. Otherwise healthy individuals become infected with this mycobacterium; clinical manifestations vary tremendously according to the host's immune response to the organism. *M. tuberculosis* complex, (consisting of *M. tuberculosis, M. bovis,* and *M. africanum*) are pathogenic in otherwise healthy individuals; however, tuberculosis is much more florid in individuals who are compromised. With the exception of *M. leprae,* the other mycobacteria are referred to as atypical mycobacteria, mycobacteria other than tuberuculosis (MOTT), or nontuberculous mycobacteria (NTM). NTM exist in the environment; identification in human tissue, unlike *M. tuberculosis* or *M. leprae,* is not a sine qua non of etiology of a disorder.

EPIDEMIOLOGY

With the advent of HIV disease, tuberculosis and NTM infections have been brought to the forefront of clinical medicine. Concurrent HIV and *M. tuberculosis* infections can result in severe infections; disseminated infections with NTM are extremely common in advanced HIV disease.

Leprosy

Leprosy is a chronic granulomatous disease caused by *Mycobacterium leprae* and principally acquired during childhood or young adulthood. The skin, mucous membrane of the upper respiratory tract, and peripheral nerves are the major sites of involvement in all forms of leprosy. The clinical manifestations, natural history, and prognosis of leprosy are related to the host response, and the various types of leprosy (tuberculoid, lepromatous, etc.) represent the spectra of the host's immunologic response (cell-mediated immunity).
Synonym: Hansen's disease.

CLINICOPATHOLOGIC CLASSIFICATION OF LEPROSY

(Based on clinical, immunologic, and bacteriologic findings)

Tuberculoid (TL) Localized skin involvement and/or peripheral nerve involvement; few organisms are present in the skin biopsies.

Lepromatous (LL) Generalized involvement including skin, upper respiratory mucous membrane, the reticuloendothelial system, adrenal glands, and testes; many bacilli are present in tissue.

Borderline (or "Dimorphic") (BL) Has features of both tuberculoid and lepromatous leprosy. Usually many bacilli present, varied skin lesions: macules, plaques; progresses to TL or regresses to LL.

Indeterminate and Transitional Forms (See Pathogenesis, below)

EPIDEMIOLOGY

Age of Onset Incidence rate peaks at 10 to 20 years; prevalence peaks at 30 to 50 years.

Sex Males>females.

Race There appears to be an inverse relationship between the skin color and the severity of the disease; in the black African, susceptibility is high, but there is predominance of milder forms of the disease, i.e., TL vis-à-vis LL.

Etiology *M. leprae* is a slender, straight, or slightly curved, acid-fast rod, about 3 by .5 μm. The organism cannot be cultured in vitro.

Hosts Humans are the main reservoirs of *M. leprae*. Wild armadillos (Louisiana) as well as mangabey monkeys and chimpanzees are naturally infected with *M. leprae;* armadillos can develop lepromatous lesions.

Transmission Mode of transmission of *M. leprae* is uncertain; however, human-to-human transmission is the norm. The main source of dissemination is individuals with multibacillary-type infection, shedding several millions of bacilli per day in nasal and upper respiratory tract secretions. Portals of entry of *M. leprae* are poorly understood but include ingestion of food or drink, inoculation into or through skin (bites, scratches, small wounds, tattoos), or inhalation into nasal passages or lungs.

Scope of Problem Worldwide (estimated 12 million); approximately 5.5 million individuals are estimated to require or are receiving chemotherapy for leprosy, of whom 2 to 3 million have significant disabilities. Fifty-three countries report endemic leprosy. India has approximately 4 million cases.

Geography At present, more prevalent in hot and humid climates (Africa, Southeast Asia, and South and Central America). New lesions may first appear or suddenly flare during the hot, rainy season. The disease is endemic in Texas, southern Louisiana, Hawaii, and California, and immigrants with leprosy are not uncommonly seen in Florida and New York City. There are approximately 2500 patients with leprosy in the continental United States.

Predisposing or Risk Factors (1) Residence in an endemic area, (2) having a blood relative with leprosy, (3) poverty (malnutrition?), and (4) contact with affected armadillos.

PATHOGENESIS

The clinical spectrum of leprosy depends exclusively on variable limitations in the host's capability to develop effective cell-mediated immunity (CMI) to *M. leprae*. The organism is capable of invading and multiplying in peripheral nerves and infecting and surviving in endothelial and phagocytic cells in many organs. Subclinical infection with leprosy is common among residents in endemic areas. Presumably the subclinical infection is handled readily by the host's CMI response, Clinical expression of leprosy is the development of a granuloma; and the patient may develop a "reactional state," which may occur in some form in >50% of certain groups of patients. The granulomatous spectrum of leprosy consists of (1) a high-resistance tuberculoid response (TT), (2) a low- or absent-resistance lepromatous pole (LL), (3) a dimorphic or borderline region (BB) and two intermediary regions: (4) borderline lepromatous (BL), and (5) borderline tuberculoid (BT). In order of decreasing resistance, the spectrum is TT, BT, BB, BL, LL.

Immunologic Responses Immune responses to *M. leprae* can produce several types of reactions associated with a sudden change in the clinical status.

Lepra Type 1 Reactions (Downgrading and Reversal Reactions) Individuals with BT and BL develop inflammation within existing skin lesions. Downgrading reactions occur before therapy; reversal reactions occur in response to therapy. Type 1 reactions can be associated with low-grade fever, new multiple small "satellite" maculopapular skin lesions, and/or neuritis.

Lepra Type 2 Reactions (Erythema Nodosum Leprosum, ENL) Seen in half of LL patients, usually occurring after initiation of antilepromatous therapy, generally within the first 2 years of treatment. Massive inflammation with erythema nodosum-like lesions.

Lucio's Reaction Individuals with diffuse LL develop shallow, large polygonal sloughing ulcerations on the legs. The reaction appears to be either a variant of ENL or secondary to arteriolar occlusion. The ulcers heal poorly, recur frequently, and may occur in a generalized distribution. Generalized Lucio's reaction is frequently complicated by secondary bacterial infection and sepsis.

HISTORY

Onset Insidious and painless, first affects the peripheral nervous system with persistent or recurrent paresthesias and numbness without any visible clinical signs. At this stage there may be transient macular skin eruptions.

Systems Review Neural involvement leads to muscle weakness, muscle atrophy, severe neuritic pain, and contractures of the hands and feet.

Lepra Type 1 Reactions Acute or insidious tenderness and pain along affected nerve(s), associated with loss of function.

PHYSICAL EXAMINATION

Tuberculoid Leprosy *Type of Lesion* A few well-defined hypopigmented anesthetic mac-

ules (Fig. 20-46) with raised edges and varying in size from a few millimeters to very large lesions covering the entire trunk. Erythematous or purple border and hypopigmented center. Sharply defined, raised. Often annular. Any site including the face.

Nerve Involvement May be a thickened nerve on the edge of the lesion; large peripheral nerve enlargement frequent (ulnar).

Lepromatous Leprosy Small erythematous or hypopigmented macules that are anesthetic; later papules, plaques (Fig. 20-47) nodules, and diffuse thickening of the skin, with loss of hair (eyebrows and eyelashes). Leonina facies (lion's face) due to thickening, nodules, and plaques distort normal facial features. Normal skin color or erythematous or slightly hypopigmented.

Distribution of Lesions Bilaterally symmetric involving earlobes, face, arms, and buttocks, or less frequently the trunk and lower extremities. Tongue: nodules, plaques, or fissures.

Borderline Leprosy Lesions are intermediate between tuberculoid and lepromatous and comprised of macules, papules, and plaques (Fig. 20-48). Anesthesia and decreased sweating are prominent in the lesions.

Reactional Phenomenon *Lepra Type 1 Reactions* Skin lesions become acutely inflamed associated with edema and pain; may ulcerate. Edema most severe on face, hands, and feet.

Lepra Type 2 Reactions (ENL) Present as painful red skin nodules, arising superficially and deeply in contrast to true erythema nodosum; lesions form abscesses or ulcerate. Lesions occur most commonly on face and extensor limbs.

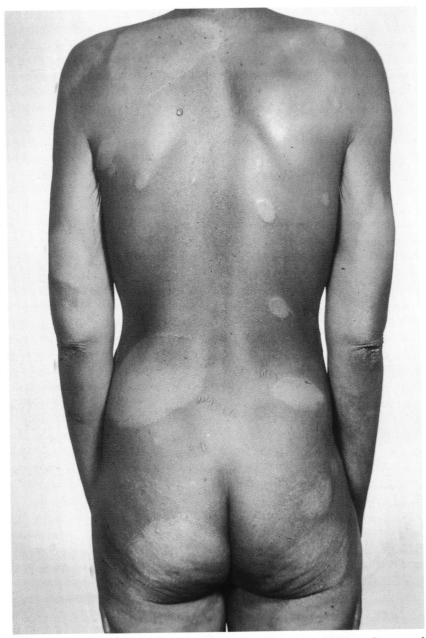

Figure 20-46   Leprosy: tuberculoid type   *Well-defined, hypopigmented, slightly scaling, anesthetic macules and plaques.*

Lucio's Reaction Presents as irregularly shaped erythematous plaques; lesions may resolve spontaneously or undergo necrosis with ulceration.

General Findings *Eye* The anterior chamber can be invaded in LL with resultant glaucoma and cataract formation. Corneal damage can occur secondary to trichiasis and sensory neuropathy, secondary infection, and muscle paralysis. Uveitis occurs in some individuals with ENL.

Testes May be involved in LL with resultant hypogonadism.

DIFFERENTIAL DIAGNOSIS

Tuberculoid Leprosy Epidermal dermatophytosis (tinea corporis), pityriasis alba, pityriasis versicolor, seborrheic dermatitis, vitiligo, morphea, yaws, onchocerciasis, nutritional dyschromia.

Lepromatous Leprosy Granuloma annulare, sarcoidosis, cutaneous tuberculosis, atypical mycobacterial infection, Wegener's granulomatosis, post-kala-azar dermal leishmaniasis, neurofibromatosis, necrobiosis lipoidica, Kaposi's sarcoma.

Borderline Leprosy Late syphilis, lupus erythematosus, gyrate erythemas, cutaneous leishmaniasis, mycosis fungoides.

Peripheral Neuropathy Peroneal muscular atrophy (Charcot-Marie-Tooth disease), Déjerine-Sottas disease (familial hypertrophic interstitial neuritis), primary amyloidosis of peripheral nerves, syringomyelia, tabes dorsalis, hereditary sensory radicular neuropathy, congenital indifference to pain, peripheral neuropathy of varied etiology.

Many Acid-Fast Bacilli in Biopsy Specimens of Skin or Other Tissues *M. avium-intracellulare* complex infection in HIV-infected individuals.

LABORATORY EXAMINATIONS

Slit-Skin Smears A small skin incision is made; the site is then scraped to obtain tissue fluid from which a smear is made and examined after Ziehl-Neelsen staining. Specimens are usually obtained from both earlobes and two other active lesions. The bacterial index (BI) is computed as shown in Table 20-7. Negative BIs are seen in paucibacillary cases, treated cases, and cases examined by an inexperienced technician.

Nasal Smears or Scrapings No longer recommended.

Culture *M. leprae* has not been cultured in vitro; however, it does grow when inoculated into the mouse foot pad. Routine bacterial cultures to rule out secondary infection.

PCR *M. leprae* DNA detected by this technique makes the diagnosis of early paucibacillary leprosy and identifies *M. leprae* after therapy.

Dermatopathology TL shows epithelioid cell granulomas forming around dermal nerves; acid-fast bacilli are sparse or absent. LL shows an extensive cellular infiltrate separated from the epidermis by a narrow zone of normal collagen. Skin appendages are destroyed. Macrophages are filled with *M. leprae,* having abundant foamy or vacuolated cytoplasm (lepra cells or Virchow cells).

DIAGNOSIS

Made if one or more of the cardinal findings are detected: skin lesions characteristic of leprosy with diminished or loss of sensation, enlarged

---

Table 20-7 BACTERIAL INDEX (BI)—RIDLEY'S LOGARITHMIC SCALE

0	No bacteria in 100 fields (oil immersion)
1+	1–10 bacteria in 100 fields
2+	1–10 bacteria in 10 fields
3+	1–10 bacteria in an average field
4+	10–100 bacteria in an average field
5+	100–1000 bacteria in an average field
6+	Many clumps of bacteria (>1000) in an average field

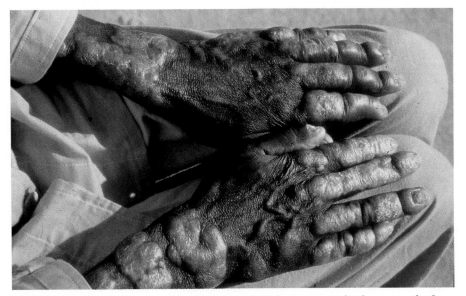

Figure 20-47   Leprosy: lepromatous type   *Nodules and thick plaques on the dorsum on the fingers, wrists, and forearms, with hypopigmentation of the overlying skin. Note the symmetry of involvement and loss of tissue of several finger tips.*

peripheral nerves, finding of *M. leprae* in skin or, less commonly, other sites.

COURSE AND PROGNOSIS

After the first few years of drug therapy, the most difficult problem is management of the changes secondary to neurologic deficits—contractures and trophic changes in the hands and feet. This requires a team of health care professionals: orthopedic surgeons, hand surgeons, podiatrists, opthalmologists, neurologists, physical medicine and rehabilitation professionals. Uncommonly, secondary amyloidosis with renal failure can complicate long-standing leprosy. Lepra type 1 reactions last 2 to 4 months in individuals with BT and up to 9 months in those with BL. Lepra type 2 reactions (ENL) occur in 50% of individuals with LL and 25% of those with BL within the first 2 years of treatment. ENL may be complicated by uveitis, dactylitis, arthritis, neuritis, lymphadenitis, myositis, orchitis. Lucio's reaction or phenomenon occurs secondary to vasculitis with subsequent infarction.

MANAGEMENT

General principles of management include: eradicate infection with antilepromatous therapy, prevent and treat reactions, reduce the risk of nerve damage, educate patient to deal with neuropathy and anesthesia, treat complications of nerve damage, rehabilitate patient into society. Management involves a broad multidisciplinary approach including orthopedic surgery, ophthalmology, and physical therapy.

Antilepromatous Therapy: Multidrug Regimens (Adult Doses)

Paucibacillary Disease (TT and BT)

Monthly, supervised	Rifampin, 600 mg
Daily, unsupervised	Dapsone, 100 mg
Duration	6 months; all treatments then stop
Follow-up after stopping treatment	Minimum of 2 years with clinical exams at least every 12 months

Multibacillary Disease (LL, BL, and BB)

Monthly, supervised medication	Rifampin, 600 mg Clofazimine, 300 mg
Daily, unsupervised medication	Dapsone, 100 mg Clofazimine, 50 mg
Duration	Minimum of 2 years, but whenever possible until slit-skin smears are negative
Follow-up after stopping treatment	Minimum of 5 years with clinical and bacteriologic examinations at least every 12 months

Therapy of Reactions

Lepra Type 1 Reactions *Prednisone,* 40 to 60 mg/d; the dosage is gradually reduced over a 2- to 3-month period. Indications for prednisone: neuritis, lesions that threaten to ulcerate, lesions appearing at cosmetically important sites (face).

Lepra Type 2 Reactions (ENL) *Prednisone,* 40 to 60 mg/d, tapered fairly rapidly; *Thalidomide* for recurrent ENL, 100 to 300 mg/d.

Lucio's Reaction Neither prednisone nor thalidomide is very effective, *Prednisone*, 40 to 60 mg/d, tapered fairly rapidly.

Systemic Antimicrobial Agents Secondary infection of ulcerations should be identified and treated with appropriate antibiotics to prevent deeper infections such as osteomyelitis.

Orthopedic Care Splints should be supplied to prevent contractures of denervated regions. Careful attention to foot care to prevent neuropathic ulceration.

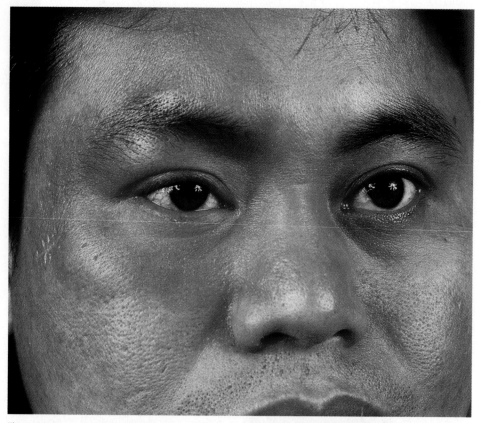

Figure 20-48 Leprosy: borderline-type *Well-demarcated, infiltrated, erythematous plaque on the left periorbicular region. The initial diagnosis was erysipelas, which did not respond to antibiotic treatment.*

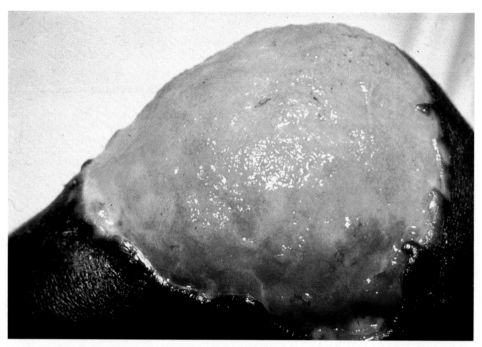

Figure 20-55 *M. ulcerans* infection (buruli ulcer) *A huge ulcer with a clean base and undermined margins extends into the adipose tissue of a Ugandan child. (Courtesy of M. Dittrich, MD)*

EPIDEMIOLOGY

Age of Onset Children, young adults.

Etiology *M. ulcerans.* An environmental habitat for the organism has not been established.

Sex Females>males.

Transmission Inoculation probably via pricks and cuts from plants, occurring in wet, marshy, or swampy sites.

Geography The tropics, most infections in Africa and Australia.

HISTORY

Incubation Period Approximately 3 months.

Symptoms The early nodule at site of trauma and subsequent ulceration are usually painless.

PHYSICAL EXAMINATION

Skin Lesions A painless subcutaneous swelling occurs at the site of inoculation. Lesion enlarges and ulcerates. The ulcer extends into the subcutaneous fat, and its margin is deeply undermined (Fig. 20-55). Ulcerations may enlarge to involve an entire extremity. Legs more commonly involved (sites of trauma). Any site may be involved.

General Findings Fever, constitutional findings are usually absent. Regional lymph nodes usually not enlarged.

DIFFERENTIAL DIAGNOSIS

Subcutaneous Induration Panniculitis, phycomycosis, nodular vasculitis, pyomyositis.

Large Cutaneous Ulceration Blastomycosis, sporotrichosis, nocardiosis, actinomycosis, mycetoma, chromomycosis, pyoderma gangrenosum, basal cell carcinoma, squamous cell carcinoma, necrotizing soft tissue infections.

LABORATORY EXAMINATIONS

Bacterial Culture Rule out secondary bacterial infection.

Mycobacterial Culture *M. ulcerans* grows optimally at 32° to 33°C.

Dermatopathology Necrosis originates in the interlobular septa of the subcutaneous fat. Ulceration is surrounded by granulation tissue with giant cells but no caseation necrosis or tubercles. Acid-fast bacilli are always demonstrable.

DIAGNOSIS

Clinical findings confirmed by isolation of *M. ulcerans* from lesional skin biopsy specimen.

COURSE AND PROGNOSIS

Ulcerations tend to persist for months to years. Spontaneous healing occurs eventually in many patients. Ulceration and healing can be complicated by scarring, contracture of the limb, and lymphedema. Secondary bacterial infection of the ulcer is an uncommon complication.

MANAGEMENT

Heat In that *M. ulcerans* prefers cooler temperatures, application of heat to the involved site has been reported to be effective.

Surgery Excision of the infected tissue, usually followed by grafting, is effective.

Antimycobacterial Chemotherapy Usually responds poorly. Combinations of sulfamethoxazole, rifampin, and minocycline may be effective.

Mycobacterium Fortuitum Complex Infection

Mycobacterium fortuitum complex (MFC) organisms cause infections at sites of inoculation, either surgical, injection, or traumatic, characterized by wound infections occurring several weeks after the insult. Cutaneous infection accounts for 60% of MFC infections.

EPIDEMIOLOGY

Age of Onset Children, young adults.

Sex Females>males.

Etiology The MFC organisms are rapid growers and include *M. fortuitum, M. chelonae,* and *M. abscessus.*

Geography *M. chelonae* is predominantly in Europe; *M. abscessus,* in the United States and Africa.

Natural Reservoirs The organisms are widely distributed in soil, dust, and water. Can be isolated from tap water, municipal water supplies, moist areas in hospitals, contaminated biologicals, aquariums, domestic animals, marine life.

Transmission Inoculation via traumatic puncture wounds (50%) or surgical procedures/injections (50%). Contaminated gentian violet used for skin marking has been the source.

HISTORY

Incubation Period Usually within 1 month (range 1 week to 2 years).

History Surgical wound infections follow augmentation mammaplasty, median sternotomy, and percutaneous catheterizations.

Symptoms Infection presents as a painful traumatic or surgical wound infection.

PHYSICAL EXAMINATION

Skin Lesions Cold postinjection abscesses. Traumatic wound infections (Fig. 20-56) present as dark red, infiltrated nodule, ±abscess formation, ±drainage of serous exudate. Linear lesions, commonly at incision sites. Traumatic infection occurs more commonly on the extremities. Surgical infections occur in scars of median sternotomy and augmentation mammaplasty. In immunocompromised individuals, infection can disseminate hematogenously to skin (multiple recurring abscesses on the extremities) and joints.

General Findings Other primary MFC infections include pneumonitis, osteomyelitis, lymphadenitis, postsurgical endocarditis.

DIFFERENTIAL DIAGNOSIS

Traumatic and Postoperative Wound Infection *Staphylococcus aureus* and group A *Streptococcus* infections, various other bacteria, foreign-body reaction, allergic contact dermatitis to topically applied agent, *Candida albicans* infection, *Aspergillus* spp. infection.

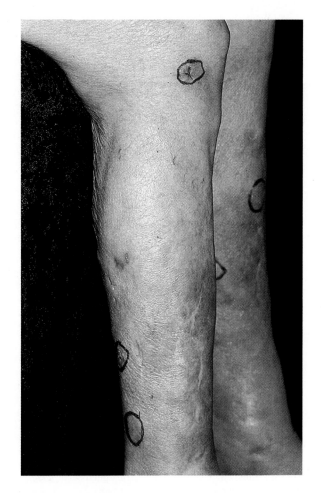

Figure 20-56 *M. chelonae* infection
Edema, erythematous nodules, scars on the lower legs of an 83-year-old female, who was taking oral glucocorticoids chronically for asthma.

LABORATORY EXAMINATIONS

Bacterial Culture Rule out secondary bacterial infection.

Mycobacterial Culture MFC organisms usually can be isolated on primary culture in 2 to 30 days; when recultured, the organisms grow well in 1 to 3 days.

Dermatopathology Polymorphonuclear microabscesses and granuloma formation with foreign-body–type giant cells (dimorphic inflammatory response) are seen. Necrosis is often present without caseation. Acid-fast bacilli can be seen within microabscesses.

DIAGNOSIS

Clinical findings confirmed by isolation of MFC from lesional skin biopsy specimen.

COURSE AND PROGNOSIS

The infection becomes chronic unless treated with antimycobacterial therapy, ±surgical debridement.

MANAGEMENT

Antimycobacterial Chemotherapy MFC organisms are resistant to all antimycobacterial agents except amikacin, and several newer agents such as fluoroquinolones and newer macrolides are frequently effective. Severe infection is usually treated with amikacin combined with another effective drug for 4 weeks, followed by 6 months of oral therapy. Mild to moderate infection is treated with an effective oral agent for 6 or more weeks.

Surgery Debridement with delayed closure is effective for localized infections.

LYME BORRELIOSIS

Lyme borreliosis (LB) is a complex, multisystem disease caused by the spirochete *Borrelia burgdorferi*, which is transmitted to humans by the bite of an infected ixodid tick. Lyme disease (LD), the syndrome occurring early in the course, is characterized by erythema migrans (EM), a local infection at the site of the tick bite. If untreated, the infection disseminates hematogenously to many different sites. Late Lyme borreliosis may manifest as involvement of the joints, nervous system, and/or heart. Chronic cutaneous LB is manifested by acrodermatitis chronica atrophicans.

EPIDEMIOLOGY

Etiology Three groups of *Borrelia burgdorferi* organisms known as *B. burgdorferi* sensu lato. In North America, most causative strains are group 1. In Europe and Asia, the most common strains isolated are group 2 (*B. garinii*) group 3 (*B. afzelii*) as well as well as group 1. Clinical variations of disease occurring in North America, Europe, and Asia may be related to differences in the various causative strains. *B. burgdorferi* has been identified in 19 of the United States.

Borrelia Burgdorferi Sensu Lato species	Geographic Range
B. burgdorferi sensu stricto	North America, Europe
B. garinii	Europe, Asia
B. afzelli	Europe, Asia

Vector Infected nymphal tick of genus *Ixodes: I. dammini* (*I. scapularis,* deer tick), *I. pacificus, I. ricinus* (sheep tick), *I. persulcatus.*

Animal Hosts White-footed mouse preferred host for immature larval and nymphal *I. dammini*. White-tailed deer, the preferred host in the adult stage of *I. dammini,* are not involved in the life cycle of the spirochete but are critical to the survival of the tick.

Transmission Ticks cling to vegetation; are most numerous in brushy, wooded, or grassy habitats; not found on open sandy beaches, *B. burgdorferi* is transmitted to humans after biting and feeding of nymphs or, less commonly, adult ticks. Transmission to humans occurs in association with hiking, camping, or hunting trips and with residence in wooded or rural areas.

Season In the midwestern and eastern United States, late May through early fall (80% of early LB begins in June and July). In the Pacific Northwest, January through May.

Risk for Exposure Strongly associated with prevalence of tick vectors and proportion of those ticks that carry *B. burgdorferi*. In the northeastern United States with endemic disease, the infection rate of the nymphal *I. scapularis* tick with *B. burgdorferi* is commonly 20 to 35%.

Distribution Worldwide, primarily in temperate climates. Correlates closely with geographic ranges of ixodid ticks. *I. dammini* is the vector in the northeastern United States (Massachusetts to Maryland); midwestern states (Wisconsin, Minnesota). *I. pacificus* is the vector in the western states (California, Oregon). *I. ricinus* is the vector in Europe and Asia (Great Britain to Scandanavia to European Russia). *I. persulcatus,* in Eastern Europe, China, and Japan.

Incidence Lyme disease is the most common vector-borne infection in the United States. In 1997, 10 states accounted for 90% of reported cases: Connecticut, Rhode Island, New Jersey, New York, Pennsylvania, Delaware, Maryland, Wisconsin, Minnesota, and Massachusetts.

PATHOGENESIS

After inoculation into the skin as the tick feeds, spirochetes replicate and migrate outward, producing the EM lesion, and invade vessels, spreading hematogenously to other organs. The spirochete has a particular trophism for tissues of the skin, nervous system, and joints. The organism persists in affected tissues during all stages of the illness. The immune response to the spirochete develops gradually. Specific IgM antibody peak between the third and sixth weeks after disease onset. The specific IgG response develops gradually over months. Proinflammatory cytokines, tumor necrosis factor-α, and interleukin 1β are produced in affected tissues.

HISTORY

Incubation Period EM: 3 to 32 days after tick bite. Cardiac manifestations: 35 days (3 weeks to >5 months after tick bite). Neurologic manifestions: average 38 days (2 weeks to months) after tick bite. Rheumatologic manifestions: 67 days (4 days to 2 years) after bite.

Prodrome With disseminated infection (stage 2), malaise, fatigue, lethargy, headache, fever, chills, stiff neck, arthralgia, myalgia, backache, anorexia, sore throat, nausea, dysesthesia, vomiting, abdominal pain, photophobia.

History Ixodid tick bites are asymptomatic. Only 14% of LB patients are aware of a preceding tick bite. Removal of the pinhead-sized tick within 18 h of attachment may preclude transmission. EM may be associated with burning sensation, itching, or pain. Only 75% of patients with LB exhibit EM. Joint complaints more common in North America. Neurologic involvement more common in Europe. With persistent disease, chronic fatigue.

PHYSICAL EXAMINATION

Skin Findings

Stage 1 Localized Infection *Erythema Migrans (EM)* Initial erythematous macule or papule enlarges within days to form an ex-

panding annular lesion with a distinct red border and partially clearing middle, i.e., a migrating erythema, at the bite site (Figs. 20-57 and 20-58). Maximum median diameter is 15 cm (range 3 to 68 cm). Center may become indurated, vesicular, or necrotic. At times, concentric rings form. When occurring on the scalp, only a linear streak may be evident on the face or neck. Multiple EM lesions are seen with multiple bite sites (Fig. 20-59). Proximal extremities, especially the axillary and inguinal areas, most common sites. Less common: central hemorrhagic vesiculation or necrosis, lymphangitic streaks. Hypersensitivity to various tick antigens, other pathogens, and outer borrelial surface proteins occur in some individuals. As EM evolves, post-inflammatory erythema or hyperpigmentation, transient alopecia, and desquamation may occur.

Borrelial Lymphocytoma Mainly in Europe; caused by *B. afzelii* and DN127 genomic group of *B. burgdorferi* sensu lato. Usually arises at the site of the tick bite. Some patients have a history of EM; others may show concomitant EM located around or near the lymphocytoma. Usually presents as a solitary bluish-red nodule (Fig. 20-60) or plaque. Sites of predilection: earlobe (children), nipple/areola (adults), areola, scrotum; 3 to 5 cm in diameter. Usually asymptomatic.

Other Cutaneous Findings Malar rash, diffuse urticaria, subcutaneous nodules (panniculitis).

Stage 2 Disseminated Infection *Secondary Lesions* Present in 17 to 50% of patients with early disseminated LB in North America; more common in Europe. Lesions range in number from 2 to >100 and thus may present as rash.

STAGING OF LYME BORRELIOSIS

Stage	Clinical Findings
Early infection: stage 1 (localized infection)	Erythema migrans (EM) Lymphocytoma
Early infection: stage 2 (disseminated infection)	Systemic sysmptoms (fever, chills, myalgia, headaches, weakness, photophobia) Secondary EM Carditis Meningitis, cranial neuritis, radiculoneuropathy Arthralgia/myalgia
Late infection: stage 3 (persistent infection)	Arthritis Encephalomyelitis Acrodermatitis chronica atrophicans (ACA)

Secondary lesions resemble EM but are smaller, migrate less, and lack central induration and may be scaly (Fig. 20-61). Lesions occur at any site except the palms and soles; can become confluent. When face, hands, feet are involved, mild swelling can occur.

Stage 3 Persistent Infection: Acrodermatitis chronica atrophicans Associated with *B. afzelii* infection in Europe and Asia. More common in elderly women.

Early Inflammatory Phase (Months to Years) Initially, diffuse or localized violaceous erythema, usually on one extremity, accompanied by mild to prominent edema (Fig. 20-62), most commonly involving the extensor surfaces and periarticular areas. Asymptomatic dull-red infiltrated plaques arise on the extremities, more commonly on lower legs than forearms, which slowly extend centrifugally over several months to years, leaving central areas of atrophy.

Endstage Skin becomes atrophic, veins and subcutaneous tissue become prominent, easily lifted and pushed into fine accordion-like folds, i.e., "cigarette paper" or "tissue paper" skin (Fig. 20-63). Lesions may be single or multiple.

Sclerotic or Fibrotic Plaques and Bands Localized fibromas and plaques are seen as subcutaneous nodules around the knees and elbows (Fig. 20-64); may involve the joint capsule with subsequent limitation of movement of joints in hand, feet, or shoulders. Fibrotic/sclerotic band along ulna is pathognomonic ("ulnar band").

General Findings

Stage 1 None.

Stage 2 Fever: in adults, low-grade; in children, may be high and persistent. Regional lymphadenopathy, generalized lymphadenopathy.

Neurologic Involvement Occurs in 10 to 20% of untreated LB cases, 1 to 6 weeks (or longer) after the tick bite. Manifested as meningitis (excruciating headache, neck pain), subtle encephalitic signs (sleep disturbances, difficulty concentrating, poor memory, irritability, emotional liability, dementia), cranial neuritis (including bilateral facial palsy), motor or sensory radiculoneuropathy, mononeuritis multiplex, or myelitis. In the United States, most common presentation is fluctuating symptoms of meningitis accompanied by facial palsy and peripheral radiculoneuropathy. In Europe and Asia, the first sign is characteristically radicular pain; meningeal and encephalitic signs are often absent. Early neurologic manifestations usually resolve within months; chronic neurologic disease may occur later.

Cardiac Involvement Occurs in 6 to 10% of untreated cases, usually within 4 weeks. Manifested by fluctuating degrees of atrioventricular block, myopericarditis, and left ventricular dysfunction. Usually transient and not associated with long-term sequelae.

Musculoskeletal Involvement Common. Migratory pain in joints, tendons, bursae, muscles, or bones. Pain lasts hours or days, affecting one or two locations at a time.

Stage 3 Fever: in adults, low-grade; in children, may be high and persistent. Regional lymphadenopathy, generalized lymphadenopathy.

Chronic Neuroborreliosis May become apparent months or years after onset of latent infection. Less common than arthritis. Most common presentation is subtle encephalopathy (altered memory, mood, or sleep), often accompanied by axonal polyneuropathy (distal paresthesias, spinal radicular pain). Prolonged course resembles that of tertiary syphilis.

Arthritis More common in United States, occuring in 60% of untreated cases. Characterized by intermittent attacks of oligoarticular arthritis in large joints (especially knees), lasting weeks to months. In a small percentage of cases, involvement of large joints (usually one or both knees) become chronic and may lead to destruction of cartilage and bone.

DIFFERENTIAL DIAGNOSIS

EM Insect bite (annular erythema cause by ticks, mosquitoes, Hymenoptera) epidermal dermatophytoses, allergic contact dermatitis, herald patch of pityriasis rosea, granuloma annulare, early inflammatory morphea, cellulitis, human granulocytic ehrlichiosis, urticaria, erythema multiforme, erythema annulare centrifugum, annular sarcoidosis, involuting psoriasis lesion, lichen simplex chronicus, subacute lupus erythematosus, fixed drug eruption.

Secondary Lesions Secondary syphilis, pityrasis rosea, erythema multiforme, urticaria.

Lymphocytoma Insect bite reaction, pseudolymphoma, cutaneous lymphoma.

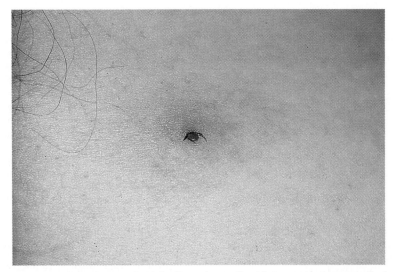

Figure 20-57   Deer tick (*Ixodes scapularis*) feeding   *A nymph with its mouth parts attached to skin with surrounding erythema; this inflammation is a response to the bite itself and is not necessarily indicative of infection. Transmission of* B. burgdorferi *usually occurs only after prolonged attachment and feeding (>18 h).*

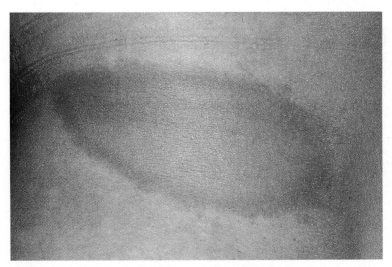

Figure 20-58   Lyme borreliosis: erythema migrans   *Solitary erythematous annular plaque on the lateral trunk at the site of an asymptomatic tick bite.*

ACA Arterial insufficiency of the lower leg, venous insufficiency with stasis dermatitis, and venous thrombosis/thrombophlebitis.

Fibrotic Nodules Rheumatic nodules, gouty tophi, and erythema nodosum.

LABORATORY EXAMINATIONS

Skin Biopsy *EM* Deep and superficial perivascular and interstitial infiltrate containing lymphocytes and plasma cells with some degree of vascular damage (mild vasculitis or hypervascular occlusion). Spirochetes can be demonstrated in up to 40% of EM biopsy specimens.

ACA Early, perivascular inflammatory infiltrate with plasma cells and dermal edema. Subsequently, infiltrate broadens to a dense middermal bandlike infiltrate. Ultimately, epidermal and dermal atrophy, dilated dermal blood vessels, plasma cell infiltrate, elastin and collagen defects.

Serology A two-test approach for active disease and for previous infection using a sensitive enzyme immunoassay (EIA) or immunofluorescent assay (IFA) followed by a Western immunoblot (WIB) is recommended. All specimens positive or equivocal by a sensitive EIA or IFA should be tested by a standardized WIB. When WIB is used during the first 4 weeks of disease onset, both IgM and IgG procedures should be performed. A positive IgM test result alone is not recommended for use in determining active disease in persons with illness of >1 months' duration. If a patient with suspected early LD has a negative serology, serologic evidence of infection is best obtained by testing paired acute- and convalescent-phase serum samples. Serum samples from persons with disseminated or late-stage LB almost always have a strong IgG response to *B. burgdorferi* antigens. It is recommended that an IgM immunoblot be considered positive if 2 of 3 bands are present and that an IgG immunoblot be considered positive if 5 of 10 bands are positive.

Positive serology indicates past infection. It does not distinguish between an abortive infection, a successfully treated past infection, or an active infection.

Culture *B. burgdorferi* can be isolated from lesional skin biopsy specimen on modified Barbour-Stoenner-Kelly medium.

PCR Detects *B. burgdorferi* DNA in lesional skin biopsy specimen, blood, or joint fluid. May be the preferred confirmatory laboratory test.

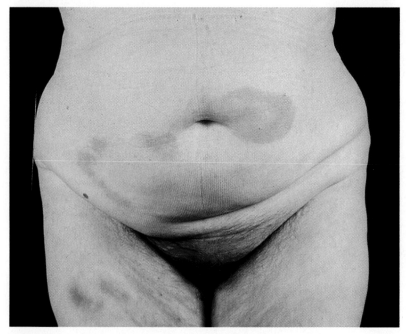

Figure 20-59 Lyme borreliosis: erythema migrans with multiple lesions *Three erythematous plaques with central clearing on the lower abdomen and thigh at multiple tick-bite sites.*

BACTERIAL INFECTIONS INVOLVING THE SKIN

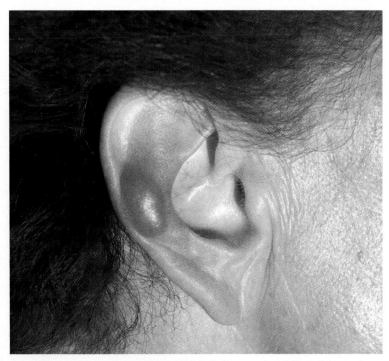

Figure 20-60   Lyme borreliosis: lymphocytoma cutis   *Solitary, red-purple nodule on the characteristic site of the ear.*

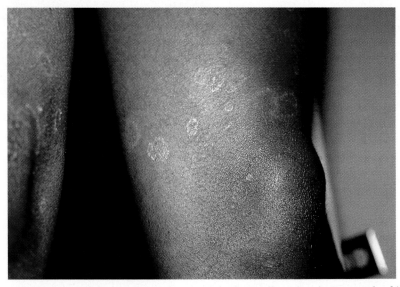

Figure 20-61   Lyme borreliosis: secondary lesions   *Multiple, small, scaling lesions on the thighs. The lesions result from spirochetemia from the primary bite size (erythema migrans) with resultant disseminated infection. These lesions are analogous to the papulosquamous lesions that occur in secondary syphilis.*

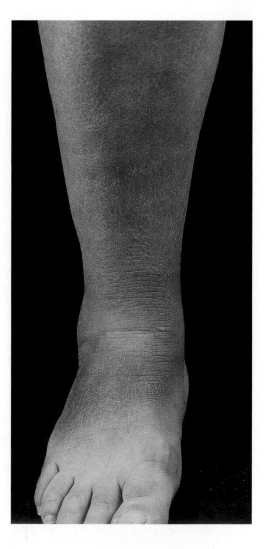

Figure 20-62 Lyme borreliosis: acrodermatitis chronica atrophicans, early *Ill-defined, violaceous erythema and edema of the leg and foot. Onset is usually several months after primary infection and is often accompanied by symptoms of peripheral sensory neuropathy.*

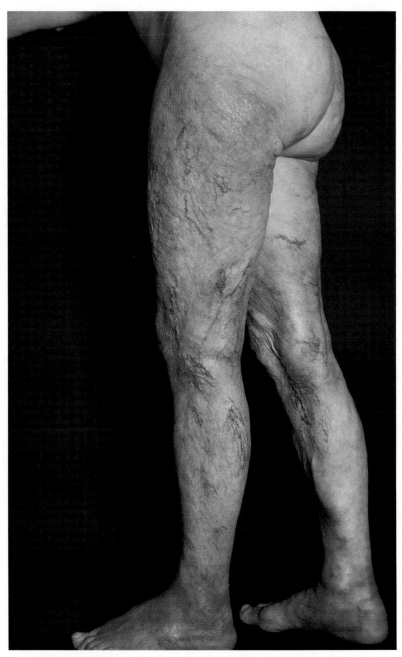

Figure 20-63 Lyme borreliosis: acrodermatitis chronica atrophicans, endstage *Advanced atrophy of the epidermis and dermis with associated violaceous erythema of legs and feet; the visibility of the superficial veins is striking.*

DIAGNOSIS

CDC surveillance criteria:

Early LB Made on characteristic clinical findings in a person living in or having visited an endemic area; does not require laboratory confirmation.

Late LB Confirmed by specific serologic tests.

ACA Made on clinical findings confirmed by lesional biopsy.

COURSE AND PROGNOSIS

Untreated EM and secondary lesions fade in a median time of 28 days, but the range is from 1 day to 14 months. Both EM and secondary lesions can fade and recur during this time. However, after adequate treatment, early lesions resolve within several days, and late manifestations are prevented. Late manifestations identified early usually clear after adequate antibiotic therapy; however, delay in diagnosis may result in permanent joint or neurologic disabilities.

ACA shows little response to adequate antibiotic therapy once atrophy has supervened. Adequately treated patients have declining titers of anti-*B. burgdorferi* antibody within 6 to 12 months.

MANAGEMENT

Prophylaxis

- Avoid known tick habitats. Other preventive measures include wearing long pants and long-sleeved shirts, tucking pants into socks.
- Apply tick repellents containing *N, N*-diethyl-*m*-toluamide ("DEET") to clothing and/or exposed skin.
- Check regularly for ticks, and promptly remove any attached ticks.
- Acaracides containing permethrin kill ticks on contact and can provide further protection when applied to clothing.
- After a recognized tick bite, the risk of infection with *B. burgdorferi* is low, and antibiotic prophylaxis is not routinely indicated. Therapy with amoxicillin or doxycycline for 10 days may be given to prevent Lyme disease in the following circumstances:

  Tick engorged (feeding for >24 h)
  Ixodes nymph from a hyperendemic area
  Pregnancy
  Immunocompromised status
  Follow-up difficult
  Patient anxious

Immunization

Immunization for prophylaxis of LB is now available for those at high risk of infection with the Lyme vaccine LYMErix™. It contains recombinant outer-surface protein A.

ANTIMICROBIAL TREATMENT OF LYME BORRELIOSIS

Oral Therapy	Drug of Choice/Dosing	Alternative Therapy
Age ≥12 years, not pregnant	Doxycycline, 100 mg bid	Amoxicillin, 500 mg tid Cefuroxime axetil, 500 mg bid Erythromycin, 250 mg qid
Age <12 years	Amoxicillin, 50 mg/kg/d	Cefuroxime axetil, 500 mg bid Erythromycin, 250 mg qid
Intravenous therapy	Ceftriaxone, 2 g qd	Cefotaxime, 2 g q8h Sodium penicillin G, 5 million U q6h

Pregnancy
  Localized early disease
	Amoxicillin, 500 mg PO
	  tid for 21 days	

Any manifestation
  of disseminated disease
	Penicillin G, 20 million units
	  (divided doses) IV qd for
	  14–28 days	

Asymptomatic seropositivity	No treatment necessary	

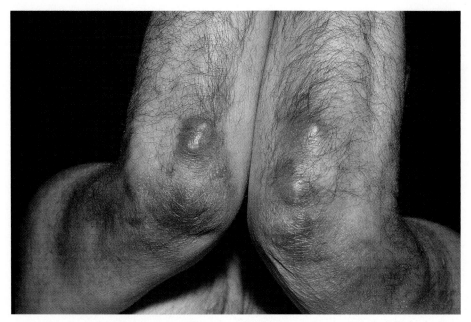

Figure 20-64 Lyme borreliosis: acrodermatitis chronica atrophicans, fibrotic nodules *Multiple, large, subcutaneous, fibrotic, violaceous nodules with surrounding erythema on the elbows.*

ROUTE AND DURATION OF THERAPY OF LYME BORRELIOSIS

Site of Infection	Route of Therapy	Duration of Therapy
Localized skin infection	Oral	10 days
Early disseminated infection	Oral	20–30 days
Cardiac involvement		
Mild involvement	Oral	30 days
High degree AV block	Intravenous	Until heart block improves, then PO for 30 days
Complete heart block/congestive heart failure	Intravenous	Until heart block improves, then PO for 30 days; may add glucocorticoid
Arthritis	Oral	30–60 days
Acrodermatitis chronica atrophicans	Oral	30 days
Neurologic involvement	Intravenous	30 days

ANTIMICROBIAL THERAPY

**Table 20-8 ORGANISMS, ANTIMICROBIAL AGENTS OF CHOICE,
AND ALTERNATIVES**

Infecting Organism	Antimicrobial Agent(s) of First Choice	Alternative Antimicrobial Agents
Staphylococcus aureus or epidermidis		
Non-penicillinase producing	Penicillin G or V	A cephalosporin; clindamycin; vancomycin; imipenem; a fluoroquinolone
Penicillinase-producing	A penicillinase-resistant penicillin. PO: dicloxacillin, cloxacillin. IV for severe infections; nafcillin, oxacillin	A cephalosporin; vancomycin; amoxicillin/clavulanic acid; ticarcillin/clavulanic acid; piperacillin/tazobactam; ampicillin/sulbactam; imipenem; clindamycin; a fluoroquinolone
Methicillin-resistant	Vancomycin ± gentamicin ± rifampin	Trimethoprim-sulfamethoxazole; a fluoroquinolone; minocycline; linezolid; quinupristin/dalfopristin
Streptococcus pyogenes (group A) and groups C and G	Penicillin G or V	An erythromycin, clarithromycin, azithromycin; a cephalosporin; vancomycin; clindamycin
Streptococcus, group B	Penicillin G or ampicillin	A cephalosporin, vancomycin, an erythromycin
Streptococcus pneumoniae (pneumococcus)	Penicillin G or V	A cephalosporin; erythromycin; azithromycin; clarithromycin; a fluoroquinolone; meropenem; imipenem; trimethoprim-sulfamethoxazole; clindamycin; a tetracycline
Penicillin-susceptible (MIC <0.1 μg/mL)		
Penicillin-intermediate resistance	Penicillin G IV (12 million U/d for adults) or ceftriaxone or cefotaxime Meningitis: vancomycin + ceftriaxone or cefotaxime ± rifampin	Levofloxacin; vancomycin; clindamycin
Penicillin-high level resistance (MIC ≥ 2 μg/mL)	Other Infections: varicomycin ± ceftriaxone or cefotaxime; or levofloxacin	Meropenem; imipenem; clindamycin
		Quinupristin/dalfopristin; linezolid
Erysipelothrix rhusiopathiae	Penicillin G	Erythromycin, a cephalosporin, a fluoroquinolone

(Continued)

Table 20-8 ORGANISMS, ANTIMICROBIAL AGENTS OF CHOICE, AND ALTERNATIVES *(Cont.'d)*

Infecting Organism	Antimicrobial Agent(s) of First Choice	Alternative Antimicrobial Agents
Haemophilus influenzae Meningitis, epiglottitis, arthritis, and other serious infections	Cefotaxime or ceftriaxone	Cefuroxime (not for meningitis); chloramphenicol; meropenem
Upper respiratory infections and bronchitis	Trimethoprim-sulfamethoxazole	Cefuroxime; amoxicillin/clavulanic acid; cefuroxime axetil; cefpodoxime; cefaclor; cefotaxime, ceftizoxime; ceftriaxone; cefixime; a tetracycline; clarithromycin; azithromycin; a fluoroquinolone; ampicillin or amoxicillin
Pasteurella multocida	Penicillin G	A tetracycline; a cephalosporin; amoxicillin/clavulanic acid; ampicillin/sulbactam
Pseudomonas aeruginosa	Ciprofloxacin; ticarcillin, mezlocillin or piperacillin + tobramycin, gentamicin or amikacin	Carbenicillin, ticarcillin, piperacillin or mezlocillin; ceftazidime; cefepime; imipenem or meropenem; aztreonam; tobramycin; gentamicin; amikacin
Vibrio vulnificus	A tetracycline	Cefotaxime
Neisseria gonorrhoeae **(gonococcus)**	Ceftriaxone or cefixime or ciprofloxacin or ofloxacin	Cefotaxime; spectinomycin; penicillin G cefotaxime; ceftizoxime; ceftriaxone
Neisseria meningitis **(meningococcus)**	Penicillin G	Chloramphenicol; a sulfonamide; a fluoroquinolone
Mycobacterium tuberculosis	Isoniazid + rifampin + pyrazinamide + ethambutol or streptomycin	Levofloxacin, ofloxacin or ciprofloxacin; cycloserine; capreomycin or kanamycin or amikacin; ethionamide; clofazimine; aminosalicylic acid
Mycobacterium fortuitum/ chelonae **complex**	Amikacin + clarithromycin	Cefoxitin; rifampin; a sulfonamide; doxycycline; ethambutol
Mycobacterium marinum (balnei)	Minocycline	Trimethoprim-sulfamethoxazole; rifampin; clarithromycin; doxycycline
Mycobacterium leprae **(leprosy)**	Dapsone + rifampin + clofazimine	Minocycline ofloxacin; sparfloxacin; clarithromycin
Actinomyces israelii **(actinomycosis)**	Penicillin G	A tetracycline; erythromycin; clindamycin
Nocardia	Trimethoprim-sulfamethoxazole	Sulfasoxazole; amikacin; a tetracycline; imipenem or meropenem; cycloser

FUNGAL INFECTIONS OF THE SKIN AND HAIR

SUPERFICIAL FUNGAL INFECTIONS

Superficial fungal infections are the most common of all mucocutaneous infections, often caused by overgrowth of transient or resident flora associated with a change in the microenvironment of the skin. The fungi causing these infection are of three genera: dermatophytes, *Candida* spp., and *Malassezia furfur*. Dermatophytes can infect any keratinized epithelium, hair follicles, and nail apparatus. *Candida* spp. require a warm humid environment. *M. furfur* require a humid microenvironment and lipids for growth.

Dermatophytoses

Dermatophytes are a unique group of fungi that are capable of infecting nonviable keratinized cutaneous epithelium including stratum corneum, nails, and hair. Dermatophytic genera include Trichophyton, Microsporum, and Epidermophyton. The term dermatophytosis thus denotes a condition caused by dermatophytes. It can be further specified according to the tissue mainly involved: epidermomycosis (epidermal dermatophytosis), trichomycosis (dermatophytosis of hair and hair follicles), or onychomycosis (dermatophytosis of the nail apparatus). The term tinea should be reserved for dermatophytoses and is modified according to the anatomic site of infection, e.g., tinea pedis. "Tinea" versicolor is better called pityriasis versicolor in that it is caused by Pityrosporum yeast and not dermatophytes.

EPIDEMIOLOGY

Age of Onset Children have scalp infections (*Trichophyton, Microsporum*), and young adults have intertriginous infections. The incidence of onychomycosis is correlated directly with age; in the United States, nearly 50% of individuals age 75 years have onychomycosis.

Sex Onychomycosis more common in males.

Race Adult blacks are said to have a lower incidence of dermatophytosis. Tinea capitis is more common in black children.

Etiology Three genera of dermatophytes: *Trichophyton, Microsporum*, and *Epidermophyton*. More than 40 species are currently recognized; approximately 10 species are common causes of human infection.

T. rubrum, which is currently the most common cause of epidermal dermatophytosis and onychomycosis in industrialized nations, was first discovered and reported in France in 1890 as a cause of tinea capitis with associated fingernail onychomycosis. The first report of *T. rubrum* infection in the United States was from Bir-mingham, AL in 1922. Currently, 70% of the population of the United States experience at least one episode of *T. rubrum* infection (usually tinea pedis). *T. rubrum* is indigenous to Southeast Asia, the Australian outback, and western Africa. Visitors/colonizers from Europe and North America became infected in these areas, developing tinea pedis and onychomycosis; these conditions did not occur in natives, who were barefoot or wore open moccasins. These visitors/colonizers and soldiers (World Wars I and II, and the Vietnam conflict) brought *T. rubrum* to North America and Europe. Soldiers wearing occlusive boots in tropical climates developed "jungle rot"—extensive tinea pedis ±secondary bacterial infection. Presently, *T. rubrum* infection can be acquired by contact with contaminated floors in public facilities such as health clubs, athletic locker rooms or hotel rooms.

The etiology of tinea capitis in children varies geographically. In North America and Europe, *T. tonsurans* is the most common cause, having replaced *M. audouinii*. In Europe, Asia, and Africa, *T. violaceum*. In adults in the United States, *T. rubrum* is the most common cause of dermatophytic folliculitis.

Geography Some species have a worldwide distribution; others are restricted to particular continents or regions. However, *T. concentricum*, the cause of tinea imbricata, is endemic to the South Pacific and parts of South America. *T. rubrum* was endemic to Southeast Asia, western Africa, and Australia but now occurs most commonly in North America and Europe.

Transmission Dermatophyte infections can be acquired from three sources: most commonly from another person (usually by fomites, less so by direct skin-to-skin contact), from animals such as puppies or kittens, and least commonly from soil. Based on their ecology, dermatophytes are also classified as follows:

Anthropophilic Person-to-person transmission by fomites and by direct contact. *Trichophyton* spp.: *T. rubrum*, *T. mentagrophytes* (var. *interdigitale*), *T. schoenleinii*, *T. tonsurans*, *T. violaceum*. *Microsporum audouinii*. *Epidermophyton floccosum*.

Zoophilic Animal-to-human by direct contact or by fomites. *Trichophyton* spp.: *T. equinum*, *T. mentagrophytes* (var. *mentagrophytes*), *T. verrucosum*. *M. canis*.

Geophilic Environmental. *Microsporum* sp.: *M. gypseum*, *M. nanum*.

Predisposing Factors Atopic diathesis for *T. rubrum* infections. *Immunosuppressed patients* have a higher incidence and more intractable dermatophytoses. With topical immunosuppression (i.e., with prolonged application of topical glucocorticoids), there can be marked modification in the usual banal character of dermatophytosis; this is especially true of the face, groin, and hands. In immunocompromised patients, abscesses and granulomas may occur.

CLASSIFICATION

Dermatophytes grow only on or within keratinized structures and, as such, involve the following:

Dermatophytoses of Keratinized Epidermis (Epidermal Dermatophytosis, Epidermomycosis) Tinea facialis, tinea corporis, tinea cruris, tinea manus, tinea pedis.

Dermatophytoses of Nail Apparatus (Onychomycosis) Tinea unguium (toenails, fingernails). Onychomycosis (here it is a more inclusive term, including nail infections caused by dermatophytes, yeasts, and molds).

Dermatophytoses of Hair and Hair Follicle (Trichomycosis) Dermatophytic folliculitis, Majocchi's (trichophytic) granuloma, tinea capitis, tinea barbae.

PATHOGENESIS

Dermatophytes synthesize keratinases that digest keratin and sustain existence of fungi in keratinized structures. Cell-mediated immunity and antimicrobial activity of polymorphonuclear leukocytes restrict dermatophyte pathogenicity.

- *Host factors that facilitate dermatophyte infections:* atopy, topical and systemic glucocorticoids, ichthyosis, collagen vascular disease
- *Local factors favoring dermatophyte infection:* sweating, occlusion, occupational exposure, geographic location, high humidity (tropical or semitropical climates)

The clinical presentation of dermatophytoses depends on several factors: site of infection, immunologic response of the host, species of fungus. Dermatophytes (e.g., *T. rubrum*) that initiate little inflammatory response are better able to establish chronic infection. Organisms such as *M. canis* cause an acute infection associated with a brisk inflammatory response and spontaneous resolution. In some individuals, infection can involve the dermis, as in kerion and Majocchi's granuloma.

LABORATORY EXAMINATIONS

Direct Microscopy (Fig. 21-1)

Sampling *Skin:* Collect scale with a no. 15 scalpel blade, edge of a glass microscope slide, brush (tooth or cervical brush). Scales are placed on center of microscope slide, swept into a small pile, and covered with a coverslip. Recent application of cream/ointment or powder often makes identification of fungal element difficult/impossible.

Nail: Keratinaceous debride is collected with a no. 15 scalpel blade or small curette. Distal lateral subungual onychomycosis (DLSO): debride from the undersurface of nail of most proximally involved site; avoid nail plate. Superficial white onychomycosis (SWO): superficial nail plate. Proximal subungual onychomycosis (PSO): undersurface of proximal nail plate; obtain sample by using a small punch biopsy tool, boring through involved nail plate to undersurface; obtain keratin from undersurface.

Hair: Remove hairs by epilation of broken hairs with a needle holder or forceps. Place on microscope slide and cover with glass coverslip. Skin scales from involved hairy site can be obtained with a brush (tooth or cervical).

Preparation Of Sample *Potassium hydroxide 5 to 20% solution* is applied at the edge of coverslip. Capillary action draws solution under coverslip. The preparation is gently heated with a match or lighter until bubbles begin to expand, clarifying the preparation. Excess KOH solution is blotted out with bibulous or lens paper. Condenser should be "racked down." Epidermal dermatophytosis: positive unless patient using antifungal therapy. DLSO: 90% of cases positive. Variations of KOH with fungal stains: Swartz-Lampkins stain, chlorazol black E stain.

Microscopy Dermatophytes are recognized as septated, tubelike structures (hyphae or mycelia) (Fig. 21-1).

Wood's Lamp Hairs infected with *Microsporum* spp. fluoresce. Greenish. Darken room and illuminate affected site with Wood's lamp. Coral red fluorescence of intertriginous site confirms diagnosis of erythrasma.

Fungal Cultures Specimens collected from scaling skin lesions, hair, nails. Scale and hair from the scalp are best harvested with tooth or cervical brush; the involved scalp is brushed vigorously; keratinaceous debride and hairs then placed into fungal culture plate. Culture on Sabouraud's glucose medium. Repeat cultures recommended monthly

Dermatopathology DLSO: periodic acid–Schiff (PAS) or methenamine silver stains are more sensitive than KOH preparation or fungal culture in identification of fungal elements in DLSO.

MANAGEMENT

Prevention	Apply powder containing miconazole or tolnaftate to areas prone to fungal infection after bathing.
Topical antifungal preparations	*These preparations may be effective for treatment of dermatophytoses of skin but not for those of hair or nails.* Preparation is applied bid to involved area optimally for 4 weeks including at least 1 week after lesions have cleared. Apply at least 3 cm beyond advancing margin of lesion. These topical agents are comparable. Differentiated by cost, base, vehicle, and antifungal activity.
Imidazoles	Clotrimazole (Lotrimin, Mycelex)
	Miconazole (Micatin)
	Ketoconazole (Nizoral)
	Econazole (Spectazole)
	Oxiconizole (Oxistat)
	Sulconizole (Exelderm)
Allylamines	Naftifine (Naftin)
	Terbinafine (Lamisil)
Naphthiomates	Tolnaftate (Tinactin)
Substituted pyridone	Ciclopirox olamine (Loprox)

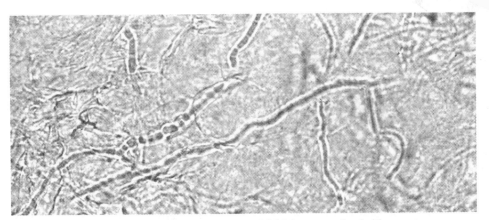

Figure 21-1 Potassium hydroxide (KOH) preparation *Multiple, septated, tubelike structures (hyphae or mycelia) and spore formation in scales from an individual with epidermal dermatophytosis. In contrast, KOH preparation in candidiasis shows elongated yeast forms (pseudohyphae) without true septations.*

None of them are reliable

Systemic antifungal agents	*For infections of keratinized skin:* use if lesions are extensive or if infection has failed to respond to topical preparations. *Usually required for treatment of tinea capitis and tinea unguium.* Also may be required for inflammatory tineas and hyperkeratotic moccasin-type tinea pedis.
Terbinafine	250-mg tablet. Allylamine. Rarely, nausea; dyspepsia, abdominal pain, loss of sense of taste, aplastic anemia. Most effective oral antidermophyte antifungal; low efficacy against other fungi.
Azole/imidazoles	Itraconazole and ketoconazole have potential clinically important interactions when administered with astemizole, calcium channel antagonists, cisapride-coumadin, cyclosporin A, oral hypoglycemic agents, phenytoin, protease inhibitors, tacrolimus, terfenadine, theophylline, trimetrexate, and rifampin.
Itraconazole	100-mg capsules; oral solution (10 mg/mL); Intravenous. Triazole. Needs acid gastric pH for dissolution of capsule. Rarely, ventricular arrhythmia when coadministered with terfenadine/astemizole. Raises levels of digoxin and cyclosporine. Approved for onychomycosis in the United States.
Fluconazole	100-, 150-, 200-mg tablets; oral suspension (10 or 40 mg/mL); 400 mg IV.
Ketoconazole	200-mg tablets. Needs acid gastric pH for dissolution of tablet. Take with food or cola beverage; antacids and H_2 blockers reduce absorption. The most hepatotoxic of azole drugs; hepatotoxicity occurs in an estimated one of every 10,00–15,000 exposed persons. Rarely, ventricular arrhythmia when coadministered with terfenadine/astemizole. Not approved for treatment of dermatophyte infections in the United States.
Griseofulvin	*Micronized:* 250- or 500-mg tablets; 125 mg/teaspoon suspension. *Ultramicronized:* 165- or 330-mg tablets. Active only against dermatophytes; less effective than triazoles. Adverse effects include headache, nausea/vomiting, photosensitivity; lowers effect of crystalline warfarin sodium. *T. rubrum* and *T. tonsurans* infection may respond poorly. Should be taken with fatty meal to maximize absorption. In children, CBC and LFTs recommended if risk factors for hepatitis exist or treatment lasts longer than 3 months. Not used in Europe.

Not only young people + old people

Dermatophytoses of Epidermis

Epidermal dermatophytoses are the most common dermatophytic infection. Epidermal dermato-phytoses may be followed/accompanied by dermatophytic infection of hair/hair follicles and/or the nail apparatus.

Synonym: "ring worm," epidermomycosis.

Tinea Pedis

Tinea pedis is a dermatophytic infection of the feet, characterized by erythema, scaling, macera-tion, and/or bulla formation. In most cases of epidermal dermatophytosis, the infection occurs ini-tially on the feet, and, in time, spreads to sites such as the inguinal area (tinea cruris), trunk (tinea corporis), hands (tinea manuum). Tinea pedis often provides breaks in the integrity of the epider-mis through which bacteria such as *Staphylococcus aureus* or group A streptococcus can invade, causing localized infection or spreading infections such as cellulitis or lymphangitis.

Synonym: Athlete's foot.

EPIDEMIOLOGY

Age of Onset Late childhood or young adult life. Most common 20 to 50 years.

Sex Males>females.

Predisposing Factors Hot, humid weather; occlusive footwear; excessive sweating.

Transmission Walking barefoot on contami-nated floors. Arthrospores can survive in human scales for 12 months.

CLASSIFICATION

Type	Clinical Features	Etiology
Interdigital (acute and chronic)	Most common type; frequently over-looked	*T. rubrum* most common cause of chronic tinea pedis; *T mentagrophytes* causes more inflammatory lesions
	Two patterns: dry and moist with maceration	
Dry	Scaling of webspace, may be erosive	*T. rubrum*
Moist (macerated)	Hyperkeratosis of webspace with maceration of stratum corneum	*T. mentagrophytes*
Moccasin (chronic hyperkeratotic or dry)	Most often caused by *T. rubrum.* More common in atopic individuals	Most often caused by *T. rubrum,* especially in atopic individuals; also *E. floccosum*
Inflammatory or bullous (vesicular)	Least common type; usually caused by *T. mentagrophytes*; resembles an allergic contact dermatitis	Least common type; usually caused by *T. mentagrophytes* var. *mentagrophytes* (granular). Resembles an allergic contact dermatitis
Ulcerative	An extension of interdigital type into dermis due to maceration and secondary (bacterial) infection	*T. rubrum, E. floccosum, T. mentagrophytes, C. albicans*
Dermatophytid	Presents as a vesicular eruption of the fingers and/or palmar aspects of the hands secondary to inflammatory tinea pedis. A combined clinical presentation also occurs. *Candida* and bacteria (*Staph-ylococcus aureus,* group *aeruginosa*) A *Streptococcus, Pseudomonus* may cause superinfection.	*T. mentagrophytes, T. rubrum*

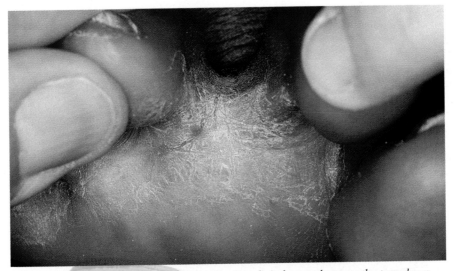

Figure 21-2   Tinea pedis: interdigital dry type *The interdigital space between the toes shows erythema and scaling; the toenail is thickened, indicative of associated distal subungual onychomycosis.*

HISTORY

Duration   Months to years. Often, prior history of tinea pedis, ±tinea unguium of toenails. May flare if in hot climate.

Skin Symptoms   Asymptomatic frequently. Pruritus. Pain with secondary bacterial infection.

PHYSICAL EXAMINATION

Skin Lesions   *Interdigital Type*   Two patterns: (1) dry scaling (Fig. 21-2); and (2) maceration, peeling, fissuring of toe webs (Fig. 21-3). Underlying skin red, ±weeping. Most common site: between fourth and fifth toes. Infection may spread to adjacent areas of feet.

Moccasin Type   Well-demarcated erythema with minute papules on margin, fine white scaling, and hyperkeratosis (Figs. 21-4 and 21-5) (confined to heels, soles, lateral borders of feet). *Distribution:* Sole, involving area covered by a ballet slipper. One or both feet may be involved with any pattern; bilateral involvement more common.

Inflammatory/Bullous Type   Vesicles or bullae filled with clear fluid (Fig. 21-6). Pus usu-ally indicates secondary *S. aureus* infection or group A streptococcus. After rupturing, erosions with ragged ringlike border. May be associated with dermatophytid. *Distribution:* Sole, instep, webspaces.

Ulcerative Type   Extension of interdigital tinea pedis onto dorsal and plantar foot. Usually complicated by bacterial infection.

DIFFERENTIAL DIAGNOSIS

Interdigital Type   Erythrasma, impetigo, pitted keratolysis, *Candida* intertrigo, *P. aeruginosa* webspace infection.

Moccasin Type   Psoriasis vulgaris, eczematous dermatitis (dyshidrotic, atopic, allergic contact), pitted keratolysis, various keratodermas.

Inflammatory/Bullous Type   Bullous impetigo, allergic contact dermatitis, dyshidrotic eczema, bullous disease.

LABORATORY EXAMINATIONS

Direct Microscopy   (Fig. 21-1). In bullous type, examine scraping from the inner aspect of bulla roof for detection of hyphae.

SUPERFICIAL FUNGAL INFECTIONS

Wood's Lamp Negative fluorescence usually rules out erythrasma in interdigital infection. Erythrasma and interdigital tinea pedis may coexist.

Culture Fungal Dermatophytes can be isolated in 11% of normal-appearing interspaces and 31% of macerated toe webs. *Candida* spp. may be copathogens in webspaces.

Bacterial In individuals with macerated interdigital space, *S. aureus, P. aeruginosa,* and diphtheroids are commonly isolated. *S. aureus* and group A streptococcus can cause superinfection.

DIAGNOSIS

Demonstration of hyphae on direct microscopy, ±isolation of dermatophyte on culture.

COURSE AND PROGNOSIS

Tends to be chronic, with exacerbations in hot weather. May provide portal of entry for lymphangitis or cellulitis, especially in patients whose leg veins have been used for coronary artery bypass surgery and have chronic low-grade edema of leg. Without secondary prophylaxis, recurrence is the rule.

MANAGEMENT

Prevention

Use of shower shoes while bathing at home or in public facility. Washing feet with benzoyl peroxide bar directly after shower. Diabetics and those who have undergone coronary artery bypass with harvesting of leg veins are especially subject to secondary bacterial infection (impetiginization, lymphangitis, cellulitis).

Special considerations by type of infection

Macerated interdigital

Acute: Burow's wet dressings; Castellani's paint. Chronical: aluminum chloride hexahydrate 20% bid to reduce sweating.

Moccasin

Most difficult to eradicate. Many patients have a minor defect in cell-mediated immune response: stratum corneum thick, making it difficult for topical antifungal agents to penetrate, often associated with tinea unguium, a source of reinfection of skin. Keratolytic agent (salicylic acid, lactic acid, hydroxy acid) with plastic occlusion useful in reducing hyperkeratosis. Nail reservoir must be eradicated to cure moccasin-type infection.

Inflammatory/bullous

Acutely, use cool compresses. If severe, systemic glucocorticoids are indicated.

Antifungal agents

Topical

See Dermatophytoses, page 685. Apply to all affected sites twice daily. Treat for 2–4 weeks.

Systemic

Indicated for extensive infection, for failures of topical treatment, or for those with tinea unguium and moccasin-type tinea.

Terbinafine
Itraconazole

250 mg qd for 14 days
200 mg bid for 7 days *or*
200 mg qd for 14 days

Fuconazole

150–200 mg qd for 4–6 weeks

Secondary prophylaxis

Important in preventing recurrence of interdigital and moccasin types of tinea pedis. Daily washing of feet while bathing with benzoyl peroxide bar is effective and inexpensive. Antifungal powders.

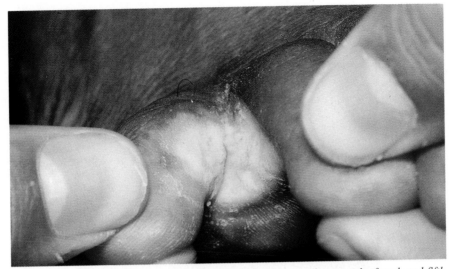

Figure 21-3   Tinea pedis: interdigital macerated type   *The webspace between the fourth and fifth toes is hyperkeratotic and macerated in a black individual with plantar keratoderma and hyperhidrosis. The greenish hue is caused by* Pseudomonas aeruginosa *superinfection of this moist intertriginous site. Erythrasma also occurs in the setting of moist intertriginous sites and may occur concomitantly with interdigital tinea pedis and/or* Pseudomonas *intertrigo.*

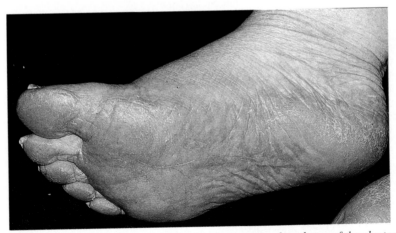

Figure 21-4   Tinea pedis: moccasin type   *Fairly sharply marginated erythema of the plantar foot with a mild keratoderma associated with distal/lateral subungual onychomycosis, typical of* T. rubrum *infection.*

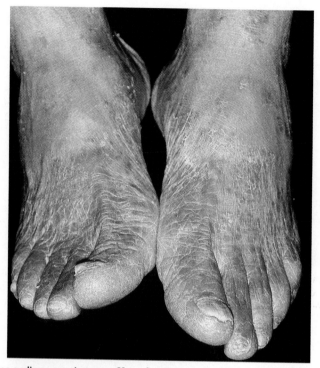

Figure 21-5   Tinea pedis: moccasin type   *Hyperkeratosis and scaling of the dorsum of the feet occurring on the portion of the foot covered by a moccasin; note the associated distal/lateral subungual onychomycosis, typical of* T. rubrum *infection.*

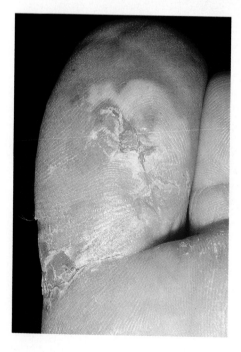

Figure 21-6   Tinea pedis: bullous type
Ruptured vesicles, bullae, erythema, and erosion on the plantar aspect of the great toe. Hyphae were detected on KOH preparation obtained from the roof of the inner aspect of the bulla. In some cases, superficial white onychomycosis may also be seen with this T. mentagrophytes *infection.*

FUNGAL INFECTIONS OF THE SKIN AND HAIR

Tinea Manuum

Tinea manuum is a chronic dermatophytosis of the hand(s), often unilateral, most commonly on the dominant hand, and usually associated with tinea pedis.

HISTORY

Duration   Month to years.

Skin Symptoms   Frequently symptomatic. Pruritus. Pain if secondarily infected or fissured.

Dyshidrotic type   Episodic symptoms of pruritus.

PHYSICAL EXAMINATION

Skin Lesions   Well-demarcated scaling patches, hyperkeratosis and scaling confined to palmar creases, fissures on palmar hand (Fig. 21-7). Borders well demarcated; central clearing. Often extends onto dorsum of hand with follic-ular papules, nodules, pustules with dermatophytic folliculitis.

Dyshidrotic type   Papules, vesicles, bullae (uncommon on the margin of lesion) on palms and lateral fingers, similar to lesions of bullous tinea pedis.

Secondary changes   Lichen simplex chronicus, prurigo nodules, impetiginization.

Distribution   Diffuse hyperkeratosis of the palms with pronounced involvement of palmar creases or patchy scaling on the dorsa and sides of fingers; 50% of patients have unilateral involvement (Fig. 21-7). Usually associated with tinea pedis, ±tinea crusis. If chronic, often associated with tinea unguium of fingernails.

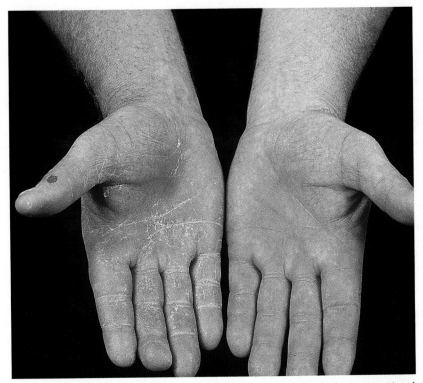

Figure 21-7   Tinea manuum   *Erythema and scaling of the right hand, which was associated with bilateral tinea pedum; the "one hand, two feet" distribution is typical of epidermal dermatophytosis of the hands and feet. In time, distal/lateral subungual onychomycosis occurs on the fingernails.*

Erythema/Scaling Hands   Atopic dermatitis, lichen simplex chronicus, allergic contact dermatitis, irritant contact dermatitis, psoriasis vulgaris, squamous cell carcinoma in situ.

COURSE

Chronic, does not resolve spontaneously. After treatment, recurs unless onychomycosis of fingernails, feet, and toenails is eradicated. Fissures and erosions provide portal of entry for bacterial infections.

MANAGEMENT

Prevention   Must eradicate tinea unguium of fingernails as well as toenails, tinea pedis ±tinea cruris as well; otherwise, tinea manuum will recur.

**Antifungal Agents   *Topical*   See Dermatophytoses, page 686. Failure common.

Systemic   Because of thickness of palmar stratum corneum, and especially if associated with tinea unguium of fingernails, tinea manuum is impossible to cure with topical agents. Oral agents eradicate dermatophytoses of hands, feet, and nails:

Terbinafine 250 mg qd for 14 days
Itraconzole 200 mg qd for 7 days
Fluconazole 150–200 mg qd for 2 to 4 weeks

Note: Eradication of fingernail onychomycosis requires longer use.

Tinea Cruris

Tinea cruris is a subacute or chronic dermatophytosis of the groin, pubic regions, and thighs. *Synonym:* "Jock itch."

EPIDEMIOLOGY

Age of Onset   Adult.

Sex   Males>females.

Etiology   *T. rubrum, T. mentagrophytes.*

Predisposing Factors   Warm, humid environment; tight clothing worn by men; obesity. Chronic topical glucocorticoid application.

HISTORY

Duration   Months to years. Often, history of long-standing tinea pedis. Often prior history of tinea cruris.

Skin Symptoms   Usually none. In some persons, pruritus causes patient to seek treatment.

PHYSICAL EXAMINATION

Skin Lesions   Usually associated with tinea pedis, ±tinea unguium of toenails. Large, scaling, well-demarcated dull red/tan/brown plaques (Fig. 21-8). ±Central clearing. Papules, pustules may be present at margins. Treated lesions: lack scale; postinflammatory hyperpigmentation in darker-skinned persons. In atopics, chronic scratching may produce secondary changes of lichen simplex chronicus.

Distribution   Groins and thighs (Fig. 21-8); may extend to buttocks. Scrotum and penis are rarely involved.

DIFFERENTIAL DIAGNOSIS

Erythema/Scaling in Groins   Erythrasma, intertrigo, *Candida* intertrigo, inverse-pattern psoriasis, pityriasis versicolor, Langerhans' cell histiocytosis.

MANAGEMENT

Prevention   After eradication of tinea cruris, ±tinea pedis, ±tinea unguium, reinfection can be minimized by wearing shower shoes when using a public or home (if family members are infected) bathing facility; using antifungal powders; benzoyl peroxide wash.

**Antifungal Agents   *Topical Treatment*   See Dermatophytoses, page 686.

Systemic Treatment   If recurrent, if dermatophytic folliculitis is present, or if it has failed to respond to adequate topical therapy. See tinea manuum.

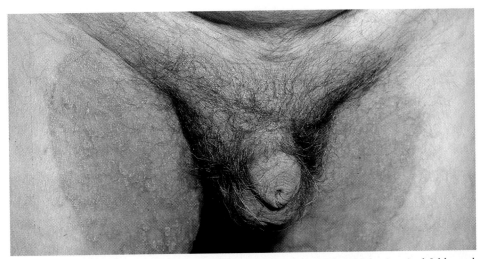

Figure 21-8 Tinea cruris *Erythematous, scaling plaques on the medial thighs, inguinal folds, and pubic area; areas of clearing are apparent within the large plaques. The margins are raised and sharply marginated.*

Tinea Corporis

Tinea corporis refers to dermatophyte infections of the trunk, legs, arms, and/or neck, excluding the feet, hands, and groin.

EPIDEMIOLOGY

Age of Onset   All ages.

Occupation   Animal (large and small) workers.

Etiology   *T. rubrum* most commonly; *M. canis*. *T. tonsurans* in parents of black children with tinea capitis.

Transmission   Autoinoculation from other parts of the body, i.e., from tinea pedis and tinea capitis. Contact with animals or contaminated soil.

Geography   More common in tropical and subtropical regions.

Predisposing Factors   Most commonly, infection is spread from dermatophytic infection of the feet (*T. rubrum, T. mentagrophytes*). Infection also can be acquired from an active lesion of an animal (*T. verrucosum, M. canis*) or rarely, from soil (*M. gypseum*).

HISTORY

Incubation Period   Days to months.

Duration   Weeks to months to years.

Symptoms   Often asymptomatic. Mild pruritus.

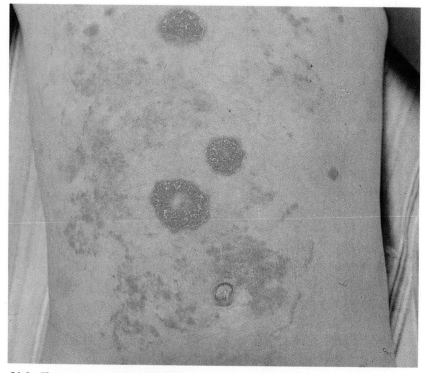

Figure 21-9   Tinea corporis: acute and subacute   *Multiple, bright red, sharply marginated lesions with only minimal scaling of several weeks' duration on the trunk of a child. Three lesions are more inflammatory and thicker.* Microsporum canis *was isolated on fungal culture, which had been contracted from a pet guinea pig.*

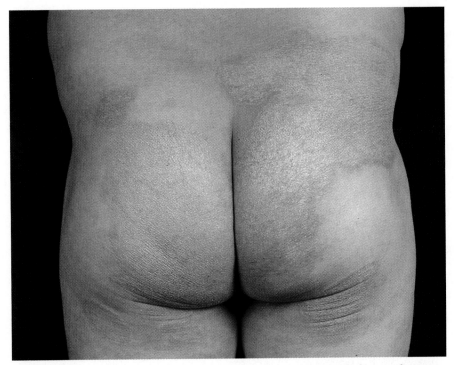

Figure 21-10 Tinea corporis: chronic *Sharply marginated, hyperpigmented plaques of many months' duration on the back, buttocks, and thighs. The lesions have a psoriasiform appearance. Associated tinea cruris and tinea pedis are usually present.*

PHYSICAL EXAMINATION

Skin Lesions Small (Fig. 21-9) to large (Fig. 21-10), scaling, sharply marginated plaques with or without pustules or vesicles, usually at margins. Peripheral enlargement and central clearing (Fig. 21-9) produces annular configuration with concentric rings or arcuate lesions; fusion of lesions produces gyrate patterns. Single and occasionally scattered multiple lesions. Bullae. Granulomatous lesions (Majocchi's granuloma). Psoriasiform plaques (Fig. 21-10). Verrucous lesions. Zoophilic infection (contracted from animals) lesions are more inflammatory with marked vesiculation and crusting at margins, bullae.

DIFFERENTIAL DIAGNOSIS

Well-Demarcated Scaling Plaque(s) Allergic contact dermatitis, atopic dermatitis, annular erythemas, psoriasis, seborrheic dermatitis, pityriasis rosea, pityriasis alba, pityriasis versicolor, erythema migrans, subacute LE mycosis fungoides.

LABORATORY EXAMINATIONS

See Dermatophytoses, page 686.

MANAGEMENT

Antifungal Agents See Dermatophytoses, page 686, for topical therapy. See Tinea manuum, page 694, for systemic antifungal therapy.

Tinea Facialis

Tinea facialis is dermatophytosis of the glabrous facial skin, characterized by a well-circumscribed erythematous patch, and is more commonly misdiagnosed than any other dermatophytosis. *Synonym:* Tinea faciei.

EPIDEMIOLOGY

Age of Onset   More common in children.

Etiology   *T. tonsurans* associated with tinea capitis in black children and their parents. *T. mentagrophytes, T. rubrum* most commonly; also *M. audouinii, M. canis.*

Predisposing Factors   Animal exposure, chronic topical application of glucocorticoids.

HISTORY

Skin Symptoms   Most commonly asymptomatic. At times, pruritus and photosensitivity.

PHYSICAL EXAMINATION

Skin Lesions   Well-circumscribed macule to plaque of variable size; elevated border and central regression (Fig. 21-11). Scaling often is minimal (Fig. 21-12) but can be pronounced. Pink to red. In black patients, hyperpigmentation. Any area of face but usually not symmetric.

DIFFERENTIAL DIAGNOSIS

Scaling Facial Patches   Seborrheic dermatitis, contact dermatitis, erythema migrans, lupus erythematosus, polymorphic light eruption, phototoxic drug eruption, lymphocytic infiltrate.

LABORATORY EXAMINATIONS

See Dermatophytoses, page 686.

MANAGEMENT

Antifungal Agents   See Dermatophytoses, page 686, for topical therapy. See Tinea manuum, page 694, for systemic antifungal therapy.

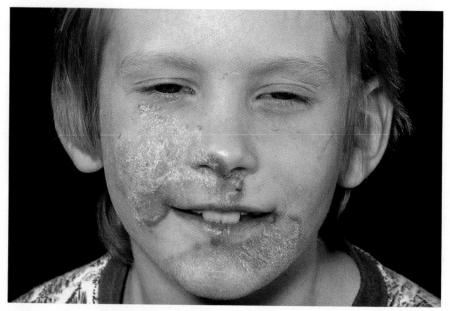

Figure 21-11   Tinea facialis   *Sharply marginated, erythematous, scaling, and crusted plaques on the face of a child. Note asymmetry.*

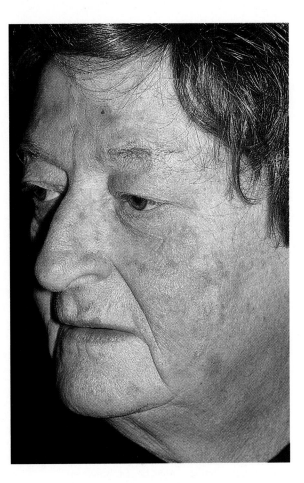

Figure 21-12 Tinea facialis: tinea incognito *Well-demarcated erythema of central face and neck in an elderly female, who had been applying topical glucocorticoid cream for presumed seborrheic dermatitis.*

Tinea Incognito

Tinea incognito is an epidermal dermatophytosis, often associated with dermatophytic folliculitis, that occurs after the topical application of a glucocorticoid preparation to a site colonized or infected with dermatophyte. It usually occurs when an inflammatory dermatophytosis is mistaken for psoriasis or an eczematous dermatitis (Fig. 21-22). Lesions are usually aymptomatic but may be very pruritic or even painful. Involved sites often often have exaggerated features of epidermal dermatophytoses, being a deep red or violaceous with follicular papules or pustules. Epidermal atrophy caused by chronic glucocorticoid application may be present. Systemic antifungal therapy may be indicated due to deep involvement of the hair apparatus.

Dermatophytoses Of Hair

Dermatophytes are capable of invading hair follicles and hair shaft, causing dermatophytic trichomycosis, with resultant tinea capitis, tinea barbae, and dermatophytic folliculitis.

Tinea Capitis

Tinea capitis is a dermatophytic trichomycosis of the scalp. Clinical presentations vary widely, ranging from mild scaling and broken-off hairs to severe, painful inflammation with painful, boggy nodules that drain pus and result in scarring alopecia.

Synonyms: Ringworm of the scalp, tinea tonsurans.

EPIDEMIOLOGY

Age of Onset Toddlers and school-aged children. Most common 6 to 10 years of age. Less common after age 16; in adults it occurs most commonly in a rural setting.

Race Much more common in blacks than in whites.

Etiology Varies from country to country and from region to region; species change in time due to immigration. Infections can become epidemic in schools and institutions, especially with overcrowding. Random fungal cultures in urban study revealed 4% positive rate and a 12.7% positive rate among black children.

United States and Western Europe 90% of cases of tinea capitis caused by *Trichophyton tonsurans;* less commonly, *Microsporum canis.* Formerly, most cases were caused by *M. audouinii.* Less commonly, *M. gypseum, T. mentagrophytes, T. rubrum.*

Eastern and Southern Europe, North Africa *T. violaceum.*

Transmission Person-to-person, animal-to-person, via fomites. Spores are present on asymptomatic carriers, animals, or inanimate objects.

Risk Factors For favus: debilitation, malnutrition, chronic disease.

CLASSIFICATION

Ectothrix Infection Invasion occurs outside hair shaft. Hyphae fragment into arthroconidia, leading to cuticle destruction. Caused by *Microsporum* species (*M. audouinii* and *M. canis*).

Endothrix Infection Infection occurs within hair shaft without cuticle destruction. Arthroconidia found within hair shaft. Caused by *Trichophyton* species (*T. tonsurans* in North America; *T. violaceum* in Europe, Asia, parts of Africa).

"Black Dot" Tinea Capitis Variant of endothrix resembling seborrheic dermatitis.

Kerion Variant of endothrix with boggy inflammatory plaques.

Favus Variant of endothrix with arthroconidia and airspaces within hair shaft. Very uncommon in western Europe and North America. In some parts of the world (Middle East, South Africa), however, it is still endemic.

PATHOGENESIS

Noninflammatory lesions Invasion of hair shaft by the dermatophytes, principally *M. audouinii* (child-to-child, via barber, hats, theater seats), *M. canis* (young pets-to-child and then child-to-child) or *T. tonsurans.* Inflammatory lesions: *T tonsurans, M. canis, T. verrucosum,* and others. Spores enter through breaks in hair shaft or scalp to cause clinical infection.

Scalp hair traps fungi from the environment or fomites. Asymptomatic colonization is common. Trauma assists inoculation. Dermatophytes initially invade stratum corneum of scalp, which may be followed by hair shaft infection. Spread to other hair follicles then occurs. Eventually, infection regresses with or without an inflammatory response. Clinical appearance varies with type of hair invasion, level of host resistance, degree of inflammatory host response: few dull-grey, broken-off hairs with little scaling to severe painful inflammatory mass covering entire scalp. Partial hair loss with

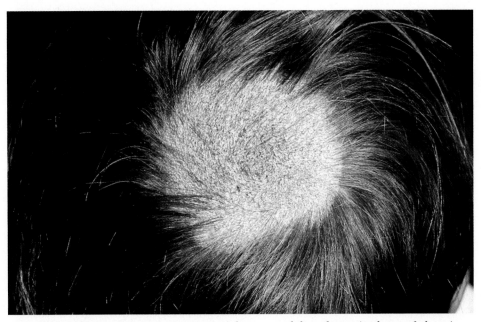

Figure 21-13 Tinea capitis: "gray patch" type *A large, round, hyperkeratotic plaque of alopecia due to breaking off of hair shafts close to the surface, giving the appearance of a mowed wheat field on the scalp of a child. Remaining hair shafts and scales exhibit a green fluorescence when examined with a Wood's lamp.* Microsporum canis *was isolated on culture.*

inflammation in all cases. Kerion is associated with a high degree of hypersensitivity to fungal hapten. Types of hair invasion:

Microsporum types: (1) Small-spored ectothrix; hair shaft is invaded in mid-follicle. Intrapiliary hyphae grow inward toward hair bulb. Secondary extrapiliary hyphae burst, growing over surface of hair shaft. (2) Large-spored ectothrix have similar arrangement.

Trichophyton types: (1) Large-spored ectothrix (in chains); arthrospores spherical, arranged in straight chains, confined to external surface of hair shaft. Spores are all larger than those of small-spored *Microsporum* ectothrix. (2) Endothrix type; intrapiliary hyphae fragment into arthroconidia within hair shaft, making it fragile, with subsequent breakage close to scalp surface.

HISTORY

Duration of Lesions Weeks to months.

Skin Symptoms In patients with inflammatory tinea capitis, pain, tenderness, and/or alopecia. With noninflammatory infection, scaling, scalp pruritus, diffuse or circumscribed alopecia, or occipital or posterior auricular adenopathy.

PHYSICAL EXAMINATION

Skin Lesions and Hair Changes *Small-Spored Ectothrix Tinea Capitis* "Gray patch" tinea capitis (Fig. 21-13). Partial alopecia, often circular in shape, showing numerous broken-off hairs, dull grey from their coating of arthrospores. Inflammation minimal. Fine scaling with fairly sharp margin. Hair shaft becomes brittle, breaking off at or slightly above scalp. Small patches coalesce, forming larger patches. Inflammatory response minimal but massive scaling. Several or many patches, randomly arranged may be present. *M. audouinii, M. ferrugineum, M. canis* infections show green fluorescence with Wood's lamp.

Endothrix Tinea Capitis

- *"Black dot" tinea capitis:* Broken-off hairs near surface give appearance of "dots" (Fig. 21-14) (swollen hair shafts) in dark-haired patients. Dots occur as affected hair breaks at surface of scalp. Tends to be diffuse and poorly circumscribed. Low-grade folliculitis may be present. Resembles seborrheic dermatitis, chronic cutaneous lupus erythematosus. Usually caused by *T. tonsurans, T. violaceum*. Onychomycosis also occurs in 2 to 3% of cases.

- *Kerion:* Inflammatory mass in which remaining hairs are loose. Characterized by boggy, purulent, inflamed nodules and plaques (Fig. 21-15). Usually extremely painful; drains pus from multiple openings, like honeycomb. Hairs do not break off but fall out and can be pulled without pain. Follicles may discharge pus; ±sinus formation; ±mycetoma-like grains. Thick crusting with matting of adjacent hairs. A single plaque is usual, but multiple lesions may occur with involvement of entire scalp. Frequently, associated lymphadenopathy is present. Usually caused by zoophilic (*T. verrucosum, T. mentagrophytes* var. *mentagrophytes*) or geophilic species. Heals with scarring alopecia.

- *Agminate folliculitis:* Less severe inflammation than kerion with sharply defined, dull-red plaques studded with follicular pustules. Caused by zoophilic species.

- *Favus:* Early cases show perifollicular erythema and matting of hair. Later, thick yellow adherent crusts (scutula) composed of skin debris and hyphae that are pierced by remaining hair shafts (Fig. 21-16). Fetid odor. In treatment, cutaneous atrophy, scar formation, and scarring alopecia. Caused by *T. schoenleinii*. Shows little tendency to clear spontaneously.

DIFFERENTIAL DIAGNOSIS

"Gray Patch" Tinea Capitis   Seborrheic dermatitis, psoriasis, atopic dermatitis, lichen simplex chronicus, alopecia areata.

"Black Dot" Tinea Capitis   Seborrheic dermatitis, psoriasis, seborrhiasis, atopic dermatitis, lichen simplex chronicus, chronic cutaneous lupus erythematosus, alopecia areata.

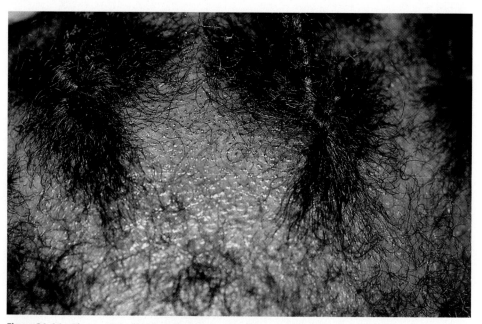

Figure 21-14   Tinea capitis: "black dot" variant   *A subtle, asymptomatic patch of alopecia due to breaking off of hairs on the frontal scalp in a 4-year-old black child. The lesion was detected because her infant sister presented with tinea corporis.* Trichophyton tonsurans *was isolated on culture.*

FUNGAL INFECTIONS OF THE SKIN AND HAIR

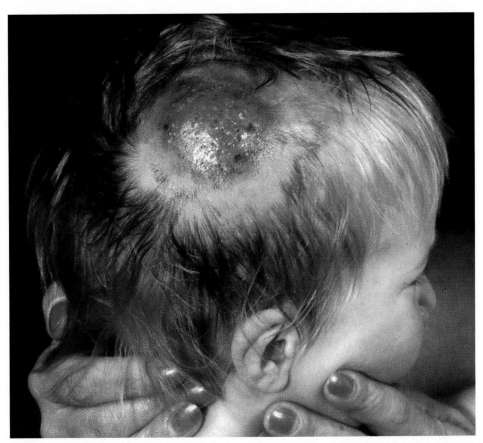

Figure 21-15 Kerion *An extremely painful, boggy, purulent inflammatory nodule on the scalp of this 4-year-old child. The lesion drains pus from multiple openings and there is retroauricular, tender lymphadenophathy. Infection was due to* T. verrucosum *contracted from an infected rabbit.*

Kerion Cellulitis, furuncle, carbuncle.

Favus Impetigo, ecthyma, crusted scabies.

LABORATORY EXAMINATIONS

Wood's Lamp Should be performed in any patient with scaling scalp lesions or hair loss of undetermined origin. *T. tonsurans,* the most common cause of tinea capitis in the United States, does not fluoresce. Formerly, *M. canis* and *M. audouinii,* which previously were the most common causes of tinea capitis, could be diagnosed by Wood's lamp examination, by bright green hair shafts with ectothrix infection.

Direct Microscopy Specimens should include hair roots and skin scales. Pluck hairs and use toothbrush to gather specimens. Skin scales contain hyphae and arthrospores. *Ectothrix:* arthrospores can be seen surrounding the hair shaft in cuticle. *Endothrix:* spores within hair shaft. *Favus:* loose chains of arthrospores and airspaces in hair shaft.

Fungal Culture With brush-culture technique, a dry toothbrush or brush used for cervical Pap testing is rubbed over area of scale or alopecia; bristles are then inoculated into fungal medium. A wet cotton swab also can be rubbed in affected area, which is then implanted into medium. The cotton-tipped swab from a bacterial culturette, moistened with tap water, can also be used to collect the specimen, and sent to a commercial laboratory. Growth of dermatophytes usually seen in 10 to 14 days.

Endothrix *T. tonsurans, T. violaceum, T. soudanense,* and *T. schoenleinii.*

Ectothrix *Microsporum* spp., *T. mentagrophytes, T. verrucosum.*

Favus *T. schoenleinii,* most commonly; also *T. violaceum, M. gypseum.*

Bacterial Culture   Rule out secondary bacterial infection, usually *Staphylococcus aureus* or group A streptococcus.

COURSE

Chronic untreated kerion and favus, especially if secondarily infected with *S. aureus,* result in scarring alopecia. Regrowth of hair is the rule if treated with systemic antifungal agents. Favus may persist until adulthood.

MANAGEMENT

Prevention	Important to examine home and school contacts of affected children for asymptomatic carriers and mild cases of tinea capitis. Ketoconazole or selenium sulfide shampoo may be helpful in eradicating the asymptomatic carrier state.
Topical antifungal agents	Topical agents are ineffective in management of tinea capitis. Duration of treatment should be extended until symptoms have resolved and fungal cultures negative.
Oral antifungal agents	Of the systemic antifungals available, terbinafine and itraconazole are superior to ketoconazole and all three to griseofulvin. Side effects in increasing order: terbinafine<itraconazole<ketoconazole< griseofulvin.
Griseofulvin	**Pediatric Dose** • Microsized: 15 mg/kg/d, maximum 500 mg/d • Ultramicrosized: 10 mg/kg/d Treatment duration: at least 6 weeks to several months; better absorption with fatty meal. **Adult Dose** • "Gray patch" ringworm: 250 mg bid for 1 or 2 months • "Black dot" ringworm: longer treatment and higher doses continued until KOH and cultures are negative *For kerion:* 250 mg bid for 4–8 weeks, hot compresses; antibiotics for accompanying staphylococcal infection
Terbinafine	250 mg qd. Reduce dosing according to weight in pediatric patients.
Itraconazole	100-mg capsules or oral solution (10 mg/mL). Treatment duration: 4 to 8 weeks. **Pediatric Dose** 5 mg/kg/d **Adult Dose** 200 mg/d
Fluconazole	100-, 150-, 200-mg tablets; oral solution (10 mg/mL, 40 mg/mL). 6–8 mg/kg/d. Treatment duration: 3–4 weeks (in some cases 2). **Pediatric Dose** 6 mg/kg/d • Daily for 2 weeks; repeat at 4 weeks if indicated **Adult Dose** 200 mg/d
Ketoconazole	200-mg tablets. Treatment duration: 4–6 weeks. **Pediatric Dose** 5 mg/kg/d **Adult Dose** 200–400 mg/d
Adjunctive therapy	
Prednisone	1 mg/kg/d for 14 days for children with severe, painful kerion.
Systemic antibiotics	For secondary *S. aureus* or group A *Streptococcus* infection, erythromycin, dicloxacillin, or cephalexin
Surgery	Drain pus from kerion lesions.

FUNGAL INFECTIONS OF THE SKIN AND HAIR

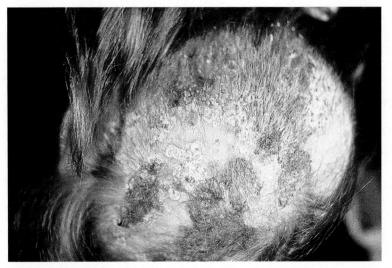

Figure 21-16   Tinea capitis: favus   *Extensive hair loss with atrophy, scarring, and so-called scutula, i.e., yellowish adherent crusts present on the scalp; remaining hairs pierce the scutula.* Trichophyton schoenleinii *was isolated on culture.*

Tinea Barbae

Tinea barbae is a dermatophytic trichomycosis involving the beard and moustache areas, closely resembling tinea capitis, with invasion of the hair shaft.
Synonym: Ringworm of the beard.

EPIDEMIOLOGY

Age of Onset Adult.

Sex Males only.

Etiology *T. verrucosum, T. mentagrophytes* var. *mentagrophytes,* most commonly. May be acquired through animal exposure. *T. rubrum* an uncommon cause.

Predisposing Factors More common in farmers.

HISTORY

Skin Symptoms Pruritus, tenderness, pain.

PHYSICAL EXAMINATION

Skin Lesions Pustular folliculitis (Fig. 21-17), i.e., hair follicles surrounded by red inflammatory papules or pustules, often with exudation and crusting. Involved hairs are loose and easily removed. With less follicular involvement, there are scaling, circular, reddish patches in which hair is broken off at the surface. Papules may coalesce to inflammatory plaques topped by pustules. Kerion: boggy purulent nodules and plaques as with tinea capitis (Fig. 21-18). Beard and moustache areas, rarely, eyelashes, eyebrows.

Systemic Findings Regional lymphadenopathy, especially if long duration and if superinfected.

DIFFERENTIAL DIAGNOSIS

Beard Folliculitis *S. aureus* folliculitis, furuncle, carbuncle, acne vulgaris, rosacea, pseudofolliculitis.

LABORATORY EXAMINATIONS

See Tinea Capitis, page 703.

MANAGEMENT

Topical Agents Ineffective.

Systemic Agents See Tinea Manuum, page 694; Tinea Capitis, page 704.

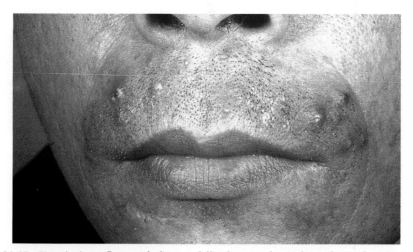

Figure 21-17 Tinea barbae *Scattered, discrete follicular pustules and papules in the moustache area, easily mistaken for* S. aureus *folliculitis.*

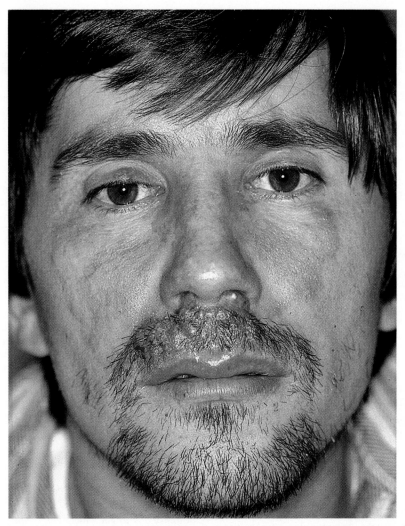

Figure 21-18   Tinea barbae and tinea facialis *Confluent, painful papules, nodules, and pustules on the upper lip. Epidermal dermatophytosis (tinea facialis) with sharply marginated erythema and scaling is present on the cheeks, eyelids, eyebrows, and forehead.* Trichophyton mentagrophytes *was isolated on culture. In this case, the organism caused two distinct clinical patterns (epidermal involvement, tinea facialis versus follicular inflammation, tinea barbae), depending on whether glabrous skin or hairy skin was infected.*

Candidiasis

Candidiasis is most frequently caused by the yeast Candida albicans, and less often by other Candida spp. Superficial infections of mucosal surface (oropharynx, genitalia) are common in otherwise healthy individuals; infections of the esophagus and/or tracheobronchial tree occur in the setting of significant immunocompromise. Cutaneous candidiasis occurs at moist occluded skin. Invasive, disseminated candidiasis occurs in immunocompromised individuals, usually after invasion of the gastrointestinal tract.
Synonyms: Candidosis, moniliasis.

EPIDEMIOLOGY

Age of Onset The young and old are more likely to be colonized.

Etiology *Candida albicans,* an oval yeast varying in size (2 to 6 μm by 3 to 9 μm). Polymorphism is displayed as yeast forms, budding yeast, pseudohyphae, and true hyphae. Besides *C. albicans,* >100 species of the genus have been identified, most of which are neither commensals nor pathogenic for humans. Other pathogenic species, usually in the setting of immunocompromise, include: *C. tropicalis, C. parapsilosis, C. guilliermondii, C. krusei, C. pseudotropicalis, C. lusitaneae, C. glabrata* (formerly, *Torulopsis glabrata*).

Ecology *Candida albicans* and other species frequently colonize the gastrointestinal tract of humans. Colonization may occur during birthing from the birth canal, during infancy, or later. Oropharyngeal colonization is present in approximately 20% of healthy individuals, the rate being higher in hospitalized patients. Fecal colonization is higher than oral, with a rate of 40 to 67%; the rate increases after treatment with antibacterial agents. Serologic and skin test studies indicate that a significant proportion of those not colonized have been exposed to *Candida* in the past. Antibiotic therapy increases the incidence of carriage, the number of organisms present, and the chances for tissue invasion. Approximately 13% of women are colonized vaginally with *C. albicans;* antibiotic therapy, pregnancy, oral contraception, and intrauterine devices increase the incidence of carriage. *C. albicans* may transiently colonize the skin but is not one of the permanent flora.

Host Factors Diabetes mellitus, obesity, hyperhidrosis, heat, maceration, polyendocrinopathies, systemic and topical glucocorticoids, chronic debilitation.

Immunologic Factors Reduced cell-mediated immunity is the most significant factor. Decreased specific anti-*Candida* IgA salivary antibody may be a factor. Defects in neutrophil or macrophage functions are factors in invasive candidiasis.

EPIDEMIOLOGY

Ecology *C. albicans* is seldom recovered from skin of normal individuals. Usually endogenous infection. *Candida* is a normal inhabitant of mucosal surfaces of oropharynx and GI tract. In males with balanitis, *Candida* may be transmitted from female sexual partner.

Occupation Persons who immerse their hands in water: housewives, mothers of young children, health care workers, bartenders, florists.

LABORATORY EXAMINATIONS

Direct Microscopy KOH preparation visualizes pseudohyphae and yeast forms. (Fig. 21-19)

Culture   Fungal Identifies species of *Candida;* however, the presence in culture of *C. albicans* does not make the diagnosis of candidiasis; *Candida* is a normal inhabitant of the GI tract. Identifying *Candida* in the absence of symptoms should not lead to treatment, because 10 to 20% of normal women harbor *Candida* spp. and other yeasts in the vagina. Sensitivities to antifungal agents can be performed on isolate in cases of recurrent infection.

Bacterial Rule out bacterial superinfection.

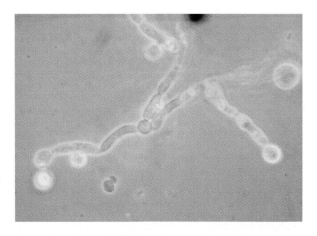

Figure 21-19 Candida albicans: KOH preparation *Budding yeast forms and sausage-like pseudohyphal forms.*

CLASSIFICATION

Type	Site	Clinical presentation
Occluded site (where occlusion and maceration create warm, moist microecology)	Body folds	Axillae, inframammary, groin, intergluteal, abdominal panniculus
		Webspace: hands (erosio interdigitale blastomycetica), feet
		Angular cheilitis; often associated with oropharyhgeal candidiasis
	Genital	Balanitis, balanoposthitis
		Vulvitis, vulvovaginitis
	Occluded skin	Under occlusive dressing, under cast, back in hospitalized patient
	Folliculitis	Back; in hospitalized patient
	Area occluded under diaper	Diaper dermatitis
Nail apparatus	Paronychium	Chronic paronychia
	Nail plate	Onychia
	Hyponychium	Onycholysis
Chronic mucocutaneous	Extensive, multiple or 20 nail	Individuals with congenital immunologic (T cell defects) or endocrinologic disorders (hypoparathyroidism, hypoadrenalism, hypothyroidism, diabetes mellitus) develop persistent or recurrent mucosal, cutaneous, and/or paronychial/ nail infections.
Genitalia	Vulva, vagina; preputial sac	Erythema, erosions, white plaques of candidal colonies
Mucosal	Oropharynx	Thrush; atrophic candidiasis; hyperplastic candidiasis
	Esophagus	Inflamed, eroded plaques
	Trachea, bronchi	Inflamed, eroded plaques
Candidemia	Skin, viscera	Skin: erythematous papules, ±hemorrhage

MANAGEMENT

Oral antifungal agents Indicated for infections resistant to topical modalities of therapy.

Fluconazole Tablets: 50, 100, 150, 200 mg. Oral suspension: 50 mg/5 mL. Parenteral: for injection or IV infusion.

Itraconazole Capsules: 100 mg. Oral solution: 10 mg/mL.

Ketoconazole Tablets: 200 mg.

Cutaneous Candidiasis

Cutaneous candidiasis is a superficial infection occurring on moist, occluded cutaneous sites; many patients have predisposing factors such as increased moisture at the site of infection, diabetes, or alterations in systemic immunity.

EPIDEMIOLOGY

Other Predisposing Factors   Diabetes, obesity, hyperhidrosis, heat, maceration, systemic and topical glucocorticoids, chronic debilitation.

HISTORY

Intertrigo   Erythema. Pruritus, tenderness, pain.

Occluded Skin   Under occlusive dressing, under cast, back in hospitalized patient.

Diaper Dermatitis   Irritability, discomfort with urination, defecation, changing diapers.

PHYSICAL EXAMINATION

Intertrigo   Initial pustules on erythematous base become eroded and confluent. Subsequently, fairly sharply demarcated, polycyclic, erythematous, eroded patches with small pustular lesions at the periphery (satellite pustulosis).

Distribution   Inframammary (Fig. 21-20), axillae, groins (Fig. 21-21), perineal, intergluteal cleft (Fig. 21-22).

Interdigital   Erosio interdigitalis blastomycetica. Initial pustule becomes eroded, with formation of superficial erosion or fissure, ±surrounded by thickened white skin (Fig. 21-23). May be associated with *Candida* onychia or paronychia.

Distribution   On hands, usually between third and fourth fingers (Fig. 21-23); on feet, similar presentation as interdigital tinea pedis.

Diaper Dermatitis   Erythema, edema with papular and pustular lesions; erosions, oozing, collarette-like scaling at the margins of lesions involving perigenital and perianal skin, inner aspects of thighs and buttocks (Fig. 21-24).

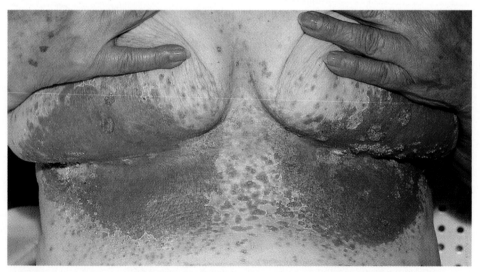

Figure 21-20   Cutaneous candidiasis: intertrigo   *Small peripheral "satellite" papules and pustules that have become confluent centrally, creating large eroded area in the submammary region.*

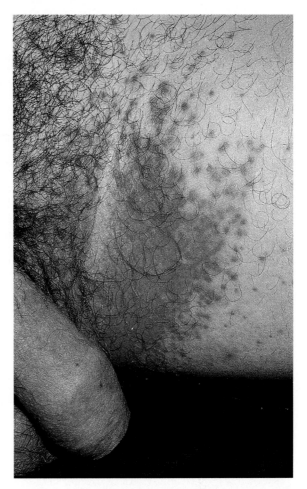

Figure 21-21 Cutaneous candidiasis: intertrigo *Erythematous papules with a few pustules, becoming confluent on the medial thigh. The lesions occurred during a holiday trip to the Caribbean.*

Follicular Candidiasis Small, discrete pustules in ostia of hair follicles.

DIFFERENTIAL DIAGNOSIS

Intertrigo/Occluded Skin Nonspecific intertrigo, inverse pattern psoriasis, erythrasma, dermatophytosis, pityriasis versicolor.

Interdigital Scabies.

Diaper Dermatitis Atopic dermatitis, psoriasis, irritant dermatitis, seborrheic dermatitis.

Folliculitis Bacterial (*Staphylococcus aureus, Pseudomonas aeruginosa*) folliculitis, *Pityrosporum* folliculitis, acne.

LABORATORY EXAMINATIONS

See Candidiasis, page 708.

DIAGNOSIS

Clinical findings confirmed by direct microscopy or culture.

MANAGEMENT

Prevention	Keep intertriginous areas dry (often difficult).
	Washing with benzoyl peroxide bar may reduce *Candida* colonization.
	Powder with miconazole applied daily.
Topical treatment	
Castellani's paint	Brings almost immediate relief of symptoms, i.e., candidal paronychia.
Glucocorticoid preparation	Judicious short-term use speeds resolution of symptoms.
Topical antifungal agents	Antiungal preparation: Nystatin, azole, or imidazole cream bid or more often with diaper dermatitis. Tolnaftate not effective for candidiasis. Torbinafine may be effective.
Nystatin cream	Effective for *Candida* only; not effective for dermatophytosis.
Azole creams	Effective for candidiasis, dermatophytosis, and pityriasis versicolor.
Oral antifungal agents	Eliminate bowel colonization. Azoles treat cutaneous infection.
Nystatin (suspension, tablet, pastille)	Not absorbed from the bowel. Eradicates bowel colonization. May be effective in recurrent candidiasis of diaper area, genitals, or intertrigo.
Systemic antifungal, agents	See Candidiasis, page 708.

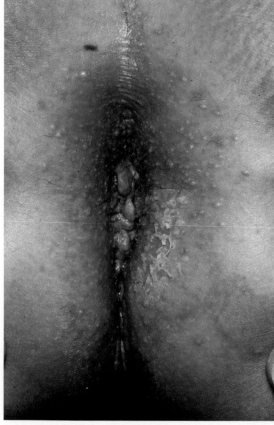

Figure 21-22   Cutaneous candidiasis: intertrigo *Vesicles, pustules, and papules becoming confluent on the perineum and perianal area. The patient had successfully undergone a bone marrow transplantation 4 weeks before the appearance of the cutaneous lesions. The initial impression by the oncologist was that the lesions were reactivated herpes simplex; KOH preparation and cultures confirmed the diagnosis of* Candida *intertrigo.*

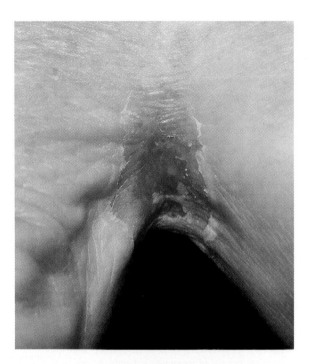

Figure 21-23 Cutaneous candidiasis: interdigital intertrigo *Erythematous eroded webspace of the hand; several other webspaces were also involved in this elderly obese diabetic.*

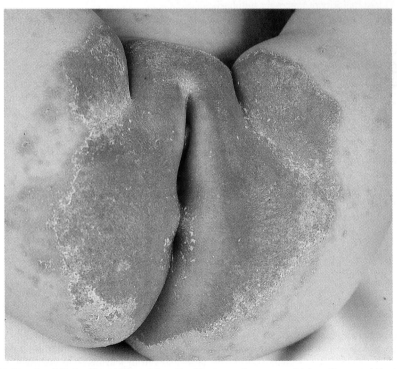

Figure 21-24 Candidiasis: diaper dermatitis *Confluent erosions, marginal scaling, and "satellite pustules" in the area covered by a diaper in an infant.*

SUPERFICIAL FUNGAL INFECTIONS

Oropharyngeal Candidiasis

Candidiasis of the oropharyngeal mucosa (OPC) occurs with minor variations of host factors such as antibiotic therapy, glucocorticoid therapy (topical or systemic), age (very young, very old) as well as with significant immunocompromise. Esophageal and/or tracheobronchial candidiasis may be associated with oropharyngeal candidiasis and always occurs in the setting of advanced immunocompromise. *Candida* can invade through eroded mucosa, with resultant fungemia and invasive candidiasis.

Synonyms: Thrush, mycotic stomatitis, *Candida* leukoplakia.

EPIDEMIOLOGY

Etiology   *C. albicans,* one of resident flora of the mouth, overgrows in association with various local or systemic factors. In some cases, an exogenous infection. After chronic antifungal therapy, especially with advanced immunocompromise, fluconazole-resistant strains of *Candida* can evolve and cause infection resistant to oral/intravenous azole therapy.

Incidence   Although a number of risk factors exist (see below) and almost obligatory involvement occurs in immunocompromised patients, the vast majority of mucosal candidiasis; occurs in otherwise healthy individuals.

HIV Disease   Untreated OPC occurs in 50% of HIV-infected and 80 to 95% of those with AIDS; 60% relapse within 3 months after treatment. Esophageal candidiasis occurs in 10 to 15% of individuals with AIDS.

Bone Marrow Transplant Recipients   30 to 40% develop superficial mucosal candidiasis; occurs in otherwise healthy individuals.

Transmission   Normal inhabitant of mucosal surfaces of the oropharynx and gastrointestinal tract; overgrowth associated with local or systemic suppression of immunity or antibiotic therapy. In neonatal OPC, *C. albicans* is acquired from the genital tract of mother. Nosocomial transmission does occur.

Risk Factors   In addition to HIV-induced immunodeficiency, other risk factors include general debilitation, diabetes mellitus, therapy with broad-spectrum antibiotics, topical or parenteral glucocorticoids, parenteral hyperalimentation.

CDC Surveillance Case Definition for AIDS Candidiasis of the esophagus, trachea, bronchi, or lungs is an AIDS-defining condition if the patient has no other cause of immunodeficiency and is without knowledge of HIV antibody status.

CLASSIFICATION

Superficial Mucosal Candidiasis   May be associated with mild to moderate impairment of cell-mediated immunity.

Oropharyngeal Candidiasis   Pseudomembranous candidiasis (thrush); erythematous (atrophic) candidiasis; candidal leukoplakia (hyperplastic candidiasis); angular cheilitis.

Deep Mucosal Candidiasis   Occurs in states of advanced immunocompromise: esophageal candidiasis, tracheobronchial candidiasis, both of which are AIDS-defining conditions. Bladder.

HISTORY

Symptoms   *Oropharynx*   Asymptomatic. Burning or pain on eating spices/acidic foods, diminished taste sensation. Cosmetic concern about white curds on tongue. Odynophagia. In HIV disease, may be the initial presentation; OPC is a clinical marker for disease progression, first noted when CD4+ cell count is 390/μL.

Esophagus   Asymptomatic. Occurs when CD4+ cell count is low (<200/μL and is an AIDS-defining condition. Dysphagia. Odynophagia, resulting in difficulty eating and malnutrition.

PHYSICAL EXAMINATION

Mucosal Lesions

Type   *Pseudomembranous Candidiasis (Thrush)*   (Figs. 21-25 and 21-26) White-to-creamy plaques on any mucosal surface; vary in size from 1 to 2 mm to extensive and widespread; removal with a dry gauze pad leaves an erythematous or bleeding mucosal surface.

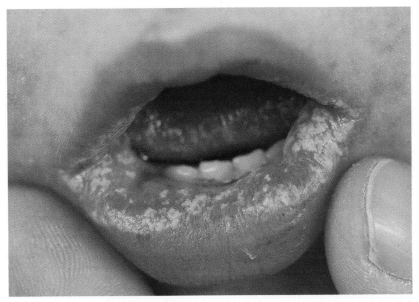

Figure 21-25 Oral candidiasis: thrush *White curd-like material on the mucosal surface of the lower lip of a child; the material can be abraded off with gauze (pseudomembranous), revealing underlying erythema.*

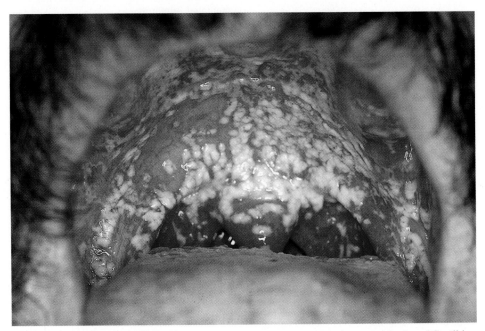

Figure 21-26 Oral candidiasis: thrush *Extensive cottage cheese-like plaques, colonies of* Candida *that can be removed by rubbing with gauze (pseudomembranous), on the palate and uvula of an individual with advanced HIV disease. Patches of erythema between the white plaques represent erythematous (atrophic) candidiasis. Involvement may extend into the esophagus and be associated with dysphagia.*

Erythematous (Atrophic) Candidiasis Smooth, red, atrophic patches (Figs. 21-26 and 21-27); may be associated with thrush.

Candidal Leukoplakia White plaques that cannot be wiped off but regress with prolonged anticandidal therapy.

Angular Cheilitis Erythema, fissuring, i.e., intertrigo at the corner of mouth (Figs. 21-25 and 21-27).

Distribution *Thrush*: dorsum of tongue, buccal mucosa, hard/soft palate, pharynx extending down into esophagus and tracheobronchial tree. *Erythematous (atrophic) candidiasis:* hard/soft palate, buccal mucosa, dorsal surface of tongue. *Leukoplakia:* buccal mucosa, tongue, hard palate.

General Findings

Invasive Candidiasis In individuals with severe prolonged neutropenia, *Candida* can invade into submucosa and blood vessels with subsequent hematogenous dissemination to skin (Fig. 21-28) and viscera. Candidemia also occurs in the setting of prolonged catheterization.

DIFFERENTIAL DIAGNOSIS

Pseudomembranous Candidiasis (Thrush) Oral hairy leukoplakia, condyloma acuminatum, geographic tongue, hairy tongue, lichen planus, bite irritation.

Atrophic (Erythematous) Candidiasis Lichen planus.

LABORATORY EXAMINATIONS

See Candidiasis, page 708.

Endoscopy Documents esophageal and/or tracheobronchial candidiasis.

DIAGNOSIS

Clinical suspicion confirmed by KOH preparation of scraping from mucosal surface.

COURSE AND PROGNOSIS

Most cases respond to correction of the precipitating cause (e.g., use of inhaled glucocorticoids). Topical agents effective in most cases. Clinical resistance to antifungal agents may be related to patient noncompliance, severe immunocompromise, drug-drug interaction (rifampin-fluconazole). Between 30 and 40% of bone marrow transplant recipients develop superficial mucosal candidiasis; 10 to 25% develop deep invasive candidiasis, of whom a quarter die from the infection and others go on to develop chronic visceral candidiasis.

In HIV disease, oropharyngeal and esophageal candidiasis have been reported with primary HIV infection. In later HIV disease [before the advent of highly active retroviral therapy (HAART)], OPC is nearly universal; esophageal infection occurs in 10 to 20% of patients. Relapse after topical or systemic treatment is expected. Virtually all HIV-infected individuals with CD4+ cell counts of ≤100/μL harbor oral *Candida;* chronic suppressive therapy is associated with changes in mouth flora rather than eradication.

MANAGEMENT

Topical Therapy These preparations are effective in the immunocompetent individual but relatively ineffective with decreasing cell-mediated immunity.

Nystatin Oral tablets, 100,000 units qid dissolved slowly in the mouth, are the most effective preparation. The oral suspension, 1 to 2 teaspoons, held in mouth for 5 min and then swallowed may be effective.

Clotrimazole Oral tablets (troche), 10 mg, one tablet 5 times daily may be effective.

HIV Disease Responds to topical and/or systemic therapy; however, recurrence is the rule. May become refractory to intermittent therapy, requiring daily chemoprophylaxis, with either topical or systemic treatment. Increase dose with resistant disease.

Fluconazole 200 mg PO once followed by 100 mg/d for 2 to 3 weeks, then discontinue. Increase the dose to 400 to 800 mg in resistant infection. Also available in IV form.

Itraconazole Capsules or oral solution. 100 mg PO qd or bid for 2 weeks. Increase dose with resistant disease.

Ketoconazole 200 mg PO qd to bid for 1 to 2 weeks.

Fluconazole-Resistant Candidiasis Defined as clinical persistence of infection after treatment with fluconazole, 100 mg/d PO for 7 days.

Occurs most commonly in HIV-infected individuals with CD4+ cell counts <50/μL who have had prolonged fluconazole exposure. Chronic low-dose fluconazole treatment (50 mg/d) facilitates emergence of resistant strains; 50% of resistant strains sensitive to itraconazole. Amphotericin B for severe resistant disease. New liposomal preparations are effective and less toxic. Recurrence is the rule; maintenance therapy is often required.

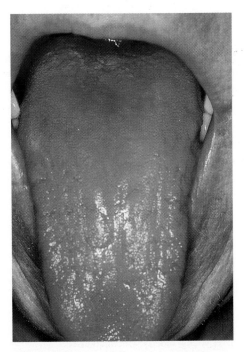

Figure 21-27 Oral candidiasis: atrophic with angular cheilitis *The surface of the tongue is atrophic and shiny; an intertrigo is present at the angles of the lips. The patient is diabetic; anogenital candidiasis was also present.*

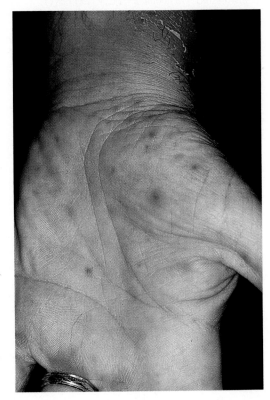

Figure 21-28 Invasive candidiasis with candidemia *Multiple erythematous papules on the hand of a febrile patient with granulocytopenia associated with treatment of acute myelogenous leukemia. The usual source of the infection is the gastrointestinal tract.* Candida tropicalis *was isolated on blood culture; candidal forms were seen on lesional skin biopsy.*

Genital Candidiasis

Genital candidiasis is a *Candida* infection of the mucosa (nonkeratinized epithelium) of the vulva, vagina, and preputial sac of the penis. Infection usually represents overgrowth of colonizing infection rather than arising from exogenous source.

EPIDEMIOLOGY

Ecology >20% of normal women have vaginal colonization with *Candida*. *C. albicans* accounts for 80 to 90% of genital isolates.

Incidence Most vaginal candidiasis (VC) occurs in the normal population. 75% of women experience at least one episode of VC during their lifetime, and 40 to 45% experience two or more episodes. Often associated with vulvar candidiasis, i.e., vulvovaginal candidiasis (VVC). A small percentage of women (probably <5%) experience recurrent VVC (RVVC).

Risk Factors Usually none. Pregnancy. Usually sexually active. But also in sexually inactive, young, elderly. Uncircumcised.

Transmission In neonatal OPC, *C. albicans* is acquired from the genital tract of mother. To males from colonized sexual partners.

HISTORY

Symptoms *Vulvitis/Vulvovaginitis* Onset often abrupt, usually the week before menstruation; symptoms may recur before each menstruation. Pruritus, vaginal discharge, vaginal soreness, vulvar burning, dyspareunia, external dysuria.

Balanoposthitis, Balanitis Burning, itching, redness.

PHYSICAL EXAMINATION

Mucosal Lesions *Vulvitis* Erosions, pustules, erythema (Fig. 21-29), swelling, removable curd-like material.

Vulvitis/Vulvovaginitis Vaginitis with white discharge; vaginal erythema and edema; white plaques that can be wiped off on vaginal and/or cervical mucosa. Often associated with vulvar candidiasis and candidal intertrigo of inguinal folds and perineum. Subcorneal pustules at periphery with fringed, irregular margins. In chronic cases, vaginal mucosa glazed and atrophic.

Balanoposthitis, Balanitis Glans and preputial sac: papules, pustules, erosions (Fig. 21-30). Maculopapular lesions with diffuse erythema. Edema, ulcerations, and fissuring of prepuce, usually in diabetic men; white plaques under foreskin.

DIFFERENTIAL DIAGNOSIS

VC/VVC Trichomoniasis (caused by *Trichomonas vaginalis*), bacterial vaginosis (caused by replacement of normal vaginal flora by an overgrowth of anaerobic microorganisms and *Gardnerella vaginalis*), lichen planus, lichen sclerosus et atrophicus.

Balanoposthitis Psoriasis, eczema.

LABORATORY EXAMINATIONS

See Candidiasis, page 708.

DIAGNOSIS

Clinical suspicion confirmed by KOH preparation of scraping from mucosal surface.

COURSE AND PROGNOSIS

RVVC Defined as three or more episodes of symptomatic VVC annually. Affects a small proportion of women (<5%). The natural history and pathogenesis of RVVC are poorly understood. The majority of women with RVVC have no apparent predisposing conditions.

MANAGEMENT

VC/VVC *Topical Therapy* Azoles/imidazoles (see page 720) are more effective than nystatin and result in relief of symptoms and negative cultures among 80 to 90% of patients after therapy is completed.

Recommended Regimens Single-dose regimens probably should be reserved for cases of uncomplicated mild to moderate VVC. Multi-day regimens (3- to 7-day) are the preferred treatment for severe or complicated VVC.

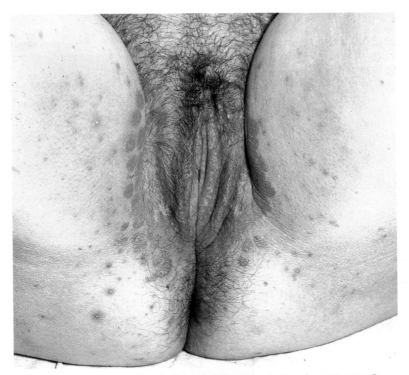

Figure 21-29   Candidiasis: vulvitis   *Psoriasiform, erythematous lesions becoming confluent on the vulva with erosions and satellite pustules on the thighs.*

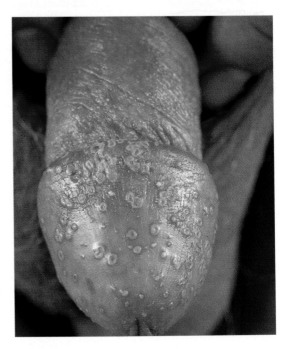

Figure 21-30   Candidiasis: balanoposthitis   *Multiple, discrete pustules on the glans penis and inner aspect of the foreskin (the preputial sac). The "umbilicated" lesions can be mistaken for genital herpes, mollusca contagiosa, or condylomata acuminata.*

SUPERFICIAL FUNGAL INFECTIONS

Butoconazole: 2% cream 5 g intravaginally for 3 days *or*

Clotrimazole: 1% cream 5 g intravaginally for 7 to 14 days *or*
   100-mg vaginal tablet for 7 days *or*
   100-mg vaginal tablet, two tablets for 3 days *or*
   500-mg vaginal tablet, one tablet in a single application *or*

Miconazole: 2% cream 5 g intravaginally for 7 days *or*
   200-mg vaginal suppository, one suppository for 3 days *or*
   100-mg vaginal suppository, one suppository for 7 days *or*

Tioconazole: 6.5% ointment 5 g intravaginally in a single application *or*

Terconazole: .4% cream 5 g intravaginally for 7 days *or*
   .8% cream 5 g intravaginally for 3 days *or*
   80-mg suppository, one suppository for 3 days

Fluconazole: 150 mg PO as a single dose

RVVC   Weekly dosing with the following may be effective:

Clotrimazole: 500-mg vaginal tablet, one tablet in a single application *or*

Fluconazole: 150 mg PO as a single dose

Itraconazole: 100 mg PO bid

Balanitis, Balanoposthitis   Azole cream bid. Treat sexual partner if recurrent.
Systemic Treatment   See above.

Candidiasis of the Nail Apparatus

See Disorders of Nail, Section 28.

Chronic Mucocutaneous Candidiasis

Chronic mucocutaneous candidiasis (CMC) is characterized by persistent/recurrent *Candida* infections of the oropharynx, skin, and nail apparatus, (Figs. 21-31 and 21-32) usually associated with underlying immunocompromise and onset in infancy or early childhood. Oropharyngeal candidiasis is refractory to conventional therapy, relapsing after successful therapy; chronic infection results in hypertrophic (leukoplakic) candidiasis. Cutaneous candidiasis manifests as intertrigo or widespread infection of the trunk and/or extremities; lesions become hypertrophic in chronic untreated cases. Infection of the nail apparatus is universal with chronic paronychia, nail plate infection, and eventually total nail dystrophy. Many patients also have dermatophytosis and cutaneous warts.

Five types of CMC have been defined: (1) autosomal recessive CMC (early onset, oral and skin affected, may have dermatophytosis as well); (3) diffuse CMC; (4) CMC with endocrinopathy (familial polyendocrinopathy syndrome with hypoparathyroidism, hypoadrenocorticalism, hypothyroidism, pernicious anemia, vitiligo); (5) late onset CMC (associated with thymoma).

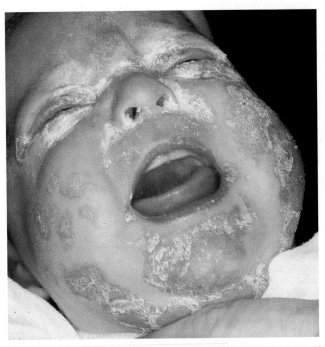

Figure 21-31 Mucocutaneous candidiasis *Persistent candidiasis in an immunocompromised infant manifesting as erosions covered by scales and crusts, oropharyngeal candidiasis, and widespread infection of the trunk.*

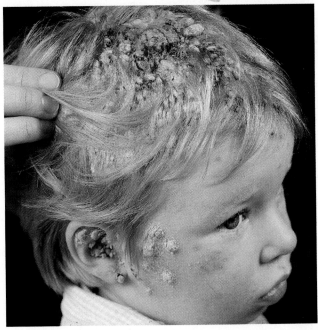

Figure 21-32 Mucocutaneous candidiasis *This 3-year-old child with hypothyroidism had oral thrush, intertriginous candidiasis, warty hyperkeratoses, and crusts on the scalp and face; and also, candidal onychomycosis. The warty growths shown in the photo consisted of dried pus, serum, and pure cultures of Candida.*

SUPERFICIAL FUNGAL INFECTIONS

721

Pityriasis Versicolor

Pityriasis versicolor (PV) is a chronic asymptomatic scaling dermatosis associated with the superficial overgrowth of the hyphal form of Pityrosporum ovale, characterized by well-demarcated scaling patches with variable pigmentation, occurring most commonly on the trunk. Synonym: Tinea versicolor.

EPIDEMIOLOGY

Age of Onset Young adults. Less common when sebum production is reduced or absent; tapers off during fifth and sixth decades.

Etiology *P. ovale* (also known as *P. orbiculare* and *Malassezia furfur*), a lipophilic yeast that normally resides in the keratin of skin and hair follicles of individuals 15 years of age or older. It is an opportunistic organism, causing pityriasis versicolor, *Pityrosporum* folliculitis, and implicated in the pathogenesis of seborrheic dermatitis. *Pityrosporum* infections are not contagious, but an overgrowth of resident cutaneous flora occurs under certain favorable conditions.

Predisposing Factors High humidity at the skin surface. High rate of sebum production. Application of grease such as cocoa butter predisposes young children to PV. High levels of cortisol appear to increase susceptibility—both in Cushing's syndrome and with prolonged administration of glucocorticoids (topical as well as systemic).

Incidence In temperate zones: 2%. In subtropical and tropical zones: 40%.

Season In temperate zones, appears in summertime; fades during cooler months. In physically active individuals, may persist year round.

PATHOGENESIS

Dicarboxylic acids formed by enzymatic oxidation of fatty acids in skin surface lipids inhibit tyrosinase in epidermal melanocytes and thereby lead to hypomelanosis. The enzyme is present in the organism.

HISTORY

Duration of Lesions Months to years.

Skin Symptoms Usually none. Occasionally, mild pruritus. Individuals with PV usually present because of cosmetic concerns about the blotchy pigmentation.

PHYSICAL EXAMINATION

Skin Lesions Macules, sharply marginated (Figs. 21-33 through 21-35), round or oval in shape, varying in size. Fine scaling is best appreciated by gently abrading lesions with a no. 15 scalpel blade or the edge of a microscope slide. Treated or burned-out lesions lack scale. Some patients have findings of *Pityrosporum* folliculitis and seborrheic dermatitis. In untanned skin, lesions are light brown. On tanned skin, white. In dark-skinned individuals, dark brown macules. Brown of varying intensities and hues (Fig. 21-33); off-white macules (Figs. 21-34 and 21-35). In time, individual lesions may enlarge, merge, forming extensive geographic areas.

Distribution Upper trunk, upper arms, neck, abdomen, axillae, groins, thighs, genitalia. Facial, neck, and/or scalp lesions occur in patients applying creams/ointments or topical glucocorticoid preparations.

DIFFERENTIAL DIAGNOSIS

Hypopigmented PV Vitiligo, pityriasis alba, postinflammatory hypopigmentation, tuberculoid leprosy.

Scaling Lesions Tinea corporis, seborrheic dermatitis, pityriasis rosea, guttate psoriasis, nummular eczema.

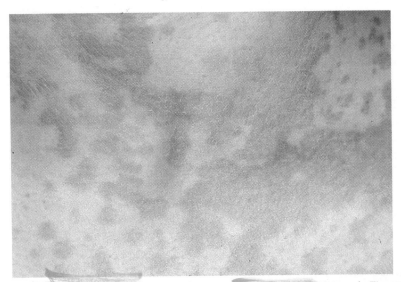

Figure 21-33 **Pityriasis versicolor** *Sharply marginated brown macules on the trunk. Fine scale was apparent when the lesions were abraded with the edge of a microscope slide.*

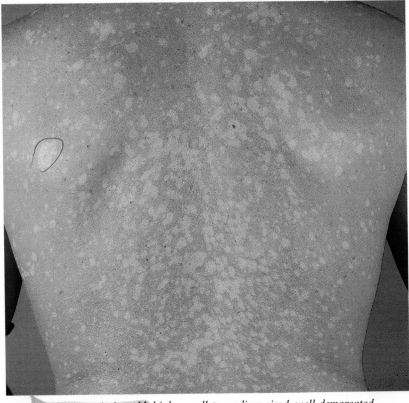

Figure 21-34 **Pityriasis versicolor** *Multiple, small-to-medium-sized, well-demarcated hypopigmented macules on the back of a tanned individual with white skin.*

SUPERFICIAL FUNGAL INFECTIONS

LABORATORY EXAMINATIONS

Direct Microscopic Examination of Scales Prepared with KOH Scale is best obtained with two microscope slides, using one to raise scale and move it onto the other. The harvested scale is moved into a small pile in the center of the slide and covered with a coverslip. KOH solution (15 to 20%) is added at the edge of the coverslip; the slide is gently heated and examined. Filamentous hyphae and globose yeast forms, termed "spaghetti and meatballs," are seen (Fig. 21-36).

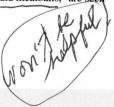

Wood's Lamp Blue-green fluorescence of scales; may be negative in individuals who have showered recently because the fluorescent chemical is water soluble. Vitiligo appears as depigmented, white, and has no scale.

Dermatopathology Budding yeast and hyphal forms in the most superficial layers of the stratum corneum, seen best with PAS stain. Variable hyperkeratosis, psoriasiform hyperplasia, chronic inflammation with blood vessel dilatation.

DIAGNOSIS

Clinical findings, confirmed by positive KOH preparation findings.

MANAGEMENT

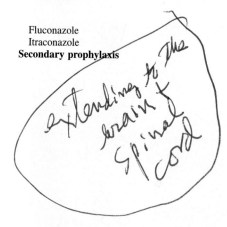

Topical agents
Selenium sulfide (2.5%) lotion or shampoo | Apply daily to affected areas for 10 to 15 min, followed by shower, for 1 week

Propylene glycol 50% solution (in water): Apply bid for 2 weeks
Ketoconazole shampoo | Applied same as selenium sulfide shampoo
Azole creams (ketoconazole, econazole, micronazole, clotrimazole) | Apply qd or bid for 2 weeks
Terbinafine 1% solution | Apply bid for 7 days
Systemic therapy (None of these agents is approved for use in PV in the United States)
Ketoconazole | 200 mg/d PO for 7–14 days or 400 mg once; repeat in 1 week *or* 400 mg stat, repeat in 1 month

Fluconazole | 400–600 mg stat; repeat in 1 week
Itraconazole | 200 mg bid for one day; 200 mg for 5–7 days
Secondary prophylaxis | Ketoconazole shampoo once or twice a week. Selenium sulfide (2.5%) lotion or shampoo. Salicylic acid/sulfur bar. Pyrithione zinc (bar or shampoo). Propylene glycol 50% solution once a month

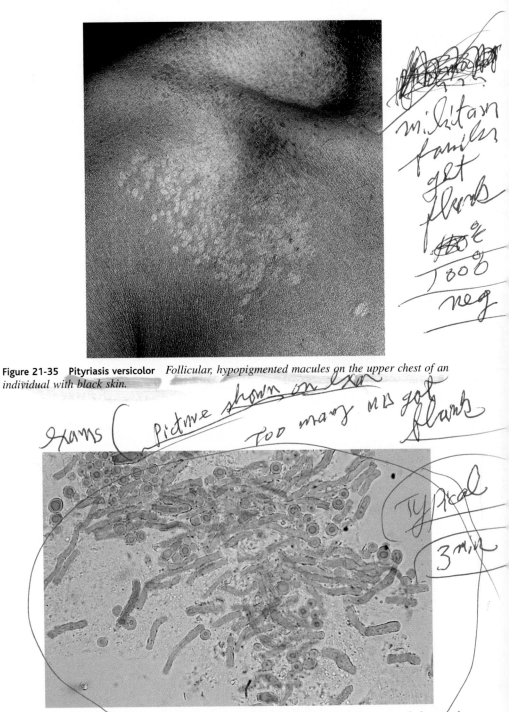

Figure 21-35   Pityriasis versicolor   *Follicular, hypopigmented macules on the upper chest of an individual with black skin.*

Figure 21-36   *Malassezia furfur* (*Pityrosporum ovale*): KOH preparation   *Round yeast and elongated pseudohyphal forms, so-called "spaghetti and meatballs."*

INVASIVE FUNGAL INFECTIONS

Invasive fungal infections can arise by deeper extension of local cutaneous infections (mycetoma, chromomycosis, and sporotrichosis) or by dissemination of a primary pulmonary infection to the skin or mucosa (cryptococcosis, blastomycosis, histoplasmosis, coccidioidomycosis). Locally invasive fungal infections can occur in otherwise healthy individuals; in the setting of immunocompromise, these infections can disseminate systemically. Many individuals with dissemination of fungal infections to the skin do have underlying immunocompromise.

Mycetoma

Mycetoma is a local, chronic, slowly progressive infection of skin, subcutaneous tissues, fascia, bone, and muscle, most commonly of the foot or hand, characterized by swelling or tumorfaction, draining sinuses, and granules; the exudate contains grains that may be yellow, white, red, brown, or black depending on the causative microorganisms.
Synonyms: Madura foot, maduromycetoma.

EPIDEMIOLOGY

Age of Onset   20 to 50 years.

Sex   90% of patients are males.

Occupation   Agricultural workers and laborers exposed to soil in tropical and subtropical regions.

Transmission   Cutaneous inoculation (thorn prick, wood splinter, stone cut) of organism, commonly with soil or plant debris, into foot or hand.

Geography   Fungi isolated from soil except *Actinomyces israelii*. Tropical and subtropical climate supports growth of organisms. In Central/South America, 90% of cases caused by *Nocardia brasiliensis*. In Africa, *M. mycetomatis* common cause. Most commonly seen in India, Mexico, Nigeria, Saudi Arabia, Senegal, Somalia, Sudan, Venezuela, Yemen, Zaire.

Risk Factors   Poor hygiene, walking barefoot, necrotic injured tissue, diminished nutrition.

PATHOGENESIS

Pathogens live in soil and enter through minor traumatic breaks in the skin. Only organisms that can survive at body temperature can produce mycetoma. Infection begins in skin and subcutaneous tissues, extending into fascial planes, destroying contiguous tissues.

HISTORY

Incubation Period   Lesion occurs at inoculation site weeks to years after trauma.

Duration of Lesion   Lesions may continue to expand for decades.

Symptoms   Relatively few, with little pain, tenderness or fever.

PHYSICAL EXAMINATION

Skin Lesions   Primary lesion: papule/nodule at inoculation site. Swelling increases slowly. Epidermis ulcerates and pus-containing granules (grains) drain. *Granules* are microbial colonies, small (<1 to ≥5mm). Skin surrounding portals of fistula drainage is heaped up (Fig. 21-37). Infection spreads to deeper tissues, into fascia, muscle, bone. Tissue becomes greatly distorted. Old mycetoma characterized by healed scars and draining sinuses.

Palpation   Usually not tender; pus drains on pressure. Central clearing gives older lesions an annular shape.

Distribution   Unilateral on the leg, foot, hand. Uncommonly on torso, arm, head, thigh, buttock, head.

General Findings   Fever with secondary bacterial infection. Regional lymphadenopathy occasionally.

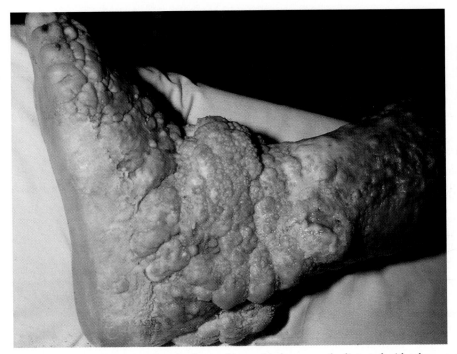

Figure 21-37   Eumycotic mycetoma *The foot, ankle, and leg are grossly distorted with edema and confluent subcutaneous nodules, cauliflower-like tumors, and ulcerations.*

ETIOLOGY AND CLASSIFICATION OF MYCETOMA-LIKE CLINICAL PRESENTATION WITH GRAIN FORMATION

Type of Mycetoma	Etiologic Agents
Botryomycosis Caused by true bacteria. Not a true mycetoma.	Most common: *Staphylococcus aureus* Also: *S. epidermidis, Pseudomonas aeruginosa, Escherichia coli, Bacteroides* spp., *Proteus* spp., *Streptococcus* spp.
Actinomycetoma (actinomycotic mycetoma) Caused by Actinomycetales organisms	*Actinomyces:* cause mycetoma and actinomycosis (cervical, thoracic, abdominal) *Nocardia:* cause mycetoma, lymphocutaneous infection (sporotrichoid pattern), superficial skin infections, disseminated infection with skin involvement *Actinomadura* *Streptomyces*
Eumycetoma (eumycotic mycetoma) Caused by true fungi	Most common: *Pseudallescheria boydii, Madurella grisea, M. mycetomatis* Also: *Phialophora jeanselmei, Pyrenochaeta romeroi, Leptosphaeria senegaliensis, Curvularia lunata, Neotestudina rosatti, Aspergillus nidulans* or *flavus, Acremonium* spp., *Fusarium* spp., *Cylindrocarpon* spp., *Microsporum audouinii*

DIFFERENTIAL DIAGNOSIS

Chronic Draining Subcutaneous Inflammatory Mass(es) Osteomyelitis, botryomycosis, chromoblastomycosis, blastomycosis, bacterial pyoderma, foreign-body granuloma, inflammatory dermatophytoses, leishmaniasis, pyoderma gangrenosum.

LABORATORY EXAMINATIONS

Smear of Pus from Lesion Granules Medlar bodies (Table 21-1) visualized on KOH preparation as microbial colonies (see below).

Dermatopathology Pseudoepitheliomatous hyperplasia of epidermis. Suppurative acute and chronic inflammation with granules within. Surrounded by dense fibrous tissue.

Culture Isolate organism. Secondary bacterial infection common.

Imaging X-ray of bone shows multiple osteolytic lesions (cavities), periosteal new bone formation.

DIAGNOSIS

Clinical suspicion confirmed by demonstration of grains in pus and/or by visualization of Medlar bodies on smear of pus or lesional biopsy specimen, and/or isolation of organism on culture. Medlar bodies (granules, grains) are white, black to gray, pinpoint globular grains that can be seen and felt in pus. Can be crushed on slide. They represent globular colonies of organism (Table 21-1).

COURSE AND PROGNOSIS

Actinomycetoma usually enlarges more rapidly than eumycetoma. Secondary bacterial infections are common. The infection runs a relentless course over many years, with destruction of contiguous bone and fascia. Infection does not spread hematogenously. Relapse after antifungal or antibiotic therapy common.

MANAGEMENT

Individuals are advised to seek medical attention early.

Surgery Smaller lesions can be cured by surgical excision. More extensive lesions often recur after incomplete excision.

Medicosurgical Approach Bulk reduction surgery is performed; amputation/disarticulation avoided. Causative agent identified, and effective antimicrobial agent given.

Systemic Antimicrobial Therapy Usually continued for ≥ 10 months.

Botryomycoses Antimicrobial agents according to sensitivities of isolated organism.

Actinomycotic Mycetoma Streptomycin sulfate combined with either dapsone or trimethoprim-sulfamethoxazole.

Eumycetoma Rarely responds to chemotherapy. Some cases caused by *M. mycetomatis* may respond to ketoconazole or itraconazole.

Table 21-1   COLOR GRAINS IN MYCETOMA AND ASSOCIATED ORGANISMS

Color of Grain	Organism
Black	*Madurella mycetomatis*
	M. grisea
	Leptosphaeria senegalensis
White	*Pseudallescheria boydii*
	Acremonium spp.
	Nocardia brasiliensis
	N. asteroides
White to yellow	*N. caviae*
Pink, white, to cream	*Actinomyces israelii*
	Actinomadura madurae
Red	*A. pelletieri*

Chromomycosis

Chromomycosis is a chronic localized invasive fungal infection of skin and subcutaneous tissues characterized by verrucous plaques on the leg or foot, caused by dematiaceous (dark-colored) fungi. *Synonym:* Chromoblastomycosis.

EPIDEMIOLOGY

Age of Onset 20 to 60 years.

Sex Males>females.

Etiology Dematiaceous fungi: *Fonsecaea pedrosoi* (most commonly); also *F. compacta, Phialophora verrucosa, Cladosporium carrionii, Rhinocladiella aquaspersa, Botryomyces caespitosus.*

Occupation Agricultural workers, mine workers, those exposed to soil while barefoot in tropical and subtropical regions.

Transmission Cutaneous inoculation. Autoinoculation to other sites may occur. Transmission to other individuals does not occur.

Geography Fungi isolated from soil and vegetation, preferring regions with >100 in of rainfall per year and mean temperatures from 12° to 24°C.

HISTORY

Duration of Lesion Lesions may continue to expand for decades.

Symptoms Relatively few, with little pain, tenderness, or fever. Patients usually present with secondary infection, cosmetic disfigurement, lymphedema.

PHYSICAL EXAMINATION

Skin Lesions Initial lesion: single scaling nodule at site of traumatic implantation (Fig. 21-38). Later (months to years), new crops of nodules appear. Subsequently, expanding verrucous plaques with central clearing and islands of normal skin between verrucous macules. Large cauliflower-like lesions often form, which, in some cases, may become pedunculated. Surface of verrucous lesion: pustules, small ulcerations, "black dots" of hemopurulent material, ±friable granulation tissue that bleeds easily is common. Extension occurs via lymphatic spread or via autoinoculation. Chronic lesions may be 10 to 20 cm in diameter, enveloping calf or foot. In areas of long-standing, lymphedema of involved extremity (elephantiasis).

Arrangement Smaller lesions coalesce to form large verrucous masses. Central clearing gives older lesions an annular shape.

Distribution Unilateral on the leg, foot. Rarely, hand, thorax.

DIFFERENTIAL DIAGNOSIS

Large Verrucous Plaques Blastomycosis, phaeohyphomycosis, lobomycosis, yaws, tertiary syphilis, tuberculosis verrucosa cutis, mycetoma, sporotrichosis, *Mycobacterium mari-num* infection, lepromatous leprosy, botryomycosis, foreign-body granuloma, inflammatory dermatophytoses, leishmaniasis, pyoderma gangrenosum, squamous cell carcinoma.

LABORATORY EXAMINATIONS

Smear of Pus from Lesion Medlar bodies (see below) visualized on 10 to 20% KOH preparation as black dots. Hyphal forms can be seen in crusts, pus, exudate.

Dermatopathology Warty granuloma: pseudoepitheliomatous hyperplasia, hyperkeratosis, intraepidermal abscesses containing inflammatory cells and Medlar bodies. Dense suppurative and granulomatous dermal response with histiocytes, giant cells, plasma cells, eosinophils, abscess formation. Medlar bodies (also known as sclerotic bodies, "copper pennies") are small brown fungal forms, which are round with thick bilaminate walls, 4 to 6 μm in diameter; occur singly or in clusters; all etiologic agents appear identical in tissue. Older lesions show dense fibrosis in and around granulomas.

Culture Organism in Sabouraud's glucose agar shows velvety green to black, restricted, slow-growing colonies. Agents grow very slowly, requiring 4 to 6 weeks for identification.

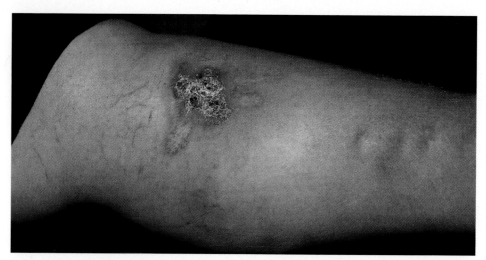

Figure 21-38 Chromomycosis *Hyperkeratotic and crusted plaque with old scars on the leg had been present for several decades.*

DIAGNOSIS

Clinical suspicion confirmed by visualization of Medlar bodies on smear of pus or lesional biopsy specimen and/or isolation of organism on culture.

COURSE AND PROGNOSIS

Secondary bacterial infections are common. Recurrence after oral triazole therapy is common. Late complication is squamous cell carcinoma arising within verrucous area.

MANAGEMENT

Adjunctive Therapy   Application of heat may be helpful in that lesions arise at cooler acral sites.

Surgery   Smaller lesions can be cured by surgical excision.

Systemic Antifungal Therapy   *Amphotericin B:* usually is not effective at usual dosing.

Oral Antifungal Agents   Treatment is usually continued for at least 1 year. The response is highly variable.

Terbinafine, 250 mg/d
Itraconazole, 200 to 600 mg/d
Ketoconazole, 400 to 800 mg/d

FUNGAL INFECTIONS OF THE SKIN AND HAIR

Sporotrichosis

Sporotrichosis commonly follows accidental inoculation of the skin and is characterized by ulceronodule formation at the inoculation site, chronic nodular lymphangitis, and regional lymphadenitis. In the immunocompromised host, disseminated infection can occur from the skin involvement or from primary pulmonary infection.

EPIDEMIOLOGY

Etiology *Sporothrix schenckii,* a dimorphic fungus commonly found in soil and on plants. The tissue form is an oval, cigar-shaped yeast.

Sex Males>females, especially disseminated disease.

Occupation Occupation exposure important: gardeners, farmers, florists, lawn laborers, agricultural workers, forestry workers, paper manufacturers, gold miners, laboratory workers. In Uruguay, 80% of cases occur after a scratch by an armadillo.

Transmission Commonly, subcutaneous inoculation by a contaminated sharp object (rose or barberry thorn, barb, wood splinter) or from sphagnum moss, straw, marsh hay, soils. Rarely, inhalation, aspiration, or ingestion causes systemic infection. Most cases isolated. Epidemics do occur. Cutaneous sporotrichosis in cats has been transmitted to humans.

Geography Ubiquitous, worldwide. More common in temperate, tropical zones.

Predisposing Factors For localized disease: diabetes mellitus, alcoholism. For disseminated disease: HIV infection, carcinoma, hematologic and lymphoproliferative disease, diabetes mellitus, alcoholism, immunosuppressive therapy.

PATHOGENESIS

After subcutaneous inoculation, *S. schenckii* grows locally. Infection can be limited to the site of inoculation (plaque sporotrichosis) or extend along the proximal lymphatic channels (lymphangitic sporotrichosis). Spread beyond an extremity is rare; hematogenous dissemination from the skin remains unproven. The portal for osteoarticular, pulmonary, and other extracutaneous forms is unknown but is probably the lung.

HISTORY

Incubation Period 3 weeks (range, 3 days to 12 weeks) after trauma or injury to site of lesion. Lesions are relatively asymptomatic, painless. Afebrile.

PHYSICAL EXAMINATION

Skin Lesions *Plaque Sporotrichosis* Subcutaneous papule, pustule, or nodule appears at inoculation site several weeks after inoculation. Surrounding skin is pink to purplish. In time, skin becomes fixed to deeper tissues. Painless indurated ulcer (Fig. 21-39) may occur, resulting in sporotrichoid chancre. Border ragged and not sharply demarcated. Draining lymph nodes become swollen and suppurative. Crusted ulcers, ecthymatous, verrucous plaques, pyoderma gangrenosum-like, infiltrated papules and plaques may also occur.

Lymphangitic Sporotrichosis Follows lymphatic extension of local cutaneous type (Fig. 21-40). Proximal to local cutaneous lesion, intervening lymphatics become indurated, nodular, thickened.

Disseminated Sporotrichosis (Fungus disseminates hematogenously to skin, as well as joints, eyes, and meninges.) Crusted nodules, ulcers. Widespread.

Distribution Primary lesion most common on dorsum of hand or finger with chronic nodular lymphangitis up arm. Fixed cutaneous—face in children, upper extremities in adults. Disseminated sporotrichosis: widespread lesions, usually sparing palms, soles.

General Examination

Lungs Primary pulmonary infection does occur and has a worse prognosis than cutaneous infection.

Joints Swelling, painful joint(s) (hand, elbow, ankle, knee), often in the absence of skin lesion. Hematogenous dissemination results in bone, muscle, joint, visceral, CNS lesions.

DIFFERENTIAL DIAGNOSIS

Plaque Sporotrichosis Cutaneous tuberculosis, atypical mycobacterial infection, tularemia, cat-scratch disease, primary syphilis, bacterial pyoderma, foreign-body granuloma, inflammatory dermatophytoses, blastomycosis, chromoblastomycosis, leishmaniasis.

Chronic Nodular Lymphangitic Sporotrichosis "Common" Infecting Agents *Mycobacterium marinum, Nocardia brasiliensis, Leishmania brasiliensis, Francisella tularensis*

Unusual Infecting Agents *N. asteroides, M. chelonei, L. major.* Rare: *M. kansasii, Blastomyces dermatitidis, Coccidioides immitis, Cryptococcus neoformans, Histoplasma capsulatum, Streptococcus pyogenes, Staphylococcus aureus, Pseudomonas pseudomallei* (melioidosis), *Bacillus anthracis* (anthrax).

LABORATORY EXAMINATIONS

Touch Preparation In disseminated sporotrichosis (usually with advanced HIV disease), KOH solution added to smear from back of lesional skin biopsy specimen helps visualize multiple yeast forms.

Gram's Stain In disseminated sporotrichosis (usually with advanced HIV disease), smear from crusted lesion shows multiple yeast forms.

Dermatopathology Granulomatous, Langhans-type giant cells, pyogenic microabscesses. Organisms rare, difficult to visualize in all except infection in immunocompromised host. Yeast appear as 1- to 3-μm by 3- to 10-μm cigar-shaped forms.

Culture Organism usually isolated within a few days from lesional biopsy specimen.

Serology Not helpful.

DIAGNOSIS

Clinical suspicion and isolation of organism on culture.

COURSE AND PROGNOSIS

Shows little tendency to resolve spontaneously. Responds well to therapy, but a significant percentage relapse after completion of therapy. Disseminated infection in HIV-infected individuals responds poorly to all forms of therapy.

MANAGEMENT

Oral antifungal agents

Itraconazole 200 to 600 mg qd. Very effective for lymphocutaneous infection; not as effective for bone/joint and pulmonary infection.

Fluconazole 200–400 mg/d reported to be effective.

Ketoconazole 400–800 mg/d reported to be effective.

Saturated solution of potassium iodide 3–4 g tid effective for lymphocutaneous infection; less effective than oral antifungal agents.

Intravenous therapy

Amphotericin B For those with pulmonary or disseminated infection or who are unable to tolerate oral therapy for lymphocutaneous disease.

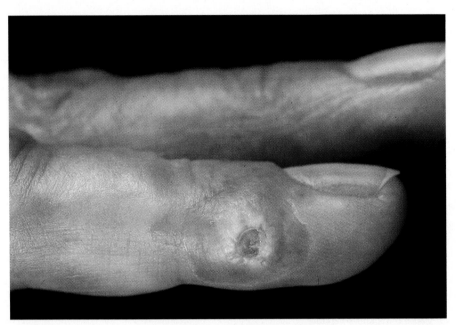

Figure 21-39 Sporotrichosis: chancriform type *An ulcerated nodule at the site of inoculation on the finger was associated with regional axillary lymphadenopathy.*

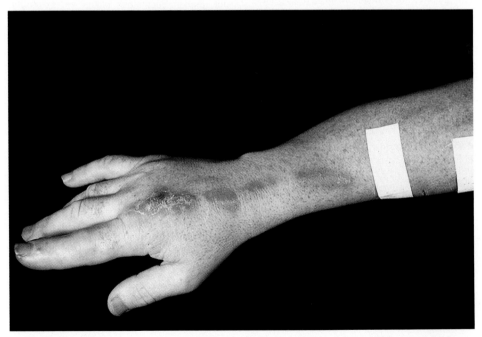

Figure 21-40 Sporotrichosis: chronic lymphangitic (sporotrichoid) type *An erythematous papule at the site of inoculation on the index finger with a linear arrangement of erythematous dermal and subcutaneous nodules extending proximally in lymphatic vessels of the dorsum of the hand and arm.*

Disseminated Cryptococcosis

Systemic cryptococcosis is a systemic mycosis acquired by the respiratory route, with the primary focus of infection in the lungs, and with occasional hematogenous dissemination, characteristically to the meninges, and on occasion to skin.

Synonyms: Torulosis, European blastomycosis.

EPIDEMIOLOGY

Age of Onset More common over the age of 40 years.

Sex Males>females 3:1.

Etiology *Cryptococcus neoformans,* a yeast, serotypes A, B, C, D causing infection in humans. Serotypes A and D designated *C. neoformans* var. *neoformans;* serotypes B and C, *C. neoformans* var. *gattii.* In tissue, encapsulated yeastlike fungi (3.5 to 7.0 μm in diameter). Bud connected to parent cell by narrow pore. Capsule thickness variable.

Incidence Globally, cryptococcosis (usually meningitis) is the most common invasive mycosis in HIV disease, occurring in 6 to 9% of HIV-infected individuals in the United States and 20 to 30% in Africa. Incidence is also high in Europe and South America. Currently, in the industrialized nations, the incidence is much less due to immune reconstitution. In untreated HIV disease, cutaneous dissemination occurs in 10 to 15% of cryptococcosis cases.

Risk Factors HIV disease, solid-organ transplantation, glucocorticoid therapy, sarcoidosis, lymphoma, diabetes mellitus.

Geography Worldwide, ubiquitous. Distribution of serotype varies in geographic areas.

PATHOGENESIS

Associated with avian feces worldwide (parakeets, budgerigars, canaries, and especially pigeons). *C. neoformans* is inhaled in dust and causes a primary pulmonary focus of infection with subsequent hematogenous dissemination to meninges, kidneys, and skin. Between 10 and 15% of patients have skin lesions. Cell-mediated immune deficiency is an important factor in pathogenesis in many patients.

HISTORY

Occurs in the setting of advanced HIV disease. Cutaneous lesions: usually asymptomatic. CNS: headache most common symptom (80%), mental confusion, impaired vision for 2 to 3 months. Lungs: pulmonary symptoms uncommon.

PHYSICAL EXAMINATION

Skin Lesions Papule(s) or nodule(s): with surrounding erythema that occasionally break down and exude a liquid, mucinous material. Can present as a solitary nodule in otherwise healthy individuals. Molluscum contagiosum–like lesions commonly occur in HIV-infected patients (Fig. 21-41). Acneform. Cryptococcal cellulitis: mimics bacterial cellulitis, i.e., red, hot, tender, edematous plaque on extremity; possibly multiple noncontiguous sites. In HIV disease, lesions occur most commonly on face/scalp.

Oral Mucosa Occur in <5% of patients, presenting as nodules/ulcers.

General Findings Meningoencephalitis. In HIV disease, cryptococcosis tends to be widespread with fungemia and infection of meninges, lungs, bone marrow, genitourinary tract including prostate, and skin. In HIV disease, hepatomegaly and splenomegaly.

DIFFERENTIAL DIAGNOSIS

Widespread Papular Eruption in Immunocompromised Patient Acne, sarcoidosis, pyoderma, other bacterial or fungal skin lesions, blastomycosis, histoplasmosis, molluscum contagiosum.

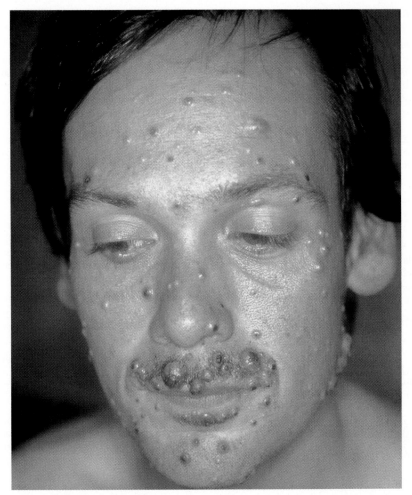

Figure 21-41 Cryptococcosis: disseminated *Multiple, skin-colored papules and nodules on the face in an HIV-infected individual represent dissemination of pulmonary cryptococcosis hematogenously to skin; meninges are also a common site of infection after fungemia. The lesions are easily mistaken for molluscum contagiosum, which occurs commonly in HIV disease. (Courtesy of Loïc Vallant, M.D.)*

LABORATORY EXAMINATIONS

Dermatopathology Two patterns of histologic reactions are seen. Gelatinous reactions show numerous organisms in aggregates with little inflammatory response. Granulomatous reactions show tissue reaction with histiocytes, giant cells, lymphoid cells, and fibroblasts, ±areas of necrosis; organisms are present in smaller numbers. Capsules stain with mucicarmine stain, differentiating *C. neoformans* from *B. dermatitidis*.

Touch Preparation Lesional skin biopsy specimen or scrapings from skin lesion smeared on microscope slide examined with KOH to identify *C. neoformans*.

CSF With meningitis, encapsulated budding yeast is seen with India ink preparations in 40 to 60% of cases, lymphocytic pleocytosis, elevated protein, decreased glucose. Intracranial pressure may be moderately to extremely elevated.

Imaging X-ray findings of chest variable.

Culture CSF. Lesional skin biopsy specimen. In HIV disease, cryptococcosis tends to be widespread, with cultures positive in blood, sputum, bone marrow, and urine. If *C. neoformans* isolated from lesional skin biopsy specimen, extent of disease should be determined by examination of CSF, bone marrow, sputum, urine, and prostate fluid.

Cryptococcal Antigens Sensitive and specific. Detect in CSF, serum, urine. Useful in following response to therapy and in formulating prognosis.

DIAGNOSIS

Confirmed by skin biopsy and fungal cultures.

COURSE AND PROGNOSIS

Acute pulmonary cryptococcosis is usually mild. Chronic cavitary forms lead to respiratory impairment. In HIV disease in the absence of immune reconstitution, cryptococcal meningitis relapses in 30% of cases after amphotericin B plus 5-flucytosine therapy; lifelong secondary prophylaxis with fluconazole reduces relapse rate to 4 to 8%. Prostate is a site of extrameningeal disease and also a source of relapse after treatment.

MANAGEMENT

Primary prophylaxis In some centers, fluconazole is given to HIV-infected individuals with low CD41 cell counts; the incidence of disseminated infection is reduced, but there is no effect on the mortality rate.

Therapy of meningitis Amphotericin B65-flucytosine for 2 to 4 weeks in uncomplicated cases and for 6 weeks in complicated cases. Fluconazole (alternative).

Infection limited to skin Fluconazole, 400–600mg/d. Itraconazole (alternative), 400 mg/d.

Secondary prophylaxis In HIV disease (without immune reconstitution), lifelong secondary prophylaxis is given. Fluconazole, 200–400 mg/d; itraconazole (alternative), 200–400 mg/d.

Histoplasmosis

Histoplasmosis is a common systemic mycosis with a primary pulmonary infection but with uncommon hematogenous dissemination, characterized by chronic infection of mucous membranes, skin, and reticuloendothelial organs (liver, bone marrow, and spleen).
Synonyms: Darling's disease, cave disease, Ohio Valley disease.

EPIDEMIOLOGY

Age of Onset For disseminated infection, very old and very young.

Etiology *Histoplasma capsulatum*, a dimorphic fungus. In Africa, *H. capsulatum* var. *duboisii*. The fungus grows well in soil enriched with bird or bat guano.

Transmission Inhalation of spores in soil contaminated with bird or bat droppings. Those at risk: farmers, construction workers, children, others involved in outdoor activities (cave exploration). Acute pulmonary histoplasmosis may occur in outbreaks in individuals with occupational or recreational exposure. In southern Kentucky, middle Tennessee, and surrounding areas, histoplasmin skin test positive in 95% of population.

Risk Factors for Dissemination Immunosuppressed host (HIV infection, post-organ transplant, lymphoma, leukemia, chemotherapy), very old. Occurs in advanced HIV disease when CD4+ cell count is very low.

Incidence Common opportunistic infection in HIV-infected individuals in highly endemic regions such as Indianapolis, IN. Early in the HIV epidemic, first cases of histoplasmosis were in immigrants from the endemic foci in the Caribbean Islands who developed AIDS while living in New York or California; disease presented as reactivation of latent foci of infection. In cities such as IN and Kansas City, 20 to 25% of patients with HIV disease have primary histoplasmosis. Incidence also increased in HIV disease in South America.

Geography North America: eastern and central United States, especially Ohio/Mississippi River valleys (Kentucky, Illinois, Indiana, Missouri, Ohio, Tennessee, and western New York); in some areas, 80% of residents are histoplasmin-positive. Caribbean Islands. Equatorial Africa.

PATHOGENESIS

In HIV disease, can present as either primary histoplasmosis or reactivation of latent infection.

HISTORY

Incubation Period For acute pulmonary infection, 5 to 18 days. For disseminated infection, ≥2 months. In severe forms of infection, presentation may be acute, resembling septicemia with associated disseminated intravascular coagulopathy.

Acute Primary Infection 90% of patients asymptomatic; if large numbers of spores inhaled, influenza-like syndrome may occur (fever ≥38.3°C, chills, night sweats, cough, headache, fatigue, myalgia).

Disseminated Infection Chronic disease syndrome. In HIV disease, can present as widely disseminated infection with symptoms of sepsis, adrenal insufficiency, diarrheal illness, or colonic mass.

PHYSICAL EXAMINATION

Skin Lesions *Acute Pulmonary Histoplasmosis* Cutaneous lesions represent hypersensitivity reactions to *Histoplasma* antigen(s): Erythema nodosum, erythema multiforme.

Disseminated Histoplasmosis to Skin Lesions caused by tissue infection. Historically, lesions of mucous membranes much more common than those on skin. However, in HIV infection, 10% of patients with disseminated histoplasmosis have cutaneous lesions; in renal transplant patients, 4 to 6%. Erythematous necrotic or hyperkeratotic papules and nodules (Fig. 21-42); erythematous macules; folliculitis, ±pustules, ±acneform ulcers; vegetative plaques; panniculitis; erythroderma. Diffuse hyperpigmentation with Addison's disease secondary to adrenal infection.

Mucous Membranes *Most common site of involvement;* nodules, vegetations, painful ulcerations of soft palate, oropharynx, epiglottis, nasal vestibule.

General Examination Disseminated disease: hepatosplenomegaly, lymphadenopathy, meningitis.

DIFFERENTIAL DIAGNOSIS

Disseminated Disease Miliary tuberculosis, coccidioidomycosis, cryptococcosis, leishmaniasis, lymphoma.

LABORATORY EXAMINATIONS

Dermatopathology Identify *H. capsulatum* in tissue by size and staining. Differentiate from *Coccidioides immitis, Blastomyces dermatitidis, Leishmania donovani, Toxoplasma gondii.*

Smear *H. capsulatum* can be identified by smears obtained from touching lesional skin biopsy specimen to microscope slide (touch preparation), sputum, or bone marrow aspirate, stained with Giemsa's stain.

Culture Identify *H. capsulatum* from biopsy specimens of skin, oral lesions, bone marrow, sputum, lung biopsy specimen, blood, urine, lymph node, liver.

Antigen Detection Determination of *H. capsulatum* polysaccharide antigen titers in serum can be used for diagnosis, assessing response to treatment, and predicting later relapse. (Histoplasmosis Reference Laboratory, 1001 W. 10th St., OPW441, Indianapolis, IN 46202-2897; Tel: 317-630-6262, Fax: 317-630-7522.)

Antibody Detection Immunodiffusion and complement-fixation tests detect antibodies to *H. capsulatum.* Positive serologic test defined as presence of M or H band on immunodiffusion or 1:32 or higher titer by complement fixation.

Bone Marrow Aspiration *H. capsulatum* can be visualized in those with disseminated infection.

Imaging Chest x-ray: interstitial infiltrates and/or hilar adenopathy (acute).

DIAGNOSIS

Clinical suspicion, confirmed by culture of organism.

COURSE AND PROGNOSIS

Primary infection resolves spontaneously in most cases. Untreated chronic cavitary pulmonary infection or progressive disseminated form has a very high mortality rate, 80% of patients dying within 1 year. Prognosis linked to underlying condition. Chronic maintenance often required. With itraconazole therapy, cure rate 80%.

MANAGEMENT

Prevention When any material contaminated with bird or bat guano is to be disturbed in an area of endemic histoplasmosis, personal protective equip-ment (respirators, eye protection, gloves, or protective clothing) should be used during potential recreational or occupational exposure. Information regarding prevention and control of histoplasmosis can be obtained from the CDC's Division of Bacterial and Mycotic Diseases, National Center for Infectious Diseases (Mailstop A-13, 1600 Clifton Rd., N.E., Atlanta, GA 30333; Tel: 404-639-3158).

Systemic antimycotic therapy Non-life-threatening infections and for those unable to tolerate amphotericin B: Itraconazole, 400 mg bid PO for 12 weeks; *or* fluconazole, 800 mg qd PO for 12 weeks. Life-threatening and meningeal infection: Amphotericin B given IV.

Secondary prophylaxis In HIV disease, itraconazole, 200 mg/d, *or* fluconazole, 400 mg/d for life

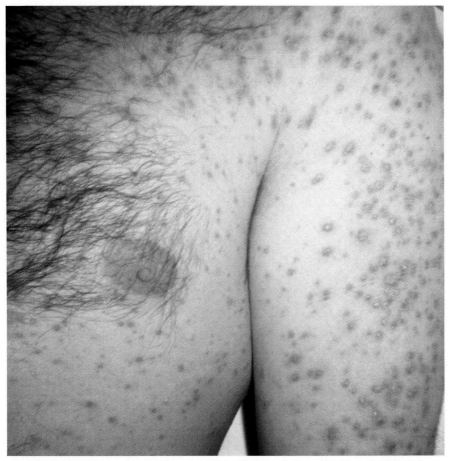

Figure 21-42 Histoplasmosis, disseminated *Multiple, erythematous, scaling papules on the trunk and upper arm occurred during a 2-week period and mimicked acute guttate psoriasis in an individual with HIV disease. The cutaneous lesions occurred after reactivation of pulmonary infection and fungemia. Multiple yeast-like* H. capsulatum *were demonstrated within macrophages in a lesional skin biopsy specimen. (Courtesy of J. D. Fallon, M.D.)*

North American Blastomycosis

Blastomycosis is a chronic systemic mycosis characterized by primary pulmonary infection, which in some cases is followed by hematogenous dissemination to skin and other organs.
Synonyms: Gilchrist's disease, Chicago disease.

EPIDEMIOLOGY

Age of Onset   Young, middle-aged.

Sex   Males>females 10:1.

Etiology   *Blastomyces dermatitidis,* a dimorphic fungus. In tissue, a yeast 10 μm in diameter with 1-μm-thick cell wall; pore of bud is wide.

Transmission   Most cases are isolated. Occupations at risk: outdoor vocation or avocation (farm workers, manual laborers). However, currently, many individuals infected during leisure activities: fishing, hunting, camping, hiking in areas of high endemicity.

Geography   Uncommon in any locality. Most cases occur in the southeastern, central, and mid-Atlantic areas of the United States. Rarely occurs in Africa, Mexico, Central America, South America.

PATHOGENESIS

B. dermatitidis infection acquired from inhalation of dust from soil, decomposed vegetation, or rotting wood. Asymptomatic primary pulmonary infection usually resolves spontaneously. Hematogenous dissemination may occur to skin, skeletal system, prostate, epididymis, or mucosa of nose, mouth, or larynx. Reactivation may occur within lung or in sites of dissemination. Risk factors for dissemination: T cell dysfunction; advanced HIV disease.

HISTORY

Incubation Period   Depends on size of inoculum and immune status. Estimated median, 45 days.

Symptoms   Primary pulmonary infection: usually asymptomatic; flulike or resembles bacterial pneumonitis. Chronic pulmonary infection: fever, cough, night sweats, weight loss. Cutaneous ulcers often painless.

PHYSICAL EXAMINATION

Skin Lesions   *Primary Infection*   Accompanied or followed by erythema nodosum or erythema multiforme.

Disseminated Infection to Skin   Initial lesion, inflammatory nodule that enlarges and ulcerates (Fig. 21-43); subcutaneous nodule, ±many small pustules on surface. Subsequently, verrucous/crusted plaque with sharply demarcated serpiginous borders. Peripheral border extends on one side, resembling a one-half to three-quarter moon. Pus exudes when crust is lifted. Central healing with thin geographic atrophic scar.

Distribution   Usually symmetrically on trunk but also face, hands, arms; multiple lesions in half of patients.

Mucous membranes   25% of patients have oral or nasal lesions, half of whom have contiguous skin lesions. Laryngeal infection.

General Examination   *Lungs*   Infiltrates, miliary, cavitary lesions. *Bones*   50% involvement; osteomyelitis in thoracolumbar vertebrae, pelvis, sacrum, skull, ribs, long bones. May extend to form large subcutaneous abscess; may occur in conjunction with cutaneous ulcer; septic arthritis and sinus tracts to skin can develop.

DIFFERENTIAL DIAGNOSIS

Verrucous Skin Lesion   Squamous cell carcinoma, pyoderma gangrenosum tumor stage of mycosis fungoides, ecthyma, tuberculosis verrucosa cutis, actinomycosis, nocardiosis, mycetoma, syphilitic gumma, granuloma inguinale, leprosy, bromoderma.

LABORATORY EXAMINATIONS

Direct Examination   KOH preparation of pus or respiratory tract secretions shows large (8- to 15-μm), single, budding cells with a thick "double-contoured" wall and a wide pore of

FUNGAL INFECTIONS OF THE SKIN AND HAIR

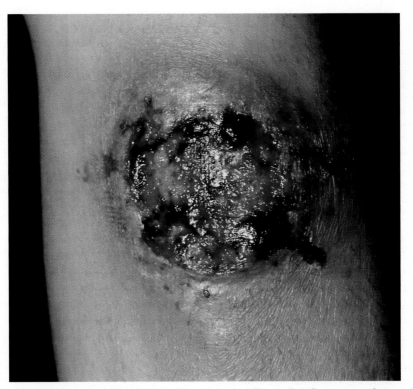

Figure 21-43   North American blastomycosis: disseminated   *Ulcerated, inflammatory plaque with surrounding erythema, edema, and fibrosis on the leg results from dissemination from pulmonary blastomycosis via blood to skin. The lesion must be differentiated from pyoderma gangrenosum. (Courtesy of Elizabeth M. Spiers, M.D.)*

attachment. Specific diagnosis can be made with antibodies to *B. dermatitidis* antigens.

Culture Of sputum, pus from skin lesion or biopsy, prostatic secretions.

Dermatopathology Pseudoepitheliomatous hyperplasia. Budding yeast with thick walls and broad-based buds in microabscess in dermis visualized by silver stain or periodic acid–Schiff stain. Mucicarmine stain differentiates *B. dermatitidis* from *Cryptococcus neoformans*.

Imaging Acute (primary) infection shows pneumonitis, ±hilar lymphadenopathy. With chronic pulmonary infection, x-ray findings highly variable.

DIAGNOSIS

Clinical suspicion, confirmed by culture of organism from skin biopsy, sputum, pus, urine.

COURSE AND PROGNOSIS

Most primary pulmonary blastomycosis cases are asymptomatic, self-limited. Cutaneous infection usually occurs months or years after primary pulmonary infection. Skin most common site of extrapulmonary infection, followed by bones, prostate, and meninges; rarely, adrenals and liver. Before amphotericin B, mortality rate in individuals with disseminated infection was 80 to 90%. Cure rate with itraconazole, 95%.

MANAGEMENT

Prevention Because of the widespread extent of *B. dermatitidis* in endemic regions, avoidance is not possible.

General Care Patients with mild to moderate acute pulmonary blastomycosis often can be followed without antifungal therapy, especially if the patient is improving at time of diagnosis. Patients with meningitis or acute respiratory distress syndrome are best treated in hospital with IV amphotericin B.

Intravenous Amphotericin B In life-threatening infections: *amphotericin B,* 120–150 mg/week with a total dose of 2 g in adults. New liposomal preparations are less toxic. After initial improvement, therapy can be continued on an outpatient basis, three times weekly.

Oral Antifungal Therapy In those whose infection is non-life-threatening and/or those unable to tolerate amphotericin B: Itraconazole, 200–400 mg/d for >2 months; ketoconazole (alternative), 800 mg/d.

Disseminated Coccidioidomycosis

Coccidioidomycosis is a systemic mycosis characterized by primary pulmonary infection that usually resolves spontaneously. Subsequently, it can disseminate hematogenously and result in chronic, progressive, granulomatous infection in skin, lungs, bone, meninges.

Synonyms: San Joaquin Valley fever, valley fever, desert fever.

EPIDEMIOLOGY

Race   Blacks, Filipinos.

Sex   Risk of dissemination greater in males, pregnant females.

Incidence   Greatly increased in southern California during the past few years. Approximately 100,000 cases in the United States per year; most asymptomatic. In endemic areas: infection rates, measured by skin test reactivity, may be 16 to 42% or higher by early adulthood. Occurs in up to 25% of HIV-infected individuals in highly endemic regions such as Arizona or Bakersfield, CA.

Etiology   *Coccidioides immitis,* a dimorphic fungus. This mold grows in soil in arid areas of the western hemisphere.

Season   Late spring through fall, i.e., dry season.

Acquisition   Inhalation of arthroconidia is followed by primary pulmonary infection. Rarely, percutaneous.

Risk Factors   Nonwhite, pregnancy, immunosuppression, HIV infection with low CD4+ cell counts.

Geography   Regions endemic for *C. immitis* include: southern California (San Joaquin Valley), southern Arizona, Utah, New Mexico, Nevada, southwestern Texas; adjacent areas of Mexico; Central and South America. Primary pulmonary coccidioidomycosis occurs in individuals living in these regions (endemic) or in visitors to the regions (nonendemic).

Classification   Asymptomatic infection, febrile illness (valley fever), acute self-limited pulmonary coccidioidomycosis, disseminated coccidioidomycosis (cutaneous, osteoarticular, meningeal).

PATHOGENESIS

Spores inhaled, resulting in primary pulmonary infection that is asymptomatic or accompanied by symptoms of coryza. Failure to develop cell-mediated immunity is associated with disseminated infection and relapse after therapy.

HISTORY

Incubation Period   1 to 4 weeks.

History   About 40% of persons infected with *C. immitis* become symptomatic. With primary pulmonary infection, influenza- or grippelike illness with fever, chills, malaise, anorexia, myalgia, pleuritic chest pain. With disseminated infection, headache, bone pain. In HIV disease, clinical presentation is quite variable: focal pulmonary lesions, meningitis, focal disseminated lesions, or widespread disease. In HIV disease, usually presents when CD4+ cell count is <200/μL; the lower the CD4+ cell count, the more diffuse and widespread the mycosis.

Travel History   Living in or visiting endemic area. Disseminated coccidioidomycosis in individuals living in an endemic area is usually diagnosed more readily than in those with remote history of travel to an endemic region.

PHYSICAL EXAMINATION

Skin Lesions   *Primary Infection*   Toxic erythema (diffuse erythema, morbilliform, urticaria); erythema nodosum.

Hematogenous Dissemination to Skin   Initially, papule evolving with formation of pustules, plaques, nodules (Fig. 21-44); abscess formation, multiple draining sinus tracts, ulcers; subcutaneous cellulitis; verrucous plaques; granulomatous nodules; scars. Central face (Fig. 21-44), especially nasolabial fold preferential site; extremities.

Primary Cutaneous Inoculation Site (Rare)
Nodule eroding to ulcer. May have sporotrichoid lymphangitis, regional lymphadenitis.

General Examination *Bone* Osteomyelitis. Psoas area produces draining abscess.

CNS Signs of meningitis.

DIFFERENTIAL DIAGNOSIS

Disseminated Papules/Pustules Warts, furuncles, ecthyma, bromoderma, rosacea, lichen simplex chronicus, prurigo nodularis, keratoacanthoma, blastomycosis, cryptococcosis, tuberculosis, tertiary syphilis, bacterial infection. In HIV-infected patient: may resemble folliculitis, molluscum contagiosum.

LABORATORY EXAMINATIONS

Dermatopathology Granulomatous inflammation; spores in tissue.

Culture Pus, biopsy specimen grows organism on Sabouraud's medium.

DIAGNOSIS

Detection of *C. immitis* sporangia containing typical sporangiospores in sputum/pus; culture; skin biopsy.

COURSE AND PROGNOSIS

About 40% of persons infected with *C. immitis* become symptomatic. Disseminated disease is rare in immunocompetent persons but occurs at a higher rate in the United States among blacks, Filipinos, pregnant women, and immunosuppressed persons, particularly those with HIV infection. Most infected residents of endemic areas heal spontaneously. Meningeal infection difficult to cure. The incidence of relapse of pulmonary or dissemiated infection is relatively high. In HIV-infected individuals with coccidioidomycosis, the mortality rate in a study of 77 patients was 43%; 60% mortality rate with diffuse pulmonary disease; relapse rate very high.

MANAGEMENT

Systemic Antifungal Therapy *Non-Life-Threatening Infection* Fluconazole, 200–400 mg/d, *or* itraconazole.

Life-Threatening Infection Amphotericin B deoxycholate.

Secondary Prophylaxis Lifelong therapy for meningeal infection may be required and is required in HIV disease.

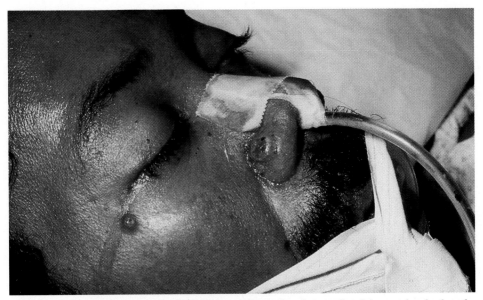

Figure 21-44   Coccidioidomycosis: disseminated   *Ulcerated and crusted nodules on the cheek and nose in an individual with pulmonary coccidioidomycosis with dissemination to the skin. (Courtesy of Francis Renna, M.D.)*

RICKETTSIAL INFECTIONS

Rickettsiae are gram-negative coccobacilli and short bacilli, characterized by their intra-cellular localization and persistence, movement through mammalian reservoirs, and trans-mission by insect vectors; except for louse-borne typhus, humans are incidental hosts. Rickettsioses are classified into five groups; an exanthem is a major clinical and diag-nostic feature of the first group, i.e., the spotted fevers.

CLASSIFICATION OF GROUPS OF RICKETTSIAL INFECTIONS AND CLINICAL FEATURES

Group of Rickettsial Infection	Cutaneous Findings
Tick-and gamasid mite-borne spotted fever group (SFG)	Exanthem is a major clinical and diagnostic feature
Flea-and louse-borne typhus group rickettsial diseases	
Flea-borne typhus (endemic murine)	Maculopapular rash occurring on the extremities and trunk, sparing the face, palms and soles, in 13% of patients
Louse-borne typhus	Generalized maculopapular rash, sparing the face, palms, and soles, possibly becoming petechial and confluent
Chigger-borne scrub typhus	Eschar at site of chigger feeding ($<$50% of cases)
	Maculopapular rash may occur, but seldom observed
Ehrlichiosis	Rash in 5% or less at onset
Q fever	Rare

SPOTTED FEVERS

The spotted fevers include Rocky Mountain spotted fever (RMSF), tick typhus, and rickettsialpox, and are characterized by an exanthem and fever. All, except for rickettsialpox, are transmitted to humans by the bite of ixodid ticks. Clinically, the spectrum of severity of clinical findings is broad, ranging from mild symptoms of general malaise and an exanthem to life-threatening illness.

EPIDEMIOLOGY

Age of Onset   More common in children and young adults, related to out-of-doors activities.

Sex   Males>females.

Etiology, Geographic Distribution   The rickettsiae causing the spotted fevers are collectively referred to as the *spotted fever group* (SFG) (Table 22-1).

Transmission   All except rickettsialpox (transmitted by mite bite) are transmitted by ixodid tick bite.

Season   Mediterranean spotted fever (MSF) occurs mainly in warmer summer months (July, August, September) when ticks are feeding.

PATHOGENESIS

Rickettsiae reproduce within endothelial cells at the bite site; the subsequent injury results in dermal and epidermal necrosis and perivascular edema, which presents clinically as a papule that evolves to a crusted ulcer at the bite site (tache noire or eschar). Rickettsiae then seed from this site into blood and systemically. In severe cases, disseminated vascular infection occurs with meningoencephalitis and vascular lesions in kidneys, lungs, GI tract, liver, pancreas, heart, spleen, and skin.

HISTORY

Incubation Period   Range, 3 to 14 days (mean, 7 days) after the tick bite.

Prodrome   Nonspecific.

Travel History   Recent travel to endemic region.

History of Tick Bite   Often not elicited in that the rickettsiae are transmitted by tiny immature larvae and nymphs.

Symptoms   Onset is sudden in 50% of patients. Most common: headache, fever. Also: chills, myalgias, arthralgias, malaise, anorexia.

Table 22-1   ETIOLOGY AND GEOGRAPHIC DISTRIBUTION OF SPOTTED FEVERS

Disease in Humans	Etiology	Distribution
Rocky Mountain spotted fever (RMSF)	*Rickettsia rickettsii*	Western hemisphere
Tick typhus		Primarily Mediterranean countries (southern Europe below 45th parallel), all of Africa, India, southwestern and south-central Asia
Mediterranean spotted fever (fievre boutonneuse, Marseilles fever), Kenya tick typhus, Israeli spotted fever, Indian tick typhus, Astrakhan spotted fever	*R. conorii*	Mediterranean Sea islands and surrounding lands; Africa
African tick-bite fever	*R. africae*	Central, eastern, southern Africa
Siberian (North Asian) tick typhus	*R. sibirica*	Siberia, Mongolia, northern China
Queensland tick typhus	*R. australis*	Australia
Flinders Island spotted fever	*R. honei*	Flinders Island (near Tasmania)
Japanese or Oriental spotted fever	*R. japonica*	Japan
Rickettsialpox	*R. akari*	United States, Russia, South Africa, Korea, Europe

PHYSICAL EXAMINATION

Skin Lesions

Types

RMSF   See Rocky Mountain Spotted Fever.

Tâche Noire   An inoculation eschar: papule forms at the bite site and evolves to a painless, black-crusted ulcer with a red areola (resembles a cigarette burn) (Fig. 22-1) in 3 to 7 days. Occurs in all spotted fevers except RMSF.

Tick Typhus   About 3 to 4 days after appearance of the tâche noire, an erythematous maculopapular eruption appears on the forearms and subsequently becomes generalized, involving the face, palms/soles. The density of the eruption heightens during the next few days. In severe cases, the lesions may become hemorrhagic.

Rickettsialpox   About 2 to 3 days after the onset of symptoms, a papulovesicular eruption appears. The initial lesions are erythematous papules (2 to 10 mm in diameter) (Fig. 22-2). Papules evolve to vesicles and then heal after crust formation.

Distribution   Similar pattern of spread and distribution in all spotted fevers—trunk→extremities→face (centrifugal)—except RMSF, which first appears at wrists and ankles and spreads centripetally.

General Findings

Conjunctivitis, pharyngitis, photophobia. CNS symptoms (confusion, stupor, delirium, seizures, coma) common in RMSF but not seen in other spotted fevers.

Lymph Nodes   Nodes proximal to tâche noire are usually enlarged and nontender.

DIFFERENTIAL DIAGNOSIS

Tick Typhus   Viral exanthems, drug eruption.

Rickettsialpox   Varicella, pityriasis lichenoides et varioliformis acuta (PLEVA), viral exanthems, disseminated gonococcal infection.

LABORATORY EXAMINATIONS

Skin Biopsy

Rickettsialpox   Basal layer of epidermis shows vacuolar degeneration; vesiculation is subepidermal. Superficial and middermal neutrophilic and mononuclear cell infiltrate is present.

Direct Immunofluorescence   Rickettsiae can be detected in lesional biopsy specimens from site of tick bite and cutaneous lesions; also in circulating endothelial cells and various tissues obtained postmortem.

PCR   Detects rickettsial DNA in lesions and blood.

Serodiagnosis

Various tests are available. Antirickettsial therapy usually blunts antibody responses. Demonstration of antibodies to SFG rickettsiae by microimmunofluorescence, latex agglutination, enzyme immunoassay, Western blot, or complement fixation. Enzyme-linked immunosorbent assay (ELISA) (IgM capture assays) among the most sensitive.

Culture

Not available as a routine test. Rickettsiae can be cultured in the guinea pig and in a shell vial cell culture system.

DIAGNOSIS

Epidemiologic and clinical findings with identification of a tâche noire confirmed by demonstration of rickettsiae by immunohistologic techniques in lesional skin biopsy specimens and/or serology. In an endemic area, patients presenting with fever, rash, and/or a skin lesion consisting of a black necrotic area or a crust surrounded by erythema should be considered to have one of the rickettsial spotted fevers.

COURSE AND PROGNOSIS

In France and Spain, the mortality rate ranges from 1.4 to 5.6%, similar to that of RMSF. Spotted fevers are usually milder in children. Morbidity and mortality rates are higher in individuals with diabetes mellitus, cardiac insufficiency, alcoholism, old age, and G6PD deficiency. In rickettsialpox, clinical symptoms are usually mild, morbidity and mortality are uncommon; in untreated cases, symptoms resolve in 2 to 3 weeks.

MANAGEMENT

Prevention   Control host animals and vectors.

Antirickettsial Therapy   Specific antirickettsial therapy abbreviates the length and severity of illness, i.e., spotted fevers, tick typhus, and rickettsialpox.

Drug of Choice   Doxycycline, 100 mg PO bid for 1 to 5 days.

Alternatives   Ciprofloxacin, 750 mg PO bid for 5 days *or* chloramphenicol, 500 mg PO qid for 7 to 10 days *or* josamycin (in pregnancy), 3 g/d PO for 5 days.

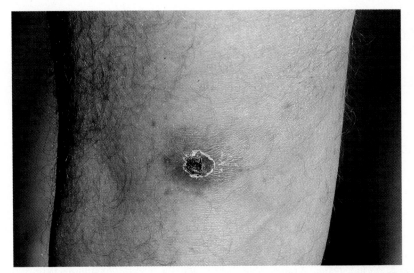

Figure 22-1 Rickettsialpox: tâche noire *A crusted, ulcerated papule (eschar) with a red halo resembling a cigarette burn at the site of a tick bite.*

Figure 22-2 Rickettsialpox: exanthem *Multiple, erythematous papules and pustules, some with central hemorrhage and crusting, on the back after hematogenous dissemination of the* R. akari *from the tick bite site.*

ROCKY MOUNTAIN SPOTTED FEVER

Rocky Mountain spotted fever (RMSF), the most severe of the rickettsial spotted fevers, is characterized by sudden onset of fever, severe headache, myalgia, and a characteristic acral exanthem; it is associated with significant morbidity and mortality rates.

EPIDEMIOLOGY

Age of Onset   Incidence of infection highest in 5- to 9-year-old children.

Sex   Case fatality highest in males.

Etiology   *Rickettsia rickettsii.*

Transmission   Occurs through bite of an infected tick or inoculation through abrasions contaminated with tick feces or tissue juices. The reservoirs and vectors are the wood tick *Dermacentor andersoni* in the western United States, the dog tick *D. variabilis* in the eastern two-thirds and California, *Rhipicephalus sanguineus* in Mexico, and *Amblyomma cajennense* in Mexico and Central and South America. Patient either lives in or has recently visited an endemic area, *but only 60% have knowledge of a recent tick bite during the 2 weeks before onset of illness.* Exposure to ticks occurs in tick-infested areas or in association with dogs who bring the dog tick into the patient's yard and home.

Season   Cases occur mainly in the spring in northern areas. In warmer southern states, most cases occur April 1 to September 30. The longest season and greatest number of wintertime cases occur further south.

Geography   Occurs only in the western hemisphere. In the United States, highest incidence in Oklahoma, North Carolina, Virginia, Maryland, Georgia, Missouri, Arkansas, Montana, and South Dakota. Although first recognized in the Rocky Mountains, currently rarely occurs in this region. Also documented in Canada, Mexico, Costa Rica, Panama, Columbia, Brazil. Travelers to the western hemisphere may import RMSF to their homeland.

Incidence   In the United States, 600 cases of RMSF are reported to the Centers for Disease Control and Prevention (CDC) annually. The actual incidence is probably significantly higher. Four states (North Carolina, Oklahoma, Tennessee, South Carolina) account for 48% of United States cases. Incidence highest in 5- to 9-year old children.

PATHOGENESIS

Feeding by ticks usually takes place for ≥6 h, after which rickettsiae are released from the salivary glands. After inoculation of rickettsiae into the pool of blood in the dermis, initial local replication of rickettsiae occurs in endothelial cells, which is followed by hematogenous and lymphatic dissemination. Organisms spread throughout the body and attach to the vascular endothelial cells, the principal target. Foci infected by *R. rickettsii* enlarge as rickettsiae spread from cell to cell, forming a network of contiguously infected endothelial cells in the microcirculation of the dermis, brain, lungs, heart, kidneys, stomach, large and small intestines, pancreas, liver, testes, skeletal muscle, and other organs and tissues. Focal infection of vascular smooth muscle causes a generalized vasculitis. Patients with severe infection of brain and lungs have a high mortality rate. Hypotension, local necrosis, gangrene, and DIC may follow. Rash results from extravasation of blood after vascular necrosis.

HISTORY

Incubation Period   Range, 3 to 14 days (mean, 7 days) after the tick bite.

Prodrome   Anorexia, irritability, malaise, chilliness, and feverish feeling.

History of Tick Bite   Given in only 60% of cases.

Symptoms   Onset of symptoms is usually abrupt with fever (94%), severe headache (86%), generalized myalgia especially the back and leg muscles (83%), a sudden shaking rigor, photophobia, prostration, nausea with occasional vomiting, all within the first 2 days. However, onset is at times less striking. Symptoms are similar to those of many acute infectious diseases, making specific diagnosis difficult during the first few days. On first day of illness, only 14% of patients have characteristic rash; during first 3 days, 49% of patients have rash. In 20% of cases, rash appears only on day 6 or after. In 13% of cases, no rash is detected (spotless RMSF).

PHYSICAL EXAMINATION

Skin Lesions The patient first seeking medical care may have no rash or a few small, pink macules that are identified only after a complete and careful examination of the skin. The temporal evolution of the rash is extremely helpful in the diagnosis. Extensive cutaneous necrosis due to DIC occurs in 4% of cases and may be associated with gangrene of extremities requiring amputation.

Types Early lesions, 2 to 6 mm, pink, blanchable macules (Figs. 22-3 and 22-4). In 1 to 3 days evolve to deep red papules (Fig. 22-5). In 2 to 4 days become hemorrhagic, no longer blanchable. Local edema. Rarely, an eschar (round crusted ulcer associated with an acute rickettsial infection) is present at the site of the tick bite. Necrosis of the skin and underlying structures. With DIC, skin infarcts (gangrene) occur.

Distribution Characteristically, rash begins on wrists, (Fig. 22-3) forearms, and ankles (Fig. 22-4) and somewhat later on palms and soles. Within 6 to 18 h rash spreads centripetally to the arms, thighs, trunk, (Fig. 22-5) and face. The hemorrhagic rash involving the palms and soles occurs in 36 to 82% of cases and appears after day 5 of illness in 43%. Necrosis occurs in acral extremities and scrotum.

General Findings Fever to 40°C. Hypotension, shock later in course. Hepatomegaly, splenomegaly, GI hemorrhage, altered consciousness, transient deafness, incontinence, oliguria, and secondary bacterial infections of the lung, middle ear, and parotid gland may occur.

Variants

Spotless fever: 13% of cases. Associated with higher mortality rate because diagnosis is overlooked.

Abdominal syndrome: Can mimic acute abdomen, acute cholecystitis, acute appendicitis. *Thrombotic thrombocytopenic purpura*

DIFFERENTIAL DIAGNOSIS

Usually of a tick-exposed patient who presents between May and September with a 1- to 3-day history of fever, headache, myalgia, malaise, and rash: meningococcemia, disseminated gonococcal infection, secondary syphilis, *Staphylococcus aureus* septicemia, toxic shock syndrome, typhoid fever, leptospirosis, other rickettsioses (ehrlichiosis, murine typhus, epidemic typhus, rickettsialpox), viral exanthem (measles, varicella, rubella, enterovirus), adverse cutaneous drug reaction, immune-complex vasculitis, idiopathic thrombocytopenic purpura, thrombotic thrombocytopenic purpura, Kawasaki's syndrome.

LABORATORY EXAMINATIONS

Skin Biopsy Necrotizing vasculitis Rickettsiae can at times be demonstrated within the endothelial cells by immunofluorescence or immunoenzyme staining techniques.

Direct Immunofluorescence Specific *R. rickettsii* antigen within endothelial cells 70% sensitive; 100% specific. Treatment with antirickettsial drugs within 48 h reduces sensitivity.

Serodiagnosis Immunofluorescent antibody test (IFA) can be used to measure both IgG and IgM anti-*R. rickettsii* antibodies. Fourfold rise in titer between acute and convalescent stages is diagnostic, with a titer of ≥64 detectable between 7 and 10 days after onset of illness.

DIAGNOSIS

Clinical and epidemiologic considerations more important than a laboratory diagnosis in early RMSF. Suspect in febrile children, adolescents, and men older than 60 years of age—particularly those who reside in or have traveled to the southern Atlantic states and South-Central states from May through September and participated in outdoor activity. Diagnosis must be made clinically and confirmed later. Only 3% of cases with RMSF present with the triad of rash, fever, and history of a tick bite during the first 3 days of illness.

COURSE AND PROGNOSIS

Death is associated with older age, delay in diagnosis and delay in treatment or no treatment, treatment with chloramphenicol (compared with tetracycline). Untreated (before the availability of effective antibiotics), the fatality rate was 23%; treated, 3% (6% if older than 40 years of age). Fatality rate 1.5% with known tick bite but 6.6% if no known tick exposure. Fulminant RMSF is defined as a fatal disease whose course is unusually rapid (i.e., ≤5 days from onset to death) and is usually characterized by early onset of neurologic signs and late or absent rash. In 1990, the case-fatality rate was 8% for individuals younger than 20 years of age and 6.8% for those older than 20 years of age. In uncomplicated cases, defervescence usually occurs within 48 to 72 h after initiation of therapy.

Long-term sequelae (complications that persist for ≥1 year after acute infection): neurologic (paraparesis; hearing loss; peripheral neuropathy; bladder and bowel incontinence; cerebellar, vestibular, and motor dysfunction; language disorders); nonneurologic (disability from limb amputation and scrotal pain after cutaneous necrosis).

MANAGEMENT

Prevention   Avoid tick bites: protective clothing, tick repellants. After possible exposure, inspect for ticks.

Antirickettsial Therapy   Specific antirickettsial therapy should be initiated as soon as the diagnosis is suspected clinically.

Drug of Choice   Doxycycline (except for pregnant patients, history of allergy to doxycycline, or possibly a child younger than 9 years of age), 200 mg/d PO or IV in two divided doses for adults. Tetracycline, 25 to 50 mg/kg/d in four divided doses.

Alternative   Chloramphenicol, 50 to 75 mg/kg/d in four divided doses.

Supportive Therapy   For acute problems of shock, acute renal failure, respiratory failure, prolonged coma.

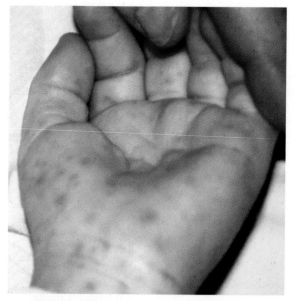

Figure 22-3   Rocky Mountain spotted fever: early   *Erythematous and hemorrhagic macules and papules appeared initially on the wrists of a young child.*

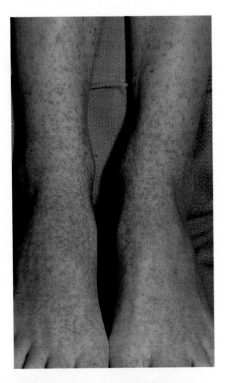

Figure 22-4　Rocky Mountain spotted fever: early　*Erythematous and hemorrhagic macules and papules appeared initially on the ankles of an adolescent.*

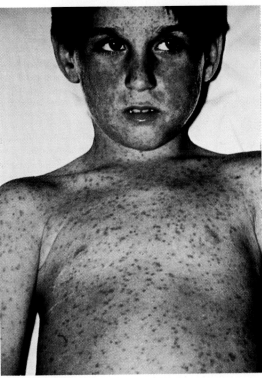

Figure 22-5　Rocky Mountain spotted fever: late　*Disseminated hemorrhagic macules and papules on the face, neck, trunk, and arms on the fourth day of febrile illness in an older child. The initial lesions were noted on the wrists and ankles, subsequently extending centripetally.*

VIRAL INFECTIONS OF SKIN AND MUCOSA

Viral infections of skin and mucosa produce a wide spectrum of clinical manifestations. Viruses such as human papillomavirus (HPV) and molluscum contagiosum virus (MCV) colonize the epidermis of most individuals without causing any clinical lesions. Benign epithelial proliferations, i.e., warts and molluscum, occur in some, are transient, and eventually resolve without therapy. In immunocompromised individuals, however, these lesions may become extensive, persistent, and refractory to therapy. Viruses that cause febrile illness with exanthems are usually self-limited, with primary infection conveying lifetime immunity. The eight human herpesviruses often have asymptomatic primary infection but are characterized by lifelong latent infection. In the setting of immunocompromise, these viruses can become active and cause disease with significant morbidity and mortality rates.

POXVIRUS INFECTIONS

Poxviruses have a large double-stranded DNA genome. They are the only DNA viruses that replicate in cytoplasm, where accumulated viral particles form eosinophilic inclusions or Guarnieri bodies, visible by light microscopy. Smallpox or variola has been eradicated as a naturally occurring infection. Cowpox is an infection of cattle and is caused by cowpox virus. The origins of vaccinia virus, which are used to immunize humans against smallpox, are uncertain. It may be derived from variola virus, cowpox virus, or be a hybrid of the two. Molluscum contagiosum virus colonizes the skin of many healthy individuals, causing molluscum contagiosum with self-limited epidermal proliferations that resolve spontaneously. Human orf and milker's nodules are zoonotic infections that can sometimes occur in exposed humans. Other poxviruses that are zoonoses in animal hosts (monkeys, cows, buffalo, sheep, goats) can also infect humans.

Molluscum Contagiosum

Molluscum contagiosum is a self-limited epidermal viral infection, characterized clinically by skin-colored papules that are often umbilicated, occurring in children and sexually active adults. In HIV-infected individuals, however, numerous large mollusca often arise on the face, causing significant cosmetic disfigurement.

EPIDEMIOLOGY

Age/Sex Children. Sexually active adults. Males>females.

Risk Factors HIV-infected individuals may have hundreds of small mollusca or giant mollusca on the face.

Etiology Molluscum contagiosum virus (MCV), a poxvirus, with 30% homology with smallpox virus. Types MCV-1 and MCV-2. The virus has not been cultivated. Not distinguishable from other poxviruses by electron microscopy. In most healthy adults, the epidermis and infundibulum of hair follicle are colonized by MCV.

Transmission Skin-to-skin contact.

Classification by Risk Groups *Children* Commonly occur on exposed skin sites. Child-to-child transmission relatively low. Resolve spontaneously. Usually caused by MCV-1.

Sexually Active Adults Occur in genital region. Virus transmitted during sexual activity. Resolve spontaneously.

HIV-Infected Individuals Most commonly occur on the face, spread by shaving. Without aggressive therapy, mollusca enlarge. Spontaneous regression does not occur. Usually caused by MCV-2. With response to highly active antiretroviral therapy (HAART), lesions often resolve.

HISTORY

Duration of Lesions In the normal host, mollusca usually persist up to 6 months and then undergo spontaneous regression. In HIV-infected individuals without HAART, mollusca persist and proliferate even after aggressive local therapy.

Skin Symptoms Usually none. Cosmetic disfigurement. Concern about having a transmissible infection. Painful if secondarily infected.

PHYSICAL EXAMINATION

Skin Lesions Papules (1 to 2 mm), nodules (5 to 10 mm) (rarely, giant) (Fig. 23-1). Pearly white or skin-colored. Round, oval, hemispherical, umbilicated (Fig. 23-1). Isolated single lesion, multiple, scattered discrete lesions, or confluent mosaic plaques. Most larger mollusca have a central keratotic plug, which gives the lesion a central dimple or umbilication, best observed after light liquid nitrogen freeze. Gentle pressure on a molluscum causes the central plug to be extruded. Autoinoculation is apparent in that mollusca are clustered at a site such as the axilla. In HIV-infected males who shave, mollusca can be confined to the beard area. Hundreds of lesions occur in HIV-infected patients (Fig. 23-2). Mollusca undergoing spontaneous regression have an erythematous halo. In dark-skinned individuals, significant postinflammatory hyperpigmentation after treatment or spontaneous regression may occur.

Distribution Face, eyelids, neck; trunk, especially axilla; anogenital area. Multiple facial mollusca suggest HIV infection.

DIFFERENTIAL DIAGNOSIS

Multiple Small Mollusca Flat warts, condylomata acuminata, syringoma, sebaceous hyperplasia.

Large Solitary Molluscum Keratoacanthoma, squamous cell carcinoma, basal cell carcinoma, epidermal inclusion cyst.

Multiple Facial Mollusca in HIV-Infected Individual Disseminated invasive fungal infection, i.e., cryptococcosis, histoplasmosis, coccidioidomycosis, penicillinosis.

LABORATORY EXAMINATIONS

Smear of Keratotic Plug Direct microscopic examination of Giemsa-stained central semisolid core reveals "molluscum bodies" (inclusion bodies).

Dermatopathology Epidermal cells contain large intracytoplasmic inclusion bodies, i.e., molluscum bodies, that appear as single, ovoid eosinophilic structures in lower cells of stratum malpighii. Epidermis grows down into dermis. Infection also occurs in epithelium and follicle.

DIAGNOSIS

Usually made on clinical findings. Biopsy lesion in HIV-infected individual if disseminated invasive fungal infection is in the differential diagnosis.

COURSE AND PROGNOSIS

In healthy individuals, mollusca resolve spontaneously. In HIV-infected individuals, mollusca often progress even with aggressive therapies, creating significant cosmetic disfigurement, especially by facial lesions. In HIV-infected individuals successfully treated with HAART, mollusca either do not occur or resolve after several months. Recurrence of mollusca usually indicates failure of HAART.

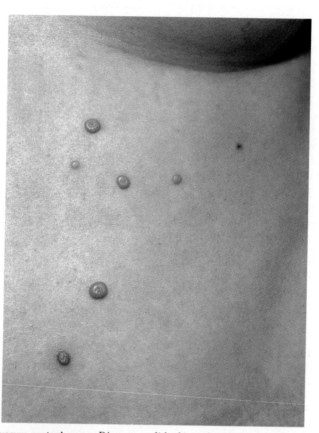

Figure 23-1 Molluscum contagiosum *Discrete, solid, skin-colored papules, 1 to 2 mm in diameter, with central umbilication on the chest of an adolescent female. The lesion with an erythematous halo is undergoing spontaneous regression.*

VIRAL INFECTIONS OF SKIN AND MUCOSA

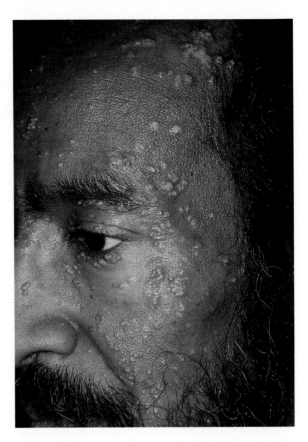

Figure 23-2   Molluscum contagiosum in advanced HIV disease   *Discrete and confluent skin-colored umbilicated papules on the face of a 52-year-old black male; note the periorbital clustering. The image is from 1990, before effective antiretroviral therapy. The lesions recurred and progressed after aggressive cryo- and electrosurgery.*

MANAGEMENT

Prevention	Avoid skin-to-skin contact with individual having mollusca. HIV-infected individuals with mollusca in the beard area should be advised to minimize shaving facial hair or grow a beard.
Supportive therapy	In immunocompetent children and sexually active adults, mollusca regress spontaneously; painful aggressive therapy is not indicated.
Treatment of lesions	
Topical patient-directed therapy	Aldara cream (5% imiquimod) applied hs 3 times per week for up to 1–3 months.
Clinician-directed therapy (office)	These procedures are painful and traumatic, especially for young children. EMLA cream applied to lesions 1 h before therapy may reduce/eliminate pain.
Curettage	Small mollusca can be removed with a small curette with little discomfort or pain.
Cryosurgery	Freezing lesions for 10–15 s is effective and minimally painful, using either a cotton-tipped applicator or liquid nitrogen spray.
Electrodesiccation	For mollusca refractory to cryosurgery, especially in HIV-infected individuals with numerous and/or large lesions, electrodesiccation or laser surgery is the treatment of choice. Large lesions usually require injected lidocaine anesthesia. Giant mollusca may require several cycles of electrodesiccation and curettage to remove the large bulk of lesions; these lesions may extend through the dermis into the subcutaneous fat.

Milker's Nodules and Human Orf

Milker's nodules (MN) and human orf (HO) are cutaneous infections caused by parapoxviruses, which normally infect animals and accidentally cause infection in humans, and are characterized clinically by nodular lesions on exposed cutaneous sites.

Milker's nodules Most common in dairy farmers. Bovine lesions occur on muzzles of calves and teats of cows. Humans can be infected by contact with bovine lesions or teat cups of milking machines. Clinically, lesions can present as solitary red-purple nodules or less commonly, multiple cherry-red papules and nodules, arising at site of inoculation (Fig. 23-3). Diagnosis is usually made on history of bovine exposure and clinical findings. Antiviral agents are not effective; treatment should be directed at treatment of bacterial superinfection and pain management.

Human orf Most common in farmers, veterinarians, sheep shearers exposed to infected ungulates (sheep, goats, yaks, etc.), usually in springtime (when lambs are born) and season of slaughter of lambs and sheep. Occurs worldwide with epidemics in Norway and other parts of Europe, New Zealand; rare in North America. Virus survives for many months on fences, feeding basins, and surfaces in barns. Only newborn lambs lacking viral immunity are susceptible. In lambs, orf is manifested as erythematous, exudative nodules around mouth that heal spontaneously in about a month, producing permanent immunity. Humans are infected either by inoculation of virus by direct contact with lambs (bottle feeding) or indirectly (knives, barbed wire, towels, other contaminated surfaces). Human-to-human infection does not occur.

Six clinical stages are described, each lasting approximately 6 days: papular, targetoid, nodular, exudative, regenerative, and regressive. Initially, papule(s) to nodule(s) to plaque(s) at site of inoculation; may appear very edematous to vesicular to bullous (Fig. 23-4). Older nodules have central crusting with purulent discharge. Ascending lymphangitis may occur. Lesions average 1.6 cm in diameter; most commonly only one lesion is present, but can be 10 or more. Heal without scar formation. Lesions occur on exposed sites (hands, arms, legs, face); most common site: dorsum of right index finger. Resolves spontaneously in 4 to 6 weeks. Antiviral agents are not effective; treatment should be directed at treatment of bacterial superinfection and pain management.

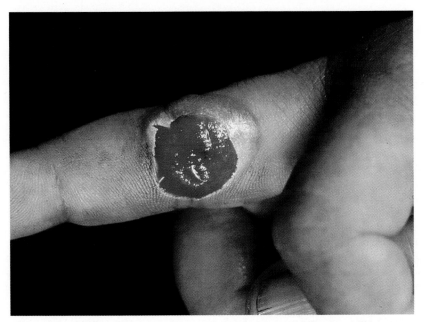

Figure 23-3 Milker's nodule *Firm, purple, eroded nodule occurred following milking a cow.*

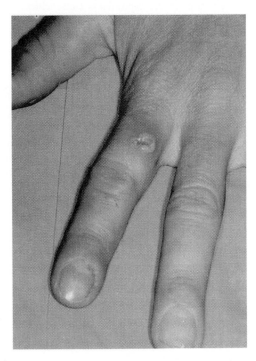

Figure 23-4 Human orf *A single erythematous nodule with a central pustule is seen on the finger at the site of inoculation.*

HUMAN PAPILLOMAVIRUS INFECTIONS

Human papillomaviruses (HPV) are very widespread-to-ubiquitous in humans, causing subclinical infection or a wide variety of benign clinical lesions on skin and mucous membranes, and have a role in the oncogenesis of cutaneous and mucosal premalignancies and malignancies. More than 150 types of HPV have been identified and are associated with various clinical lesions (Table 23-1).

Three clinical manifestations of cutaneous HPV infections occur commonly in the general population: common warts, plantar warts, and flat warts. Common warts represent approximately 70% of all cutaneous warts, occurring in up to 20% of all school-aged children. Plantar warts are common in older children and young adults, accounting for 30% of cutaneous warts. Flat warts occur in children and adults, accounting for 4% of cutaneous warts. Common in butchers, meat packers, and fish handlers are butcher's warts.

The most common presentation of mucosal HPV infection is condyloma acuminatum (genital wart), which is the most prevalent sexually transmitted disease. Some HPV types have a major etiologic role in the pathogenesis of in situ as well as invasive squamous cell carcinoma of the anogenital epithelium. During delivery, maternal genital HPV infection can be transmitted to the neonate, resulting in anogenital warts or recurrent respiratory papillomatosis (RRP) after aspiration of the virus into the upper respiratory tract.

EPIDEMIOLOGY

Etiology Papillomaviruses are double-stranded DNA viruses of the papovavirus class, which infect most vertebrate species with exclusive host and tissue specificity. They infect squamous epithelia of skin and mucous membranes. Clinical lesions induced by HPV and its natural history are largely determined by HPV type.

HPV are normally grouped according to their pathologic associations and tissue specificity—either cutaneous or mucosal. The 23 mucosal-associated HPV can be further subgrouped according to their risk of malignant transformation. New types of HPV are defined as possessing <90% homology to known types in six specified early and late genes.

Human Papillomavirus: Cutaneous Infections

Certain human papillomavirus (HPV) types commonly infect keratinized skin. Cutaneous warts are a discrete benign epithelial hyperplasia with varying degrees of surface hyperkeratosis manifested as minute papules to large plaques; lesions may become confluent forming a mosaic. The extent of lesions is determined by the immune status of the host.
Synonym: Verruca, myrmecia.

EPIDEMIOLOGY

Etiology (Table 23-1)

Transmission Skin-to-skin contact. Minor trauma with breaks in stratum corneum facilitates epidermal infection. Contagion occurs in groups—small (home) or large (school gymnasium).

Other Factors Immunocompromise, such as occurs in HIV disease or after iatrogenic immunosuppression with solid organ transplantation, is associated with an increased incidence of and more widespread cutaneous warts. Occupational risk associated with meat handling.

Inheritance Epidermodysplasia verruciformis (EDV): most commonly autosomal recessive.

Duration of Lesions Warts often persist for several years if not treated.

Symptoms Cosmetic disfigurement. Plantar warts act as a foreign body and can be quite painful during normal daily activities such as walking if located over pressure points. More aggressive therapies such as cryosurgery often result in much more pain than that caused by the wart itself. Bleeding, especially after shaving.

PHYSICAL EXAMINATION

Skin Lesions *Verruca Vulgaris (Common Warts)* Firm papules, 1 to 10 mm or rarely larger (Fig. 23-5), hyperkeratotic, clefted surface, with vegetations (Fig. 23-6). Palmar lesions disrupt the normal line of fingerprints. Return of fingerprints is a sign of resolution of the wart. Characteristic "red or brown dots" (thrombosing capillary loops) (Figs. 23-5 and 23-6) are better seen with hand lens, are pathognomonic, representing thrombosed capillary loops. Isolated lesion, scattered discrete lesions. Annular at sites of prior therapy. Occur at sites of trauma: hands, fingers, knees. Butcher's warts: large cauliflower-like lesions on hands of meat handlers. Filiform warts have relatively small bases, extending out with elongated cap (Fig. 23-7).

Verruca Plantaris (Plantar Warts) Early small, shiny, sharply marginated papule (Fig. 23-8)→plaque with rough hyperkeratotic surface, studded with brown-black dots (thrombosed capillaries). As with palmar warts, normal dermatoglyphics are disrupted. Return of dermatoglyphics is a sign of resolution of the wart. Warts heal without scarring. Therapies such as cryosurgery and electrosurgery can result in lifelong scarring at treatment sites. Tenderness may be marked, especially in certain acute types and in lesions over sites of pressure (metatarsal head). Confluence of many small warts results in a mosaic wart (Fig. 23-8). "Kissing" lesion may occur on opposing surface of two toes. Plantar foot, often solitary but may be three to six or more. Pressure points, heads of metatarsal, heels, toes.

Verruca Plana (Flat Warts) Sharply defined, flat papules (1 to 5 mm); "flat" surface; the thickness of the lesion is 1 to 2 mm (Fig. 23-9). Skin-colored or light brown. Round,

Table 23-1   HPV TYPES AND ASSOCIATED CLINICAL LESIONS

HPV Type	Most Common Clinical Lesions	Less Frequent Lesions	Potential Oncogenicity
1	Deep plantar/palmar warts	Common warts	None
2, 4, 27, 29	Common warts	Plantar, palmar, mosaic, oral, anogenital warts	None
3, 10, 28, 49	Flat warts	Flat warts in EV	None
7	"Butchers" warts		
13, 32	Oral focal epithelial hyperplasia (Heck's disease)		None
5, 8, 9, 12, 14, 15, 17, 19–26, 36, 47, 50	Epidermodysplasia verruciformis (EV); warts in immunosuppression	Normal skin(?)	HPV -5, -8, -9 isolated from SCC
6, 11	Anogenital warts, cervical condylomas	Squamous intraepithelial lesion, SCC in situ; common warts; respiratory papillomatosis	"Lock risk" Bushke-Lowenstein tumor (giant condyloma); rare in penile, vulvar, cervical, and other urogenital tumors
16, 18 31, 33, 35, 39, 45, 51–53, 55, 56, 59, 63, 66, 68	Cervical condylomata; anogenital warts; SCC in situ	Common warts	"High risk" Genital and cervical dysplasias and carcinomas; rare in cutaneous SCC

oval, polygonal, linear lesions (inoculation of virus by scratching). Lesions that arise after trauma may have a linear arrangement. Occur on face, beard area, dorsa of hands, shins.

Epidermodysplasia Verruciformis Flat-topped papules. Pityriasis versicolor-like lesions, particularly on the trunk. Color: skin-colored, light brown, pink, hypopigmented. Lesions may be numerous, large, and confluent. Seborrheic keratosis-like lesions. Actinic keratosis-like lesions. Squamous cell carcinoma (SCC), in situ and invasive. Lesions often become confluent, forming large maplike areas. Linear arrangement after traumatic inoculation. Distribution: face, dorsa of hands, arms, legs, anterior trunk. Premalignant and malignant lesions arise most commonly on face.

DIFFERENTIAL DIAGNOSIS

Verruca Vulgaris Molluscum contagiosum, seborrheic keratosis, actinic keratosis, keratoacanthoma, SCC in situ, invasive SCC.

Verruca Plantaris Callus, corn (keratosis), exostosis.

Verruca Plana Syringoma (facial), molluscum contagiosum.

Epidermodysplasia Verruciformis Pityriasis versicolor, actinic keratoses, seborrheic keratoses, SCC, basal cell carcinoma.

LABORATORY STUDIES

Dermatopathology Acanthosis, papillomatosis, hyperkeratosis. Characteristic feature is foci of vacuolated cells (koilocytosis), vertical tiers of parakeratotic cells, foci of clumped keratohyaline granules.

DIAGNOSIS

Usually made on clinical findings. In the immunocompromised host, HIV-induced SCC at periungual sites or anogenital region should be ruled out by lesional biopsy.

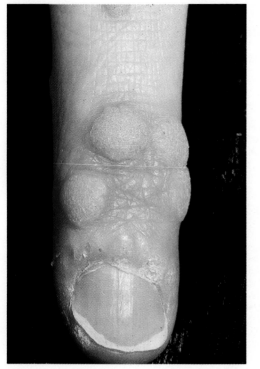

Figure 23-5   Verruca vulgaris: periungual
Hyperkeratotic papules located periungually on the dorsum of a finger. Similar lesions were present on all fingers of both hands. All modalities of therapy had failed. The warts resolved with microinjections of bleomycin.

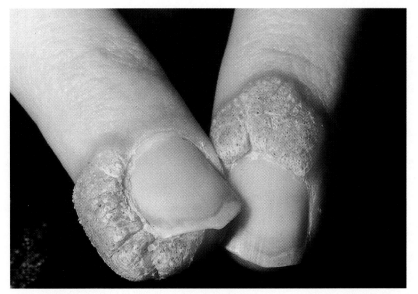

Figure 23-6 Verruca vulgaris in an immunocompromised individual *Large, very thick, fissured, painful periungual and subungual warts are present on two fingers of a 20-year-old male treated with immunosuppressive drugs after renal transplantation. Similar lesions were also present on multiple toes.*

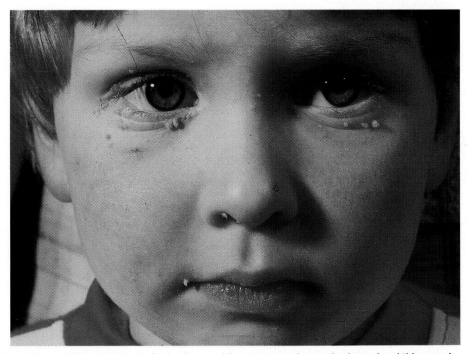

Figure 23-7 Filiform warts *Multiple elongated keratotic papules on the face of a child; note the clustering on the eyelids.*

COURSE AND PROGNOSIS

In immunocompetent individuals, cutaneous HPV infections usually resolve spontaneously, without therapeutic intervention. In immunocompromised individuals, cutaneous HPV infections may be very resistant to all modalities of therapy. In EDV, disease starts at 5 to 7 years of age; lesions appear progressively, becoming widespread in some. 30 to 50% of individuals with EDV develop malignant cutaneous lesions on areas of skin exposed to sunlight.

MANAGEMENT

Goal	Aggressive therapies, which are often quite painful and may be followed by scarring, are usually to be avoided in that the natural history of cutaneous HPV infections is for spontaneous resolution in months or a few years. Plantar warts that are painful because of their location warrant more aggressive therapies.
Patient-initiated therapy	Minimal cost; no/minimal pain.
For small lesions	10–20% salicylic acid and lactic acid in collodion.
For large lesions	40% salicylic acid plaster for 1 week, then application of salicylic acid–lactic acid in collodion.
Imiquimod cream	At sites that are not thickly keratinized, apply hs 3 times per week. Persistent warts may required occlusion. Hyperkeratotic lesions on palms/soles should be debrided frequently; Imiquimod used alternately with a topical retinoid such as tararotene topical gel may be effective.
Hyperthermia for verruca plantaris	Hyperthermia with hot water (113°F) immersion for 1/2 to 3/4 h two or three times weekly for 16 treatments is effective in some patients.
Clinician-initiated therapy	Costly, painful.
Cryosurgery	If patients have tried home therapies and liquid nitrogen is available, light cryosurgery using a cotton-tipped applicator or cryospray, freezing the wart and 1 to 2 mm of surrounding normal tissue for approximately 30 s, is quite effective. Freezing kills the infected tissue but not HPV. Cryosurgery is usually repeated about every 4 weeks until the warts have disappeared. Painful.
Electrosurgery	More effective than cryosurgery, but also associated with a greater chance of scarring. EMLA cream can be used for anesthesia for flat warts. Lidocaine injection is usually required for thicker warts, especially palmar/plantar lesions.
CO_2 laser surgery	May be effective for recalcitrant warts, but no better than cryosurgery or electrosurgery in the hands of experienced clinician.
Surgery	Single, nonplantar verruca vulgaris:curettage after freon freezing; surgical excision of cutaneous HPV infections is not indicated in that these lesions are epidermal infections.

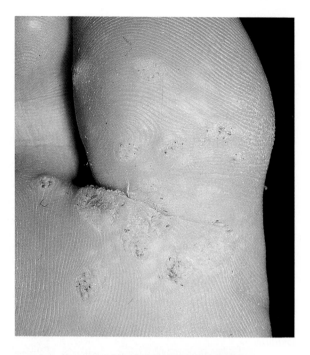

Figure 23-8   Verruca plantaris
Confluent, skin-colored, verrucous papules, forming a mosaic, disrupting the normal dermatoglyphics of the plantar foot. The thrombosed capillaries (brown dots) differentiate the lesion from a corn (an often painful, translucent, yellowish, keratotic granule) and a callus (a poorly demarcated, hyperkeratotic plaque with normal dermatoglyphics at pressure sites).

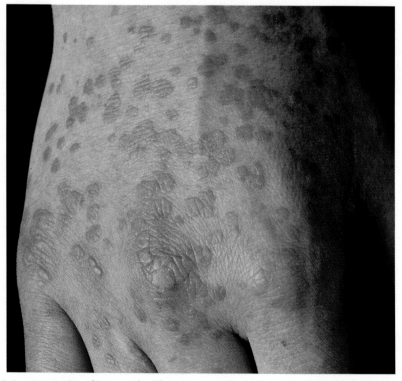

Figure 23-9   Verruca plana (flat warts)   *Flat-topped, pink papules with sharp margination and minimal hyperkeratosis on the dorsum of the hands and fingers.*

HUMAN PAPILLOMAVIRUS INFECTIONS

INFECTIOUS EXANTHEMS

An infectious exanthem is a generalized cutaneous eruption associated with a primary systemic infection; it is often accompanied by oral mucosal lesions, i.e., an enanthem. Most often it is of viral nature but can be caused by *Rickettsia,* bacteria, and parasites.

EPIDEMIOLOGY

Age of Onset   Usually younger than 20 years.

Etiology *Viral* Rubella virus, attenuated rubella virus in vaccine; paramyxovirus (measles); parvovirus B19 (erythema infectiosum); rhinovirus; respiratory syncytial virus; adenoviruses; herpesviridae: cytomegalovirus (CMV), Epstein-Barr virus (EBV), human herpesvirus 6 and 7 (exanthem subitum, roseola infantum); enteroviruses (e.g., coxsackieviruses, echo virus); flavivirus (dengue); hepatitis B virus; HIV (acute retroviral syndrome); orbivirus (Colorado tick fever); reoviruses; rotaviruses.

Bacterial Group A streptococcus (scarlet fever); *Staphylococcus aureus* (toxic shock syndrome); *Legionella, Leptospira, Listeria,* meningococci.

Mycoplasmal

Rickettsial Rocky Mountain spotted fever, other spotted fevers, rickettsialpox, murine and epidemic typhus.

Miscellaneous Mycoplasma pneumoniae, Strongyloides, Toxoplasma, Treponema pallidum.

Transmission   Respiratory, food, sexual, blood.

Season   Enterovirus infections, summer months.

Geography   Worldwide.

PATHOGENESIS

Skin lesions may be produced by the direct effect of microbial replication in infected cells, the host response to the microbe, or the interaction of these two phenomena.

HISTORY

Incubation Period   Usually less than 3 weeks; hepatitis B virus several months.

Prodrome   Fever, malaise, coryza, sore throat, nausea, vomiting, diarrhea, abdominal pain, headache.

PHYSICAL EXAMINATION

Skin Lesions *Scarlitiniform* Erythema. Diffuse to generalized. May be more prominent in body folds. May be associated with erythema of oropharynx and/or genitalia. Desquamation may occur with resolution of exanthem.

Exanthematous [Morbilliform (Measles-Like)] Erythematous macules and/or papules (Figs. 23-10A and 23-10B); less frequently, vesicles, petechiae, Usually central, i.e., head, neck, trunk, proximal extremities. Diffuse erythema of cheeks, i.e., "slapped cheek" with erythema infectiosum.

Vesicular Initially, vesicles with clear fluid; may evolve to pustules. In a few days to a week, roof of vesicle sloughs, resulting in erosions. In varicella, lesions are disseminated and may involve oropharynx. In hand-foot-and-mouth disease, vesicles/erosion occur in oropharynx; painful linear vesicles on palms/soles.

Mucous Membranes Koplik's spots in measles; microulcerative lesions in herpangina due to coxsackievirus A (Fig. 23-11); palatal petechiae in mononucleosis syndrome of EBV or CMV; conjunctivitis.

General Examination   Lymphadenopathy, hepatomegaly, splenomegaly.

DIFFERENTIAL DIAGNOSIS

Exanthematous Eruption Drug eruption, systemic lupus erythematosus, Kawasaki's syndrome.

LABORATORY STUDIES

Cultures   If practical.

Serology   Acute and convalescent titers most helpful in specific diagnosis.

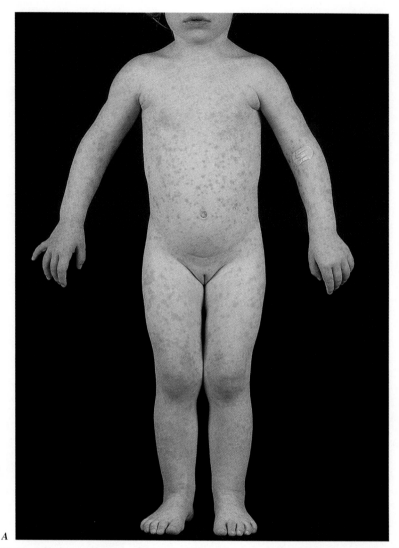

A

Figure 23-10 Infectious exanthem *Disseminated, erythematous macules and papules, typical of the cutaneous changes with many acute infections. The eruption must be differentiated from an exanthematous (morbilliform) drug eruption.* **A.** *Typical distribution of lesions on the trunk and extremities.*

DIAGNOSIS

Usually made on history and clinical findings.

COURSE AND PROGNOSIS

Usually resolves in less than 10 days. Patients with primary EBV or CMV infection very of-ten develop an exanthematous eruption if given ampicillin or amoxacillin.

MANAGEMENT

Symptomatic.

Antimicrobial Therapy Specific antimicro-bial therapy when available.

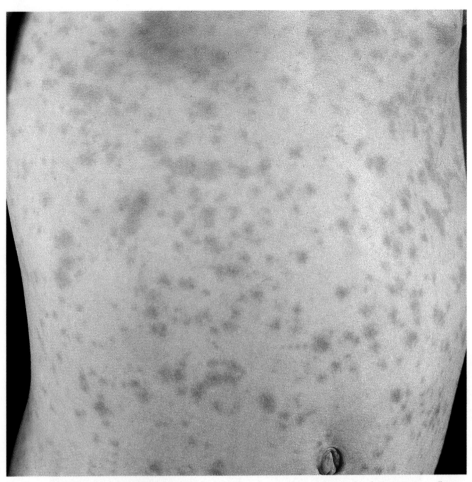

B

Figure 23-10   Infectious exanthem   B. *Close-up of pink macules and papules becoming confluent in some areas.*

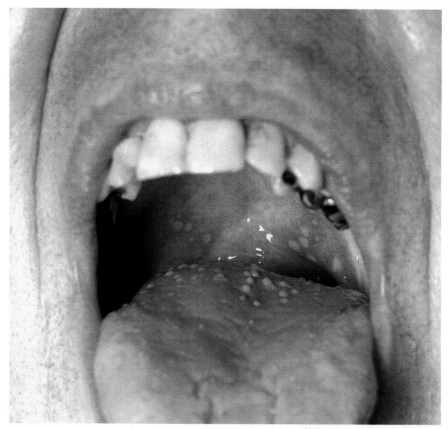

Figure 23-11 Infectious enanthem herpangina *Multiple, small vesicles and erosions with erythematous halos on the soft palate; some taste buds on the posterior tongue are inflamed and prominent.*

Rubella

Rubella is a common benign childhood infection manifested by a characteristic exanthem and lymphadenopathy. Rubella virus infecting a pregnant female, while causing a benign illness in the mother, may result in the congenital rubella syndrome with serious chronic fetal infection and malformation. Childhood immunization is highly effective at preventing infection.

Synonyms: German measles, "3-day measles."

EPIDEMIOLOGY

Age of Onset Before widespread immunization, children younger than 15 years. Currently, young adults.

Etiology Rubella virus. Attenutated rubella virus used in immunization can cause an illness with rubella-like rash, lymphadenopathy, and arthritis.

Occupation Young adults in hospitals, colleges, prisons, prenatal clinics.

Transmission Inhalation of aerosolized respiratory droplets; moderately contagious; 10 to 40% of cases asymptomatic; period of infectivity from end of incubation period to disappearance of rash.

Risk Factors Lack of active immunization, lack of natural infection. After immunization begun in 1969, incidence has decreased by 99%.

Season Before 1969, epidemics in the United States every 6 to 9 years, occurring in spring.

Geography Worldwide. Marked reduction in incidence in developed countries after immunization.

HISTORY

Incubation Period 14 to 21 days.

Prodrome Usually absent, especially in young children. In adolescents and young adults: anorexia, malaise, conjunctivitis, headache, low-grade fever, mild upper respiratory tract symptoms.

History Arthralgia, especially in adult women after immunization.

Immune Status In women, rubella-like illness frequently follows administration of attenuated live rubella virus.

PHYSICAL EXAMINATION

Skin Lesions Pink macules, papules (Fig. 23-12A). Initially on forehead, spreading inferiorly to face, trunk, and extremities during first day. By second day, facial exanthem fades. By third day, exanthem fades completely without residual pigmentary change or scaling. Trunkal lesions may become confluent, creating a scarlatiniform eruption (Fig. 23-12B).

Mucous Membranes Petechiae on soft palate (Forchheimer's sign) during prodrome (also seen in infectious mononucleosis).

General Examination *Lymph nodes*: enlarged during prodrome. Postauricular, suboccipital, and posterior cervical lymph nodes enlarged and possibly tender. Mild generalized lymphadenopathy may occur. Enlargement usually persists for 1 week but may last for months. *Spleen:* may be enlarged. *Joints:* arthritis in adults; possible effusion.

DIFFERENTIAL DIAGNOSIS

Exanthem Other viral exanthems, drug eruption, scarlet fever.

Exanthem with Arthritis Acute rheumatic fever, rheumatoid arthritis, erythema infectiosum.

LABORATORY STUDIES

Serology Acute and convalescent rubella antibody titers show fourfold or greater rise.

Culture Virus can be isolated from throat, joint fluid aspirate.

DIAGNOSIS

Clinical diagnosis; can be confirmed by serology.

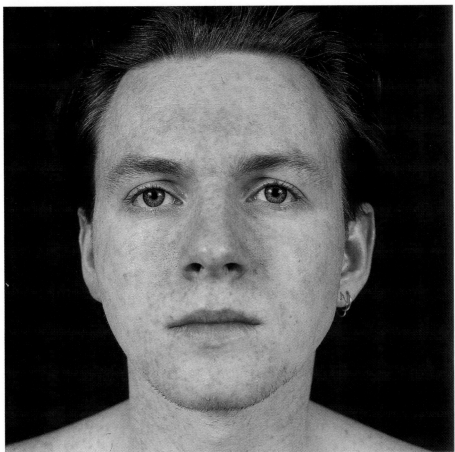

A

Figure 23-12 Rubella A. *Erythematous macules and papules appearing initially on the face and spreading inferiorly to the trunk and extremities, usually within the first 24 h. Postauricular and posterior cervical lymph nodes were enlarged. Lesions becoming confluent on the cheeks while clearing on the forehead.*

COURSE AND PROGNOSIS

In most persons, rubella is a mild, inconsequential infection. However, when rubella occurs in a pregnant woman during the first trimester, the infection can be passed transplacentally to the developing fetus. Approximately half of infants who acquire rubella during the first trimester of intrauterine life will show clinical signs of damage from the virus. Manifestations of the congenital rubella syndrome are congenital heart defects, cataracts, microphthalmia, deafness, microcephaly, hydrocephaly.

MANAGEMENT

Prevention   Rubella is preventable by immunization. Previous rubella should be documented in young women; if antirubella antibody titers are negative, rubella immunization should be given.

Acute Infection   Symptomatic.

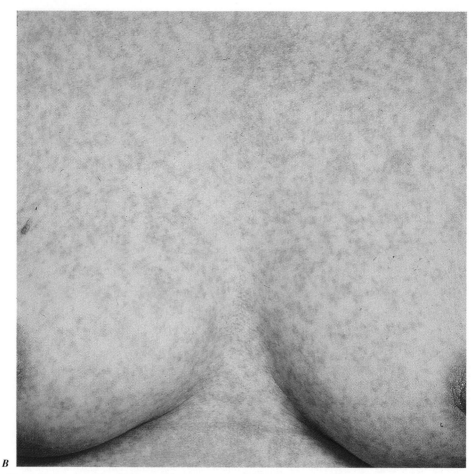

B

Figure 23-12   Rubella   B. *Truncal lesions appear 24 h after onset of facial lesions.*

Measles

Measles is a highly contagious childhood viral infection characterized by fever, coryza, cough, conjunctivitis, pathognomonic enanthem (Koplik's spots), and an exanthem. It can be complicated, acutely and chronically, by significant morbidity and mortality. Childhood immunization is highly effective at preventing infection.

Synonym: Rubeola, morbilli.

EPIDEMIOLOGY

Age of Onset Before measles immunization: 5 to 9 years of age in the United States. In underdeveloped countries, up to 45% of cases occur before the age of 9 months.

Etiology Measles virus, a paramyxovirus.

Incidence United States: greater than fourfold increase, 1988 to 1989. Since 1993, an historic low of 312 cases were reported. In 1994, 92% of cases were indigenous and 8% imported from other countries. *Worldwide:* hyperendemic in many underdeveloped countries, resulting in >1.5 million deaths annually.

Risk Factors After immunization begun in 1963, incidence has decreased by 98%. Current outbreaks in the United States occur in innercity unimmunized preschool-aged children, school-aged persons immunized at early age, and imported cases. Most outbreaks are in primary or secondary schools, colleges or universities, day-care centers.

Transmission Spread by respiratory droplet aerosols produced by sneezing and coughing. Infected persons contagious from several days before onset of rash up to 5 days after lesions appear. Attack rate for susceptible contacts exceeds 90 to 100%. Asymptomatic infection rare.

Season Before widespread use of vaccine, epidemics occurred every 2 to 3 years, in late winter to early spring.

Geography Worldwide.

PATHOGENESIS

Virus enters cells of respiratory tract, replicates locally, spreads to local lymph nodes, and disseminates hematogenously to skin and mucous membranes. Viral replication also occurs on skin and mucosa. Modified measles, a milder form of the illness, may occur in individuals with preexisting partial immunity induced by active or passive immunization.

HISTORY

Incubation Period 10 to 15 days.

Symptoms Upper respiratory infection with coryza and hacking, barklike cough, photophobia, malaise, fever. As exanthem progresses, systemic symptoms subside.

PHYSICAL EXAMINATION

Skin Lesions *Exanthem* On the fourth febrile day, erythematous macules and papules. Initial discrete lesions may become confluent, especially on face (Fig. 23-13), neck, and shoulders. Lesions gradually fade in order of appearance with subsequent residual yellow-tan stain or faint desquamation. Exanthem resolves in 4 to 6 days. Periorbital edema in prodrome. Appear on forehead at hairline, behind ears; spread centrifugally and inferiorly to involve the face, trunk (Fig. 23-13), and extremities, reaching the feet by third day.

Mucous Membranes (Enanthem) Koplik's spots: cluster of tiny bluish-white papules with an erythematous areola, appearing on or after second day of febrile illness, on buccal mucosa opposite premolar teeth. Bulbar conjunctivae: conjunctivitis.

General Examination Generalized lymphadenopathy common. Otherwise unremarkable.

Variants

Modified Measles Milder clinical findings.

Atypical Measles Occurs in individuals immunized with formalin-inactivated measles vaccine, subsequently exposed to measles virus. Exanthem begins peripherally and moves centrally; can be urticarial, maculopapular, hemorrhagic, and/or vesicular. Systemic symptoms can be severe.

Measles in Compromised Host Rash may not occur. Pneumonitis, encephalitis more common.

DIFFERENTIAL DIAGNOSIS

Disseminated Maculopapular Eruption Drug eruption, other viral exanthems (e.g., rubella), secondary syphilis, scarlet fever.

LABORATORY EXAMINATIONS

Cultures Isolate virus from blood, urine, pharyngeal secretions.

Serology Demonstrates fourfold or greater rise in measles titer.

PCR Detects genomic sequences of measles virus DNA in serum, throat swabs, and CSF.

DIAGNOSIS

Clinical diagnosis, at times, confirmed by serology.

COURSE AND PROGNOSIS

Self-limited infection in most patients. Mortality rate: in the United States, .3%; in develop-ing countries, 1 to 10%. Complications more common in malnourished children, the unimmunized, and those with congenital immunodeficiency, and leukemia. Acute complications (9.8% of cases): otitis media, pneumonia (bacterial or measles), diarrhea, measles encephalitis (1 in 800 to 1000 cases), thrombocytopenia. In unimmunized HIV-infected children, fatal measles pneumonia has occurred without rash. Chronic complication: subacute sclerosing panencephalitis.

MANAGEMENT

Prevention Prophylactic immunization. The goal of eliminating indigenous measles transmission in the United States is based on four components: (1) maintaining high coverage with a single dose of measles-mumps-rubella vaccine (MMR) among preschool-aged children, (2) achieving coverage with two doses of MMR for all school and college attendees, (3) enhancing surveillance and outbreak response, and (4) increasing efforts to develop and implement strategies for global measles elimination.

Acute Infection Symptomatic.

Secondary Bacterial Infections Administration of appropriate antibiotics.

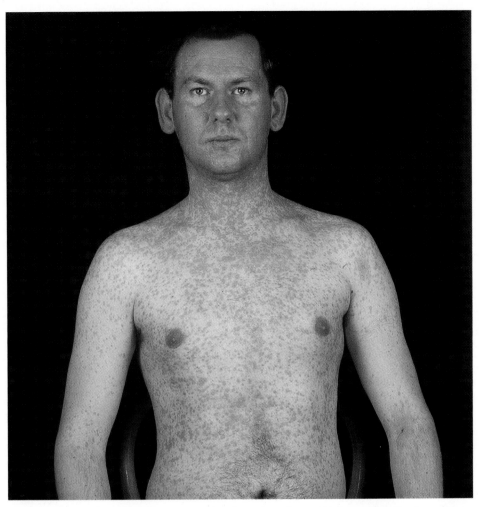

Figure 23-13 Measles *Erythematous papules, first appearing on the face and neck where they become confluent, spreading to the trunk and arms in 2 to 3 days where they remain discrete. In contrast, rubella also first appears initially on the face but spreads to the trunk in 1 day. Koplik's spot on the buccal mucosa were also present.*

Hand-Foot-and-Mouth Disease

Hand-foot-and-mouth disease (HFMD) is a systemic infection caused by coxsackievirus A16, characterized by ulcerative oral lesions and a vesicular exanthem on the distal extremities in association with mild constitutional symptoms.

EPIDEMIOLOGY

Age of Onset Most commonly children younger than 10 years of age, but also young and middle-aged adults.

Etiology Coxsackievirus A16. Sporadic cases have been reported with coxsackieviruses A4–7, A9, A10, B2, and B5 and enterovirus 71.

Season Epidemic outbreaks every 3 years. In temperate climates, outbreaks during warmer months.

Transmission Highly contagious, spread from person to person by oral-oral and fecal-oral routes.

PATHOGENESIS

Enteroviral implantation in the GI tract (buccal mucosa and ileum) leads to extension into regional lymph nodes, and 72 h later a viremia occurs with seeding of the oral mucosa and skin of the hands and feet.

HISTORY

Incubation Period 3 to 6 days.

Prodrome 12 to 24 h of low-grade fever, malaise, and abdominal pain or respiratory symptoms.

Symptoms Frequently 5 to 10 *painful* ulcerative oral lesions, leading to refusal to eat in children. Few to 100 cutaneous lesions appear together or shortly after the oral lesions and may be asymptomatic or *tender* and *painful.*

PHYSICAL EXAMINATION

Skin Lesions Lesions begin as 2- to 8-mm *macules* or *papules* that quickly evolve to *vesicles* (Fig. 23-14). Lesions on palms and soles usually do not rupture (Fig. 23-15). At other cutaneous sites, vesicles can rupture, with formation of *erosions* and *crusts.* Lesions heal without scarring. Early papules, pink to red. Vesicles have clear fluid with a watery appearance or yellowish hue. Cutaneous lesions have a characteristic "linear" shape on the palms and soles. Characteristically, lesions arise on palms and soles, especially on sides of fingers, toes, and buttocks.

Mucosal Lesions 5- to 10-mm, small, punched-out painful ulcers preceded by macules→grayish vesicles, arising on the hard palate, tongue, buccal mucosa.

General Findings Typically, HFMD is accompanied by low-grade fever, malaise, and a sore mouth. In some patients, it may be associated with high fever, severe malaise, diarrhea, and joint pains. Enterovirus 71 infections may have associated CNS and lung involvement.

DIFFERENTIAL DIAGNOSIS

A sudden outbreak of oral and distal extremity lesions is pathognomonic for HFMD. However, if only the oral lesions are present, the differential diagnosis would include herpes simplex virus infection, aphthous stomatitis, herpangina, erythema multiforme major.

LABORATORY EXAMINATIONS

Histopathology Epidermal reticular degeneration leads to an intraepidermal vesicle filled with neutrophils, mononuclear cells, and proteinaceous eosinophilic material. The dermis reveals a perivascular mixed cell infiltrate.

Electron Microscopy Intracytoplasmic particles in crystalline array characteristic of coxsackie viral infections.

Serology In acute serum, neutralizing antibodies may be detected but disappear rapidly. In convalescent serum, elevated titers of complement-fixing antibodies are found.

Tzanck Preparation Negative for both multinucleated giant cells and inclusion bodies.

Viral Culture Virus may be isolated from vesicles, throat washings, and stool specimens.

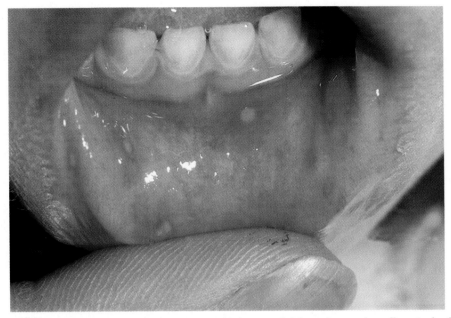

Figure 23-14 Hand-foot-and-mouth disease   *Multiple, superficial erosions and small, vesicular lesions surrounded by an erythematous halo on the lower labial mucosa; the gingiva is normal. In primary herpetic gingivostomatitis, which presents with similar oral vesicular lesions, a painful gingivitis usually occurs as well.*

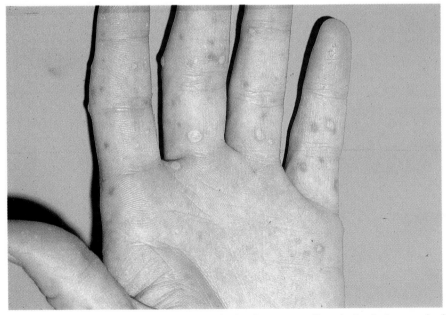

Figure 23-15 Hand-foot-and-mouth disease   *Multiple, discrete, small, vesicular lesions on the fingers and palms; similar lesions were also present on the feet. Some vesicles are typically linear.*

DIAGNOSIS

Usually made on clinical findings.

COURSE AND PROGNOSIS

Most commonly, HFMD is self-limited; and a rise in serum antibodies eliminates the viremia in 7 to 10 days. A few cases have been more prolonged or recurrent. Serious sequelae rarely occur, however, coxsackievirus has been implicated in cases of myocarditis, meningoencephalitis, aseptic meningitis, paralytic disease, and a systemic illness resembling rubeola. Enterovirus 71 infections have higher morbidity/mortality rates due to CNS involvement and pulmonary edema. Infection acquired during the first trimester of pregnancy may result in spontaneous abortion.

MANAGEMENT

Symptomatic treatment, including topical application of dyclonine HCl solution or lidocaine gel, may reduce oral discomfort.

Erythema Infectiosum

Erythema infectiosum (EI) is a childhood exanthem occurring with primary parvovirus B19 infection, characterized by edematous erythematous plaques on the cheeks ("slapped cheeks") and an erythematous lacy eruption on the trunk and extremities.
Synonym: Fifth disease.

EPIDEMIOLOGY

Age of Onset   All ages, but more common in young. Up to 60% of adolescents and adults are seropositive for anti-HPV B19 IgG. Symptomatic rheumatic involvement is more common in adults.

Sex   Symptomatic illness with arthralgias more common in adult women.

Etiology   Parvovirus, a small single-stranded DNA virus. Human infection caused by B19 (HPV B19) species.

Season   Occurs year-round; common as outbreaks in schools in late winter, early spring.

Transmission   Virus present in respiratory tract during the viremic stage of HPV B19 infection and spreads via droplet aerosol. Secondary attack rate among close contacts 50%.

PATHOGENESIS

Viremia develops 6 days after intranasal inoculation of B19 into volunteers who lack serum antibodies to the virus. Nonspecific symptoms occur during this time. IgM and then IgG antibodies develop after a week and clear viremia. Significant bone marrow depression can occur at this time. The exanthem begins 17 to 18 days after inoculation and may be accompanied by arthralgia and/or arthritis; these findings are mediated by immune complexes. In compromised hosts, B19 can destroy erythroid precursor cells, causing severe aplastic crisis in adults and hydrops fetalis in the fetus.

HISTORY

Incubation   Period 4 to 14 days.

Contacts   Exposure to classmates or siblings with EI.

Symptoms   20 to 60% of individuals are symptomatic; remainder asymptomatic.

Children   Prodrome of fever, malaise, headache, coryza 2 days before rash. Headache, sore throat, fever, myalgias, nausea, diarrhea, conjunctivitis, cough may coincide with rash. Uncommonly arthralgias. Pruritus is variably present.

Adults   Constitutional symptoms more severe, with fever, adenopathy, arthritis/arthralgias involving small joints of hand, knees, wrists, ankles, feet. Numbness and tingling of fingers. Pruritus±rash. Rash usually absent in adults.

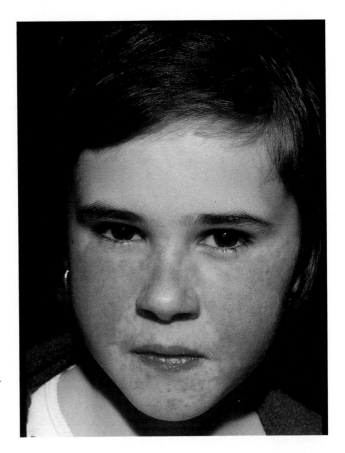

Figure 23-16 Erythema infectiosum *Diffuse erythema and edema of the cheeks with "slapped cheek" facies in a child.*

PHYSICAL EXAMINATION

Skin Lesions Edematous, confluent plaques on malar face ("slapped cheeks") (Fig. 23-16). Nonfacial lesions: erythematous macules and papules that become confluent, giving a lacy or reticulated appearance (Fig. 23-17). Less commonly, morbilliform, confluent, circinate, annular. Rarely, purpura, vesicles, pustules, palmoplantar desquamation. Face: erythematous plaques giving a "slapped cheeks" appearance. Extensor surface of extremities, trunk, neck: confluent macules/papules creating reticulated erythema. In adults with rash, "slapped cheeks" usually absent, reticulated macules on extremities.

Mucosal Lesions Uncommonly, enanthem with glossal and pharyngeal erythema; red macules on buccal and palatal mucosa.

General Findings Acute arthritis; symmetric, peripheral.

DIFFERENTIAL DIAGNOSIS

Children with Erythema Infectiosum Childhood exanthems—rubella, measles, scarlet fever, erythema subitum, enteroviral infection, *Haemophilus influenzae* cellulitis, adverse cutaneous drug reaction.

Adults with Arthritis Lyme arthritis, rheumatoid arthritis, rubella.

LABORATORY EXAMINATIONS

Serology Demonstration of IgM anti-HPV B19 antibodies or IgG seroconversion. Demonstration of HPV B19 in serum.

Electron Microscopy Infected erythroid precursor cells show parvovirus-like particles.

Hematology During aplastic crisis: absence of reticulocytes, falling hemoglobin, hypoplasia or aplasia of erythroid series in bone marrow.

DIAGNOSIS

Usually made on clinical findings.

COURSE AND PROGNOSIS

Erythema Infectiosum "Slapped cheeks" are noted first. As these lesions fade over 1 to 4 days, reticulated rash appears on the trunk, neck, and extensor extremities. Eruption lasts 5 to 9 days but characteristically can recur for weeks or months, triggered by sunlight exposure, exercise, temperature change, bathing, emotional stress.

Arthralgias Self-limited, lasting 3 weeks; but may persist for several months or years.

Aplastic Crisis In patients with chronic hemolytic anemias (sickle cell anemia, hereditary spherocytosis, heterozygous β-thalassemia, pyruvate kinase deficiency, autoimmune hemolytic anemia), transient aplastic crisis may occur, manifested by fatigue, pallor, worsening anemia.

Fetal B19 Infection Intrauterine infection may be complicated by nonimmune fetal hydrops secondary to infection of erythroid precursors, hemolysis, severe anemia, tissue anoxia, high-output heart failure. Risk <10% after maternal infection.

MANAGEMENT

Symptomatic.

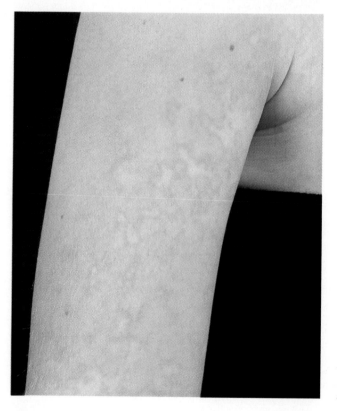

Figure 23-17 Erythema infectiosum *Discrete, erythematous macules with ring formation on the upper arm.*

VIRAL INFECTIONS OF SKIN AND MUCOSA

HUMAN HERPESVIRUSES

Human herpesviruses (HHV) (family Herpesviridae) are defined by the architecture of the virion, which has a core containing a linear double-stranded DNA and an icosahedral capsid 100 to 110 nm in diameter composed of 162 capsomers with an envelope containing viral glycoprotein spikes on the surface. Eight HHV have been identified: herpes simplex virus (HSV)-1 (HHV-1), HSV-2 (HHV-2), varicella-zoster virus (VZV or HHV-3), Epstein-Barr virus (EBV or HHV-4), cytomegalovirus (CMV or HHV-5), HHV-6, HHV-7, HHV-8 (Kaposi's sarcoma-associated virus). Primary HHV infections are usually asymptomatic with the exception of VZV, which nearly always presents with symptomatic varicella. After primary infection, HHV remain latent in neural or lymphoid cells and reactivate if an adequate immune response does not exist.

HHV are categorized into three groups: alpha-, beta-, and gammaherpesvirinae (Table 23-2). *Alphaherpesvirinae* [HSV-1, HSV-2, VZV (HHV-3)] are characterized by a variable host range, relatively short reproductive cycle, rapid spread in culture, rapid destruction of infected cells, and latent infection primarily, but not exclusively, of sensory ganglia. *Betaherpesvirinae* [CMV (HHV-5)] have a restricted host range and spread slowly in cultures. *Gammaherpesvirinae* [EBV (HHV-4), HHV-6, HHV-7, HHV-8, and herpesvirus saimiri] are lymphotropic, specific for either T or B lymphocytes. The HHV-8 DNA sequences are closely homologous to minor capsid and tegument protein genes of gammaherpesvirinae EBV and herpesvirus saimiri.

Herpes Simplex Virus Infection

Herpes simplex virus (HSV) infection, whether primary or recurrent, may "typically" present clinically with grouped vesicles arising on an erythematous base on keratinized skin or mucous membrane. Many HSV infections are "atypical," with patch(es) of erythema, small erosions, fissures, or subclinical lesions that shed HSV. Once an individual is infected, HSV persists in sensory ganglia for the life of the patient, recurring with lessening in immunity. In healthy individuals, recurrent infections are asymptomatic or minor, resolving spontaneously or with antiviral therapy. In the immunocompromised host, mucocutaneous lesions can be extensive, chronic, or disseminate to skin or viscera.

Synonyms: Herpes, herpes simplex, cold sore, fever blister, herpes febrilis, herpes labialis, herpes gladiatorum, scrum pox, herpetic whitlow, genital herpes progenitalis.

EPIDEMIOLOGY

Age of Onset Most commonly young adults; range, infancy to senescence.

Etiology Labialis: HSV-1 (80 to 90%), HSV-2 (10 to 20%). Urogenital: HSV-2 (70 to 90%), HSV-1 (10 to 30%). Herpetic whitlow in patients younger than 20 years of age usually HSV-1; older than 20 years of age, usually HSV-2. Neonatal: HSV-2 (70%), HSV-1 (30%).

Transmission Usually skin-skin, skin-mucosa, mucosa-skin contact. Herpes gladiatorum transmitted by skin-to-skin contact in wrestlers. Increased HSV-1 transmission associated with crowded living conditions and lower socioeconomic status.

Precipitating Factors for Recurrence Approximately one-third of persons who develop herpes labialis will experience a recurrence; of these, one-half will experience at least two recurrences annually. Usual factors for herpes

Table 23-2 HUMAN HERPESVIRUSES AND ASSOCIATED DISEASES IN IMMUNOCOMPETENT AND IMMUNOCOMPROMISED INDIVIDUALS

Human Herpes-Virus	Disease in Immunocompetent Individuals	Disease in Immunocompromised Individuals	Management
Herpes simplex virus-1 (HSV-1) (HHV-1)	Primary infection often asymptomatic Primary herpetic gingivostomatitis Herpes labialis Herpetic whitlow Aseptic meningitis HSV encephalitis	Widespread local infection Chronic ulcers Disseminated cutaneous infection Disseminated visceral infection	Immunization: vaccine promising Antiviral agents Acyclovir Valacyclovir Famciclovir Foscarnet
Herpes simplex virus-2 (HSV-2) (HHV-2)	Primary infection often asymptomatic Herpes genitalis, primary and recurrent Herpetic whitlow Aseptic meningitis	Widespread local infection Chronic ulcers Disseminated cutaneous infection Disseminated visceral infection	Immunization: vaccine promising Antiviral agents Acyclovir Valacyclovir Famciclovir Foscarnet
Varicella-zoster virus (VZV) (HHV-3)	Primary infection nearly always symptomatic Varicella (primary infection) herpes zoster	Disseminated cutaneous infection Disseminated visceral infection Chronic herpes zoster Chronic ecthymatous VZV infection	Immunization: vaccine available Antiviral agents Acyclovir Valacyclovir Famciclovir Foscarnet
Cytomegalovirus (CMV) (HHV-5)	Primary infection often asymptomatic CMV mononucleosis (primary CMV infection)	Retinitis Pneumonitis Colitis	Immunization: vaccine promising Antiviral agents Ganciclovir Foscarnet Cidofovir
Epstein-Barr virus (EBV) (HHV-4)	Primary infection often asymptomatic EBV mononucleosis (primary EBV infection) Nasopharyngeal carcinoma Burkitt's lymphoma, nasal T cell lymphoma, and other lymphomas	Oral hairy leukoplakia Lymphoma	Immunization: none Antiviral agents Acyclovir Ganciclovir
Human herpesvirus-6 (HHV-6)	Primary infection often asymptomatic Exanthem subitum	???	???
Human herpesvirus-7 (HHV-7)	Primary infection often asymptomatic Exanthem subitum	???	???
Human herpesvirus-8 (HHV-8)	Symptoms, if any, of primary infection unknown Kaposi's sarcoma	Kaposi's sarcoma Body cavity–lymphoma in HIV-infected individuals	???

labialis: skin/mucosal irritation (UV radiation), altered hormonal milieu (menstruation), fever, common cold, altered immune states, site of infection (genital herpes recurs more frequently than labial).

Immunocompromising Factors Predisposing to HSV Reactivation HIV infection, malignancy (leukemia/lymphoma), transplantation (bone marrow, solid organ), chemotherapy, systemic glucocorticoids and other immunosuppressive drugs, radiotherapy.

PATHOGENESIS

Primary HSV infection occurs through close contact with a person shedding virus at a peripheral site, mucosal surface, or secretion. HSV is inactivated promptly at room temperature; aerosol or fomitic spread unlikely. Infection occurs via inoculation onto susceptible mucosal surface or break in skin. After exposure of skin sites to HSV, the virus replicates in parabasal and intermediate epithelial cells, causing lysis of infected cells, vesicle formation, and local inflammation. After primary infection at inoculation site, HSV ascends peripheral sensory nerves and enters sensory (trigeminal or sacral) or autonomic nerve root ganglia (vagal), where latency is established. Latency can occur after both symptomatic and asymptomatic primary infection. Recurrences result from viral reactivation and synthesis and migration of virus through sensory nerves. Usually occur in the vicinity of the primary infection, may be clinically symptomatic or asymptomatic.

CLINICAL MANIFESTATIONS

Classification of Mucocutaneous HSV Infections

Primary infection
  Primary herpetic gingivostomatitis
  Primary genital herpes
  Primary infection at other inoculation sites
  Neonatal HSV infection
  Widespread cutaneous herpes associated with cutaneous immunocompromise
  Primary herpes in systemically immunocompromised host
Recurrent infection
  First symptomatic infection
  Herpes labialis
  Herpes genitalis

Recurrent herpes at other sites
  Recurrent widespread cutaneous herpes associated with cutaneous immunocompromise
  Recurrent herpes in systemically immunocompromised host
  Chronic herpetic ulcers
Disseminated HSV infection
  Disseminated cutaneous HSV infection
  Disseminated visceral HSV infection, ± cutaneous involvement

LABORATORY EXAMINATIONS

Direct Microscopy *Tzanck Smear* (Fig. 23-18). Optimally, fluid from intact vesicle is smeared thinly on a microscope slide, dried, and stained with either Wright's or Giemsa's stain. Positive, if acantholytic keratinocytes or multinucleated giant acantholytic keratinocytes are detected (Fig. 23-18). Positive in 75% of early cases, either primary or recurrent.

Antigen Detection Monoclonal antibodies, specific for HSV-1 and HSV-2 antigens, detect and differentiate HSV antigens on smear from lesion.

Dermatopathology Ballooning and reticular epidermal degeneration, acantholysis, and intraepidermal vesicles; intranuclear inclusion bodies, multinucleate giant keratinocytes; multilocular vesicles. Immunoperoxidase techniques can be used to identify HSV-1 and HSV-2 antigens in formalin-fixed tissue samples.

Cultures Positive HSV cultures from involved mucocutaneous site or tissue biopsy specimens.

Serology Primary HSV infection can be documented by demonstration of seroconversion. Recurring herpes can be ruled out if seronegative for HSV antibodies. Detection of type-specific antibodies to HSV-1 and HSV-2 detected by Western blot testing is the best serologic method to determine HSV infection.

Polymerase Chain Reaction (PCR) To determine HSV-DNA sequences in tissue, smears, or secretion.

DIAGNOSIS

Clinical suspicion confirmed by viral culture or antigen detection.

MANAGEMENT

Prevention   Skin-to-skin contact should be avoided during outbreak of
                                              cutaneous HSV infection.

Topical Antiviral Therapy   Approved for herpes labialis; minimal efficacy.

Acyclovir 5% ointment   Apply q3h, 6 times daily for 7 days. Approved for initial genital
                                              herpes and limited mucocutaneous HSV infections in
                                              immunocompromised individuals.

Penciclovir 1% Cream   Apply q2h while awake for recurrent orolabial infection in
                                              immunocompetent individuals.

Oral Antiviral Therapy   Currently, anti-HSV agents are approved for use in genital herpes
                                              Presumably, similar dosing regimens are effective for nongenital
                                              infections. Drug for oral HSV therapy include acyclovir,
                                              valacyclovir, and famciclovir. Valacyclovir, the prodrug of
                                              acyclovir, has a better bioavailability and is nearly 85%
                                              absorbed after oral administration. Famciclovir is equally
                                              effective for cutaneous HSV infections.

First episode   Antiviral agents more effective in treating primary infections
                                              than recurrences.

Acyclovir   400 mg tid or 200 mg 5 times daily for 7–10 days
Valacyclovir   1 g bid for 7–10 days
Famciclovir   250 mg tid for 5–10 days

Recurrences   Most episodes of recurrent herpes do not benefit from pulse
                                              therapy with oral acyclovir. In severe recurrent disease, patients
                                              who start therapy at the beginning of the prodrome or within 2
                                              days after onset of lesions may benefit from therapy by
                                              shortening and reducing severity of eruption; however,
                                              recurrences cannot be prevented.

Acyclovir   400 mg PO tid for 5 days *or*
                                              800 mg PO bid for 5 days
Valacyclovir   500 mg bid for 5 days *or*
                                              2 g bid for day 1, then 1 g bid on day 2
Famciclovir   125 mg bid for 5 days

Chronic suppression   Decreases frequency of symptomatic recurrences and
                                              asymptomatic HSV shedding. After 1 year of continuous daily
                                              suppressive therapy, acyclovir should be discontinued to
                                              determine the recurrence rate.

Acyclovir   400 mg bid
Valacyclovir   500–1000 mg qd
Famciclovir   250 mg bid

Mucocutaneous disease in   Neither the need for nor the proper increased dosage of acyclovir
Immunocompromised individuals   has been established conclusively. Patients with herpes who do
                                              not respond to the recommended dose of acyclovir may require
                                              a higher oral dose of acyclovir, IV acyclovir, or be infected with
                                              an acyclovir-resistant HSV strain, requiring IV foscarnet. The
                                              roles of valacyclovir and famciclovir are not yet established.

Acyclovir   5 mg/kg IV q8h for 7–14 days *or* 400 mg 5 times daily: for
                                              7–14 days

Oral valacyclovir *or* famciclovir   Reduces the necessity for IV acyclovir therapy.
Neonatal
Acyclovir   20 mg/kg IV q8h for 14–21 days

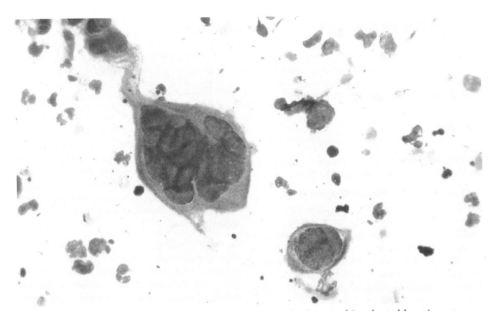

Figure 23-18   Herpes simplex virus: positive Tzanck smear   *A giant, multinucleated keratinocyte on a Giemsa-stained smear obtained from a vesicle base. Compare size of the giant cell to that of neutrophils also seen in this smear. Another smaller multinucleated acantholytic keratinocyte is seen as well as acantholytic keratinocytes. Identical findings are present in lesions caused by varicella-zoster virus.*

Acyclovir-Resistance	Extremely rare in immunocompetent host. Usually occurs in immunocompromised individuals with large herpetic lesions with high HSV viral load. Resistant HSV strains are thymidine-kinase deficient. Alternative drugs: foscarnet, cidofovir. In HIV-infected patients, chronic HSV infections are mucocutaneous, rarely invasive.
Foscarnet	40 mg/kg IV q8h for 14–21 days
Imiquimod Cream	May be effective.
HIV Infections	Lesions caused by HSV are relatively common among HIV infected persons. For severe disease, IV acyclovir therapy may be required. If lesions persist among patients undergoing acyclovir treatment, resistance to acyclovir should be suspected.
Acyclovir	Intermittent or suppressive therapy with oral acyclovir may be needed. 400 mg PO 3–5 times daily may be useful. Therapy should continue until clinical resolution is attained.
Foscarnet	For severe disease caused by proven or suspected acyclovir-resistant strains, hospitalization should be considered. Foscarnet, 40 mg/kg body weight q8h until clinical resolution is attained. Appears to be the best available treatment.

Nongenital Herpes Simplex Virus Infection

Nongenital HSV infection, whether primary or recurrent, is often asymptomatic. Lesions may present as group vesicles on an erythematous base, or as a recurrent erythematous plaque ±erosions. *Synonyms:* Herpes, herpes simplex, cold sore, fever blister, herpes febrilis, herpes labialis, herpes gladiatorum, scrum pox, herpetic whitlow.

HISTORY

Incubation Period 2- to 20-day (average 6) incubation period for primary infection.

Systems Review *Primary Herpes* Many individuals with primary HSV infection are either asymptomatic or have only trivial symptoms. Symptomatic primary herpes, which is uncommon, is characterized by vesicles at the site of inoculation associated with regional lymphadenopathy, at times accompanied by fever, headache, malaise, myalgia, peaking within the first 3 to 4 days after onset of lesions, resolving during the subsequent 3 to 4 days. Primary herpetic gingivostomatitis is the most common symptom complex accompanying primary HSV infection in children, in young women, primary herpetic vulvovaginitis, (See also Section 25).

Recurrent Herpes Prodrome of tingling, itching, or burning sensation usually precedes any visible skin changes by 24 h. Systemic symptoms are usually absent.

PHYSICAL EXAMINATION

Primary Herpes *Skin Findings* Erythemas are often noted initially, followed soon by grouped, often umbilicated vesicles, which may evolve to pustules (Fig. 23-19); these become eroded as the overlying epidermis sloughs. Erosions may enlarge to ulcerations, which may be crusted or moist. These epithelial defects heal in 2 to 4 weeks, often with resultant postinflammatory hypo- or hyperpigmentation, uncommonly with scarring. The area of involvement may be circumferential around the mouth. Location: oropharyngeal, labial, perioral; distal fingers; other sites.

Mucous Membranes Oral mucosa usually involved only in primary HSV infection with vesicles that quickly slough to form erosions (Fig. 23-19) at any site in the oropharynx, scanty to numerous; gingivitis with gingival tenderness, edema, violaceous color. Sialorrhea. Documented recurrent intraoral HSV is uncommon.

General Findings Fever is often present during symptomatic primary herpetic gingivostomatitis. Regional lymph nodes enlarged, firm, nonfluctuant, tender; usually unilateral. Signs of aseptic meningitis: headache, fever, nuchal rigidity, CSF pleocytosis with normal sugar content and positive HSV CSF culture.

Recurrent Herpes Lesions similar to primary infection but on a reduced scale. Often a 1- to 2-cm patch of erythema, ± vesicles (Fig. 23-20), ±erosions (Fig. 23-21). Heals in 1 to 2 weeks. May be associated with regional lymphadenitis. May occur at any mucocutaneous site. Most common sites are perioral, cheek, nose tip, distal finger (herpetic whitlow) (Fig. 23-22). Periocular localization requires examination of the cornea. Herpes gladiatorum occurs on the head, neck, or shoulder.

DIFFERENTIAL DIAGNOSIS

Primary Intraoral HSV Infection Aphthous stomatitis, hand-foot-and-mouth disease, herpangina, erythema multiforme.

Recurrent Lesion Fixed drug eruption.

LABORATORY EXAMINATIONS

See Herpes Simplex Virus Infection, page 784.

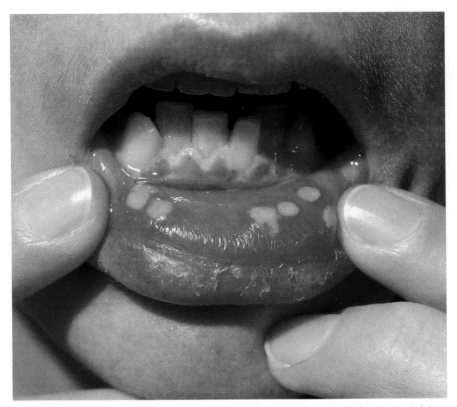

Figure 23-19   Herpes simplex virus infection: primary gingivostomatitis *Multiple, very painful erosions on the lower labial mucosa with erythema and edema of the gingiva; fibrin deposits on teeth and gingiva. Fever and tender submandibular lymphadenopathy were also present.*

DIAGNOSIS

Clinical suspicion confirmed by Tzanck smear, viral culture, or antigen detection.

COURSE AND PROGNOSIS

Recurrences of HSV tend to become less frequent with the passage of time. Eczema herpeticum (See also Widespread Cutaneous Infection Associated with Cutaneous Immunocompromise, page 791) may complicate atopic dermatitis (eczema herpeticum), keratosis follicularis (Darier's disease), and second- and third-degree thermal burns. Patients with immunodeficiency may experience cutaneous and systemic dissemination of HSV and chronic herpetic ulcers (See also Infections Associated with Systemic Immunocompromise, page 794). Erythema multiforme may complicate herpes, occurring 1 to 2 weeks after an outbreak.

MANAGEMENT

See Herpes Simplex Virus Infection, page 784.

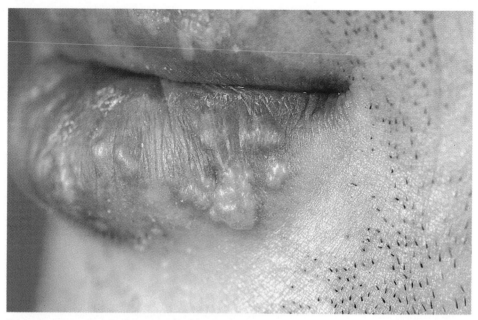

Figure 23-20   Herpes simplex virus infection: recurrent herpes labialis   *Grouped and confluent vesicles with an erythematous rim on the lips, 24 h after onset of symptoms.*

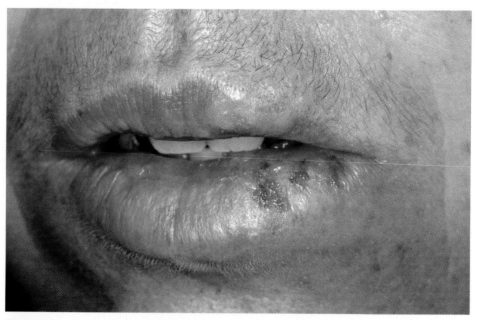

Figure 23-21   Herpes simplex virus infection: recurrent herpes labialis   *Edema with crusting of the lips that followed sun exposure, 48 to 72 h after onset of symptoms; vesiculation is present but difficult to detect because of confluence of lesions. In some cases, crusting is the only finding.*

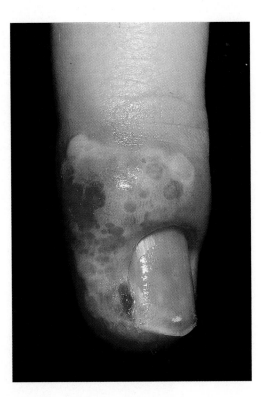

Figure 23-22   Herpes simplex virus infection: herpetic whitlow   *Painful, grouped, confluent vesicles on an erythematous edematous base on the distal finger were the first (and presumed primary) symptomatic infection.*

Neonatal Herpes Simplex Virus Infection

Neonates may be infected during delivery or in the perinatal period, usually from the mother, but also from individuals around the infant after birthing. The majority of infections are caused by HSV-2; HSV-1 is more virulent in the newborn and associated with higher morbidity and mortality rates. 70% of infants with neonatal HSV infection are born to mothers with asymptomatic genital herpes; 70% of cases occur in the first-born child. Eruption occurs on the mucous membranes (Fig. 23-23) or on the intact skin at inoculation sites (such as monitoring sensors) (Fig. 23-24). Disseminated HSV infection in neonates is difficult to diagnose in that up to 70% of infants have no mucocutaneous lesions. IV acyclovir therapy is mandatory in these cases.

MANAGEMENT

Prophylaxis   Many experts recommend sero-testing for HSV-1 and HSV-2 (Western blot) at the first prenatal visit. Infants born to women who asymptomatically shed HSV have reduced birth weight and increased prematurity. Acyclovir suppressive therapy at the end of pregnancy probably (but not documented) reduces the risk of transmission to the neonate.

Pregnancy   The safety of systemic acyclovir for pregnant women and the fetus has not yet been established, although acyclovir appears to completely safe in last months of pregnancy. Acyclovir, valacyclovir, and famciclovir are active only in cells with active viral infection. If HSV is acquired late in pregnancy, cesarean section is indicated.

Perinatal Infections   Most mothers of infants who acquire neonatal herpes lack histories of clinically evident genital herpes. The risk for transmission to the neonate from an infected mother appears highest among women with first-episode genital herpes near the time of delivery and is low (<3%) among women with recurrent herpes. The results of viral cultures during pregnancy do not predict viral shedding at the time of delivery, and such cultures are not routinely indicated.

At the time of labor, all women should be questioned carefully about symptoms of genital herpes and should be examined. Women without symptoms or signs of genital herpes infection (or prodrome) may deliver babies vaginally.

Among women who have a history of genital herpes or who have a sex partner with genital herpes, cultures of the birth canal at delivery may aid in decisions relating to neonatal management.

Infants delivered through an infected birth canal (proven by virus isolation or presumed by observation of lesions) should be followed carefully, including virus cultures obtained 24 to 48 h after birth. Treatment should be reserved for infants who develop evidence of clinical disease and for those with positive postpartum cultures.

Antiviral Therapy   Acyclovir, 20 mg/kg IV q8h for 14 to 21 days.

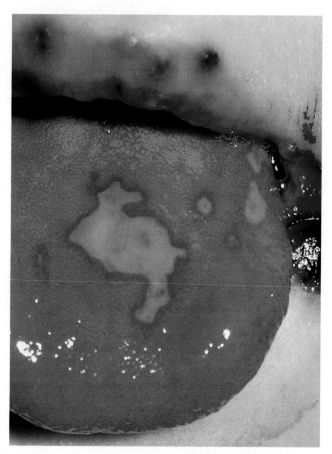

Figure 23-23   Herpes simplex virus infection: neonatal   *Vesicles and crusted erosions on the upper lip and large geographic ulcerations of the tongue were the clinical findings in this neonate with herpetic gingivostomatitis.*

VIRAL INFECTIONS OF SKIN AND MUCOSA

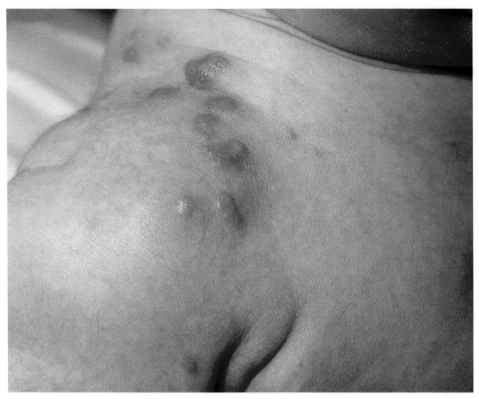

Figure 23-24   Herpes simplex virus infection: neonatal   *Grouped and confluent vesicles with underlying erythema and edema on the shoulder of a newborn infant, arising at the inoculation site.*

Herpes Simplex Virus: Widespread Cutaneous Infection Associated with Cutaneous Immunocompromise

Widespread HSV cutaneous infection in underlying dermatoses occurs most commonly in atopic dermatitis (eczema herpeticum) and is characterized by widespread vesicles and erosions; it may occur as a primary or recurrent infection.
Synonym: Kaposi's varicelliform eruption.

EPIDEMIOLOGY

Age of Onset   Children>adults.

Etiology   HSV-1>HSV-2.

Transmission   Commonly from parental herpes labialis.

Risk Factors   Most commonly, atopic dermatitis; more serious infections occur in erythrodermic atopic dermatitis. Also, Darier's disease, thermal burns, pemphigus vulgaris, bullous pemphigoid, ichthyosis vulgaris, cutaneous T cell lymphoma (mycosis fungoides), Wiscott-Aldrich syndrome.

PATHOGENESIS

See Herpes Simplex Virus Infection, page 784.

HISTORY

Primary eczema herpeticum often associated with fever, malaise, irritability. When recurrent, history of prior similar lesions; systemic symptoms less severe. Primary skin disease may be pruritic; onset of eczema herpeticum associated with pain and tenderness. Lesions begin in abnormal skin and may extend peripherally for several weeks during the primary infection or secondary eruption.

PHYSICAL EXAMINATION

Skin Lesions   Umbilicated vesicles evolving into "punched-out" erosions (Fig. 23-25). Vesicles are first confined to eczematous skin and are, in contrast to primary or recurrent HSV eruptions, not grouped but disseminated. Common sites: face, neck, trunk. May later spread to normal-appearing skin. Erosions may become confluent, producing large denuded areas (Fig. 23-25). Larger crusted lesions and follicular pustules occur with staphylococcal superinfection. Successive crops of new vesiculation may occur.

General Examination   Primary infection may be associated with fever and lymphadenopathy.

DIFFERENTIAL DIAGNOSIS

Widespread Vesiculopustules/Erosions   Varicella zoster virus (VZV) infection with dissemination, disseminated (systemic) HSV infection, widespread bullous impetigo, staphylococcal folliculitis, pseudomonal ("hot tub") folliculitis,

Candida folliculitis, Kaposi's varicelliform eruption caused by vaccinia virus.

LABORATORY EXAMINATIONS

See Herpes Simplex Virus Infection, page 784.

DIAGNOSIS

Clinical, confirmed by detection of HSV on culture or antigen detection.

COURSE AND PROGNOSIS

Primary episode of eczema herpeticum runs course with resolution in 2 to 6 weeks. Recurrent episodes tend to be milder and not associated with systemic symptoms. Systemic dissemination can occur, especially in immunocompromised patients; reported mortality rates range from 10 to 50%. Widely distributed cutaneous HSV infection in burn patients can be difficult to detect clinically.

MANAGEMENT

Management of Underlying Dermatosis   For atopic dermatitis, see Eczema/Dermatitis, Section 2.

Antiviral Therapy   See Herpes Simplex Virus Infection, page 784.

Antibacterial Therapy   Treat associated bacterial infection. See Bacterial Infections Involving the Skin, Section 20.

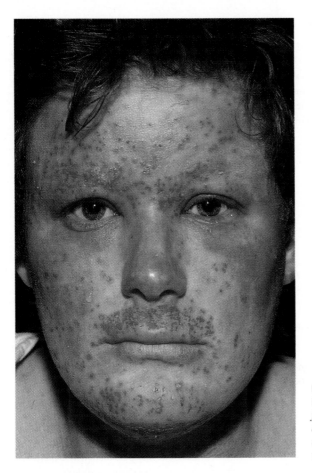

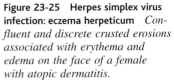

Figure 23-25   Herpes simplex virus infection: eczema herpeticum   *Confluent and discrete crusted erosions associated with erythema and edema on the face of a female with atopic dermatitis.*

Herpes Simplex Virus: Infections Associated with Systemic Immunocompromise

In the immunocompromised host, HSV is capable of causing local infection, characterized by extensive local involvement (e.g., eczema herpeticum) or chronic herpetic ulcers, or widespread systemic infection, characterized by widespread mucocutaneous vesicles, pustules, erosions, and ulcerations, associated with signs of pneumonia, encephalitis, hepatitis, as well as involvement of other organ systems, usually occurring in an immunocompromised host. (See also Nongenital Herpes Simplex Virus Infection, above; Sexually Transmitted Diseases: Herpes Simplex Virus: Genital Infections.

EPIDEMIOLOGY

Age of Onset   Any age.

Etiology   HSV-1 and -2.

Incidence   Rising due to an increasing population of immunocompromised individuals: 80% in bone marrow transplant recipients, 65% in solid organ transplant recipients, 60% of those with lymphoma and 55% of those with leukemia, 25% in individuals with HIV disease. Incidence of symptomatic outbreaks has decreased markedly because of the primary prophylaxis of HSV-seropositive immuncompromised individuals with acyclovir.

Risk Factors   *Immunodeficiency: HIV Infection*   Frequency and duration increase sharply as CD4+ T cell count falls below 50/μL. In most HIV-infected individuals, frequency, duration, and severity of HSV outbreaks similar to those in immunocompetent individuals. Disseminated cutaneous and visceral HSV infections are less common than in other immunocompromised states. CDC Surveillance Case Definition for AIDS: HSV infection causing a mucocutaneous ulcer that persists longer than 1 month, or HSV infection causing bronchitis, pneumonitis, or esophagitis for any duration in a patient older than 1 month, is an AIDS-defining condition if the patient has no other cause of immunodeficiency and is without knowledge of HIV antibody status. In industrialized nations, immune stabilization or restoration with highly active antiretroviral therapy (HAART) has markedly reduced the incidence of serious HSV infections.

Leukemia/Lymphoma   HSV reactivation typically occurs during induction or reinduction within 20 days in HSV-seropositive individuals.

Bone Marrow Transplantation (BMT)   HSV reactivation occurs within the first 5 weeks after BMT (median, day 8 posttransplantation). Untreated, 3% of patients die from disseminated HSV infection.

Chemotherapy   For solid organ or BMT, congenital or acquired cellular immune defects. Cytotoxic cancer chemotherapy, glucocorticoid therapy.

Other   Autoimmune diseases, malnutrition; rarely, pregnancy. Radiotherapy. Instrumentation such as nasogastric tube in debilitated patient associated with HSV esophagitis.

PATHOGENESIS

60 to 80% of HSV-seropositive transplant recipients and patients undergoing chemotherapy for hematologic malignancies will experience reactivation of HSV. After viremia, disseminated cutaneous or visceral HSV infection may occur. Factors determining whether severe localized disease, cutaneous dissemination, or visceral dissemination will occur are not well defined.

HISTORY

General   Patients often hospitalized with underlying condition or disease.

Skin Symptoms   Tender and painful mucocutaneous ulcers.

Recurrent Herpetic Lesion   Mild pain in ulcers.

Chronic Herpetic Ulcers   Mild to moderate pain (Fig. 23-27).

Herpetic Whitlow   Severe pain.

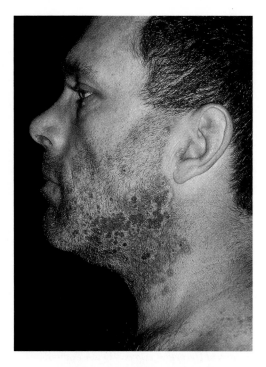

Figure 23-26 Herpes simplex virus infection: primary infection in HIV disease *Confluent vesicles and erosions with underlying erythema and edema (5 to 6 days' duration) in the beard area of a 35-year-old HIV-infected male (CD4 cell count, 400/mL). Gingivostomatitis and acute lymphadenopathy were also present, with onset 5 days after orogenital sex.*

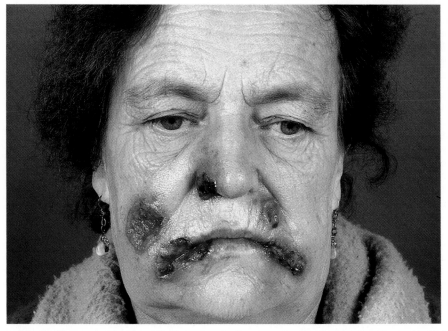

Figure 23-27 Herpes simplex virus infection: chronic ulcer in an immunocompromised host *Multiple, slowly spreading, deep ulcers with central necrosis and hemorrhagic crusts on the lips, cheeks, and nose of a female with leukemia.*

Oropharyngeal Ulcers   Oral pain on eating.

Esophageal Ulcers   Retrosternal pain and/or painful swallowing (odynophagia) and/or dysphagia.

Anorectal Ulcers   Perianal/anal ulcers are usually quite painful. Anorectal ulcers are associated with pain, constipation, pain on defecation, discharge, tenesmus, and at times, sacral radiculopathy, impotence, neurogenic bladder.

Mucocutaneous Dissemination   Fever.

Visceral Dissemination   Fever, deterioration of clinical status.

PHYSICAL EXAMINATION

Skin Lesions   *Primary infection*   Local infection may be widespread on the face (Fig. 23-26), oropharynx, anogenital region with initial vesiculation followed by crusted erosions. Without antiviral therapy, lesions may persist to become chronic herpetic ulcers.

Recurrent Herpetic Lesions   In most immunocompromised individuals, lesions appear as in the immunocompetent host. However, outbreaks may present with recurrent lesions (grouped crusts, erosions, ulcers) in a much larger area of involvement than usual. In HIV-infected individuals, large, necrotic, eroded lesions may appear over a period of a few days without apparent vesicle formation.

Chronic Herpetic Ulcers   Recurrent lesions enlarge over weeks to months, forming large ulcers, 10 to 20 cm in diameter (Fig. 23-27). Margins may be slightly rolled, hyperplastic. Coalescence of ulcerations may result in linear ulcers in intergluteal cleft or inguinal fold. Base of ulcer may be crusted or moist. Painful on palpation. Perianal and/or rectal > genital > orofacial > digital (Fig. 23-28A). Uncommonly, ulcer on face and perineum simultaneously.

Oropharyngeal Ulcers   Large ulcerations occur on the hard palate, often at the site of dental extraction. Linear ulcerations occur on the tongue (Fig. 23-28B).

Esophageal Ulcers   Usually associated with oropharyngeal herpetic ulcer and swallowing HSV-infected saliva. Esophagoscopy: mucosal erosions/ulceration.

Genital, Perineal, Perianal, Anorectal Ulcers   Acute ulceration of the vulva (Fig. 23-29), penis, scrotum, and/or perineum may become chronic ulcers unless effectively treated. In individuals infected with acyclovir-resistant HSV, ulcerations do not respond to usual antiviral therapies. Anal ulcers usually occur via enlargement of perianal ulcers. Herpetic proctitis: Sigmoidoscopy shows friable mucosa and ulcerations.

Mucocutaneous Dissemination   Disseminated (nongrouped) vesicles and pustules often hemorrhagic with inflammatory halo; quickly rupture, resulting in "punched-out" erosions. Lesions may be necrotic and then ulcerate (Fig. 23-30). Ulcers may become confluent with polycyclic well-demarcated borders; edges may be slightly raised, rolled.

Infarctive Skin Lesions   If complicated by purpura fulminans.

Mucous Membranes   Oropharyngeal erosion: necrotizing gingivitis, palatal ulcers, glossitis.

General Examination   Oropharyngeal infection can occur in the absence of external facial lesions. HSV esophagitis, tracheobronchitis, and focal pneumonitis can be local infection associated with spread by aspirated or swallowed secretions. Diffuse interstitial pneumonitis can be a manifestation of hematogenous infection. HSV pneumonitis often results from endogenous reactivation. Widespread visceral involvement (liver, lungs, adrenals, GI tract, CNS) can occur in immunocompromised individuals.

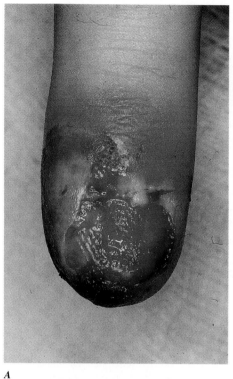

A

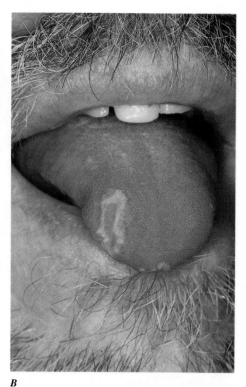

B

Figure 23-28   Herpes simplex virus infection: chronic ulcers in HIV disease   *The patient with advanced HIV disease presented to the surgical service with subacute ulceration of the distal finger **A**. He was treated with debridement and intravenous antibiotic. When seen by the dermatology service, chronic ulcers were also noted on the tongue **B**. and left nares. All lesions resolved with oral acyclovir with minimal scarring.*

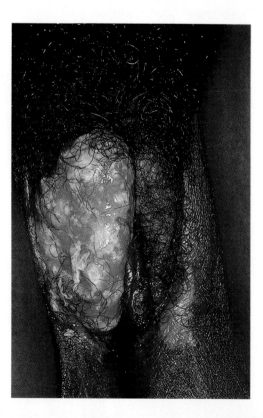

Figure 23-29   Herpes simplex virus infection: chronic ulcer in HIV disease   *The entire right labium majus is edematous and ulcerated; the lesion had been present for 6 months. CD4 cell count was 325/mL. The patient was noncompliant with her antiretroviral drug regimen. There was no response to any oral antiviral agent. The ulceration resolved in 6 weeks with 5% imiquimod cream applied three times weekly. Highly active antiretroviral therapy was reinstituted; the ulceration did not recur.*

Variations with Specific States of Immunocompromise

Leukemia/Lymphoma HSV infection is often atypical, with extensive lesions on lips or nasolabial skin; oropharyngeal infection manifested as necrotic gingival papillae, intraoral ulcerations that mimic thrush, or mucositis from chemotherapy or radiotherapy.

HIV Disease HSV reactivation is usually local, with chronic herpetic ulcers on the face or anogenital region. HSV esophagitis may coexist with candidal esophagitis. Persistent perianal herpes and herpetic proctitis. Disseminated visceral disease is uncommon.

DIFFERENTIAL DIAGNOSIS

Recurrent Herpetic Lesions Fixed drug eruption.

Chronic Herpetic Ulcers Chronic VZV infection, impetigo, ecthyma, ecthyma gangrenosum, pressure ulcer, syphilitic chancre, deep mycotic (cryptococcal, histoplasmal, blastomycotic, coccidioidal) ulcer, fixed drug reaction.

Herpetic Whitlow Acute *Staphylococcus aureus* paronychia, chronic (*Candida*) paronychia.

Oropharyngeal Ulcers Aphthous ulcers, lymphoma, histoplasmosis with oral ulcer.

Esophageal Ulcers Cytomegalovirus ulcers, aphthous (idiopathic) ulcers, *Candida* esophagitis, histoplasmosis with esophageal ulcer.

Anorectal Ulcers HPV-induced squamous cell carcinoma (in situ or invasive), Crohn's disease; amebiasis, chronic rectal abuse of ergot alkaloids.

Mucocutaneous Dissemination VZV infection (varicella, disseminated herpes zoster), eczema herpeticum, eczema vaccinatum, disseminated vaccinia in immunosuppressed patients.

LABORATORY EXAMINATIONS

See Herpes Simplex Virus Infection, page 784.

Urinalysis Hematuria due to HSV cystitis.

DIAGNOSIS

Clinical suspicion confirmed by Tzanck smear, positive HSV antigen detection, or isolation of HSV on viral culture.

COURSE AND PROGNOSIS

In most immunocompromised individuals with reactivation of HSV, clinical manifestations differ little from infections in healthy hosts. In renal transplant recipients, HSV is excreted in throat washings of 80% of patients shortly after grafting; two-thirds of those excreting HSV develop lesions shortly after excretion is detected. In some immunocompromised individuals, however, large ulcerations can persist for weeks to years. Herpetic ulcers provide a break in the epithelium, facilitating superinfection with bacteria or fungi.

When widespread, HSV may disseminate to liver, lungs, adrenals, GI tract, CNS. Visceral spread can be complicated by disseminated intravascular coagulation, which has a very high mortality rate. Factors determining whether severe localized disease, cutaneous involvement,

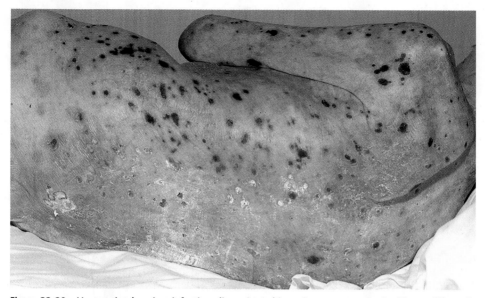

Figure 23-30 Herpes simplex virus infection: disseminated in an immunocompromised host *Disseminated erosion, ulcerations, vesicles with hemorrhagic crusts and necrotic bases in an individual with advanced lymphoma. Patients often have infection of lungs, liver, and brain.*

or visceral dissemination will occur in an individual are not well defined. Disseminated HSV infection with visceral involvement in neonates has a 50 to 80% mortality rate if untreated.

In HIV disease, individuals successfully treated with HAART usually experience reduction in frequency and severity of HSV recurrences. Chronic herpetic ulcers that fail to respond to acyclovir should be evaluated promptly for the presence of resistant virus. Infection with acyclovir-resistant strains results in chronic, progressive ulcerations that persist and/or continue to enlarge despite oral and IV acyclovir treatment. These ulcers can enlarge to 20 to 30 cm in diameter and are associated with major morbidity and pain.

MANAGEMENT

Prevention *Acyclovir prophylaxis* for seropositive patients undergoing bone marrow transplantation. induction therapy for leukemia, or solid organ transplantation: acyclovir, 5 mg/kg IV q8h or 400 mg PO tid, from the day of conditioning, induction, or transplantation for 4 to 6 weeks suppresses both HSV and VZV reactivation.

Systemic Antiviral Therapy See Herpes Simplex Virus Infection, page 784.

VARICELLA-ZOSTER VIRUS INFECTIONS

Varicella-zoster virus (VZV) is a human herpesvirus that infects 98% of adult populations. Primary VZV infection, i.e., varicella or chickenpox, is nearly always symptomatic and characterized by disseminated pruritic vesicles. During primary infection, VZV establishes lifelong infection in sensory ganglia. When immunity to VZV declines, VZV reactivates within the nerve cell, traveling down the neuron to the skin, where it erupts in a dermatomal pattern, i.e., herpes zoster (HZ) or shingles. In the immunocompromised host, primary and reactivated VZV infection is often more severe, associated with higher morbidity rates and some mortality.

EPIDEMIOLOGY

Age of Onset 90% of cases occur in children younger than 10 years of age, <5% in persons younger than 15 years of age.

Etiology VZV, a herpesvirus. Structurally similar to other herpesviruses: lipid envelope surrounding nucleocapsid with icosahedral symmetry, a total diameter of approximately 150 to 200 nm, centrally located double-stranded DNA with a molecular weight of 80 million.

Transmission Airborne droplets as well as direct contact; indirect contact uncommon. Patients are contagious several days before exanthem appears and until last crop of vesicles. Crusts are not infectious. VZV can be aerosolized from skin of individuals with herpes zoster, which is about one-third as contagious as varicella, causing varicella in susceptible contacts.

Season In metropolitan areas in temperate climates, varicella epidemics occur in winter and spring.

PATHOGENESIS

In varicella, VZV is thought to enter through mucosa of upper respiratory tract and oropharynx, followed by local replication and primary viremia; VZV then replicates in cells of reticuloendothelial system with subsequent secondary viremia and dissemination to skin and mucous membranes. Localization of VZV in the basal cell layer is followed by virus replication, vacuole formation, ballooning degeneration of epithelial cells, and accumulation of edema fluid. Second episodes of varicella have been documented but are rare. During the course of varicella, VZV passes from the skin lesions to the sensory nerves, travels to the sensory ganglia, and establishes latent infection.

In HZ, humoral and cellular immunity to VZV established with primary infection ebbs naturally or because of an underlying cause of immunocompromise, resulting in VZV replication in sensory ganglia. VZV then travels down the sensory nerve, resulting in initial dermatomal pain followed by skin lesions. Since the neuritis precedes the skin involvement, pain appears before the skin lesions are visible. The locations of pain are varied and relate directly to the ganglion where VZV has emerged from latency to active infection. Prodromal symptoms may appear initially in the trigeminal, cervical, thoracic, lumbar, or sacral dermatome. Postherpetic neuralgia (PHN) is caused by reflex sympathetic dystrophy.

LABORATORY EXAMINATIONS

VZV Antigen Detection Smear of vesicle fluid or scraping from ulcer base/margin is made on a glass microscope slide. Direct fluorescent antibody test (DFA) detects VZV-specific antigens. Sensitive and specific method for identifying VZV-infected lesions. Higher yield than VZV cultures.

Viral Cultures Isolation of virus on viral culture (human fibroblast monolayers) from vesicular skin lesions, biopsy specimens, corneal scraping, and CSF is possible but more difficult than for HSV. Distinctive cytopathic effects usually appear in 3 to 10 days. Vesicle fluid can be cultured.

Tzanck Smear Cytology of fluid or scraping from base of vesicle or pustule shows both giant and multinucleated acantholytic epidermal cells (as does that of HSV infections) (see Fig. 23-18). Cytologists and dermatopathologists are most experienced in interpretation of smear.

Serology Seroconversion documents primary VZV infection.

Dermatopathology Lesional skin or visceral biopsy specimen shows multinucleated giant epithelial cells indicating HSV-1, HSV-2, or VZV infection. Immunoperoxidase stains specific for HSV-1, HSV-2, or VZV antigens can identify the specific herpesvirus.

Varicella

Varicella is the highly contagious primary infection caused by varicella-zoster virus. It is characterized by successive crops of pruritic vesicles that evolve to pustules, crusts, and at times, scars. This infection is often accompanied by mild constitutional symptoms; the primary infection occurring in adulthood may be complicated by pneumonia and encephalitis.
Synonym: Chickenpox.

EPIDEMIOLOGY

Age of Onset 90% of cases occur in children younger than 10 years of age, <5% in persons older than 15 years of age.

Incidence 3 to 4 million cases in the United States annually.

Transmission Airborne droplets as well as direct contact; indirect contact uncommon. Patients are contagious several days before exanthem appears and until last crop of vesicles. Crusts are not infectious. VZV also aerosolized from skin of individuals with herpes zoster and can cause varicella.

Season In metropolitan areas in temperate climates, varicella epidemics occur in winter and spring.

HISTORY

Incubation Period 14 days (range, 10 to 23 days).

Prodrome Characteristically absent or mild. Uncommon in children, more common in adults: headache, general aches and pains, severe backache, malaise. Exanthem appears within 2 to 3 days.

History Exposure at day care, school, to older sibling; relative with zoster.

Skin Symptoms Exanthem usually quite pruritic.

PHYSICAL EXAMINATION

Skin Lesions In most children, illness begins with appearance of exanthem, vesicular lesions evident in successive crops. Often single, discrete lesions or scanty in number in children, and much more dense in adults. Initial lesions are *papules* (often not observed) that may appear as *wheals* and quickly evolve to *vesicles* and initially appear as small "drops of water" or "dewdrops on a rose petal" (Fig. 23-31), superficial and thin-walled with surrounding erythema. Vesicles become umbilicated and rapidly evolve to *pustules* and *crusts* over an 8- to 12-h period. With subsequent crops, all stages of evolution may be noted simultaneously, i.e., papules, vesicles, pustules, crusts.

Distribution First lesions begin on face (Fig. 23-31) and scalp, spreading inferiorly to trunk (Fig. 23-32) and extremities; most profuse in areas least exposed to pressure, i.e., back between shoulder blades, flanks, axillae, popliteal and anticubital fossae; density highest on trunk and face, less on extremities; palms and soles usually spared.

Crusts fall off in 1 to 3 weeks, leaving a pink, somewhat depressed base. Characteristic punched-out permanent scars may persist. Uncommonly, hemorrhage into pustular lesion occurs in otherwise healthy children, i.e., hemorrhagic varicella. Complicated by superinfection by staphylococci or streptococci; impetigo, furuncles, cellulitis, and gangrene may occur.

Mucous Membranes Vesicles (not often observed) and subsequent shallow erosions (2 to 3 mm) most common on palate but also occur on mucosa of nose, conjunctivae, pharynx, larynx, trachea, GI tract, urinary tract, vagina.

General Examination Low-grade fever. Vesicopustules may occur in respiratory, GU, and GI tracts.

Variants

Varicella Gangrenosa Cutaneous gangrene in varicella lesions may follow secondary infection (usually *Staphylococcus aureus*), but rarely extensive local gangrene may occur in the absence of bacterial superinfection, sometimes during a mild episode of varicella.

"Malignant" Varicella Immunosuppressed or glucocorticoid-treated individuals may develop pneumonitis, hepatitis, encephalitis, hemorrhagic complications, which may be severe with disseminated intravascular coagulation and purpura fulminans. Continued VZV replication and dissemination results in prolonged high-level viremia, more extensive rash, longer period of new vesicle formation.

DIFFERENTIAL DIAGNOSIS

Widespread Vesicles/Crusts Disseminated herpes simplex virus (HSV) infection, cutaneous dissemination of zoster, eczema herpeticum, eczema vaccinatum, disseminated vaccinia in immunosuppressed patients (smallpox vaccination still given in the U.S. military), rickettsialpox, enterovirus infections, bullous form of impetigo.

LABORATORY EXAMINATIONS

See Varicella-Zoster Virus Infections, page 800.

Bacterial Cultures Rule out superinfection with *S. aureus* or group A streptococcus.

Serology Seroconversion, i.e., fourfold or greater rise in VZV titers.

DIAGNOSIS

Usually made on clinical findings alone.

COURSE AND PROGNOSIS

In healthy children, the course is self-limited; however, a mortality rate of 1 per 50,000 cases in the United States is reported (100 deaths annually in the 3 to 4 million cases). 6500 hospitalizations annually (U.S.) for varicella. The most common complication of varicella in children younger than 5 years is bacterial (*S. aureus,* group A streptococcus) superinfection; severe infection of pox can occur with bacteremia. In children 5 to 11 years of age, the most common complications are varicella encephalitis and Reye's syndrome.

In adults, prodromal symptoms are common and may be severe; exanthem may last for a week or more, with prolonged period of recovery. Primary varicella pneumonia, which presents 1 to 6 days after appearance of rash, is relatively common in adults, with 16% of adults showing x-ray evidence of pneumonitis; however, only 4% have clinical signs of pneumonitis. VZV encephalitis also may complicate varicella in adults. Less common complications of varicella include viral arthritis, uveitis, conjunctivitis, carditis, inappropriate antidiuretic hormone syndrome, nephritis, and orchitis. The mortality rate in adults is 15 per 50,000 cases; 25% of varicella-associated deaths occur in adults.

Maternal varicella during the first trimester of pregnancy may result in fetal varicella syndrome (limb hypoplasia, eye and brain damage, skin lesions) in 2% of exposed fetuses. Neonatal varicella has higher associated incidence of pneumonitis and encephalitis than occur in older children. Immunocompromised or glucocorticoid-treated patients with varicella may manifest dissemination, hepatitis, encephalitis, and hemorrhagic complications. If varicella occurs at an early age when maternal antibody is still present, an individual can have a second episode of varicella. In HIV-infected patients, reactivation of VZV may result in chronic painful ecthymatous varicella.

In immunocompromised individuals, VZV hepatitis and pneumonitis are relatively common and are associated with significant mortality.

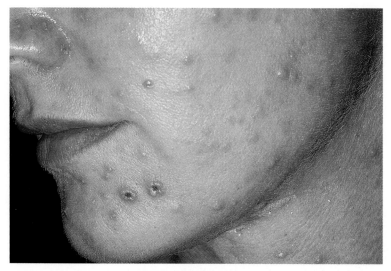

Figure 23-31 Varicella-zoster virus infection: varicella *Multiple, very pruritic, erythematous papules, vesicles ("dewdrops on a rose petal"), and crusted papules on erythematous, edematous bases on the face and neck of a young female. The spectrum of lesions, arising over 7 to 10 days, is typical of varicella.*

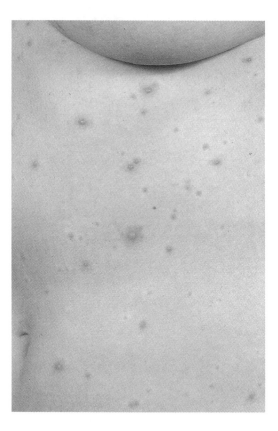

Figure 23-32 Varicella-zoster virus infection: varicella *Multiple papules and vesicles on erythematous bases in a random pattern of dissemination on the trunk.*

MANAGEMENT

Prevention

Immunization — VZV immunization is now available (Varivax) and is 80% effective in preventing symptomatic primary VZV infection. 5% of newly immunized children develop rash. Those at high risk for varicella, who should be immunized, include: normal VZV-negative adults, children with leukemia, and immunocompromised individuals (immunosuppressive treatment, HIV infection, cancer). VZV vaccine results in both cell-mediated immunity and antibody production against the virus. Immunization with VZV vaccine may boost humoral and cell-mediated immunity and decrease the incidence of zoster in populations with declining VZV-specific immunity.

Symptomatic therapy — Directed at reducing pruritus.

Lotions — Application gives short-term relief of pruritus.

Oral antihistamines

Caution re antipyretic agents — Antipyretic administration is of concern because of a possible link between aspirin and Reye's syndrome in children with varicella.

Antiviral agents

Otherwise healthy patients — If begun within 24 h after onset of varicella, decreases the severity of varicella and reduces secondary cases.

Acyclovir — 20 mg/kg (800 maximum) qid for 5 days

Valacyclovir — Effective but not an approved use; dosing same as for herpes zoster.

Famciclovir — Effective but not an approved use; dosing same as for herpes zoster.

VZV infection (varicella or zoster) in immunocompromised patients

Acyclovir — 10 mg/kg IV q8h for 7 days

Acyclovir-resistant

Foscarnet — 40 mg/kg IV q8h for 7 days

Treatment of bacterial superinfection — Directed at *S. aureus* and/or group A streptococcus.

Mupirocin ointment — Applied twice daily to lesions.

Oral antibiotics — See Table 20-2.

Herpes Zoster

Herpes zoster (HZ) is an acute dermatomal infection associated with reactivation of varicella-zoster virus (VZV) and is characterized by unilateral pain and a vesicular or bullous eruption limited to a dermatome(s) innervated by a corresponding sensory ganglion. The major morbidity is postherpetic neuralgia (PHN).

Synonym: Shingles.

EPIDEMIOLOGY

Age of Onset More than 66% are older than 50 years of age; 5% of cases in children younger than 15 years of age.

Incidence In the United States, nearly 100% of adults are seropositive for anti-VZV antibodies by the third decade of life and are thus at risk for reactivation of latent VZV. More than 500,000 cases of HZ annually. Cumulative lifetime incidence: 10 to 20%. In one cohort, 5% of individuals with HZ were HIV-infected and 5% had cancer. Recurrent HZ <1% of cases. Occurs in 25% of HIV-infected individuals, an eight times higher incidence than the general population, aged 20 to 50 years; 7 to 9% of renal and cardiac transplant recipients. Recurrent HZ more common in immunocompromised individuals.

Risk Factors Most common factor is diminshing immunity to VZV with advancing age, with most cases occurring in those ≥55 years old. Malignancy. Immunosuppression, especially from lymphoproliferative disorders and chemotherapy. Radiotherapy. HIV-infected individuals have an eightfold increased incidence of zoster.

Classification HZ manifests in three distinct clinical stages: prodromal, active, and chronic.

HISTORY

Duration of Symptoms Prodromal stage: neuritic pain or paresthesia precedes for 2 to 3 weeks. Acute vesiculation: 3 to 5 days. Crust formation: days to 2 to 3 weeks. PHN: months to years.

Skin Symptoms *Prodromal Stage* Pain (stabbing, pricking, sharp, boring, penetrating, lancinating, shooting), tenderness, paresthesia (itching, tingling, burning, freeze-burning) in the involved dermatome precedes the eruption. Allodynia: heightened sensitivity to mild stimuli.

Active Vesiculation Skin lesions may be pruritic but in themselves are not painful.

Zoster Sine Zoster Nerve involvement can occur without cutaneous zoster.

Chronic Stages PHN, described as "burning," "ice-burning," "shooting," or "lancinating," can persist for weeks, months, or years after the cutaneous involvement has resolved.

Constitutional Symptoms Prodromal stage and active vesiculation: flu-like symptoms such as headache, malaise, fever. Chronic stages: depression is very common in individuals with PHN.

PHYSICAL EXAMINATION

Skin Lesions Papules (24 h)→vesicles-bullae (Fig. 23-33) (48 h)→pustules (96 h)→crusts (7 to 10 days). New lesions continue to appear for up to 1 week. Necrotic and gangrenous lesions sometimes occur. Erythematous, edematous base (Figs. 23-34 and 23-35) with superimposed clear vesicles, sometimes hemorrhagic. The vesicle-bulla is oval or round, may be umbilicated. Some scarring is very common after healing of HZ; the dermatomal pattern is pathognomonic of HZ.

Distribution Unilateral, dermatomal (Fig. 23-36). Two or more contiguous dermatomes may be involved (Fig. 23-34). Noncontiguous dermatomal zoster is rare. Hematogenous dissemination to other skin sites in 10% of healthy individuals (Fig. 23-35).

Site of predilection Thoracic (>50%), trigeminal (10 to 20%), lumbosacral and cervical (10 to 20%).

Mucous Membranes Vesicles and erosions occur in mouth, vagina, and bladder depending on dermatome involved.

General Examination *Lymphadenopathy* Regional nodes draining the area are often enlarged and tender.

Sensory or Motor Nerve Changes Detectable by neurologic examination. Sensory defects (temperature, pain, touch) and (mild) motor paralysis, e.g., facial palsy.

Eye In ophthalmic zoster, nasociliary involvement of VI (ophthalmic) branch of the trigeminal nerve occurs in about one-third of cases and is heralded by vesicles on the side and tip of the nose. Complications include uveitis, keratitis, conjuctivitis, retinitis, optic neuritis, glaucoma, proptosis, cicatricial lid retraction, and extraocular muscle palsies. *An ophthalmologist should always be consulted.*

DIFFERENTIAL DIAGNOSIS

Prodromal Stage/Localized Pain Can mimic migraine, cardiac or pleural disease, an acute abdomen, or vertebral disease.

Dermatomal Eruption Zosteriform herpes simplex virus infection, phytoallergic (poison ivy, poison oak) contact dermatitis, erysipelas, bullous impetigo, necrotizing fasciitis.

LABORATORY EXAMINATIONS

See Varicella-Zoster Virus Infections, page 800.

Electrocardiogram In prodromal stage with individuals with chest pain, rule out ischemic heart disease.

Imaging In prodromal stage, rule out organic, pleural, pulmonary, or abdominal disease.

DIAGNOSIS

Prodromal Stage Suspect HZ in older or immunocompromised individual with unilateral pain.

Active Vesiculation Clinical findings usually adequate; may be confirmed by Tzanck test and possible DFA or viral culture to rule out HSV infection.

PHN By history and clinical findings.

COURSE AND PROGNOSIS

In immunocompetent host, rash usually resolves in 2 to 3 weeks. Complications can be local: hemorrhage, gangrene; or general: meningoencephalitis, cerebral vascular syndromes, cranial nerve syndromes [trigeminal (ophthalmic) branch (herpes zoster ophthalmicus), facial and auditory nerves (Ramsay Hunt syndrome)], peripheral motor weakness, transverse myelitis, visceral involvement (pneumonitis, hepatitis, pericarditis/myocarditis, pancreatitis, esophagitis, enterocolitis, cystitis, synovitis), cutaneous dissemination, and superinfection of skin lesions. Pain with HZ is associated with neural inflammation, nerve infection during the acute reactivation, and neural inflammation and scarring with PHN. In most cases of HZ, 50% of individuals are pain-free 50 days after onset of symptoms; 95% pain-free at 6 months. Only 1 to 2% have PHN after 6 months.

The course in HIV-infected, renal and cardiac transplant recipients is usually uncomplicated without significant dissemination. Dissemination generally occurs 6 to 10 days after onset of localized lesions and is most often limited to cutaneous involvement. In immunosuppressed individuals, visceral dissemination can occur, involving CNS, lung, heart, and GI tract. The risk of PHN is 40% in patients older than 60 years of age. In one large follow-up study, PHN was present 1 month after onset of the rash in 60%, by 3 months there was some pain in 24%, and by 6 months 13% of the patients still had pain. The highest incidence of PHN is in ophthalmic zoster. Dissemination of zoster—20 or more lesions outside the affected or adjacent dermatomes—occurs in up to 10% of patients, usually in immunosuppressed patients. Motor paralysis occurs in 5% of patients, especially when the virus involves the cranial nerves.

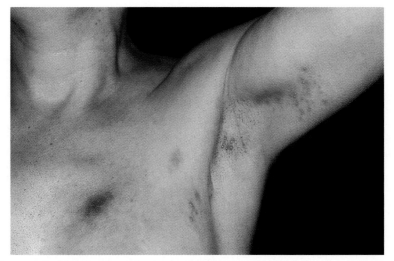

Figure 23-33 Varicella-zoster virus infection: herpes zoster in T2 dermatome *Grouped and confluent papules, vesicles, and crusted erosions arising in the fourth left cervical dermatome in a healthy 41-year-old female. Pruritus and a burning sensation accompanied the clinical findings. The involvement is relatively mild and can be mistaken for other dermatoses, such as allergic contact dermatitis.*

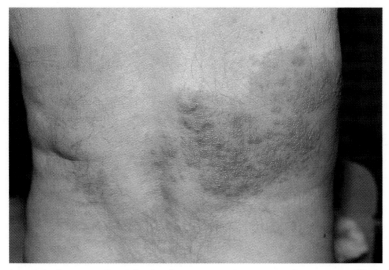

Figure 23-34 Varicella-zoster virus infection: herpes zoster in T8 to T10 dermatomes *Typical grouped vesicles and pustules with erythema and edema of three contiguous thoracic dermatomes on the posterior chest wall.*

MANAGEMENT

Prevention

Immunization	Immunization with VZV vaccine may boost humoral and cell-mediated immunity and decrease the incidence of zoster in populations with declining VZV-specific immunity.
Goals of management	Relieve constitutional symptoms; minimize pain; reduce viral shedding; prevent secondary bacterial infection; speed crusting of lesions and healing; ease physical, psychological, emotional discomfort; prevent viral dissemination or other complications; prevent or minimize PHN.
Antiviral therapy	In individuals at high risk for reactivation of VZV infection, oral acyclovir can reduce the incidence of HZ. In prodromal stage: begin antiviral agent if diagnosis is considered likely; analgesics. With active vesiculation: antiviral therapy begun ≤72 h accelerates healing of skin lesions, decreases the duration of acute pain, and may decrease the frequency of PHN when given in adequate dosage.
Acyclovir	800 mg PO qid for 7–10 days. The 50% viral inhibitory concentration of acyclovir is three to six times higher for VZV than for HSV in vitro, and drug dose must be increased appropriately. The bioavailability of acyclovir is only 15 to 30% of the orally administered dose. For ophthalmic zoster and HZ in the immuno compromised host, acyclovir should be given intravenously. Acyclovir hastens healing and lessens *acute* pain if given within 48 h of the onset of the rash.
Valacyclovir	1000 mg PO tid for 7 days, 70 to 80% bioavailable.
Famciclovir	500 mg PO tid for 7 days, 77% bioavailable. Reduce dose in individuals with diminished renal function.
Acyclovir-resistant VZV	
Foscarnet	IV.
Immunosuppressed patients	IV acyclovir and recombinant interferon α-2a to prevent dissemination of HZ is indicated.
Supportive therapy for acute HZ	
Constitutional symptoms	Bed rest, NSAIDs.
Sedation	Pain often interferes with sleep. Sleep deprivation and pain commonly result in depression. Doxepin, 10 to 100 mg hs, is an effective agent.
Oral glucocorticoids	Prednisone given early in the course of HZ relieves constitutional symptoms but has not been proven to reduce PHN.
Dressings	Application of moist dressings (water, saline, Burow's solution) to the involved dermatome is soothing and alleviates pain.
Pain management	Early control of pain with narcotic analgesics is indicated; failure to manage pain can result in failure to sleep, fatigue, and depression: Best to begin with more potent analgesics and then reduce potency as pain lessens.
Chronic stages (PHN)	Pain is that of reflex sympathetic dystrophy.
Pain management	Severe prodromal pain or severe pain on the first day of rash is predictive of severe PHN. Gabapentin: 300 mg tid. Tricyclic antidepressants such as doxepin, 10 to 100 mg PO hs. Capsaicin cream every 4 h. Topical anesthetic such as EMLA or 5% lidocaine patch for allodynia. Nerve block to area of allodynia. Analgesics.

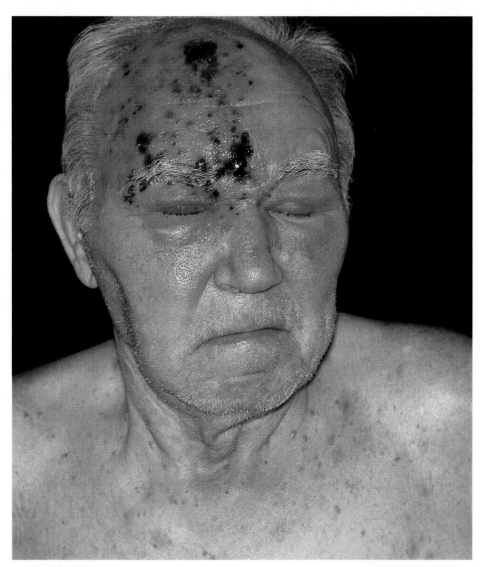

Figure 23-35   Varicella-zoster virus infection: necrotizing ophthalmic herpes zoster with cutaneous dissemination   *Hemorrhagic, crusted ulcerations and vesicles on the right forehead and periorbital area in the ophthalmic branch of the trigeminal nerve; note the bilateral facial edema and erythema. Hematogenous cutaneous dissemination has occurred with hundreds of vesicles and erythematous papules on the trunk. In spite of the extensive cutaneous infection, this immunocompetent patient was relatively pain free.*

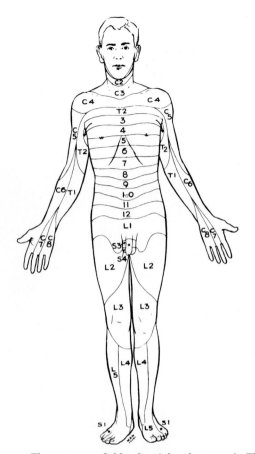

A

Figure 23-36 Dermatomes *The cutaneous fields of peripheral nerves.* **A.** *The segmental innervation of the skin from the anterior aspect. The uppermost dermatome adjoins the cutaneous field of the mandibular division of the trigeminal nerve. The arrow indicate the lateral extensions of dermatome T3.* **B.** *The dermatomes from the posteriour view. Note the absence of cutaneous innervation by the first cervical segment. Arrows in the axillary regions indicate the lateral etent of dermatome T3; those in the region of the vertebral column point to the first thoracic, the first lumbar, ad the first sacral spinous pocesses. (After Foerster in Haymaker W, Woodhall B: Peripheral Nerve Injuries, 2d ed. Saunders, Philadelphia/London, 1953.)* **C.** *Dermatomes of head. (Modified from Steergmann AT: Examination of the nervous System, 2d. ed. Year Book Medical Publishers, Chicago, 1962.)*

VIRAL INFECTIONS OF SKIN AND MUCOSA

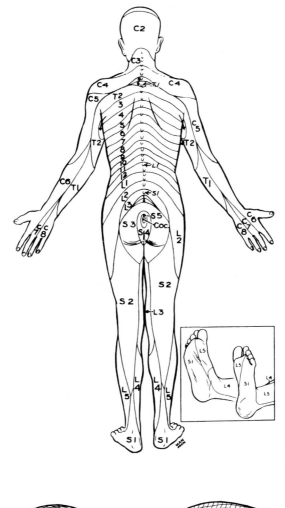

B

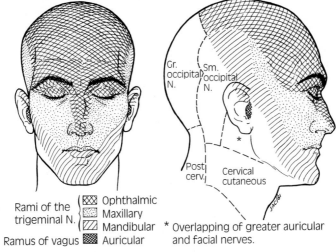

Rami of the trigeminal N. { ⊠ Ophthalmic
                        { ▢ Maxillary
                        { ▨ Mandibular
Ramus of vagus ▨ Auricular

* Overlapping of greater auricular and facial nerves.

C

Varicella-Zoster Virus Infections in the Immunocompromised Host

In immunocompromised individuals, varicella-zoster virus (VZV) infections can be more severe in primary infections (varicella) and reactivated infections [herpes zoster (HZ)]. In individuals with varicella, cutaneous and visceral involvement can be more severe. In those with HZ, the infection may involve several contiguous dermatomes, have more extensive cutaneous necrosis, wide hematogenous dissemination to mucocutaneous structures as well as to the viscera, and often be associated with high morbidity and mortality rates.

EPIDEMIOLOGY

Incidence Population of immunocompromised individuals is increasing. Most cases of recurrent HZ occur in immunocompromised individuals.

Risk Factors Immunosuppression, especially from lymphoproliferative disorders, and cancer chemotherapy.

Visceral dissemination of varicella: children undergoing cancer chemotherapy; solid organ and bone marrow transplant recipients; HIV infection; certain cell-mediated immunodeficiency disorders of childhood. HZ: often the first sign of HIV infection, preceding oral candidiasis and oral hairy leukoplakia by 1 year. Visceral dissemination of HZ: Hodgkin's disease (risk of developing zoster is 13 to 15% compared with 7 to 9% for non-Hodgkin's lymphoma patients and 1 to 3% for patients with solid tumors).

CLASSIFICATION OF VZV INFECTION IN THE IMMUNOCOMPROMISED HOST

- Primary varicella with visceral dissemination
- HZ with cutaneous dissemination
- HZ with visceral and cutaneous dissemination
- Reactivated VZV with hematogenous dissemination but without HZ
- HZ with persistent dermatomal infection
- Chronic cutaneous VZV infection after hematogenous dissemination

HISTORY

Skin Symptoms Symptoms of varicella and zoster. Chronic cutaneous VZV infections following hematogenous dissemination are often associated with significant lesional pain requiring narcotic analgesia for pain management.

Constitutional Symptoms Visceral dissemination usually accompanied by fever

PHYSICAL EXAMINATION

Skin Lesions *Varicella and Cutaneous Dissemination of Reactivated VZV Infection* (See Varicella, page 801.) Reactivated VZV without HZ with dissemination cannot be distinguished clinically from varicella.

Herpes Zoster In HIV disease and leukemia, involvement of several contiguous dermatomes is common (Fig. 23-28).

Herpes Zoster with Cutaneous Dissemination A variable number of vesicles or bullae are seen at any mucocutaneous site, which evolve into crusted erosions (Fig. 23-37). Lesions are disseminated and range from a few to hundreds. The condition thus appears clinically as zoster plus varicella.

Herpes Zoster with Persistent Dermatomal Infection Papules and nodules, which can become hyperkeratotic or verrucous, persisting in a dermatomal pattern (single or multiple contiguous) after an outbreak of zoster (Fig. 23-39).

Chronic Cutaneous VZV Infection After Hematogenous Dissemination Lesions on the palms or soles may present initially as bullae. Continual appearance of vesicles/bullae in a dermatomal or generalized distribution. Dissemination can occur without dermatomal HZ. Chronic lesions present as nodules, ulcers, (Fig. 23-40) crusted nodules/ulcers (ecthymatous). ±Postinflammatory hyper- or hypopigmentation.

Systemic Findings *Eye* In HIV disease, retinal VZV infection (acute retinal necrosis) can occur in the absence of apparent conjunctival or cutaneous involvement with subsequent

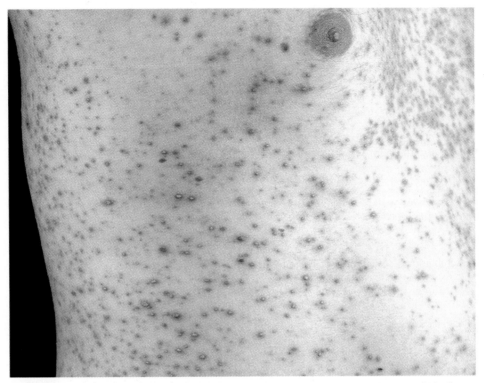

Figure 23-37   Varicella-zoster virus infection: disseminated cutaneous, in an immunocompromised patient   *Hundreds of vesicles and pustules on erythematous bases of the trunk of a patient with lymphoma. Note the absence of grouping of lesions seen in herpes simplex or herpes zoster. The eruption is indistinguishable from varicella and must be differentiated from disseminated HSV infection.*

loss of vision. Bilateral involvement in one-third of cases with subsequent loss of vision. VZV optic neuritis is rare.

CNS In HIV disease, VZV is the etiologic agent of up to 2% of CNS disease (encephalitis, polyneuritis, myelitis, vasculitis).

DIFFERENTIAL DIAGNOSIS

Primary Varicella with Visceral Dissemination Pneumonia must be distinguished from *Pneumocystis carinii* pneumonia associated with varicella.

Herpes Zoster with Cutaneous Dissemination Zosteriform herpes simplex virus (HSV) infection with dissemination.

Herpes Zoster with Visceral and Cutaneous Dissemination Zosteriform HSV infection with dissemination. Pneumonia must be distinguished from *P. carinii* pneumonia associated with varicella.

Herpes Zoster with Persistent Dermatomal Infection Chronic zosteriform HSV infection. Hypertrophic scars or keloids.

Chronic Cutaneous VZV Infection After Hematogenous Dissemination Ecthyma, ecthyma gangrenosum, disseminated mycobacterial infection, deep fungal infection, syphilis.

LABORATORY EXAMINATIONS

See Varicella-Zoster Virus Infection, page 800.

Antiviral Sensitivities When isolated, VZV from cultured lesion can be tested for sensitivity to acyclovir and other antiviral agents.

Bacterial Culture Rule out secondary bacterial infection, most commonly caused by *Staphylococcus aureus* or group A streptococcus.

Chemistries Abnormalities of liver function tests with VZV hepatitis.

COURSE AND PROGNOSIS

Approximately 2 to 35% of children with varicella who are undergoing cancer chemotherapy experience visceral dissemination; the associated mortality rate is 7 to 30%. Dissemination is more common in those with a peripheral blood lymphocyte count of $<500/\mu L$.

Children with Varicella Visceral involvement most commonly affects lungs; less often, liver and brain. Varicella pneumonia occurs 3 to 7 days after onset of skin lesions; can progress rapidly over a few days or remain indolent with gradual improvement over 2 to 4 weeks. Neurologic complications present 4 to 8 days after onset of rash; associated with poor prognosis.

Adults with HZ In HIV-infected adults, recurrent episodes occur in same or different dermatome(s); disseminated zoster infrequent. Between 15 and 30% of patients with Hodgkin's disease experience significant dissemination (most often cutaneous). Mortality rates for disseminated zoster much lower than for children with disseminated varicella. Postherpetic neuralgia does not appear to be more common in immunocompromised individuals than in the general population.

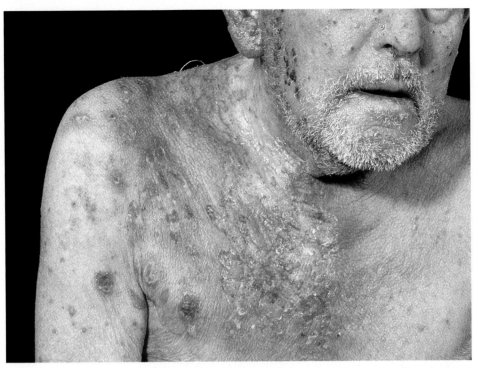

Figure 23-38 Varicella-zoster virus infection: necrotizing herpes zoster with cutaneous dissemination in an immunocompromised patient *Confluent, crusted ulcerations on an inflammatory base in multiple contiguous dermatomes (right face, ear, neck, and upper chest) with vesicles, crusts, and ulcers at sites of hematogenous, cutaneous dissemination in an elderly male with leukemia.*

Prevention

Immunization

VZV immunization is available and is 80% effective in preventing symptomatic primary VZV infection. About 5% of newly immunized children develop rash. Those at high risk for varicella who should be immunized include normal adults, children with leukemia, neonates, and immunocompromised individuals (immunosuppressive treatment, HIV infection, cancer).

Antiviral agents for VZV- and/or HSV-seropositive individuals Undergoing BMT

Acyclovir

400 mg PO bid, from the day of conditioning, induction, or transplantation for 4 to 6 weeks, suppresses both HSV and VZV reactivation.

Systemic antiviral therapy

Oral acyclovir, valacyclovir, famciclovir may be effective in some patients.

In individuals with mild to moderate immunocompromise

High-dose oral acyclovir, 800 mg five times daily for 7 days, hastens healing and lessens *acute* pain if given within 48 h of the onset of the rash. Large controlled studies in patients over 60 years of age have not, however, demonstrated any effect on the incidence and severity of *chronic* postherpetic neuralgia of high-dose oral acyclovir. A recent preliminary study of older patients (age 60) demonstrated a reduced frequency of persistent pain when IV acyclovir, 10 mg/kg q8h for 5 days, was given within 4 days of the onset of the pain or within 48 h after the onset of the rash.

In individuals with advanced immunocompromise or severe or

IV acyclovir or recombinant interferon α-2a to prevent dissemination of HZ is indicated.

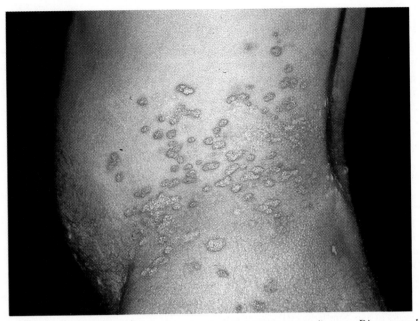

Figure 23-39 Varicella-zoster virus infection: chronic herpes zoster in HIV disease *Discrete and confluent hyperkeratotic papules in several contiguous dematomes persistent for 2 years in a male with advanced untreated HIV disease. The lesions were minimally symptomatic.*

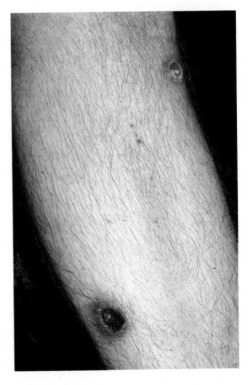

Figure 23-40 Varicella-zoster virus infection: chronic ulcers *Two large, deep ulcers, present for 6 months, on the lower leg of a 31-year-old male with advanced HIV disease. A severe neuritis pain accompanied the ulcers. There was an associated transverse myelitis. The ulcers and myelitis resolved with oral famciclovir and highly active antiretroviral therapy (HAART). Chronic suppression with oral famciclovir was continued for 3 years; when discontinued, V2 herpes zoster occurred in 5 days in spite of a high CD4 cell count.*

HUMAN HERPESVIRUS-6 AND -7 INFECTIONS

Exanthema subitum (ES) (sudden rash) is a childhood exanthem associated with primary human herpesvirus type 6 (HHV-6) and HHV-7 infection, characterized by the sudden appearance of rash as high-fever lysis in a healthy-appearing infant.

Synonym: Roseola infantum.

EPIDEMIOLOGY

Age of Onset   6 to 24 months.

Etiology   HHV-6 and HHV-7. They share genetic, biologic, and immunologic features; primary T cell tropic. At birth, most children have passively transferred anti-HHV-6 and -7 IgG. Primary infection is acquired via oropharyngeal secretions. HHV-6 antibodies reach a nadir at 4 to 7 months and increase throughout infancy. By 12 months, two-thirds of children become infected, with peak antibody levels reached at 2 to 3 years of age. Similarly, HHV-7 antibodies reach nadir at 6 months, with level peaking at 3 to 4 years of age. Latent infection may persist for the lifetime of individual.

PATHOGENESIS

Pathogenesis of ES rash is not known.

HISTORY

Incubation Period   5 to 15 days.

Prodrome   High fever ranging from 38.9° to 40.6°C. Remains consistently high, with morning remission, until the fourth day, when it falls precipitously to normal, coincident with the appearance of rash. Infant remarkably well despite high fever. Asymptomatic primary HHV-6 and HHV-7 infection is common.

Symptoms   Usually absent.

PHYSICAL EXAMINATION

Skin Lesions   Small blanchable pink macules and papules, 1 to 5 mm in diameter (Fig. 23-41). Lesions may remain discrete or become confluent.

Distribution   Trunk and neck.

General Findings   Absent in presence of high fever. Febrile seizures are common.

DIFFERENTIAL DIAGNOSIS

Morbilliform Exanthem   See Viral Infections of Skin and Mucosa: Infectious Exanthems, Section 23.

LABORATORY EXAMINATIONS

Serology   Demonstration of IgM anti-HHV-6 or anti-HHV-7 antibodies or IgG seroconversion.

Other   Viral culture and isolation from peripheral blood mononuclear cells. Demonstration or HHV-6 or HHV-7 DNA by PCR.

DIAGNOSIS

Usually made on clinical findings.

COURSE AND PROGNOSIS

Course self-limited with rare sequelae. In some cases, high fever may be associated with seizures. Intussusception associated with hyperplasia of intestinal lymphoid tissue, and hepatitis has been reported. As with other human herpesvirus infections, HHV-6 and HHV-7 persist throughout the life of the patient; however, clinical manifestations associated with HHV-6 and HHV-7 reactivation have not yet been identified. An infant with HHV-6 ES may experience a second clinical syndrome, HHV-7 ES, and vice versa.

MANAGEMENT

Symptomatic.

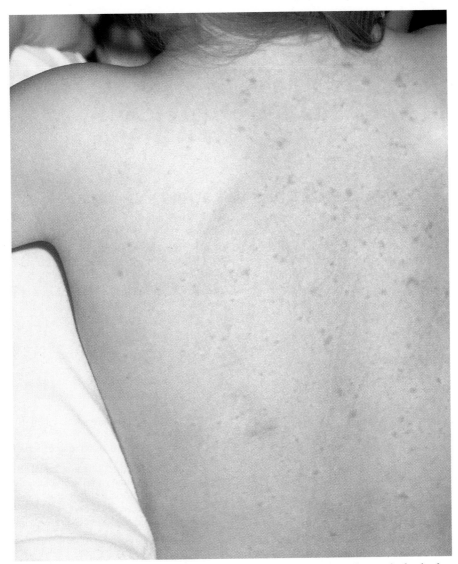

Figure 23-41 Exanthema subitum *Multiple, blanchable macules and papules on the back of a febrile child, which appeared as the temperature fell. (Courtesy of Karen Wiss, MD)*

INSECT BITES AND INFESTATIONS

CUTANEOUS REACTIONS TO ARTHROPOD BITES

Cutaneous reactions to arthropod bites (CRAB) are inflammatory and/or allergic reactions, characterized by an intensely pruritic eruption at the bite sites hours to days after the bite, manifested by solitary or grouped urticarial papules, papulovesicles, and/or bullae that persist for days to weeks; patients are often unaware of having been bitten. In some cases, systemic symptoms may occur, ranging from mild to severe, with death occurring from anaphylactic shock. Arthropod bites are also the method of transmission of many systemic infections and infestations.

EPIDEMIOLOGY

Season Summer in temperate climates.

Etiology 5 of 9 classes of arthropods cause local and systemic reactions associated with their bites: Arachnida, Chilopoda, Diplopoda, Crustacea, Insecta.

Arthropods That Infest, Bite, or Sting

I. Arachnida (four pairs of legs): mites, ticks, spiders, scorpions
   A. Acarina
      1. Mites: follicle (*Demodex*), food, fowl, grain, harvest, murine, scabies (*Sarcoptes*)
      2. Ticks
   B. Araneae: spiders
   C. Scorpionida
II. Chilopoda and Diplopoda: centipedes, millipedes
III. Insecta (three pairs of legs)
   A. Anoplura: lice (*Phthirius* and *Pediculus*)
   B. Coleoptera: beetles
   C. Diptera: mosquitoes, black flies, midges (punkies, no seeums, sand flies), Tabandae (horseflies, deerflies, clegs, breeze flies, greenheads, mango flies); botflies, *Callitroga americana, Dermato-*
bia hominis, phlebotomid sand flies, tsetse flies
   D. Hemiptera: bedbugs, kissing bugs
   E. Hymenoptera: ants, bees, wasps, hornets
   F. Lepidoptera: caterpillars, butterflies, moths
   G. Siphonaptera: fleas, chigoe or sand flea

Arthropod-Borne Infections and Infestations

Scrub typhus, endemic (murine) typhus, Lyme borreliosis, babesiosis, ehrlichiosis, spotted fever groups, Q fever, tick-borne encephalitis, malaria, filariasis, onchocerciasis (river blindness), tularemia, leishmaniasis, loiasis, cutaneous myiasis, trypanosomiasis (sleeping sickness, Chagas' disease), bubonic plague.

Geographic Distribution Worldwide.

PATHOGENESIS

• **Mites** Produce pruritus and/or allergic reactions through salivary proteins deposited during feeding. Harvest mites (chiggers) may present as intense pruritus on the ankles, legs, belt line; mites usually fall off after feeding or may be scratched off. In nonsensitized individuals, 1 to 2 mm pruritic papules are seen. In sensitized individuals, CRAB may be papular urticaria, vesiculation, or granulomatous reaction with fever and lymphadenopathy.

- **Ticks** Reactions include foreign body reactions, reactions to salivary secretions, reactions to injected toxins, and hypersensitivity reactions. Tick paralysis is caused by a toxin secreted in the saliva of the tick.

- **Spiders** Brown recluse spider (*Loxosceles reclusa*) bite causes reactions ranging from mild urticaria to full-thickness necrosis (loxoscelism). "Widow" spiders (*Latrodectus*) inject a venom that contains a neurotoxin (α-latrotoxin) producing reactions at the bite site as well as varying degrees of systemic toxicity.

- **Scorpion** Venom also contains a neurotoxin that can cause severe local and systemic reactions.

- **Blister Beetles** Contain the chemical cantharidin, which produces blister when the beetle is crushed on the skin.

- **Black Flies** Bites produce local reactions as well as black fly fever, characterized by fever, headache, nausea, generalized lymphadenitis.

- **Nonbiting Flies** Flies commonly feed on open wounds, exudates, and skin ulcers and may deposit eggs at these sites, resulting in wound myiasis. Fly larvae can burrow into injured or normal skin, invading through the epidermis into the dermis, resulting in furuncular myiasis. In some cases, larvae move about the subcutis (migratory myiasis), mimicking the pattern of cutaneous larva migrans.

- **Bedbugs** Nocturnal feedings produce a linear arrangement of papular urticaria.

- **Hymenoptera** Bees, hornets, wasp bites can produce painful stings, and anaphylaxis in the sensitized individual.

- **Caterpillars and Moths** Hairs can produce local irritant and allergic reactions.

- **Fleas (Cat, Dog, Bird)** Bites tend to cause more local reactions than human flea bites.

- **Chigoe or Sand Fleas** (*Tunga penetrans*) Recently impregnated female flea penetrates skin of a human host, burrows into epidermis to dermal-epidermal junction, where she feeds on blood drawn from host vessels in superficial dermis. Enlargement of the buried flea to 5 to 8 mm causes local pain in the infested skin. Mature eggs (150 to 200) are

extruded singly from a terminal abdominal orifice during a period of 7 to 10 days. The female dies shortly after egg extrusion, and the infested tissues collapse around it; ulcerations can occur at the site. Inflammation and secondary infection can arise if parts of the flea are retained in the tissue.

HISTORY

Incubation Period CRAB appears hours to days after the bite.

Duration of Lesions Days, weeks, months.

Skin Symptoms Pruritus, pain at bite site. Systemic symptoms with systemic reaction.

PHYSICAL EXAMINATION

Skin Findings

Erythematous Macules Occur at bite sites and are usually transient.

Papular Urticaria Persistent (>48 h) urticarial papules (Figs. 24-1 and 24-2), often surmounted by a vesicle, usually < 1 cm. Excoriations and excoriated urticarial papules, vesicles. Crusted painful lesions, usually purulent, may represent impetigo, ecthyma, or cutaneous diphtheria. Excoriated or secondarily infected lesions may heal with hyper- or hypopigmentation, and/or raised or depressed scars, especially in more darkly pigmented individuals.

Bullous Lesions Tense bullae with clear fluid on a slightly inflamed base. Excoriation results in large erosion.

Erythema Migrans Enlarging plaque occurring at site of tick bite, characteristic of Lyme borreliosis (see Section 20).

Spiders Brown recluse and black widow bites can result in mild local urticarial reactions to full-thickness skin necrosis, associated with a maculopapular exanthem, fever, headache, malaise, arthralgial, nausea/vomiting.

Diptera *Mosquitoes* Bites usually present as papular urticaria on exposed sites; reactions can be urticaria, eczematous, or granulomatous.

Black Flies Anesthetic is injected, resulting in painless initial bite; may subsequently become painful with itching, erythema, and edema. Black fly fever characterized by fever, nausea, generalized lymphadenitis.

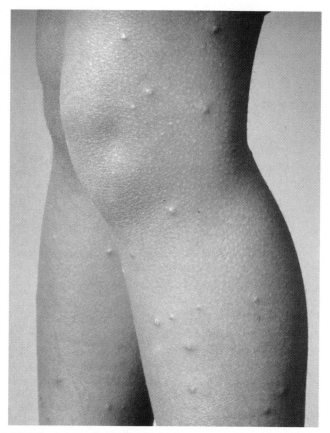

Figure 24-1 Papular urticaria from flea bites *Multiple, very pruritic, urticaria-like papules at the sites of flea bites on the knees and legs of a child; these persistent urticaria-like papules are usually <1cm in diameter and may have a vesicle on the top. When scratched, they exhibit erosions or crusts.*

Midges Bites produce immediate pain with erythema at bite site with 2 to 3-mm papulovesicles, followed by indurated nodules (up to 1 cm) persisting for many months.

Tabandae Bites painful with papular urticaria, rarely associated anaphylaxis.

Botfly Larvae penetrate skin or are deposited on open wounds producing cutaneous myiasis. Larvae may be fixed or migrate resembling larva migrans (compare Fig. 24-19). *Callitroga americana* most common in United States. *Dermatobia hominis* in tropical regions causes furuncular myiasis, painful lesions that resemble pyogenic granuloma or abscess; a pruritic papule develops at the site, slowly enlarging over several weeks into a domed nodule (resembles a furuncle) with a central pore (Fig. 24-3) through which the posterior end of the larve intermittently protrudes.

House Flies Larvae deposited into any exposed skin site (ear, nose, paranasal sinuses, mouth, eye, anus, and vagina) or at any wound site (leg ulcers, ulcerated squamous and basal cell carcinomas, hematomas, umbilical stump) and grow into maggots, which can be seen on surface of wound (Fig. 24-4); although repulsive for the patient, maggots are very effective at debriding nonviable tissue and debris.

Hemiptera Bedbug bites produce papular urticaria (Fig. 24-2) that have a characteristic linear array. Reduvid (kissing bugs, assassin bugs, conenosed bugs) bites usually present as papular urticaria; severe reactions can produce necrosis and ulceration resembling spider bites.

INSECT BITES AND INFESTATIONS

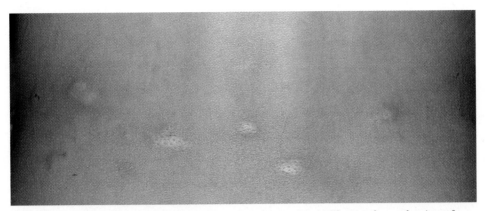

Figure 24-2 Papular urticaria from bedbug bites *Pruritic, urticaria-like papules at the sites of bedbug bites on the lower back at the waist. Bedbugs (Cimex lectularius) share human domains, residing in crevices of floors and walls, in bedding, and in furniture. They usually feed only once a week, and less often in cold weather. Bedbugs can travel long distances in search of a human host and can survive for 6 to 12 months without feeding. Bite reactions occur on exposed sites such as the face, neck, arms, and hands, with two to three lesions in a row ("breakfast, lunch, dinner"). In previously unexposed individuals, bite sites appear as erythematous, pruritic macules. In sensitized individuals, intensely pruritic papules, papular urticaria, or vesicles/bullae may arise at the bite sites. Changes secondary to scratching include excoriations, eczematous dermatitis, and secondary infections.*

Fleas Papular pruritic urticaria (Fig. 24-1) at exposed bite site.

Tungiasis Papule or vesicle (6 to 8 mm in diameter) with central black dot produced by posterior part of the flea's abdominal segments. As eggs mature and abdomen swells, papule becomes a white, pea-sized nodule. With intralesional hemorrhage, it becomes black (Fig. 24-5). With severe infestation, nodules and plaques with a honeycombed appearance. If lesions are squeezed, eggs, feces, and internal organs are extruded through pore. Sites: feet, especially under toenails, between toes, plantar aspect of the feet, sparing weight-bearing areas; in sunbathers, any area of exposed skin.

Hymenoptera Stings by female bee, hornet, or wasp from modified ovipositor (stinger apparatus) produces immediate burning/pain, followed by intense, local, erythematous reaction with swelling and urticaria. Severe systemic reactions occur in .4 to .8% of individuals with angioedema/generalized urticaria and/or respiratory insufficiency from laryngeal edema or bronchospasm and/or shock. Fire ants and harvester ants produce local skin necrosis and systemic reactions to sting; bite reaction begins as an intense local inflammatory reaction that evolves to a sterile pustule.

Lepidoptera Contact with hairs of caterpillars/moths can produce burning/itching sensation, papular urticaria, irritation due to histamine release, allergic contact dermatitis, and/or systemic reactions. Wind-borne hairs can cause keratoconjunctivitis.

Systemic Findings

Systemic findings may occur associated with toxin or allergy to substance injected during bite. Many varied systemic infections can be injected during bite.

DIFFERENTIAL DIAGNOSIS

Bite Site Reactions (Erythematous Papules, Blisters) Allergic contact dermatitis, especially to plants such as poison ivy or poison oak.

Furuncular Myiasis/Tungiasis *Staphylococcus aureus* paronychia, *Candida* paronychia, cercarial dermatitis, scabies, fire ant bite, folliculitis.

Cutaneous Necrosis Necrotizing soft tissue infection, vascular insufficiency, adverse cutaneous drug reaction.

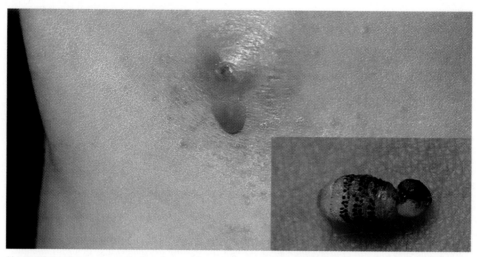

Figure 24-3   Furuncular myiasis   *A pruritic papule at the site of deposition of a botfly larva, slowly enlarging over several weeks into a domed nodule (resembles a furuncle). The lesion has a central pore through which the posterior end of the larva intermittently protrudes and thus respires. The larva (inset) can be induced to exit the lesion by occluding it with petrolatum or fat.*

LABORATORY EXAMINATIONS

Dermatopathology

Bite Site Reactions   In acute phase, variable epidermal necrosis, spongiosis, parakeratosis with plasma exudate; dermal inflammatory infiltrate extends into deep dermis in a wedge-shaped pattern, surrounding vessels with some extension into dermal collagen. The dermal infiltrate is mixed, composed of eosinophils, neutrophils, lymphocytes, and histiocytes. Eosinophils are usually prominent; neutrophils may predominate in reactions to fleas, mosquitoes, fire ants, and brown recluse spiders. Bullae forms secondary to marked edema. Insect parts are rarely seen except in scabies and in tick bites where removal is incomplete.

In chronic phase, lesions result from retained arthropod parts or hypersensitivity. Chronic lesions can appear as a pseudolymphoma.

Infection at Bite Site   In infestations such as leishmaniasis, the pathogen can be demonstrated in the lesional biopsy specimen by special stains.

Bacterial Culture   Rule out secondary infection with *S. aureus* or group A streptococcus (GAS). Rule out systemic infection.

Serology   Rule out systemic infection/infestation.

DIAGNOSIS

Clinical diagnosis, at times confirmed by lesional biopsy.

COURSE AND PROGNOSIS

Excoriation of CRAB commonly results in secondary infection of the eroded epidermis by GAS and/or *S. aureus* causing impetigo or ecthyma. This is especially common in humid tropical climates. Less common is secondary infection with *Corynebacterium diphtheriae,* with resultant cutaneous diphtheria. Streptococcal skin infections are, at times, complicated by glomerulonephritis.

MANAGEMENT

Prevention   Avoid contact with arthropods. Apply insect repellent such as diethyltoluamide (DEET) to skin. Apply permethrin spray (Permanone [USA]) to clothing. Use passive measures such as screens, nets, clothing. Treat flea-infested cats and dogs; spray household with insecticides (e.g., malathion, 1 to 4% dust) with special attention to baseboards, rugs, floors, upholstered furniture, bed frames, mattresses, and cellar.

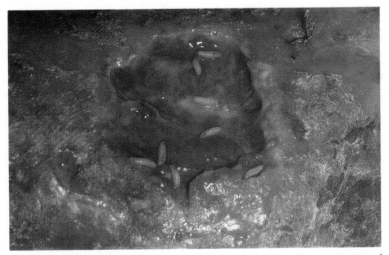

Figure 24-4 Wound myiasis *Multiple larvae or maggots of the housefly are seen in a chronic stasis ulcer on the ankle. The leg had been treated with Castellani's paint and Unna boot for 1 week. When the dressing was removed, the maggots were visible; the base of the ulcer was red and clean, having been debrided by the maggots.*

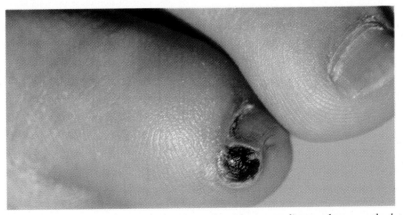

Figure 24-5 Tungiasis *A necrotic, periungual papule with surrounding erythema on the lateral margin of the fifth toe; the larva is visualized by removing the overlying crust.*

Larvae in Skin Tungiasis: remove flea with needle, scalpel, or curette, attempting to remove all flea parts; oral thiabendazole, (25 mg/kg/d) or albendazole (400 mg/d for 3 days), effective for heavy infestations. Furuncular myiasis: suffocate larvae by covering the larvae with vaseline; remove the following day when dead.

Glucocorticoids Potent topical glucocorticoids given for a short time are helpful for intensely pruritic lesions. In some cases, a short tapered course of oral glucocorticoids can be given for extensive CRAB that are persistent.

Antimicrobial Agents *Secondary Infection* Antibiotic treatment with topical agents such as mupirocin ointment or antistaphylococcal/antistreptococcal agents if secondary infection is present.

Systemic Infection/Infestation Treat with appropriate antimicrobial agent.

PEDICULOSIS

Two species of blood sucking lice of the order Anoplura have evolved to be obligate ectoparasites of humans: *Pediculus humanus* and *Phthirius pubis*. The two variants of *Pediculus,* the head louse and the body louse, are similar morphologically but distinct in ecologic niches on the body and the clinical manifestations of infestation. The body louse may have evolved from the head louse after humans began to wear clothes.

EPIDEMIOLOGY

Etiology *Pediculus humanus* var. *capitis* live on the head (head lice). *P. humanus* var. *corporis* live in clothing, benefiting from warmth and feeding on the body (body lice). *Phthirius pubis* (pubic or crab lice) lives in the pubic area as well as other hair-bearing areas. Lice are 1 to 3 mm long, are flattened dorsoventrally, and have three pairs of legs that end in powerful claws of a diameter adapted to the region colonized. The female lives for 1 to 3 months; it dies in <24 h when separated from the host (head lice). A female louse lays up to 300 eggs (nits) during her lifetime. Nits are <1 mm in diameter and, when viable, are opalescent. Nits are deposited on hair shafts emerging from the skin and hatch 6 to 10 days after laying, giving rise to nymphs that become adults in 10 days. Empty egg cases remain on the hair shaft after hatch; demonstration of empty egg cases away from the skin is not diagnostic of active infestation.

Incidence Hundreds of millions of cases worldwide annually.

Transmission Most commonly by direct contact between individuals or indirectly by contact with bedding, brushes, or clothing, according to species. Pediculosis and scabies may coexist in the same individual.

Body Lice Associated with poor socioeconomic conditions, when clothing is not changed or washed frequently: indigent, homeless, refugee-camp populations.

Pubic Lice Typically transmitted sexually, frequently coexisting with another STD. Nonsexual transmission occurs in homeless persons who have pubic lice in hair on head and back. In children, contracted from an infested parent and rarely sexually transmitted.

Associated Infections *Scabies, Head and Crab Lice* S. aureus and Group A Streptococcus: Excoriation may become secondarily infected. Infection can extend, resulting in cellulitis, lymphangitis, and/or bacteremia.

Body Lice Bartonella Quintana: Causes trench fever. Body lice are vector. Trench fever characterized by fever, myalgias, headache, meningoencephalitis, chronic lymphadenopathy, transient maculopapular eruption. Homeless chronic alcoholic persons at risk; may be complicated by endocarditis. In United States, 15% of homeless persons tested had *B. quintana* bacteremia. Rickettsia Prowazekii: Causes epidemic typhus. Large outbreaks (1995–1997) in Burundi, first affecting prison inmates, then >45,000 camp refugees. Small outbreak occurred in Russia in 1998. Characterized by fever, headache, rash, confusion. Brill-Zinsser disease is recrudescence of epidemic typhus fever occurring in mild forms years after primary infection.

SYMPTOMS

Pruritus occurs in a variable proportion. Excoriations can become secondarily infected.

DIAGNOSIS

Head Lice Demonstration of live adult lice, nymphs, or viable-appearing nits that are close to scalp, especially in hair above the ears. Detection combs may help. Dead nits are not diagnostic of active infection.

Pubic Lice Demonstration of live adult lice, nymphs, or nits in pubic area. Must carefully examine hair for nits as there may be only one or two. Also colonize other hairy areas, including axillae of adolescents, eyelashes of children, hair of head.

Body Lice Lice and eggs are found in clothing seams.

MANAGEMENT

Topically Applied Insecticides Ideally, should have 100% activity against louse and egg. Malathion kills all lice after 5 min of exposure, and more than 95% of eggs fail to hatch after 10 min of exposure. Synthetic pyrethroids, synergized pyrethrins, and malathion are most efficacious and safe. Lotion preparations are preferred; creams, foams, gels are also available. Shampoos should be avoided in that contact time is short, drug concentration low, insecticide penetration reduced when lice are immersed in water, and inappropriate applications favor emergence of resistance. The product should be applied to dry hair for various specified times in sufficient quantity; reapplication is recommended 7 to 10 days later.

Recommended Regimen

Permethrin or Pyrethrins Over-the-counter preparation include Nix, RID, A-200. Preparation applied to infested area(s) and washed off after 10 min. Not totally ovicidal, lacks residual activity; in that the incubation period of louse eggs is 6 to 10 days, should be reapplied in 7 to 14 days.

Malathion .5% in 78% isopropyl alcohol (Ovide). Applied to involved site for 8 to 12 h; binds to hair providing residual protection. Indicated in lindane-resistant cases. Should not be used in children younger than 6 months.

Alternative Regimen

Pyrethrins with Piperonyl Butoxide Applied to scalp and washed off after 10 min.

Lindane 1% shampoo applied for 4 min and then thoroughly washed off. (Not recommended for pregnant or lactating women.) Not totally ovicidal and lacks residual activity; in that the incubation period of louse eggs is 6 to 10 days, the agents should be reapplied in 7 to 14 days. Retreatment may be necessary if lice are found or eggs are observed at the hair-skin junction.

Ivermectin .8% lotion or shampoo.

Systemic Therapy *Oral Ivermectin* 200 μg/kg; repeat on day 10.

Acquired Resistance to Insecticides Occurs worldwide, mainly to pyrethrins and pyrethroids; also to malathion. If resistance is suspected, an alternative agent should be used. Other alternatives include newer insecticides and oral ivermectin in cases of resistance to both pyrethroids and malathion.

PEDICULOSIS CAPITIS

Pediculosis capitis is an infestation of the scalp by the head louse, which feeds on the scalp and neck and deposits its eggs on the hair; presence of head lice is associated with few symptoms but much consternation.

EPIDEMIOLOGY

Age of Onset More common in children age 3 to 11 years, but all ages.

Etiology The subspecies of *Pediculus humanus* var. *capitis*. Unlike *P. humanus* var. *corporis,* the head louse is not a vector of infectious diseases.

Predisposing Factors School-age children and their mothers. Promiscuity, age, sex (female >males), hair traits (color, quantitity). More common in warmer months. In United States, more common in whites than blacks; claws have adapted to grip cylindrical hair. In Africa, pediculosis capitis is relatively uncommon; however, lice easily grip non-cylindrical hair.

Transmission Shared hats, caps, brushes, combs; head-to-head contact. Epidemics in schools; classrooms are the main source of infestations. Head lice can survive off the scalp for up to 55 h.

Incidence The most common pediculosis. Estimated that 6 to 12 million people in the United States are infested annually. Bordeaux, France: up to 49% of schoolchildren. Jerusalem, Israel: 20% in 1991. Bristol, UK: 25% in 1998. Ilorin, Nigeria: 3.7% in 1987.

HISTORY

Skin Symptoms   Children said to be distracted, restless, and inattentive at school. Pruritus of the back and sides of scalp. Scratching and secondary infection associated with occipital and/or cervical lymphadenopathy.

PHYSICAL EXAMINATION

Skin Findings   *Head lice* are identified with eye or with hand lens but are difficult to find. Most patients have a population of <10 head lice. Nits are the oval grayish-white egg capsules (1 mm long) firmly cemented to the hairs (Fig. 24-6); vary in number from only a few to thousands. Nits are deposited by head lice on the hair shaft as it emerges from the follicle. With recent infestation, nits are near the scalp; with infestation of long standing, nits may be 10 to 15 cm from the scalp. In that scalp hair grows .5 mm daily, the presence of nits 15 cm from the scalp indicates that the infestation is approximately 9 months old. New viable eggs have a creamy-yellow color; empty eggshells are white.
Eczema and lichen simplex chronicus occur on the occipital scalp and neck secondary to chronic scratching and rubbing. *Excoriations, crusts, and secondarily impetiginized lesions* are seen commonly and mask the presence of lice and nits; may extend onto neck, forehead, face, ears. In the extreme, scalp becomes a confluent, purulent mass of matted hair, lice, nits, crusts, and purulent discharge. Papular urticaria occur at site of the lice bite, sometimes apparent on neck.

Sites of Predilection   Head lice nearly always confined to scalp, especially occipital and postauricular regions. Rarely, head lice infest beard or other hairy sites. Although more common with crab lice, head lice also can infest the eyelashes (pediculosis palpebrarum).

Wood's Lamp   Live nits fluoresce with a pearly fluorescence; dead nits do not.

Regional Lymph Nodes   Postoccipital lymphadenopathy secondary to impetiginization of excoriated sites.

DIFFERENTIAL DIAGNOSIS

Small White Hair "Beads"   Hair casts, hair lacquer, hair gels, dandruff (epidermal scales).

Scalp Pruritus   Impetigo, lichen simplex chronicus.

LABORATORY EXAMINATIONS

Microscopy   The louse or a nit on a hair shaft (Fig. 24-7) can be examined to confirm the gross examination of the scalp and hair.

Nits   .5-mm oval, whitish eggs. Nonviable nits show an absence of an embryo or operulum.

Louse   Insect with six legs, 1 to 4 mm in length, wingless, translucent grayish-white body that is red when engorged with blood.

Culture   If impetiginization is suspected, bacterial cultures should be obtained.

DIAGNOSIS

Clinical findings, confirmed by detection of nits and/or lice.

MANAGEMENT

Prevention   Avoid contact with possibly contaminated items such as hats, headsets, clothing, towels, combs, hair brushes, bedding, upholstery. The environment should be vacuumed. Bedding, clothing, and head gear should be washed and dried on the hot cycle of a dryer. Combs and brushes should be soaked in rubbing alcohol or Lysol 2% solution for 1 h. Families should look for lice routinely. Many schools in the United States adhere to a "no-nit" policy before children can return after infestation.

Contacts   All children and adults in the household should be examined. All infested individuals should be treated. Clothing, bedding, and fomites should be machine-washed. Other items (brushes, combs, pillow, mattresses, and toys) can be decontaminated with insecticidal powders.

Pediculocide Therapy   See Pediculosis, page 827.

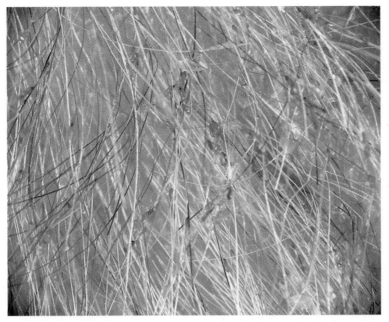

Figure 24-6   Pediculosis capitis: multiple nits on scalp hair   *Myriads of nits (oval, grayish-white egg capsules) are firmly attached to the hair shafts, visualized with a lens. On close examination these have a bottle shape.*

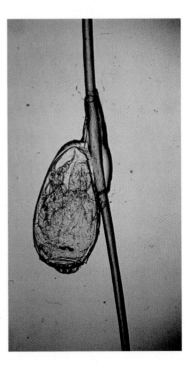

Figure 24-7   Pediculosis capitis: nit on hair shaft   *Under a microscope, an egg with a developing head louse, attached to a hair shaft, is seen.*

Causes of Therapeutic Failure Misunderstanding of instructions; noncompliance; inappropriate instructions on head-lice products or from health professionals; high cost of products; misdiagnosis; psychogenic itch; incomplete ovicidal activity; inappropriate preparation (e.g., shampoo); insufficient dose-time, frequency, and/or quantity of product applied; failure to retreat; reinfestation; live eggs not removed; acquired resistance to insecticides.

Removal of Nits After treatment and neutral shampoo, the hair is wet-combed with a fine-toothed comb to remove nits. Complete nit removal depends on comb structure, duration/ technique of combing, and thoroughness. Overnight application of petroleum jelly or HairClean 1-2-3 may facilitate removal of nits.

Pediculosis Palpebrarum Apply petrolatum to lashes twice daily for 8 days, followed by removal of nits, *or* physostigmine ophthalmic preparations applied twice daily for 1 or 2 days.

Secondary Bacterial Infection Should be treated with appropriate doses of erythromycin *or* dicloxacillin *or* cephalexin.

PEDICULOSIS PUBIS (PHTHIRIASIS)

Pediculosis pubis is an infestation of hair-bearing regions, most commonly the pubic area; but at times the hairy parts of the chest and axillae and the upper eyelashes. It is manifested clinically by mild to moderate pruritus, papular urticaria, and excoriations.
Synonyms: Crabs, crab lice, pubic lice.

EPIDEMIOLOGY

Age of Onset Most common in young adults; range from childhood to senescence.

Sex More extensive infestation in males.

Etiology *Phthirus pubis,* the crab or pubic louse. The life cycle from egg to adult is 22 to 27 days; the incubation period for the egg is 7 to 8 days; the rest of the life cycle is taken up with larval and nymphal development. The average life span is 17 days for the female and 22 days for the male. Lives exclusively on humans. Prefers a humid environment; tends not to wander.

Transmission Close physical contact such as sexual intercourse; sleeping in same bed; possibly exchange of towels.

HISTORY

Skin Symptoms May be asymptomatic. Mild to moderate pruritus for months. Patient may detect a nodularity to hairs (nits or eggs) while scratching. With excoriation and secondary infection, lesions may become tender and be associated with enlarged regional, e.g., inguinal, lymph node.

PHYSICAL EXAMINATION

Skin Findings *Lice* appear as 1- to 2-mm, brownish-gray specks (Figs. 24-8 and 24-9) in the hairy areas involved. Remain stationary for days; mouth parts embedded in skin; claws grasping a hair on either side. Usually few in number. *Eggs (nits)* attached to hair appear as tiny white-gray specks (Fig. 24-9). Few to numerous. Eggs found at hair-skin junction indicate active infestation.
Papular urticaria, (small erythematous papules) at sites of feeding, especially periumbilical (Fig. 24-10); rarely, feeding sites may become bullous. Secondary changes of *lichenification, excoriations,* and *impetiginized excoriations* detected in patients with significant pruritus. Serous crusts may be present along with lice and nits when eyelids are infested; occasionally, edema of eyelids with severe infestation. *Maculae cerulea (taches bleues)* are slate-gray or bluish-gray macules .5 to 1 cm in diameter, irregular in shape, nonblanching. Pigment thought to be breakdown product of heme affected by louse saliva.

Distribution Most common in pubic and axillary areas; also, perineum, thighs, lower legs, trunk, especially periumbilical (Fig. 24-10). In hairy males: nipple areas, upper arms, rarely wrists; rarely, beard and moustache area. In

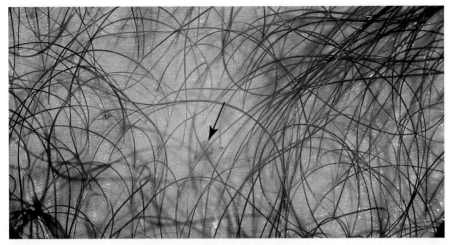

Figure 24-8 Pediculosis pubis: crab louse in pubis *A crab louse (arrow) on the skin in the pubic region.*

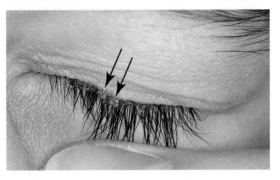

Figure 24-9 Pediculosis pubis: crab lice in eyelashes of a child *Crab lice (arrows) and nits on the upper eyelashes of a child; this was the only site of infestation.*

children, eyelashes (Fig. 24-9) and eyebrows may be infested without pubic involvement. *M. cerulea* most common on lower abdominal wall, buttocks, upper thighs.

General Findings With secondary impetiginization, regional lymphadenopathy.

DIFFERENTIAL DIAGNOSIS

Pruritic Dermatosis Eczema, seborrheic dermatitis, tinea cruris, folliculitis, molluscum contagiosum, scabies.

Tache Bleuâtres Ashy dermatosis.

LABORATORY EXAMINATIONS

Microscopy Lice (Fig. 24-11) and nits may be identified with hand lens or microscope.

Cultures Bacterial cultures if excoriation impetiginized.

Serology Sexually transmitted. Testing for other STDs may be indicated in some individuals.

DIAGNOSIS

Clinical diagnosis with demonstration of lice and/or viable nits.

COURSE AND PROGNOSIS

Patients should be evaluated after 1 week if symptoms persist. Retreatment may be necessary if lice are found or if eggs are observed at hair-skin junction. Patients not responding to one regimen should be retreated with an alternative.

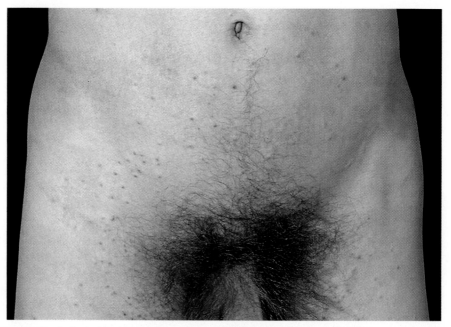

Figure 24-10 Pediculosis pubis: papular urticaria *At this magnification only inflammatory papules (sites of crab lice bites), which are extremely pruritic, are seen on the abdomen and the inner aspects of the thighs. Closer examination reveals nits on the pubic hairs.*

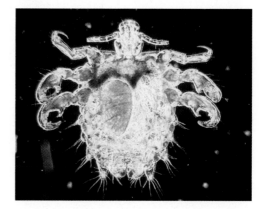

Figure 24-11 Pediculosis pubis: adult female *Under a microscope, a female crab louse containing an egg is seen suspended in mineral oil.*

MANAGEMENT

Prevention Patient and sexual partners should be treated.

Topical Insecticides The hair of the head/beard should be treated as well as pubic, axillary, and other body hair.

Pediculocides See Pediculosis, page 826.

Infestation of Eyelids 1% Permethrin or vaseline if infestation is present.

Decontamination of Environment Bedding and clothing should be decontaminated (machine-washed or machine-dried using heat cycle or dry-cleaned) or removed from body contact for at least 72 h.

Management of Sex Partner(s) Sex partners within last month should be treated. Screening for other STDs may be indicated.

INSECT BITES AND INFESTATIONS

Pediculosis Corporis

Pediculus humanus var. corporis (body louse) and nits are seen in the seams of clothing, where they live (Fig. 24-12, inset); may also live in bedding. Visits the human host only to feed. The host invariably has very poor hygiene. Sites of feeding may present as red macules, papules, or papular urticaria with central hemorrhagic punctum. Because of the associated pruritus, primary lesions are commonly scratched, resulting in excoriations, eczematous dermatitis, and lichen simplex chronicus, which, in turn, can become secondarily infected (Fig. 24-12). Diagnosis is made by demonstration of lice/eggs in clothing (Fig. 24-12, inset). In management, bedding and clothing must be systematically decontaminated. Washing the body with soap followed by application of pyrethrins/pyrethroids or malathion for 8 to 24 h is recommended in some cases. Outbreaks necessitate delousing of individuals with 1% permethrin dusting powder, basic sanitation measures, and hygiene measures to assure changes of clean clothing, body washing, and sometimes shaving. Antibiotics are indicated if louse-borne infectious disease (trench fever, epidemic typhus) exists.

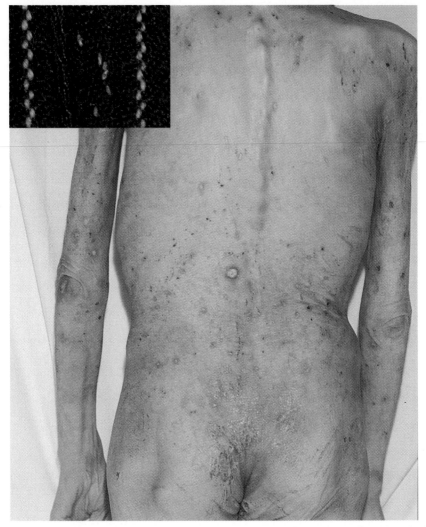

Figure 24-12 Pediculosis corporis *Severely malnourished, ill-kept, homeless male with multiple excoriations, erosions and crusted papules and nodules and eczematized lesions. Lice and nits are seen in the seams of clothing (inset).*

SCABIES

Scabies is an infestation by the mite *Sarcoptes scabiei,* usually spread by skin-to-skin contact, and characterized by generalized intractable pruritus often with minimal cutaneous findings. The diagnosis may be missed easily and should be considered in a patient of any age with persistent generalized severe pruritus.

Synonym: Chronic undiagnosed scabies is the basis for the colloquial expression, "the 7-year itch."

EPIDEMIOLOGY

Etiology *S. scabiei* var. *hominis*. Thrive and multiply only on human skin. Mites of all developmental stages burrow/tunnel into epidermis shortly after contact, not deeper than stratum granulosum; deposit feces in tunnels. Females lay eggs in tunnels. Burrow 2 to 3 mm daily. Usually burrow at night and lay eggs during the day. The female lives 4 to 6 weeks, laying 40 to 50 eggs. Eggs hatch after 72 to 96 h. In classic scabies, about a dozen females per patient are present. In hyperkeratotic or crusted scabies, >1 million mites may be present or up to 4700 mites/g skin.

Age of Onset Young adults (usually acquired by body contact); elderly and bedridden patients in the hospital (contact with mite-infested sheets); children (often 5 years or younger). Nodular scabies more common in children.

Incidence Estimated at 300 million cases in the world each year. In the past, epidemics occur in cycles every 15 years; the latest epidemic began in the late 1960s but has continued to the present.

Geography Scabies is a major public health problem in many less-developed countries. In some areas of South and Central America, prevalence is about 100%. In Bangladesh, the number of children with scabies exceeds that of children with diarrheal and upper-respiratory disease. In countries where human T cell leukemia/lymphoma virus (HTLV-I) infection is common, generalized crusted scabies is a marker of this infection, including cases of adult T cell leukemia/lymphoma.

Transmission Mites transmitted by skin-to-skin contact as with sex partner, children playing, or health care workers providing care. Mites can remain alive for longer than 2 days on clothing or in bedding; and, therefore, scabies can be acquired without skin-to-skin contact. Patients with crusted scabies shed many mites into their environment daily and pose a high risk of infecting those around them, including health care professionals.

Risk Factors In nursing homes, risk factors include age of institution (>30 years), size of institution (>120 beds), ratio of beds to health care workers (<10:1).

PATHOGENESIS

Hypersensitivity of both immediate and delayed types occur in the development of lesions other than burrows. For pruritus to occur, sensitization to *S. scabiei* must take place. Among persons with their first infection, sensitization takes several weeks to develop; after reinfestation, pruritus may occur within 24 h. Various immunocompromised states or individuals with neurologic disease predisposed to crusted Norwegian scabies. Infestation is usually by only approximately 10 mites. In contrast, the number of infesting mites in crusted scabies may exceed a million.

HISTORY

Patients are often aware of similar symptoms in family members or sexual partners. Patients with crusted scabies usually are immunocompromised (HIV disease, organ transplant recipient) or have neurologic disorders (Down's syndrome, dementia, strokes, spinal cord injury, neuropathy, leprosy).

Incubation Period Onset of pruritus varies with immunity to the mite: first infestation, about 21 days; reinfestation, immediate, i.e., 1 to 3 days.

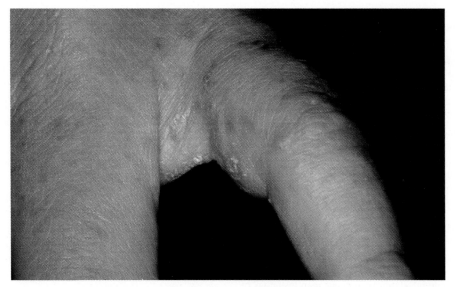

Figure 24-13 Scabies *Papules and burrows in typical location on the finger webs. Burrows are tan or skin-colored ridges with linear configuration with a minute vesicle or papule at the end of the burrow; they are often difficult to locate.*

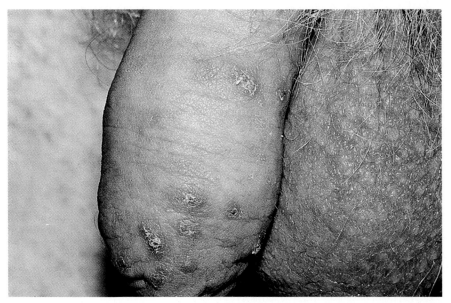

Figure 24-14 Scabies *Multiple, crusted, and excoriated papules and burrows on the penile shaft.*

Duration of Lesions Weeks to months unless treated. Crusted scabies may be present for years.

Skin Symptoms *Pruritus* Intense, widespread, usually sparing head and neck. Itching often interferes with or prevents sleep. Often present in family members. Half of patients with crusted scabies do not itch.

Rash Ranges from no rash to generalized erythroderma. Patients with atopic diathesis scratch, producing eczematous dermatitis. Other individuals experience pruritus for many months with no rash. Tenderness of lesions suggests secondary bacterial infection.

PHYSICAL EXAMINATION

Skin Findings Common cutaneous findings can be classified: lesions occurring at the sites of mite infestation, cutaneous manifestations of hypersensitivity to mite, lesions secondary to chronic rubbing and scratching, secondary infection. Variants of scabies in special hosts including those with an atopic diathesis, nodular scabies, scabies in infants/small children, scabies in the elderly, crusted (Norwegian) scabies, scabies in HIV disease, animal transmitted scabies (zoonosis), scabies of the scalp, dyshidrosiform scabies, urticarial/vasculitis scabies, and bullous scabies.

Lesions at Site of Infestation

Intraepidermal Burrows Gray or skin-colored ridges, .5 to 1 cm in length (Figs. 24-13 and 24-14), either linear or wavy (serpiginous), with minute vesicle or papule at end of tunnel. Each infesting female mite produces one burrow. Mites are about .5 mm in length. Burrows average 5 mm in length but may be up to 10 cm. In light-skinned individuals, burrows have a whitish color with occasional darks specks (due to fecal scybala). Fountain-pen ink applied to infested skin concentrates in tunnels, highlighting and marking the burrow. Blind end of burrow where mite resides appears as a minute elevation with tiny halo of erythema or as a vesicle.

Distribution Areas with few or no hair follicles, usually where stratum corneum is thin and soft, i.e., interdigital webs of hands > wrists > shaft of penis > elbows > feet (Fig. 25-15) > genitalia > buttocks > axillae > elsewhere (Fig. 24-I.) In infants, infestation may occur on head and neck.

Scabietic (Scabious) Nodule Inflammatory papule or nodule (Fig. 24-16); burrow sometimes seen on the surface of a very early lesion.

Hyperkeratosis/Crusting Psoriasiform In areas of heavily infested crusted scabies, well-demarcated plaques covered by a very thick crust or scale. Warty dermatosis of hands/feet with nail bed hyperkeratosis. Erythematous scaling eruption on face, neck, scalp, trunk.

Cutaneous Manifestations of Hypersensitivity to Mite

Pruritus Some individuals experience only pruritus without any cutaneous findings.

"Id" or Autosensitization-Type Reactions Characterized by widespread small urticarial edematous papules mainly on anterior trunk, thighs, buttocks, and forearms.

Urticaria Usually generalized.

Eczematous Dermatitis At sites of heaviest infestation: hands, axillae.

Lesions Secondary to Chronic Rubbing and Scratching Excoriation, lichen simplex chronicus, prurigo nodules. Generalized eczematous dermatitis. Erythroderma.

Atopy In individuals with atopic diathesis, atopic dermatitis occurs at sites of excoriation, most commonly on the hands, webspaces of hands, wrists, axillae, areolae, waist, buttocks, penis, scrotum. In adults, the scalp, face, and upper back are usually spared; but in infants, the scalp, face, palms, and soles are involved.

Postinflammatory hyper- and hypopigmentation Especially in more deeply pigmented individuals.

Secondary Infection

S. aureus or Group A Steptococcus Infection (Fig. 24-17) Impetiginized excoriations (crusted, tender, surrounding erythema), ecthyma, folliculitis, abscess formation; lymphangitis, lymphadenitis; cellulitis; bacteremia, septicemia. Acute post-streptococcal glomerulonephritis has been reported associated with streptococcal impetiginization of scabies.

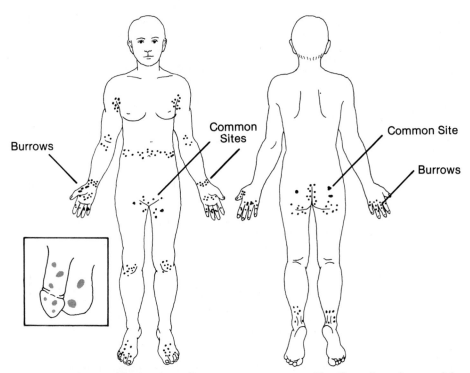

Figure 24-I   Scabies: Predilection sites   *Burrows are most easy to identify on the webspace of the hands, wrists, lateral aspects of the palms. Scabietic nodules occur uncommonly, arising on the genitalia, especially the penis and scrotum, waist, axillae, and areolae.*

Variants of Scabies in Special Hosts

Infants/Young Children Atypical lesions: vesicles, pustules, nodules; generalized; lesions concentrated on hands/feet/body folds. Head, palms, soles are not spared. Difficult to differentiate from infantile acropustulosis, which may be a post-scabietic nonspecific reaction.

Elderly Altered inflammatory response may delay diagnosis. In bedridden patients, lesions may be concentrated on the back. Bullous scabies can mimic bullous pemphigoid.

Nodular Scabies Nodular lesions develop in 7 to 10% of patients with scabies. Nodules are 5 to 20 mm in diameter, red, pink, tan, or brown in color, smooth (Fig. 24-16). A burrow may be seen on the surface of early nodule.

Distribution Penis, scrotum, axillae, waist, buttocks, areolae. Resolve with postinflammatory hyperpigmentation. May be more apparent after treatment, as eczematous eruption resolves. Upper back, lateral edge of foot (infants). Nodules are usually countable.

Crusted or Norwegian Scabies Predisposing factors: glucocorticoid therapy, Down's syndrome, HIV disease, HTLV-I infection, organ transplant recipients, elderly. May begin as ordinary scabies. In others, clinical appearance is of chronic eczema, psoriasiform dermatitis (Fig. 24-17), seborrheic dermatitis, or erythroderma. Lesions often markedly hyperkeratotic and/or crusted.

Distribution Generalized (even involving head and neck in adults) or localized. Scale/crusts found on dorsal surface of hands, wrists, fingers, metacarpophalangeal joints, palms, extensor aspect of elbows, scalp, ears, soles, and toes. In patients with neurologic deficit, crusted scabies may occur only in affected limb. May be localized only to scalp, face, finger, toenail bed, or sole.

General Findings Lymphadenopathy in some cases.

DIFFERENTIAL DIAGNOSIS

Pruritus, Localized or Generalized, Rash Adverse cutaneous drug reaction, atopic dermatitis, contact dermatitis, fiberglass dermatitis, dyshidrotic eczema, dermatographism, physical urticaria, pityriasis rosea, dermatitis herpetiformis, animal scabies, pediculosis corporis, pediculosis pubis, lichen planus, delusions of parasitosis, metabolic pruritus.

Pyoderma Impetigo, ecthyma, furunculosis.

Nodular Scabies Urticaria pigmentosa (in young child), papular urticaria (insect bites), Darier's disease, prurigo nodularis, secondary syphilis, pseudolymphoma, lymphomatoid papulosis, vasculitis.

Crusted Scabies Psoriasis, eczematous dermatitis, seborrheic dermatitis, erythroderma, Langerhans cell histiocytosis.

LABORATORY EXAMINATIONS

Microscopy

Finding the Mite A healthy adult with scabies has an average of 6 to 12 adult mites infesting the body. The highest yield in identifying a mite is in typical burrows on the finger webs, flexor aspects of wrists, and penis. A drop of mineral oil is placed over a burrow, and the burrow is scraped off with a no. 15 scalpel blade and placed on a microscope slide.

Conventional Microscopy A drop immersion of mineral oil is placed on the scraping, which is then covered by a coverslip. Three findings are diagnostic of scabies: *S. scabiei* mites, their eggs, and their fecal pellets (scybala) (Fig. 24-18).

Epiluminescence Microscopy Characteristic image of scabies, "jet-with-contrail" image.

Dermatopathology *Scabietic burrow:* located within stratum corneum; female mite situated in blind end of burrow. Body round, 400 μm in length. Spongiosis near mite with vesicle formation common. Eggs also seen. Dermis shows infiltrate with eosinophils. *Scabietic nodules:* dense chronic inflammatory infiltrate with eosinophils. In some cases, persistent arthropod reaction resembling lymphoma with atypical mononuclear cells. *Crusted scabies:* thickened stratum corneum riddled with innumerable mites.

Hematology Eosinophilia in crusted scabies.

Cultures *S. aureus* and group A streptococcus cause secondary infection.

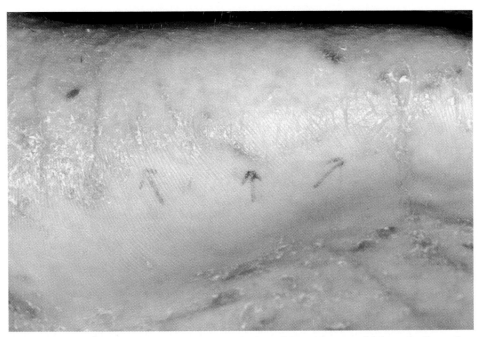

Figure 24-15 Scabies *Papules and burrows on the lateral foot; in young children, the feet and neck are often infested, sites usually spared in older individuals. In this adult case, there was massive infestation of the foot.*

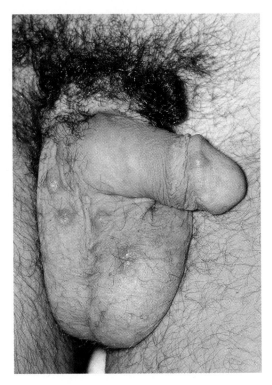

Figure 24-16 Scabietic nodules *Red-brown papules and nodules on the penis and scrotum; these lesions are pathognomonic for scabies, occurring at sites of infestation in some individuals.*

DIAGNOSIS

Clinical findings, confirmed, if possible, by microscopy (identification of mites, eggs, or mite feces). Assiduous search for burrows or papules should be made in every patient with severe generalized pruritus. Sometimes when the mite cannot be demonstrated, a "therapeutic test" will clinch the diagnosis.

COURSE AND PROGNOSIS

Pruritus Often persists up to several weeks after successful eradication of mite infestation, understandable in that the pruritus is a hypersensitivity phenomenon to mite antigen(s). If reinfestation recurs, pruritus becomes symptomatic within a few days. Most cases resolve after recommended regimen of therapy. Glomerulonephritis has followed group A streptococcal secondary infection. Bacteremia and death have followed secondary *S. aureus* infection of crusted scabies in an HIV-infected patient. Delusions of parasitosis can occur in individuals who have been successfully treated for scabies or have never had scabies.

Crusted Scabies May be impossible to eradicate in HIV-infected individuals. Recurrence more likely to be relapse than reinfestation.

Nodular Scabies In treated patients, 80% resolve in 3 months, but may persist up to 1 year.

MANAGEMENT

Principles of Treatment Infested individuals and close physical contacts should be treated at the same time, whether or not symptoms are present. Topical agents are more effective after hydration of the skin, i.e., after bathing. Application should be to all skin sites, especially the groin, around nails, behind ears, including face and scalp. Sexual partners and close personal or household contacts within last month should be examined and treated prophylactically.

Scabicides Choice of scabicide based on effectiveness, potential toxicity, cost, extent of secondary eczematization, and age of patient. Permethrin is effective and safe but costs more than lindane. Lindane is effective in most areas of the world, but resistance has been reported. Seizures have occurred when lindane was applied after a bath or used by patients with extensive dermatitis. Aplastic anemia after lindane use was also reported. No controlled studies have confirmed that two applications are better than one. Clean clothing should be put on afterwards. Clothing and bedding are decontaminated by machine-washing at 60°C. Pruritus can persist for up to 1 to 2 weeks after the end of effective therapy. After that time, cause of persistent itching should be investigated.

Recommended Regimens

Permethrin 5% Cream Applied to all areas of the body from the neck down. Wash off 8–12 h after application. Adverse events very low.

Lindane (g-Benzene Hexachloride) 1% Lotion or Cream Applied thinly to all areas of the body from the neck down; wash off thoroughly after 8 h. *Note:* Lindane should not be used after a bath or shower, and it should not be used by persons with extensive dermatitis, pregnant or lactating women, and children younger than 2 years. Mite resistance to lindane has developed in North, Central, and South America and Asia. Low cost makes lindane a key alternative in many countries.

Alternative Regimens

Crotamiton 10% Cream Applied thinly to the entire body from the neck down, nightly for 2 consecutive nights; wash off 24 h after second application.

Sulfur 2 to 10% in Petrolatum Applied to skin for 2 to 3 days.

Benzyl Benzoate 10 and 25% Lotions Several regimens are recommended: swabbing only once; two applications separated by 10 min, or two applications with a 24-h or 1-week interval. 24 h after application, preparation should be washed off and clothes and bedding changed. The compound is an irritant and can induce pruritic irritant dermatitis, especially on face and genitalia.

Benzyl Benzoate with Sulfiram Several regimens are recommended: swabbing only once:

Esdepallethrine .63%
Malathion .5% lotion
Sulfiram 25% lotion Can mimic effect of disulfiram; no alcoholic drinks should be consumed for at least 48 h.
Ivermectin .8% lotion

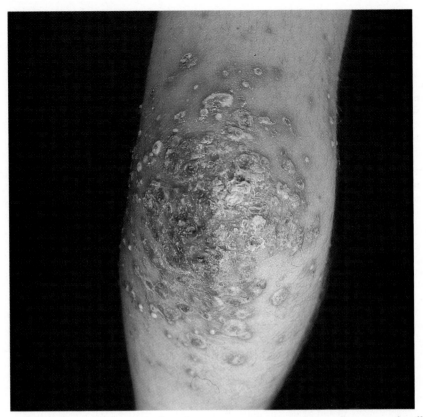

Figure 24-17 Crusted scabies *Crusted erythematous papules becoming confluent over the elbow; numerous pustules are seen associated with secondary* S. aureus *infection.*

Systemic Ivermectin Ivermectin, 200 μg/kg PO; single dose reported to be very effective for common as well as crusted scabies in 15 to 30 days. Two to three doses, separated by 1 to 2 weeks, usually required for heavy infestation or in immunocompromised individuals. May effectively eradicate epidemic or endemic scabies in institutions such as nursing homes, hospitals, and refugee camps. Not approved by USFDA or European Drug Agency.

Infants, Young Children, Pregnant/Lactating Women Permethrin or crotamiton regimens or precipitated sulfur ointment should be used with application to all body areas. Lindane and ivermectin should not be used.

Crusted Scabies *Scabicides* Lindane should be avoided because of risk of CNS toxicity. Multiple scabicide applications are required to all the skin. Treatment also should also be directed at removing scale/crusts that protect mites from scabicide; nails should be trimmed. Oral ivermectin combined with topical therapy is most effective. Control of dissemination is essential and includes isolation of patient, avoidance of skin-to-skin contact, use of gloves/gowns by staff, prophylactic treatment of contacts (entire institution and visitors or family members).

Decontamination of Environment Bedding, clothing, and towels should be decontaminated (machine washed or machine dried using heat cycle or dry-cleaned) or removed from body contact for at least 72 hours. Thorough cleaning of patient's room or residence.

Treatment of Eczematous Dermatitis *Antihistamines* Systemic sedating antihistamine such as hydroxyzine hydrochloride, doxepin, or diphenhydramine at bedtime.

Topical Glucocorticoid Ointment Applied to areas of extensive dermatitis associated with scabies.

Systemic Glucocorticoids Prednisone 70 mg, tapered over 1 to 2 weeks, gives symptomatic relief of severe hypersensitivity reaction.

Postscabietic Itching Generalized itching that persists a week or more is probably caused by hypersensitivity to remaining dead mites and mite products. Nevertheless, a second treatment 7 days after the first is recommended by some physicians. For severe, persistent pruritus, especially in individuals with history of atopic disorders, a 14-day tapered course of prednisone (70 mg on day 1) is indicated.

Secondary Bacterial Infection Treat with mupirocin ointment or systemic antimicrobial agent.

Scabietic Nodules May persist in association with pruritus for up to a year after eradication of infestation. Intralesional triamcinolone, 5 to 10 mg/ml into each lesion, is effective; repeat every 2 weeks if necessary.

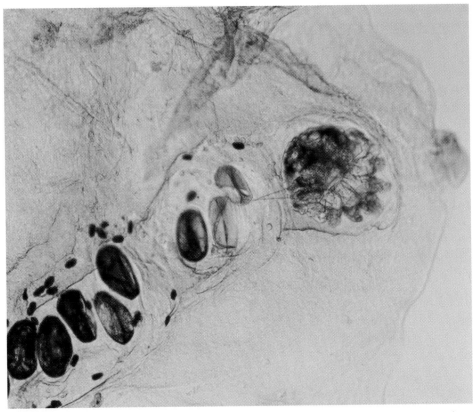

Figure 24-18 Burrow with Sarcoptes scabiei (female), eggs, and feces *Under a microscope, a mite at the end of a burrow with eight eggs and smaller fecal particles obtained from a papule on the webspace of the hand.*

CUTANEOUS LARVA MIGRANS

Cutaneous larva migrans (CLM) is a cutaneous lesion produced by percutaneous penetration and migration of larvae of various nematode parasites, characterized by erythematous, serpiginous, papular, or vesicular linear lesions corresponding to the movements of the larvae beneath the skin.

Synonyms: Creeping eruption, creeping verminous dermatitis, sandworm eruption, plumber's itch, duckhunter's itch.

EPIDEMIOLOGY

Etiology (see Table 24-1)

CLM Most common cause of *Ancylostoma braziliense* in central and southeastern United States. Other penetrating nematode larvae: *A. caninum, Uncinaria stenocephala* (hookworm of European dogs), *Bunostomum phlebotomum* (hookworm of cattle).

Larva Currens Filariform larvae of *Strongyloides stercoralis* can penetrate skin (usually on buttocks), producing similar lesions, i.e., *larva currens*.

Other Migrating Cutaneous Parasitic Infestations Other parasites (*Gnathostoma spinigerum, Strongyloides procyonis, Dirofilaria repens, Fasciola hepatica*) and some forms of myiasis can cause migratory skin lesions.

Epidemiology Ova of hookworms are deposited in sand and soil in warm, shady areas, hatching into larvae that penetrate human skin. Activities and occupations that pose risk include contact with sand/soil contaminated with animal feces: playing in sandbox, walking barefoot or sitting on beach, working in crawl spaces under houses, gardeners and plumbers, farmers, electricians, carpenters, pest exterminators.

Geographic Distribution Tropical and subtropical areas, especially southeastern United States, Caribbean, Africa, Central/South America, Southeast Asia.

PATHOGENESIS

Humans are aberrant, dead-end hosts who acquire the parasite from environment contaminated with animal feces. Larvae remain viable in soil/sand for several weeks. Third-stage larvae penetrate human skin and migrate up to several centimeters a day, usually between stratum germinativum and stratum corneum. Parasite induces localized eosinophilic inflammatory reaction. Most larvae are unable to develop further or invade deeper tissues and die after days or months.

HISTORY

Incubation Period 1 to 6 days from time of exposure to onset of symptoms.

Skin Symptoms Local pruritus begins within hours after larval penetration.

PHYSICAL EXAMINATION

Skin Lesions Serpiginous, thin, linear, raised, tunnel-like lesion 2 to 3 mm wide containing serous fluid (Fig. 24-19). Several or many lesions may be present depending on the number of penetrating larvae. Larvae move a few to many millimeters daily, confined to an area several centimeters in diameter. If multiple larvae are present, multiple tracts are seen.

Distribution Exposed sites, most commonly the feet, lower legs, buttocks, hands.

Variant *Larva Currens* Caused by *S. stercoralis*. Papules, urticaria, papulovesicles at the site of larval penetration (Fig. 24-20). Associated with intense pruritus. Occurs on skin around anus, buttocks, thighs, back, shoulders, abdomen. Pruritus and eruption disappear when larvae enter blood vessels and migrate to intestinal mucosa.

Systemic Findings Visceral larva migrans characterized by persistent hypereosinophilia, hepatomegaly, and frequently pneumonitis. Caused by *Toxocara canis, T. cati, A. lumbricoides.*

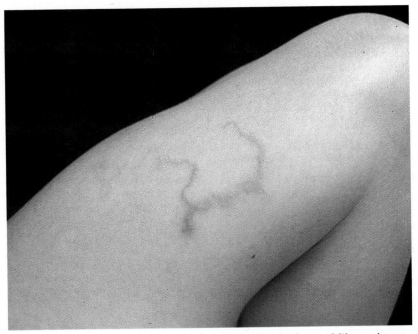

Figure 24-19 Cutaneous larva migrans *A serpiginous, linear, raised, tunnel-like erythematous lesion outlining the path of migration of the larva. Upon palpation, it feels like a thread within the superficial layers of the skin.*

Table 24-1 HELMINTHIC CAUSES OF MIGRATORY DERMATOLOGIC LESIONS

Infestation	Helminth(s)	Comments
Cutaneous larva migrans	Primarily *Ancylostoma braziliense* and *A. caninum*	Larvae of dog/cat hookworms
Dracunculiasis	*Dracunculus medinensis*	Movement of worm just below dermis before eruption
Fascioliasis	*Fasciola hepatica* and *F. gigantica*	Migratory areas of inflammation, especially with *F. gigantica*
Gnathostomiasis	*Gnathostoma spinigerum* and other *Gnathostoma* species	Migratory inflammatory lesions, 1 cm/h or faster when subcutaneous
Hookworm	*Ancylostoma duodenale, Necator americanus, A. ceylanicum*	
Loiasis	*Loa loa*	Migratory inflammatory swellings; worm may be visible crossing conjunctivae
Paragonimiasis	Primarily *Paragonimus westermani*	Subcutaneous migratory swelling or subcutaneous nodules
Sparganosis	*Spirometra erinaceri, S. mansoni, S. mansonides, S. proliferum*	
Strongyloidiasis	*Strongyloides stercoralis*	Migratory, serpiginous lesions (larva currens), 5–10 cm/h

DIFFERENTIAL DIAGNOSIS

Curvilinear Inflammatory Lesion Larva currens, migratory lesions from other parasites, phytoallergic contact dermatitis, phytophotodermatitis, erythema migrans of Lyme borreliosis, jelly fish sting, bullous impetigo, epidermal dermatophytosis, granuloma annulare, scabies, loiasis.

LABORATORY EXAMINATIONS

Hematology Peripheral eosinophilia.

Dermatopathology Part of the parasite can be seen on biopsy specimens from the advancing point of the lesion(s).

DIAGNOSIS

Clinical findings.

COURSE

Self-limited; humans are "dead-end" hosts. Most larvae die and the lesions resolve within 2 to 8 weeks; rarely, up to 2 years.

MANAGEMENT

Prevention Avoid direct skin contact with fecally contaminated soil.

Symptomatic Therapy Topical application of a glucocorticoid preparation under occlusion to lesion.

Anthelmintic Agents

Topical Agents Thiabendazole, ivermectin, albendazole are effective topically.

Systemic Agents Thiabendazole, orally 50 mg/kg/d in two doses (maximum 3 g/d) for 2 to 5 days; also effective when applied topically under occlusion. *Ivermectin,* 6 mg bid. *Albendazole,* 400 mg/d for 3 days; highly effective.

Cryosurgery Liquid nitrogen to advancing end of larval burrow.

Removal of Parasite Do not attempt to extract; parasite not in visible lesion.

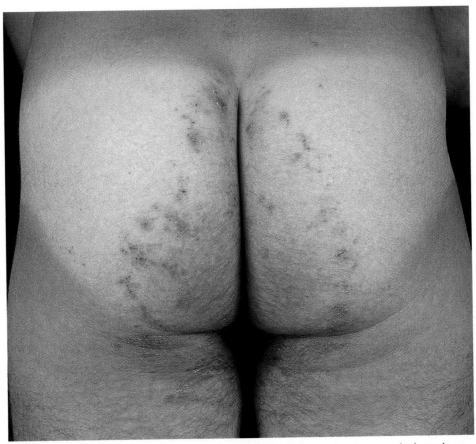

Figure 24-20 Larva currens *Multiple pruritic serpiginous, inflammatory lines on the buttocks at sites of penetration of* S. stercoralis *larvae.*

WATER-ASSOCIATED INFECTIONS AND INFESTATIONS

Various organisms normally live in aqueous environments and can cause soft tissue infections after exposure: *Aeromonas hydrophila, Edwardsiella tarda, Erysipelothrix rhusiopathiae, Mycobacterium marinum, Pfisteria piscicida, Pseudomonas* species, *Streptococcus iniae, Vibrio vulnificus,* other *Vibrio* species, *Prototheca wickerhamii.* Localized cutaneous infestations, including cercarial dermatitis and seabather's eruption, can also occur after exposure to microscopic marine animals (Table 24-2).

Table 24-2 COMPARISON OF CERCARIAL DERMATITIS AND SEABATHER'S ERUPTION

Factor	Cercarial Dermatitis	Seabather's Eruption
Type of water	Fresh and salt	Salt
Body part involved	Uncovered	Covered and hairy areas
Geographic locale	Northern USA, Canada	Florida, Cuba
Etiology	Cercarial forms of schistosomes	Larval forms of marine coelenterates: *L. unquiculata, E. lineata*

INSECT BITES AND INFESTATIONS

Cercarial Dermatitis

Cercarial dermatitis (CD) (known also as swimmer's itch, clam digger's itch, schistosome dermatitis, sedge pool itch) is an acute pruritic papular eruption at the sites of cutaneous penetration by Schistosoma cercariae (larvae) of nonhuman schistosomes, whose usual hosts are birds and small mammals. Nonhuman schistosomes implicated: Trichobilharzia, Gigantobilharzia, Ornithobilharzia, Microbilharzia, Schistosomatium. Exposure can be to fresh, brackish, or salt water. Eggs produced by adult schistosomes living in animals are shed with animal feces into environment; on reaching water, schistosome eggs hatch, releasing miracidia (fully developed larvae). Snails are the appropriate hosts for miracidia, from which they emerge as cercariae. These must penetrate the skin of a vertebrate host to continue development. Humans are dead-end hosts. Cercariae penetrate human skin, elicit an inflammatory response, and die without invading other tissues. CD occurs worldwide in areas with fresh and salt water inhabited by appropriate molluscan hosts.

CD is acquired by skin exposure to fresh/salt water infested by cercariae. Pruritus and rash begin within hours after exposure. A pruritic macular, papular, papulovesicular, and/or urticarial eruption develops at exposed sites with marked pruritus (Fig. 24-21), sparing parts of the body covered by clothing. (In contrast, seabather's eruption occurs on areas of the body covered by swimsuits.) Papular urticaria occurs at each site of penetration in previously sensitized individuals. In highly sensitized persons, lesions may progress to eczematous plaques, urticarial wheals, and/or vesicles, reaching a peak 2 to 3 days after exposure. Schistosomes capable of causing invasive disease in humans (Schistosoma mansoni, S. haematobium, S. japonicum) may cause a similar skin eruption shortly after penetration as well as late visceral complications. Lesions usually resolve within a week. Topical and/or systemic glucocorticoids may be indicated in more severe cases.

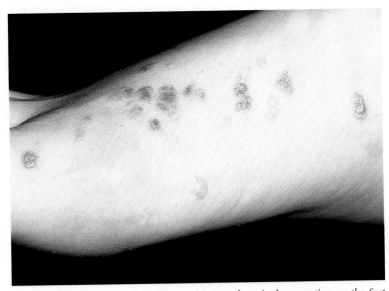

Figure 24-21 Cercarial dermatitis *A highly pruritic papulovesicular eruption on the feet and lower legs acquired after the patient waded through a slow-flowing creek.*

Seabather's Eruption

Seabather's eruption is caused by exposure to two marine animals: larvae of the thimble jellyfish, Linuche unquiculatum in waters off the coast of Florida and in the Caribbean, and planula larvae of the sea anemone, Edwardsiella lineata, Long Island, NY. Nematocysts of coelenterate larvae sting the skin of hairy areas or under swimwear, presumably causing an allergic reaction. Some affected individuals recall a stinging or prickling sensation while in the water. Lesions present clinically as inflammatory papules 4 to 24 h after exposure. A monomorphous eruption of erythematous papules or papulovesicles is seen most commonly: vesicles, pustules, and papular urticaria which may progress to crusted erosions. In comparison with cercarial dermatitis, which occurs on exposed sites, seabather's eruption occurs at sites covered by bathing apparel (Fig. 24-22) while bathing in salt water. On average, lesions persist for 1 to 2 weeks. In sensitized individuals, the eruption can become progressively more severe with repeated exposures and may be associated with systemic symptoms. Topical or systemic glucocorticoids provide symptomatic relief.

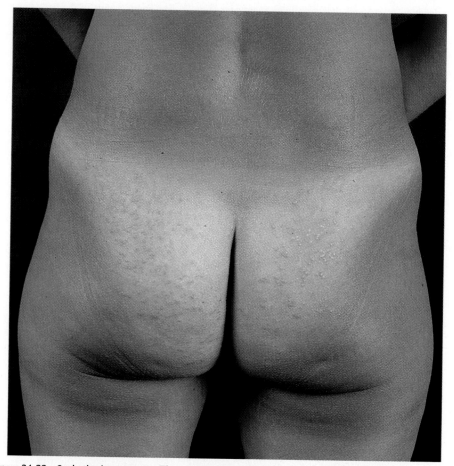

Figure 24-22 Seabather's eruption *This papulovesicular rash occurred in a swimmer while on vacation in the Caribbean. During swimming the patient experienced slight stinging in the regions covered by her bikini; later that evening she noticed the eruption. The rash is characteristically confined to the areas covered by swimwear.*

CUTANEOUS AND MUCOCUTANEOUS LEISHMANIASIS

Leishmaniasis is a parasitic infection caused by many species of the protozoa *Leishmania*, manifested clinically as four major syndromes—cutaneous leishmaniasis (CL) of Old and New World types, mucocutaneous leishmaniasis (MCL), diffuse cutaneous leishmaniasis (DCL), and visceral leishmaniasis (VL). CL is characterized by development of single or multiple cutaneous papules at the site of a sandfly bite, often evolving into nodules and ulcers, which heal spontaneously with a depressed scar.

Synonyms: Old World leishmaniasis: Baghdad/Delhi boil or button, oriental/Aleppo sore, *bouton d'Orient.* Mucocutaneous leishmaniasis: Espundia. Visceral leishmaniasis: Kala-azar.

CLASSIFICATION OF LEISHMANIASIS

Clinical Form	Species	Major Localities
Cutaneous leishmaniasis (CL)		
Old World (OWCL)	*L. major*	Near East, Africa
	L. tropica	Near East, former USSR
	L. aethiopica	Ethiopia, Kenya
	L. infantum	Mediterranean rim
New World (NWCL)	*L. mexicana* complex	Mexico, Central America
	L. braziliensis complex	Brazil, Bolivia
	L. amazonensis	Brazil
Mucocutaneous leishmaniasis (MCL)		
Diffuse (anergic) cutaneous leishmaniasis (DCL)		
Old World	*L. aethiopica*	Ethiopia
New World	*L. braziliensis* complex	South America
Visceral leishmaniasis (VL)	*L. donovani*	India, Kenya
	L. infantum	Mediterranean rim
	L. chagasi	South America
Uncommon forms of leishmaniasis		
Leishmaniasis recidivans (LR)	*L. tropica*	Middle East, former USSR
Post-kala-azar dermal leishmaniasis (PKADL)	*L. donovani*	India, Nepal, China

EPIDEMIOLOGY

Incidence Estimated 12 million people infected worldwide; 400,000 new cases reported annually; 350 million individuals are at risk of infection. 75,000 individuals die annually of MCL and ML.

Etiology The clinical symptomatology, whether cutaneous, mucocutaneous, or visceral, depends on the infecting species.

Life Cycle *Leishmania* dimorphic. In mammalian host: amastigote (leishmanial) form—2 to 3 μm in length, oval/round, aflagellate; lives intracellularly in cells of reticuloendothelial system. In GI tract of sandfly/in culture: promastigote (leptomonad) form—10 to 15 μm in length, spindle-shaped, flagellated; extracellular. Speciation: isoenzyme patterns, kinetoplast DNA buoyant densities, specific phlebotomine vectors, monoclonal antibodies, DNA hybridization, DNA restriction endonuclease fragment analysis.

Reservoir Varies with geography and leishmanial species. Zoonosis involves rodents/canines. Mediterranean littoral—dogs. Southern Russia—gerbils. For *L. major,* desert rodents. For *L. tropica,* rats. For *L. infantum,* wild canines, dogs; in endemic areas of Spain, up to 20% of dogs tested harbored parasites in skin and viscera.

Vector Female sandflies of genus *Phlebotomus* (Old World) and genera *Lutzomyia* and *Psychodopygus* (New World). Breed in cracks in buildings, rubbish, rubble; rodent burrows, termite hills, rotting vegetation. Weak fliers; remain close to ground near breeding site, Ingest amastigotes while feeding on infected mammals, converting to promastigotes in the gut of the sandfly; replicate in gut.

Transmission Promastigotes deposited on skin of host into a small pool of blood drawn by probing sandfly.

Geography All inhabited continents except Australia.

OWCL Asia Minor, Middle East, southern Russia, China, the Mediterranean littoral, India, Africa (Sudan, Ethiopia, Congo Basin).

ACL, MCL Forests of South and Central America. *L. mexicana* endemic in south-central Texas.

DCL South America, Dominican Republic, Africa.

PATHOGENESIS

The clinical and immunologic spectrum of leishmaniasis parallels that of leprosy. CL occurs in a host with good protective immunity. MCL occurs in those with an intense inflammatory reaction. DCL occurs with extensive and widespread proliferation of the organism in the skin but without much inflammation or tendency for visceralization. VL occurs in the host with little immune response and/or in immunosuppression. Unlike leprosy, extent and pattern are strongly influenced by the specific species of *Leishmania* involved. Additional factors that affect the clinical picture: number of parasites inoculated, site of inoculation, nutritional status of host, nature of the last non-blood meal of vector. Infection and recovery are followed by lifelong immunity to reinfection by the same species of *Leishmania.* In some cases, interspecies immunity occurs.

HISTORY

Incubation Period Inversely proportional to size of inoculum: shorter in visitors to endemic area. OWCL: *L. tropica major,* 1 to 4 weeks; *L. tropica,* 2 to 8 months; acute CL: 2 to 8 weeks or more.

Symptoms Noduloulcerative lesions usually asymptomatic. With secondary bacterial infection, may become painful.

PHYSICAL EXAMINATION

Skin Findings

Types of Lesions Primary lesions occur at site of sandfly bite, usually on exposed site.

Old World CL

L. major Asia, Africa, Europe in tropical and subtropical zones; Middle East (Iran, Iraq, eastern Saudi Arabia, Jordan Valley of Israel and Jordan, Sinai Peninsula). More common in rural areas. Begins as small erythematous papule, which may appear immediately after sandfly bite but usually 2 to 4 weeks later. Papule slowly enlarges to ≥2 cm over a period of several weeks and assumes a dusky violaceous hue. Eventually, lesion becomes crusted in center with a shallow ulcer and raised indurated border (Fig. 24-23). In some cases, the center of the nodule becomes hyperkeratotic, forming a cutaneous horn. Small satellite papules may develop at periphery of lesion, and occasionally subcutaneous nodules along the course of proximal lymphatics. Rarely, lesions become locally invasive and extend into subcutaneous tissue and muscle. Peripheral extension usually stops after 2 months and ulcerated nodule persists for another 3 to 6 months, or longer. The lesion then heals with a slightly depressed scar. In some cases, CL remains active with positive smears for ≥24 months (nonhealing chronic cutaneous leishmaniasis). The number of lesions depends on the circumstances of the exposure and extent of infection within the sandfly vector. May result in multiple lesions, up to 100 or more (Figs. 24-24 and 24-25).

L. tropica Southern Europe, Iran, Iraq, Middle East, southern republics of former USSR. More common in urban areas. Clinical pattern similar to that of *L. major,* although lesions caused by *L. tropica* are more apt to be solitary, more inflammatory, last longer, and be more difficult to treat.

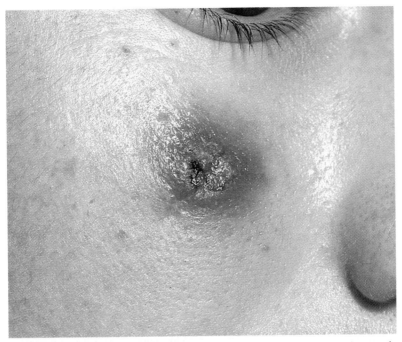

Figure 24-23 Old World cutaneous leishmaniasis *A solitary, inflamed nodule with central necrosis and ulceration on the cheek for 1 month arising at the site of a sandfly bite.*

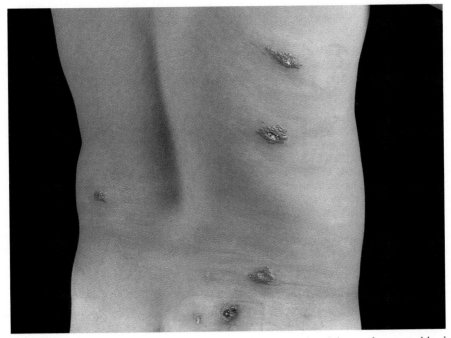

Figure 24-24 Old World cutaneous leishmaniasis *Multiple, crusted nodules on the exposed back, arising at sites of sandfly bites. Many of the lesions resemble a volcano with a central depressed center, i.e., volcano sign.*

CUTANEOUS AND MUCOCUTANEOUS LEISHMANIASIS

L. infantum Countries bordering Mediterranean, including southern Europe and northern Africa. Lesions are similar to those in *L. major* form but duration shorter.

L. aethiopica Kenya, Sudan, Ethiopia. The common form of CL in these areas is similar to CL caused by *L. major*. In approximately 20% of individuals, widespread skin involvement develops (DCL) that resembles lepromatous leprosy.

New World CL

L. mexicana complex Mexico, Central America, as far north as Texas, as far south as Brazil. Lesions develop in similar fashion to those caused by *L. major*. Small erythematous papule develops at sandfly bite site, evolving into ulcerated nodule. Eventually lesion heals with a depressed scar. Enlarges to 3 to 12 cm with raised border. Nonulcerating nodules may become verrucous. ± Lymphangitis, ± regional lymphadenopathy. Isolated lesions on hand or head usually do not ulcerate; heal spontaneously. Ear lesions may persist for years, destroying cartilage (chiclero ulcers) (Fig. 24-26).

L. braziliensis complex Clinical lesions similar to those of OWCL. Some strains can invade mucous membranes of mouth, nose, pharynx, larynx to cause MCL.

Mucocutaneous Leishmaniasis Characterized by skin and upper respiratory tract involvement. Caused by *L. braziliensis* complex in South America; *L. aethiopica* in Africa. In form caused by *L. braziliensis braziliensis,* mucosal lesions develop from cutaneous lesions in > 75% of infected individuals. In infections caused by *L. braziliensis guyanensis,* nasal involvement develops in 5% of cases. MCL begins with typical lesions of CL; rather than showing eventual resolution, infection spread to mucosa (Fig. 24-27) and eventually to cartilages of upper respiratory tract, especially nose, oral pharynx, larynx. Edema and inflammatory changes lead to epistaxis and coryzal symptoms. In time, nasal septum, floor of mouth, and tonsilar areas destroyed. Results in marked disfigurement (referred to as *espundia* in South America). Death may occur due to super-imposed bacterial infection, pharyngeal obstruction, or malnutrition. Diagnosis usually made on clinical findings; parasites are difficult to demonstrate in mucosa.

Diffuse Cutaneous Leishmaniasis

Resembles lepromatous leprosy; large number of parasites in macrophages in dermis; no visceral involvement. In Old World, occurs in 20% of individuals with leishmaniasis in Ethiopia and Sudan. In South America, attributed to a member of *L. braziliensis* complex. Presents as a single nodule, which then spreads locally, often through extension from satellite lesions, and eventually by metastasis. In time, lesions become widespread with nonulcerating nodules appearing diffusely over face, trunk. Responds poorly to treatment.

Less Common Forms of Leishmaniasis

Leishmaniasis Recidivans (LR) Complication of *L. tropica* infection. Dusky-red plaques with active, spreading borders and healing centers, giving rise to gyrate and annular lesions. Most commonly affects face; can cause tissue destruction and severe deformity.

Post-Kala-Azar Dermal Leishmaniasis (PKADL) Sequel to VL that has resolved spontaneously or after adequate treatment. Lesions appear a year or so after course of therapy with macular, papular, nodular lesions, and hypopigmented macules/plaques on face, trunk, extremities. Resemble lepromatous leprosy when lesions are numerous. Develops in 20% of Indian patients treated for VL caused by *L. donovani,* and to small percentage of Ethiopian patients with VL caused by *L. aethiopica.*

General Examination

In VL (kala-azar), bone marrow, liver, spleen are involved. Occurs in China, India, former USSR, Middle East, east Africa through Sudan to west Africa, and South America. Patients present with fever, splenomegaly, pancytopenia, wasting. Diagnosis made by demonstration of parasites from bone marrow or spleen aspirates.

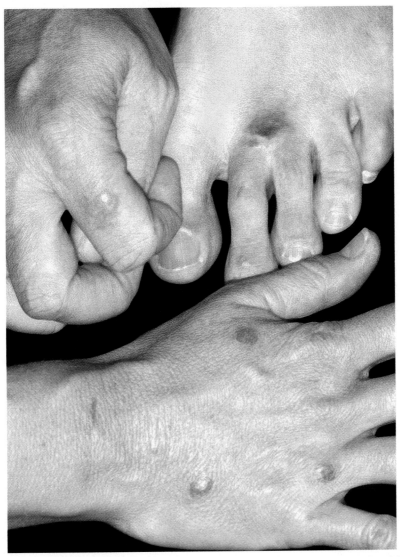

Figure 24-25   Old World cutaneous leishmaniasis   *Multiple erythematous papules and nodules on the dorsum of hands and foot in a husband and wife who had been camping in Israel. A facial papule was present in the wife. All lesions resolved spontaneously within 2 to 3 months.*

DIFFERENTIAL DIAGNOSIS

Acute CL   Insect bite reaction, impetigo, furuncle, carbuncle, ecthyma, anthrax, orf, milker's nodule, tularemia, swimming pool granuloma, tuberculosis cutis, syphilitic gumma, yaws, sporotrichosis, blastomycosis, kerion, myiasis, dracunculosis, molluscum, warts, pyogenic granuloma, tropical ulcer, foreign-body granuloma, keratoacanthoma, basal cell carcinoma, squamous cell carcinoma, metastases, lymphoma, leukemia.

Chronic CL and Relapsing CL   Lupus vulgaris, leprosy, sarcoidosis, granuloma faciale, Jessner's lymphocytic infiltrate, lymphocytoma cutis, discoid lupus erythematosus, psoriasis, acne, rosacea, cellulitis, erysipelas, keloids, Wegener's granulomatosis, syphilitic gumma.

LABORATORY EXAMINATIONS

Leishmanin (Montenegro) Skin Test   Of no use in endemic areas. Negative in DCL.

Serology   Lacks specificity.

Dermatopathology   Large macrophages filled with 2- to 4-μm amastigotes (Leishman-Donovan bodies); mixed lymphocytic, plasmacytic infiltrate. In Wright- and Giemsa-stained preparations, the amastigote cytoplasm appears blue, nucleus relatively large and red, distinctive kinetoplast rod-shaped and stains intensely red.

Culture   Novy-MacNeal-Nicolle medium at 22°C to 28°C for 21 days grows motile promastigotes.

Touch Preparation   Macrophages containing organisms: dark, slightly flattened nucleus and rod-shaped kinetoplast observed.

Needle Aspiration   Visualize amastigote within macrophages.

PCR   Can detect different species of *Leishmania*.

DIAGNOSIS

Clinical suspicion, confirmed by demonstrating amastigotes on smear or in skin biopsy specimen or promastigotes on culture of aspirates or tissue.

COURSE AND PROGNOSIS

CL   Whether caused by *L. tropica* or *L. mexicana,* CL is self-limited. Scarring is increased by secondary bacterial infection.

MCL   May extend to secondary sites. Secondary infection common. Death from pneumonia.

DCL   Progressive; refractory to treatment; cures rare.

MANAGEMENT

Prophylaxis   No chemoprophylaxis for travelers exists. OWCL: Delay specific treatment until ulceration occurs, allowing protective immunity to develop, unless lesions are disfiguring, disabling, persist ± 6 months.

Lesional Therapy   Local injection of antimonials (Pentostam), usually at weekly intervals; up to 1 mg/kg may be injected in borders of lesions. Also cryosurgery, ultrasound-induced hyperthermia, excision, electrosurgery. Topical 15% paramomycin sulfate, 12% methylbenzethonium chloride in white paraffin twice daily for 10 days.

Systemic Therapy   Depends on clinical form. OWCL is usually self-limited and in most cases does not require specific treatment. Treatment should be given for extensive lesions, especially involving face, or for those lesions that invade deeper tissues.

For selected CL, MCL, DCL   Sodium antimony gluconate (Pentostam) IV or IM In single daily dose of 10 mg/kg for adults and 20 mg/kg for patients <18 years of age for 10 days. Meglumine antimonate (Glucantime) 20 mg/kg/d for 10 days, ECG control. Amphotericin B, pentamidine, or sodium antimony gluconate *plus* interferon gamma for resistant cases. Ketoconazole.

Indian VL   Milfefosine PO 100 mg qd for 4 weeks.

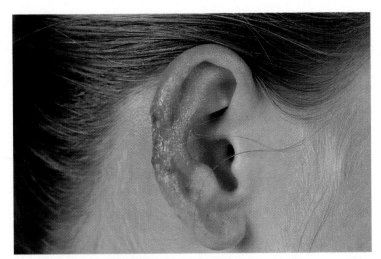

Figure 24-26 New World cutaneous leishmaniasis: chiclero ulcer *A deep ulcer on the helix at the site of a sandfly bite. This variant typically occurs in leishmaniasis acquired in Central and South America.*

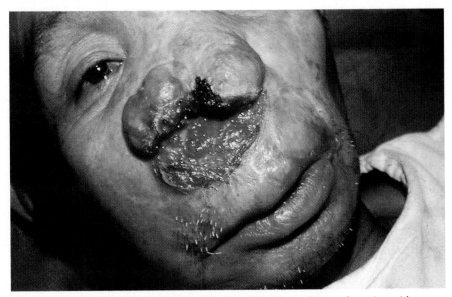

Figure 24-27 Mucocutaneous leishmaniasis: espundia *Painful, mutilating ulceration with destruction of portions of the nose. (Courtesy of Eric Kraus, M.D.)*

SEXUALLY TRANSMITTED DISEASES

Sexually transmitted diseases (STDs) are caused by a broad range of pathogens (Table 25-1). The syndromes caused by these pathogens affect both the sexually active couple and neonates born to an infected mother (Table 25-2).

Bacterial STDs such as gonorrhea, syphilis, chancroid, donovanosis, and lymphogranuloma venereum can easily be cured with antimicrobial therapy. In contrast, viral STDs, such as those caused by human immunodeficiency virus (HIV), human papillomavirus (HPV), and herpes simplex virus 2 (HSV-2), are chronic, uncurable infections, characterized by prolonged viral shedding and opportunity for infecting a sexual partner; these cannot be cured by antiviral therapy. Nearly all sexually active individuals are at risk for these viral STDs. HPV persists in the anogenital mucosa for months, years, or decades after primary infection. HSV-2 infection is chronic and lifelong. Prevention offers the best approach to managing STDs.

Many STDs can be transmitted perinatally to the neonate. In developing nations, where STDs are more common, lack of funds for health care often limit detection and treatment of STDs as well as immunizations. Syphilis can be a lifelong infection with severe long-term morbidity. Transmission of HIV to neonates occurs commonly in developing nations, where the prevalence of infection is high; zidovudine treatment of mother and neonate markedly reduces neonatal infection. Transmission of HSV has more immediate effects on the neonate, who is more susceptible to acute visceral infection. Transmission of HPV infection to the neonate can result in anogenital condyloma, and, later in life, respiratory papillomatosis.

LABORATORY EXAMINATIONS

All individuals being evaluated for STDs should have a culture for gonorrhea and serology for syphilis. HIV testing is strongly advised. Serologic testing for HPV infections is not available. Type-specific serologic tests (TSST) for HSV infection, such as the Western blot, are very reliable, detecting previous infection with HSV-1, HSV-2, or both.

MANAGEMENT

The most effective way to prevent sexual transmission of STDs is to avoid sexual intercourse with an infected partner. Both new partners should get tested for STDs before initiating sexual intercourse. If a person chooses to have sexual intercourse with a partner whose infection status is unknown or who is infected with HIV or another STD, a new condom should be used for each act of intercourse. Vaccines for STDs are limited at this time. Immunization for hepatitis A and hepatitis B is advised to prevent transmission of these viral infections during intercourse. The prospects for development of a vaccine for HSV-2 and HPV are excellent.

Table 25-1 SEXUALLY TRANSMISSIBLE PATHOGENS AND ASSOCIATED DISEASE SYNDROMES

Pathogen	Associated Disease or Syndrome
Bacteria	
Neisseria gonorrhoeae	Urethritis, epididymitis, proctitis, cervicitis, endometritis, salpingitis, perihepatitis, bartholinitis, pharyngitis, conjunctivitis, prepubertal vaginitis, prostatitis, accessory gland infection, disseminated gonococcal infection (DGI), chorio-amnionitis, premature rupture of membranes, premature delivery, amniotic infection syndrome
Chlamydia trachomatis	All of the above except DGI, plus otitis media, rhinitis, and pneumonia in infants, and Reiter's syndrome
Ureaplasma urealyticum	Nongonococcal urethritis (NGU)
Mycoplasma genitalium	(?) Nongonococcal urethritis
M. hominis	Postpartum fever, salpingitis (?)
Treponema pallidum	Syphilis
Gardnerella vaginalis	Bacterial ("nonspecific") vaginosis (in conjunction with *Mycoplasma hominis* and vaginal anaerobes, such as *Mobiluncus* spp.)
Mobiluncus curtisii	Bacterial vaginosis
M. mulieris	Bacterial vaginosis
Haemophilus ducreyi	Chancroid
Calymmatobacterium granulomatis	Donovanosis (granuloma inguinale)
Shigella spp.	Shigellosis in men who have sex with men (MSM)*
Campylobacter spp.	Enteritis, proctocolitis in MSM*
Helicobacter cinaedi	(?) Proctocolitis; dermatitis, bacteremia in AIDS
H. fenneliae	(?) Proctocolitis; dermatitis, bacteremia in AIDS
Viruses	
HIV	HIV disease, AIDS
HSV types 1 and 2	Initial and recurrent genital herpes, aseptic meningitis, neonatal herpes
HPV	Condyloma acuminata; laryngeal papilloma; intraepithelial neoplasia and carcinoma of the cervix, vagina, vulva, anus, penis
Hepatitis A virus (HAV)	Acute hepatitis A
Hepatitis B virus (HBV)	Acute hepatitis B, chronic hepatitis B, hepatocellular carcinoma, polyarteritis nodosa, chronic membranous glomerulonephritis, mixed cryoglobulinemia (?), polymyalgia rheumatica (?)
Hepatitis C virus (HCV)	Acute hepatitis C, chronic hepatitis C, hepatocellular carcinoma, mixed cryoglobulinemia, chronic glomerulonephritis
Cytomegalovirus (CMV)	Heterophil-negative infectious mononucleosis; congenital CMV infection with gross birth defects and infant mortality, cognitive impairment (e.g., mental retardation, sensorineural deafness); protean manifestations in the immunosuppressed host
Molluscum contagiosum virus (MCV)	Genital molluscum contagiosum
Human T cell lymphotrophic virus (HTLV-1)	Human T cell leukemia or lymphoma, tropical spastic paraparesis
Human herpes virus type 8 (HHV-8)	Kaposi's sarcoma, body cavity lymphoma, multicentric Castleman's disease, (?) multiple myeloma
Protozoa	
Trichomonas vaginalis	Vaginal trichomoniasis, NGU
Entamoeba histolytica	Amebiasis in MSM*
Giardia lamblia	Giardiasis in MSM*
Fungi	
Candida albicans	Vulvovaginitis, balanitis
Ectoparasites	
Phthirus pubis	Pubic lice infestation
Sarcoptes scabiei	Scabies

*Men who have sex with men (MSM).

Table 25-2 SELECTED SYNDROMES AND COMPLICATIONS OF SEXUALLY TRANSMITTED PATHOGENS

Syndrome or Complication	Associated Sexually Transmitted Pathogen
In men	
HIV disease	HIV
Urethritis	*Neisseria gonorrhoeae, Chlamydia trachomatis,* HSV, *Ureaplasma urealyticum,* (?) *Mycoplasma genitalium, T. vaginalis*
Epididymitis	*C. trachomatis, N. gonorrhoeae*
Intestinal infections	
Proctitis	*N. gonorrhoeae,* HSV, *C. trachomatis*
Proctocolitis or enterocolitis	*Campylobacter* spp., *Shigella* spp., *Entamoeba histolytica,* (?) *Helicobacter* spp.
Enteritis	*Giardia lamblia*
In women	
HIV disease	HIV
Lower genitourinary tract infection	
Vulvitis	*Candida albicans,* HSV
Vaginitis	*Trichomonas vaginalis, C. albicans*
Vaginosis	*Gardnerella vaginalis, Mobiluncus* spp., other anaerobes, *Mycoplasma hominis*
Cervicitis	*N. gonorrhoeae, C. trachomatis,* HSV
Pelvic inflammatory disease	*N. gonorrhoeae, C. trachomatis, M. hominis,* anaerobes, group B streptococcus
Infertility	
Postsalpingitis, postobstetrical, postabortion	*N. gonorrhoeae, C. trachomatis, M. hominis* (?)
Pregnancy morbidity	Several STDs implicated in one or more of these conditions
Chorioamnionitis, amniotic fluid infection, prematurity, premature rupture of membranes, preterm delivery, postpartum endometritis, ectopic pregnancy	
In men and women	
Neoplasia	HPV
Cervical, vulvar, vaginal, anal, and penile, intraepithelial neoplasia, carcinoma	
Hepatocellular carcinoma	HBV, HCV
Kaposi's sarcoma, body cavity lymphoma, Castleman's disease	HHV-8
	T cell lymphoma/leukemia (HTLV-I)
Genital ulceration	HSV, *T. pallidum, Haemophilus ducreyi, Calymmatobacterium granulomatis, C. trachomatis* (LGV strains)
Acute arthritis with urogenital or intestinal infection	*N. gonorrhoeae, C. trachomatis, Shigella* spp., *Campylobacter* spp.
Hepatitis	HAV, HBV, HCV, CMV, *Treponema pallidum*
Genital warts	HPV
Molluscum contagiosum	MCV
Ectoparasite infestations	*Sarcoptes scabiei, Phthirus pubis*
Heterophil-negative mononucleosis	CMV, Epstein-Barr virus (some evidence for sexual transmission)
Tropical spastic paraparesis	HTLV-I

(Continued)

In neonates and infants

Neonatal systemic infection, with potential cognitive impairment, deafness, death	Cytomegalovirus, HSV, *T. pallidum*, HIV
Conjunctivitis	*C. trachomatis, N. gonorrhoeae*
Pneumonia, (?) chronic pulmonary disease	*C. trachomatis, U. urealyticum* (?)
Otitis media	*C. trachomatis*
Sepsis, meningitis	Group B streptococcus
Laryngeal papillomatosis	HPV

NOTE: For each of the above syndromes, some cases cannot yet be ascribed to any cause and must currently be considered idiopathic. "?" indicates a possible associated syndrome.

SOURCES (Tables 25-1 and 25-2): Adapted from Cates W Jr, KK Holmes: Sexually transmitted diseases, In J M Last, RB Wallace (eds): *Maxcy-Rosenau-Last Public Health and Preventive Medicine*, 14th ed. Norwalk, CT, Appleton & Lange, 1998, pp 137–155; and Holmes KK, HH Handsfield: Sexually transmitted diseases: Overview and clinical approach, In A Fauci et al. (eds): Harrison's Principles of Internal Medicine, 14th ed. New York, McGraw-Hill, 1998, pp 801–812.

HUMAN PAPILLOMAVIRUS: MUCOSAL INFECTIONS

Mucosal human papillomavirus (HPV) infections are the most common sexually transmitted disease (STD). When clinically symptomatic, lesions are barely visible papules to nodules to confluent masses occurring on anogenital or oral mucosa or skin, caused by infection with a mucosal type of HPV. Only 1 to 2% of HPV-infected individuals have any visibly detectable clinical lesion. HPV present in the birth canal can be transmitted to a newborn during vaginal delivery and can cause external genital warts (EGW) and respiratory papillomatosis. HPV dysplasia of the anogenital skin and mucosa ranging from mild to severe to squamous cell carcinoma (SCC) in situ (SCCIS); invasive SCC can arise within SCCIS, most commonly in the cervix and anal canal.

Synonyms: Condylomata acuminata, external genital warts (EGW), anogenital warts, venereal warts.

EPIDEMIOLOGY

Etiology HPV is a DNA papovavirus that multiplies in the nuclei of infected epithelial cells. More than 20 types of HPV can infect the genital tract: types 6, 11 most commonly; also types 16, 18, 31, 33 (see Table 25.1). Types 16, 18, 31, 33, and 35 are strongly associated with genital dysplasia and carcinoma. In individuals with multiple sexual partners, subclinical infection with multiple HPV types is common.

Age of Onset Young, sexually active adults.

Risk Factors for Acquiring HPV Infection
Number of sexual partners/frequency of sexual intercourse; sexual partner with EGW, sexual partner's number of sexual partners, infection with other STDs.

Transmission Through sexual contact: genital-genital, oral-genital, genital-anal. Microabrasions occur on epithelial surface allowing virions from infected partner to gain access to basal cell layer of noninfected partner. Digital transmission of nongenital warts probably accounts for few cases of EGW. During delivery, mothers with anogenital warts can transmit HPV to neonate, resulting in EGW and laryngeal papillomatosis in children.

Incidence Most sexually active individuals are subclinically infected with HPV; most HPV infections are asymptomatic, subclinical, or unrecognized. 1% of sexually active adults (15 to 19 years of age) develop EGW. Increased many fold during the past two decades.

Psychosexual Impact of Genital Warts Of less effect than genital herpes, which has had much more coverage in the lay press as the incurable STD. Few patients are aware of the role of HPV in anogenital cancer. Diagnosis of genital warts may result in fears about transmission and recurrence, sexual lifestyle changes (abstinence, caution, condoms), depression or low self-esteem, relationships becoming strained and/or breaking down, anxiety related to partner disclosure.

PATHOGENESIS

"Low-risk" and "high-risk" HPV types both cause EGW. *HPV infection probably persists throughout a patient's lifetime in a dormant state and becomes infectious intermittently.* Exophytic warts are probably more infectious than subclinical infection.

Immunosuppression results in new expression of HPV lesions, progression of HPV lesions, no increased rate of HPV infection but an increased risk of transmission, increased multifocal intraepithelial neoplasia. Immunosuppressed renal transplant recipients have a 17-fold greater incidence of genital HPV infection.

All HPV types replicate exclusively in host's cell nucleus. In benign HPV-associated lesions, HPV exists as a plasmid in cell's cytoplasm, replicating extrachromosomally. In malignant HPV-associated lesions, HPV integrates into host's chromosome, following a break in the viral genome (around E1/E2 region). E1 and E2 function is deregulated, resulting in cellular transformation.

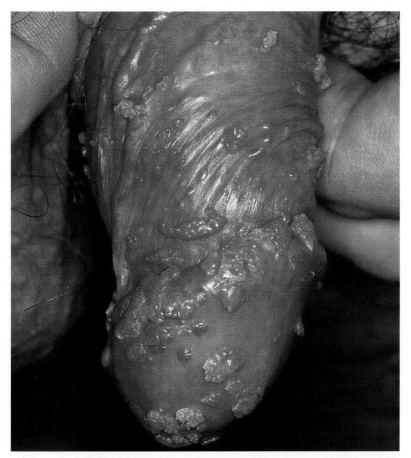

Figure 25-1 Condylomata acuminata: penis *Multiple, soft, filiform papules, discrete with some coalescing to raspberry-like lesions, on the glans penis and prepuce.*

HISTORY

Incubation Period Several weeks to months to years.

Duration of Lesions Months to years.

Skin Symptoms Usually asymptomatic, except for cosmetic appearance. Itching, burning, bleeding, vaginal or urethral discharge, dyspareunia. Obstruction if large mass.

PHYSICAL EXAMINATION

Mucocutaneous Lesions

Four clinical types of genital warts occur: small papular, cauliflower-floret (acuminate or pointed) lesions (Figs. 25-1 through 25-3), keratotic warts, and flat-topped papules/plaques (most common on cervix). Lesions are skin-colored, pink, red, tan, brown. Lesions may be solitary, scattered, and isolated, or form voluminous confluent masses. In immunocompromised individuals, lesions may be huge. (Fig. 25-4 *A* and *B*) Acetic acid is helpful in visualizing lesions on the cervix and anus but is of little help in defining small EGW.

Sites of Predilection *Male* Frenulum, corona, glans penis, prepuce, shaft, scrotum.

Female Labia, clitoris, periurethral area, perineum, vagina, cervix (flat lesions) (Fig. 25-5).

Both Sexes Perineal, perianal, anal canal, rectal; urethral meatus, urethra, bladder; oropharynx.

Laryngeal Papillomas

Relatively uncommon; associated with HPV-6 and -11. Arise most commonly on true vocal cords of larynx. Age: children <5 years of age; adults >20 years of age.

DIFFERENTIAL DIAGNOSIS

Papular/Nodular External Genital Lesions Normal anatomy (e.g., sebaceous glands, pearly penile papules, vestibular papillae), squamous intraepithelial lesions, SCCIS, invasive SCC, benign neoplasms (moles, seborrheic keratoses, skin tags, pilar cyst, angiokeratoma), inflammatory dermatoses (lichen nitidus, lichen planus), molluscum contagiosum, condylomata lata, folliculitis, scabietic nodules.

LABORATORY EXAMINATIONS

Acetowhitening Helpful in defining the extent of cervical and anal HPV infection. Acetowhitening of external genital lesions is not specific for warts. (See Appendix B.)

Pap Smear All women should be encouraged to have an annual Pap smear, in that HPV is the major etiologic agent in pathogenesis for cancer of cervix. Anal Pap test with a cervical brush and fixative solution is helpful in detecting anal dysplasia.

Dermatopathology Biopsy is indicated if diagnosis is uncertain; the lesions do not respond to standard therapy; the lesions worsen during therapy; the patient is immunocompromised; warts are pigmented, indurated, fixed, and/or ulcerated; all suspect cervical lesions. Indicated in some cases to confirm diagnosis and/or rule out SCCIS or invasive SCC.

Detection of HPV DNA Presence of HPV DNA and specific HPV types can be determined on smears and lesional biopsy specimens by in situ hybridization. However, no data support the use of type-specific HPV nucleic acid tests in the routine diagnosis or management of visible genital warts.

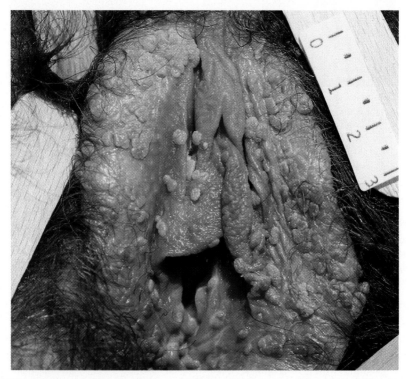

Figure 25-2   Condylomata acuminata: vulva   *Multiple, pink-brown, soft papules on the labia.*

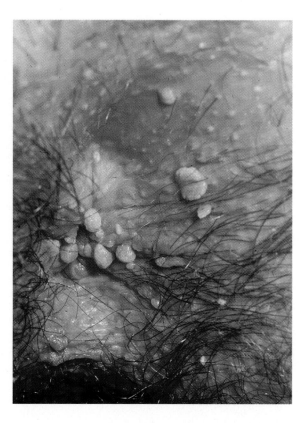

Figure 25-3 Condylomata acuminata: perianal *Fleshy papules becoming a confluent cauliflower-like mass on the perineum.*

Serology Occurrence of genital warts is a marker of unsafe sexual practices. Serologic tests for syphilis should be obtained on all patients to rule out coinfection with *Treponema pallidum*, and all patients offered HIV testing.

DIAGNOSIS

Clinical diagnosis, occasionally confirmed by biopsy.

COURSE AND PROGNOSIS

HPV is highly infectious, with an incubation period of 3 weeks to 8 months. Most HPV-infected individuals who develop EGW do so 2 to 3 months after becoming infected. Spontaneous regression occurs in 10 to 30% of patients within 3 months and is associated with an appropriate cell-mediated immune response. After regression, *subclinical infection may persist for life*. Recurrence may occur in individuals with normal immune function as well as with immunocompromise.

Condylomata recur even after appropriate therapy in a high percentage of patients, due to persistence of latent HPV in normal-appearing perilesional skin (see Transmission, above). Recurrences more commonly result from reactivation of subclinical infection than from reinfection by a sex partner. If left untreated, genital warts may resolve on their own, remain unchanged, or grow. In placebo-treated cases, genital warts clear spontaneously in 20 to 30% of patients within 3 months.

In pregnancy, genital warts may increase in size and number, show increased vaginal involvement, and have an increased rate of secondary bacterial infection of vaginal warts. Children delivered vaginally of mothers with genital HPV infection are at risk for developing recurrent respiratory papillomatosis in later life.

The major significance of HPV infection is its oncogenicity. HPV types 16, 18, 31, and 33 are the major etiologic factors for cervical dysplasia and cervical SCC; bowenoid papulosis, in situ and invasive carcinoma of both the vulva and penis; anal SCC of homosexual/bisexual males. Treatment of external genital warts is not likely to influence the development of cervical cancer. The importance of the annual Pap test must be stressed for women with genital warts.

MANAGEMENT

Prevention Use of condoms reduces transmission to uninfected sex partners. Goal of treatment is removal of exophytic warts and amelioration of signs and symptoms—not eradication of HPV. No therapy has been shown to eradicate HPV. Treatment is more successful if warts are small and have been present for <1 year. Risk of transmission might be reduced by "debulking" genital warts. Selection of treatment should be guided by preference of patient—expensive therapies, toxic therapies, and procedures that result in scarring avoided.

Indications for Therapy Cosmetic; reduce transmissiblity; provide relief of symptoms; improve self-esteem.

Primary Goal of Treating Visible Genital Warts Removal of symptomatic warts. Treatment can induce wart-free periods in most patients. Genital warts are often asymptomatic. No evidence indicates that currently available treatments eradicate or affect the natural history of HPV infection. Removal of warts may or may not decrease infectivity. If untreated, visible genital warts may resolve on their own, remain unchanged, or increase in size and number. No evidence indicates that treatment of visible warts affects the development of cervical or anal cancer.

Subclinical Genital HPV Infection (without exophytic warts) Subclinical genital HPV infection in much more common than exophytic warts among both men and women. Infection is often indirectly diagnosed on the cervix by Pap smear, colposcopy, or biopsy and on the penis, vulva, and other genital skin by the appearance

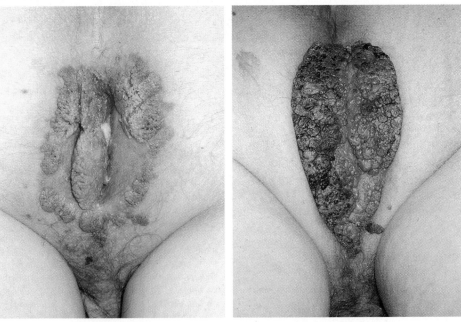

A　　　　　　**B**

Figure 25-4　Condylomata acuminata in an immunosuppressed individual　*A 21-year-old male, who underwent liver transplantation 2 years previously, noted the appearance of extragenital warts several months after the operation. Perianal and perineal condyloma were removed surgically, and immunosuppressive therapy was reduced; lesions recurred several months later. **A.** Very large perianal/perineal condylomata. **B.** Several months later, the mass of condylomata had increased in size many fold; the mass of tissue was painful and hygiene was difficult.*

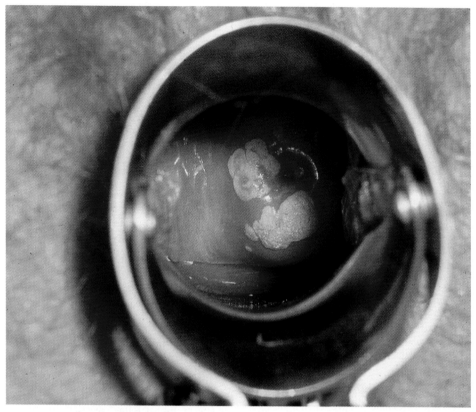

Figure 25-5 Condylomata acuminata: uterine cervix *Sharply demarcated, whitish, flat plaques* becoming confluent around the cervix.

of white areas after application of acetic acid. Treatment is not indicated.

External genital/perianal warts

Patient-applied agents

Imiquimod, 5% cream (Aldara) Mechanism of action is via local cytokine release (interferon, tumor necrosis factor, interleukin). No direct antiviral activity. The cream, which is supplied in single dose packets, is applied to the involved site by the patient, three times per week, usually at bedtime. Some patients experience local irritation. Treatment duration up to 16 weeks.

Podofilox (Condylox) .5% solution and gel. A purified and stable preparation of the active agent in podophyllin. Solution applied with a cotton swab and gel with a finger to condylomata and/or site involved (including normal-appearing skin between lesions) twice daily for

3 days, followed by 4 days of no therapy. This cycle may be repeated as necessary for a total of four cycles. Total area of treatment should not exceed 10 cm², and total volume should not exceed .5 mL/d. The health care provider should apply the initial treatment to demonstrate the proper application technique and identify lesions and sites to be treated. Podofilox is contraindicated during pregnancy.

Clinician-administered Therapy

Cryosurgery with liquid nitrogen Apply with cotton swab or cryospray. Repeat weekly or biweekly. Relatively inexpensive, does not require anesthesia, and does not result in scarring.

Podophyllin, 10 to 25% In compound tincture of benzoin. Limit the total volume of podophyllin solution applied to ≤.5 mL or ≤10 cm² per session. Thoroughly wash off in 1 to 4 h. Treat <10 cm² per session. Repeat weekly if necessary. If warts persist after six applications,

---

other therapeutic methods should be considered. Podophyllin contraindicated during pregnancy. Repeated application may cause irritation.

Trichloroacetic Acid (TCA) or Bichloroacetic acid bicarbonate (BCA), 80 to 90% Apply only to warts: powder with talc or sodium (baking soda) to remove unreacted acid. Repeat weekly if necessary. If warts persist after six applications, other therapeutic methods should be considered.

Surgical Removal Either by tangential scissor excision, tangential shave excision, curettage, or electrosurgery.

Electrodesiccation/electrocautery Highly effective in destruction of infected tissue and HPV. Should be attempted only by clinicians trained in the use of this modality. Electrodesiccation is contraindicated in patients with cardiac pacemakers.

Carbon Dioxide Laser and Electrodesiccation Useful in management of extensive warts, particularly for those patients who have not responded to other regimens; not appropriate for treatment of limited lesions.

Cervical Warts

For women who have exophytic cervical warts, high-grade squamous intraepithelial lesions (SIL) must be excluded before treatment is begun. Management of exophytic cervical warts should include consultation with an expert.

Vaginal Warts

Cryosurgery with Liquid Nitrogen This modality is difficult due to "fog" formation, which restricts visualization of lesions.

TCA or BCA, 80 to 90% Applied to warts only, powder with talc or sodium bicarbonate to remove unreacted acid if an excess amount is applied. Repeat weekly if necessary.

Podophyllin, 10 to 25% In compound tincture of benzoin. Treated area must be dry before the speculum is removed. Treat with ≤2 cm² per session. Repeat application at weekly intervals. Systemic absorption is a concern.

Urethral Meatus Warts

Cryosurgery with Liquid Nitrogen As above.

Podophyllin, 10 to 25% In compound tincture of benzoin. Treated area must be dry before contact with normal mucosa. Wash off in 1–2 h.

Repeat weekly if necessary. If warts persist after six applications, other therapeutic methods should be considered.

Anal Warts

Management of warts on rectal mucosa should be referred to an expert.

Cryosurgery with Liquid Nitrogen As above.

TCA or BCA, 80 to 90% Apply to warts only, powder with talc or sodium bicarbonate (baking soda) to remove unreacted acid. Repeat weekly if necessary. If warts persist after six applications, other thera peutic methods should be considered.

Surgical removal As above.

Oral Warts

Cryosurgery with Liquid Nitrogen As above.

Surgical Removal As above.

Follow-up After visible warts have cleared, a follow-up evaluation is not mandatory. Patients should be cautioned to watch for recurrences, which occur most frequently during the first 3 months. Because the sensitivity and specificity of self-diagnosis of genital warts are unknown, patients concerned about recurrences should be offered a follow-up evaluation 3 months after treatment. Earlier follow-up visits also may be useful to document a wart-free state, to monitor for or treat complications of therapy, and to provide the opportunity for patient education and counseling. Women should be counseled about the need for regular cytologic screening as recommended for women without genital warts. The presence of genital warts is not an indication for cervical colposcopy.

Immunosuppressed Patients Persons who are immunosuppressed because of HIV or other reasons may not respond as well as immunocompetent persons to therapy for genital warts and may have more frequent recurrences after treatment. SCC arising in or resembling genital warts might occur more frequently among immunosuppressed persons, requiring more frequent biopsy for confirmation of diagnosis.

Management of Sex Partners Examination of sex partners is not necessary because role of reinfection is probably minimal. Most partners are probably already subclinically infected with HPV, even if no warts are visible.

Human Papillomavirus: Squamous Cell Carcinoma In Situ, and Invasive Squamous Cell Carcinoma of the Anogenital Skin

Human papillomavirus (HPV) infection of the anogenital epithelium can result in a spectrum of changes referred to as squamous intraepithelial lesions (SILs), ranging from mild dysplasia to squamous cell carcinoma (SCC) in situ (SCCIS). Over time, these lesions can regress, persist, progress, or recur, in some cases to invasive SCC. Clinically, lesions appear as multifocal macules, papules, plaques on the external anogenital region. Lesions involving the cervix and anus have the highest risk for transformation to invasive SCC; however, lesions can transform at any site.

Synonyms: Vulvar intraepithelial neoplasia, penile intraepithelial neoplasm, bowenoid papulosis.

EPIDEMIOLOGY

Terminology
The Bethesda System (National Cancer Institute) is currently used as terminology for "dysplastic" lesions caused by HPV on anogenital sites (Table 25-3). The terminology applies to both cytologic (Pap test) and histologic assessments. Intraepithelial neoplasia are designated as cervical (CIN), vulvar (VIN), penile (PIN), and anal (AIN). VIN is classified as VIN1 (mild dysplasia), VIN2 (moderate dysplasia), VIN3 (severe dysplasia or carcinoma in situ), and VIN3 differentiated type, basaloid, bowenoid (warty).

Etiology HPV types 16, 18, 31, and 33 (See Table 23-1)

Transmission HPV transmitted sexually. Autoinoculation. Rarely, HPV-16 transmitted from mother to newborn with subsequent development of bowenoid papulosis (BP) on penis.

Incidence Marked increase during past two decades associated with increased sexual promiscuity. Cervical SCC is the second most common female malignancy worldwide, second only to breast cancer. It is the most frequent malignancy in developing countries—500,000 new cases and 200,000 deaths worldwide attributed to it annually.

Risk Factors Immunocompromised state, cigarette smoking are risk factors for more dysplastic lesions and invasive SCC.

PATHOGENESIS

HPV-16 and -18 infected cells may not be able to differentiate fully as a result of either (a) functional interference of cell cycle–regulating proteins, caused by viral gene expression (e.g., interaction between HPV-16 E6 with cellular protein p53, interaction between HPV-16 E7 with cellular protein pRB) or (b) over-production of E5, E6, and E7. When this occurs, the host DNA synthesis continues unchecked and leads to rapidly dividing undifferentiated cells with morphologic characteristics of intraepithelial neoplasias. Accumulated chromosomal breakages, rearrangements, deletions, and other genomic mutations in these cells lead to cells with invasion capability and, ultimately, to cervical malignancy.

HISTORY

Duration of Lesions Weeks to months to years to decades.

Incubation Period Months to years.

Systems Review Prior history of condylomata acuminata. Female partners of males may have CIN.

PHYSICAL EXAMINATION

Skin Lesions Erythematous macules. Lichenoid (flat-topped) or pigmented papules (called bowenoid papulosis) (Figs. 25-6 and 25-7); may show some confluence or form plaque(s) (Fig. 25-8). Leukoplakia-like plaque. Surface usually smooth, velvety. Nodule or ulceration in field of SIL suggests invasive SCC (Figs. 25-9 and 25-10). Tan, brown, pink, red, violaceous, white. Characteristically clusters, i.e., commonly multifocal. May be solitary.

Distribution Males: glans penis, prepuce (75%) (flat lichenoid papules or erythematous macules); penile shaft (25%) (pigmented papules) (Fig. 25-6). Females: labia majora and minora, clitoris. Multicentric involvement of the cervix, vulva, perineum, and/or anus occurs not infrequently. Both sexes: inguinal folds, perineal/perianal skin (Fig. 25-7). Oropharyngeal mucosa.

Acetowhitening Application of 3 to 5% acetic acid to the area of involvement for 5 min may facilitate visualization of lesions on the cervix or in the anal canal.

Other May be associated with cervical dysplasia, CIN, cervical SCC. Rarely, SCCIS of other sites, i.e., periungual, intraoral.

DIFFERENTIAL DIAGNOSIS

Multiple Skin Colored Papules ± Hyperkeratosis External genital warts, psoriasis vulgaris; lichen planus.

Pigmented Anogenital Macule(s)/Papule(s) Genital lentiginosis, melanoma (in situ or invasive), pigmented basal cell carcinoma, angiokeratomas.

LABORATORY EXAMINATIONS

Dermatopathology Epidermal proliferation with numerous mitotic figures, abnormal mitoses, atypical pleomorphic cells with large hyperchromatic, often clumped nuclei, dysker-

atotic cells; basal membrane intact. Koilocytosis. Recent application of podophyllin to condyloma acuminatum may cause changes similar to SCCIS.

Southern Blot Analysis Identifies HPV type.

Pap Smear Koilocytotic atypia.

Exfoliative Cytology Cervical Pap smears have been recommended annually for women 50 years of age or older. Cytology of the anal canal may also be helpful in management of individuals with a history of anal HPV infection, especially if immunocompromised (HIV disease, renal transplant recipients). Anal Pap tests are obtained with a cervical brush and ThinPrep solution. By The Bethesda System, these cytologic findings are reported as atypical squamous cells of undetermined significance (ASCUS), low-grade squamous intraepithelial lesion (LSIL), high-grade (SILH), and SCC.

Diagnosis Clinical suspicion, confirmed by biopsy of lesion.

COURSE AND PROGNOSIS

Invasive SCC develops only through well-defined precursor lesions. Over time, these lesions can regress, persist, recur, or progress,

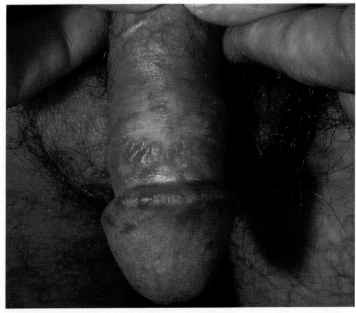

Figure 25-6 HPV-induced squamous cell carcinoma in situ: penis *Multiple red papules, discrete and confluent, on the distal shaft and glans penis. Diagnosis is made on lesional biopsy.*

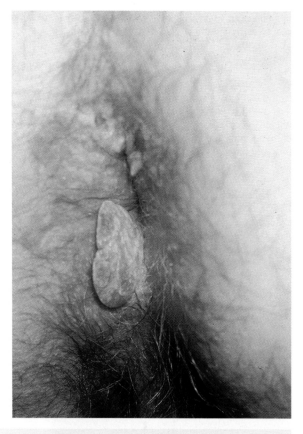

Figure 25-7 HPV-induced squamous cell carcinoma in situ: perianal/perineal *Asymptomatic well-demarcated perianal/perineal pink plaque. The rudder-like lesion is a skin tag at the site of an old hemorrhoid. The lesions resolved with 5% imiquimod cream. Although the individual was apparently healthy, underlying immunodeficiency was present; lymphoma was diagnosed one year after the SCCIS was detected.*

Table 25-3   BETHESDA SYSTEM FOR CLASSIFICATION OF ANOGENITAL DYSPLASIA

Histologic Findings		Older Terminology/ Replaced	Still Older Terminology
Atypical proliferating suprabasal cells present in the lower one-third of the epithelium, although cytopathic changes of HPV are full thickness	Low-grade squamous intraepithelial lesion (LSIL)	Intraepithelial 1 (IN1)	Mild dysplasia
Atypical proliferating suprabasal cells present in the lower two-thirds of the epithelium, although cytopathic changes of HPV are full thickness	High-grade SIL (HSIL)	IN2 and IN3	
Atypical proliferating suprabasal cells present in the full thickness of the epithelium	Squamous cell carcinoma in situ (SCCIS)	Squamous cell carcinoma in situ (SCCIS)	Erythroplasia of Querat, Bowen's disease, bowenoid papulosis
Invasive SCC present, usually arising in a field of HSIL	Invasive SCC	Invasive SCC	

in some cases to invasive SCC. Natural history of CIN is best studied: progression to invasive SCC occurs in 36% of cases over a 20-year period. Rate of progression of AIN is not known but appears to be increasing. AIN may develop deep in glands and, although detected cytologically, can exist before visible lesions are detected with colposcopy. Patients with intraepithelial neoplasias, which often occurs in immunocompromised individuals, should be followed indefinitely, with monitoring by exfoliative cytology and lesional biopsy specimens.

MANAGEMENT

Colposcopy A colposcope is a binocular microscope used to examine the cervix, providing magnification (6- to 40-fold) and illumination. The most common indication for colposcopy is abnormal exfoliative cytology. Acetic acid, 3 to 5%, is applied to the cervix, which causes columnar and abnormal epithelium to become edematous. Abnormal (atypical) epithelium adopts a white or opaque appearance that can be distinguished from the normal pink epithelium. Abnormal epithelium is then biopsied. Colposcopy can also be performed on individ-

uals with abnormal anal exfoliative cytology, and biopsy specimens obtained from abnormal site(s).

Biopsy of Lesions In cases of documented SIL or SCCIS, biopsy specimens should be obtained from rapidly enlarging lesions, areas of ulceration or bleeding, exuberant tissue with abnormal vascularity.

Local Therapy of SIL The only way of possibly reducing the potential risk of invasive SCC with its morbidity and mortality is diagnosis and eradication of intraepithelial disease. In that lesions are relatively uncommon, cases are often best managed by a dermatologist with clinical experience in the care of these patients, an oncologic gynecologist, or a colorectal surgeon. If lesion biopsy specimens do not show early invasion, lesions can be treated medically or surgically.

Medical Management 5-fluorouracil cream has been used but is difficult to use because of erosions. Imiquimod cream 5% is also effective.

Surgical Management Surgical excision, Mohs' surgery, electrosurgery, laser vaporization, cryosurgery.

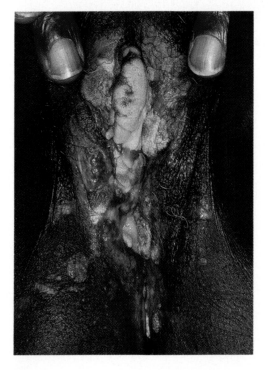

Figure 25-8 HPV-induced squamous cell carcinoma in situ: vulva/perineum *Huge verrucous lesions on the vulva and perineum recurred several times after laser surgery in a HIV-infected female; SCCIS was also present on the cervix. The vulvar lesion evolved into invasive SCC, so-called verrucous carcinoma (giant condyloma of Buschke and Lowenstein).*

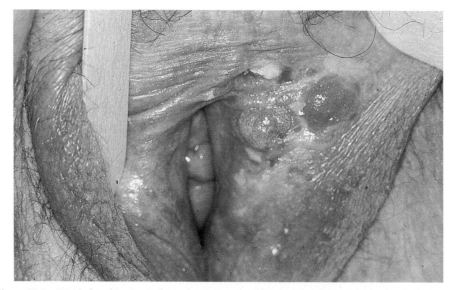

Figure 25-9 HPV-induced in situ and invasive squamous cell carcinoma: vulva *Several red, flesh nodules (invasive SCC) arising within a white plaque (SCCIS) on the left labium.*

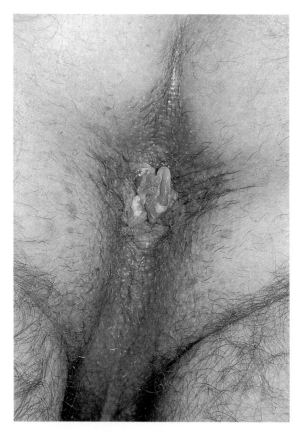

Figure 25-10 HPV-induced in situ and invasive squamous cell carcinoma: perineal/perianal *Brown perineal and perianal macules and papules (SCCIS) with a pink nodule arising at the anal verge in an HIV-infected male. The patient presented when he detected the nodule, which he thought was a hemorrhoid. Excisional biopsy of the nodule detected invasive SCC arising within SCCIS.*

HERPES SIMPLEX VIRUS: GENITAL INFECTIONS

Genital herpes (GH) is a chronic sexually transmitted viral infection, characterized by asymptomatic viral shedding. In most cases, both primary infection and recurrences are asymptomatic. When symptomatic, primary GH may present with grouped vesicles at the site of inoculation associated with significant pain and regional lymphadenopathy. When aware of GH, individuals may notice mild symptoms, uncommonly of recurring outbreaks of vesicles at the same site. Most symptoms from GH relate to the psychological stigma of having a chronic transmissible STD. (See also HSV Infections.) Neonates are susceptible to HSV infection when exposed perinatally, with risk of significant morbidity and mortality.

Synonyms: Herpes progenitalis, herpes genitalis, genital herpes simplex.

EPIDEMIOLOGY

Age of Onset   Young, sexually active adults.

Etiology   Herpes simplex virus (HSV)-2 > HSV-1. Currently in the United States, 30% of new cases of GH are caused by HSV-1.

Incidence   >600,000 new infections in the United States annually; 30 million Americans are HSV-2 infected, i.e., approximately 1 in 5 adults. Incidence has increased by 30% during the past 13 years, in spite of awareness of "safe sex" practices. Older studies report the presence of antibodies to HSV-2 varies with the sexual history of the individual: nuns, 3%; middle class, 25%; heterosexuals at an STD clinic, 26%; homosexuals, 46%; lower classes, 46 to 60%; prostitutes, 70 to 80%.

Race and Sex   By HSV-2 seropositivity studies in the United States, more common in blacks: 3 in 5 men, 4 in 5 women; in whites: 1 in 5 men, 1 in 4 women. In whites, prevalence levels off after age 30 years. In blacks/Hispanics, prevalence continues to increase after age 30.

Transmission   Usually skin-to-skin contact. In most cases, 70% of transmission occurs during times of asymptomatic HSV shedding, which occurs during 1% of days when no identifiable lesion is present. Transmission rate in discordant couples (one partner infected, the other not) approximately 10% per year; 25% of females become infected, compared with only 4 to 6% of males. Prior HSV-1 infection is protective; in females with anti-HSV-1 antibodies, 15% become infected with HSV-2, but in those without anti-HSV-1 antibodies, 30% become infected with HSV-2.

Risk Factors for Transmission   Risk increases with number of sex partners. 40% of those with ≥50 different partners have genital HSV infection.

Diseases Characterized by Genital Ulcers   In the United States, most patients with genital ulcers have GH, syphilis, or chancroid. The relative frequency varies by geographic area and patient population, but in most areas GH is the most common of these diseases. More than one of these diseases may be present among at least 3 to 10% of patients with genital ulcers. Each disease has been associated with an increased risk for HIV infection.

Impact of GH   The physical symptoms of GH are minor in most individuals. The major symptoms are psychological, i.e., social stigmatization and fear of harming someone through sexual intercourse.

Pregnancy and GH   Asymptomatic HSV shedding occurs in .35 to 1.4% of women in labor in the United States. 32% of pregnant women have anti-HSV antibodies. 10% of pregnant women are at risk for primary HSV-2 infection from HSV-2 infected partners. Incidence of neonatal herpes: 1 in 2000 to 1 in 15,000 births. 95% of newborns with HSV infection contract it during labor and delivery. Transmission can occur intrauterine, perinatally, or postnatally. Risk factors for neonatal HSV infection: primary GH in mother at time of delivery, absent maternal anti-HSV antibody, procedures on fetus, father with HSV infection. Treatment of mother with GH at time of delivery is an option to cesarean section (not approved).

PATHOGENESIS

HSV infection is transmitted through close contact with a person shedding virus at a peripheral site, mucosal surface, or secretion. HSV is inactivated promptly at room temperature; aerosol or fomitic spread unlikely. Infection occurs via inoculation onto susceptible mucosal surface or break in skin. Subsequent to primary infection at inoculation site, HSV ascends peripheral sensory nerves and enters sensory or autonomic nerve root ganglia, where latency is established. Latency can occur after both symptomatic and asymptomatic primary infection. Recrudescences may be clinically symptomatic or asymptomatic.

HISTORY

Incubation Period   2- to 20-day (average 6) incubation period.

Symptoms   Only 9.2% of HSV-2 seropositive individuals are aware symptoms are those of GH; 90.8% do not recognize symptoms of GH.

Primary GH   Most individuals with primary infection are asymptomatic. Those with symptoms report fever, headache, malaise, myalgia, peaking within the first 3 to 4 days after onset of lesions, resolving during the subsequent 3 to 4 days. Depending on location, pain, itching, dysuria, lumbar radiculitis, vaginal or urethral discharge are common symptoms. Tender inguinal lymphadenopathy occurs during second and third weeks. Deep pelvic pain associated with pelvic lymphadenopathy. Some cases of first clinical episode of GH are manifested by extensive disease that requires hospitalization.

Recurrent GH   New symptoms may result from old infections. Most individuals with GH do not experience "classic" findings of grouped vesicles on erythematous base. Common symptoms are itch, burning, fissure, redness, irritation prior to eruption of vesicles. Dysuria, sciatica, rectal discomfort.

Systemic Symptoms   Symptoms of aseptic HSV-2 meningitis can occur with primary or recurrent GH.

PHYSICAL EXAMINATION

Skin Lesions

Most clinical lesions are minor breaks in the mucocutaneous epithelium, presenting as erosion, "abrasions," fissures. The classically described findings are uncommon.

Primary GH   An erythematous plaque is often noted initially, followed soon by grouped vesicles, which may evolve to pustules; these become eroded as the overlying epidermis sloughs (Fig. 25-11). Erosions are punched out and may enlarge to ulcerations, which may be crusted or moist. These epithelial defects heal in 2 to 4 weeks, often with resulting postinflammatory hypo- or hyperpigmentation, uncommonly with scarring. The area of involvement may be circumferential around the penis, or the entire vulva may be involved (Fig. 25-11).

Recurrent GH   Lesions may be similar to primary infection but on a reduced scale. Often a 1- to 2-cm plaque of erythema surmounted with vesicles (Fig. 25-12), which rupture with formation of erosions (Fig. 25-13). Heals in 1 to 2 weeks.

Distribution   *Males*   Primary infection: glans, prepuce, shaft, sulcus, scrotum, thigh, buttocks. Recurrences: penile shaft (Fig. 25-13), glans, buttocks.

Females   Primary infection: labia majora/minora (Fig. 25-11), perineum, inner thighs. Recurrences: labia majora/minora (Fig. 25-14), buttocks.

Anorectal infection   Occurs in male homosexuals (often HSV-1); characterized by tenesmus, anal pain, proctitis, discharge, and ulcerations (Fig. 25-15) as far as 10 cm into anal canal.

General Findings

Regional Lymph Nodes   Inguinal/femoral lymph nodes enlarged, firm, nonfluctuant, tender; usually unilateral.

Signs of Aseptic Meningitis   Fever, nuchal rigidity. Can occur in the absence of GH. Pain along sciatic nerve.

DIFFERENTIAL DIAGNOSIS

Anogenital erosive(s)/ulcer(s) Trauma, candidiasis, syphilitic chancre, fixed drug eruption, chancroid, gonococcal erosion.

LABORATORY STUDIES

Diagnosis can be confirmed by tests that detect HSV or antibodies to HSV.

HSV Detection *Viral Culture/Modified Culture* Gold standard of diagnosis. Documents the presence of HSV in 1 to 10 days. Positive in 70% of active lesions.

HSV Antigen Detection Direct fluorescent antibody (DFA) is sensitive and specific method of identifying HSV-1 and -2 on a smear from vesicle fluid or ulcer base. EIA (Herpchek): rapid, sensitive.

PCR Specific, sensitive, but expensive.

Antibodies to HSV Primary HSV infection documented by obtaining acute and convalescent sera that show seroconversion for HSV antibodies (seroconversion occurs at approximately 13 days after becoming infected), as well as indicating whether HSV-1 or -2. In a patient with recurrent genital lesions, GH can be ruled out if HSV type specific serologic test (TSST)

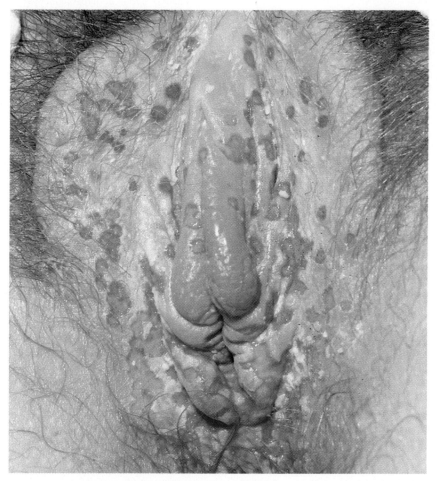

Figure 25-11 Genital herpes: primary vulvar infection *Multiple, extremely painful, punched-out, confluent, shallow ulcers on the vulva and perineum. Micturition is often very painful. Associated inguinal lymphadenopathy is common.*

SEXUALLY TRANSMITTED DISEASES

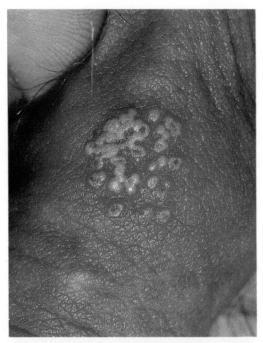

Figure 25-12 Genital herpes: recurrent infection of the penis *Group of vesicles with early central crusting on a red base arising on the shaft of the penis. This "textbook" presentation, however, is much less common than small asymptomatic erosions or fissures.*

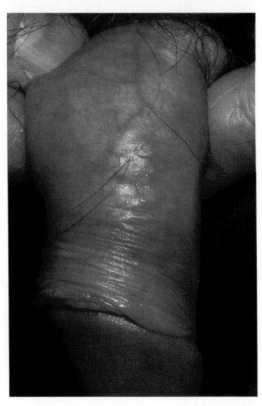

Figure 25-13 Genital herpes: recurrent infection of the penis *A cluster of small erosive lesions on the shaft of the penis associated with a mild burning and pruritic sensation. These types of lesions are the most common presentation of recurrent genital herpes and are often unnoticed by the patient.*

is negative. The most specific serologic tests are type-specific antibodies detected by Western blot technique.

Type-specific serologic test (TSST) Does not influence treatment but can influence counseling.

(ELISA) Enzyme-linked Immunosorbent Assay Of no value in diagnosis of HSV infection.

Sensitivity of Diagnostic Tests With HSV with blisters: viral culture positive, 70 to 80%; Herpchek, 90%; DFA, 90%. With ulcerated lesions: viral culture positive, 30 to 40%; Herpchek, 50%; DFA, 30 to 70%. With crusted lesions, viral culture positive, 20 to 30%; Herpchek, 60%; DFA, 10%.

Tzanck Smear Optimally, fluid from intact vesicle and/or base is smeared thinly on a microscope slide, dried, and stained with either Wright's or Giemsa's stain. Positive if giant keratinocytes or multinucleated giant keratinocytes are detected but not specific.

Dermatopathology Ballooning and reticular epidermal degeneration, acanthosis, acantholysis, and intraepidermal vesicles; intranuclear inclusion bodies, multinucleate giant keratinocytes; multilocular vesicles.

DIAGNOSIS

Because in most cases intermittent asymptomatic shedding is occurring and lesions are "atypical" (not grouped vesicles on erythematous base), GH must be confirmed by viral culture or DFA.

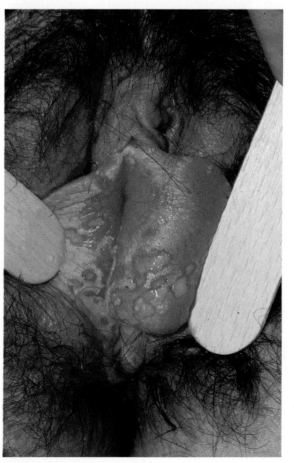

Figure 25-14 Genital herpes: recurrent vulvar infection *Large painful erosions on the labia. Extensive lesions such as these are uncommon in recurrent genital herpes in an otherwise healthy individual.*

SEXUALLY TRANSMITTED DISEASES

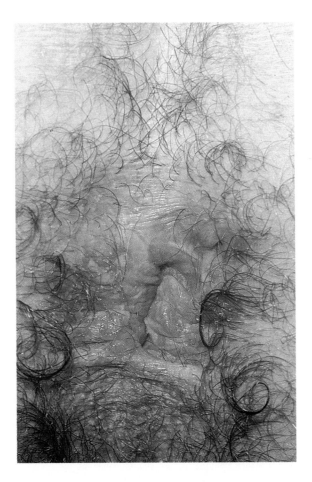

Figure 25-15 Genital herpes: recurrent infection of the anus and perineum *Multiple, painful, sharply demarcated ulcers in an HIV-infected male.*

COURSE AND PROGNOSIS

GH may be recurrent and has no cure. 70% of HSV-2 infections are asymptomatic. HSV-2 GH recurs approximately 6 times/year; HSV-1 GH usually recurs, on the average, only once per year. Of individuals with initially symptomatic genital HSV-2 infection, almost all have symptomatic recurrences; recurrence rates are high in those with an extended first episode of infection, regardless of whether antiviral therapy is given. The rate of recurrence is 20% higher in men than women. Chronic suppressive therapy does not completely suppress viral shedding; it is reduced by 95% as detected by viral culture, and by 80% by PCR. Chronic suppressive therapy may reduce transmission, but this has not been documented. The incidence of primary infection with acyclovir-resistant HSV strains in individuals never exposed to acyclovir is 2.7% in the United States.

Erythema multiforme may complicate GH, occurring 1 to 2 weeks after an outbreak.

MANAGEMENT

PREVENTION OF GH

Sexual transmission

- Patients should be advised to abstain from sexual activity while lesions are present.
- Use of condoms should be encouraged during all sexual exposures.
- Efficacy of chronic suppressive therapy not proven.
- Patients with GH should be told about the natural history of the disease, with emphasis on the potential of recurrent episodes, asymptomatic viral shedding, and sexual transmission.
- Sexual transmission of HSV has been documented to occur during periods without evidence of lesions. In discordant couples, transmission usually occurs during period of asymptomatic shedding.
- Risk for neonatal infection should be explained to all patients—male and female—with GH.

Perinatal transmission

Many experts recommend serotesting for HSV-1 and HSV-2 (Western blot) at the first prenatal visit. Infants born to women who asymptomatically shed HSV have reduced birth weight and increased prematurity.

Topical Antiviral Therapy

No significant efficacy.

Oral Antiviral Therapy

Antiviral agents provide partial control of symptoms and signs of herpes episodes when used to treat first clinical episode or when used as suppressive therapy. They neither eradicate latent virus nor affect subsequent risk, frequency, or severity of recurrences after drug is discontinued. Even after laboratory testing, at least a quarter of patients with GH have no laboratory-confirmed diagnosis. Many experts recommend treatment for chancroid and syphilis as well as GH if the diagnosis is unclear or if the patient resides in a community in which chancroid is present.

First clinical episode (primary or first symptomatic)

Antiviral agents are more effective in treating primary infections than recurrences. Most effective when initiated ≤ 48 h after onset of symptoms.

Acyclovir

400 mg tid or 200 mg 5 times daily for 7–10 days or until clinical resolution occurs.

Valacyclovir

1 gm bid for 10 days.

Famciclovir

250 mg bid for 10 days.

First clinical episode of herpes proctitis

Acyclovir

400 mg PO 5 times daily for 10 days or until clinical resolution occurs.

Recurrent episodes

When treatment is instituted (by patient) during the prodrome or within 2 days of onset of lesions, patients with recurrent disease experience limited benefit from therapy in that the severity of the eruption is reduced. If early treatment cannot be administered, most immunocompetent patients with recurrent disease do not benefit from acyclovir treatment; and for these patients it is not generally recommended.

Acyclovir

400 mg PO tid for 5 days *or* 800 mg PO bid for 5 days.

Valacyclovir	500 mg bid for 5 days.
Famciclovir	250 mg bid for 5 days.
Daily suppressive therapy	Reduces frequency of recurrences by at least 75% among patients with frequent (more than 6–9 per year) recurrences. Suppressive treatment with oral acyclovir does not totally eliminate symptomatic or asymptomatic viral shedding or the potential for transmission. Safety and efficacy have been documented among persons receiving daily therapy for as long as 5 years. Acyclovir-resistant strains of HSV have been isolated from some persons receiving suppressive therapy, but these strains have not been associated with treatment failure among immunocompetent patients. *After 1 year of continuous therapy, acyclovir should be discontinued to allow assessment of the patient's rate of recurrent episodes.*
Acyclovir	400 mg bid.
Valacyclovir	500–1000 mg/d.
Famciclovir	250 mg bid.
Severe disease/immuno-compromise	Patients with herpes who do not respond to the recommended dose of acyclovir may require a higher oral dose of acyclovir, IV acyclovir, or may be infected with an acyclovir-resistant HSV strain, requiring IV foscarnet. The role of valacyclovir and famciclovir are not yet established. IV therapy should be provided for patients with severe disease or complications necessitating hospitalization (e.g., disseminated infection that includes encephalitis, pneumonitis, or hepatitis).
Acyclovir	5 mg/kg body weight IV every 8 h for 5–7 days or until clinical resolution is attained *or* 400 mg PO 5 times a day for 7–14 days.
Oral valacyclovir *or* famciclovir	Have reduced the necessity for IV acyclovir therapy.
Neonatal	See Neonatal HSV Infection.
Acyclovir-resistant	See HSV Infections.
Foscarnet	40 mg/kg IV q8h for 14–21 days.
Imiquimod cream 5%	May be effective.

NEISSERIA GONORRHOEAE INFECTIONS

Approximately 600,000 new infections with *Neisseria gonorrhoeae* occur each year. Most infections among men produce symptoms that cause them to seek curative treatment soon enough to prevent serious sequelae—but this may not be soon enough to prevent transmission to others. Many infections among women do not produce recognizable symptoms until complications [e.g., pelvic inflammatory disease (PID)] have occurred. In males, the most common presentation is an acute urethritis; in females, cervicitis. Others sites in the genitourinary tract may become infected as well as the rectum, pharynx, and conjunctiva. Both symptomatic and asymptomatic cases of PID can result in tubal scarring that leads to infertility or ectopic pregnancy. Because gonococcal infections among women are often asymptomatic, an important component of gonorrhea control continues to be the screening of women at high risk for STDs. Gonococcemia results in seeding of multiple sites, most commonly the joints and skin, resulting in disseminated gonococcal infection (DGI).

EPIDEMIOLOGY

Age of Onset   Young, sexually active. In newborns, conjunctivitis.

Sex   Young females; males who have sex with males. Symptomatic infection more common in males. Pharyngeal and anorectal in homosexual males.

Race   Incidence higher in whites than in blacks.

Incidence   Decreasing in the United States. Current estimates are that slightly: >1 million new infections with *N. gonorrhoeae* occur in the United States each year, half of which go unreported.

Etiology   *N. gonorrhoeae,* the gonococcus, a gram-negative diplococcus. Humans are the only natural reservoir of the organism. Strains that cause DGI tend to cause minimal genital inflammation. In the United States, these strains have occurred infrequently during the past decade.

Transmission   Sexually, from partner who either is asymptomatic or has minimal symptoms. Neonate exposed to infected secretions in birth canal. About 1% of patients with untreated mucosal gonococcal infection develop DGI.

Geography   Worldwide. Incidence of DGI varies with local incidence of DGI strains of gonococcus.

PATHOGENESIS

Gonococcus has affinity for columnar epithelium, while stratified and squamous epithelia are more resistant to attack. Epithelium is penetrated between epithelial cells, causing a submucosal inflammation with PMN reaction with resultant purulent discharge. Strains of gonococcus that cause DGI tend to cause little genital inflammation and thereby escape detection. These strains have become uncommon in the United States during the past decade. Most signs and symptoms of DGI are manifestations of immune-complex formation and deposition. Multiple episodes of DGI may be associated with abnormality of terminal complement component factors.

LABORATORY STUDIES

Gram's Stain   Gram-negative diplococci intracellularly in PMNs in exudate (Fig. 25-16)

Culture   Isolation on gonococcal-selective media, i.e., chocolatized blood agar, Martin-Lewis medium, Thayer-Martin medium. Antimicrobial susceptibility testing important due to resistant strains.

Specimen Collection Sites   *Heterosexual men*: Urethra, oropharynx. *Homosexual men*: Urethra, rectum, oropharynx. *Women*: Cervix, rectum, oropharynx. *DGI*: Blood.

Serologic Tests   None available for gonorrhea. All patients should have a serologic test for syphilis and should be offered HIV testing.

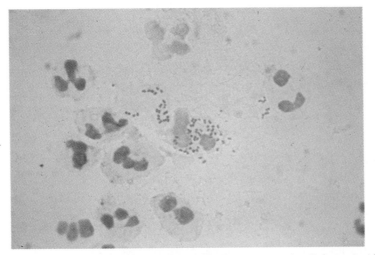

Figure 25-16 *Neisseria gonorrhoeae:* **Gram's stain**   *Multiple, gram-negative diplococci within polymorphonuclear leukocytes as well as in the extracellular areas of a smear from a urethral discharge.*

MANAGEMENT

Prevention

Use of condoms should be encouraged.

Antimicrobial regimens

Most patients with incubating syphilis may be cured by any of the regimens containing ceftriaxone or doxycycline. There is a high frequency of chlamydial infections in persons with gonorrhea, and treatment regimens cover this possibility.

Uncomplicated urethral, endocervical, or rectal infections

Recommended regimens

Cefixime	400 mg PO in a single dose *or*
Ceftriaxone	250 mg IM in a single dose *or*
Ciprofloxacin	500 mg PO in a single dose *or*
Ofloxacin	400 mg PO in a single dose *or*
Azithromycin	1 g PO in a single dose *or*
Doxycycline	100 mg PO bid for 7 days

Alternative regimens

Spectinomycin	2 g IM in a single dose *or*
Injectable cephalosporin	Given with probenecid 1 g PO
Ceftizoxime	500 mg IM in a single dose
Cefotaxime	500 mg IM in a single dose
Cefotetan	1 g IM in a single dose
Cefoxitin	2 g IM in a single dose

Single-dose quinolone

Enoxacin	400 mg PO
Lomefloxacin	400 mg PO
Norfloxacin	800 mg PO

Pharyngeal infection

More difficult to eradicate than infections at urogenital and anorectal sites. Few regimens can reliably cure pharyngeal infections >90% of the time. Although chlamydial coinfection of the pharynx is unusual, coinfection at genital sites sometimes occurs. Therefore, treatment for both gonorrhea and chlamydia is suggested.

Recommended regimens

Ceftriaxone	250 mg IM in a single dose *or*
Ciprofloxacin	500 mg PO in a single dose *or*
Oflaxacin	400 mg PO in a single dose *or*
Azithromycin	1 g PO in a single dose *or*
Doxycycline	100 mg PO bid for 7 days

Disseminated infection

Hospitalization recommended for initial therapy, especially for patients who cannot reliably comply with treatment, have uncertain diagnoses, or have purulent synovial effusions or other complications. Patients should be examined for clinical evidence of endocarditis or meningitis. Patients treated for DGI should be treated presumptively for concurrent *C. trachomatis* infection unless appropriate testing excludes this infection.

Recommended initial regimen

Ceftriaxone	1 g IM or IV q 24 h

Alternative initial regimen

Cefotaxime	1 g IV q 8 h *or*
Ceftizoxime	1 g IV q 8 h *or*
For persons allergic to β-lactam drugs	
Ciprofloxacin	500 mg IV q 12 h
Ofloxacin	400 mg IV q 12 h
Spectinomycin	2 g IM q 12 h

Recommended completion of therapy

All regimens should be continued for 24 to 48 h after improvement begins; then therapy may be switched to one of the following regimens to complete a full week of antimicrobial therapy:

Cefixime	400 mg PO bid *or*
Ciprofloxacin	500 mg PO bid *or*
Ofloxacin	400 mg PO bid

SEXUALLY TRANSMITTED DISEASES

Persons with uncomplicated gonorrhea who are cured with any of the preceding regimens need not return for test-of-cure. Persons with persisting symptoms after treatment should be evaluated by culture for *N. gonorrhoeae*, and any gonococci isolated should be evaluated for antimicrobial susceptibility. Infections detected after treatment with one of the recommended regimens more commonly occur because of reinfection rather than treatment failure, indicating a need for improving sex partner referral and patient education. Persistent urethritis, cervicitis, or proctitis also may be caused by *C. trachomatis* and other organisms.

Management of sex partners

Sex partners should be referred for evaluation and treatment. Gonococcal infection is often asymptomatic in sex partners of patients with DGI. As for uncomplicated infections, patients should be instructed to refer sex partner(s) for evaluation and treatment.

Localized Infection (Gonorrhea)

Gonorrhea affectes the mucocutaneous surfaces of the lower genitourinary tract, anus, and rectum, and the oropharynx. The most common presentation in males is a purulent urethral discharge. In females, cervical infection is most common and is often asymptomatic; if untreated, infection can spread to deeper structures with abscess formation and disseminated gonococcal infection (DGI). *Synonyms:* Clap, blennorrhagia, blennorrhea.

HISTORY

Incubation Period

Males 90% of males develop urethritis within 5 days of exposure.

Females Usually >2 weeks when symptomatic; however, up to 75% of women are asymptomatic.

Skin Symptoms Urethral discharge, dysuria. Vaginal discharge; deep pelvic or lumbar pain. Copious purulent anal discharge; burning or stinging pain on defecation; tenesmus; blood in/on stool. Mild sore throat.

PHYSICAL EXAMINATION

Site of Infection

External Genitalia

Males Urethral discharge ranging from scanty and clear to purulent and copious (Fig. 25-17); meatal edema; preputial or penile edema. Balanoposthitis with subpreputial discharge in uncircumcised men; balanitis in circumcised men. Folliculitis or cellulitis of thigh or abdomen. Rare complications of anterior urethritis include infection of parafrenal sebaceous glands of Tyson, paraurethral ducts, Littré's glands, lacunae of Morgagni, subepithelial and periurethral tissue of the urethra, median raphe, Cowper's ducts, and glands.

Females Periurethral edema, urethritis. Purulent discharge from cervix but no vaginitis. In prepubescent females, vulvovaginitis. Bartholin's abscess.

Deeper Structures *Males* Prostatitis, epididymitis, vesiculitis, cystitis.

Females Pelvic inflammatory disease with signs of peritonitis, endocervicitis, endosalpingitis, endometritis.

Anorectum In females and homosexual males, proctitis with pain and purulent discharge

Oropharynx In females and homosexual males, pharyngitis with erythema.

Eye *Conjunctivitis* In newborn, organism is transmitted as newborn passes through birth canal. In adults, rare in industrialized nations but in epidemics in third world countries such as Ethiopia. Usually occurs in the absence of genital infection, copious purulent conjunctival discharge. Can be complicated by corneal ulceration and perforation.

General Examination

DGI Acral hemorrhagic pustules.

DIFFERENTIAL DIAGNOSIS

Urethritis Genital herpes with urethritis, *Chlamydia* trachomatis urethritis, *Ureaplasma urealyticum* urethritis, *Trichomonas vaginalis* urethritis, Reiter's syndrome.

Cervicitis *Chlamydia trachomatis* or herpes simplex virus cervicitis.

LABORATORY EXAMINATIONS

See *Neisseria Gonorrhoeae* Infections, page 882.

DIAGNOSIS

Clinical suspicion, confirmed by laboratory findings, i.e., presumptively by identifying gram-negative diplococci intracellularly in PMNs in smears, confirmed by culture.

COURSE AND PROGNOSIS

Most infections among men produce symptoms that cause the person to seek curative treatment soon enough to prevent serious sequelae—but not soon enough to prevent transmission to others. If not treated, complications due to ascending infection occur: prostatitis—pain on defecation; epididymitis—swelling of epididymis and pain in walking; cystititis. Many infections among women do not produce recognizable symptoms until complications such as pelvic inflammatory disease (PID) occur. PID, whether symptomatic or asymptomatic, can cause tubal scarring, leading to infertility or ectopic pregnancy. Because gonococcal infections among women are often asymptomatic, a primary measure for controlling gonorrhea in the United States has been the screening of high-risk women. DGI more common in women with asymptomatic cervical, endometrial, or tubal infection and in homosexual men with asymptomatic rectal or pharyngeal gonorrhea.

MANAGEMENT

See *Neisseria Gonorrhoeae* Infections, page 882.

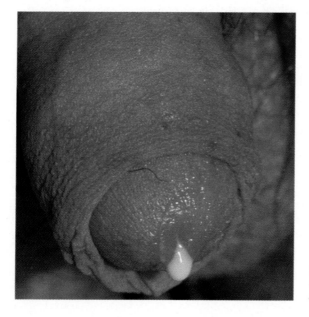

Figure 25-17 Gonorrhea *Purulent, creamy urethral discharge from the distal urethra of a male.*

Disseminated Gonococcal Infection

Disseminated gonococcal infection (DGI) is a systemic infection that follows the hematogenous dissemination of the gonococcus from infected mucosal sites to skin, tenosynovium, and joints and is characterized by fever, petechial or pustular acral lesions, asymmetric arthralgias, tenosynovitis, or septic arthritis. It is occasionally complicated by perihepatitis and, rarely, endocarditis or meningitis. *Synonyms:* Gonococcemia, gonococcal arthritis-dermatitis syndrome.

HISTORY

Incubation Period   7 to 30 days of mucosal infection (range, from a few days to 1 year). Varies with host factors such as menstruation, invasiveness of infecting organism.

Prodrome   Fever, anorexia, malaise, ±shaking chills.

Other Factors   Recurring symptoms around menses, migratory polyarthralgias.

PHYSICAL EXAMINATION

Skin Findings   1- to 5-mm erythematous macules evolving to hemorrhagic pustules (Fig. 25-18) within 24 to 48 h. Centers at times hemorrhagic/necrotic. Rarely, large hemorrhagic bullae, 3 to 20 in number.

Distribution   Acral (Fig. 25-18), arms more often than legs, near small joints of hands or feet. Difficult to detect in black patients; look in web spaces. Face spared.

Mucous Membranes   Usually asymptomatic colonization of oropharynx, urethra, anorectum, endometrium.

General Examination   Fever 38°C to 39°C usual. Severity varies: DGI with skin lesions alone, classic DGI with skin lesions and tenosynovitis, DGI with septic arthritis, DGI with metastatic infection at other sites.

Tenosynovitis   Common. Single or few sites, acrally. Extensor/flexor tendons and sheaths of hands/feet. Erythema, tenderness, swelling along tendon sheath aggravated by moving tendon.

Septic Arthritis   Joint—red, hot, tender with effusion; asymmetric. Most commonly involved: knee, elbow, ankle, metacarpophalangeal/interphalangeal joints of hand, shoulder, hip. Usually only one to two joints involved.

Other   Hepatitis, perihepatitis (Fitz-Hugh-Curtis syndrome), myopericarditis, endocarditis, meningitis, perihepatitis. Rarely, pneumonitis, adult respiratory distress syndrome, osteomyelitis.

DIFFERENTIAL DIAGNOSIS

Scant, Acral, Hemorrhagic Pustules   Bacteremia: meningococcemia, other bacteremias, endocarditis. Tenosynovitis/arthritis: infectious arthritis, infectious tenosynovitis, Reiter's syndrome, psoriatic arthritis, SLE.

LABORATORY STUDIES

Dermatopathology   Immunofluorescence of skin lesion biopsy shows gonococcus in 60%.

Gram's Stain   From the male urethra or cervix, may show gonococci.

Culture   Mucosal sites yield 80 to 90% positive cultures. Skin biopsy, joint fluid, blood have only a 10 to 30% chance of positive culture.

DIAGNOSIS

Made on clinical criteria, confirmed by culture of gonococcus from mucosal sites.

COURSE AND PROGNOSIS

Untreated, skin/joint lesions often gradually resolve; endocarditis usually fatal.

MANAGEMENT

See *Neisseria Gonorrhoeae* Infections, page 882.

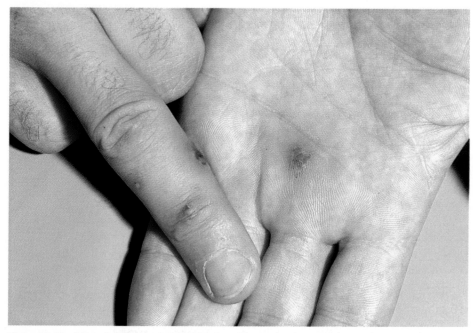

Figure 25-18 Disseminated gonococcal infection *Hemorrhagic, painful pustules on erythematous bases on the palm and the finger of the other hand. These lesions occur at acral sites and are few in number.*

SEXUALLY TRANSMITTED DISEASES

SYPHILIS

Syphilis is a sexually transmitted infection caused by *Treponema pallidum* and characterized by the appearance of a painless ulcer or chancre at the site of inoculation, associated with regional lymphadenopathy; shortly after inoculation, syphilis becomes a systemic infection with characteristic secondary and tertiary stages. During the past few years, the incidence of syphilis has increased and the clinical course and response to standard therapy may be altered in HIV-infected patients.
Synonyms: Lues, the great imitator.

EPIDEMIOLOGY

Age of Onset   In decreasing order: 20 to 39 years, 15 to 19 years, 40 to 49 years.

Race   All races; in the United States, incidence increasing in African Americans and Hispanics.

Sex   Males outnumber females 2:1 to 4:1.

Other Factors   Until recently, nearly half of all males with syphilis in the United States were homosexual, but this percentage has decreased due to safer sexual practices. The incidence of syphilis, however, has markedly increased in minorities and is associated with exchange of sex for drugs. Associated with the increase in sexually transmitted syphilis is a marked increase in the number of cases of congenital syphilis.

Etiology   *T. pallidum.*

PATHOGENESIS

T. pallidum does not live or cause disease outside the human body. It is spread from person to person through direct contact with an infectious lesion. The spirochetes, passing through intact mucous membrane and abraded skin, divide locally, with resulting host inflammatory response and chancre formation, either a single lesion or, less commonly, multiple lesions. Primary syphilis is the most contagious stage of the disease. Shortly after invasion, spirochetes are then carried by the blood stream to every organ in the body. Later syphilis is essentially a vascular disease, lesions occurring secondary to obliterative endarteritis of terminal arterioles and small arteries and by the resulting inflammatory and necrotic changes.

LABORATORY EXAMINATIONS

Detection of *T. pallidum*

Dark-Field Examination   Dark-field examination is a simple and reliable test to demonstrate the causative agent. The chancre is debrided from crusts and cleaned with saline swabs and, if not primarily eroded or ulcerated, scarified with a scalpel by gentle scraping, blotted until bleeding stops, and then squeezed between fingers (gloves!) until serous fluid emerges on surface or base of the ulcer. Serous exudate is removed by a glass capillary and pipetted onto microscopic slide, covered with a coverslip, and examined in a dark-field microscope. *T. pallidum* is recognized as a corkscrew-like organism, 5 to 20 μm in length, showing rotatory, pocket knife-like kinking and harmonica-like contractile movements. In contrast to saprophytic spirochetes, it does not, however, exhibit locomotion. Dark-field examination is positive in primary chancre and papular lesions of secondary syphilis, in particular condylomata lata. Unreliable in oral cavity because of the presence of saprophytic spirochetes, and negative in patients treated systemically or topically with antibiotics. In the latter case the regional lymph node is punctured and the aspirate is examined in the dark-field microscope.

Direct Fluorescent Antibody Test   Fluorescent antibodies are used to detect *T. pallidum* in exudate from lesion, lymph node aspirate, or tissue. Identification of *T. pallidum* makes a definitive diagnosis.

Serologic Tests   Presumptive diagnosis is possible with the use of two types of serologic tests for syphilis (STS): (1) nontreponemal (cardiolipin-VDRL, RPR) and (2) treponemal (FTA-ABS, TPHA). The use of one type of test alone is not sufficient for diagnosis. Nontreponemal test antibody titers usually correlate with disease activity; results are reported quantitatively. A fourfold change in titer is necessary to demonstrate a substantial difference between two nontreponemal test results. A positive treponemal test usually remains so for a lifetime, regardless of treatment or disease activity (15 to 25% of patients treated during primary stage may revert to being serologically nonreactive after 2 to 3 years). Treponemal test antibody titers correlate poorly with disease activity and should not be used to assess response to treatment.

Primary Syphilis Positive reactions develop in the third to fourth week after infection or concomitantly and up to 1 week after appearance of the chancre. Untreated primary syphilis has a positive FTA-ABS *T. pallidum* hemagglutination (TPHA) test (91%) 6 weeks after infection, compared with VDRL (88%). Cardiolipin tests become nonreactive 1 year after adequate treatment. Specific *Treponema* antigen tests (FTA-ABS, TPHA) usually remain positive at low titers.

Secondary Syphilis Nontreponemal STS (e.g., VDRL) are always positive (>1:32). FTA-ABS is 99.2% positive, as is TPHA. HIV-infected individuals with secondary syphilis rarely may have negative STS. Beware of false-negative STS resulting from *prozone phenomenon* (presence of excess antibody results in failure of the flocculation reaction and thus a false nonreactive test). Nontreponemal serologic tests become nonreactive 24 months after adequate treatment; treponemal serologic tests usually remain reactive.

Tertiary Syphilis STS is usually highly reactive, but false-negative nontreponemal tests are possible.
Note: Testing for HIV infection is advised for all patients with syphilis.

False-Positive STS *False-Positive Reactions Occur with FTA-ABS for the Following Reasons* Technical error, inefficient sorbents, genital herpes simplex, pregnancy, lupus erythematosus (systemic or skin only), alcoholic cirrhosis, scleroderma, mixed connective tissue disease.

False-Positive Reactions of Nontreponemal Tests Are Associated with the Following *Transient reactors:* technical error (low titer), *Mycoplasma* pneumonia, enterovirus infection, infectious mononucleosis, pregnancy, injecting drug use (IVDU), and less common causes (advanced tuberculosis, scarlet fever, viral pneumonia, brucellosis, rat-bite fever, relapsing fever, leptospirosis, measles, mumps, lymphogranuloma venereum, malaria, trypanosomiasis, varicella). *Chronic reactors:* malaria, leprosy, SLE, IDVU, other connective tissue disorders, elder population, Hashimoto's thyroiditis, rheumatoid arthritis, reticuloendothelial malignancy, familial false-positives, idiopathic. *Note:* If no history of possible early lesions, or no evidence of congenital syphilis based on patient's history, or no sexual exposure except

CLASSIFICATION OF THE CLINICAL STAGES

Stage	Characterization
Primary syphilis	Localized infection at site of inoculation (chancre)
Secondary syphilis	Disseminated infection (exanthem, maculopapules, condylomata lata)
Latent syphilis	No clinical signs or symptoms of infection (seropositive)
Early	Less than one-year duration; any period between primary and secondary stage
Late	More than one year since patient became infected
Syphilis of unknown duration	
Late (tertiary) syphilis	Cutaneous, vascular, neurologic findings
Congenital syphilis	Acquired perinatally; early and late clinical findings

to individuals who are known to have a negative STS, then diagnosis of false-positive is probably correct. False-positive reactions to *both* treponemal and nontreponemal tests are highly unlikely.

Dermatopathology In primary and secondary syphilis, lesional skin biopsy shows central thinning or ulceration of epidermis. Lymphocytic and plasmacytic dermal infiltrate. Proliferation of capillaries and lymphatics with endarteritis; may have thrombosis and small areas of necrosis. Dieterle stain demonstrates spirochetes.

COURSE AND PROGNOSIS

Even without treatment, chancre heals completely in 4 to 6 weeks, the infection either becoming latent or clinical manifestations of secondary syphilis appearing. Secondary syphilis usually manifests as macular exanthem initially; after weeks, lesions resolve spontaneously and recur as maculopapular or papular eruptions. In 20% of untreated cases, up to three to four such recurrences followed by periods of clinical remission may occur over a period of 1 year. The infection then enters a latent stage, in which there are no clinical signs or symptoms of the disease. After untreated syphilis has persisted for more than 4 years, it is rarely communicable, except in the case of pregnant women, who, if untreated, may transmit syphilis to their fetuses, regardless of the duration of their disease. Gummas hardly ever heal spontaneously. Noduloulcerative syphilides undergo spontaneous partial healing, but new lesions appear at the periphery.

MANAGEMENT

ANTIMICROBIAL THERAPY

Primary and Secondary Syphilis

Recommended regimen

Benzathine penicillin G	2.4 million units IM in one dose

Alternative regimen for penicillin-allergic patients (nonpregnant)

Doxycycline	100 mg PO bid for 2 weeks *or*
Tetracycline	500 mg PO qid for 2 weeks *or*
Erythromycin	500 mg PO qid for 2 weeks *or*
Ceftriaxone	250 mg IM once a day for 10 days

Children

Benzathine penicillin G	50,000 units/kg IM, up to adult dose of 2.4 million units in a single dose

Latent syphilis

Early	2.4 million units IM in one dose
Late or unknown duration	7.2 million units total, administered as 3 doses of 2.4 million units IM each at 1-week intervals

Tertiary syphilis

	7.2 million units total, administered as 3 doses of 2.4 million units IM each at 1-week intervals

Neurosyphilis

Recommended regimen

Aqueous crystalline penicillin G	12 to 24 million units, administered as 6 doses of 2 to 4 million units every 4 h IV for 10–14 days

Alternative regimen (if outpatient compliance can be ensured)

	Procaine penicillin, 2–4 million units IM daily, and probenecid, 500 mg PO qid, both for 10–14 days

Penicillin regimens should be used whenever possible for all stages of syphilis in HIV-infected patients. Some authorities advise CSF examination and/or treatment with a regimen appropriate for neurosyphilis for all patients coinfected with syphilis and HIV, regardless of the clinical stage of syphilis. Patients should be followed clinically and with quantitative nontreponemal STS (VDRL, RPR) at 1, 2, 3, 6, 9 and 12 months after treatment. Patients with early syphilis whose titers increase or fail to decrease fourfold within 6 months should undergo CSF examination and be re-treated. In such patients, CSF abnormalities could be due to HIV-related infection, neurosyphilis, or both.

Jarisch-Herxheimer reaction

An acute febrile reaction, often accompanied by chills, fever, malaise, nausea, headache, myalgia, arthralgia, that may occur after any therapy for syphilis. May occur within hours after treatment, subsiding within 24 h. More common in patients with early syphilis; developing lesions of secondary syphilis may first appear at this time. Treatment: reassurance, bed rest, aspirin. Pregnant patients should be warned that early labor may occur.

Management of sex partners

Sex partners should be referred for evaluation and treatment.

Primary Syphilis

HISTORY

Symptoms   A genital or extragenital sore may be noted. Ulcers are usually not painful unless superinfected.

Incubation Period   21 days (average); range, 10 to 90 days.

PHYSICAL EXAMINATION

Skin Lesions

Chancre   Button-like papule that develops at the site of inoculation into a painless erosion and then ulcerate with raised border and scanty serous exudate (Figs. 25-19 and 25-20). Surface may be crusted. Size: few millimeters to 1 or 2 cm in diameter. Border of lesion may be raised. Palpation: most commonly, firm with indurated border; painless. Extragenital chancres, particularly on the fingers, may be painful. Atypically, genital chancres painful, especially if secondarily infected with *Staphylococcus aureus.* Arrangement: single lesion; less commonly, few, multiple, or kissing lesions.

Sites of Predilection   Genital sites are most common. Male: inner prepuce (Fig. 25-19), coronal sulcus of the glans penis, shaft, base. Female: cervix, vagina, vulva (Fig. 25-20), clitoris, breast; chancres observed less frequently in women because of their location within vagina or on cervix. Extragenital chancres (Fig. 25-21): anus or rectum, mouth, lips, tongue, tonsil, fingers (painful!), toes, breast, nipple.

General Findings   Syphilis is a systemic infection; all patients should have a thorough clinical examination. Regional lymphadenopathy appears within 1 week. Nodes are discrete, firm, rubbery, nontender, more commonly unilateral.

DIFFERENTIAL DIAGNOSIS

Genital erosion/ulcer: Genital herpes, traumatic ulcer, furuncle, aphthous ulcer, fixed drug eruption. Also, chancroid, lymphogranuloma venereum, donovanosis.

DIAGNOSIS

Clinical suspicion, confirmed by dark-field examination or serologically.

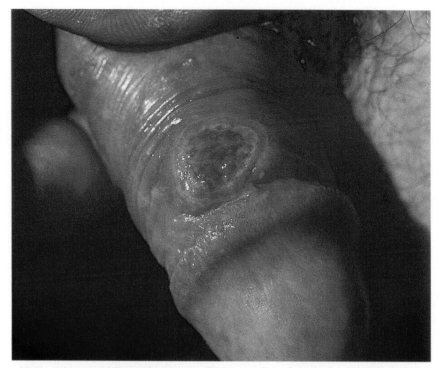

Figure 25-19 Primary syphilis: penile chancre *Large, painless ulcer on the distal shaft of the penis. On palpation, the area surrounding the ulcer is strikingly indurated. The chancre arises at the site of inoculation of T. pallidum.*

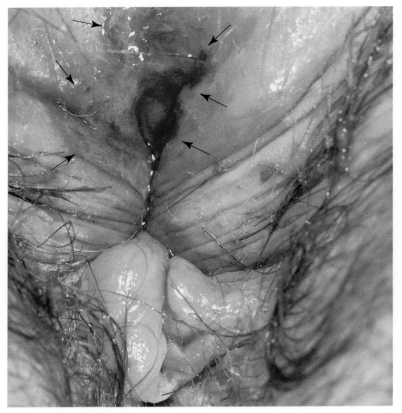

Figure 25-20 Primary syphilis: vulvar chancre *Large, painless erosion with jagged margins on the anterior introitus.*

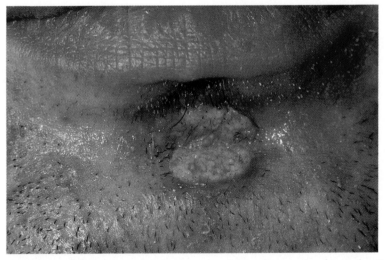

Figure 25-21 Primary syphilis: extragenital chancre *A painless ulcer on the chin at the site of inoculation of* T. pallidum *after orogenital sex.*

SEXUALLY TRANSMITTED DISEASES

Secondary Syphilis

HISTORY

Secondary syphilis appears 2 to 6 months after primary infection and 2 to 10 weeks after appearance of the primary chancre. Chancre may still be present when secondary lesions appear. Concomitant HIV infection may alter course of secondary syphilis. "Acute illness" syndrome: headache, chills, feverishness, arthralgia, myalgia, malaise, photophobia. Mucocutaneous lesions are asymptomatic.

Duration of Lesions   Weeks.

PHYSICAL EXAMINATION

Skin Lesions   Macules (Fig. 25-22) and papules .5 to 1 cm, round to oval; pink brownish-red. First exanthem always macular. Later eruptions may be papulosquamous (Fig. 25-23 and 25-24), pustular, or acneform. Vesiculobullous lesions occur only in neonatal congenital syphilis (palms and soles). Uncommonly, lesions of secondary syphilis and chancre of primary syphilis occur concomitantly. On palpation, papules are firm; condylomata lata, soft. The shape of lesions may be annular or polycyclic, especially on face in dark-skinned individuals. In relapsing secondary syphilis, arciform lesions. Always sharply defined except for macular exanthem. Lesions are scattered, tend to remain discrete, and usually symmetric.

Condylomata lata: soft, flat-topped, moist, red-to-pale papules, nodules, or plaques (Fig. 25-24), which may become confluent.

Distribution   Generalized eruption on the trunk; localized eruptions most commonly are scaling and papular localizing, especially on the head (hairline, nasolabial, scalp), neck, palms, and soles (Fig. 25-24). Here they are often hyperkeratotic–psoriasiform. Condylomata lata (Fig. 25-25): most commonly in anogenital region and mouth; can be seen on any body surface where moisture can accumulate between intertriginous surfaces, i.e., axillae or toe webs.

Hair   Two types: diffuse hair loss, including temples and parietal scalp; or patchy, "moth-eaten" alopecia on the scalp and beard area. Loss of eyelashes, lateral third of eyebrows.

Mucous Membranes   *Mucous patches,* i.e., small, asymptomatic, round or oval, slightly elevated, flat-topped macules and papules .5 to 1 cm in diameter, covered by hyperkeratotic white to gray membrane, occurring on the oral or genital mucosa; *split papules* at the angles of the mouth.

General Examination   ±Fever. Generalized lymphadenopathy (cervical, suboccipital, inguinal, epitrochlear, axillary) and splenomegaly.

Associated Findings   Diffuse pharyngitis. Acute bacterial iritis. Periostitis of long bones, particularly tibia (nocturnal pain) and arthralgia or hydrarthrosis of knees or ankles without x-ray changes. Meningovascular reaction (CSF positive for inflammatory markers). Hepatosplenomegaly, cardiac arrhythmia, nephritis, cystitis, prostatitis, gastritis.

COURSE

In secondary syphilis there may be only one or several recurrent eruptions that appear after month-long asymptomatic intervals. The first secondary syphilis eruption is a relatively faint exanthem (Fig. 25-22), always macular, pink, and lesions are ill-defined; later lesions of early syphilis are papular, brownish (Fig. 25-23), and tend to be more localized (Figs. 25-24). Symptoms may last 2 to 6 weeks (4 weeks average) and may recur in untreated or inadequately treated patients.

DIFFERENTIAL DIAGNOSIS

Exanthem/enanthem   Adverse cutaneous drug eruption (e.g., captopril), pityriasis rosea, viral exanthem, infectious mononucleosis, tinea corporis, tinea versicolor, scabies, "id" reaction, condylomata acuminata, acute guttate psoriasis, lichen planus.

DIAGNOSIS

Clinical suspicion confirmed by dark-field examination and/or serology. Dark-field is positive in all secondary syphilis lesions except for macular exanthem.

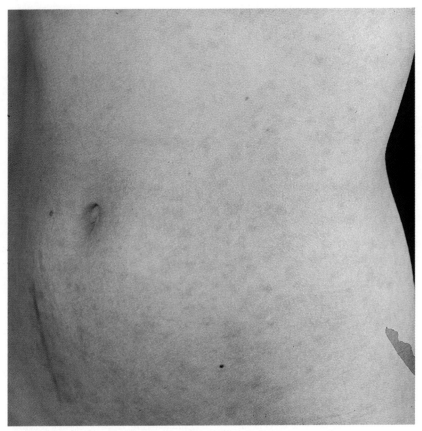

Figure 25-22   Secondary syphilis: early exanthem   *An asymptomatic morbilliform (measles-like) exanthem on the trunk associated with very early dissemination of* T. pallidum *from the site of inoculation. A chancre of primary syphilis may be coexistent with this finding.*

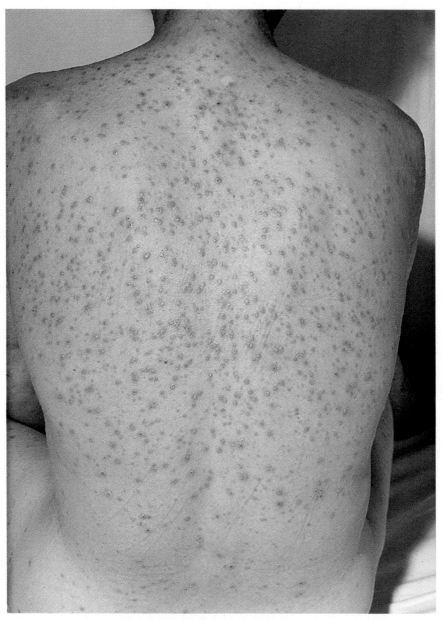

Figure 25-23   Secondary syphilis: papulosquamous eruption on trunk   *Asymptomatic, scaling, erythematous papules and macules on the back. The eruption must be differentiated from guttate psoriasis and pityriasis rosea.*

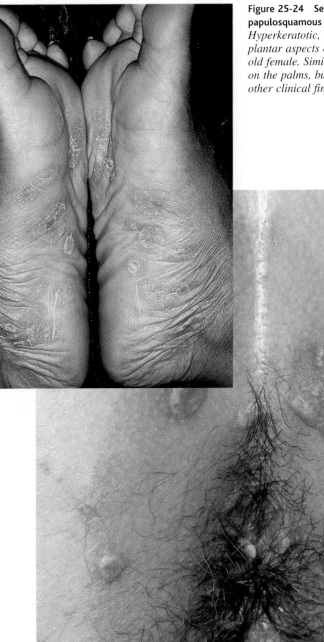

Figure 25-24   Secondary syphilis: annular papulosquamous eruption on soles   *Hyperkeratotic, scaling plaques on the plantar aspects of both feet in a 20-year-old female. Similar lesions were present on the palms, but to a lesser extent. No other clinical findings were detected.*

Figure 25-25   Secondary syphilis: condylomata lata   *Soft, flat-topped, moist, pink-tan papules and nodules on the perineum and perianal area. The lesions are teeming with* T. pallidum.

Latent Syphilis

Latent syphilis is that stage in which there are no clinical signs or symptoms of the infection. The diagnosis is made only after a careful history and physical examination have ruled out symptoms and signs of active infection. The serologic tests for syphilis (STS) are positive; CSF is normal. Early latent syphilis (<2 years) is distinguished from late latent disease (>2 years). All patients with syphilis have latent disease at some time during the course of the illness; some patients have only latent-stage syphilis and are diagnosed by a positive STS. Latent disease does not preclude infectiousness or the development of gummatous skin lesions, cardiovascular lesions, or neurosyphilis. A pregnant woman with latent disease can infect her fetus, with congenital syphilis occurring in the baby.

Tertiary Syphilis

HISTORY

Duration of Lesions In *untreated* syphilis, 15% of patients developed late benign syphilis, mostly skin lesions; tertiary syphilis is now very rare. Previously, patients presenting with tertiary syphilis gave a history of lesions of 3 to 7 years' duration (range, 2 to 60 years); gumma develop by fifteenth year.

PHYSICAL EXAMINATION

Skin Lesions

Noduloulcerative Syphilides Simulate lupus vulgaris (cutaneous tuberculosis). Plaques and nodules with scars healed in the center with or without psoriasiform scales and with or without ulceration (Fig. 25-26). Typically, and in contrast to lupus vulgaris, syphilides do not recur in scars but rather on their periphery and are not soft but firm. Grouped, serpiginous (snake-like), annular, polycyclic, scalloped borders. Solitary isolated lesions (Fig. 25-26): arms (extensor aspects), back, or face.

Gumma The term *gumma* (Latin: "gum") describes the rubbery lump or deep granulomatous lesion found in the subcutaneous tissue, having a tendency for necrosis and ulceration. Nodule, with ulceration, "punched out." Solitary. Anywhere, but especially on scalp, face, chest (sternoclavicular), calf.

General Examination 25% of patients have neurosyphilis or cardiovascular syphilis.

DIFFERENTIAL DIAGNOSIS

Plaque(s) ±Ulceration, ±Granulomatous Cutaneous tuberculosis, cutaneous atypical mycobacterial infection, malignancy such as lymphoma, deep fungal infections, furuncle.

DIAGNOSIS

Clinical findings, confirmed by STS and lesional skin biopsy; dark-field examination always negative, silver impregnation of histologic sections for demonstration of spirochetes only very rarely positive.

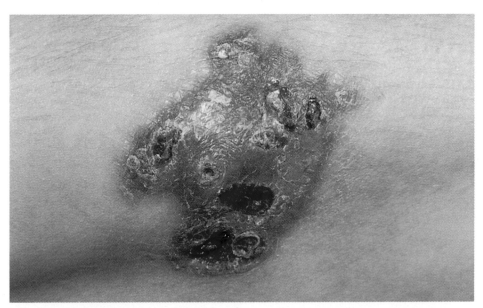

Figure 25-26   Tertiary syphilis: noduloulcerative type   *Asymptomatic, red-brown, translucent, crusted, ulcerated plaque with serpiginous borders.*

Syphilis In HIV Disease

HIV-infected individuals with neurosyphilis are more likely to present with uveitis or retinitis and have significantly higher RPR titers. Some, however, fail to respond immunologically to *T. pallidum* infection with antibody formation (i.e., negative STS).

DIAGNOSIS

HIV testing is advised for all patients with syphilis. Neurosyphilis should be considered in the differential diagnosis of neurologic disease in HIV-infected persons. When clinical findings suggest syphilis but STS are negative or confusing, alternative tests such as biopsy of lesions, dark-field examination, and direct fluorescent antibody (DFA) staining of lesional material should be used.

CHANCROID

Chancroid is an acute STD characterized by a *painful* ulcer at the site of inoculation, usually on the external genitalia, and the development of suppurative regional lymphadenopathy.

Synonyms: Soft chancre, ulcus molle, chancre mou.

EPIDEMIOLOGY

Sex Young males. Lymphadenitis more common in males.

Etiology *Hemophilus ducreyi,* a gram-negative streptobacillus.

Transmission Most likely during sexual intercourse with partner who has *H. ducreyi* genital ulcer. Chancroid is a cofactor for HIV transmission; high rates of HIV infection among those who have chancroid. 10% of individuals with chancroid have syphilis or genital herpes.

Incidence Underreported. In 1994, 773 cases reported to CDC in the United States.

Geography Uncommon in industrialized nations; microepidemics introduced sporadically from tropical countries. Endemic in tropical and subtropical third-world countries, especially in poor, urban, and seaport populations.

PATHOGENESIS

Poorly studied. *H. ducreyi* is inoculated through small breaks in the epidermis or mucosa. Primary infection develops at the site of inoculation, followed by lymphadenitis. Bubo formation occurs with scant organisms and an exuberant acute inflammatory response. The role of the immune response is unknown. Cofactor for HIV transmission: chancroid is the STD most strongly associated with increased risk for HIV transmission. About 10% of patients with chancroid may be coinfected with *T. pallidum* or HSV.

HISTORY

Incubation Period 4 to 7 days.

Prodrome None.

Travel History Sexually active during visit to country where chancroid is endemic. Possible contact with prostitute.

PHYSICAL EXAMINATION

Skin Lesions Primary lesion: tender papule with erythematous halo that evolves to pustule, erosion, and ulcer. Ulcer is usually quite *tender* or *painful*. Its borders are sharp, undermined, and not indurated (Fig. 25-27). Its base is friable with granulation tissue and covered with gray to yellow exudate (Fig. 25-28). Edema of prepuce common. Ulcer may be singular or multiple, merging to form large or giant ulcers (>2 cm) with a serpiginous shape.

Distribution Multiple ulcers (Figure 25-28) develop by autoinoculation. Male: prepuce, frenulum, coronal sulcus, glans penis, shaft. Female: fourchette, labia, vestibule, clitoris, vaginal wall by direct extension from introitus, cervix, perianal. Extragenital lesions: breast, fingers, thighs, oral mucosa.

General Examination Painful inguinal lymphadenitis (usually unilateral) occurs in 50% of patients 1 to 2 weeks after primary lesion. Buboes occur with overlying erythema and may drain spontaneously.

DIFFERENTIAL DIAGNOSIS

Genital Ulcer Genital herpes, primary syphilis, donovanosis, lymphogranuloma venereum, secondarily infected human bites or traumatic lesions.

Tender Inguinal Mass Genital herpes, syphilis, incarcerated hernia, plague, tularemia.

LABORATORY EXAMINATIONS

Gram's Stain Of scrapings from ulcer base or pus from bubo, attempt to see small clusters or parallel chains of gram-negative rods. Interpretation difficult due to presence of contaminating organisms in ulcers.

Culture Special growth requirements; isolation difficult. Using special media, sensitivity is no higher than 80%.

Serologic Tests None available. Patients should be tested for HIV infection at time of diagnosis. Patients also should be tested 3 months later for both syphilis and HIV infection if initial results are negative.

Dermatopathology May be helpful. Organism rarely demonstrated.

PCR Detects *H. ducreyi* DNA sequences.

DIAGNOSIS

The combination of a painful ulcer with tender lymphadenopathy (which occurs in one-third of patients) is suggestive of chancroid and, when accompanied by suppurative inguinal lymphadenopathy, is almost pathognomonic.

Definitive Diagnosis Made by isolation of *H. ducreyi* on special culture media (not widely available). Sensitivity ≤80%.

Probable Diagnosis Made if patient has following criteria: (1) ≥1 painful genital ulcers, (2) no evidence of *T. pallidum* infection by dark-field examination of ulcer exudate or by STS performed at least 7 days after onset of ulcers, and (3) clinical presentation, appearance of genital ulcers, and lymphadenopathy, if present, are typical for chancroid and a test for HSV is negative. The combination of a painful ulcer and

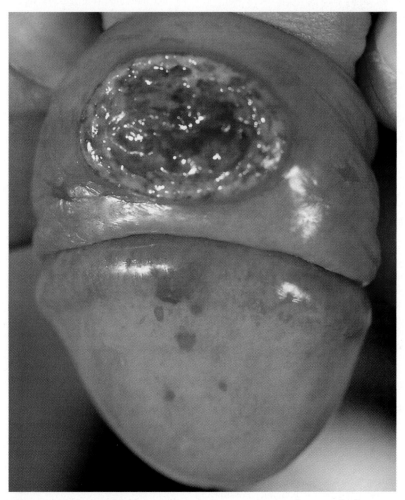

Figure 25-27   Chancroid   *Painful ulcer with marked surrounding erythema and edema. (Courtesy of Prof. Alfred Eichmann, M.D.)*

SEXUALLY TRANSMITTED DISEASES

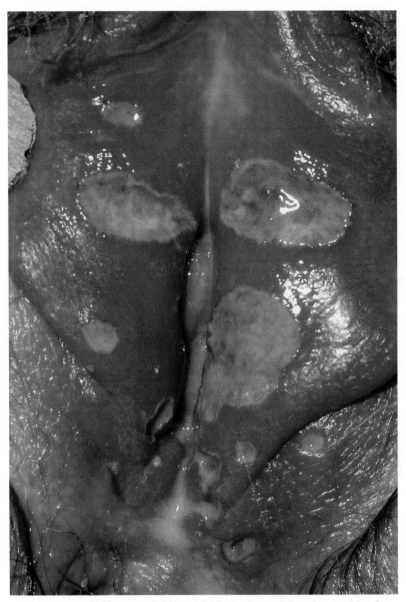

Figure 25-28 Chancroid *Multiple, painful, punched-out ulcers with undermined borders on the vulva occurring after autoinoculation.*

tender inguinal adenopathy, which occurs in about one-third of patients, suggests a diagnosis of chancroid; when accompanied by suppurative inguinal lymphadenopathy, these signs are pathognomonic.

COURSE AND PROGNOSIS

Patients should be reexamined 3 to 7 days after initiation of therapy. If treatment is successful, ulcers improve symptomatically within 3 days and improve objectively within 7 days after therapy is begun. If no clinical improvement is evident, diagnosis may be incorrect, coinfection with another STD agent exists, the patient is HIV-infected, treatment was not taken as instructed, or the *H. ducreyi* strain causing infection is resistant to the prescribed antimicrobial. The time required for complete healing is related to the size of the ulcer; large ulcers may require ≥2 weeks. Complete resolution of fluctuant lymphadenopathy is slower than that of ulcers and may require needle aspiration through adjacent intact skin—even during successful therapy. In HIV-infected persons, healing may be slower, and treatment failures may occur; longer treatment regimens may be advisable.

MANAGEMENT

Antimicrobial therapy

Azithromycin	1 g PO in a single dose, *or*
Ceftriaxone	250 mg IM in a single dose *or*
Ciprofloxacin	500 mg PO bid for 3 days *or*
Erythromycin base	500 mg PO qid for 7 days
Management of sex partners	Sex partners should be referred for evaluation and treatment.

DONOVANOSIS

Donovanosis is a mildly contagious, chronic, indolent, progressive, autoinoculable, ulcerative disease involving the skin and lymphatics of the genital and perianal areas.
Synonyms: Granuloma inguinale, granuloma venereum.

EPIDEMIOLOGY

Sex Young males.

Etiology *Calymmatobacterium granulomatis,* an encapsulated intracellular gram-negative rod.

Transmission Poorly studied. Venereal but also nonvenereal transmission occurs.

Geography Endemic foci in tropical and subtropical environments (India; Papua, New Guinea; southern Africa; central Australia). Rare in United States, Canada, Europe.

PATHOGENESIS

Poorly understood. Mildly contagious. Repeated exposure necessary for clinical infection to occur. In most cases, lesions cannot be detected in sexual contacts.

HISTORY

Incubation Period Most lesions appear within 30 days after sexual exposure (range, 8 to 80 days).

Travel History Sexual exposure in endemic area.

Characterization Genital ulcers are relatively painless.

PHYSICAL EXAMINATION

Skin Lesions

Primary Lesion Button-like papule or subcutaneous nodule that ulcerates within a few days. Ulcers have beefy-red friable granulation tissue base with sharply defined irregular margins. Spreads by continuity or by autoinoculation of approximated skin surfaces. Anaerobic superinfection may produce pain and foul-smelling exudate. Less common complications: deep ulcerations, chronic cicatricial lesions, phimosis, lymphedema (elephantiasis of penis, scrotum, vulva), exuberant epithelial proliferation that grossly resembles carcinoma.

Distribution *Males:* prepuce or glans, penile shaft, scrotum. *Females:* labia minora, mons veneris, fourchette. Ulcerations then spread by direct extension or autoinoculation to inguinal and perineal skin. Extragenital lesions occur in mouth, lips, throat, face, GI tract, and bone.

Variants *Ulcerovegetative* (Fig. 25-29) Develops from the nodular variant; large, spreading, exuberant ulcers.

Nodular Soft, red nodules that eventually ulcerate with bright red granulating bases.

Hypertrophic Proliferative reaction; formation of large vegetating masses.

Cicatricial Spreading scar tissue formation associated with spread of infection.

Late Sequela Squamous cell carcinoma of genital skin.

General Examination

Regional lymph node enlargement is uncommon. Large subcutaneous nodule may mimic a lymph node, i.e., pseudobubo.

DIFFERENTIAL DIAGNOSIS

Genital Ulcer(s) Syphilitic chancre, chancroid, lymphogranuloma venereum, cutaneous tuberculosis, cutaneous amebiasis, filariasis, squamous cell carcinoma.

Perianal Hypertrophic Donovanosis Condylomata acuminata, condylomata lata.

LABORATORY STUDIES

Culture The organism cannot be cultured on standard microbiologic media. Bacterial superinfection does occur. Coinfection with other STD may be present.

Touch or Crush Preparation Of punch biopsy stained with Wright's or Giemsa's stain shows Donovan bodies in cytoplasm of macrophages. Clinical variants differ in quantity of organisms.

Dermatopathology Extensive acanthosis and dense dermal infiltrate, mainly plasma cells and histiocytes. Large mononuclear cells containing cytoplasmic inclusions (Donovan bodies), i.e., *C. granulomatis,* are pathognomonic.

DIAGNOSIS

Clinical diagnosis excluding other causes of genital ulcer(s) and identifying organism with touch preparation or crush preparation of biopsied tissue.

COURSE AND PROGNOSIS

Little tendency toward spontaneous healing. After antibiotic treatment, lesions often heal with depigmentation of reepithelialized skin. Relapse can occur 6 to 18 months later despite effective initial therapy.

MANAGEMENT

ANTIMICROBIAL THERAPY

Recommended regimens	Treatment appears to halt progressive destruction of tissue, although prolonged duration of therapy often is required to enable granulation and re-epithelialization of ulcers.
Trimethoprim-sulfamethoxazole	One double-strength tablet bid for at least 3 weeks
Doxycycline	100 mg bid for at least 3 weeks
Alternative regimens	
Sulfamethoxazole	750 mg bid for at least 3 weeks
Erythromycin base	500 mg qid for at least 3 weeks
Parenteral therapy	If lesions do not respond within the first few days of therapy, the addition of an aminoglycoside (gentamicin, 1 mg/kg IV q8h) should be considered.
Follow-up	Patients should be followed clinically until signs and symptoms have resolved.

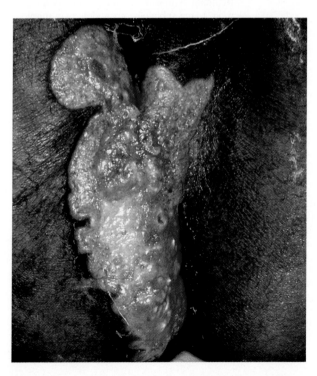

Figure 25-29 Donovanosis: ulcerovegetative type *Extensive granulation tissue formation, ulceration, and scarring of the perineum, scrotum, and penis.*

LYMPHOGRANULOMA VENEREUM

Lymphogranuloma venereum (LGV) is an STD caused by *Chlamydia trachomatis*. Acute LGV in heterosexual men is characterized by a transient primary genital lesion followed by multilocular suppurative regional lymphadenopathy. Women, homosexual men, and— in occasional instances—heterosexual men may develop hemorrhagic proctitis with regional lymphadenitis. After a latent period of years, late complications include genital elephantiasis due to lymphatic involvement; strictures; and fistulas of penis, urethra, rectum. *Synonym:* Lymphogranuloma inguinale.

EPIDEMIOLOGY

Age of Onset   Third decade, while most sexually active.

Sex   Acute infection much more common in heterosexual males, presenting as inguinal syndrome. In women and homosexual men, anogenitorectal syndrome most common.

Etiology   *C. trachomatis*, invasive serovars (immunotypes) L_1, L_2, L_3. In the United States, L_2 most common.

Transmission   *C. trachomatis* in purulent exudate is inoculated onto the skin or mucosa of a sexual partner and gains entry through minute lacerations and abrasions.

Geography   Sporadic/rare in North America, Europe, Australia, and most of Asia and South America. Endemic in East and West Africa, India, parts of southeastern Asia, South America, and the Caribbean.

PATHOGENESIS

Primarily an infection of lymphatics and lymph nodes. Lymphangitis and lymphadenitis occur in drainage field of the inoculation site with subsequent perilymphangitis and periadenitis. Necrosis occurs, and loculated abscesses, fistulas, and sinus tracts develop. As the infection subsides, fibrosis replaces acute inflammation with resulting obliteration of lymphatic drainage, chronic edema, and stricture. Inoculation site determines affected lymph nodes: penis, anterior urethra—superficial, deep inguinal; posterior urethra—deep iliac, perirectal; vulva—inguinal; vagina, cervix—deep iliac, perirectal, retrocrural, lumbosacral; anus—inguinal; rectum—perirectal, deep iliac.

HISTORY

Incubation Period   3 to 12 days or longer for primary stage; 10 to 30 days (but up to 6 months) for secondary stage.

Travel History   In North America and Europe, most cases occur in patients who have traveled to endemic areas, where they were sexually active.

Symptoms

Primary Stage

Acute LGV usually associated with systemic symptoms: fever, chills, headache, meningismus, anorexia, myalgias, arthralgias., leukocytosis. Painless herpetiform erosion or ulceration at the site of inoculation noted in fewer than one-third of men and rarely in women.

Secondary Stage

Inguinal Syndrome   Constitutional symptoms (fever, malaise) associated with inguinal buboes. Severe local pain in buboes. Lower abdominal and back pain.

Anogenitorectal Syndrome   Anal pruritus, rectal discharge, fever, rectal pain, tenesmus, constipation, " pencil" stools, weight loss.

PHYSICAL EXAMINATION

Skin Lesions

Primary Stage   Papule, shallow erosion or ulcer, grouped small erosions or ulcers (herpetiform), or nonspecific urethritis. In heterosexual males, cordlike lymphangitis of dorsal penis may follow. Lymphangial nodule (bubonulus) may occur. Bubonuli may rupture, resulting in sinuses and fistulas of urethra and deforming scars of penis. In females, cervicitis, perimetritis, salpingitis may occur. After receptive anal intercourse, primary anal or rectal infection.

Distribution At the site of inoculation. *Males:* coronal sulcus, frenulum, prepuce, penis, urethra, glans, scrotum. *Females:* posterior vaginal wall, fourchette, posterior lip of cervix, vulva. When primary lesion occurs intraurethrally, presentation is of a nonspecific urethritis with a thin, mucopurulent discharge.

Other Erythema nodosum in 10% of cases. Primary inoculation of mouth or pharynx results in lymphadenitis of submaxillary or cervical lymph nodes.

Secondary Stage *Inguinal Syndrome* Unilateral bubo in two-thirds of cases (most common presentation) (Fig. 25-30). Marked edema and erythema of skin overlying node. One-third of inguinal buboes rupture; two-thirds slowly involute. " Groove" sign: inflammatory mass of femoral and inguinal nodes separated by depression or groove made by Poupart's ligament. 75% of cases have deep iliac node involvement with a pelvic mass that seldom suppurates.

Anogenitorectal Syndrome Associated with receptive anal intercourse, proctocolitis, hyperplasia of intestinal and perirectal lymphatic tissue. Resultant perirectal abscesses, ischiorectal and rectovaginal fistulas, anal fistulas, rectal stricture. Overgrowth of lymphatic tissue results in lymphorrhoids (resembling hemorrhoids) or perianal condylomata.

Esthiomene Elephantiasis of genitalia, usually females, which may ulcerate, occurring 1 to 20 years after primary infection.

General Examination

Anogenitorectal Syndrome Lower abdominal tenderness, pelvic colon thickened, enlarged perirectal nodes.

DIFFERENTIAL DIAGNOSIS

Primary Stage Genital herpes, primary syphilis, chancroid.

Inguinal Syndrome Incarcerated inguinal hernia, plague, tularemia, tuberculosis, genital herpes, syphilis, chancroid, Hodgkin's disease.

Anogenitorectal Syndrome Rectal stricture caused by rectal cancer, trauma, actinomycosis, tuberculosis, schistosomiasis.

Esthiomene Filariasis, mycosis.

LABORATORY EXAMINATIONS

Detection of *C. trachomatis*

PCR Most specific and sensitive.

Culture *C. trachomatis* can be cultured on tissue-culture cell lines in up to 60 to 80% of cases.

DFA Examine exudate for antigens.

Antibodies to *C. trachomatis* *ELISA test* 60 to 80% sensitive and specific; 97 to 99% in high-risk populations.

DNA-RNA Hybridization As sensitive and specific as ELISA test. Chlamydial DNA in urine is diagnostic.

Complement-Fixation (CF) Test Acute LGV usually has titer ≥1:64. Microimmunofluorescence test most sensitive and specific test, identifying infecting serovar.

Imaging MRI may show massive pelvic lymphadenopathy in women and homosexual men.

Dermatopathology Not pathognomonic. *Primary stage:* small stellate abscesses surrounded by histiocytes, arranged in palisade pattern. *Late stage:* epidermal acanthosis/papillomatosis; dermis—edematous; lymphatics—dilated with fibrosis and lymphoplasmocytic infiltrate.

DIAGNOSIS

By DFA, culture, serologic tests, and exclusion of other causes of inguinal lymphadenopathy or genital ulcers.

COURSE AND PROGNOSIS

Natural history is highly variable. Complications of untreated anorectal infection: perirectal abscess; fistula in ano; rectovaginal, rectovesical, ischiorectal fistulas. Bacterial superinfections contribute to complications. Rectal stricture is a late complication. Spontaneous remission is common.

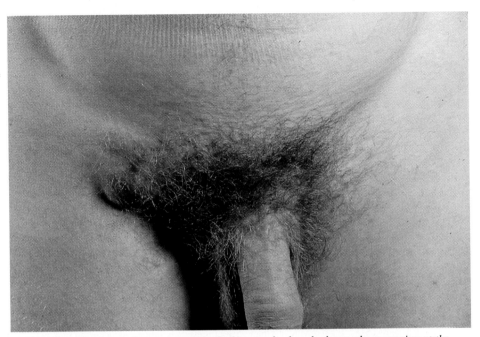

Figure 25-30 Lymphogranuloma venereum *Striking tender lymphadenopathy occurring at the femoral and inguinal lymph nodes separated by a groove made by Poupart's ligament (groove sign).*

MANAGEMENT

Antimicrobial Therapy Cures infection and prevents ongoing tissue damage, although tissue reaction can result in scarring.

Recommended regimen

Doxycycline 100 mg PO bid for 21 days.

Alternative regimens

Erythromycin 500 mg PO qid for 21 days.

Sulfisoxazole 500 mg PO qid for 21 days, or equivalent sulfonamide course.

Surgery Buboes may require aspiration through intact skin or incision and drainage.

Follow-up Patients should be followed clinically until signs and symptoms have resolved.

Management of Sex Partners Sex partners should be referred for evaluation and treatment.

MUCOCUTANEOUS MANIFESTATIONS OF HUMAN IMMUNODEFICIENCY VIRUS DISEASE

THE HIV EPIDEMIC

At the dawn of the twenty-first century, the HIV pandemic has been in existence for at least 30 years. The world first became aware of this new disease in the summer of 1981. By the end of 1998, more than 33 million people worldwide were HIV-infected, 43% of them female. An estimated 5.8 million new HIV infections occurred worldwide during 1998—approximately 16,000 each day. More than 95% of these new infections occurred in developing nations. In 1998, HIV infection was the fourth leading cause of death worldwide, resulting in an estimated 2.3 million deaths. More than 40 million people are estimated to have been infected with HIV worldwide.

In the United States, 40,000 new HIV infections occurred annually during the 1990s. The number of annual deaths has sharply declined due to the availability of highly active antiretroviral therapy (HAART). An estimated 650,000 to 900,000 people are currently infected with HIV, of whom 200,000 are unaware of their infection. Through 1998, 688,200 cumulative cases of AIDS and 410,800 AIDS-related deaths had been reported to the Centers for Disease Control and Prevention (CDC). Early in the epidemic, homosexual men were nearly exclusively infected; today new cases of HIV infection result predominantly from injecting-drug use and heterosexual contact, with a disproportionate representation among minority populations. Women are increasingly affected; the proportion of cases in the United States reported among women and adolescent girls more than tripled between 1985 and 1998, from 7 to 23%. In Canada, Australia, and western Europe, the epidemiology is similar to that in the United States. Currently, sub-Saharan Africa is bearing the greatest burden of the epidemic worldwide. The number of new infections is escalating in the former Soviet Union, India, and China.

Nearly all HIV-infected individuals exhibit some dermatologic disorder attributable to progressive immunodeficiency during the course of the infection. Some disorders are highly associated with HIV infection, and their diagnosis often warrants HIV serotesting (Table 26-1); these disorders include the exanthem of acute retroviral syndrome, Kaposi's sarcoma, oral hairy leukoplakia, proximal subungual onychomycosis, bacillary angiomatosis, eosinophilic folliculitis, chronic herpetic ulcers (>1 month duration), any sexually transmitted disease, multiple facial molluscum contagiosum in an adult, and skin findings of injecting drug use. Other findings are common in HIV disease and may be indications for serotesting in some patients: herpes zoster, mucosal candidiasis (oropharyngeal, recurrent vulvovaginal), seborrheic dermatitis, and severe persistent aphthous ulcers.

Table 26-1 MUCOCUTANEOUS FINDINGS ASSOCIATED WITH HIV INFECTION AND INDICATIONS FOR HIV SEROTESTING

Risk for HIV Infection	Mucocutaneous Finding
High—HIV serotesting always indicated	Acute retroviral syndrome Kaposi's sarcoma Oral hairy leukoplakia Proximal subungual onychomycosis Bacillary angiomatosis Eosinophilic folliculitis Chronic herpetic ulcers (>1 month duration) Any sexually transmitted disease Skin findings of injecting drug use
Moderate—HIV serotesting may be indicated	Herpes zoster Molluscum contagiosum: multiple facial in an adult Candidiasis: oropharyngeal, esophageal, or recurrent vulvovaginal
Possible—HIV serotesting may be indicated	Generalized lymphadenopathy Seborrheic dermatitis Aphthous ulcers (recurrent, refractory to therapy)

Early diagnosis is critical in the management of HIV disease for several reasons. Given the knowledge of their HIV infection and its contagiousness, most patients will reduce or eliminate behaviors associated with transmission of HIV. Early treatment with HAART retards progression of HIV-induced immunodeficiency and, in many cases, reduces immunocompromise. In patients with low CD4+ cell counts, many of the opportunistic infections such as *Pneumocystis carinii* pneumonia (PCP) are better treated by primary prophylactic regimens before development of clinical disease.

ACUTE HIV SYNDROME

The acute HIV syndrome is characterized by an infectious mononucleosis-like syndrome or aseptic meningitis syndrome with fever, lymphadenopathy, meningitis, GI symptoms, and a characteristic infectious exanthem, an enanthem, and genital ulceration.
Synonym: Symptomatic primary HIV infection, acute retroviral syndrome (ARS).

EPIDEMIOLOGY

Age of Onset   Commonly young, but any age.

Sex   Initially in the United States and Europe, much more common in males due to male-male sexual intercourse; currently, incidence in females increasing due to heterosexual transmission. Worldwide, heterosexual transmission is the most common mode of infection, particularly in developing countries, and the incidence of HIV disease is about equal in sexes.

Etiology   Nearly all cases in the United States and western Europe caused by HIV-1; some cases in western Africa caused by HIV-2. Both HIV-1 and HIV-2 can have a similar ARS; clinical findings with HIV-2 infection are usually less severe.

Incidence   In the United States, approximately 40,000 new HIV infections occurring annually. Of these individuals, 50 to 70% experience significant symptoms.

Transmission of HIV

Sexual Exposure   *Predominant* mode of transmission worldwide: heterosexual and homosexual contact.

Injecting-Drug Use (IDU)   Needle sharing transmits HIV.

Blood or Blood Products   Recipients of blood or blood products after 1978 but before 1985 were inadvertently infected with HIV. Currently, blood is screened for p24 antigen and anti-HIV antibody. Risk of HIV infection after transfusion of HIV-contaminated blood: 90 to 100%.

Organ Transplant Recipients   Prior to HIV testing, HIV was transmitted during transplantation of solid organs, bone marrow, and corneae.

Semen   Occurred during artificial insemination from HIV-infected donor.

Health Care Workers   HIV can be transmitted by needle sticks and cuts contaminated with HIV-infected blood during medical procedures. Risk for HIV infection after puncture with HIV-contaminated blood is .3%.

Perinatal Transmission   Child born to mother with HIV infection, i.e., intrapartum, perinatally, or by breast feeding, may become infected.

Risk Factors   Genital ulcer disease, such as genital herpes, chancroid, or syphilis, increases the risk of HIV transmission. HIV is concentrated in seminal fluid, particularly in genital inflammatory states such as other sexually transmitted diseases. HIV-infected individuals with higher viral loads may transmit the virus more efficiently. Strong association of HIV transmission with receptive anal intercourse.

PATHOGENESIS

After primary HIV infection, billions of virions are produced and destroyed each day; a concomitant daily turnover of actively infected CD4+ cells is also in the billions. HIV infection is relatively unique among human viral infections in that, despite robust cellular and humoral immune responses that are mounted after primary infection, the virus is not cleared completely from the body (with a few exceptions). Chronic infection develops that persists with varying degrees of virus replication for a median of 10 years before an individual becomes clinically ill.

HISTORY

Incubation Period   3 to 6 weeks (from presumed exposure to development of acute febrile illness); varies according to route and size of virus inoculation. Between 50 and 70% of recently infected individuals experience symptomatic primary infection.

Skin Symptoms   Exanthem, usually appears 2 to 3 days after onset of fever, lasting 5 to 8 days; exanthem asymptomatic; ulcers, painful in mouth and/or anogenital region.

Systems Review   *General* fever/rigors, malaise/lethargy, anorexia/weight loss, sore throat, arthralgias/myalgias, abdominal cramps, nausea/vomiting/diarrhea, headache/retroorbital pain. *Neurologic*: meningitis, encephalitis, peripheral neuropathy, myelopathy.

PHYSICAL EXAMINATION

Skin Lesions   Morbilliform rash, i.e., infectious exanthem (Fig. 26-1) with pink macules, papules up to 1 cm in diameter. Ulcers occur on penis and/or scrotum. Less common: urticaria. Also reported: vesicular and pustular exanthems, desquamation of palms/soles. Lesions remain discrete. Most common site of exanthem is upper thorax and collar region (100%)>face (60%)>arms (40%)>scalp, thighs (20%). Palms.

Mucous Membranes   Pharyngitis. Enanthem, spotty, on hard and soft palate. Ulcers: 5 to 10 mm in diameter, round to oval, shallow with white bases surrounded by a red halo, arising on the tonsils, palate, and/or buccal mucosa; esophageal ulcers. Uncommonly, oral candidiasis.

Anogenitalia   Ulcers: prepuce of penis, scrotum, anus, anal canal.

General Examination

Lymph Nodes   Lymphadenopathy.

Neurologic Findings   Acute meningitis; acute reversible encephalopathy with loss of memory, alteration of consciousness, and personality change.

DIFFERENTIAL DIAGNOSIS

Fever, Exanthem, and Lymphadenopathy in Individuals at Risk for HIV Infection   Primary Epstein-Barr virus (EBV) infection (infectious mononucleosis), primary cytomegalovirus (CMV) infection, rubella, toxoplasmosis, hepatitis, secondary syphilis, primary HSV infection.

Fever, Exanthem, and Aseptic Meningitis in Individuals at Risk for HIV Infection   Lymphocytic (aseptic) meningitis, disseminated gonococcal infection.

LABORATORY EXAMINATIONS

Hematology   Leukopenia, elevated ESR.

CD4+ T Lymphocytes   Usually dip down by several hundred (normal in adults, approximately 1000/μL), occasionally as low as 200/μL, but return to normal levels within several weeks. After a latent period, CD4+ cell levels again fall. CD4+ cell counts are used to monitor degree of immunodeficiency and response to antiretroviral therapy.

Detection of HIV

Viral Load Levels (VLL)   Usually extremely high initially. Subsequently reduced to low or undetectable levels. After a hiatus of years, the viral load eventually increases as immune function declines. Individuals with low VLL and relatively high CD4+ cell counts are usually not treated with HAART. VLL are used to monitor response to HAART.

HIV Antigen   p24 antigen is detectable in serum during ARS before HIV seroconversion. Becomes undetectable after immune response. Recurs as immune function declines.

Viral Cultures   HIV isolation from blood or CSF during ARS. Virus is undetectable after immune response. Viremia recurs as immune function declines.

Serologic Testing

Acute Retroviral Syndrome   Demonstrate seroconversion of anti-HIV-1 antibodies by ELISA, confirmed by Western blot, within 3 weeks of illness. HIV-2 infection is rare in industrialized countries.

Asymptomatic HIV Infection   HIV antibody is detectable in 95% or more of individuals within 6 months of infection. Although a negative antibody test usually means an individual is not infected, antibody tests cannot rule out infection that occurred less than 6 months before the test.

Dermatopathology   Lesion biopsy specimens from exanthem of primary HIV infection show sparse lymphohistiocytic infiltrate around blood vessels of the superficial dermal plexus and between collagen bundles in upper dermis.

DIAGNOSIS

Demonstrated seroconversion of anti-HIV antibodies by ELISA, confirmed by Western blot, confirms diagnosis of primary HIV infection. Established HIV infection can be confirmed by these serologic tests as well as by isolation of HIV from blood or CSF or demonstration of p24 antigen.

COURSE AND PROGNOSIS

The spectrum of symptoms associated with primary HIV infection is broad; most individuals experience no or mild symptoms that do not prompt medical consultation. In those with symptomatic illness, the mean duration of illness in one study was 13 days (range 5 to 44 days). Long-term illness of >2 weeks is associated with an eight times higher risk of developing AIDS within 3 years of seroconversion.

After an asymptomatic or symptomatic primary infection, HIV infection becomes latent with no clinical symptoms or findings. With disease progression and diminution of immune function, criteria for diagnosis of AIDS occur. The pace of disease progression is variable. The median time between primary HIV infection (seroconversion) and the development of AIDS among young homosexual men is >10 years (in the United States), with a range from a few months to ≥12 years. Most adults and adolescents infected with HIV remain symptom-free for long periods, but with viral replication occurring at a high rate. Factors that correlate with more rapid disease progression are HIV infection transmitted from someone with advanced HIV disease rather than an asymptomatic individual, older individuals (>30 years), and severe ARS. Essentially all HIV-infected individuals will eventually have symptoms related to the infection: 70 to 85% of infected adults develop symptoms and 55 to 62% develop AIDS within 12 years of seroconversion. Additional cases occur among those who have remained AIDS-free for >12 years.

MANAGEMENT

HIV Prevention Counseling

Sex Education The most common mode of HIV transmission is during sexual intercourse. Currently, in terms of numbers of new HIV infections, female-to-male and male-to-female transmission is much more common than male-to-male. Safer sexual practices must be taught at an early age.

Transfusions and Transplantation Blood and blood by-products must be tested before administration. HIV infection must be ruled out in donors of any transplanted organ.

Treatment of ARS Symptomatic. Efficacy of antiretroviral therapy at this stage still controversial.

Treatment of Asymptomatic HIV Infection Early diagnosis offers the opportunity for counseling and for assistance in preventing the transmission of HIV infection to others.

Antiretroviral Therapy Combinations of zidovudine/didanosine and zidovudine/zalcitabine are preferred to zidovudine monotherapy. Protease inhibitors such as indinavir and ritonavir reduce viral load by 2 to 3 logs in some individuals. Combinations of two or more drugs are currently recommended. Recent data on HIV pathogenesis, the development of methods for quantitation of plasma HIV RNA, clinical trial data, and the availability of new drugs have resulted in profound changes of therapeutic approaches.

It is now evident that in all stages of the infection the virus replicates at high levels in the lymphoid tissue, as reflected by the amount of HIV RNA in the plasma. This large amount of virus turns over rapidly with a virion half-life of less then 6 h and an estimated 10 billion virus particles produced daily. Shortly after infection, each individual establishes his or her own quasi-steady-state level of plasma HIV RNA, which largely determines the rate of CD4 cell destruction and ultimately the natural history of this infection. At any time point of the infection this set-point of plasma HIV RNA correlates inversely with prognosis and, in fact, can be used to predict the natural course of the disease.

Inhibition of viral replication with even potent antiretroviral agents either at suboptimal doses and/or as monotherapy by about 70 to 90% is gradually lost within a few months, coincident with the development of resistance. Nevertheless, when antiretroviral agents of different classes with nonoverlapping genetic patterns are used in combination, their genetic barrier to simultaneous resistance is significantly increased.

Antiretroviral agents approved for treatment of HIV in one or more countries can be divided

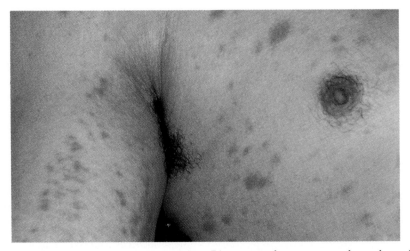

Figure 26-1 Acute retroviral syndrome: exanthem *Discrete, erythematous macules and papules on the trunk and arm; associated findings were fever, scrotal ulcers, erythematous macules on palate, and lymphadenopathy.*

into three classes of drugs: nucleoside reverse transcriptase inhibitors (NRTI), nonnucleoside reverse transcriptase inhibitors (NNRTI), and protease inhibitors (PI) (Table 26-2). They are directed against two target-enzymes—HIV reverse transcriptase and HIV protease—thereby interfering with formation of proviral DNA and virus assembly, respectively.

Combination therapy can slow down or even prevent selection of drug-resistant strains and is associated with significant clinical benefit. Current treatment recommendations favor the combined usage of two NRTI and one PI (preferably Indinavir, nelfinavir, or ritonavir) or two NRTI and one NNRTI.

Treatment is now recommended for all patients with HIV RNA levels above 5000 to 10,000 copies/mL plasma. For patients at low risk of progression (low plasma HIV RNA level and high CD4+ cell count), particularly those who are not committed to complex antiretroviral regimens, therapy might be safely deferred. These patients should be reevaluated every 3 to 6 months. HAART, with a combination of 3 to 4 drugs, has become the standard of care for treatment of HIV infection. None of the drugs currently available can eradicate HIV infection; but used in combination, the drugs can decrease viral replication, improve immunologic status, and prolong life.

Table 26-2 ANTIRETROVIRAL DRUGS, PRINCIPAL ACTIVITIES, AND DOSING

Generic Name	Other Names	Principal Activities	Usual Adult Dose
Nucleoside reverse transcriptase inhibitors (NRTI)			
Didanosine	ddI	HIV-1, HIV-2	20 mg bid
Lamivudine	3TC	HIV-1, HIV-2, HBV	150 mg bid
Stavudine	d4T	HIV-1, HIV-2	40 mg bid
Zalcitabine	ddC	HIV-1, HIV-2	.75 mg tid
Zidovudine	ZDV	HIV-1, HIV-2	300 mg bid
Nonnucleoside reverse transcriptase inhibitors (NNRTI)			
Delavirdine	DLV	HIV-1	400 mg tid
Nevirapine	NVP	HIV-1	200 mg bid
Protease inhibitor (PI)			
Indinavir	IDV	HIV-1, HIV-2	800 mg tid
Nelfinavir	NFV	HIV-1, HIV-2	750 mg tid or 1250 mg bid
Ritonavir	RTV	HIV-1, HIV-2	600 mg bid
Saquinavir	SQV	HIV-1, HIV-2	600 mg tid

EOSINOPHILIC FOLLICULITIS

Eosinophilic folliculitis (EF) is an idiopathic, extremely pruritic, papular follicular eruption of the upper trunk, face, neck, and proximal extremities occurring in advanced HIV disease and/or after initiation of highly active antiretroviral therapy, often associated with peripheral eosinophilia. EF occurring in HIV disease is different from that of Ofuji's disease. *Synonym*: Eosinophilic pustular folliculitis.

EPIDEMIOLOGY

Unknown.

PATHOGENESIS

Unknown.

HISTORY

Symptoms   Moderate to intense itching unrelieved by many therapies. Pruritus may be severe, especially in those with atopic diathesis, disturbing sleep.

Systems Review   Occurs in HIV disease. Until recently, all individuals have had an AIDS-defining criterion. Recently, many cases are seen in persons who have recently begun highly active antiretroviral therapy; thought to associate with immune reconstitution.

PHYSICAL EXAMINATION

Skin Lesions   The primary lesions are 3- to 5-mm erythematous, edematous, follicular papules and pustules (Fig. 26-2*A* and 2*B*). Most patients have hundreds of lesions. Frequently, changes secondary to scratching/rubbing are seen: excoriations/crusting; atopic dermatitis, lichen simplex chronicus, prurigo nodularis. Secondary infections of excoriated sites include impetiginization, deep infections such as furuncles, and/or cellulitis. Postinflammatory hyperpigmentation occurs in more darkly pigmented individuals and can be quite disfiguring.

Distribution   Trunk; head and neck; proximal extremities. In some individuals, lesions present only on face or on trunk.

DIFFERENTIAL DIAGNOSIS

Allergic contact dermatitis, adverse cutaneous drug reaction, atopic dermatitis, scabies, papular urticaria (insect bites), acne vulgaris, dermatophytic folliculitis, bacterial folliculitis (*Staphylococcus aureus*), fungal folliculitis (*Pityrosporum ovale*).

LABORATORY EXAMINATIONS

Serology   HIV ELISA and Western blot positive.

Cultures   Negative for pathogenic organisms. Many patients with longstanding untreated EF have secondary colonization or infection with *S. aureus*.

Dermatopathology   Perifollicular and perivascular infiltrate with varying numbers of eosinophils. Epithelial spongiosis of follicular infundibulum and/or sebaceous glands associated with a mixed cellular infiltrate. Eosinophilic pustules uncommon. Special stains for bacteria, fungi, and parasites are negative.

Hematology   Many patients have either absolute or relative peripheral eosinophilia. CD4+ cell count usually <100 μL.

DIAGNOSIS

Clinical diagnosis confirmed by skin biopsy, with cultures ruling out infectious causes. A new primary lesion (follicular papule) should be marked with a pen and biopsied with a 2-mm punch.

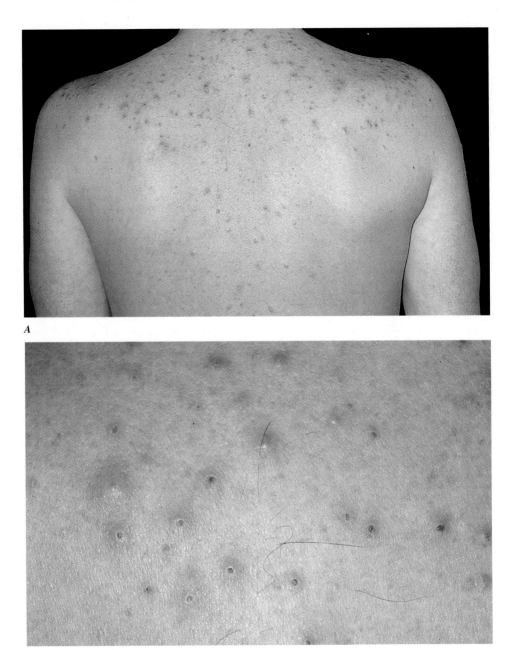

A

B

Figure 26-2   Eosinophilic folliculitis   *Multiple, very pruritic, edematous papules and a few pustules in a male with advanced HIV disease (CD4+ cell count < 50/μL):* **A.** *Distribution on the upper trunk; lesions were also present on the face and neck.* **B.** *Closeup showing urticarial papules, pustules, and erosion secondary to rubbing; the primary lesions resemble papular urticaria (insect bites), but are follicular.*

COURSE AND PROGNOSIS

In untreated HIV disease, the course of EF tends to be chronic and persistent. In patients in whom EF occurs after initiation of HAART, symptoms often persist for months if untreated.

Pruritus is moderate to severe, significantly affecting quality of life. Changes secondary to chronic scratching such as secondary infections and lichen simplex chronicus also should be identified and treated. The most predictably effective therapy is a short tapered course of oral glucocorticoid such as prednisone.

Antihistamines	Those causing sedation are more effective for symptomatic relief of pruritus. Doxepin, 10–100 mg, is especially effective at bedtime.
Topical Agents	
Glucocorticoids	Class I (superpotent) glucocorticoids applied to affected areas produce fair to moderate improvement in pruritus and lesions. Patients using these agents on the face should be closely monitored for atrophic changes.
Systemic Agents	
Prednisone	Initial dose of 70 mg, followed by a taper of 5–10 mg/d (14 → 7 days) provides rapid symptomatic improvement as well as resolution of EF. EF gradually recurs after completion of course.
Isotretinoin (Accutane)	1–2 mg/kg/d (about 80 mg) very effective in causing resolution of EF. Once symptoms and skin findings have resolved, dose is reduced to 40 mg/d for 2–4 weeks and then tapered to 40 mg qod. Dosing may be discontinued in 1–2 months if symptoms do not recur. Many HIV-infected individuals treated with HAART have elevated triglyceride levels; isotretinoin can further increase triglyceride levels.
Itraconazole	400 mg/d for 4 weeks reported to be effective.
Phototherapy	
UVB	Treatments are usually given three times a week, tapering as symptoms of EF resolve. Moderately effective.
Natural sunlight	Many individuals cannot tolerate natural sunlight because of treatment with photosensitizing drugs such as trimethoprim-sulfamethoxazole (Bactrim), which are photosensitizing in the UVA spectrum.

ORAL HAIRY LEUKOPLAKIA

Oral hairy leukoplakia (OHL) is a benign, virally induced hyperplasia of the oral mucosa, most commonly of the inferolateral surface of the tongue, characterized by white, corrugated, verrucous plaques, occurring in patients with symptomatic HIV disease.

Synonym: Oral viral leukoplakia.

EPIDEMIOLOGY

Etiology   Epstein-Barr virus (EBV).

PATHOGENESIS

Many adults have asymptomatic EBV infection of the oral mucosa. EBV is thought to emerge from latency as HIV-induced immunocompromise progresses and to cause the epidermal hyperplasia in OHL. In those patients who do not carry the diagnosis of AIDS at the time of detection of OHL, the probability of developing AIDS has been reported to be 48% by 16 months after detection and 83% by 31 months.

HISTORY

Risk Groups   HIV-infected individuals.

Incubation Period   Usually 5 to 10 years after primary HIV infection.

Symptoms   Lesions are asymptomatic. In some patients, OHL is bothersome in that it is a visible manifestation of their HIV disease. In some cases, OHL lesions are large and a cosmetic disfigurement for the patient.

PHYSICAL EXAMINATION

Oral Mucosa   White or grayish-white, well-demarcated verrucous plaque (Fig. 26-3). Surface appears irregular, with corrugated or hairy texture. Often present bilaterally, but size of plaques usually not equal. Some individuals may have oropharyngeal candidiasis and/or condyloma in addition to OHL.

Distribution   Most commonly on the lateral and inferior surfaces of the tongue. Rarely on the buccal and soft palatal mucosa.

DIFFERENTIAL DIAGNOSIS

Oral candidiasis, condyloma acuminatum, geographic or migratory glossitis, lichen planus, tobacco-associated leukoplakia, mucous patch of secondary syphilis, squamous cell carcinoma either in situ or invasive, occlusal trauma.

LABORATORY EXAMINATIONS

Dermatopathology   Acanthotic epithelium with hyperkeratosis, hairlike projections of keratin, areas of koilocytes (ballooned cells with clear cytoplasm).

Electron Microscopy   Herpes viral structures in epithelial cells; positive for Epstein-Barr virus markers; often also HPV viral particles.

Cultures   Not helpful. *Candida albicans* is commonly isolated.

DIAGNOSIS

Clinical diagnosis. Does not rub off; does not clear with adequate anticandidal therapy.

COURSE AND PROGNOSIS

The severity of OHL varies spontaneously from day to day. OHL is much less common in HIV-infected individuals treated and responding to HAART. May also clear completely during a course of treatment with acyclovir (oral or topical), IV ganciclovir, or foscarnet.

MANAGEMENT

OHL is asymptomatic, but its presence may cause anxiety in patients with the lesion. Reassurance that OHL is a benign viral infection is usually adequate to reduce patients' concerns.

Topical Therapy Podophyllin 25% in tincture of benzoin applied to the lesion with a cotton-tipped applicator for 5 min is very effective in most individuals. OHL usually recurs in weeks to months.

Systemic Antiviral Drugs Concomitant use of acyclovir, valacyclovir, famciclovir, ganciclovir, foscarnet for other indications often results in regression/clearing of OHL.

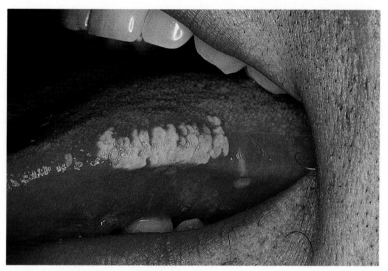

Figure 26-3 Oral hairy leukoplakia *White plaque on the lateral tongue with corduroy-like pattern. The finding is essentially pathognomonic for HIV infection and in this case, was the indication for HIV serotesting. CD4+ cell count was 223 cell/µL at the time of diagnosis.*

HIV-ASSOCIATED LIPODYSTROPHY SYNDROME

HIV-associated lipodystrophy syndrome occurs in individuals treated with antiretroviral drugs (usually a protease inhibitor), and is characterized by cosmetically disfiguring lipohypertrophy in the dorsocervical fat pad (buffalo hump), circumferentially around the neck, the breasts, and the abdomen (central adiposity), and lipoatrophy of the cheeks and proximal extremities (peripheral wasting); some cases are associated with increase in serum triglyceride and glucose levels.

EPIDEMIOLOGY

Incidence 83% of individuals treated with protease inhibitor (21 months); 4% of treatment-naïve patients. Lipodystrophy is severe in only 10% of these patients.

Etiology Ritonavir-saquinavir combination most strongly associated with syndrome>indinavir or nelfinavir. Also occurs in HIV-infected individuals who have never taken these drugs.

PATHOGENESIS

Unknown, but protease inhibitors may inhibit proteins involved in lipid metabolism, with the primary event being apoptosis and reduced differentiation of peripheral adipocytes. HIV protease has 60% homology with two human regulatory proteins that affect lipid metabolism, i.e., the cytoplasmic retinoic-acid binding protein type I (CRABP-1) and the low-density lipoprotein-receptor-related protein (LPR). Inhibition not only of HIV protease but also of CRABP-1 would impair the metabolism of retinoic acid, leading to fat-cell death and consequent lipid release and/or reduced lipid storage. Inhibition of LPR may result in the failure to remove fatty acids from circulating triglycerides into the vascular endothelium and in a reduced hepatic uptake of chylomicrons.

HISTORY

Lipodystrophy is progressive, the severity worsening with the duration of protease-inhibitor treatment. Lipoatrophy of the face results in a characteristic facies that stigmatizes the individual as having HIV disease. Lipohypertrophy of the dorsothoracic fat pad and neck can also be quite disfiguring. The incidence of atherosclerotic cardiovascular disease is increased.

PHYSICAL EXAMINATION

Skin Findings

Lipohypertrophy The dorsothoracic fat pad becomes hypertrophied to a variable extent (Fig. 26-4). With early mild involvement, the skin over the vertebral spinous processes becomes thickened due to increase in the subcutaneous fat, even in a thin individual. With severe involvement, the fat pad can become 5 to 10 cm thick. Lipohypertrophy can also occur circumferentially around the neck. Breasts may become enlarged in males and females. Abdominal girth can increase due to accumulation of intraabdominal fat (Fig. 26-5).

Lipoatrophy Subcutaneous fat is lost and/or disappears in the cheeks, giving a gaunt characteristic appearance (Fig. 26-6). The upper arms, shoulders, thighs, and buttocks become depleted of subcutaneous fat; superficial veins are visible in these sites. There is also generalized loss of body fat.

DIFFERENTIAL DIAGNOSIS

Lipohypertrophy Cushing's disease, glucocorticoid therapy, Launois-Bensaude syndrome, scleredema of diabetes mellitus.

Lipoatrophy Wasting of chronic disease, malnutrition.

LABORATORY EXAMINATIONS

Blood Chemistries

Hyperlipidemia 74% of protease-inhibitor recipients; 28% in treatment-naïve patients.

Glucose Tolerance Impaired in 16% of protease-inhibitor recipients and type 2 diabetes mellitus in 7%.

Glucocorticoid Metabolism Normal.

DIAGNOSIS

Clinical diagnosis. In some cases, rule out Cushing's disease.

COURSE AND PROGNOSIS

Lipodystrophy becomes progressively more severe as protease-inhibitor therapy is continued, and is, to some extent, reversible when therapy is discontinued.

MANAGEMENT

For most individuals with mild to moderate lipodystrophy, the changes in body habitus are not significant. However, with more severe involvement, patients may request change in protease-inhibitor therapy in spite of excellent response of HIV disease.

Lipohypertrophy Discontinuing and/or changing antiretroviral drugs may result in regression. Administration of recombinant human growth factor. Liposuction has been helpful in some cases, but recurrence is common.

Lipoatrophy For the cheeks, lipotransfer with a syringe may be effective. Implantation of Gore-Tex.

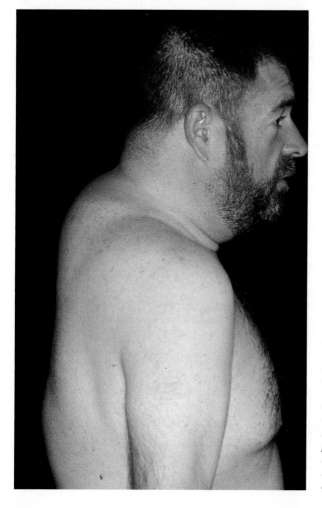

Figure 26-4   HIV-associated lipodystrophy syndrome: lipohypertrophy *Increase in subcutaneous fat is seen on the upper back creating a "buffalo hump," neck, and breast of an otherwise thin middle-aged HIV-infected male, who is on highly active antiretroviral therapy (HAART). Liposuction of the fat had been performed two years previously, however, the lipohypertrophy recurred. Mild lipoatrophy of the cheek is also apparent.*

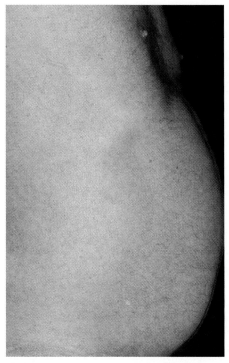

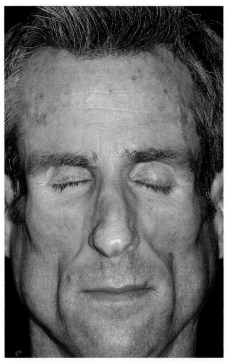

Figure 26-5   HIV-associated lipodystrophy syndrome: lipohypertrophy   *Increased abdominal girth is seen in an otherwise thin middle-aged HIV-infected male on highly active antiretroviral therapy (HAART).*

Figure 26-6   HIV-associated lipodystrophy syndrome: lipoatrophy   *Striking lipoatrophy of the face (mainly the cheeks) of a middle-aged HIV-infected male. Enlargement of the parotid glands is also apparent. Several aggressive invasive squamous cell carcinomas have occurred (note excision scar with graft on nose), associated with his immunocompromised state, as well as multiple basal cell carcinomas and actinic keratoses.*

PROPOSED CASE DEFINITION FOR PROTEASE-INHIBITOR-RELATED LIPODYSTROPHY SYNDROME

Clinical features
- Fat wasting of the face, arms, legs, or buttocks (possibly with prominence of leg and arm veins)
- Fat accumulation in the abdomen or over the dorsocervical spin *and*

Metabolic features
One or more of the following since start of HIV-1 protease-inhibitor therapy:
- Fasting hyperlipidemia (cholesterol ≥5.5 mmol/L or triglyceride ≥2 mmol/L)
- Fasting C-peptide >2.5 mmol/L
- Impaired fasting glucose (6.1 to 7 mmol/L) or diabetes mellitus (≥7 mmol/L) on fasting blood glucose
- Impaired glucose tolerance (7.8 to 11.1 mmol/L) or diabetes mellitus (≥11.1 mmol/L) on 2-h blood glucose by oral glucose tolerance test

Patients should not have any of the following within 3 months of assessment:
- AIDS-defining event or other severe clinical illness
- Anabolic steroids, glucocorticoids, immune modulators

VARIATIONS OF COMMON MUCOCUTANEOUS DISORDERS IN HIV DISEASE

Early in HIV disease when immune function is relatively intact, common dermatoses and infections present in typical ways, have the usual course, and respond to standard therapies. However, with progressive decline in immune function, each of these characteristics of a disease can be strikingly altered, such that the correct diagnosis is not considered nor is correct treatment instituted.

Kaposi's Sarcoma (See also Kaposi's Sarcoma, Section 17)   Early in the HIV epidemic in the United States and Europe, 50% of homosexual men at the time of initial diagnosis of AIDS had Kaposi's Sarcoma (KS); currently, the incidence is 18% within this risk group.

In HIV-infected individuals, the risk for KS is 20,000 times that of the general population, 300 times that of other immunosuppressed individuals. KS in HIV-infected individuals shows rapid progression and is characterized by extensive systemic involvement.

Nonmelanoma Skin Cancers   As in renal transplant recipients, the incidence of ultraviolet light–induced basal cell carcinomas and invasive squamous cell carcinoma (SCC) appears to be increased in HIV-infected individuals. SCC can be quite aggressive, invading locally, growing rapidly, and metastasizing by lymphatics and blood, with increased morbidity and mortality.

Aphthous Stomatitis (See also Aphthous Ulcers, Section 29)   Recurrent aphthous ulcerations may occur more frequently, become larger (often >1 cm), and/or become chronic in persons with advanced HIV disease. Ulcers may be quite extensive and/or multiple, commonly involving the tongue, gingiva, lips, and esophagus, at times causing severe odynophagia with rapid weight loss. Intralesional triamcinolone and/or a one- to two-week tapered course of prednisone (70 to 0 mg). In resistant cases, thalidomide is an effective agent.

Drug Eruptions (See also Exanthematous Drug Reactions, Section 18)   The incidence of cutaneous drug eruptions is greatly increased in HIV disease and may be correlated with the decline and dysregulation of immune function. Between 50 and 60% of patients with AIDS treated with trimethoprim-sulfamethoxazole develop a morbilliform eruption 1 to 2 weeks after starting therapy. Other drugs associated with an increased incidence of cutaneous reactions include sulfadiazine, trimethoprim-dapsone, and aminopenicillins. The incidence of toxic epidermal necrolysis caused by sulfonamides is also increased. Lipodystrophy and chronic paronychia have been associated with protease-inhibitor therapy. After immune restoration by antiretroviral therapy, some patients who had previously tolerated the drug may develop allergic cutaneous drug reactions.

Staphylococcus aureus Infection (See also Impetigo and Ecthyma; Abscess, Furuncle, and Carbuncle; and Cellulitis, Section 20)   S. aureus is the most common cutaneous bacterial pathogen in HIV disease. The nasal carriage rate of S. aureus is 50%, twice that of HIV-seronegative control groups. In most instances, S. aureus infections are typical, presenting as primary infections (folliculitis, furuncles, carbuncles), secondarily impetiginized lesions (excoriations, eczema, scabies, herpetic ulcer, Kaposi's sarcoma), cellulitis, or venous access device infections, all of which can be complicated by bacteremia and disseminated infection.

Dermatophytoses (See also Dermatophytoses, Section 21, and Onychomycosis, Section 28)   Epidermal dermatophytosis in HIV-infected individuals can be extensive, recurrent, and difficult to eradicate. Proximal subungual onychomycosis, which is common in untreated HIV disease, presents as a chalky-white discoloration of the undersurface of the proximal nail plate and is an indication for HIV serotesting.

Mucosal Candidiasis (See also Candidiasis, Section 21)   Mucosal candidiasis affecting the upper aerodigestive tracts and/or vulvovagina is common in HIV disease. Oropharyngeal candidiasis, the most common presentation, is often the initial manifestation of HIV disease and a marker for disease progression. Four patterns are commonly seen: erythematous/atrophic, pseudomembranous/thrush, hyperplastic/Candida leukoplakia, and angular cheilitis. Esophageal and tracheobronchial candidiasis occur in advance of HIV disease and are AIDS-defining conditions. The incidence of recurrent candidal vulvovaginitis appears to be increased in HIV-infected women compared with non-HIV-infected controls. The incidence of cutaneous candidiasis may be somewhat increased in HIV disease. In young children with HIV disease, chronic candidal paronychia and nail dystrophy are seen frequently.

Invasive Fungal Infection with Cutaneous Dissemination (See also Disseminated Cryptococcosis, Histoplasmosis, and Disseminated Coccidioidomycosis, Section 21) Latent pulmonary fungal infections with *Cryptococcus neoformans, Coccidioides immitis, Histoplasma capsulatum,* and *Penicillium marneffei* can be reactivated in HIV-infected individuals and disseminated to the skin. The most common cutaneous presentation of disseminated infection is molluscum contagiosum–like lesions on the face; other lesions such as nodules, pustules, ulcers, abscesses, or a papulosquamous eruption resembling guttate psoriasis (seen with histoplasmosis) also occur.

Herpes simplex Virus Infection (See also *Herpes simplex* Virus Infections Associated Immunocompromise with, Section 23) Reactivated herpes simplex virus type 1 (HSV-1) or HSV-2 infection is one of the most common viral complications of HIV disease. With increasing immunodeficiency, early lesions present with erosions or ulcerations due to epidermal necrosis without vesicle formation. Untreated, these lesions may evolve to large, painful ulcers with raised margins. In contrast to its effect in healthy individuals, reactivated HSV in those with advanced HIV disease can cause large, chronic ulceration in the oropharynx, esophagus, and anogenitalia. HSV should be considered in the differential diagnosis of any ulcerative or crusted lesion on the face, mouth, anogenitalia, or fingers in an individual with advanced HIV disease. Ulcers persisting after adequate acyclovir therapy may be caused by acyclovir-resistant HSV strains.

Varicella-Zoster Virus Infection (See also Varicellar-zoster Virus Infections in the Immunocompromised Host, Section 23) Primary varicella-zoster virus (VZV) infection (chickenpox) in HIV-infected individuals can be severe, prolonged, and complicated by parenchymal infection, bacterial superinfection, and death. Herpes zoster occurs in 25% of HIV-infected persons during the course of their HIV disease, associated with modest decline in immune function. Cutaneous dissemination of herpes zoster is relatively common; however, visceral involvement is rare. With increasing immunodeficiency, VZV infection can present clinically as chronic dermatomal verrucous lesions; one or more chronic painful ulcers or ecthymatous lesions within a dermatome; ecthymatous lesion(s), ulcer(s), or nodule(s) resembling basal cell carcinoma or squamous cell carcinoma. Untreated, these lesions persist for months or the lifetime of the patient. Herpes zoster can be recurrent within the same dermatome(s) or in other dermatomes. VZV can cause a rapidly progressive chorioretinitis with acute retinal necrosis, often bilaterally, in the absence of any cutaneous involvement and must be differentiated from cytomegalovirus chorioretinitis.

Molluscum contagiosum (See also Molluscum Contagiosum, Section 23) In HIV-infected individuals, molluscum contagiosum has up to an 18% prevalence; the severity of the infection is a marker for advanced immunodeficiency. Patients may have multiple small papules or nodules or large tumors, >1 cm in diameter, most commonly arising on the face, especially the beard area, the neck, and intertriginous sites. Shaving is a major factor in the facial spread of mollusca and should be avoided if possible. Cystlike mollusca occur on the ears. Occasionally, mollusca can arise on the non-hair-bearing skin of the palms/soles. Multiple facial mollusca must be differentiated from the cutaneous lesions of disseminated fungal infection (cryptococcosis, histoplasmosis, coccidioidomycosis, and penicillinosis). With HAART, multiple mollusca either do not occur or resolve after immune restoration.

Human Papilloma Virus (HPV) infection (See also Human Papilloma Virus Infections, Section 25) With advancing immunodeficiency, cutaneous and/or mucosal warts can become extensive and refractory to treatment. Of more concern, however, HPV-induced intraepithelial neoplasia, more recently termed squamous intraepithelial lesion (SIL), is a precursor to invasive squamous cell carcinoma (SCC), arising most often on the cervix, vulva, penis, perineum, and anus. In HIV-infected females, the incidence of cervical SIL is six to eight times that of controls. The current trend toward longer median survival of patients with advanced HIV disease may lead to an increased incidence of HPV-associated neoplasia and invasive SCC in the future. SIL on the external genitalia, perineum, or anus is best managed with local therapies such as imiquimod cream, cryosurgery, electrosurgery, or laser surgery rather than with aggressive surgical excision.

Syphilis (See also Syphilis, Section 25) The clinical course of syphilis in HIV-infected individuals is most often the same as in the normal host, with a painless chancre in primary syphilis or a macular or papular eruption in secondary syphilis. However, an accelerated course with the development of pneurosyphilis or tertiary syphilis has been reported within months of initial syphilitic infection.

DISORDERS OF HAIR FOLLICLES AND RELATED DISORDERS

DISORDERS OF HAIR GROWTH

Loss of hair is termed *effluvium* or *defluvium,* and the resulting condition is called *alopecia* (baldness, from Latin). Patients have a different perception of balding from that of the dermatologist; they often are aware and very concerned about subtle thinning of the hair. Disorders characterized by loss of hair are conveniently classified into *noncicatricial alopecia,* where, at least clinically, there is no sign of tissue inflammation, scarring, or atrophy of skin, and *cicatricial alopecia,* where evidence of tissue destruction such as inflammation, atrophy, and scarring is apparent.

Biology of Hair

1. Hair growth on the scalp occurs in cycles of intermittent activity (Fig. 27-1); periods of growth are followed by periods of quiescence. The period of active growth is referred to as *anagen,* which is followed normally by a brief transition phase, called *catagen,* during which growth stops and follicles, enter the resting, or *telogen,* phase. The total duration of anagen determines the length of the hair. The anagen phase is short and the telogen phase is prolonged in the eyebrows, eyelashes, and axillary and pubic hair compared with the relatively long anagen phase in the scalp and beard areas. At birth there are 100,000 terminal scalp hair follicles that are genetically determined to produce long, thick pigmented hairs. Other hairs over most of the body are genetically predestined to produce "vellus" (from Latin: *wool*) hairs that are short, fine, and nonpigmented.

2. The hair follicles can vary in size under the influence of androgens, which increase the size of hair follicles in the beard, chest, legs, and arms but decrease the size of the hair follicles in the temporal regions of the scalp; this shapes the hair line in men and many women.

3. The response of the hair follicle to testosterone (Te) and dihydrotestosterone (DHT) is under genetic control. DHT causes growth of the prostate, growth of terminal hair, androgenetic alopecia, and acne. Te causes growth of axillary hair and lower pubic hair, as well as sex drive, growth of the phallus and scrotum, and spermatogenesis.

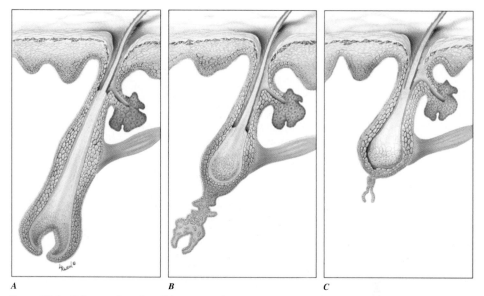

Figure 27-1 Hair growth cycle *Diagrammatic representation of the changes that occur to the follicle and hair shaft during the hair growth cycle.* **A.** *Anagen (growth stage);* **B.** *Catogen (degenerative stage);* **C.** *Telogen (resting stage). (Courtesy of Lynn M. Klein, MD).*

NONSCARRING ALOPECIA

Alopecia Areata

Alopecia areata is a localized loss of hair in round or oval areas without any visible inflammation of the skin in hair-bearing areas; the most common presenting site is the scalp. *Alopecia totalis* is loss of all scalp hair and eyebrows. *Alopecia universalis,* the end stage of alopecia areata, is complete loss of all body hair.

EPIDEMIOLOGY

Age of Onset   Young adults (<25 years); children are affected more frequently.

Sex   Equal in both sexes, although the male:female ratio is reported to be 2:1 in Italy and Spain.

Prevalence   Relatively common. About 1% of the U.S. population has at least one episode of alopecia areata by age 50.

Etiology   Unknown. Association with other autoimmune diseases suggests an anti-hair bulb autoimmune process.

PATHOGENESIS

Alopecia areata is considered an autoimmune disease. The rationale for this disorder being autoimmune is the presence of CD4 and CD8 lymphocytes around affected hair bulbs and the fact that the T lymphocytes from the involved scalp can be transferred to explants of human scalp in mice with severe combined immunodeficiency where they induce hair loss. Also, there is an association of alopecia areata with certain HLA class II alleles, DQB1*03 and DRB1*1104, which are markers of general susceptibility to alopecia areata. Two other alleles, DRB1*0401 and DQB1*1301, are increased in patients with alopecia totalis. Although the course of alopecia areata is not altered, treatment with immunomodulating therapies such as glucocorticoids, cyclosporine, and topical immunotherapy can induce remission of alopecia areata.

Not a sign of any multisystem disease but may be associated with other autoimmune disorders such as vitiligo, familial autoimmune polyendocrinopathy syndrome (hypoparathyroidism, Addison's disease, and mucocutaneous candidiasis), and thyroid disease (Hashimoto's disease).

HISTORY

Duration of Hair Loss   Gradual over weeks to months. Patches of alopecia areata can be stable and often show spontaneous regrowth over a period of several months; new patches may appear while others resolve.

Skin Symptoms   No pain or itching. However, patients are often very concerned about a single area of hair loss and prognosis of continued, progressive balding.

Associated Findings   Hashimoto's thyroiditis, vitiligo, myasthenia gravis.

PHYSICAL EXAMINATION

Skin Findings   Usually none. Possibly erythema in the area of hair loss. The absence of clinical signs of inflammation is remarkable in that histopathologically there is always an inflammatory infiltrate around hair follicles in active lesions.

Hair   Alopecia, normal-appearing skin with follicular openings present (Figs. 27-2 through 27-4). No scarring, no atrophy; occasionally, with diagnostic broken-off stubby hairs called *exclamation point hairs,* sharp margins (Fig. 27-2). With regrowth of hair, new hairs are thin and often white or gray. Alopecia always sharply defined. Scattered, discrete areas of alopecia (Fig. 27-2) or confluent (Fig. 27-3) with total loss of scalp hair (alopecia areata totalis) (Fig. 27-4), or generalized resulting in generalized loss of body hair (including vellus

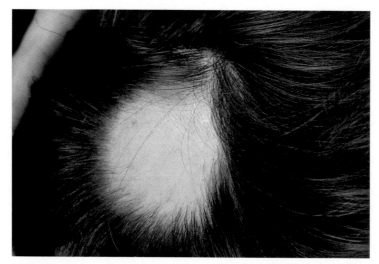

Figure 27-2 Alopecia areata of scalp: solitary lesion *A sharply outlined portion of the scalp with complete alopecia without scaling, erythema, atrophy, or scarring. Empty follicles can still be seen on the involved scalp. The short, broken-off hair shafts (so-called exclamation point hair) appear as very short stubs emerging from the bald scalp.*

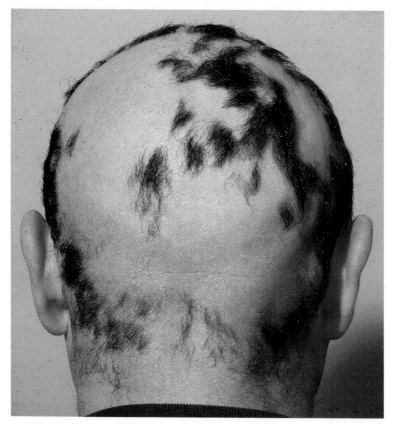

Figure 27-3 Alopecia areata of scalp: multiple, extensive lesions *Multiple, confluent, involved sites on the scalp with "exclamation point hairs" and evidence of regrowth in some areas. Newly regrowing hairs may be fine and gray-white in color.*

hair), termed *alopecia areata universalis.* Sometimes hair loss in alopecia areata totalis may follow a diffuse (noncircumscribed) pattern.

Sites of Predilection Scalp, eyebrows, eyelashes, pubic hair, beard.

Nails The dorsal nail plate may have hundreds of tiny depressions simulating "hammered brass."

DIFFERENTIAL DIAGNOSIS

Nonscarring Alopecia Secondary syphilis ("moth-eaten" appearance in beard or scalp), white-patch tinea capitis, trichotillomania, traction alopecia, early chronic cutaneous lupus erythematosus, androgenetic alopecia.

LABORATORY EXAMINATIONS

Serology Antinuclear antibodies (to rule out lupus erythematosus); rapid plasma reagin (RPR) test (to rule out secondary syphilis).

KOH Preparation To rule out tinea capitis.

Dermatopathology Follicles are reduced in size and lie high in the dermis; perifollicular lymphocytic infiltrate with dilated vessels followed by degenerative changes in the blood vessels that lead to the hair papillae. Hair roots have typical club shape; proximal portion of shaft shows dystrophic taper (exclamation point hairs). Dystrophic anagen hairs. Increase of telogen hair from normal (<20%) to 40% or more.

COURSE

If occurring after puberty, 80% of patients regrow hair. Alopecia universalis is rare. After the first episode of hair loss, about 33% completely regrow the hair within a year. Recurrences of alopecia, however, are frequent. Repeated attacks, nail changes, and total alopecia before puberty are poor prognostic signs. Another poor prognostic sign is confluence of lesions in the occipital region (ophiasis).

MANAGEMENT

No curative treatment is currently available. Efficacy of treatment in individual patients is difficult to assess in light of spontaneous regrowth. All in all, treatment for alopecia areata is unsatisfactory. In many cases, the most important factor in management of the patient is psychological support from the dermatologist, family, and support groups (The National Alopecia Areata Foundation, Tel. 1-415-456-4644).

Glucocorticoids

Topical Superpotent agents may be effective.

Intralesional Injection Few and small spots of alopecia areata can be treated with intralesional triamcinolone acetonide, 3.5 mg/mL, which can be very effective temporarily.

Systemic Glucocorticoids Usually induce regrowth, but alopecia recurs on discontinuation; risks of long-term therapy therefore preclude their use.

Systemic Cyclosporine Induces regrowth, but alopecia recurs when drug is discontinued.

Induction of Allergic Contact Dermatitis Dinitrochlorobenzene, squaric acid dibutylester, or diphencyprone can be used successfully, but local discomfort due to allergic contact dermatitis and swelling of regional lymph nodes poses a problem.

Oral PUVA (Photochemotherapy) Variably effective, as high as 30%, and worth a trial in patients who are highly distressed about the problem. The entire body must be exposed, in that the therapy is believed to be a form of systemic immune suppression.

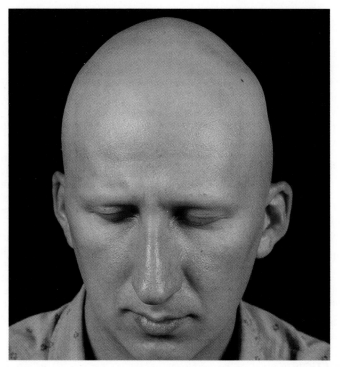

Figure 27-4   Alopecia universalis   *This patient has lost all scalp hair (alopecia totalis), eyebrows, eyelashes, beard, and all body hair (alopecia universalis), and has dystrophic ("hammered brass") nails.*

Androgenetic Alopecia

Androgenetic alopecia (AGA) is the common progressive balding that occurs through the combined effect of a genetic predisposition and the action of androgen on the hair follicles of the scalp. Pattern of hair loss in males varies from bitemporal recession, to frontal and/or vertex thinning, to loss of all hair except that along the occipital and temporal margins. In males, diffuse thinning occurs, worse centrally.

Synonyms: Male-pattern baldness, common baldness (males), hereditary thinning (females).

EPIDEMIOLOGY

Age of Onset *Males:* May begin any time after puberty, as early as the second decade; often fully expressed in forties. *Females:* Later—in about 40% occurs in the sixth decade.

Sex Males much more commonly than females.

Heredity Polygenic or autosomal dominant in males; autosomal recessive in females.

Etiology Combined effects of androgen on genetically predisposed hair follicles.

CLASSIFICATION

Hamilton (Am J Anat 71:451, 1941) classified male-pattern hair loss into stages (Fig. 27-5): type I, loss of hair along the frontal margin; type II, increasing frontal hair loss as well as onset of loss on the occipital scalp (crown); and types III, IV, and V, increasing hair loss in both regions with eventual confluent and complete balding of the top of the scalp with sparing of the sides. (See Fig. 27-5.)

PATHOGENESIS

The mechanism of action of androgen on follicular cellular processes that results in AGA is unclear, but in most cases it is a local phenomenon (increased expression of androgen receptors, changes in androgen metabolism) of the scalp hair follicles. *Consequently, most patients (male and female) are endocrinologically normal.* Terminal follicles are transformed into vellus-like follicles, which in turn undergo atrophy. During successive follicular cycles, the hairs produced are of shorter length and of decreasing diameter. Conversely, androgens induce vellus-to-terminal follicle production of secondary sexual hair. Males castrated before or during puberty do not develop AGA despite a strong family history; administration of androgen can produce baldness that does not progress if the drug is withdrawn. Dihydrotestosterone, an intracellular hormone, causes growth of androgen-dependent hair (e.g., pubic, beard) and loss of non-androgen-dependent scalp hair. In males, testosterone produced by the testes is the major androgen. In females, androstenedione and dehydroepiandrosterone sulfate are the major peripheral androgens, and these two hormones are very slowly converted to dihydrotestosterone in the target cell (hair keratinocyte) by 5α-testosterone reductase. The serum testosterone levels in men are much higher than in women, and there are higher tissue levels and greater conversion to dihydrotestosterone.

HISTORY

Skin Symptoms Most patients present with complaints of gradually thinning hair or baldness. In males (Fig. 27-6), there is a receding anterior hair line, especially in the parietal regions, which results in an M-shaped recession. Following this, a bald spot may appear on the posterior crown. If AGA progresses rapidly, some patients also complain of increased falling out of hair. In females, parietal and temporal recession is not usually a major feature, and effluvium follows a pattern depicted in Fig. 27-5; severe thinning is not common. The cosmetic appearance of AGA is very disturbing to many patients owing to the high value that our society places on a "healthy head of hair."

Systems Review In young women, manifestations of androgen excess should be sought as significant: acne, hirsutism, irregular menses, or virilization. However, most women with AGA are endocrinologically normal.

DISORDERS OF HAIR FOLLICLES AND RELATED DISORDERS

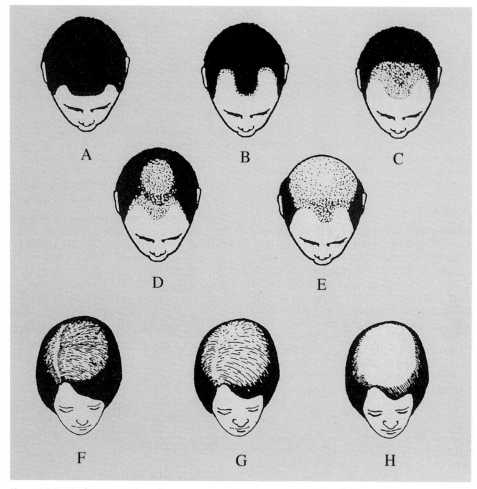

Figure 27-5 Androgenetic alopecia: patterns in males and females *The different patterns as they appear in males (A–E corresponding to types I–V, classification according to Hamilton) and in females (F–H corresponding to types I–III, classification according to Ludwig).*

PHYSICAL EXAMINATION

Skin Findings No skin lesions are seen in AGA except seborrhea that may be present in severe cases. In young women, other signs of virilization should be sought, such as acne and excess facial or body hair or a male-pattern escutcheon.

Hair (Figs. 27-6 and 27-7) Hair in areas of AGA becomes finer in texture, i.e., shorter in length and of reduced diameter. In time, hair becomes vellus and eventually atrophies completely. With complete alopecia, scalp is smooth and shiny; orifices of follicles are barely perceptible with the unaided eye.

Distribution Males usually exhibit patterned loss in the frontotemporal and vertex areas (Fig. 27-6). The end result may be only a rim of residual hair on the lateral and posterior scalp (Fig. 27-5E). In these regions hair never falls out in AGA. Paradoxically, males with extensive AGA may have excess growth of secondary sexual hair, i.e., axillae, pubic area, chest, and beard.

Females, including those who are endocrinologically normal, also lose scalp hair according to the male pattern, but hair loss is far less pronounced (Fig 27-7). Often hair loss is more diffuse in women following a pattern first described by Ludwig (Br J Dermatol 97:249, 1977) (Fig. 27-5).

Systemic Findings In young women with AGA, signs of virilization such as clitoral hypertrophy, acne, and facial hirsutism should be sought to rule out endocrine dysfunction.

DIFFERENTIAL DIAGNOSIS

Diffuse Nonscarring Scalp Alopecia Diffuse pattern of hair loss with alopecia areata, telogen defluvium, secondary syphilis, systemic lupus erythematosus, iron deficiency, hypothyroidism, hyperthyroidism, trichotillomania, seborrheic dermatitis.

LABORATORY EXAMINATIONS

Trichogram A trichogram determines the number of anagen and telogen hairs and is made by epilating (plucking) 50 hairs or more from the scalp with a needleholder and counting the number of anagen hairs (growing hairs with a long encircling hair sheath) and the number of club or telogen hairs (resting hairs with an in-

ner root sheath and roots usually largest at the base). Normally, 80 to 90% of hairs are in anagen phase. In AGA, the earliest changes are an increase in the percentage of telogen hairs.

Dermatopathology Abundance of telogen-stage follicles is noted, associated with hair follicles of decreasing size and eventually nearly complete atrophy.

Hormone Studies In women with hair loss and evidence of increased androgens (menstrual irregularities, infertility, hirsutism, severe cystic acne, virilization), total testosterone, free testosterone, dehydroepiandrosterone sulfate (DHEAS), and prolactin should be determined.

Other Studies Treatable causes of thinning hair should be excluded with measurement of TSH, T_4, serum iron, serum ferritin, and/or total iron-binding capacity (TIBC), CBC.

DIAGNOSIS

Clinical diagnosis is made on the history, pattern of alopecia, and family incidence of AGA. Skin biopsy may be necessary in some cases.

COURSE

The progression of alopecia is usually very gradual, over years to decades.

MANAGEMENT

Oral Finasteride An oral prescription drug available in the United States, finasteride, at 1 mg/d, competitively inhibits type 2 5α-reductase and thus the conversion of testosterone to dihydrotestosterone; this results in lower serum and scalp levels of dihydrotestosterone. Finasteride has no affinity for androgen receptors and therefore does not block the important actions of testosterone cited previously (sex drive, growth of the phallus and scrotum, and spermatogenesis). Finasteride was developed to treat male pattern hair loss in two sites only: the vertex (at the top of the head) and the anterior mid-scalp area. It is now approved for use only in men. Finasteride has been proved to maintain or increase hair count in most men. In large double-blind clinical studies of men (18 to 41 years) with mild to moderate hair loss, hair count was maintained in those men taking finasteride, while men taking a placebo exhibited progressive hair loss. According to large clini-

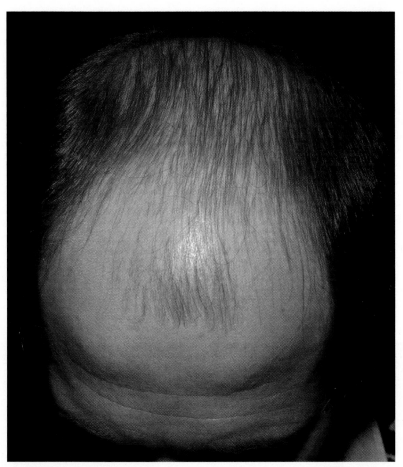

Figure 27-6 Androgenetic alopecia: male *Loss of hair in the frontotemporal and vertex areas in a male corresponding to Hamilton types IV and V.*

cal studies in 1850 men, finasteride starts immediately to block the formation of dihydrotestosterone, but because the hair is slow growing, visible results from finasteride takes time. Most men may begin to see the first benefit of finasteride in slowing hair loss as early as 3 months. After 6 months there is a regrowth of terminal hair on the vertex and anterior midscalp. If the drug is stopped, however, the hair that had grown will be lost within 12 months. The side effects of finasteride are minimal, and in only 2% of men taking finasteride was there a decrease in libido and erectile function; these effects were reversible when the drug was stopped and, in fact, disappeared in two-thirds of those who continued taking finasteride.

Topical Minoxidil Topically applied minoxidil 5% solution is helpful in reducing the rate of hair loss or in partially restoring lost hair in some patients; in large clinical trials, moderate growth has been noted at 4 and 12 months in 40% of males. The efficacy of minoxidil in females is not yet known from large clinical trials. Combinations of higher concentrations of minoxidil with topical retinoic acid are promising improvements.

Antiandrogens Spironolactone, cyproterone acetate, flutamide, and cimetidine, which bind to androgen receptors and block the action of dihydrotestosterone, have been reported to be effective in treating women with AGA who have elevated adrenal androgens; these must not be used in men.

Wigs Many types of hair pieces are used.

Hair Transplantation Moving multiple punch grafts of follicles taken from androgen-insensitive hair sites (peripheral occipital and parietal hairy areas) to bald androgen-sensitive scalp areas is effective in some patients with AGA. These micrografts are a successful technique in many patients and help restore more normal appearance.

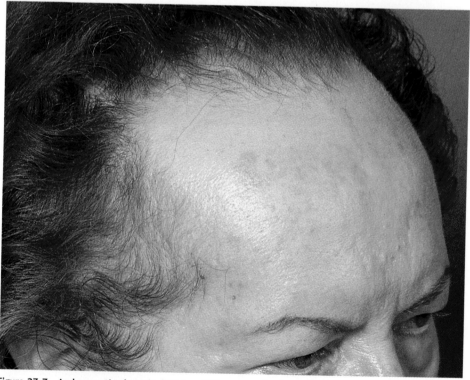

Figure 27-7 Androgenetic alopecia: female *This woman had pronounced diffuse thinning of hair on the crown, but in addition, also had thinning of the hair in the frontotemporal region of the scalp after treatment with androgens.*

Telogen Effluvium

Telogen effluvium is the transient increased shedding of normal club hairs (telogen) from resting scalp follicles secondary to accelerated shift of anagen (growth phase) into catagen and telogen (resting phase), which results clinically in increased daily hair loss and, if severe, thinning of hair. *Synonym:* Telogen defluvium.

EPIDEMIOLOGY AND ETIOLOGY

Age of Onset Any age.

Sex More common in women due to parturition, cessation of an oral contraceptive, and "crash" dieting.

Incidence Second most common cause of alopecia after androgenetic alopecia.

Etiology Factors that affect follicle growth resulting in telogen effluvium include pregnancy followed by either abortion or parturition, discontinuing or changing type of oral contraceptive, major surgical procedure, major traumatic injury, "crash" dieting with significant weight loss in a short period of time, and significant medical illness (especially with high fever). Profound emotional stress.

PATHOGENESIS

In the normal scalp, 80 to 90% of hairs are in anagen phase, 5% in catagen phase, and 10 to 15% in telogen phase; 50 to 100 hairs are shed as they are replaced daily. With telogen effluvium, many more hairs than normal are shed daily. The precipitating stimulus for telogen effluvium results in a premature shift of anagen follicles into the telogen phase.

HISTORY

Skin Symptoms Patient presents with complaint of increased hair loss on the scalp that may be accompanied by varying degrees of hair thinning. Most patients are very anxious, fearing they will become bald. The physician is often presented with a plastic bag containing the shed hair. The precipitating event precedes the telogen effluvium by 6 to 16 weeks.

PHYSICAL EXAMINATION

Skin Lesions No abnormalities of the scalp are detected.

Hair (Fig. 27-8) Diffuse shedding of the scalp hair is seen. In running the fingers through the patient's hair, several to many hairs may be shed with each passage. These hairs are all telogen or club hairs.

Distribution Hair loss occurs diffusely throughout the scalp and includes the sides and back of the head. If hair loss is significant enough to result in thinning of hair, alopecia is noted diffusely throughout the scalp. Short regrowing new hairs are present close to the scalp; these hairs are finer than older hairs and have tapered ends.

Site of Predilection Scalp.

Nails The precipitating stimulus for telogen effluvium also may affect the growth of nails, resulting in Beau's lines, which appear as transverse lines or grooves on the fingernail and toenail plates.

DIFFERENTIAL DIAGNOSIS

Increased Shedding of Scalp Hair ± Alopecia
Nonscarring, noninflammatory alopecia: androgenetic alopecia, diffuse-pattern alopecia areata, hyperthyroidism, hypothyroidism, systemic lupus erythematosus, secondary syphilis, drug-induced alopecia (Table 27-1).

LABORATORY EXAMINATIONS

Trichogram Compared with the normal trichogram, in which 80 to 90% of hair is in the anagen phase, telogen effluvium is characterized by a reduced percentage of anagen hairs, varying with the intensity of hair shedding. See "Androgenetic Alopecia" for an explanation of the trichogram.

Table 27-1 DRUG-INDUCED ALOPECIA[a]

Drugs	Features of Alopecia
ACE Inhibitors	
Enalapril	Probable telogen effluvium
Anticoagulants	
Heparin	Few reports
Warfarin	Reported incidence ranges from 19 to 70% but is probably much lower; diffuse shedding with increased number of hairs in telogen phase.
Antimitotic Agents	
Colchicine	Diffuse hair loss; increased number of telogen hairs
Antineoplastic Agents	
Bleomycin	Anagen effluvium
Cyclophosphamide	Anagen effluvium
Cytarabine	Anagen effluvium
Dacarbazine	Anagen effluvium
Dactinomycin	Anagen effluvium
Daunorubicin	Anagen effluvium
Doxorubicin	Anagen effluvium
Etoposide	Anagen effluvium
Fluorouracil	Anagen effluvium
Hydroxyurea	Anagen effluvium
Ifosfamide	Anagen effluvium
Mechlorethamine	Anagen effluvium
Melphalen	Anagen effluvium
Methotrexate	Anagen effluvium
Mitomycin	Anagen effluvium
Mitoxantrone	Anagen effluvium
Nitrosourea	Anagen effluvium
Procarbazine	Anagen effluvium
Thiotepa	Anagen effluvium
Vinblastine	Anagen effluvium
Vincristine	Anagen effluvium
Antiparkinsonian Agents	
Levodopa	Probable telogen effluvium
Antiseizure Agents	
Trimethadione	Probable telogen effluvium
Beta Blockers	
Metoprolol	Probable telogen effluvium
Propranolol	Probable telogen effluvium
Birth Control Agents	
Oral contraceptives	Diffuse hair loss (telogen effluvium) 2 to 3 months after cessation of oral contraceptive.
Drugs Used in Treatment of Bipolar Disorders	
Lithium	Probable telogen effluvium
Ergot Derivatives (used in treatment of prolactinemia)	
Bromocriptine	Probable telogen effluvium
H₂ Blockers	
Cimetidine	Onset 1 week to 11 months; probable telogen effluvium.
Heavy Metals (Poisoning)	
Thallium	Diffuse shedding of abnormal anagen hair 10 days after ingestion; complete hair loss in 1 month; characteristic is pronounced hair loss on sides of head, also of lateral eyebrows.
Mercury and lead	Diffuse hair loss with acute and chronic exposure.

(continued)

Cholesterol-Lowering Drugs
Clofibrate   Occasionally associated with hair loss.

Pesticides
Boric acid   Total scalp alopecia reported after acute intoxication; with chronic exposure hair becomes dry and falls out.

Retinoids
Etretinate   Increased hair shedding and plucked telogen count; decreased duration of anagen phase.

Isotretinoin   Diffuse loss; probably same mechanism as above.

*a*Prepared by Suzanne Virnelli-Grevelink, M.D.

CBC   Rule out iron deficiency anemia.

Chemistry   Serum iron, iron-binding capacity.

TSH   Rule out thyroid disease.

Serology   Antinuclear antibodies, RPR (to rule out syphilis).

Histopathology   No abnormality other than an increase in the proportion of follicles in telogen.

DIAGNOSIS

Made on history, clinical findings, and trichogram, excluding other causes.

COURSE AND PROGNOSIS

Complete regrowth of hair is the rule. In postpartum telogen effluvium, if hair loss is severe and recurs after successive pregnancies, regrowth may never be complete. Telogen effluvium may continue for up to a year after the precipitating cause.

MANAGEMENT

No intervention is needed or required. The patient should be reassured that the process is part of a normal cycle of hair growth and shedding and that full regrowth of the hair is to be expected in most cases.

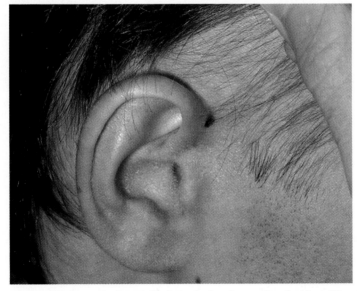

Figure 27-8 Telogen effluvium *A clump of hair in the hand, associated with striking thinning of scalp hair. The patient was HIV-infected and experienced* Pneumocystis carinii *pneumonia 10 weeks previously. Using the fingers as shown, 30 to 40 hairs could be removed with each "hair pull."*

Anagen Effluvium

In anagen effluvium, the pattern of hair loss follows that of telogen effluvium—it is diffuse and involves the entire scalp—but is usually more rapid in onset and far more pronounced. It results from a rapid growth arrest or damage to anagen hairs that skip catagen and telogen phases and are shed. In most cases, anagen effluvium is caused by drugs, intoxication, or chemotherapy (Fig. 27-9).

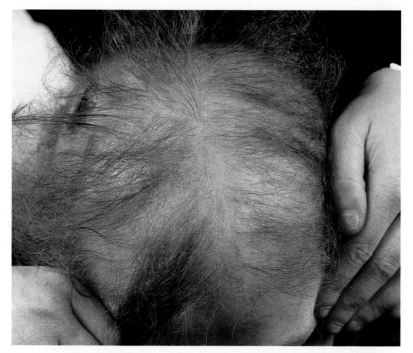

Figure 27-9 Anagen efluvium *Massive, diffuse hair loss of the scalp following initiation of cancer chemotherapy.*

SCARRING ALOPECIA

Scarring (cicatricial) alopecias result from damage or destruction of the hair follicles by inflammatory (infectious and noninfectious) or other pathologic processes, and healing occurs with scarring. A large number of dermatologic conditions, mostly inflammatory, that also occur on glabrous skin lead to cicatricial alopecia; these conditions are listed in Table 27-2, which has been restricted to conditions described elsewhere in this volume.

Practically all these bald (hairless) lesions are characterized by scarring and atrophy and complete loss of hair follicles. Skin lesions within or at the periphery of the alopecia may be characteristic for that given disease (e.g., chronic cutaneous lupus erythematosus or tinea capitis). Idiopathic conditions (where the etiology or pathogenesis is unknown) confined to nonglabrous skin also can result in scarring and cicatricial alopecia, and most of these are exceedingly rare. Five conditions are a little more common and are therefore described briefly here.

Pseudopelade of Brocq

This cicatricial alopecia is slowly progressive and may represent the end stage of other inflammatory follicular diseases, such as lichen planus (Fig. 27-10) or lupus erythematosus (Fig. 27-11). It does, however, occur as a primary noninflammatory scarring process without known cause. The scalp is usually smooth with atrophic or mildly scarred patches devoid of hair that may coalesce. Hair follicles are absent, but nonsuppurative inflammation may be present around persisting follicles in the periphery of the lesions. Several hairs are often seen emerging from a single orifice within the scarred area (Fig. 27-10).

Folliculitis Decalvans (Fig. 27-12) This condition is a circumscribed cicatricial alopecia on the scalp or beard area resulting from coalescing inflammation of hair follicles with pustulation that leads to crusting and atrophic or scarred areas devoid of hair.

Dissecting Perifolliculitis of the Scalp (Perifolliculitis Capitis Abscedens et Suffodiens)

Manifested by deep and superficial abscess formation and extensive scarring (Fig. 27-13). The disease is primarily not of bacterial etiology. Scarring leads to permanent alopecia.

Acne Keloidalis

Occurs most commonly in black men. Usually occurs on the nape of the neck, starting with a chronic papular or pustular eruption (Fig. 27-14) localized to the nape of the neck and occipital area and eventuating in hypertrophic keloidal scar formation.

Pseudofolliculitis Barbae

Because of the tight curls in beard of black men, hair often grows back into the skin, causing an inflammatory response, a pseudofolliculitis. *Staphylococcus aureus* secondary infection is common (Fig. 27-15).

Table 27-2 CLASSIFICATION OF CICATRICIAL ALOPECIAS

Developmental Defects and Hereditary Disorders
  Recessive X-linked ichthyosis
  Epidermal nevi
  Epidermolysis bullosa (GAREB)
  (recessive dystrophic type)
Infections
  Staphylococcus aureus
  Tinea capitis: follows kerion or favus
  Varicella zoster virus (VZV): follows
  severe herpes zoster
Neoplasms
  Basal cell carcinoma
  Squamous cell carcinoma
  Metastatic tumors
  Lymphomas
  Adnexal tumors
Physical/Chemical Agents
  Mechanical trauma (including factitial:
  trichotillomania)
  Burns
  Radiation
  Caustic agents
  Other chemicals/drugs

Dermatoses of Uncertain Origin and Clinical Syndromes
  Lupus erythematosus: chronic
  cutaneous
  Lichen planus
  Sarcoidosis
  Scleroderma/morphea
  Lichen sclerosus et atrophicus
  Necrobiosis lipoidica diabeticorum
  Dermatomyositis
  Cicatricial pemphigoid
  Follicular mucinosis
  Acne keloidalis/sycosis nuchae
  Pseudofolliculitis barbae
  Pseudopelade of Brocq
  Folliculitis decalvans
  Dissecting perifolliculitis of the scalp
  (perifolliculitis capitis abscedens et
  suffodiens)
  Amyloidosis

[1]Angela Wong and Ann E. Taylor, M.D. were responsible for the major portion of this précis.
[2]Associated virilization.

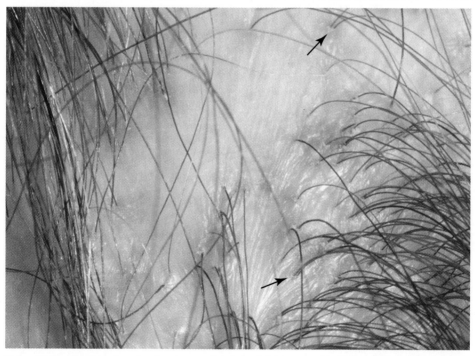

Figure 27-10 Scarring alopecia of scalp: pseudopelade of Brocq caused by lichen planus *The scalp is smooth, shiny, devoid of hair and hair follicles in many areas; some of the remaining follicles are inflamed with perifollicular erythema and scale. Several hairs are seen emerging from a single site within the area of alopecia (arrows).*

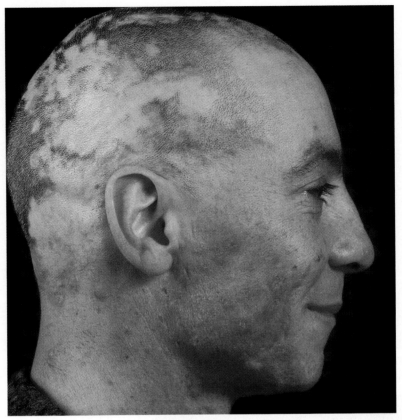

Figure 27-11 **Scarring alopecia of scalp and beard: chronic cutaneous lupus erythematosus** *Active inflammatory plaques and burned out lesions with white depressed scars and scarring alopecia on scalp. Similar findings are also present in the beard area.*

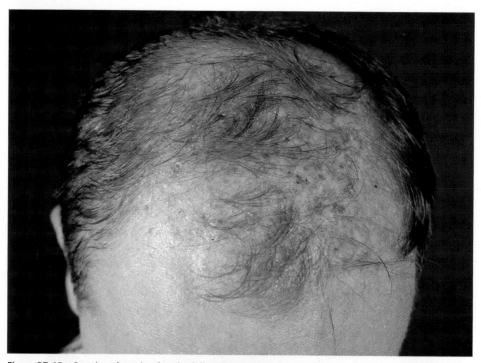

Figure 27-12 Scarring alopecia of scalp: folliculitis decalvans *Erythema, inflammatory papules, crusts, and scarring in a male who also has androgenetic alopecia.*

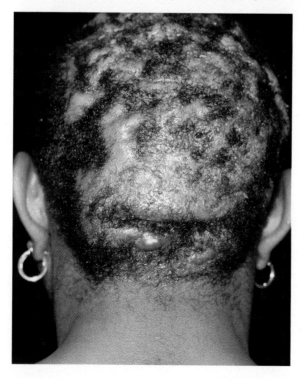

Figure 27-13 Scarring alopecia of scalp: dissecting perifolliculitis *Longstanding abscess formation of the scalp has resulted in very severe keloidal scarring. There was associated cystic acne and hidradenitis suppurativa. The scalp lesions were treated with surgical "scalping," split thickness skin grafts, and scalp reduction.*

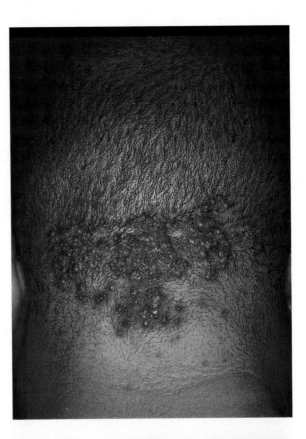

Figure 27-14 Scarring alopecia of scalp: follicular keloids *Papular scars, of 3 years' duration, becoming confluent on the occipital scalp of a black male. The condition is chronic and progressive, resulting in significant hair loss.*

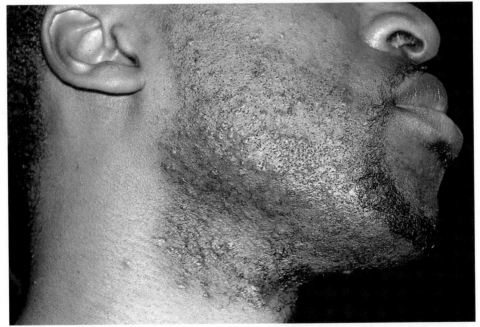

Figure 27-15 Pseudofolliculitis barbae *Multiple follicular papular scars in the beard area of a black male; the presence of follicular pustules usually is indicative of secondary* Staphylococcus aureus *folliculitis.*

HIRSUTISM[*]

Hirsutism is excessive hair growth in androgen-dependent hair patterns (i.e., face, chest, areolae, linea alba, lower back, buttocks, inner thighs, and external genitalia) secondary to increased androgenic activity.

EPIDEMIOLOGY

- Familial, ethnic, and racial influences
- Hirsuteness: white>black>Asian
- College survey of women showed that 25% had easily noticeable facial hair, 33% had hair along the linea alba below the umbilicus, and 17% had periareolar hair.
- Series of 100 patients: 15% idiopathic, 3% late-onset CAH (varies within ethnic group)

ETIOLOGY

Adrenal Causes

ACTH-dependent Cushing's syndrome
   Cushing's disease
   Ectopic ACTH production
Androgen-producing adrenal tumors
Congenital adrenal hyperplasia (CAH)
   Classic
   Late-onset

Ovarian Causes

Ovarian hyperthecosis
Ovarian neoplasms (only 1% of all ovarian tumors cause virilization)
Polycystic ovarian (PCO) syndrome
   Acne, alopecia, acanthosis nigricans, obesity, menorrhagia, oligomenorrhea, amenorrhea, infertility
Elevated LH levels, increased LH/FSH ratio
Insulin resistance/obesity (triggers excess ovarian androgen production)

Exogenous Medications

Androgens
Anabolic steroids
Birth control pills (uncommon with current low-dose oral contraceptives)

Hyperprolactinemia/Prolactinoma (Galactorrhea, Amenorrhea)

Gonadal Dysgenesis

Idiopathic

PATHOGENESIS

- Androgens promote conversion of vellus hairs to terminal hairs in androgen-sensitive hair follicles (pubis, axillae, back, face, chest, abdomen).
- 5α-Dihydrotestosterone, derived from conversion of testosterone by 5α-reductase at the hair follicle, is the hormonal stimulus for hair growth.
- 50 to 70% of circulating testosterone in normal women is derived from precursors, androstenedione, and DHEA; the rest is secreted directly, mostly by the ovaries. In hyperandrogenic women, a greater percentage of androgens may be secreted directly.
- In women, adrenal glands secrete androstenedione, DHEA, DHEA sulfate, and testosterone; ovaries secrete mainly androstenedione and testosterone.

HISTORY

- Virilization symptoms: androgenic alopecia, acne, deepened voice, increased muscle mass, clitoromegaly, increased libido, personality change
- Amenorrhea or changes in menstruation
- New-onset hypertension
- Family history
- Drug history
- Relatively recent or rapid onset of symptoms and signs *not* associated with puberty

[*]Drs. Angela Wang and Ann E. Taylor were responsible for the details of this precis.

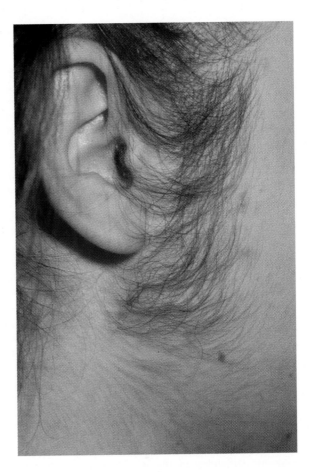

Figure 27-16   Hirsuitism: face of female   *Increased hair growth in androgen-dependent hair follicles of the beard area in a female, associated with androgen excess.*

PHYSICAL EXAMINATION

Careful documentation of the amount and all sites of hair is important in order to evaluate progression and therapy.

- Skin and hair changes: androgenic alopecia, acne, acanthosis nigricans, striae
- New growth of terminal hair (Fig. 27-16), especially on chest (Fig. 27-17), abdomen, upper back, shoulders
- Suspect Cushing's syndrome if centripetal obesity, muscle wasting (especially peripheral muscle weakness), and violaceous striae are found.
- If suspicious for polycystic ovary (PCO) syndrome, perform pelvic examination.
- Ferriman-Gallwey scale rates hair growth in each of 11 androgen-sensitive areas (upper lip, chin, chest, upper back, lower back, upper abdomen, lower abdomen, arm, forearm, thigh, leg) from 0 (no hair growth) to 4. Score of 8 or more is considered hirsutism.

LABORATORY EVALUATION

Urinary 17-ketosteroid measurement helpful in evaluating the overall amount of androgen secretion. (The results should be checked against age-appropriate normal levels; peak levels occur at age 30, and there is a significant decline with age thereafter.)

- If menstrual dysfunction (oligomenorrhea or amenorrhea): minimal evaluation: prolactin, FSH, and total testosterone.
- If (+) virilization:
     Serum testosterone: 200 ng/dL in women with ovarian or adrenal tumor
     Urinary 17-ketosteroids: elevated adrenal androgens.
     Serum DHEA sulfate: most specific to adrenals (>90% arising in adrenals); if >800 μg/d, suggestive of adrenal tumor.
- If CAH (late onset) is suspected: refer patient to endocrinologist.
- If Cushing's syndrome is suspected: refer patient to endocrinologist.
- If tumor suspicion is high: refer patient to endocrinologist.

MANAGEMENT

Cosmetic   Shaving, waxing, electrolysis, hydrogen peroxide bleaching. Removal with laser, effective and the best method.

Systemic Antiandrogen Therapy   *Cyproterone Acetate (CPA)*   Potent progestogen (not available in the United States). Both antiandrogen and inhibitor of secretion of gonadotropin. Decreases androgen production. Increases testosterone clearance. Decreases 5α-reductase activity. Administered with cyclical estrogens to maintain regular menstruation.

Regimen: 50 to 100 mg CPA for 10 days per cycle.
Side effects: weight gain, fatigue, loss of libido, mastodynia, nausea, H/A, depression.
Contraindications: smoking, obesity, hypertension.

Spironolactone   An antihypertensive diuretic. Decreases testosterone biosynthesis. Binds to androgen receptor. Decreases 5α-reductase activity.
Regimen: begin at 50 mg bid from day 4 through day 22 of each menstrual cycle; dose can be given as high as 100 mg bid.

Cimetidine   Histamine-2 receptor antagonist; competes for target tissue binding with androgens; less effective than spironolactone.

Glucocorticoid   First-line therapy for classic CAH. *Regimen:* 1 mg dexamethasone qhs. For late-onset, nonclassic CAH, use antiandrogens or oral contraceptives.

Oral Contraceptives   Suppress ovarian and adrenal androgen production by decreasing LH and FSH. Recommend an oral contraceptive with the lowest tolerable dose of ethinyl estradiol (30 to 35 μg) and a low dose of a progestin with low androgenic potential (less than 1 mg of norethindrone, norgestimate, desogestrel, ethynodiol diacetate).

Avoid levonorgestrel, norgestrel, and high doses of norethindrone acetate.

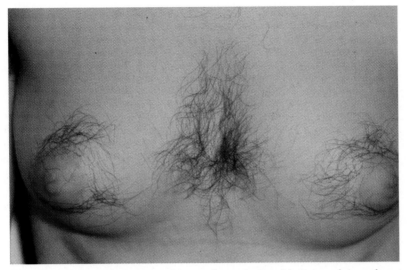

Figure 27-17 Hirsuitism: chest of female *Increased constitutional hair growth in androgen-dependent hair follicles of the presternal and periareolar regions in a female. In this case, no androgen excess was detected, the finding occurring in other female relatives. Removal of these black hairs can be done with a laser.*

HYPERTRICHOSIS

Hypertrichosis is excessive hair growth also in areas that are not androgen-sensitive.

Drug-Induced Hypertrichosis

HISTORY/PHYSICAL EXAMINATION

Uniform growth of fine hair in a pattern unrelated to androgen sensitivity.

Drugs

Diphenylhydantoin: after 2 to 3 months of treatment, affects extensor regions of limbs, face, trunk; clears by 1 year of drug cessation
Diazoxide: cosmetic problem in 50%
Minoxidil
Cyclosporine: affects over 80% (Fig. 27-18)
Benoxaprofen: after a few weeks of treatment, fine downy hair on face and exposed extremities
Streptomycin
Oral glucocorticoids: forehead, temples, cheeks; sometimes back and extensor aspects of limbs
Penicillamine: lengthening and coarsening of hair on trunk and limbs
Psoralens: transient hypertrichosis of light-exposed areas

Other Conditions Associated with Hypertrichosis

Porphyria (variegate, cutanea tarda, congenital erythropoietic porphyria)
Epidermolysis bullosa
Hurler's syndrome and other mucopolysaccharidoses
Cornelia de Lange syndrome
Trisomy 18
Post-shock/head injuries
Fetal alcohol syndrome
Dermatomyositis
Malnutrition
Anorexia nervosa
At sites of trauma/scar/occupation-related sites of irritation

Hypertrichosis Lanuginosa

In *congenital hypertrichosis lanuginosa,* vellus and terminal hairs do not replace white, blond fetal pelage; fetal pelage grows excessively and may be >10 cm long. In *acquired hypertrichosis lanuginosa,* there is a production of lanugo hair in follicles previously producing vellus hair.

EPIDEMIOLOGY

Usually harbinger of malignancy; of all cases of acquired hypertrichosis lanuginosa reported, 98% had malignancy of the gastrointestinal tract, bronchus, breast, gallbladder, uterus, or bladder. Hypertrichosis can precede a neoplastic diagnosis by several years.

PHYSICAL EXAMINATION

- Hair may be >10 cm in length in nonscalp areas.
- Can involve entire body, except for palms and soles.
- Fine, downy hair covers large areas of the body.
- In mild types, downy hair is limited to the face; hair on previously hairless areas such as the nose and eyelids is usually noticed first.
- Scalp, beard, and pubic hair may not be replaced.

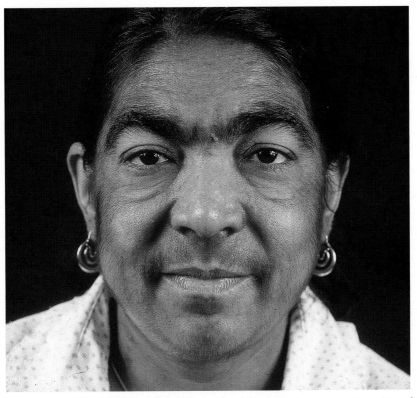

Figure 27-18   Hypertrichosis of face   *Excessive hair grow in nonandrogen-sensitive areas of the face in a female treated with cyclosporine.*

DISORDERS OF THE NAIL APPARATUS

NORMAL NAIL APPARATUS

The nail apparatus, composed of the nail plate and surrounding soft tissue structures, adds function, especially fingernails, and protects the terminal digits. Nail apparatus disorders can be primary, manifestations of cutaneous disease (e.g., psoriasis), manifestations of systemic diseases (e.g., lupus erythematosus), traumatic or structural, or infectious.

Components of the Nail Apparatus (Fig. 28-1)

Nail Plate   The hard protective tool, the product of the nail apparatus. Rests on and firmly attached to nail bed, which is attached to underlying bone. Surrounded on three sides by nail folds. Made of three horizontal layers: thin dorsal lamina, thicker intermediate lamina, ventral layer from nail bed. Hardness of nail plate due to high sulfur matrix protein. Nail plate shape relates to shape of underlying phalangeal bone.

Proximal Nail Fold   Covers proximal one-quarter of the nail plate. Has two epithelial surfaces, dorsal and ventral. Devoid of dermatoglyphic markings and sebaceous glands.

Cuticle   Junction of two epithelial surfaces of proximal nail fold, projects distally onto nail surface, sealing proximal nail fold and nail: Protects structures at base of nail (germinative matrix) from irritants, allergens, bacterial/fungal pathogens. Loss of cuticle produces potential space or pocket: infection of this pocket results in chronic paronychia.

Lateral Folds   Usually cover lateral edges of plate.

Lunula   Underlies proximal fold. Normally is white. Represents most distal region of the matrix.

Free Margin   Distal nail. Natural shape same as contour of distal lunula.

Nail Matrix   Proximal matrix underlies nail plate to distal border of lunula. Distal matrix is that portion distal to distal border of lunula. Produces the major part of nail plate. As in epidermis, possesses a dividing basal cell layer producing keratinocytes, which differentiate, harden, die, and contribute to nail plate—analogous to epidermal stratum corneum. Keratinocytes mature and keratinize without keratohyalin (granular layer) formation. Melanocytes are present in lower layers and produce melanin. Linear longitudinal pigmented bands may be seen in black-skinned individuals.

Nail Bed   Consists of epidermal part (ventral matrix) (no more than two to three cells thick) and underlying dermis closely aposed to periosteum of distal phalanx. Within connective tissue network lie blood vessels, lymphatics, a fine network of elastic fibers, and scattered fat cells. Subcutaneous fat layer is absent. Normally pink due to vasculature as seen through the translucent nail plate.

Hyponychium   Space under free margin of nail plate, from point of separation of nail plate from nail bed to the distal end of the nail plate.

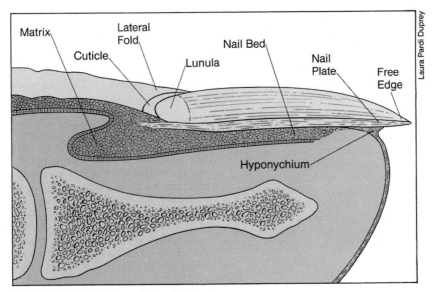

Figure 28-1   Schematic drawing of normal nail.

CUTANEOUS NAIL DISORDERS

Onycholysis Detachment of nail from its bed at distal and/or lateral attachments (Fig. 28-2). Onycholysis creates a subungual space that collects dirt and keratinous debris; grayish-white color due to presence of air under nail, but color varies from yellow to brown; area may be malodorous. In psoriasis, yellowish-brown margin is visible between pink normal nail and white separated areas. In "oil spot" or "salmon-patch" variety, nail plate–nail bed separation may start in middle of nail. *Pseudomonas aeruginosa* growing on undersurface of onycholytic nail gives a greenish discoloration. Etiologies: idiopathic; systemic (e.g., thyrotoxicosis); congenital/hereditary; cutaneous diseases (e.g., psoriasis, drug-induced photo-onycholysis); local causes (e.g., trauma, onychomycosis, chemicals).

Onychogryphosis Hypertrophy of nail plate and subungual hyperkeratosis (Fig. 28-3). Mainly seen on the great toe nails of elderly. Probably due to trauma, footwear pressure, poor peripheral circulation.

Central Longitudinal Grooved Dystrophy *Onychodystrophia mediana canaliformis.* Washboard nail plate (Fig. 28-4). Caused by chronic, mechanical injury. Cuticle is pushed back with inflammation ± thickening of proximal nail fold. Occurs most commonly on thumbnail(s), as compulsive disorders (tic habit), caused by the index finger repeatedly picking at cuticle of thumbnail.

Myxoid Pseudocysts (See Benign Neoplasms and Hyperplasias, Section 7.)

Psoriasis Most common dermatosis affecting the nail apparatus. Up to 50% of persons with psoriasis have nail involvement at one point in time; lifetime involvement up to 80 to 90%. Findings in the nail plate include: nail pits (tiny, fairly uniform, punctate surface depressions), transverse furrows, crumbling nail plate, punctate leukonychia, roughened nails (trachyonychia) (Fig. 28-5). Findings in the nail bed and hyponychium include: "oil spot," distal onycholysis, distal subungual hyperkeratosis, splinter hemorrhages, false nail following onychomadesis (spontaneous separation of nail plate from matrix area), *Pseudomonas* colo-

nization of the under surface of onycholytic nail plate causing green discoloration.

Lichen Planus Nail involvement occurs in 10% of individuals with disseminated lichen planus, but may be the only manifestation. Matrix involvement results in thinning, onychorrhexis, brittleness, crumbling or fragmentation, accentuation of surface longitudinal ridging, melanonychia, or leukonychia (Fig. 28-6). Severe chronic inflammation results in loss of nail plate, either partial or complete; pterygium formation occurs with partial loss of the central nail plate, which presents as a distal notch or entire split nail. Nail bed involvement results in onycholysis, distal subungual hyperkeratosis, bulla formation, permanent anonychia. One, several, or all 20 nails may be involved (twenty nail syndrome, where there is loss of all 20 nails without any other evidence of lichen planus elsewhere on the body). Similar changes are seen in lichenoid graft-versus-host disease.

Squamous Cell Carcinoma Squamous cell carcinoma (SCC) in situ (SCCIS) occurring periungually is usually caused by the oncogenic human papillomavirus (HPV) types 16 and 18. Lesions are skin-colored or hyperpigmented, keratotic, hyperkeratotic, or warty papules and plaques that arise on the proximal and lateral nails folds as well as the hyponychium (Fig. 28-7). SCCIS, in time, may extend to the nail bed, causing onycholysis. Invasive SCC arises within SCCIS, presenting with pain if periosteal invasion has occurred. Lesions are much more common on fingers (thumb and index finger most often) than toes. A solitary lesion is most common, but multiple fingers may be involved in the immunocompromised host. Lesions are best treated with CO_2 laser ablation, Mohs' surgery, or amputation of digit for more deeply invasive lesions.

Nail Matrix Nevomelanocytic Nevus May be congenital or acquired, presenting as a subungual longitudinal melanonychia (LM) (Fig. 28-8). The differential diagnosis of LM includes focal activation of nail matrix (e.g., trauma), hyperplasia of nail matrix melanocytes, nevome-

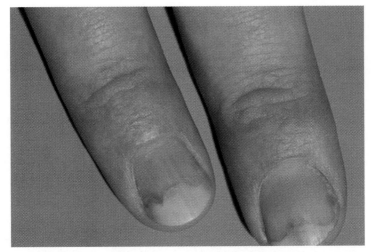

Figure 28-2 Onycholysis *The distal nail bed is separated from the nail plate in two nails. In this case, the distal nail bed has a pink-tan color, a so-called "oil-stain," which is indicative of psoriasis. In onycholysis associated with psoriasis, the subungual space may or may not be filled with hyperkeratotic debris.*

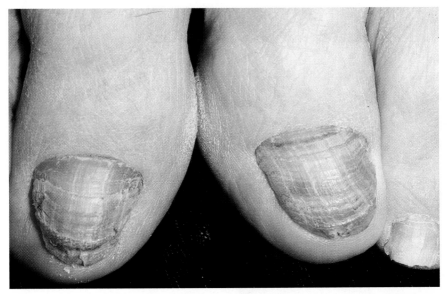

Figure 28-3 Onychogryphosis *The nail plate of both great toes is greatly thickened. In some cases, usually associated with trauma, onycholysis occurs. The nails grow very slowly, requiring clipping infrequently. Pressure on the nail bed may compromise the circulation of those with reduced arterial blood flow.*

lanocytic nevus, drug-induced [e.g., zidovudine (AZT)], or melanoma of nail matrix. Matrix nevi are usually junctional.

Acrolentiginous Melanoma (ALM) Arises subungually or periungually, presenting with pigmentation and/or nail plate dystrophy (Fig. 28-9). Matrix lesions usually present as ALM in whites or broadening of an existing ALM in blacks. ALM after puberty in whites require biopsy. ALM accounts for 2 to 3% of melanomas in whites and 15 to 20% in blacks. Most common sites: thumbs, great toes. Mean age: 55 to 60 years. Usually asymptomatic. Most patients notice pigmented lesion, especially after trauma. Hutchinson's sign: periungual extension of brown-black pigmentation from ALM onto proximal and lateral nail folds (Fig. 28-9). 25% of ALM may be amelanotic (pigmentation not obvious or prominent). For lesions within ventral portion of nail plate, a punch biopsy can be obtained if ALM is <3 mm; a transverse matrix biopsy, if ALM is >3 mm. Nail apparatus melanoma has a poor prognosis: 5-year survival rates from 35 to 50%.

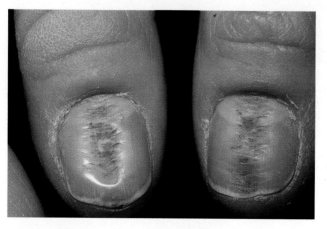

Figure 28-4   Central longitudinal grooved dystrophy *A central groove is seen in the thumbnails bilaterally. The patient had picked at the proximal nail fold with the index fingernail of the same hand as a compulsive habit for many years. Once aware of the cause of the nail dystrophy, the patient stopped picking and both nails grew normally.*

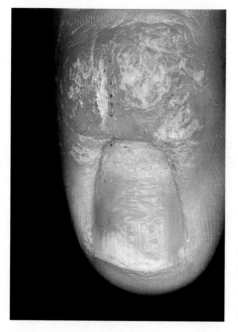

Figure 28-5   Psoriasis vulgaris *All nail changes associated with psoriasis are seen in this finger. A psoriatic plaque is present on the periungual skin. The adjacent nail matrix is involved with transverse ridging and pits. There is distal onycholysis. "Oil staining" of the adjacent distal nail bed is present.*

DISORDERS OF THE NAIL APPARATUS

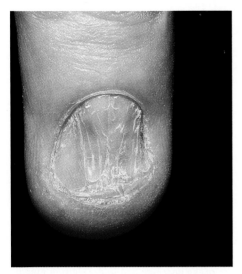

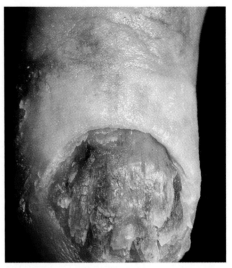

Figure 28-6 Lichen planus *The nail bed is inflamed, affecting the matrix with resultant thinning of the nail plate and longitudinal ridging. Two other fingernails were similarly involved. Untreated, the matrix can be destroyed with pterygium formation where the skin of the cuticle grows over and merges with the thinned nail plate. Typically, the area of the lunula is more elevated than the more distal portion. Typical lichen planus was present on the buccal mucosa. All findings resolved with triamcinolone injection into the proximal nail fold.*

Figure 28-7 HPV-induced in situ and invasive squamous cell carcinoma *A 32-year-old HIV-infected male presented with severe pain of the left index finger. The nail folds are verrucous. The nail plate is absent. The nail bed is markedly hyperkeratotic. All ten fingers had similar periungual findings. Biopsy of the nail bed showed invasive SCC involving the periostium. The finger was amputated. The HPV infections of the hands were associated with SCCIS of the perineum and anus.*

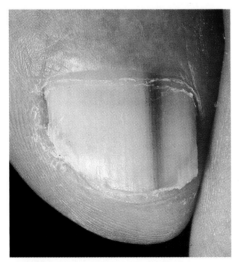

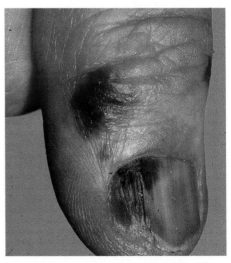

Figure 28-8 Junctional nevomelanocytic nevus of the nail matrix *A junctional nevus is present in the nail matrix resulting in a longitudinal brown stripe in the nail bed.*

Figure 28-9 Acrolentiginous melanoma *The melanoma arose in the nail matrix of the thumb with resultant nail plate dystrophy, subungual melanosis, and extension into the proximal nail fold and beyond it (Hutchinson's sign).*

INFECTIONS OF THE NAIL APPARATUS

Dermatophytes are the most common pathogens infecting the nail apparatus. *Staphylococcus aureus* and group A streptococcus cause soft tissue infection of the nail fold. *Candida* and *S. aureus* can cause secondary infection of chronic paronychia. Recurrent herpes simplex virus infection.

Acute Paronychia Inflammation of the nail fold produces erythema, swelling, and throbbing pain (Fig. 28-10) and may extend into the proximal nail fold and eponychium.

Felon A subcutaneous infection of the pulp space of the distal phalanx of a digit (Fig. 28-11); considered a closed space infection of the multiple compartments created by fibrous septa passing between the skin and the periosteum. History of a penetrating injury. The course may be rapid and severe. Contained by the unyielding skin of the fingertip, the infection creates tension with microvascular compromise, necrosis, and abscess formation. The abscess may break in the center of the pulp space and decompress spontaneously, with slough of necrotic skin over the pulp space. May be complicated by osteitis, osteomyelitis of the distal phalanx, sequestration of the diaphysis of the phalanx. Rupture into the distal interphalangeal joint with septic arthritis can occur, or extension into the distal end of the flexor tendon sheath, producing tenosynovitis.

Pseudomonas on Onycholytic Nail Plate *Pseudomonas aeruginosa* does not infect the nail apparatus but can grow on the undersurface of an onycholytic nail as well as in the nail of chronic paronychia, presenting as a greenish discoloration of the nail plate (Fig. 28-12). Management includes debridement of the onycholytic nail and treatment of the underlying cause of onycholysis (e.g., psoriasis) or paronychia.

Candidiasis *Candida albicans* infections of the nail unit occur most often on fingers, most commonly as secondary infection of chronic paronychia. *Candida* can cause distal and lateral onycholysis, especially in diabetics (Fig. 28-13). Invasion of the nail plate usually occurs only in immunocompromised indviduals, i.e., chronic mucocutaneous candidiasis (CMC) or HIV disease. In CMC, many or all nails become thick (nail plate and subungual hyperkeratosis) (i.e., total nail dystrophy associated with periungual inflammation and hyperkeratosis.

Chronic Paronychia An inflammatory disorder of the proximal nail fold occurring in individuals whose hands are in a wet environment. Repeated minor trauma damages cuticle, allowing irritants to further damage the nail fold. In children, chronic paronychia occurs as a result of thumb sucking. During the course of chronic paronychia, proximal and lateral nail folds show erythema and edema; cuticle is lost and ventral portion of proximal nail fold separates from nail plate. Microorganisms, especially *C. albicans* infect this newly formed space. In time, the nail fold retracts and becomes thickened and rounded. Chronic paronychia is interspersed with self-limiting episodes of painful acute inflammation, which is often due to *Candida* or *S. aureus* infection of the space between proximal nail fold and nail plate. Pus may drain from this fold (Fig. 28-13). In time, one or both lateral edges of nail plate develops irregularities and yellow, brown, or blackish discoloration; eventually the entire nail plate becomes involved with numerous transverse grooves. *Pseudomonas* may colonize the dystrophic nail plate, causing a greenish discoloration. Chronic paronychia responds to removal or protection of the nail apparatus from chronic irritation, topical application of triamcinolone/clotrimazole cream to the nail folds and into the pocket, and weekly doses of 100 to 200 mg fluconazole until the normal anatomy has been restored.

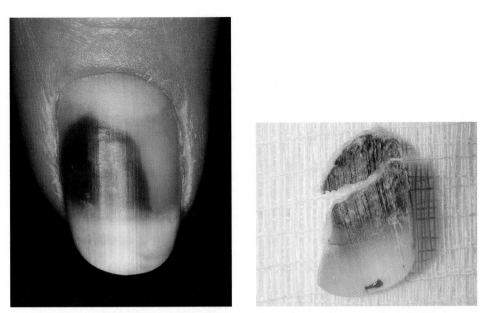

Figure 28-10 Acute paronychia *The nail fold is erythematous, edematous, with early abscess formation, and is very painful. (left)* Staphylococcus aureus *was isolated on culture from dislodged nail (right).*

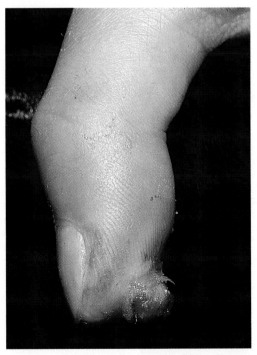

Figure 28-11 Felon *A puncture wound of the fingertip resulted in formation of a pyogenic granuloma and* Staphylococcus aureus *infection of the subcutaneous tissue of the distal phalanx; early abscess formation is seen.*

INFECTIONS OF THE NAIL APPARATUS

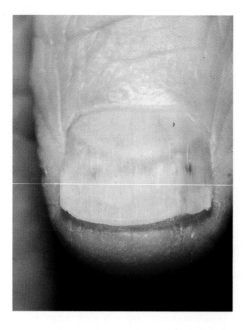

Figure 28-12 *Pseudomonas* **colonization of onycholytic nail plate** *Psoriasis has resulted in distal onycholysis of the thumbnail. The nail plate has a dark green discoloration of the onycholytic portion. After debridement of the onycholytic nail, the undersurface of the nail plate is discolored. This is not a pseudomonal infection but rather colonization of a moist surface. The onycholysis resolved following the debridement and treatment of the nail bed with corticosteroid cream.*

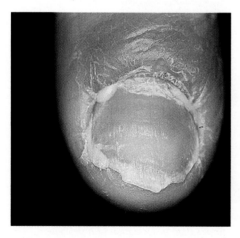

Figure 28-13 **Chronic paronychia** *The paronychial tissue is erythematous and edematous; on probing, a "pocket" has formed following separation of the undersurface of the proximal nail fold and the proximal dorsal nail plate draining pus. The multiple transverse ridges on the dorsal nail plate are the result of recurrent acute episodes of* Candida *infection of the "pocket." The paronychia resolved with weekly dosing of fluconazole (150 mg) and a topical preparation containing clotrimazole and triamcinolone.*

ONYCHOMYCOSIS

Onychomycosis is a chronic progressive infection of the nail apparatus, caused by dermatophytes most commonly, and less often by *Candida* sp. and molds. Tinea unguium refers to onychomycosis caused by the dermatophytes. *Trichophyton rubrum* has been imported into industrialized nations during the last century, resulting in an epidemic of onychomycosis, tinea pedis, and other types of epidermal onychomycosis. In addition to appearance, onychomycosis of toenails can cause pain, predispose to secondary bacterial infections, and ulcerations of underling nail bed. These complications occur more commonly in the growing population of immunocompromised individuals and diabetics.

CLASSIFICATION BY THE ANATOMIC SITE INVOLVED

Distal and Lateral Subungual Onychomycosis (DLSO) (Fig. 28-14) Most common type of onychomycosis. Nearly always caused by dermatophytes. Infection begins in stratum corneum of hyponychial area or nail fold, extending subungually, and progressively involves the nail centripetally and medially. May be either primary, i.e., involving a healthy nail, or secondary (e.g., psoriasis). Characterized by onycholysis, subungual hyperkeratosis, and yellow-brown discoloration of nail plate. Usually associated with tinea pedis.

Superficial White Onychomycosis (SWO) Pathogen invades surface of dorsal nail plate (Fig. 28-15). Mainly caused by *T. mentagrophytes* or *T. rubrum* (children). Much less commonly, mold: *Acremonium, Fusarium, Aspergillus terreus.*

Proximal Subungual Onychomycosis (PSO) Pathogen enters by way of the posterior nail fold–cuticle area and then migrates along the proximal nail groove to involve the underlying matrix, proximal to the nail bed, and finally the underlying nail plate (Fig. 28-16). Caused by *T. rubrum.* Characterized by leukonychia that extends distally from under proximal nail fold. Usually 1 or 2 nails involved. Always associated with immunocompromise.

***Candida* Onychomycosis** Three types: (1) *Candida* paronychia: primarily caused by *C. albicans;* chronic candidal paronychia : characterized by erythema and swelling of proximal and lateral nail folds with secondary involvement of nail plate. (2) DLSO: occurs in setting of onycholysis. (3) Total nail dystrophy (Fig. 28-17): usually with chronic mucocutaneous candidiasis (CMC) with many or all nails involved. Organism directly invades nail plate and proximal/lateral nail folds become thick until nail apparatus is totally dystrophic. May also occur in HIV disease with single nail involved.

EPIDEMIOLOGY

Age of Onset Children or adults. Once acquired, usually does not remit spontaneously. Therefore, the incidence increases with advancing age. 1% of individuals younger than 18 years affected; almost 50% of those older than 70 years affected.

Sex *Tinea Unguium* Somewhat more common in men.

Etiology *Dermatophytes* >95 to 97% caused by *T. rubrum* and *T. mentagrophytes.* Much less common causes are *Epidermophyton floccosum, T. violaceum, T. schoenleinii, T. verrucosum* (usually infects only fingernails).

Yeasts 2%, most commonly *Candida albicans.*

Molds Rarely, primary pathogens in onychomycosis, but rather secondarily colonize already dystrophic nails/nail apparatus. *Acremonium, Fusarium,* and *Aspergillus* spp. can rarely cause SWO. Dermatosis such as psoriasis, which results in onycholysis and subungual hyperkeratosis, or dermatophytic onychomycosis, can be secondarily infected by molds. More than 40 mold species have been reported to be isolated from dystrophic nails, including *Scopulariopsis brevicaulis, Aspergillus* spp., *Alternaria* sp., *Acremonium* spp., *Fusarium* spp., *Scytalidium dimidiatum (Hendersonula toruloidea), S. hyalinum.*

Etiology of Anatomic Types of Onychomycosis DLSO: most commonly, *T. rubrum, T. mentagrophytes.* PSO: most commonly, *T. rubrum.* SWO: most commonly, *T. mentagrophytes.*

Geographic Distribution Worldwide. The etiologic agent varies in different geographic areas. More common in urban than in rural areas (associated with wearing occlusive footwear).

Prevalence Incidence varies in different geographic regions. In the United States and Europe, up to 10% of adult population affected (related to occlusive footwear). In developing nations where open footwear is worn, onychomycosis uncommon.

Candida Onychomycosis More common in women.

Transmission *Dermatophytes* Anthropophilic dermatophyte infections are transmitted from one individual to another, by fomite or direct contact, commonly among family members. Some spore forms (arthroconidia) remain viable and infective in the environment for up to 5 years.

Candida Part of the normal flora, which usually causes infection if the local ecology is changed in favor of the yeast or associated with altered immune status.

Molds These organisms are ubiquitous in the environment and are not transmitted between humans.

Risk Factors Atopics are at increased risk for *T. rubrum* infections. Diabetes mellitus, treatment with immunosuppressive drugs, HIV disease. For toenail onychomycosis, the most important factor is wearing of occlusive footwear.

PATHOGENESIS

Primary Onychomycosis Invasion occurs in an otherwise healthy nail. The probability of nail invasion by fungi increases with defective vascular supply (i.e., with increasing age, CVI, peripheral arterial disease), in posttraumatic states (lower leg fractures), or disturbance of innervation (e.g., injury to brachial plexus, trauma of spine).

Secondary Onychomycosis Infection occurs in an already altered nail, such as psoriatic or traumatized nail. Toenail onychomycosis usually occurs after tinea pedis; fingernail involvement is usually secondary to tinea manuum, tinea corporis, or tinea capitis. Infection of the first and fifth toenails probably occurs secondary to damage to these nails by footwear.

DLSO (Fig. 28-14) The nail bed produces soft keratin stimulated by fungal infection that accumulates under the nail plate, thereby raising it, a change that clinically gives the involved nail an altered cream color rather than the normal transparent appearance. The dense keratin of the nail plate is not involved primarily. The accumulated subungual keratin promotes further fungal growth and keratin production. The nail matrix is usually not invaded, and production of normal nail plate remains unimpaired despite fungal infection. In time, dermatophytes create air-containing tunnels within the nail plate; where the network is sufficiently dense, the nail is opaque. Often the invasion follows the longitudinal ridges of the nail bed. The subungual location of the infection could block effective topical antifungal agents.

HISTORY

PSO Previously a rare pattern, it occurs commonly on toenails in persons with HIV disease or other immunocompromised states.

Candidal Onychia and Paronychia History of frequent immersion in water is common. Occurs more commonly on the dominant hand, especially on the first and third fingers; infection of toenails uncommon. In comparison with other types of onychomycosis, *Candida* paronychia is intermittently painful and tender. Candidal onychia and paronychia are common in children with HIV disease and are usually associated with mucosal candidiasis.

Chronic Mucocutaneous Candidiasis (CMC) In patients with CMC with multiple endocrine gland failure, candidiasis at mucosal sites and paronychia occur in childhood followed by endocrinopathies, with hypoparathyroidism presenting first. CMC is associated with thymomas, myasthenia gravis, myositis, aplastic anemia, neutropenia, and hypogammaglobulinemia; onset is usually in adulthood.

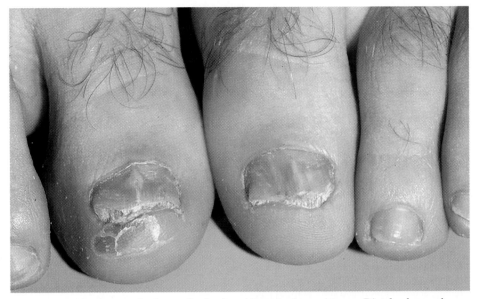

Figure 28-14 Onychomycosis of toenails: distal and lateral subungual type *Distal subungual hyperkeratosis and onycholysis involving most of the nail bed of the great toenails; these findings are usually associated with tinea pedis.*

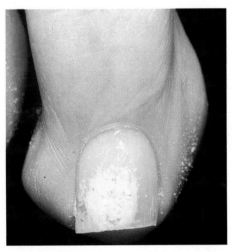

Figure 28-15 Onychomycosis of toenails: superficial white type *The dorsal nail plate is chalky white. White nail dystrophy can easily be treated by curettage; KOH preparation of the curetting shows hyphae.*

CLINICAL FINDINGS

Skin Findings Approximately 80% of onychomycosis occurs on the feet, especially on the big toes; simultaneous occurrence on toe- and fingernails is not common.

DLSO A white patch is noted on the distal or lateral undersurface of the nail and nail bed, usually with sharply demarcated borders. In time, the whitish color can become discolored to a brown or black hue. Progressive involvement of the nail can occur in a matter of weeks, as in HIV disease, or more slowly over a period

of months or years. With progressive infection, the nail becomes opaque, thickened cracked, friable, raised by underlying hyperkeratotic debris in the nail bed (Fig. 28-14). Sharply marginated white streaks beginning at the distal nail margin and extending proximal are filled with keratinaceous debris and air. DLSO caused by dermatophytes or mold is indistinguishable on clinical findings. Toenails are involved much more commonly than fingernails. The first and fifth toenails are infected most frequently. Involvement of the fingernails is usually unilateral. When fingernails are involved, pattern is usually two feet and one hand.

SWO   A white chalky plaque is seen on the proximal nail plate, which may become eroded with loss of the nail plate (Fig. 28-15). Diagnostically, the involved nail can be removed easily with a curette in comparison with a traumatized nail, which has white, air-containing areas. In some cases, the entire superficial nail plate may become involved. SWO may coexist with DLSO. Occurs almost exclusively on the toenails, rarely on the fingernails.

PSO (Fig. 28-16)   A white spot appears from beneath the proximal nail fold. In time the white spot fills the lunula, eventually moving distally to involve much of the undersurface of the nail plate. Patients treated with oral azoles show interruption of the involved nail. Occurs more commonly on the toenails.

Candidal Onychomycosis Candida paronychia: Begins with a proximal and later lateral paronychia, which appears clinically as edema, erythema, and pain of the nail fold; at times pus can be expressed (Fig. 28-13). Secondary to paronychial infection, nail plate becomes dystrophic with areas of opacification, white, yellow, green, or black discoloration, with transverse furrowing Fig. 28-17). *Pressure on the nail is often painful*. About 70% of cases occur on the fingernails, most commonly the middle finger. Uncommon presentation:subungual abscess. DLSO: occurs in setting of onycholysis; see DLSO above. Total nail dystrophy: Proximal/lateral nail folds become thick until nail apparatus is totally dystrophic (Fig. 28-17). In HIV disease, solitary nails may be involved. In CMC, 20 nails may be involved in time.

General Findings   In patients with CMC, oropharyngeal and vulvovaginal candidiasis is often present. In those with CMC and endocrinopathy, vitiligo and alopecia areata also may be present, as well as polyglandular failure (hypoparathyroidism, hypoadrenalism, hypothyroidism, and diabetes mellitus).

DIFFERENTIAL DIAGNOSIS

Paronychial Disease   *Candida* paronychia, herpetic whitlow, eczematous dermatitis, allergic contact dermatitis, lichen planus.

DLSO   Psoriatic involvement of the nails ("oil drop" staining of the distal nail bed and nail pits are seen in psoriasis but not onychomycosis), paronychial involvement of eczema, Reiter's syndrome and keratoderma blennorrhagicum, onychogryphosis, pincer nails, congenital nail dystrophies, pseudomonal nail infection (black-green discoloration).

SWO   Traumatic injury to nail, psoriasis with leukonychia.

LABORATORY EXAMINATIONS

All clinical diagnoses of onychomycosis should be confirmed by laboratory testing. (See Dermatophytoses, Section 21.)

Nail Samples   For DLSO: distal portion of involved nail bed. SWO: involved nail surface. PSO: punch biopsy through nail plate to involved nail bed.

Direct Microscopy   Direct microscopic examination of nail samples is used to confirm the clinical diagnosis. Keratinaceous material from the involved nail scrapings is placed on a glass slide, covered with a glass coverslip, suspended in a solution of potassium hydroxide (KOH), and gently heated. Addition of dimethyl sulfoxide and/or Parker Quink ink to the KOH solution may facilitate identification of fungal elements. Specific identification of the pathogen is usually not possible by microscopy but, in most cases, yeasts can be differentiated from dermatophytes by morphology.

Fungal Culture   Isolation of the pathogen permits better use of oral antifungal agents. Samples of the infected nail are inoculated onto Sabouraud's agar with or without cyclohexaimide.

Histology of Nail Clipping   Indicated if clinical findings suggest onychomycosis even after three KOH wet mounts and three cultures performed at weekly intervals have not detected pathogen. PAS stain is used to detect fungal elements in the nail. Probably the most reliable technique for diagnosing onychomycosis.

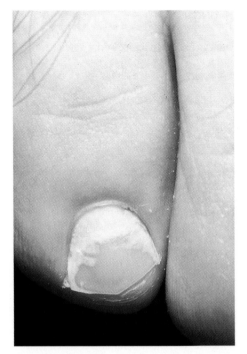

Figure 28-16 Tinea unguium: proximal subungual onychomycosis type *The proximal nail plate is a chalky white color due to invasion from the undersurface of the nail matrix. The patient had advanced HIV disease.*

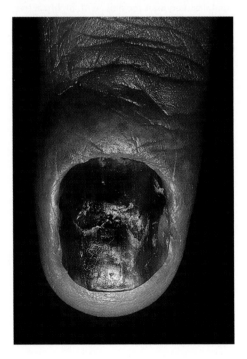

Figure 28-17 *Candida* onychomycosis: total dystrophic type *The entire fingernail plate is thickened and dystrophic and is associated with a paronychial infection; both findings were caused by* C. albicans *in an individual with advanced HIV disease.*

DIAGNOSIS

Clinical findings confirmed by finding fungal forms in KOH preparation and/or isolation of pathogenic fungus on culture.

COURSE AND PROGNOSIS

Without effective therapy, onychomycosis does not resolve spontaneously; progressive involvement of multiple toenails is the rule. DLSO persists after topical treatment of tinea pedis and often results in repeated episodes of epidermal dermatophytosis of feet, groin, and other sites. Tinea pedis and/or DLSO provide portal of entry for recurrent bacterial infections (*S. aureus,* group A streptococcus), especially cellulitis of lower leg after venous harvesting. Prevalence in diabetics estimated to be 33%; DLSO contributes to severity of foot problems: superficial bacterial infection, ulceration, cellulitis, osteomyelitis, necrosis, amputation. *Diabetics need early intervention and should be screened regularly by a dermatologist.* Untreated HIV disease is associated with an increased prevalence of dermatophytoses; PSO, DLSO, and SWO may occur in the small nail, leading to rapid destruction of the nail. With highly active antiretroviral therapy (HAART), dermatophytic infections may not be more common than in the non-HIV-infected population.

Long-term relapse rate with newer oral agents such as terbinafine or itraconazole reported to be 15 to 21% two years after successful therapy; long-term follow-up studies not yet reported. Causes of relapse/reinfection uncertain: reinfection, immunologic incompetence, persistent trauma, unknown causes. Mycologic cultures may be positive without any clinically apparent disease. Nail/foot hygiene is important: benzoyl peroxide soap in shower or antifungal preparation.

MANAGEMENT

Indications for Systemic Therapy Fingernail involvement, limitation of function, pain (thickened great toenails with pressure on nail bed, ingrowing toe nails), physical disability, potential for secondary bacterial infection, source of recurrent epidermal dermatophytosis, quality of life issues (poorer perceptions of general and mental health, social functioning, physical appearance, difficulty in trimming nails, discomfort in wearing shoes). Early onychomycosis easier to cure in younger, healthier individuals than in older individuals with more extensive involvement and associated medical conditions. It is essential to prove (fungal) infection before starting systemic treatment.

Debridement	Dystrophic nails should be trimmed. In DLSO, the nail and the hyperkeratotic nail bed should be removed with nail clippers. In SWO, the abnormal nail can be debrided with a curette.
Topical agents	Available as lotions and lacquer. Usually not effective except for early DLSO and SWO after prolonged use (months).
	Amorolfine nail lacquer: reported to be effective when applied >12 months (available in Europe). Penlac: monthly professional nail debridement recommended.
Systemic agents	*Note:* In systemic treatment of onychomycosis, nails usually do not appear normal after the treatment times recommended because of slow growth of nail. If cultures and KOH preparations are negative after these time periods, medication can nonetheless be stopped and nails will usually regrow normally.
Allylamines	Most effective against dermatophyte infections; also efficacious against selected other fungi.
Terbinafine	250 mg/d for 6 weeks for fingernails and 12 weeks for toenails.
Azoles	Drugs in this category are usually effective in treatment of nail infections caused by dermatophytes, yeasts, and molds.
Itraconazole: approved (USA) for onychomycosis. Effective in dermatophytes and *Candida* only.	200 mg/d for 6 weeks (fingernails), 12 weeks (toenails) (continuous therapy).
	200 mg bid for first 7 days of each month for 2 months (fingernails) (pulse dosing). Although not approved for toenail onychomycosis, pulse dosing is used, given for 3–4 months.
Fluconazole: not approved (USA) for onychomycosis. Effective in dermatophytes and *Candida.*	Reported effective at dosing of 150–400 mg 1 day per week or 100–200 mg/d until the nails grow back normally. Effective in yeasts and less so in dermatophytes.
Ketoconazole: not approved for onychomycosis. Prolonged therapy as for onychomycosis has highest incidence of liver function abnormalities.	Effective at 200 mg/d; more effective for *Candida* than dermatophytes; however, infrequently hepatotoxicity and antiandrogen effect have limited its long-term use for onychomycosis.
Secondary prophylaxis	Recommended for all patients. The entirety of both feet should be treated. Prophylaxis should be simple to use and inexpensive:

- Benzoyl peroxide soap for washing feet when bathing
- Antifungal cream daily
- Miconazole lotion/powder on feet
- Antifungal sprays or powders in shoes.
- Discard old, moldy shoes
- Pedicures/manicures: make sure instruments are sterilized or individuals have their own.

NAILS AS CLUES TO MULTISYSTEM DISEASES

Systemic disorders can affect the nail apparatus.

Apparent Leukonychia *Terry's Nail* White opacity of nails in patients with cirrhosis. Opaque white color obscures lunula. Discoloration stops abruptly 1 to 2 mm from distal edge of nail, leaving a pink area corresponding to onychodermal band (Fig. 28-18). Involves all nails evenly. *Muehrcke's bands* Parallel to lunula, separated from one another, and from lunula, by strips of pink nail (Fig. 28-19). Associated with hypoalbuminemia, which produces edema of connective tissue in front of lunula just below epidermis of nail bed. Also appears during chemotherapy.

Half-and-Half Nail of Lindsay Proximal area is dull white, resembling ground glass, obscuring lunula; distal area is pink, reddish, or brown, occupying 20 to 60% of length of nail. Observed in uremic patients.

Yellow Nail Syndrome Color due to thickening of nail plate (Fig. 28-20). Increased transverse and longitudinal curvature; loss of cuticle. Usually accompanied by lymphedema at one or more sites and respiratory (bronchiectasis, chronic bronchitis, malignant neoplasms) or nasal sinus disease. Nails grow at a greatly reduced rate. All 20 nails are involved.

Periungual Fibroma Koenen tumors are associated with tuberous sclerosis, presenting at puberty. Usually multiple, small to large, elongated to nodular; produce a longitudinal groove in nail plate due to matrix compression (Fig. 28-21).

Splinter Hemorrhages Subungual epidermal ridges extend from lunula distally to hyponychium, fitting in a "tongue-and-groove" fashion between similarly arranged dermal ridges. Rupture of fine capillaries along these longitudinal dermal ridges results in splinter hemorrhages. Grossly, splinter hemorrhages appear as tiny linear structures, usually ≥ 2 to 3 mm long, arranged in the long axis of nail. The majority originate within distal one-third of nail about 4 mm proximal to tip of finger. Splinter hemorrhages are plum-colored when formed, darkening to brown or black within 1 to 2 days; they subsequently move superficially and distally with nail growth. Trauma is the most common

cause of splinter hemorrhages, occurring in up to 20% of normal population (Fig. 28-22). Other associated conditions include dermatologic disorders (psoriasis, atopic dermatitis), systemic disorders (arterial emboli, antiphospholipid antibody syndrome, vasculitis, blood dyscrasias, scurvy), and systemic infections (trichinosis, endocarditis) (Fig. 28-23).

Nail Fold Telangiectasia and Erythema Linear wiry vessels perpendicular to nail base overlie proximal nail fold. Usually bright red; may be black if thrombosed. In lupus erythematosus and dermatomyositis, usually an associated periungual erythema (Fig. 28-24). In scleroderma, dilated vessels develop on normally colored skin. Also seen in rheumatoid arthritis.

Transverse or Beau's Lines Transverse, bandlike depressions in nail plate, extending from one lateral edge to the other, affecting all nails at corresponding levels (Fig. 28-25). Systemic disease implicated if all 20 nails involved. Occur after any severe, sudden, acute, particularly febrile illness. Thumb nails (lines present for 6 to 9 months) and big nails (lines present for up to 2 years) are most reliable markers. If duration of disease completely inhibits matrix activity for 1 to 2 weeks, transverse depression results in total division of nail plate (onychomadesis).

Etiology commonly, high fever, postnatal, menstrual cycle (multiple), measles, trauma, chronic paronychia, local inflammation, chronic eczema; less commonly, cytotoxic drugs, Stevens-Johnson syndrome, Kawasaki's disease, acrodermatitis enteropathica and zinc deficiency, hypoparathyroidism.

Koilonychia Spoon-shaped nails (Fig. 28-26). More often due to local rather than systemic factors. In early stages, nail plate becomes flattened. Later, edges become everted upwards and nail appears concave.

Main types physiologic (early childhood); thin nails (old age, peripheral vascular disease); soft nails (mainly occupational); hereditary and congenital; manifestation of rare Plummer-Vinson syndrome (associated with anemia, dysphagia, glossitis).

Clubbed Nails Characteristic changes include overcurvature of nails in the proximal to distal and transverse planes with enlargement of periungual soft tissue structures confined to the tip of each digit (Fig. 28-27). Increased curvature usually affects all 20 nails. Three types of clubbing occur: simple type, hypertrophic pulmonary osteoarthropathy (HPO), idiopathic hypertrophic osteoarthropathy (IHO) pachydermoperiostosis. The degree of deformity is measured by Lovibond's "profile sign," which measures the angle between the curved nail plate and proximal nail fold when finger is viewed from the radial aspect. Normally 160° but exceeds 180° in clubbing. Simple clubbing may be congenital, familial, or associated with obstructed circulation with edema of soft tissues. HPO characterized by clubbing of nails; hypertrophy of upper/lower extremities similar to deformity in acromegaly; joint changes with pseudo-inflammatory, symmetric, painful arthropathy of large limb joints, especially legs (almost pathognomonic of malignant chest tumors); bone changes (bilateral, proliferative periostitis, and modified, diffuse decalcification); peripheral neurovascular disorders such as local cyanosis/paresthesia. IHO characterized by bulbous distal fingers with hyperhidrosis.

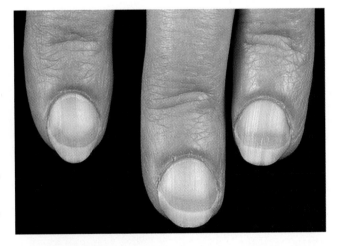

Figure 28-18 Apparent leukonychia: Terry's nails *The proximal two-thirds of the nail plate is white, whereas the distal third shows the red color of the nail bed.*

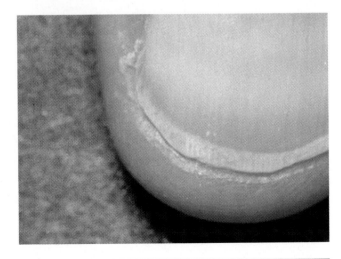

Figure 28-19 Apparent leukonychia: Muehrcke's bands *Paired narrow horizontal white bands, separated by normal color, that remain immobile as the nail grows.*

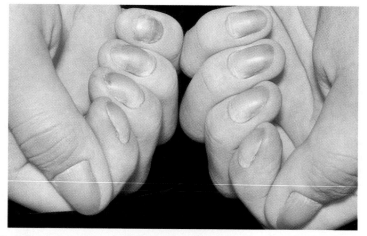

Figure 28-20 Yellow nail syndrome *Diffuse yellow-to-green color of the fingernails, nail thickening, slowed growth, and excessive curvature from side to side of all ten fingernails.*

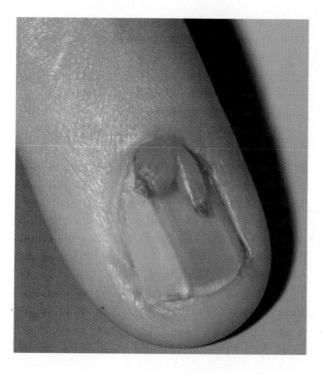

Figure 28-21 Periungual fibroma *A skin-colored tumor is seen emerging from beneath the proximal nail fold associated with a longitudinal groove in the nail plate.*

DISORDERS OF THE NAIL APPARATUS

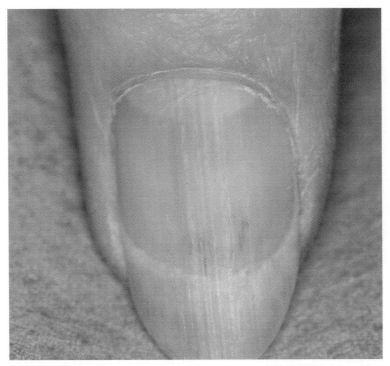

Figure 28-22   Splinter hemorrhages, traumatic   *The brown linear streaks in the nail bed arising distally are usually traumatic in origin.*

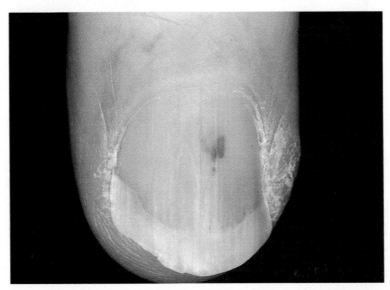

Figure 28-23   Splinter hemorrhages, embolic   *Subungual hemorrhages in the midportion of the nail bed (quite different in comparison to traumatic splinter hemorrhages) was noted in several fingernails in a 60-year-old female with enterococcal endocarditis, who had associated subconjunctival hemorrhage.*

NAILS AS CLUES TO MULTISYSTEM DISEASES

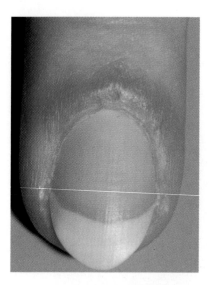

Figure 28-24 Nail fold erythema *The proximal nail fold is inflamed (erythematous and edematous) in a patient with systemic lupus erythematosus.*

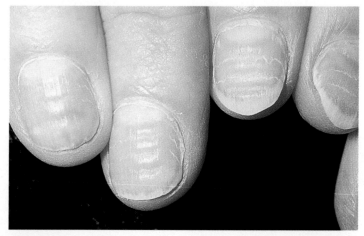

Figure 28-25 Beau's lines *Multiple transverse ridging of multiple fingernails was associated with chemotherapy for breast cancer.*

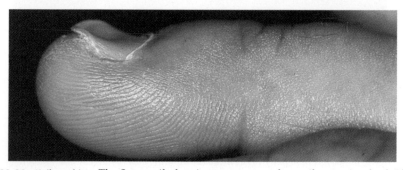

Figure 28-26 Koilonychia *The fingernail plate is concave; no other nails were involved. There were no associated systemic factors.*

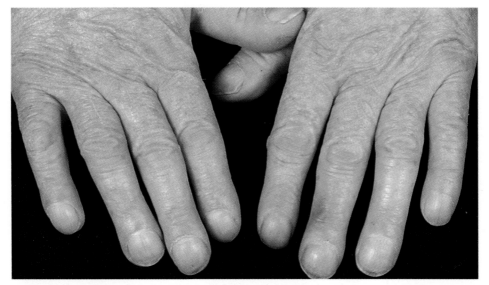

Figure 28-27   Clubbed fingers   *Bulbous enlargement and broadening of the fingertips. The angle made by the proximal nail fold and the nail plate exceeded 180°. The tissue between the nail and underlying bone had a spongy quality giving a "floating" sensation when pressure is applied downward and forward at the junction between the plate and proximal fold.*

DISORDERS OF OROPHARYNX

DISORDERS OF THE TONGUE

Hairy Tongue

Hairy tongue is a common disorder in which the "hairlike" filiform papillae that make up most of the dorsal surface of the tongue become increased in length and thickness as a result of the slowing of the normal removal of "squames" (i.e., scales) from the tips of the filiform papillae. Hairy tongue is also usually pigmented ("black") due to overgrowth of pigment-forming organisms. Precipitating factors are fever, dehydration, reduction in the normal salivary flow and the oral movements that promote desquamation; also, ingestion of antibiotics that can lead to an imbalance in the normal bacterial flora. There are usually no symptoms, but some patients note a bad taste or gagging with swallowing. The filiform papillae are hyperkeratotic and "coated" on the middorsal surface (Fig. 29-1). When the precipitating factors are eliminated, the condition disappears. However, to speed the recovery, local measures can be used such as treatment with antimicrobial mouthwashes and using a toothbrush to dislodge the adherent material.

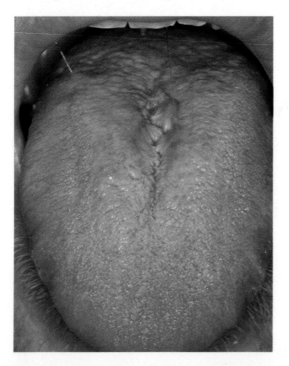

Figure 29-1 Hairy tongue *Filiform hyperkeratoses of the papillae result in a brownish coating on the dorsum of the tongue in this 31-year-old cigarette smoker.*

Fissured Tongue

A common benign asymptomatic disorder in which there are changes in the surface morphology of the dorsum of the tongue; the tongue has numerous linear "valleys," resulting in a corrugated appearance. "Fissures" (Fig. 29-2), linear patterns are related to the deep valleys in the dorsal tongue that do not involve the mucosal epithelium and are therefore not painful. Persists and becomes more exaggerated throughout life.

Synonym: "Scrotal" tongue.

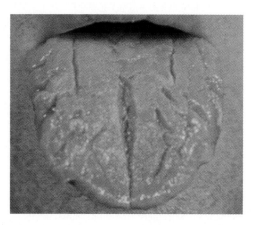

Figure 29-2   Fissured (scrotal) tongue   *Deep furrows on the dorsum of the tongue are asymptomatic.*

Migratory Glossitis

Migratory glossitis is the most common of several conditions that have been termed *psoriasiform* lesions. This disorder presents as reddish-white areas on the tongue that change shape and thus appear to migrate (Fig. 29-3). In the majority of patients, it is idiopathic and need not be associated with psoriasis. About 40% of patients also have a fissured tongue.

Synonyms: Glossitis migrans, geographic tongue.

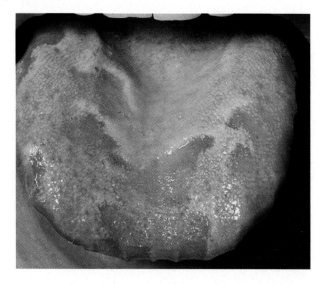

Figure 29-3   Migratory glossitis
Areas of hyperkeratosis alternate with areas of normal pink epithelium, creating a geographic pattern in a female with psoriasis.

DISORDERS OF THE BUCCAL AND GINGIVAL MUCOSA

Aphthous Ulcer

Aphthous ulcers (AU) are painful mucosal ulcerations of idiopathic etiology occurring commonly in the oropharynx and less commonly in the esophagus, upper and lower GI tract, and anogenital epithelium, characterized clinically by pain and sharply marginated gray-based, red-rimmed ulcer(s). AU occur in otherwise healthy people.

Synonyms: Aphthous (ancient Greek word for "ulcer") stomatitis, "canker sore." *Minor AU:* recurrent aphthae of Mikulicz. *Major AU:* Sutton's disease, periadenitis mucosa necrotica recurrens.

EPIDEMIOLOGY

Age of Onset Any age; often during second decade, persisting into adulthood, and becoming less frequent with advancing age.

Sex Females > males.

Etiology Unknown.

Incidence Extremely common; most adults experience AU at some time during their lives.

Risk Factors Local trauma, heredity.

Associated Disorders Behçet's disease, cyclic neutropenia, HIV disease.

Classification Minor (MiAU), <1 cm in diameter. Major (MaAu) up to 3 cm. Herpetiform (HAU), up to 100 tiny erosions.

PATHOGENESIS

Unknown; probably immune-mediated tissue damage.

HISTORY

AU may occur at the site of minor mucosal injury, such as a minor bite by teeth.

Symptoms Even though small, AU can be quite painful, which may impair nutrition. A burning or tingling sensation may be felt before ulceration. In persons with severe AU, malaise: weight loss associated with persistent, painful AU.

PHYSICAL EXAMINATION

Mucous Membranes At times, small, painful red macule or papule before ulceration. More commonly, ulcer(s) <1 cm (Fig. 29-4), covered with fibrin (gray-white), with sharp, discrete, and at times edematous borders. White-gray base with an erythematous rim. Most commonly single; at times, multiple or numerous small, shallow, grouped—i.e., herpetiform. MaAU may heal with white, depressed scars.

Distribution Oropharyngeal, anogenital, any site in the GI tract. Oral lesions most commonly on the buccal and labial mucosae, less commonly on tongue, sulci, floor of mouth. MiAU rarely occur on the palate or gums. MaAU often occur on soft palate and pharynx.

Number MiAU, 1 to 5; MaAU, 1 to 10; HAU up to 100.

General Findings With MaAU, occasionally tender cervical lymphadenopathy. Findings of Behçet's disease, cyclic neutropenia, HIV disease.

DIFFERENTIAL DIAGNOSIS

Oropharyngeal Ulcer(s) Primary herpetic gingivostomatitis, herpangina, hand-foot-and-mouth disease, bullous diseases (erythema multiforme, pemphigus vulgaris, bullous pemphigoid, cicatricial pemphigoid), lichen planus, Reiter's syndrome, adverse drug reaction (fixed eruption, systemic chemotherapy, gold), squamous cell carcinoma, Behçet's disease.

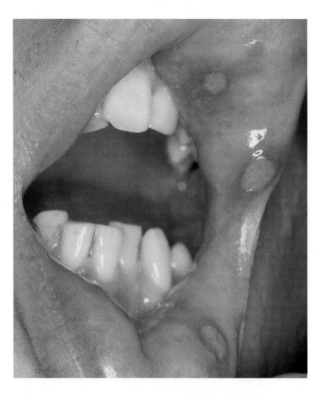

Figure 29-4 Aphthous ulcers
Multiple, very painful, gray-based ulcers with erythematous halos on the labial mucosa.

LABORATORY EXAMINATIONS

Dermatopathology The findings are not diagnostic, showing varying degrees of epithelial ulceration and inflammatory response; specific causes of epithelial ulceration can be ruled out by histologic findings, including infection (syphilitic chancre, histoplasmosis), inflammatory disorders (lichen planus), or cancers (squamous cell carcinoma).

DIAGNOSIS

Usually by clinical findings.

COURSE AND PROGNOSIS

In many persons, MiAU tend to recur during adulthood. Uncommonly, may be almost constant in the oropharynx or anogenitalia, referred to as *complex aphthosis*. MiAU heal spontaneously in 1 to 2 weeks. MaAU may persist for 6 weeks or more, healing with scarring. HAU usually heal in 1 to 2 weeks. Behçet's disease should be considered in patients with persistent oropharyngeal AU, with or without anogenital AU, associated with systemic findings (eye, nervous system). See Section 12.

MANAGEMENT

Topical Modalities Topical glucocorticoids in a base suited for mucous membranes. Topical anesthetics (diphenhydramine EMLA, viscous lidocaine).

Intralesional triamcinolone Injection 3 to 10 mg/mL.

Systemic Therapy In persons with large, persistent, painful AU interfering with nutrition, a brief course of oral glucocorticoids is effective. Thalidomide particularly has been used successfully in persons with HIV disease, Behçet's disease, and large painful AU.

Mucocele

Mucocele is a painless, translucent, blister-like swelling of the mucous membrane that is easily ruptured, drains a clear fluid, and then refills. It develops at sites where minor salivary glands are easily traumatized: mucous membranes of the lip and floor of the mouth. May be chronic, recurrent, and then it presents as a firm, inflamed nodule.
Synonym: Ranula.

Duration of Lesions   Weeks, but may recur in same site for months, and chronic lesions may be present for a year or longer.

PHYSICAL EXAMINATION

Mucus-filled cavity, with a thick roof (Fig. 29-5); chronic lesions are firm, inflamed, poorly circumscribed nodules; bluish, translucent; fluctuant. Occur in areas in the mouth where salivary glands are exposed to trauma, i.e., floor of the mouth, lower lip.

Dermatopathology   Cavity in the connective tissue that is filled with mucoid material and contained in a capsule of granulation tissue; polymorphonuclear leukocytes and "foamy" macrophages are present in the mucoid material.

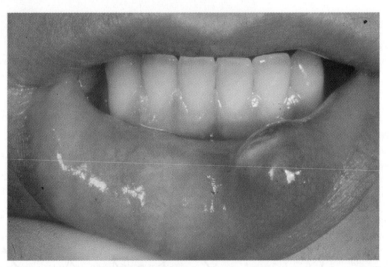

Figure 29-5   Mucocele   *A well-defined, soft bluish submucosal fluctuant nodule on the lip. Thick clear mucus drained when the lesion was incised.*

Oral Fibroma

Oral fibroma is a common circumscribed mass of dense submucosal connective tissue, sessile or pedunculated, ranging in size from a few millimeters to several centimeters, presenting as pink to pink-red, firm to hard submucosal nodule (Fig. 29-6).
Synonyms: Irritation fibroma, traumatic fibroma, fibrous nodule, focal fibrous hyperplasia.

PHYSICAL EXAMINATION

Lesions Sessile or pedunculated, well-demarcated nodule, usually ≤2 cm in diameter, but may be large if neglected. Normal color of the mucous membrane to pink-red. Firm to hard.

Distribution Buccal mucosa along bite line. Also tongue, gingiva, labial mucosa.

DIFFERENTIAL DIAGNOSIS

Giant cell fibroma, granular cell tumor, epulis fissuratum, peripheral ossifying fibroma, mucous retention cyst (mucocele), pyogenic granuloma, lymphangioma, traumatic neuroma, neurilemmoma (schwannoma), neurofibroma, leiomyoma, angiomyoma (vascular leiomyoma), lipoma, Kaposi's sarcoma, fibrosarcoma.

LABORATORY EXAMINATIONS

Dermatopathology A nodule composed of mature fibrous connective tissue surrounded by stratified squamous epithelium. Management: Excision.

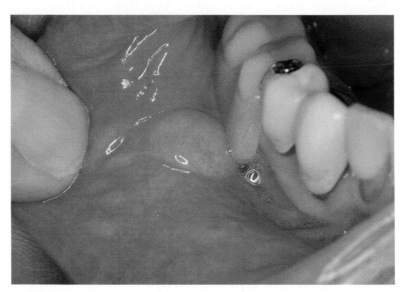

Figure 29-6   Submucosal fibroma *A rubbery pink nodule at the reflection of the buccal mucosa.*

BULLOUS DISEASES WITH ORAL MANIFESTATIONS

Pemphigus Vulgaris (See also Section 4)

Pemphigus vulgaris usually starts in the oral mucosa and may be confined to this site for months before generalized bullae occur. Since blisters are very fragile, they easily rupture and are therefore rarely seen. Sharply marginated erosions of the mouth (buccal mucosa, hard and soft palate and gingiva) are the presenting symptoms (Fig. 29-7). Lesions are extremely painful and may thus considerably interfere with nutrition. The clinical diagnosis is confirmed by cytology (Tzanck test) showing acantholytic cells, biopsy, direct and indirect immunofluorescence (see Pemphigus, Vulgaris, Section 4, and Paraneoplastic Pemphigus, Section 15).

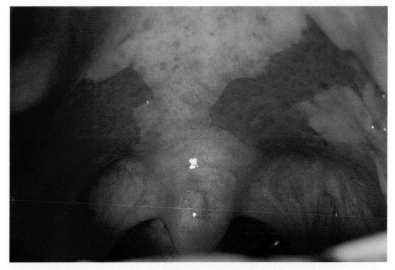

Figure 29-7 Pemphigus vulgaris: erosions *Well-demarcated, painful erosions on the soft palate were the presenting complaint of this 55-year-old female.*

Bullous Pemphigoid (See also Section 4)

In contrast to pemphigus vulgaris, mucosal lesions in bullous pemphigoid are rare. Blisters which initally are tense, erupt on the buccal mucosa and the palate, rupture and leave sharply defined erosions which are then practically indistinguishable from those of pemphigus vulgaris. However, lesions are less painful and erosions are less extensive than in pemphigus. Such erosions may also occur in cicatricial pemphigoid (see Section 4) where they may be the only lesions. Diagnosis is made histopathologically and by direct and indirect immunofluorescence and immunoblotting.

DISORDERS OF OROPHARYNX

Lichen Planus (See also Section 5)

From 40 to 60% of individuals with lichen planus have oropharyngeal involvement. Lesions may present as milky-white papules or as reticular LP, with reticulate net-like patterns of lacy-white hyperkeratosis on the buccal mucosa (Fig. 29-8), the lips, tongue, and gingiva. Hypertrophic LP presents as leukoplakia with Wickham's striae usually on the buccal mucosa; atrophic LP presents as a shiny plaque often with Wickham's striae in the surrounding mucosa, and erosive or ulcerative LP consists of superficial erosions with overlying fibrin clots that are seen on the tongue and buccal mucosa or the bright red gingiva (desquamative gingivitis) (Fig. 29-9). Erosive and ulcerative LP is painful.

Bullous LP may also arise on the oral mucous membranes presenting as intact blisters up to several centimeters in diameter that rupture and result in erosive LP.

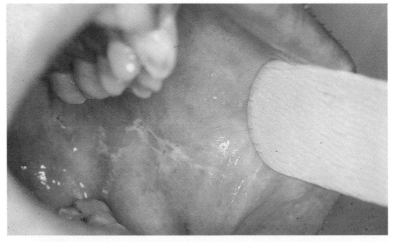

Figure 29-8   Lichen planus: buccal mucosa   *Poorly defined violaceous plaque with lacy-white pattern (Wickham's striae).*

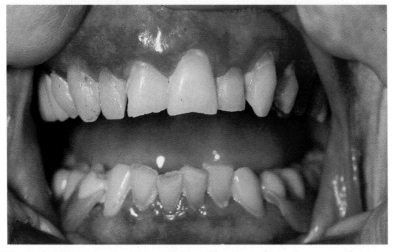

Figure 29-9   Lichen planus: desquamative gingivitis   *The gingival margins are erythematous, edematous, and retracted in a 72-year-old female. The lesions were painful, making dental hygiene difficult, resulting in plaque formation of the teeth.*

Lupus Erythematosus (See also Section 12)

Mucosal discoid lupus erythematosus occurs in approximately 25% of patients with chronic cutaneous lupus erythematosus (CCLE). The buccal mucosal surfaces are the most commonly involved, with the palate (Fig. 29-10), alveolar process and tongue being sites of less frequent involvement. Lesions are painless erythematous patches that evolve to chronic plaques which are sharply marginated and have irregularly scalloped white borders with radiating white striae and telangiectasia. Central depression can occur in older lesions and painful ulceration may develop (Fig. 29-10). Chronic plaques may also appear on the vermilion border of the lips. Mucosal lupus is easily confused with oral lichen planus. In systemic lupus erythematosus (SLE) similar CCLE lesions can be found in the oral mucosa; in acute lupus, ulcers arising in purpuric necrotic lesions of the palate (80%), buccal mucosa, or gums are common.

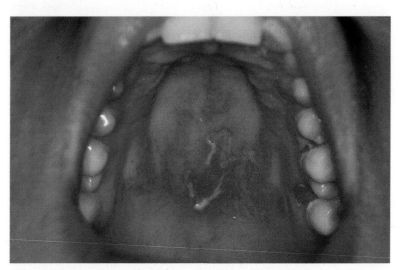

Figure 29-10   Lupus erythematosus: hard palate   *Erythematous eroded plaques were associated with chronic cutaneous LE.*

PRECANCEROUS AND CANCEROUS LESIONS

Leukoplakia and Squamous Cell Carcinoma in Situ (Erythroplasia) (See also Section 9)

Leukoplakia is defined as a white adherent patch or plaque on the mucosa that cannot be rubbed off. This is a clinical diagnosis that does not imply anything about dysplasia. The white plaque may appear homogeneously white, verrucous, or may be speckled with red spots (erythroplakia) (Fig. 29-11). When associated with erythroplakia, it is classified as a premalignant lesion (with histologic dysplasia) with its unfavorable prognosis; and when it develops on the high risk sites for oral squamous cell carcinoma (floor of the mouth, ventrolateral tongue), it should be viewed within an increased index of suspicion. Oral leukoplakia may occur as a benign lesion and may be associated with a variety of other conditions (lichen planus, secondary syphilis, ill-fitting dentures, tobacco smoking and chewing, HPV). It can also be a forerunner of verrucous carcinoma (Fig. 29-11).

Squamous cell carcinoma in situ of the oral mucous membranes corresponds to Bowen's disease of the skin and is called "erythroplasia." It represents a red patch of the mucosal surface which may or may not have a white colored component. It has a reddish velvety appearance with either stippled or patchy regions of leukoplakia (Fig. 29-11) or may be a smooth patch with minimal or no leukoplakia. It is most frequently seen on the floor of the mouth in men, whereas in women the tongue and buccal mucosa are more common sites. Lesions may be relatively small (<2 cm). The condition progresses to invasive squamous cell carcinoma. Biopsy is mandatory. (For squamous carcinoma of the anogenital skin, see Section 30.)

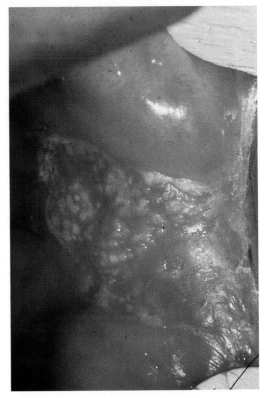

Fugure 29-11   Squamous cell carcinoma in situ (erythroplasia): buccal mucosa   *A well-demarcated white/red plaque in a 45-year-old tobacco smoker.*

Invasive Squamous Cell Carcinoma (See also Section 9)

Oral SCC is a significant killer accounting for about 5% of all neoplasms in men and 2% of those in women. Invasive squamous cell carcinoma usually appears as a granulating velvety, plaque or nodule with stippled hyperkeratosis±ulceration (lips, floor of the mouth, central and lateral sides of the tongue). Verrucous carcinoma is a low-grade squamous cell carcinoma starting with extensive hyperkeratotic white leukoplakia that evolves into warty papillomatous clefted nodules and plaques (previously called florid oral papillomatosis) (Fig. 29-12). It is associated with HPV and metastasizes late.

In both types of squamous cell carcinoma a biopsy is mandatory and aggressive surgical intervention is indicated.

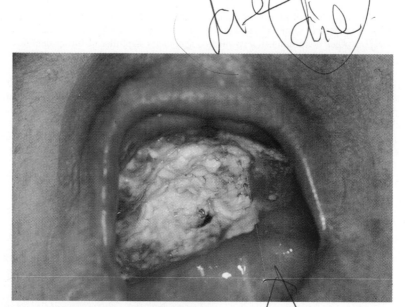

Figure 29-12 Invasive squamous cell carcinoma: palate *An advanced tumor on the hard palate of a cigarette smoker.*

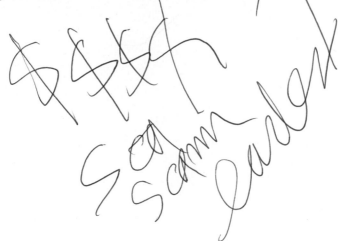

Oral Melanoma (See also Section 10)

Melanoma arising in the oropharynx is uncommon but accounts for 4% of primary oral malignancies. Many but not all lesions are pigmented. Approximately 80% arise on the pigmented mucosa of the palate and gingiva. More deeply pigmented individuals (Africans) have higher proportional incidence rates of mucosal melanoma than whites (because of the lower incidence of cutaneous melanoma). Oral melanoma presents as a pigmented lesion (Fig. 29-13), with variegation of color and irregular borders. In situ lesions are macular; sites of invasion are usually raised within the in situ lesion. For the most part, lesions are asymptomatic and may be advanced when first detected.

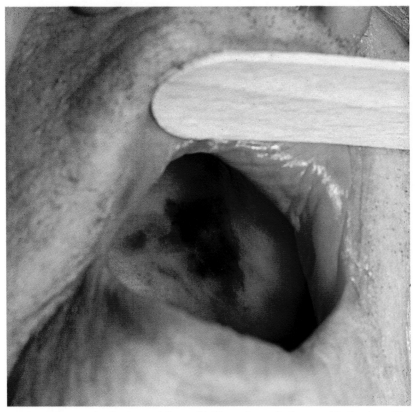

Figure 29-13   Melanoma: hard palate   *A large, highly variegated pigmented lesion in a 63-year-old male. Lesional biopsy of a raised part showed invasive acrolentiginous melanoma.*

Condyloma Acuminatum (See also Section 25)

Condyloma acuminatum may occur in oral mucous membranes (Figs. 29-14 and 29-15), sometimes associated with genital condylomata. HPV DNA has been demonstrated in these lesions. They can result from oral genital sexual contact and usually present as flat papillomatous plaques or nodules with a granular surface (Fig. 29-14). Early lesions can be visualized as white elevated patches by using 5% acetic acid.

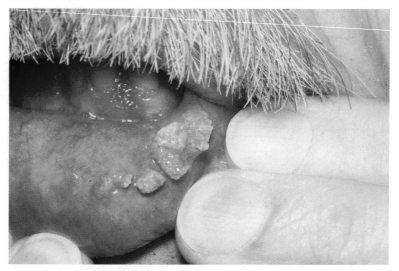

Figure 29-14   Condylomata acuminata: lip   *Cauliflower-like lesions on the mucosal surface.*

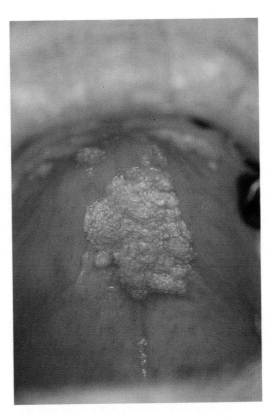

Figure 29-15 Condylomata acuminata: hard palate *Huge mosaic cauliflower floret-like lesions in a 35-year-old male with HIV infection.*

DISORDERS OF THE GENITALIA, PERINEUM, AND ANUS

Anogenital skin and mucosa are subject to unique disorders because of their special anatomy. Dermatologic and systemic disorders occur in the anogenital region, often with associated extragenital involvement. Primary neoplasms arise in these areas, most commonly associated with chronic human papillomavirus (HPV) infection. Sexually transmitted as well as other infections also occur commonly in these sites.

GENITAL LENTIGINOSES

Genital (penile and vulvar) lentiginoses are acquired multiple or single light brown, brown, dark brown, or black, oval or round, often fairly large (15 mm) macules (Figs. 30-1 and 30-2) that appear on the anogenital areas of women and men. These lesions have an adult onset and persist for years without change in size. The pathology does not show significant melanocytic hyperplasia, and nevus cells are not present; the pigmentation is the result of increased melanin in the basal cell layer. Onset during adulthood. Clinically, lesions are tan, brown, intense blue-black; usually variegated, 5- to 15-mm macules occurring in clusters on vulva (labia minora), penis (glans, shaft), and perianal areas.

Differential diagnosis: melanoma in situ, PUVA lentigo, fixed drug reaction, lentiginosis as part of the LAMB syndrome (lentigo, atrial myxoma, myxoid neurofibromas, and blue nevi), HPV-induced squamous cell carcinoma in situ.

In women, these lesions are almost always a source of concern for the patient; they may indicate vulvar melanoma. Penile lentiginosis—especially a single lesion—also suggests the possibility of melanoma; epiluminescence microscopy rules out in situ melanoma, but, since experience is still limited, a biopsy should nevertheless be performed to establish that there are no nevus or melanoma cells present. These patients should be examined at regular intervals. Extensive lesions that cannot be easily removed should be followed photographically; areas that show significant change should be biopsied.

Synonyms: Penile lentigo, vulvar melanosis.

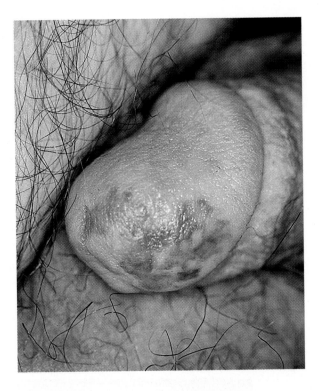

Figure 30-1   Genital lentiginoses: penis   *Variegated tan-brown macules on the glans of a 70-year-old male; lesions were present for many years. With these clinical findings, acrolentiginous melanoma in situ must be ruled out.*

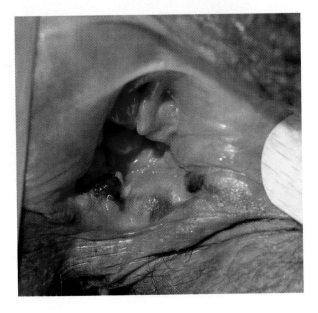

Figure 30-2   Genital lentiginoses: vulva   *Multiple, variegated dark brown macules, bilateral on the labia minora. Lesions had been present for >5 years and are multifocal in origin. Acrolentiginous melanoma in situ must be ruled out.*

VITILIGO AND LEUKODERMA (SEE ALSO SECTION 11)

Vitiligo may occur on the anogenital region as the initial presentation or as part of more widespread processes of depigmentation. Chemically induced leukoderma involving the penis and scrotum can occur with occupational leukoderma. Depigmentation occurs by direct contact with the chemical; depigmentation of the genital skin may occur as part of a systemic effect, without direct contact of the chemical with the genital skin. Chemically induced leukoderma has also been reported to occur after exposure to rubber-containing devices such as condoms and pessaries. The isomorphic phenomenon occurs in vitiligo (depigmentation at sites of injury); an individual with vitiligo may develop depigmentation on the genital skin after infections such as genital herpes or gonorrhea, or inflammatory disorders. Hypopigmentation is best differentiated from vitiligo (depigmentation) with a Wood's lamp. Vitiligo, either idiopathic or chemically induced, appears as sharply demarcated, macular, white lesions (Fig. 30-3); the entire cutaneous surface should be examined for other depigmented areas. Differential diagnosis of genital leukoderma: sclerotic disorders in which there is a loss of the dermal vasculature resulting in avascular white plaques such as in lichen sclerosus; inflammatory disorders such as genital herpes; or iatrogenic disorders after cryo-, electro-, or laser surgery.

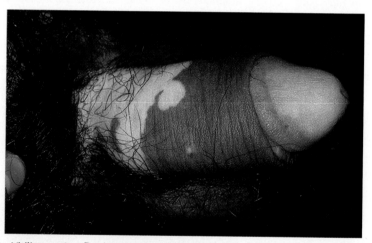

Figure 30-3   Vitiligo: penis   *Depigmentation of the proximal penile shaft. Multiple macules have become confluent. The lesions were an isolated finding.*

PSORIASIS VULGARIS (SEE ALSO SECTION 3)

Psoriasis vulgaris on the anogenital region, when occurring on nonoccluded skin, appears as erythematous plaques with various accumulations of scale. In normally occluded anogenital skin (preputial sac, labia minor, inguinal folds, intergluteal cleft) as well as umbilicus, and axillae, psoriatic lesions appear as well-demarcated erythematous plaques without scale, so-called inverse-pattern psoriasis. The most common noninfectious dermatosis occurring on the glans penis is psoriasis. Genital psoriasis may be the initial presentation of psoriasis. In circumcised males, genital psoriasis most commonly presents as a well-demarcated erythematous plaque(s) with varying degrees of scale (Fig. 30-4); similarly, inverse-pattern psoriasis occurs on the opposing aspects of the labia majora and minor. In uncircumcised males, psoriatic plaques occur on both the glans and inner aspect of the foreskin and lack any scale. Genital psoriasis is frequently accompanied by asymptomatic, unrecognized inverse-pattern psoriasis, perianally and in the intergluteal cleft, which appears as an elongated well-demarcated erythematous plaque. Inverse-pattern psoriasis also occurs in the inguinal folds (Fig. 30-5). Differential diagnosis of well-demarcated anogenital plaque(s): lichen planus, fixed drug eruption, condyloma acuminata, squamous intraepithelial lesion, squamous cell carcinoma in situ, and invasive squamous cell carcinoma. Hydrocortisone or other mild topical glucocorticoid ointments are usually effective. Patients should be advised that the nature of psoriasis is to recur and that topical glucocorticoids should be applied only during symptomatic periods, rather than on a daily basis. Topical calcipotriol is effective in some individuals but can cause irritation, especially of occluded skin or mucosa.

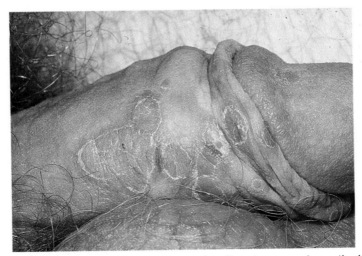

Figure 30-4   Psoriasis vulgaris: penis   *Well-demarcated scaling plaques on the penile shaft of a 25-year-old male. "Pinking" of the intergluteal cleft and nail findings of psoriasis were also present. The patient presented to a clinic for sexually transmitted diseases.*

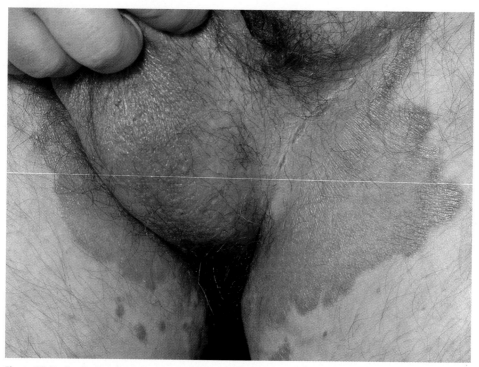

Figure 30-5 Psoriasis vulgaris: inverse pattern *Well-demarcated erythematous plaques on the intertriginous skin at the junction of the scrotum and the medial thigh. Candidiasis at this site always has satellite pustules. Tinea cruris usually has marginal scaling and often, central clearing.*

LICHEN PLANUS (SEE ALSO SECTION 5)

Lichen planus (LP) affects both mucosal and keratinized epithelium, and it is characterized by polygonal, violaceous, flat-topped papules on skin and lacy or erosive lesions on mucosa. LP involving the genitalia is commonly associated with LP at other sites; however, it may occur as the initial or sole manifestation. Symptomatically, genital LP is usually not pruritic, but eroded lesions may be painful (Fig. 30-6). The appearance of lesions often generates anxiety in the patient, raising concern about a sexually transmitted disease. Clincally, violaceous flat-topped papules, discrete or confluent, occur on the glans and the shaft of the penis; the typical lacy white surface pattern seen in some cases, most commonly on the glans. Older lesions may have a grayish hue associated with melanin incontinence into the dermis. Annular lesions occur on the glans and penile shaft (Fig. 30-7). In some individuals, involvement of mucosa of the glans results in erosions, similar to the erosive LP of the oropharyngeal mucosa. Squamous cell carcinoma is a rare complication of chronic lichen planus. Diagnosis can often be made on clinical findings, especially if similar findings are noted also on the oral mucosa and on the skin; less common variants include lichen planopilaris, i.e., lichen planus involving hair follicles, or hypertrophic lichen planus. In the majority of cases, genital LP undergoes spontaneous remission after several years with a residual postinflammatory hyperpigmentation in darker-skinned individuals. Erosive LP, as with the oral involvement, may persist for decades. Reassurance that LP is not a sexually transmitted disease is sufficient for many individuals. Papular lesions can be treated with mild topical glucocorticoid ointment; erosive lesions respond to intralesional triamcinolone injection (3 to 5 mg/mL).

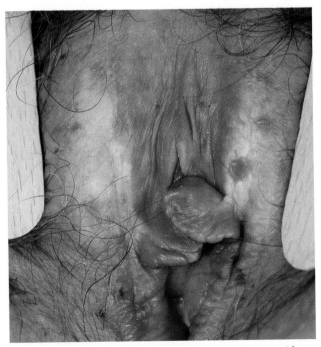

Figure 30-6 Lichen planus: vulva *White bilateral hyperkeratotic plaques with areas of painful erosion. Vulvar lentiginoses are also present, posteriorly.*

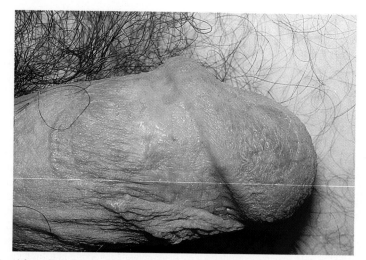

Figure 30-7 Lichen planus: penis *Violaceous annular plaques on the distal shaft and glans of a 26-year-old patient, present for > one year. White lacelike plaques were also present on the buccal mucosa.*

ALLERGIC CONTACT DERMATITIS (SEE ALSO SECTION 2)

Allergic contact dermatitis (ACD) occurring on the penis, scrotum, or vulva is often more florid and symptomatic than at any other site. In nonsensitized individuals, a minimum of 5 to 7 days elapses from the time of contact to onset of symptoms. In a previously sensitized individual, however, the time varies with the quantity of allergen and the individual reactivity, but can be as short as 4 to 6 h. The extreme reactivity and tremendous vascularity of the penis maximizes the intensity of the ACD. The most common type of ACD that occurs predominantly on the male genitalia is a phytodermatitis. Symptomatically, acute ACD is heralded by intense pruritus and a burning sensation, at times before any visible changes. Within hours or days, marked edema occurs (Fig. 30-8), accompanied by diffuse erythema and microvesiculation. Disruption of epidermal integrity is associated with exudation. Secondary bacterial infection with *Staphylococcus aureus,* group A streptococcus, or other pathogens colonizing the anogenital region may be associated with pain and tenderness. The initial presentation is erythema and marked edema, and, in time, with microvesiculation and exudation. Older lesions may become crusted. Intense pruritus often causes the patient to scratch, resulting in excoriations and larger erosions. Finding eczematous dermatitis, such as on the inguinal area, thighs, perianal area, axillae, hands, or face, is helpful in making a diagnosis of an ACD. Differential diagnosis of pruritic genital plaques: atopic dermatitis, seborrheic dermatitis, genital herpes, inguinal dermatophyte infection, balanoposthitis, intertrigo, psoriasis, lichen planus, and balanitis circinata (Reiter's syndrome).

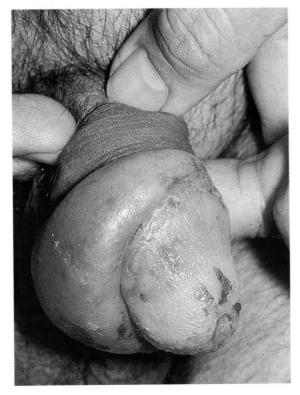

Figure 30-8   Allergic contact dermatitis: penis   *Striking edema of the distal penile shaft associated with severe pruritus in a 21-year-old patient. He had touched poison ivy with his hands, transferring the resin to his penis while urinating; pruritus and then edema occurred within 24 hours of exposure. The magenta-colored pigment is Castellani's paint. The patient was initially seen in an urgent care unit where a diagnosis of cellulitis was made. Pruritus is the distinguishing feature of allergic contact dermatitis.*

ATOPIC DERMATITIS, LICHEN SIMPLEX CHRONICUS, PRURITUS ANI

Atopic dermatitis of the genitals can present as an isolated lesion as part of either flexural or generalized dermatitis. Chronic rubbing and scratching can result in a single plaque of lichen simplex chronicus (LSC) on the scrotum (Fig. 30-9) or vulva, persisting for years or decades. In dark-skinned individuals, areas of hypo- and hyperpigmentation are often present in the plaque of LSC. LSC is best treated with Castellani's paint, intralesional injection of triamcinolone, combined with application of a mild to moderate glucocorticoid ointment for a very limited time, and oral antipruritic agents. (See also Section 2.)

Pruritus ani (Fig. 30-10) is a common symptom, defined as an unpleasant cutaneous sensation that induces the desire to scratch the skin around the anal orifice, occurring in the absence of any identifiable dermatologic disorder. The pathogenesis is often multifactorial: atopic diathesis (most common), fecal contamination and irritation, poor hygiene, anorectal disease (fissures, hemorrhoids, chronic diarrhea, fistulas, impaction or partial obstruction), diet (excessive liquids, spicy foods), anal sphincter dysfunction. The normal pH of the perianal skin and feces is acidic; factors that make it more alkaline may cause pruritus. Various infectious agents and disorders may be a factor in pruritus ani and include: *Staphylococcus aureus,* groups A and B streptococci, erythrasma, dermatophytes, *Candida albicans,* and herpes simplex virus. Two imperatives in the treatment include discontinuation of compulsive rubbing and scratching of the area and strict maintenance of perianal hygiene, especially after evacuation.

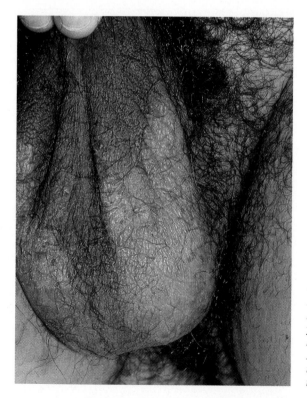

Figure 30-9 Lichen simplex chronicus: scrotum *Pruritic bilateral erythematous hyperpigmented plaques in a 46-year-old Hispanic male. Lesions had been present for >20 years. Lesions resolved following an injection of intralesional triamcinolone (3 mg/ml).*

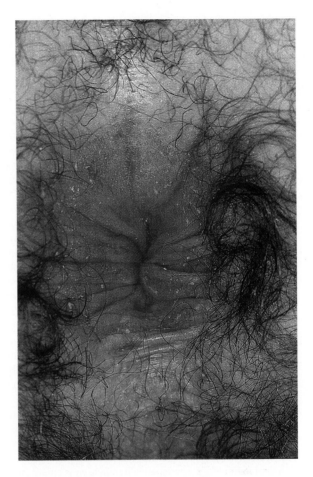

Figure 30-10 Pruritus ani *The patient had experienced intense anal pruritus for many years. Perianal erythema with mild lichen simplex chronicus and fissure is associated with chronic rubbing of the skin.*

LICHEN SCLEROSUS (SEE ALSO SECTION 5)

Lichen sclerosus (LS) [a.k.a. lichen sclerosus et atrophicus (LSA)] is a chronic dermatosis, characterized by atrophic white papules or plaques, occurring most commonly on the anogenital skin of both sexes. More common in females than males (10:1). Penile LS is diagnosed most commonly in middle age. Symptomatic individuals report itching, burning with urination, painful erections, diminished sensation of the glans, or diminution in the caliber and force of the urinary stream. In uncircumcised males, a sclerotic, constricting band forms 1 to 2 cm from the distal end of the prepuce; in time, phimosis may occur. Urinary flow may be obstructed if the urethral orifice is involved, or if phimosis becomes severe. If the sclerotic process progresses, the endstage condition of balanitis xerotica obliterans (BXO) occurs. Early LS shows nonspecific findings of erythema with or without hypopigmentation; diagnosis is made by the findings of a lesional skin biopsy. In time, if untreated, the typical ivory- or porcelain-white macules and plaques (Figs. 30-11 and 30-12) occur, the anemic color caused by a loss of dermal vasculature as well as depigmentation. The surface of lesions is usually smooth, but in some patients may be hyperkeratotic, and may be elevated above or in the same plane as normal skin. Hemorrhage may occur beneath the surface of macules and plaques, resulting in ecchymotic sites or hemorrhagic bullae within the lesions. The epidermis of atrophic lesions may sheer off, resulting in eroded or ulcerated loci within the lesions. Differential diagnosis of a white plaque on the penis/vulva: vitiligo, postinflammatory hypopigmentation, i.e., after repeated episodes of genital herpes, and posttraumatic or surgical scar. Rarely, in situ and invasive squamous cell carcinoma can arise with areas of chronic LS. High-potency topical glucocorticoids provide significant resolution of sclerosis. BXO is also the end stage of some cases of chronic balanoposthitis, but the most common disorder associated with BXO is LS. The onset and evolution of BXO is insidious, evolving over many years. Patients usually seek medical consultation because of a reduced urinary stream or an acute, painful exacerbation of balanoposthitis with resultant phimosis or paraphimosis. Clinically, the prepuce is thickened, contracted, fissured, and fixed over the glans, and cannot be retracted even with moderate tension, i.e., phimosis. Patients with LSA may have associated urethral narrowing and stricture. Circumcision is curative in patients with phimosis secondary to chronic balanoposthitis.

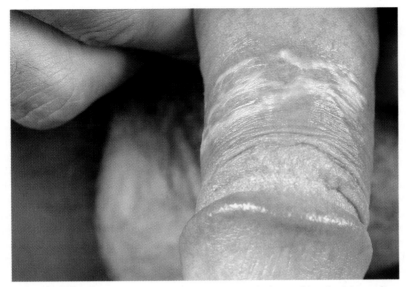

Figure 30-11   Lichen sclerosus: penis   *Early involvement with shiny white plaques on the prepuce of a 40-year-old patient.*

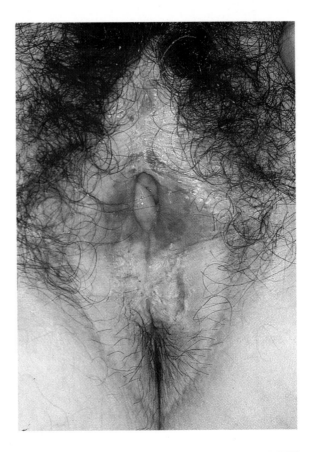

Figure 30-12   Lichen sclerosus: vulva and perineum   *A larger white sclerotic plaque extensively involving the anogenital region. The clitoral region is completely atrophic (agglutination). Ecchymoses are noted in association with atrophy. Ulcerations can occur and are painful. Sclerosis was improved with clobetasol ointment therapy.*

Squamous Cell Carcinoma in Situ

Squamous cell carcinoma (SCC) in situ (SCCIS) can arise at any location on the anogenital region. A solitary plaque of genital SCCIS is also referred to as erythroplasia of Queyrat. The most common etiologic factors in the pathogenesis of SCCIS are human papillomavirus (HPV) infection and chronic low-grade balanoposthitis (poor hygeine, LS) in older individuals. SCCIS associated with chronic inflammation appears as a solitary, well-defined, irregularly bordered, red patch with a glazed-to-velvety surface ± hyperkeratosis on the glans (Fig. 30-13) or vulva (Fig. 30-14). In contrast, HPV-associated lesions are usually multifocal, occurring at any sites of the anogenital region. Appearance of a nodule or ulcer within SCCIS suggests progression to invasive SCC. Diagnosis is made by lesional biopsy. In HPV-associated squamous intraepithelial lesion or SCCIS, the rate of transformation to invasive SCC is relatively low; the rate is higher for vulvar SCCIS. In cases associated with poor hygiene and chronic balanoposthitis, the rate of invasiveness appears to be higher as is the incidence of metastasis. (See also Sections 9 and 25.)

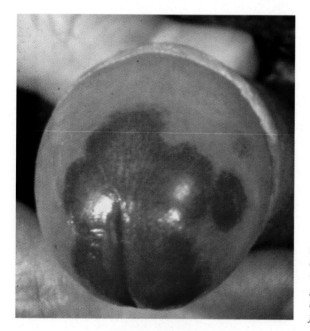

Figure 30-13   Squamous cell carcinoma in situ: glans penis   *A well-demarcated, erythematous, glistening plaque of an elderly male, which had been present for >5 years.*

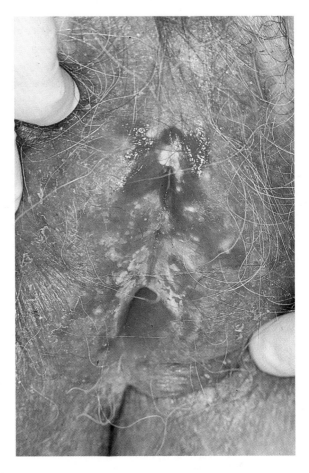

Figure 30-14 Squamous cell carcinoma in situ arising in lichen sclerosus: vulva *A 60-year-old patient with longstanding genital lichen sclerosus, characterized by erythema and erosions with marked atrophy of the labia minora and clitoris. Lesional biopsy of a white hyperkeratotic area shows associated SCC in situ arising in lichen sclerosus.*

HPV-Induced Squamous Intraepithelial Lesion and Squamous Cell Carcinoma in Situ (See also Section 25)

HPV-induced squamous intraepithelial lesion (SIL) of the anogenital skin is characterized by solitary or multifocal maculopapular lesions (Fig. 30-15) on the mucosa and anogenital and ingŭinocrural skin, exhibiting histologic epithelial atypicality. In low-grade SIL (LSIL), the atypicality is confined to the lower one-third of the epithelium; in high-grade SIL (HSIL), the atypicality is present in the lower two-thirds; in SCCIS, the entire thickness of the epithelium is atypical. (The term bowenoid papulosis has been used for SCCIS presenting with multiple brown papules. Bowenoid papulosis and erythroplasia of Queyrat are terms describing SCCIS.) SIL and SCCIS are caused most commonly by the HPV type 16, but also by types 18, 31, and 33. Immunosuppression, occurring in HIV disease, prolonged glucocorticoid therapy, systemic lupus erythematosus, and iatrogenically induced immunosuppression in solid organ transplant patients, has been linked with an increased incidence of SIL and SCCIS. Clinically, SIL and SCCIS appear as erythematous macules, lichenoid (flat-topped), or pigmented papules (several millimeters), which may show some confluence or form plaque(s). The surface of lesions is usually smooth or velvety; the color: tan, brown, pink, red, violaceous, or white. A clustering arrangement is commonly seen, but solitary lesions do occur. In some individuals, condylomata acuminata, SIL, and/or SCCIS may coexist. The course of SIL and SCC of the external anogenital region is more that of a chronic infection than a premalignant disorder with inexorable progression to invasive SCC. In many individuals, spontaneous resolution occurs; however, lesions may persist for years, with the appearance of multiple new lesions, or may progress to invasive SCC. The cervix and anus should be monitored by periodic Pap testing (cytology) to detect dysplastic changes; the incidence of invasive SCC is much higher at these sites than at external anogenital sites.

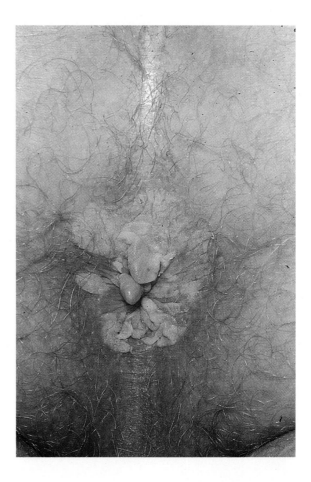

Figure 30-15   HPV-induced squamous cell carcinoma in situ: perianal   *A well-demarcated pink perianal plaque in a 35-year-old HIV-infected male. Anal Pap test showed low-grade squamous intraepithelial lesion (LSIL). All clinical findings resolved with 5% imiquimod cream applied three times a week followed by weekly applications.*

Invasive Anogenital Squamous Cell Carcinoma

The most common etiologic factor is HPV infection. Phimosis and the associated inability to cleanse the preputial sac are associated with penile cancer. Invasive genital SCC presents as a warty, exophytic papule or nodule and usually feels indurated, often arising in an area of SCCIS (Figs. 30-16 and 30-17). The invasive SCC can, in some cases, also be seen arising within areas of condylomata acŭminata, chronic balanoposthitis, or lichen sclerosus. Less commonly, lesions may be flat and ulcerative. Inguinal lymphadenopathy is indicative of secondary bacterial infection of the tumor or metastatic disease.

Genital verrucous carcinoma (GVC) (previously considered to be a benign giant condyloma acuminatum of Buschke-Löwenstein) is a slow-growing SCC arising on the anogenital region, associated with HPV infection. Verrucous carcinoma arises in three sites: anogenital region (GVC), oral mucosa (oral verrucous carcinoma or florid papillomatosis), and the plantar surface of the foot (plantar verrucous carcinoma or epithelioma cuniculatum).

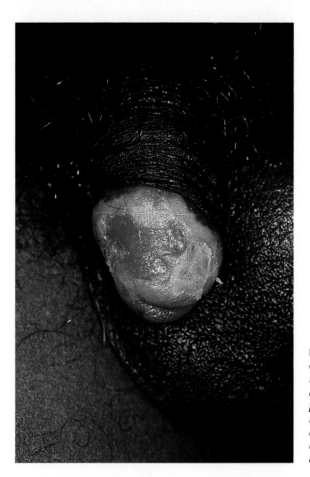

Figure 30-16 Invasive squamous cell carcinoma: glans penis *An eroded indurated plaque on the glans in a 45-year-old black male. The patient had a history of chronic balanoposthitis for >5 years; circumcision had been performed one year previously. Treatment was amputation.*

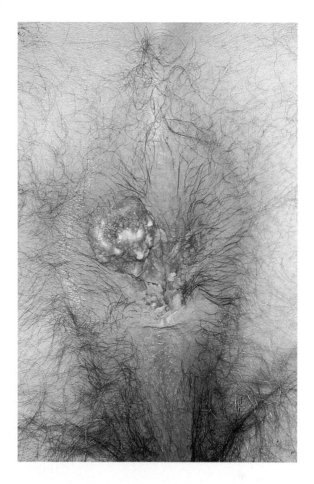

Figure 30-17   HPV-induced invasive squamous cell carcinoma: perineum   *A 32-year-old HIV-infected male presented with a perineal tumor of several months duration. Histology of the excised specimen showed invasive SCC.*

Malignant Melanoma of the Anogenital Region (See also Section 9)

Malignant melanoma of the anogenital region is rare. As with melanoma at other sites, melanoma on anogenital skin can arise either from a preexisting pigmented lesion or de novo from epidermal melanocytes. Lesions appear as macules or papules with variegation of brown-black color, irregular borders, and often with papular elevation (Fig. 30-18) or ulceration. The most common sites in males: glans (67%), prepuce (13%), urethral meatus (10%), penile shaft (7%), and coronal sulcus (3%). (Fig. 30-18). In females, most common sites are the labia minora and the clitoris (Fig. 30-19) Differential diagnosis: genital lentiginosis, an old site of fixed drug eruption, SCC, and hemangioma. Histologically, the most common type of genital melanoma is acral lentiginous melanoma, but rarely, desmoplastic melanoma. The prognosis is poor because of early metastases via lymphatic vessels; most patients die within 1 to 3 years.

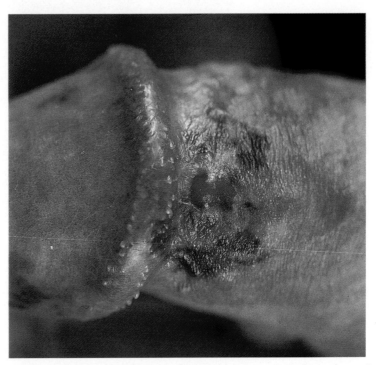

Figure 30-18   Melanoma: penis *A violaceous nodule arising in an area of macular variegated hyperpigmentation in a 60-year-old male. The macular lesions had been present for 5 years and resembled genital lentiginosis. The most common histologic type of genital melanoma is the acrolentiginous melanoma.*

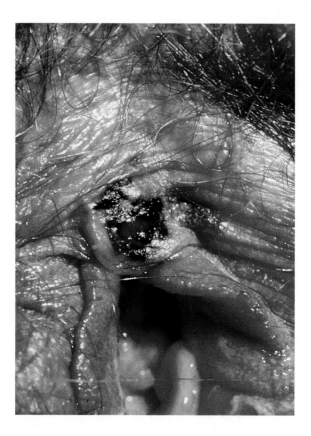

Figure 30-19 Melanoma: vulva
A violaceous nodule in a black plaque in a 52-year-old female.

APPENDICES

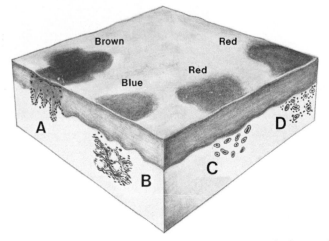

Figure A-1 Macule *(Latin:* macula, *"a spot")* *A macule is a circumscribed area of change in normal skin color without elevation or depression. It is not palpable. Lesions may appear as macules but can be shown to be elevated (i.e., papular) by oblique lighting. A rash consisting of macules is called a macular exanthem. Macules may be of any size or color. White, as in vitiligo, brown, as in café-au-lait spots (A), or blue, as in Mongolian spots (B), red, as in permanent vascular abnormalities such as port-wine stains (C), or transient capillary dilatation due to inflammation (erythema, D). Pressure of a glass slide (diascopy) on the border of a red lesion is a simple and reliable method for detecting the extravasation of red blood cells. If the redness remains under pressure from the slide, the lesion is purpuric; if the redness disappears, the lesion is erythematous and is due to vascular dilatation.*

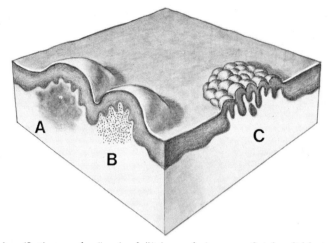

Figure A-2   Papule *(Latin:* papula, *"a pimple") A papule is a superficial, solid lesion, generally considered less than .5 cm in diameter. Most of it is elevated above, rather than deep within, the plane of the surrounding skin. A papule is palpable. In papules the elevation is caused by metabolic, or locally produced deposits (A), or by localized cellular infiltrates (B), or by hyperplasia of local cellular elements (C). Superficial papules are sharply defined. Deeper dermal papules resulting from cellular infiltrates have indistinct borders. Papules with distinct borders are seen when the lesion is the result of an increase in the number of epidermal cells (C). The topography of a papule may consist of multiple, small, closely packed, projected elevations that are known as a vegetation (C). A rash consisting of papules is called a papular exanthem. Papular exanthems may be grouped ("lichenoid") or disseminated (dispersed). Confluence of papules leads to the development of larger, usually flat-topped, circumscribed, plateau-like elevations known as plaques (French:* plaque, *"plate"). See Figure A-3.*

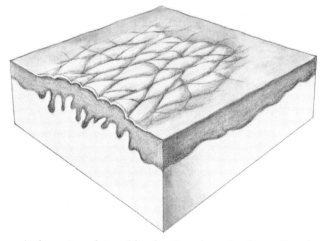

Figure A-3   Plaque *A plaque is a plateau-like elevation above the skin surface that occupies a relatively large surface area in comparison with its height above the skin. It is usually well-defined. Frequently it is formed by a confluence of papules as in psoriasis and mycosis fungoides. Lichenification is a less well-defined, large plaque where the skin appears thickened, and the skin markings are accentuated (as shown in this figure). The process results from repeated rubbing of the skin and most frequently develops in persons with atopy. Lichenification occurs also in eczematous dermatitis, psoriasis, and mycosis fungoides.*

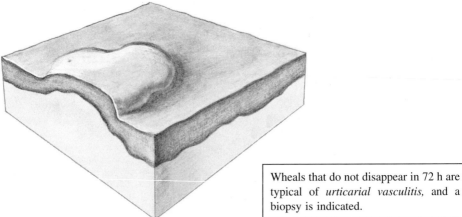

Wheals that do not disappear in 72 h are typical of *urticarial vasculitis*, and a biopsy is indicated.

Figure A-4 Wheal *A wheal is a rounded or flat-topped, pale red papule or plaque that is characteristically evanescent, disappearing within 24 to 48 h. Wheals may be round, gyrate, or irregular with pseudopods—changing rapidly in size and shape due to shifting edema in the papillary body of the dermis. A rash consisting of wheals is called an urticarial exanthem or urticaria.*

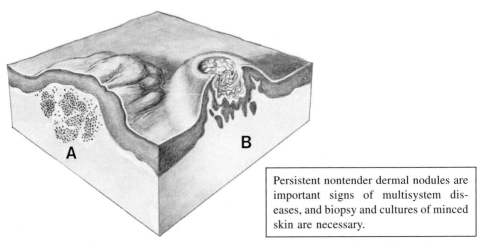

Persistent nontender dermal nodules are important signs of multisystem diseases, and biopsy and cultures of minced skin are necessary.

Figure A-5 Nodule *(Latin:* nodulus, *"small knot") A nodule is a palpable, solid, round or ellipsoidal lesion and may involve the epidermis (B), dermis (A), or subcutaneous tissue. The depth of involvement and the size differentiate a nodule from a papule. Nodules result from infiltrates (A), neoplasms (B), or metabolic deposits in the dermis or subcutaneous tissue and in such case indicate systemic disease. Tuberculosis, the deep mycoses, lymphoma, and metastatic neoplasms, for example, can present as cutaneous nodules. Nodules can develop as a result of a benign or malignant proliferation of keratinocytes, as in keratoacanthoma (B) and squamous cell and basal cell carcinoma.*

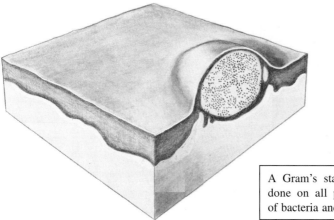

> A Gram's stain and culture should be done on all pustules for identification of bacteria and fungi.

Figure A-6 Pustule *(Latin:* pustula, *"pustule") A pustule is a circumscribed, superficial cavity of the skin that contains a purulent exudate that may be white, yellow, greenish-yellow, or hemorrhagic. This process may arise in a hair follicle or independently. Pustules may vary in size and shape; follicular pustules, however, are always conical and usually contain a hair in the center. The vesicular lesions of herpes simplex and varicella zoster virus infections may become pustular. A rash consisting of pustules is called a pustular exanthem.*

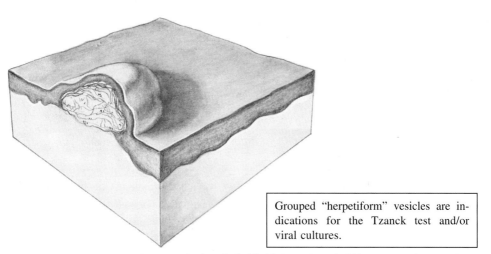

> Grouped "herpetiform" vesicles are indications for the Tzanck test and/or viral cultures.

Figure A-7 Vesicle-Bulla *(Latin:* vesicula, *"little bladder";* bulla, *"bubble") A vesicle (less than .5 cm) or a bulla (more than .5 cm) is a circumscribed, elevated, superficial cavity containing fluid. Often the walls are so thin that they are transparent, and the serum or blood can be seen. Vesicles and bullae arise from a cleavage at various levels of the skin; the cleavage may be within the epidermis (i.e., intraepidermal vesication) or at the epidermal-dermal interface (i.e., subepidermal), as in this figure. A rash consisting of vesicles is called a vesicular exanthem.*

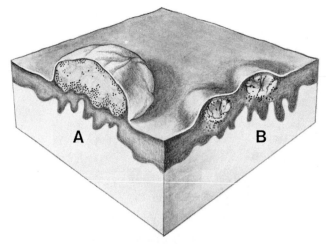

Figure A-8   Vesicle-Bulla [(A) Subcorneal, (B) Spongiotic]   *When the cleavage is just beneath the stratum corneum, a subcorneal vesicle or bulla results (A), as in impetigo. Intraepidermal vesication may result from intercellular edema or spongiosis (B), as characteristically seen in delayed hypersensitivity reactions of the epidermis (e.g., in contact eczematous dermatitis) and in dyshidrotic eczema (B). Spongiotic vesicles may or may not be observed clinically as vesicles.*

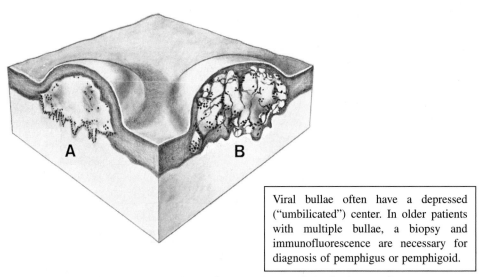

Viral bullae often have a depressed ("umbilicated") center. In older patients with multiple bullae, a biopsy and immunofluorescence are necessary for diagnosis of pemphigus or pemphigoid.

Figure A-9   Vesicle [(A) Acantholytic, (B) Viral]   *Loss of intercellular bridges, or desmosomes, is known as acantholysis (A), and this type of intraepidermal vesication is seen in the vesicles or bullae of pemphigus. Viruses cause a curious "ballooning degeneration" of epidermal cells (B) followed by acantholysis, as in herpes zoster, herpes simplex, and varicella. Viral bullae often have a depressed ("umbilicated") center.*

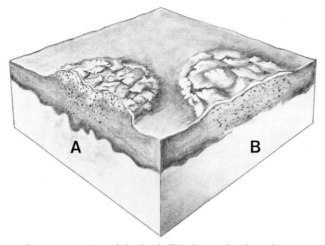

Figure A-10 Crusts *(Latin:* crusta, *"rind, bark, shell") Crusts develop when serum, blood, or purulent exudate dries on the skin surface. Crusts may be thin, delicate, and friable (A) or thick and adherent (B). Crusts are yellow when formed from dried serum, green or yellow-green when formed from purulent exudate, or brown, dark red or black when formed from blood. Superficial crusts occur as honey-colored, delicate, glistening particulates on the surface (A) and are typically found in impetigo. When the exudate involves the entire epidermis, the crusts may be thick and adherent, and if it is accompanied by necrosis of the deeper tissues (e.g., the dermis), the condition is known as* ecthyma.

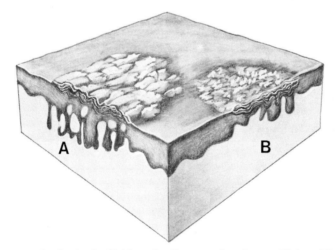

Figure A-11 Desquamation (scaling) *Epidermal cells are replaced every 27 days. The end product of this holocrine process is the stratum corneum. This outermost layer of skin, the stratum corneum, normally does not contain nuclei and is imperceptibly lost. With an increased rate of proliferation of epidermal cells, as in psoriasis, the stratum corneum is not formed normally, and the outermost layers of the skin retain the nuclei (parakeratosis). These desquamating layers of skin are seen clinically as scales (A). Scales are thus flakes of stratum corneum. They may be large (like membranes) or tiny (like dust), adherent or loose. Densely adherent scales that have a gritty feel (like sandpaper) result from a localized increase in the stratum corneum and are a characteristic of solar keratosis (B).*

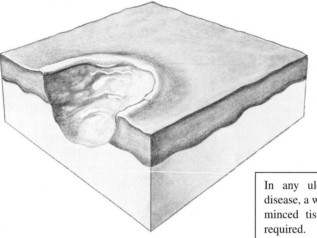

In any ulcer not related to vascular disease, a wedge biopsy for histology and minced tissue for microbial culture is required.

Figure A-12   Ulcer   *(Latin: ulcus, "sore") An ulcer is a skin defect in which there has been loss of epidermis and the upper papillary layer of the dermis. It may extend into the subcutis and always occurs within pathologically altered tissue. (This differentiates an ulcer from a wound, which is a defect inflicted on normal tissue.) An* **erosion** *is a defect only of the epidermis, not involving the dermis; in contrast to an ulcer, which always heals with scar formation, an erosion heals without a scar. Certain features that are helpful in determining the cause of ulcers include location, borders, base, discharge, and any associated topographic features, such as nodules, excoriations, varicosities, hair distribution, presence or absence of sweating, and arterial pulses. In any ulcer not related to vascular disease, a wedge biopsy for histology and minced tissue for microbial culture is required.*

APPENDIX B: SPECIAL CLINICAL AND LABORATORY AIDS TO DERMATOLOGIC DIAGNOSIS

SPECIAL TECHNIQUES USED IN CLINICAL EXAMINATION

1. *Magnification with hand lens.* To examine lesions for fine morphologic detail, it is necessary to use a magnifying glass (hand lens) (7×) or a binocular microscope (5× to 40×). Magnification is especially helpful in the diagnosis of lupus erythematosus (follicular plugging), lichen planus (Wickham's striae), carcinomas (translucence and telangiectasia), and malignant melanoma (subtle changes in color, especially gray or blue; this is best visualized after application of a drop of mineral oil). Hand lenses with built-in lighting and a magnification of 10× to 30× (dermatoscope) are now available that permit observation of lesions covered with a drop of oil (oil-immersion effect) and thus allow inspection of deeper layers of the skin (dermal-epidermal junction.) This is called *epiluminescence microscopy* and allows the distinction of benign and malignant growth patterns in pigmented lesions.
2. *Oblique lighting* of the skin lesion, done in a darkened room, is often required to detect slight degrees of elevation of depression, and it is useful in the visualization of the surface configuration of lesions and in estimating the extent of the eruption.
3. *Subdued lighting* in the examining room enhances the contrast between circumscribed hypopigmented or hyperpigmented lesions and normal skin.
4. *Wood's lamp* (ultraviolet long-wave light, "black" light) is valuable in the diagnosis of certain skin and hair diseases and of porphyria. Long-wave ultraviolet radiation can be obtained by fitting a high-pressure mercury lamp with a specially compounded filter made of nickel oxide and silica (Wood's filter); this filter is very opaque to light, except for a band between 320 and 400 nm. When the ultraviolet waves emitted by Wood's lamp (360 nm) impinge on the skin, fluorescent pigments and subtle color differences of melanin pigmentation can be visualized. Wood's lamp is particularly useful in the detection of the fluorescence of dermatophytosis in the hair shaft (green to yellow) and of erythrasma (coral red). A presumptive diagnosis of porphyria can be made if a pinkish-red fluorescence is demonstrated in urine examined with the Wood's lamp; addition of dilute hydrochloric acid intensifies the fluorescence. Wood's lamp also helps to estimate variation in the lightness of lesions in relation to the normal skin color in both dark-skinned and fair-skinned peoples; e.g., the lesions seen in tuberous sclerosis and tinea versicolor are hypomelanotic and are not as white as the lesions seen in vitiligo, which are amelanotic. Circumscribed hypermelanosis, such as a freckle and melasma, is much more evident (darker) under Wood's lamp. By contrast, dermal melanin as in a Mongolian sacral spot does not become accentuated under Wood's lamp. Therefore, it is possible to localize the site of melanin by use of the Wood's lamp; *this, however, is more difficult or not possible in patients with brown skin.*
5. *Diascopy* consists of firmly pressing a microscopic slide over a skin lesion. The examiner will find this procedure of special value in determining whether the red color of a macule or papule is due to capillary dilatation (erythema) or to extravasation of blood (purpura) that does not blanch. Diascopy is also useful for the detection of the glassy yellow-brown appearance of papules in sarcoidosis, tuberculosis of the skin, lymphoma, and granuloma annulare.
6. *Acetowhitening* facilitates detection of subclinical penile or vulvar warts. Gauze saturated with 5% acetic acid (white vinegar) is wrapped around the glans penis or used only in the cervis and anus. After 5 to 10 min, the penis or vulva is inspected with a 10× hand lens. Warts appear as small white papules.

CLINICAL SIGNS AND TESTS

1. *Darier's sign* is "positive" when a brown macular or a slightly papular lesion of urticaria pigmentosa (mastocytosis) becomes a palpable wheal after being vigorously rubbed with the blunt end of an instrument such as the blunt end of a pen. The wheal may not appear for 5 to 10 min.

2. *Auspitz's sign* is "positive" when slight scratching or curetting of a scaly lesion reveals punctate bleeding points within the lesion. This suggests psoriasis, but it is not specific.

3. The *Nikolsky phenomenon* is positive when the epidermis is dislodged from the dermis by lateral, shearing pressure with a finger, resulting in an erosion. It is an important diagnostic sign in acantholytic disorders such as pemphigus or the SSS syndrome or other blistering or epidermonecrotic disorders, such as toxic epidermal necrolysis.

4. *Patch testing* is used to document and validate a diagnosis of allergic contact sensitization and identify the causative agent. Substances to be tested are applied to the skin in shallow cups (Finn chambers), affixed with a tape and left in place for 24 to 48 hours. Contact hypersensitivity will result in a papular-vesicular reaction that develops within 48 to 72 hours when the test is read. It is a unique means of in vivo reproduction of disease in diminutive proportions, for sensitization affects all the skin and may therefore be elicited at any cutaneous site. The patch test is easier and safer than a "use test" with a questionable allergen, for test items can be applied in low concentrations in small areas of skin for short periods of time. See textbooks on contact dermatitis for a list of antigens used in patch testing.

5. *Photopatch testing* is a combination of patch testing and UV irradiation of the test site and is used to document photoallergy.

MICROSCOPIC EXAMINATION OF SCALES, CRUSTS, SERUM, AND HAIR

1. *Gram's stains* and *cultures of exudates and of tissue minces* should be made in lesions suspected of being bacterial or yeast (*Candida albicans*) infections. Ulcers and nodules require a scalpel biopsy in which a wedge of tissue consisting of all three layers of skin is obtained; the biopsy specimen is minced in a sterile mortar and is then cultured for bacteria (including typical and atypical mycobacteria) and fungi.

2. *Microscopic examination* for mycelia should be made of the roofs of vesicles or of the scales (the advancing borders are preferable) or of the hair. The tissue is cleared with 10 to 30% KOH and warmed gently (Fig. 21-1). Fungal cultures with Sabouraud's medium should be made.

3. *Microscopic examination of cells obtained from the base of vesicles* (Tzanck preparation) may reveal the presence of acantholytic cells in the acantholytic diseases (e.g., pemphigus or SSS syndrome) or of giant epithelial cells and multinucleated giant cells (containing 10 to 12 nuclei) in herpes simplex, herpes zoster, and varicella. Material from the base of a vesicle obtained by *gentle* curettage with a scalpel is smeared on a glass slide, stained with Giemsa's stain, Wright's stain, or methylene blue, and examined to determine whether there are acantholytic or giant epithelial cells, which are diagnostic. In addition, culture, immunofluorescent tests or PCR for herpes are now easily available.

4. *Laboratory diagnosis of scabies.* The diagnosis of scabies is usually considered immediately in a patient with intractable generalized pruritus and with papules and excoriations distributed in characteristic locations—on the flexor aspects of the wrists, in the finger webs, and on the buttocks and genitalia; the diagnosis is established by identification of the mite, or ova or feces, in skin scrapings removed from the papules or burrows (Fig. 24-18). The burrow, a unique lesion, is a linear or serpiginous elevation of skin in the form of a ridge, up to 5 mm in length. These occur on the anterior surface of the wrists, in the webs of the fingers, or on the ulnar border of the hands.

If burrows are not present, select a papule or the roof of a vesicle on the hand. The mineral oil technique is excellent for isolating the mite. Using a sterile scalpel blade on which a drop of sterile mineral oil has been placed, apply oil to the surface of the burrow or papule. Scrape the papule or burrow vigorously to remove the entire top of the papule; tiny flecks of blood will appear in the oil. Transfer the oil to a microscopic slide and examine for mites, ova, and feces. The mites are .2 to .4 mm in size and have four pairs of legs (Fig. 24-18).

BIOPSY OF THE SKIN

Biopsy of the skin is one of the simplest, most rewarding diagnostic techniques because of the easy accessibility of the skin and the variety of techniques for study of the excised specimen (e.g., histopathology, immunopathology, electron microscopy).

Selection of the site of the biopsy is based primarily on the stage of the eruption, and early lesions are usually more typical; this is especially important in vesiculobullous eruptions (e.g., pemphigus, herpes simplex), in which the lesion should be no more than 24 h old. However, older lesions (2 to 6 weeks) are often more characteristic in discoid lupus erythematosus.

A common technique for diagnostic biopsy is the use of a 3- to 4-mm punch, a small tubular knife much like a corkscrew, which by rotating movements between the thumb and index finger cuts through the epidermis, dermis, and subcutaneous tissue; the base is cut off with scissors. If immunofluorescence is indicated (as, for example, in bullous diseases or lupus erythematosus), a special medium for transport to the laboratory is required.

For nodules, however, a large wedge should be removed by excision including subcutaneous tissue. Furthermore, when indicated, lesions, regardless of size, should be bisected, one half for histology and the other half sent in a sterile container for bacterial and mycotic cultures or in special fixatives, cell culture media, or frozen for immunopathologic examination.

Specimens for light microscopy should be fixed immediately in buffered neutral formalin. A brief but detailed summary of the clinical history and description of the lesions should accompany the specimen. Biopsy is indicated in *all* skin lesions that are suspected of being neoplasms; in all bullous disorders with immunofluoresence used simultaneously; and in all dermatologic disorders in which a specific diagnosis is not possible by clinical examination alone.

APPENDIX C: INFECTIOUS DISEASES WITH DERMATOLOGIC MANIFESTATIONS, LISTED BY GEOGRAPHIC AREA

With the marked increase in international travel in the past decade among people of all walks of life and all ages, it is necessary to ask patients with skin lesions where they have lived and traveled. In the following tables, diseases with skin lesions are presented by areas of acquisition to facilitate diagnosis and thus appropriate treatment.

While there are many other infections associated with skin lesions that are found in the geographic areas listed here, the selected infections are rare or sporadic or are not uniformly distributed. The tables show sites of acquisition, not just where the diseases are diagnosed. The tables exclude diseases that have a worldwide distribution, those without skin manifestations, and sexually transmitted diseases that can be acquired in any geographic location. A more detailed description of geographic distribution of these and other infections can be found in M.E. Wilson, *A World Guide to Infections: Diseases, Distribution, Diagnosis* (New York, Oxford University Press, 1991).

It is important to keep in mind that a patient with an infection acquired in one geographic location may undergo medical evaluation in another location where the infection is not endemic. Also, many infections may be rare or sporadically acquired in regions outside of endemic areas. An example is anthrax. Sporadic infection may be acquired in any geographic location by way of contact with imported contaminated animal products.

Equally important to note is that infections that require a specific arthropod vector for transmission have a distribution limited by the vector distribution. Presence of the vector is not sufficient for disease to occur. For example, a mosquito competent to transmit dengue is found in many states in the southern United States. In recent years, transmission of dengue has been documented only rarely within the United States (Texas).

These tables were compiled by Leslie C. Lucchina, M.D., and Mary E. Wilson, M.D.

INFECTIOUS DISEASES WITH DERMATOLOGIC MANIFESTATIONS IN THE UNITED STATES

	Northeast	South	Midwest	West
Anthrax	*	X	*	X
Blastomycosis	X	X	X	
Cercarial dermatitis	X	X	X	X
(Note: Found in freshwater lakes and saltwater coast lines)				
Coccidioidomycosis		X		X
Colorado tick fever			*	X
Cutaneous larva migrans	*	X	*	*
Dengue fever		*		
Dirofilariasis	*	*	*	*
(Note: More cases reported from coastal areas)				
Ehrlichiosis	X	X	X	X
Histoplasmosis	X	X	X	*
Hookworm		X	*	
Leishmaniasis (cutaneous)		*(Texas)		
Leprosy	*	*	*	*
(Note: Most cases are imported)				
Leptospirosis	X	X	X	X
(Note: Especially Hawaii and warmer regions)				
Lyme disease	X	X	X	X
Myiasis	*	*	*	*
Orf			X	X
Plague				X
Relapsing fever				X
Rhinoscleroma		*(Texas)		
Rickettsial infections:				
Rickettsialpox due to *Rickettsia akari*	*	*	*	*
Spotted fever due to *R. rickettsii* (Rocky Mountain spotted fever)	X	X	X	X
Typhus fever due to *R. prowazekii* (epidemic typhus)		X	*	*
Typhus fever due to *R. typhi* (murine or endemic typhus)	*	X	*	*
Seabather's eruption	X	X		
(Note: Especially along Atlantic coast, though may be more widespread)				
Sparganosis		X		
Strongyloidiasis	*	X	*	*
(Note: Most cases are imported)				
Trypanosomiasis (American)		*		*
Tularemia	*	X	X	*
Vibrio species infections of skin	X	X	X	X
(Note: Especially associated with saltwater coast lines)				

KEY: x = Infection may be acquired in this geographic location. * = Infection is rare and sporadic in this geographic location.

INFECTIOUS DISEASES WITH DERMATOLOGIC MANIFESTATIONS BY AREA OF ACQUISITION

	Africa	North America (Except Mexico)	Mexico, Central America
Anthrax	x	x	x
Bartonellosis due to *Bartonella bacilliformis*			*
Blastomycosis	*	x	*
Buruli ulcer due to *Mycobacterium ulcerans*	x		x
Cercarial dermatitis	x	x	x
Chancroid	x	x	x
Coccidioidomycosis		x	x
Colorado tick fever		x	
Cutaneous larva migrans	x	x	x
Dengue fever	x	*	x
Dirofilariasis	x	x	x
Ehrlichiosis	x	x	
Histoplasmosis	x	x	x
Hookworm	x	x	x
Leishmaniasis (cutaneous)	x	*	x
Leprosy	x	x	x
Leptospirosis	x	x	x
Loiasis	x		
Lyme disease	x	x	x
Myiasis	x	x	x
Onchocerciasis	x		x
Orf	x	x	x
Paracoccidioidomycosis	*		x
Penicilliosis marneffei			
Plague	x	x	*
Relapsing fever	x	x	x
Rhinoscleroma	x	x	x
Rickettsial infections			
Boutonneuse fever due to *Rickettsia conorii*	x		
Rickettsialpox due to *R. akari*	x	x	
Scrub typhus due to *R. tsutsugamushi*			
Spotted fever due to *R. rickettsii* (Rocky Mountain spotted fever)		x	x
Spotted fevers due to *R. australis, R. japonicum, R. sibirica*			
Typhus fever due to *R. prowazekii* (epidemic typhus)	x	x	x
Typhus fever due to *R. typhi* (murine or endemic typhus)	x	x	x
Schistosomiasis	x		
Seabather's eruption		x	x
Sparganosis	x	x	x
Strongyloidiasis	x	x	x
Trypanosomiasis (African)	x		
Trypanosomiasis (American)		*	x
Tularemia	x	x	x
Tungiasis	x		x
Vibrio sp. infections of skin	x	x	x

KEY: x = Infection may be acquired in this geographic location. * = Infection is rare and sporadic in this geographic location.

INFECTIOUS DISEASES WITH DERMATOLOGIC MANIFESTATIONS BY AREA OF ACQUISITION

Caribbean	South America	Asia	Europe	Australia, New Zealand, Oceania	Comment
X	X	X	X	X	
	X				See note below.
	*	*	*		
	*	X		X	
X	X	X	X	X	Associated with fresh and salt water.
X	X	X	X	X	More common in tropics.
	X				
X	X	X	X	X	Especially in tropics and subtropics.
X	X	X		X	Especially in tropics and subtropics.
X	X	X	X	X	
		X	X		Probably more widespread than indicated.
X	X	X	X	X	
X	X	X	X	X	Especially in rural areas and tropics.
X	X	X	X		
X	X	X	X	X	
X	X	X	X	X	Especially in tropics.
		X	X	X	
X	X	X	X	X	Especially in tropics.
	X	*			
X	X	X	X	X	Sheep- and goat-raising countries.
	X				
		X			
	X	X	X		
	X	X	X		
	X	X	X	X	
		X	X		
		X	X		
		X		X	
	X				
		X	X	X	
	X	X	X	*	
X	X	X	X	X	
X	X	X	*		
X	X	X			May be more widespread than indicated.
X	X	X	X	X	
X	X	X	X	X	Especially in tropics and subtropics.
*	X				
X		X	X		
X	X	X			
X	X	X	X	X	

Many of the infections listed may be acquired only in focal regions within the area indicated.

NOTE: *Bartonella henselae* and *B. quintana* have been associated with infection in the United States and in other geographic areas.

INDEX

Recognize these skin alterations during the routine physical examination

(Numbers in parentheses refer to pages where disorder is discussed.)

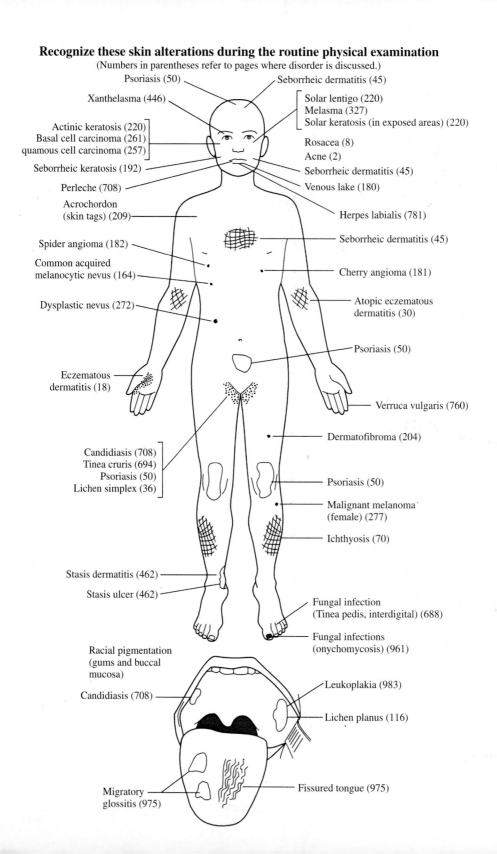

Psoriasis (50)

Xanthelasma (446)

Actinic keratosis (220)
Basal cell carcinoma (261)
quamous cell carcinoma (257)

Seborrheic keratosis (192)

Perleche (708)

Acrochordon
(skin tags) (209)

Spider angioma (182)

Common acquired
melanocytic nevus (164)

Dysplastic nevus (272)

Eczematous
dermatitis (18)

Candidiasis (708)
Tinea cruris (694)
Psoriasis (50)
Lichen simplex (36)

Stasis dermatitis (462)

Stasis ulcer (462)

Racial pigmentation
(gums and buccal
mucosa)

Candidiasis (708)

Migratory
glossitis (975)

Seborrheic dermatitis (45)

Solar lentigo (220)
Melasma (327)
Solar keratosis (in exposed areas) (220)

Rosacea (8)
Acne (2)

Seborrheic dermatitis (45)

Venous lake (180)

Herpes labialis (781)

Seborrheic dermatitis (45)

Cherry angioma (181)

Atopic eczematous
dermatitis (30)

Psoriasis (50)

Verruca vulgaris (760)

Dermatofibroma (204)

Psoriasis (50)

Malignant melanoma
(female) (277)

Ichthyosis (70)

Fungal infection
(Tinea pedis, interdigital) (688)

Fungal infections
(onychomycosis) (961)

Leukoplakia (983)

Lichen planus (116)

Fissured tongue (975)